Essentials of General Surgery

FIFTH EDITION

Senior Editor

Peter F. Lawrence, MD
Wiley Barker Endowed Chair in Vascular Surgery
Director, Gonda (Goldschmied) Vascular Center
David Geffen School of Medicine at UCLA
Los Angeles, California

Editors

Richard M. Bell, MD
Professor of Surgery
University of South Carolina School of Medicine
Columbia, South Carolina

Merril T. Dayton, MD
Professor and Chairman
Department of Surgery
State University of New York at Buffalo
Buffalo, New York

Questions Editor

James C. Hebert, MD
Albert G. Mackay and H. Gordon Page Professor of Surgery
University of Vermont College of Medicine
Burlington, Vermont

Content Editor

Mohammed I. Ahmed, MBBS, MS (Surgery)
Department of Surgery
Affiliated Institute for Medical Education
Chicago, Illinois

 Wolters Kluwer | Lippincott Williams & Wilkins
Health

Philadelphia · Baltimore · New York · London
Buenos Aires · Hong Kong · Sydney · Tokyo

Acquisitions Editor: Susan Rhyner
Product Manager: Angela Collins
Freelance Editor: Catherine Council
Marketing Manager: Joy Fisher-Williams
Vendor Manager: Bridgett Dougherty
Design & Art Direction: Teresa Mallon, Doug Smock
Compositor: SPi Global

Library of Congress Cataloging-in-Publication Data

Essentials of general surgery / [edited by] Peter F. Lawrence. — 5th ed.
    p. ; cm.
  Includes bibliographical references and index.
  ISBN 978-0-7817-8495-5
I. Lawrence, Peter F.
  [DNLM: 1. Surgical Procedures, Operative. WO 500]
  617—dc23
                                                        2011051080

DISCLAIMER

Care has been taken to confirm the accuracy of the information present and to describe generally accepted practices. However, the authors, editors, and publisher are not responsible for errors or omissions or for any consequences from application of the information in this book and make no warranty, expressed or implied, with respect to the currency, completeness, or accuracy of the contents of the publication. Application of this information in a particular situation remains the professional responsibility of the practitioner; the clinical treatments described and recommended may not be considered absolute and universal recommendations.

The authors, editors, and publisher have exerted every effort to ensure that drug selection and dosage set forth in this text are in accordance with the current recommendations and practice at the time of publication. However, in view of ongoing research, changes in government regulations, and the constant flow of information relating to drug therapy and drug reactions, the reader is urged to check the package insert for each drug for any change in indications and dosage and for added warnings and precautions. This is particularly important when the recommended agent is a new or infrequently employed drug.

Some drugs and medical devices presented in this publication have Food and Drug Administration (FDA) clearance for limited use in restricted research settings. It is the responsibility of the health care provider to ascertain the FDA status of each drug or device planned for use in their clinical practice.

Essentials of
General Surgery

FIFTH EDITION

About the Cover:

Portrait of Dr. Samuel D. Gross (The Gross Clinic)
Thomas Eakins
Oil on canvas, 1875
8 feet × 6 feet 6 inches (243.8 × 198.1 cm)
Philadelphia Museum of Art: Gift of the Alumni Association to Jefferson Medical College in 1878 and purchased by the Pennsylvania Academy of the Fine Arts and the Philadelphia Museum of Art in 2007 with the generous support of more than 3,600 donors, 2007

Preface

"What do *all* medical students need to know about surgery to be effective clinicians in their chosen fields?"

The primary responsibility of medical schools is to educate medical students to become competent clinicians. Because most physicians practice medicine in a nonacademic setting, clinical training is paramount. The 3rd year of medical school, which focuses on basic clinical training, is the foundation for most physicians' clinical training. These realities do not diminish the other critical functions of medical school, including basic science education for MD and PhD candidates, basic and clinical research, and the education of residents and practicing physicians. However, the central role of providing clinical education for medical students cannot be overemphasized.

The education of students, residents, and practicing surgeons should be a continuum, although it may seem fragmented at times to students. Because of the length of time needed to completely train surgeons, surgical residents remain "students" for 3 to 9 years beyond medical school. As a result of this extensive training period, most medical schools have large numbers of surgical residents, and resident training makes up the bulk of their educational efforts. Student education is part of the continuum that starts in the 1st or 2nd year of medical school, continues through residency, and never ends, because continuing education and lifelong learning are essential for all physicians.

NOT JUST FOR SURGEONS

This textbook and its companion volume, *Essentials of Surgical Specialties*, were produced to start that continuum of education for medical students, and to focus on medical students who are *not* planning a surgical career. We believe that all physicians need to have a fundamental understanding of the options provided by surgery to be competent, so the book asks the question, "What do all medical students need to know about surgery to be effective clinicians in their chosen field?" Rather than using traditional textbook-writing techniques to address this question, members of the Association for Surgical Education (ASE), an organization of surgeons dedicated to undergraduate surgical education, have conducted extensive research to define the content and skills needed for an optimal medical education program in surgery. Somewhat surprisingly, there has been consensus among practicing surgeons, internists, and even psychiatrists about the knowledge and skills in surgery needed by all physicians. The information from this research has become the basis for this textbook. The research process also identified technical skills, such as suturing skin, that should be mastered by all physicians and that are best taught by surgeons.

FIFTH EDITION ENHANCEMENTS

The fifth edition of this textbook has continued the approach that has resulted in its use by many medical students in the United States, in Canada, and throughout the world:

1. This edition has been extensively revised to provide the most current and up-to-date information on general surgery. Additionally, the entire interior has been refreshed and is now full-color for an even more enjoyable reading experience.
2. Our authors are surgeons devoted to teaching medical students and understand the appropriate depth of knowledge for a 3rd-year student to master.
3. We do not attempt to provide an encyclopedia of surgery. We include only information that 3rd- and 4th-year students need to know—and explain it well.
4. We intentionally limit the length of each section, so that it can reasonably be read during the clerkship.
5. Through problem solving, clinical cases, and sample exam questions, we provide numerous opportunities to practice and test new knowledge and skills, as well as features to aid in review and retention. We believe that this approach best prepares students to score high on the National Board of Medical Examiners surgery shelf exam and also prepares them for residency training.

PEDAGOGICAL FEATURES

- Learning objectives
- Full-color art program
- New and updated tables, algorithms, and charts
- New Appendix including 40 four-color burn figures
- Sample questions, answers, and rationales for every chapter

MORE TOOLS ONLINE

- Bonus chapters
- Question bank
- Patient management problems and oral exam questions
- Glossary
- Fully searchable e-book

- Chapter outlines
- Image bank

COMPANION TEXTBOOK

A companion textbook on the surgical specialties, *Essentials of Surgical Specialties*, is based on an approach similar to that of *Essentials of General Surgery* and trains you in specialty and subspecialty fields of surgery. This text is separate from *Essentials of General Surgery* because some medical schools teach the specialties in the 3rd year and others teach them in the 4th year. Students who complete both the general surgery and specialty programs and practice oral and multiple-choice questions will acquire the essential surgical knowledge and problem-solving skills that all physicians need.

SUCCESS!

You are entering the most exciting and dynamic phase of your professional life. This educational package is designed to help you achieve your goal of becoming an adept clinician and developing lifelong learning skills. It will also help you get into the residency of your choice. Best wishes for success in your endeavor.

Acknowledgments

Many members of the Association for Surgical Education (ASE) provided advice and expertise in starting the first edition of this project nearly 25 years ago. Since that time, ASE members have volunteered to assist in writing chapters and editing the textbook. At its annual meetings, the ASE provides an excellent forum to discuss and test ideas about the content of the surgical curriculum and methods to teach and evaluate what has been learned.

We would like to thank our student editors, Tamera Beam and Jason Rogers, who reviewed many of the chapters and provided valuable student perspective on the material presented. We would like to extend our thanks to Cathy Council, our editor in Salt Lake City, who coordinated all components of this project. I also would like to thank our editors at Lippincott Williams & Wilkins, Susan Rhyner, Jennifer Verbiar, and Angela Collins.

Contributors

Mohammed I. Ahmed, MBBS, MS (Surgery)
Clinical Instructor in Surgery
Affiliated Institute for Medical Education
Chicago, Illinois

James Alexander, MD
Associate Professor of Surgery
Vice Chief for Education
Cooper Medical School of Rowan University
Camden, New Jersey

Adnan A. Alseidi, MD
Program Director Surgery Residents
Co-Director HPB Fellowship Program
Hepato-Pancreato-Biliary Surgery Division
Virginia Mason Medical Center
Seattle, Washington

Gina L. Andrales, MD
Associate Professor of Surgery
Dartmouth Medical School
Lebanon, New Hampshire

David Antonenko, MD
Professor of Surgery
University of North Dakota School of Medicine and Health
Sciences
Grand Forks, North Dakota

Lecia Apantaku, MD
Associate Professor of Surgery
Chicago Medical School
Rosalind Franklin University of Medicine and Science
North Chicago, Illinois

Tracey D. Arnell, MD
Assistant Professor of Surgery
Columbia University College of Physicians & Surgeons
Memorial Sloan-Kettering Cancer Center
New York, New York

Dimitrios Avgerinos, MD
Clinical Fellow
Department of Cardiothoracic Surgery
New York Presbyterian – Weill Cornell Medical Center
New York, New York

Melinda Banister, MD
General Surgeon
Lubbock, Texas

Richard M. Bell, MD
Professor of Surgery
University of South Carolina School of Medicine
Columbia, South Carolina

Juliane Bingener, MD
Associate Professor of Surgery
Mayo Clinic
Rochester, Minnesota

H. Scott Bjerke, MD
Clinical Professor of Surgery
Kansas City University of Medicine and Biosciences
Clinical Associate Professor of Surgery at UMKC
Kansas City, Missouri

Karen R. Borman, MD
Clinical Professor (Adjunct), Surgery
Temple University School of Medicine
Senior Associate Program Director, General Surgery Residency
Abington Memorial Hospital
Abington, Pennsylvania

Mary-Margaret Brandt, MD
Trauma Director and Surgical Intensivist
St. Joseph Mercy Hospital
Ann Arbor, Michigan

Karen Brasel, MD, MPH
Professor of Surgery, Bioethics and Medical Humanities
Medical College of Wisconsin
Milwaukee, Wisconsin

Melissa Brunsvold, MD
Assistant Professor of Surgery
University of Minnesota
Minneapolis, Minnesota

Kenneth W. Burchard, MD
Professor of Surgery
Dartmouth-Hitchcock Medical Center
Lebanon, New Hampshire

Arnold Byer, MD
Clinical Professor of Surgery
UMDNJ—New Jersey Medical School
Newark, New Jersey

Michael Cahalane, MD
Associate Professor of Surgery
Harvard Medical School
Acting Chief, Division of Acute Care Surgery
Beth Israel Deaconess Medical Center
Boston, Massachusetts

Jeannette Capella, MD
Medical Director, Trauma/Surgical ICU
Assistant Medical Director, Trauma
Altoona Regional Medical Center
Altoona, Pennsylvania

Frederick D. Cason, MD
Associate Professor
Residency Program Director
Section of Gastrointestinal and Minimally Invasive Surgery
Department of Surgery
The University of Toledo College of Medicine
Toledo, Ohio

William C. Chapman, MD
Professor and Chief, Section of Transplantation
Chief, Division of General Surgery
Washington University in St. Louis
St. Louis, Missouri

Gregory S. Cherr, MD
Associate Professor of Surgery
Chief of Vascular Surgery, Buffalo General Hospital
Director, Medical Student Surgical Education
Associate Program Directory, General Surgery Program
State University of New York at Buffalo
Buffalo, New York

Jeffrey G. Chipman, MD
Associate Professor of Surgery
University of Minnesota Medical School
Minneapolis, Minnesota

Nicholas P.W. Coe, MD
Professor of Surgery
Tufts University School of Medicine
Department of Surgery
Baystate Medical Center
Springfield, Massachusetts

Annesley W. Copeland, MD
Assistant Professor of Surgery
Uniformed Services University of the Health Sciences
Bethesda, Maryland

Julia Corcoran, MD
Associate Professor of Surgery
Feinberg School of Medicine
Northwestern University
Chicago, Illinois

Wendy R. Cornett, MD
Associate Professor of Clinical Surgery
University of South Carolina School of Medicine—Greenville
Greenville, South Carolina

Gail Cresci, PhD, RD
Research Staff
Digestive Disease and Lerner Research Institutes
Departments of Gastroenterology and Pathobiology
The Cleveland Clinic
Cleveland, Ohio

Brian J. Daley, MD
Professor, Department of Surgery
University of Tennessee Medical Center at Knoxville
Knoxville, Tennessee

Dale A. Dangleben, MD
Associate Surgery Residency Program Director
Lehigh Valley Health Network
Allentown, Pennsylvania

Debra A. DaRosa, PhD
Professor of Surgery
Vice Chair for Education
Northwestern University Feinberg School of Medicine
Chicago, Illinois

Merril T. Dayton, MD
Professor and Chairman
Department of Surgery
State University of New York at Buffalo
Buffalo, New York

Chris de Gara, MBBS, MS
Professor of Surgery
Director, Division of General Surgery
Department of Surgery, University of Alberta
Director, Department of Surgical Oncology
Cross Cancer Institute, Alberta Cancer Board
Edmonton, Alberta, Canada

Matthew O. Dolich, MD
Professor and Director, General Surgery Residency Program
University of California, Irvine
Orange, California

Serge Dubé, MD
Professor of Surgery
Faculty of Medicine
University of Montreal
Montreal, Quebec, Canada

Gary L. Dunnington, MD
J. Roland Folse Professor and Chair of Surgery
Southern Illinois University School of Medicine
Springfield, Illinois

Virginia A. Eddy, MD
Director, Undergraduate Surgical Education
Maine Medical Center
Portland, Maine

Michael Edwards, MD
Associate Professor of Surgery
Georgia Health Sciences University
Augusta, Georgia

Timothy M. Farrell, MD
Professor of Surgery
University of North Carolina at Chapel Hill
Chapel Hill, North Carolina

Patrick Forgione, MD
Associate Professor of Surgery
University of Vermont College of Medicine
Fletcher Allen Healthcare
Burlington, Vermont

Kevin N. Foster, MD
Vice Chair for Education and Research
Director Arizona Burn Center
Program Director, General Surgery residency
Department of Surgery
Maricopa Integrated Health Systems
Phoenix, Arizona

Glen A. Franklin, MD
Associate Professor of Surgery
University of Louisville School of Medicine
Louisville, Kentucky

Shannon Fraser, MD, MSc
Assistant Professor
McGill University
Chief General Surgery
Jewish General Hospital
Montreal, Quebec, Canada

Charles M. Friel, MD
Associate Professor of Surgery
University of Virginia
Charlottesville, Virginia

Gregory J. Gallina, MD
Associate Director of Surgical Education
Hackensack University Medical Center
Hackensack, New Jersey

R. Neal Garrison, MD
Professor of Surgery
University of Louisville School of Medicine
Louisville, Kentucky

Jonathan Gefen, MD
Clinical Assistant Professor of Surgery
Jefferson Medical College
Wynnewood, Pennsylvania

Bruce L. Gewertz, MD
Surgeon-in-Chief
Chair, Department of Surgery
Cedars-Sinai Health System
Los Angeles, California

Steven B. Goldin, MD, PhD
Associate Professor of Surgery
Vice Chairman of Surgical Education
University of South Florida
Tampa, Florida

Mitchell H. Goldman, MD
Professor and Chairman
Department of Surgery
Assistant Dean for Research
University of Tennessee Graduate School of Medicine
Knoxville, Tennessee

Oscar H. Grandas, MD
Associate Professor of Surgery
University of Tennessee at Knoxville
Surgical Director
Transplant Surgery Service and Vascular Access Center
University of Tennessee Medical Center at Knoxville
Knoxville, Tennessee

James S. Gregory, MD
Director Intensive Care Services
Department of Surgery
Conemaugh Memorial Hospital
Johnstown, Pennsylvania

Oscar D. Guillamondegui, MD, MPH
Assistant Professor of Surgery
Vanderbilt University Medical Center
Medical Director, Surgical Intensive Care
Department of Surgery
Tennessee Valley Healthcare System, Veterans Affairs
Nashville, Tennessee

Kenneth A. Harris, MD
Director of Education
Royal College of Physicians and Surgeons of Canada
Ottawa, Ontario, Canada

Alan E. Harzman, MD
Assistant Professor of Surgery
The Ohio State University
Columbus, Ohio

Imran Hassan, MD
Assistant Professor of Surgery
Southern Illinois University School of Medicine
Springfield, Illinois

James C. Hebert, MD
Albert G. Mackay and H. Gordon Page Professor of Surgery
University of Vermont College of Medicine
Burlington, Vermont

Jonathan R. Hiatt, MD
Professor and Chief
Division of General Surgery
Vice Chair for Education
Department of Surgery
David Geffen School of Medicine at UCLA
Los Angeles, California

O. Joe Hines, MD
Assistant Professor
Director, Surgery Residency Program
Department of Surgery
David Geffen School of Medicine at UCLA
Los Angeles, California

Mary Ann Hopkins, MD
Associate Professor of Surgery
Director of Education for the Clinical Sciences
NYU School of Medicine
New York, New York

Hwei-Kang Hsu, MD
Assistant Professor of Surgery
State University of New York at Buffalo
Buffalo, New York

Gerald A. Isenberg, MD
Professor of Surgery
Director, Surgical Undergraduate Education
Jefferson Medical College
Program Director, Colorectal Residency, TJUH
Philadelphia, Pennsylvania

Ted A. James, MD
Associate Professor of Surgery
Division of Surgical Oncology
Director of Surgery Clerkship and Student Education
University of Vermont College of Medicine
Burlington, Vermont

Daniel B. Jones, MD
Professor, Harvard Medical School
Chief, Section of Minimally Invasive Surgery
Beth Israel Deaconess Medical Center
Boston, Massachusetts

Susan Kaiser, MD, PhD
Division of General Surgery
Jersey City Medical Center
Jersey City, New Jersey

Lewis J. Kaplan, MD
Associate Professor of Surgery
Yale University School of Medicine
New Haven, Connecticut

Alysandra Lal, MD
Clinical Assistant Professor
Medical College of Wisconsin
Columbia St. Mary's Hospital
Milwaukee, Wisconsin

Peter F. Lawrence, MD
Wiley Barker Endowed Chair in Vascular Surgery
Director, Gonda (Goldschmied) Vascular Center
David Geffen School of Medicine at UCLA
Los Angeles, California

Jong O. Lee, MD
Assistant Professor of Surgery
University of Texas Medical Branch
Galveston, Texas

Susan Lerner, MD
Assistant Professor of Surgery
The Mount Sinai Medical Center
New York, New York

Carlos M. Li, MD
Assistant Professor of Surgery
State University of New York at Buffalo
Buffalo, New York

D. Scott Lind, MD
Professor and Chairman
Department of Surgery
Drexel University College of Medicine
Philadelphia, Pennsylvania

Kimberly D. Lomis, MD
Associate Professor of Surgery
Associate Dean for Undergraduate Medical Education
Vanderbilt University School of Medicine
Nashville, Tennessee

Fred A. Luchette, MD
The Ambrose and Gladys Bowyer Professor of Surgery
Medical Director, Cardiothoracic Critical Care Services
Department of Surgery
Stritch School of Medicine
Maywood, Illinois

John Maa, MD
Assistant Professor of Surgery
University of California, San Francisco
San Francisco, California

Bruce V. MacFadyen Jr, MD
Moretz-Mansberger Professor of Surgery
Department of Surgery
Georgia Health Sciences University
Augusta, Georgia

Barry D. Mann, MD
Chief Academic Officer, Main Line Health
Program Director, The Lankenau Surgical Residency Program
Professor of Surgery, Jefferson Medical College
Wynnewood, Pennsylvania

Alan B. Marr, MD
Professor of Surgery
Vice Chairman of Education
Department of Surgery
Louisiana State University Health Science Center
New Orleans, Louisiana

James A. McCoy, MD, PhD
Professor of Surgery
Morehouse School of Medicine
Atlanta, Georgia

James F. McKinsey, MD
Associate Professor and Chief
Division of Vascular Surgery
Columbia University
New York, New York

John D. Mellinger, MD
Professor and Chair of General Surgery
Department of Surgery
Southern Illinois University School of Medicine
Springfield, Illinois

David W. Mercer, MD
McLaughlin Professor and Chairman
Department of Surgery
University of Nebraska Medical Center
Omaha, Nebraska

Hollis W. Merrick III, MD
Professor, Surgery
Chief, Division of General Surgery
Director, Undergraduate Surgical Education
The University of Toledo
Toledo, Ohio

James E. Morrison, MD
Assistant Professor of Surgery
University of South Carolina School of Medicine
Columbia, South Carolina

Russell J. Nauta, MD
Professor of Surgery
Harvard Medical School
Chairman, Department of Surgery
Mt. Auburn Hospital
Cambridge, Massachusetts

Peter R. Nelson, MD
Assistant Professor of Surgery
Director, Surgery Clerkship
University of Florida College of Medicine
Gainesville, Florida

Leigh Neumayer, MD, MS
Professor of Surgery
University of Utah Health Sciences Center
Salt Lakc City, Utah

John T. Paige, MD
Associate Professor of Clinical Surgery
Louisiana State University School of Medicine
New Orleans, Louisiana

Tina L. Palmieri, MD
Associate Professor and Director
University of California Davis Regional Burn Center
Assistant Chief of Burns
Shriners Hospital for Children Northern California
Sacramento, California

Alexander A. Parikh, MD
Assistant Professor
Division of Surgical Oncology
Vanderbilt University Medical Center
Nashville, Tennessee

Lisa A. Patterson, MD
Associate Professor of Surgery
Tufts University School of Medicine
Trauma Director
Department of Surgery
Baystate Health
Springfield, Massachusetts

Elizabeth Peralta, MD
Associate Professor of Surgery
Southern Illinois University School of Medicine
Springfield, Illinois

Timothy A. Pritts, MD, PhD
Associate Professor of Surgery
Division of Trauma and Critical Care
Department of Surgery
University of Cincinnati College of Medicine
Cincinnati, Ohio

Jan Rakinic, MD
Associate Professor of Surgery
Chief, Section of Colorectal Surgery
Program Director, SIU Program in Colorectal Surgery
Vice Chair for Clinical Operations, Department of Surgery
Southern Illinois University School of Medicine
Springfield, Illinois

H. David Reines, MD
Professor of Surgery
Virginia Commonwealth University
Vice Chair Surgery
InovaFairfax Hospital
Falls Church, Virginia

Melanie L. Richards, MD
Professor of Surgery
Associate Dean of Graduate Medical Education
Mayo Clinic
Rochester, Minnesota

Jeffrey R. Saffle, MD
Professor of Surgery
Director, Burn-Trauma ICU
University of Utah Health Sciences Center
Salt Lake City, Utah

Hilary Sanfey, MD
Professor of Surgery
Vice Chair for Education
Southern Illinois University School of Medicine
Springfield, Illinois

Kennith H. Sartorelli, MD
Professor of Surgery
The University of Vermont College of Medicine
Burlington, Vermont

Kimberly D. Schenarts, PhD
Affiliate Professor of Surgery
Brody School of Medicine at East Carolina University
Greenville, North Carolina

Paul J. Schenarts, MD
Vice Chair, Department of Surgery
University of Nebraska Medical Center
Omaha, Nebraska

Mohsen Shabahang, MD, PhD
Director, General Surgery
Geisinger Medical Center
Danville, Pennsylvania

Saad Shebrain, MD
Assistant Professor of Surgery
Michigan State University/Kalamazoo Center for Medical Studies
Kalamazoo, Michigan

Timothy R. Shope, MD
General Surgery
Hershey, Pennsylvania

Ravi S. Sidhu, MD, PhD
Assistant Professor
Department of Surgery
University of British Columbia
Vancouver, British Columbia, Canada

Mary R. Smith, MD
Professor of Medicine and Pathology
Associate Dean for Graduate Medical Education
The University of Toledo College of Medicine
Toledo, Ohio

David A. Spain, MD
Professor of Surgery
Chief, Trauma/Critical Care Surgery
Stanford University School of Medicine
Stanford, California

Kimberley E. Steele, MD
Assistant Professor of Surgery
Director of Adolescent Bariatric Surgery
The Johns Hopkins Center for Bariatric Surgery
Baltimore, Maryland

Michael D. Stone, MD
Professor of Surgery
Boston University School of Medicine
Chief of the Section of Surgical Oncology
Boston Medical Center
Boston, Massachusetts

John P. Sutyak, MD
Associate Professor of Surgery
Director, Southern Illinois Trauma Center
Southern Illinois University School of Medicine
Springfield, Illinois

Glenn E. Talboy Jr, MD
Professor of Surgery
Program Director, General Surgery Residency
University of Missouri—Kansas City School of Medicine
Kansas City, Missouri

J. Scott Thomas, MD
Assistant Professor of Surgery
Program Director, General Surgery Residency
Texas A&M Health Science Center
Scott & White Memorial Hospital
Temple, Texas

Areti Tillou, MD
Associate Professor
Associate Program Director
Department of Surgery
David Geffen School of Medicine at UCLA
Los Angeles, California

Samuel A. Tisherman, MD
Professor
Departments of Critical Care Medicine and Surgery
University of Pittsburgh
Pittsburgh, Pennsylvania

Judith L. Trudel, MD
Clinical Professor of Surgery
Division of Colon and Rectal Surgery
Department of Surgery
University of Minnesota Medical School
St. Paul, Minnesota

Richard B. Wait, MD, PhD
Professor of Surgery
Tufts University School of Medicine
Chairman, Department of Surgery
Baystate Medical Center
Springfield, Massachusetts

James Warneke, MD
Associate Professor of Surgery
University of Arizona College of Medicine
Tucson, Arizona

Jeremy Warren, MD
Instructor
Department of Surgery
Georgia Health Sciences University
Augusta, Georgia

Warren D. Widmann, MD
Associate Chair, Education and Training
Program Director, Department of Surgery
Staten Island University Hospital
Clinical Professor of Surgery
State of New York Downstate Medical Center
New York, New York

Christopher Wohltmann, MD
Clinical Associate Professor of Surgery
Southern Illinois University School of Medicine
Springfield, Illinois

Contents

CHAPTER 24   505

Surgical Oncology: Malignant Diseases of the Skin and Soft Tissue

D. Scott Lind, M.D.
Mohammed I. Ahmed, M.B.B.S., M.S. (Surgery)
Chris de Gara, M.B.B.S., M.S.
James Warneke, M.D.

Introduction: Transitioning to the Role as a Junior Member of the Surgical Health Care Team

DEBRA A. DAROSA, PH.D.

You are about to embark on an immersive clinical experience in surgery. It does not matter if you plan to be a surgeon; your surgery clerkship will provide you with learning opportunities that will help you hone clinical skills important to a physician, regardless of chosen specialty. During your career as a doctor, you will undoubtedly encounter patients and family members who require surgical intervention, and the surgery clerkship can equip you with the knowledge and skills necessary to identify surgical diseases, recognize the type of surgical consult needed, and position yourself to better understand and empathize with the emotional, physiological, and logistical experiences they will have, should an operation or consult be required. How you approach your role and responsibilities as a junior member of the surgical health care team will determine the extent to which you enjoy and benefit from this incredible educational experience.

You are already a well-seasoned learner or you would not be in medical school. But the first day as a junior member on a health care team, typically begun in your 3rd year of medical school, is a profound transition and requires rethinking how you approach learning and studying. It is no longer just about memorizing facts and then repeating them on a test. You now have real patients who need your understanding of their presenting complaints and disease entities. You also have serious time constraints on reading, voluminous information needing to be learned, and the challenge of determining the scope and detail level of information needed to help your patients. These challenges are not insurmountable. Variables that typically affect clinical performance include

1. Preparatory coursework and experience—new knowledge is constructed from existing knowledge. Learning is about linking new information with what you already know. Students who worked hard to do more than just memorize and accomplished a deep knowledge of anatomy, for example, will more easily associate what they are hearing, feeling, or seeing for the first time with this prior knowledge, to further form solidly constructed understanding. Remembering follows understanding.

2. Quality of study methods—active learning requires students to take responsibility for their learning. Disciplined students recognize how they best learn and maintain an ongoing study plan that meets their learning style and needs.

3. Organizational skills—successful lifelong learners know how to arrange their time and priorities so as to avoid stressful situations such as last-minute cramming.

4. Motivation and emotion—students' enthusiasm and feelings about the content to be learned, the people involved, and the learning environment can have a significant effect on how a student experiences a clerkship and how their patients and team experiences and perceives them.

5. Physical health—there is an undeniable link between how a person feels physically and how well he or she learns. Students need to pay attention to their own health needs.

6. Distractibility and concentration skills—students must be active learners. Whether reading or listening to a lecture, students who can't be fully attentive and engaged will have difficulties deeply processing information and translating it into useful knowledge. It's hard to learn when you are not cognitively present or are sleeping!

Your aim should be to take full advantage of every teachable moment in your surgery clerkship. Here is how:

MAXIMIZE YOUR INTELLECTUAL CAPABILITIES

- Prepare, practice, and review
- Organize your knowledge
- Know expectations and thyself
- Ask! Ask! Ask! Ask! Ask! Ask!

Prepare, Practice, and Review

You need to **prepare** for your clinical and didactic learning experiences by activating prior knowledge. This can be done by prereading about the topics you'll be exposed to the next day, for example in a lecture session, in the operating room, or on rounds. Although few students read textual material before a lecture, empirical evidence shows that prereading increases comprehension and puts information into longer-term memory. It is somewhat akin to looking at a map before going on a trip. You will know ahead of time where the route changes and landmarks along the way. Just as looking at a map before a trip is an advanced organizer for your journey, prereading is an advanced organizer for the topic to be learned or the operation to be seen. You'll glean the most from seeing a thyroid nodule or acute cholecystitis if you've read about it beforehand—make the most of these learning opportunities by preparing for them.

Practice is applied thinking and requires engaged learners. Be an active listener, carry an electronic or paper notebook, and jot down one or two learning issues or questions that surface during the day and then read about them with a purpose that evening. Note taking doesn't mean the transfer of the attending's lecture to your notebook without its passing through your brain! Studies have demonstrated that students who make their own notes have better retention than students who do not. Jotting notes and self-generating questions about the topic being addressed in a lecture or whatever learning environment embeds information into memory.

Reviewing information on an ongoing basis is critical to retention. Use the test questions and patient management problems provided in this book to assess your understanding of the material read. It is also helpful to create your own tests by listing open-ended questions or copying charts or tables and then blanking out portions to see if you can "fill in the blanks." Review notes, flowcharts, tables and diagrams, and test questions while looking for patterns. Re-review throughout the clerkship. Spending as little as 30 minutes per day can help reinforce information and significantly affect recall capabilities.

Organize Your Knowledge

You can organize your knowledge by taking three steps to studying.

1. Get the big picture first. Prior to reading a book chapter, review the learning objectives listed at the start of the chapter. Review the headings and subheadings to get a sense of how the author organized the information presented and what s/he thinks is important for you to learn. Also, review the questions before you read to get an additional sense of what the author finds important. You can also list questions you have about the topic and then read the chapter with this purpose in mind.
2. Review the charts, tables, and diagrams. Authors emphasize key information in these and are an excellent source for study. As noted above, it is excellent practice to eliminate parts of the table, chart, and diagram and test yourself to see if you know the missing information.
3. Emphasize integration. As you read each chapter, examine the information to see how it relates to a patient you may have seen, a lecture you attended, an image you may have reviewed, etc. Create your own mind maps or concept maps that help to organize the information in your mind and create patterns where appropriate. Many senior faculty use memories of former patients to fix surgical principles in their minds.

Search for relationships between ideas and concepts, and note anything confusing or difficult to comprehend for follow-up through reading or discussions with peers, residents, or faculty.

Know Expectations and Thyself

Read the provided syllabus or Web site provided from the clerkship director and carefully listen at orientation. Be crystal clear as to your role and responsibilities. If this can't be ascertained using the syllabus materials, then talk with students who did well in prior clerkships, residents, or faculty. Most surgeons value commitment, timeliness, and work ethic as highly as intelligence. Once you know what you are expected to do and what you expect from yourself, you are set up to succeed. Secondly, think about what you want to glean from this clerkship and outline your own learning goals. Don't be a reactive learner; instead be an active adult learner and have a learning agenda in mind. For example, if assigned to attend a breast surgeon's clinic, reflect in advance and write what you'd like to learn from that experience. Lastly, know your learning style. For example, if you are someone who learns better by talking through topics and issues, find a like-minded study partner and do it. On the other hand, if you are a learner who does best by sequestering yourself somewhere with no distractions, find study spaces inside and outside the hospital to accommodate yourself. The point is to be reflective about this and plan your study approaches in advance.

Ask! Ask! Ask!

Persistence and assertiveness are necessary in all clerkships including surgery. If you have a question, need performance feedback, or have unresolved learning issues, ask someone. Most faculty and residents are happy to help a medical student who shows interest and is invested in their learning. And if they are too busy at the time and you happen to be told "no"… just say to yourself "next" and go to someone else. It is not personal. Everyone who works with you knows things you don't know. If you are wise, you'll learn from everyone on or near the surgery team including nurses, physician assistants, pharmacists, social workers, and technicians. They can't read your mind though, so even timid individuals will need to reach out and ask for feedback, for assistance, or for answers as needed.

MAXIMIZE YOUR EMOTIONAL INTELLIGENCE

- Focus forward with a positive attitude
- Set goals and celebrate successes
- Promote a supportive learning environment

Focus Forward with a Positive Attitude

It is not what happens to you in the clerkship that matters, it is how you respond to it that determines the outcome. Make decisions about how you respond to situations or challenges with the end in mind. You can't always control situations, but you can control your response to them. If a resident or faculty member is having a bad or overly intense day, seek to have enough situational awareness to maintain a positive perspective. Anticipate in the operating room when questions might be welcome and when a surgeon needs to concentrate. A student with high emotional intelligence maintains an open mind, approaches responsibilities with positive energy and enthusiasm, and seeks to make a constructive difference in his or her patients' and team members' days. This doesn't mean we should maintain an artificial positive attitude when things are going awry, because focus forward is not about denying what we feel. Forward focus is about managing energy and focusing on solutions and not just problems. We go toward what we focus on.

Set Goals and Celebrate Successes

Mature-minded learners are specific about what they want to achieve. They dream big dreams and are committed to achieving them. Surgery clerks should start their clerkship by defining goals of what they desire to glean from the clerkship experience and how achievement of these goals will move them toward their long-range mission. I encourage all students to document their short- and long-range goals—goals that are achievable, believable, conceivable, desirable, measurable, growth facilitating, and life enhancing! What we write tends to manifest itself internally rather than serving as passing thoughts. Goals should address what one wants to accomplish as a learner, but can also include financial goals, relationship goals, as well as goals about the values you want to reflect and practice. Goals set direction—if you don't know where you are going, you are not likely to get there! The notebook should also include a section for documenting successes—large and small. Overachievers and leaders tend to meet a goal and simply move to the next one without taking the time to appreciate and honor what they accomplished. Being able to reread written accomplishments serves as a useful reminder of all you've done well, which can be especially lifting and reinforcing to one's self-confidence and sense of accomplishments when needed.

Promote a Positive Learning Environment

You are going to make mistakes. A good thing about being the junior member of a patient care team is that you have many layers of expertise to help defray them. Your team members will have made mistakes themselves. The key is to take responsibility for mistakes by owning up to them, and learning from them so they aren't repeated.

Avoid keeping company with negative people or "negaholics." These individuals are not unique to surgery, and are important to be aware of, as they can create serious chaos for the team. Negaholics are individuals who are beset with negative attitudes and behaviors. They constantly are complaining about someone or something, and can suck the positive energy out of anyone or team. They are rigid in their thinking and highly judgmental. If their negativity is fed, it becomes contagious and results in reduced productivity, lower morale, and frustration. Negaholism creates a pessimistic learning environment and is damaging to the team's esprit de corps and functionality. It is important to not get caught up in their negativity net—avoiding these individuals helps neutralize their effect.

An important element to creating a supportive learning environment is to take care of those learners behind you, beside you, and in front of you. This establishes trust among team members, which is what makes a team productive and effective and the learning environment supportive.

The electronic portion of this book includes a chapter entitled "Maximally Invasive Learning" that includes specific suggestions on how to address five common questions faced by students in the surgery clerkship including

Problem One: What exactly is my role? What are the expectations?

Problem Two: There is not enough time to read.

Problem Three: I am getting little or no feedback.

Problem Four: How can I do well on examinations?

Problem Five: What does it take to be an honors student?

Although there is overlap between this Introduction and the electronic chapter, since they are mutually based on learning principles, I'd encourage students who want to do well in their surgery clerkship to read both for a more comprehensive overview on successful learner practices.

In summary, approach the surgery clerkship with a fire in your belly! Do all you can to earn your credibility as a junior member of the surgery health care team by taking measures to maximize your intellectual capabilities and advance your emotional intelligence. Lastly, keep in mind John Wooden's sage advice. He advised that although tempting when you are in a competitive, busy, and complex environment, never try to be better than anyone else, but never cease to be the best you can be. That is all you need to be successful in the surgery clerkship, and frankly, in life as well.

1

Perioperative Evaluation and Management of Surgical Patients

VIRGINIA A. EDDY, M.D. • TRACEY D. ARNELL, M.D. • KENNETH A. HARRIS, M.D. •
IMRAN HASSAN, M.D. • JAMES E. MORRISON, M.D.

Objectives

1. Describe the value of the preoperative history, physical examination, and selected diagnostic and screening tests.

2. Describe the important aspects of communication skills.

3. Discuss the role of outside consultation in evaluating a patient undergoing an elective surgical procedure.

4. Discuss the elements of a patient's history that are essential in the preoperative evaluation of surgical emergencies.

5. Discuss the appropriate preoperative screening tests.

6. Discuss the assessment of cardiac and pulmonary risk.

7. Discuss the effect of renal dysfunction, hepatic dysfunction, diabetes, adrenal insufficiency, pregnancy, and advanced age on preoperative preparation and postoperative management.

8. Describe the documentation required in the medical record of a surgical patient, including physician's orders and daily progress notes.

9. Describe the most commonly used surgical tubes and drains.

10. Discuss common postoperative complications and their treatment.

PREOPERATIVE EVALUATION

Surgery and anesthesia profoundly alter the normal physiologic and metabolic states. Estimating the patient's ability to respond to these stresses in the postoperative period is the task of the preoperative evaluation. Perioperative complications are often the result of failure, in the preoperative period, to identify underlying medical conditions, maximize the patient's preoperative health, or accurately assess perioperative risk. Sophisticated laboratory studies and specialized testing are *no* substitute for a thoughtful and careful history and physical examination. Sophisticated technology has merit primarily in confirming clinical suspicion.

This chapter is not a review of how to perform a history and physical examination. Instead, this discussion is a review of the elements in the patient's history or findings on physical examination that may suggest the need to modify care in the perioperative period. Other chapters discuss the signs and symptoms of specific surgical diagnoses.

PHYSICIAN–PATIENT COMMUNICATION

Interviewing Techniques

The physician–patient relationship is an essential part of surgical care. The relationship between the surgeon and patient should be established, maintained, and valued. Good interviewing techniques are fundamental in establishing a good relationship. The basis for good interviewing comes from a genuine concern about people, although there are interviewing skills that can be learned and that can improve the quality of the interaction. Medical students should also acknowledge their own special role in the patient's care. Students should not be ashamed of their status, or feel that they are ineffective members of the team. Patients commonly view medical students as more accessible and will often share details with them that they might withhold from the more senior members of the team. Also, the intensity and enthusiasm of the intelligent novice is a definite asset that can be brought to the patient's great advantage. The role of the student is to discover the patient's chief medical complaint, perform a focused history and physical examination, and present the findings to the resident or faculty member. Interviewing a patient well requires communicating to the patient who you are and how you fit into the team.

Effective interviewing can be challenging because of the variety of settings in which interviews occur. These settings include the operating room, the intensive care unit, a private office, a hospital bedside, the emergency room, and an outpatient clinic. Each setting presents its own challenges to effective communication. To achieve good physician–patient relationships, surgeons adjust their styles to the environment and to each patient's personality and needs. Some basic rules are common to all professional interviews. The first rule is to make clear to the patient that during the history and examination, nothing short of a life-or-death emergency will assume greater importance than the interaction between the surgeon and the patient at that moment. This is our first, and best, chance to connect with the patient. The patient must come to understand that a caring, knowledgeable, and dedicated surgeon will be the patient's partner on the journey through the treatment of surgical disease. The surgeon should observe certain other rules, including giving adequate attention to personal appearance to present a professional image that inspires confidence; establishing eye contact; communicating interest, warmth, and understanding; listening nonjudgmentally; accepting the patient as a person; listening to the patient's description of his or her problem; and helping the patient feel comfortable in communicating.

When the patient is seen in an ambulatory setting, the first few minutes are spent greeting the patient (using the patient's formal name); shaking hands with the patient; introducing himself or herself and explaining the surgeon's role; attending to patient privacy; adjusting his or her conversational style and level of vocabulary to meet the patient's needs; eliciting the patient's attitude about coming to the clinic; finding out the patient's occupation; and determining what the patient knows about the nature of his or her problem.

The next step involves exploring the problem. To focus the interview, one moves from open-ended to closed-ended questions. Important techniques include using transitions; asking specific, clear questions; and restating the problem for verification. At this point, it is important to determine whether the patient has any questions. Near the end of the interview, the surgeon explains what the next steps will be and that he or she will examine the patient. Last, the surgeon should verify that the patient is comfortable.

Most of the techniques used in the ambulatory setting are also appropriate for inpatient and Emergency Department encounters. Often, more time is spent with the patient in the initial and subsequent interviews than in an outpatient setting. At the initial interview, patients are likely to be in pain, worried about financial problems, and concerned about lack of privacy or unpleasant diets. They may also have difficulty sleeping, be fearful about treatment, or feel helpless. It is important to gently and confidently communicate the purpose of the interview and how long it will take.

The patient is not only listening, but also is observing the physician's behavior and even attire. The setting also affects the interview. For example, a cramped, noisy, crowded environment can affect the quality of communication. Patients may have negative feelings because of insensitivities on the part of the physician or others. Examples include speaking to the patient from the doorway, giving or taking personal information in a crowded room, speaking about a patient in an elevator or another public space, or speaking to a patient without drawing the curtain in a ward.

Informed Consent

The relationship between a patient and his or her surgeon is one of the strongest in any professional endeavor. The patient comes to the surgeon with a problem, the solution to which may include alteration of the patient's anatomy while he or she is in a state of total helplessness. There is an immense duty on the part of the surgeon to merit this level of trust. Part of earning this trust involves honest discussions with patients and their families about available choices (including the choice to not operate) and their consequences.

Once the surgeon has gathered information sufficient to identify the likely problem and its contributory factors, the surgeon then identifies a number of reasonable courses of action to pursue the evaluation or treatment of the patient's problem. These strategies are discussed in layman's terms with the patient (and family where appropriate). Together, the patient and the surgeon select the course of action that seems best. This is what is meant by ***informed consent***. Informed consent is a process, not an event, and not a form. It is the process wherein the patient and surgeon together decide on a plan. *Informed consent* is different from a *consent form*. A consent form is intended to serve as legal documentation of these discussions between the physician and the patient. It is an unfortunate reality that consent forms must serve as a shield behind which care providers may take shelter should a tort claim be filed against them. The process of informed consent serves the more noble cause; consent forms serve the more mundane cause. Informed consent often takes place not just in one session, but over time, in multiple sessions, as the patient has time to digest the information and formulate further questions.

Sometimes, patients cannot speak for themselves. In these situations, the health care team will turn to those who might reasonably be thought to be able to speak on behalf of the patient. Usually, but not always, this is the next of kin. (The reader is strongly encouraged to become familiar with pertinent state law on this matter.) These individuals are known as ***surrogate decision makers***. Another concept that arises in this context is ***advance directives***. *Advance directives* are legal documents that inform care providers about the general wishes of the patient regarding level of care to be delivered should the patient not be able to speak for himself or herself. Most people wish to receive enough medical care to alleviate their suffering and to give them a reasonable chance of being able to enjoy the remainder of their life in a functional manner. The definitions of "reasonable" and "functional" will vary among individuals, but these are the causes that advance directive documents are intended to serve.

Finally, there will be times when there is nobody present who can speak for the patient in a time frame that permits acceptable medical care. In these circumstances, the physician must remember that the first duty is to the patient, and that duty is to improve the patient's life. Improving life is not always the same thing as prolonging life. It is the duty of the physician to manage this aspect of the patient's care in a reverential and respectful manner. There will be times when Physician's must make difficult judgments about matters of life and death. The responsible physician does so, expeditiously and thoughtfully, without attempting to evade the painful dilemmas that arise.

It is important to begin to address the issues of informed consent and end-of-life care early on in the relationship between surgeon and patient. This is not so much a legal issue as one of matching the care offered to the specific situation of the patient. For example, if a patient with end-stage cardiomyopathy is felt to be too fragile for elective aortic aneurysmorrhaphy, that patient is almost certainly a terrible candidate for emergent repair of a ruptured aneurysm. Conversely, an otherwise healthy 18-year-old patient who comes in for an elective herniorrhaphy will not require the same degree of delicate issue exploration as the first patient mentioned. However, they should be informed that unexpected complications could sometimes arise, including death. They should also be informed that the treating team will manage any unusual events to the best of their ability. In all cases, the surgeon must be careful to explain that while they are competent and compassionate, they are also human.

The student is referred to any number of excellent sources for further information on the subject of medical ethics. (See bonus chapter on medical ethics at http://thepoint.lww.com). Another example is *The Hastings Center Report*, a journal devoted to ethical issues.

History

A careful history is fundamental to the preoperative evaluation of the surgical patient, whether for an elective or emergent operation. It is here that the doctor learns about comorbidities that will influence the patient's ability to withstand and recover from the operation. This understanding begins with a careful review of systems intended to elicit problems that, although perhaps not the focus of the patient's surgical experience, are nonetheless important to his or her ability to recover from the operation. The following sections will consider the ways in which certain historical findings can influence a patient's perioperative risk, and what further evaluation should be prompted by the discovery of certain aspects of the patient's history.

The *history of the present illness* (HPI) will obviously direct the lines of inquiry. Within the context of the HPI, a history of the events that preceded the accident or onset of illness may give important clues about the etiology of the problem or may help to uncover occult injury or disease. For example, the onset of severe substernal chest pain before the driver of a vehicle struck a bridge abutment may suggest that the hypotension that the driver exhibited in the emergency department may be related to acute cardiac decompensation from a myocardial infarction as well as from blood loss associated with a pelvic fracture. Such a situation might require modification of hemodynamic monitoring and volume restoration. Although such scenarios sound extreme, they are encountered in emergency departments on a daily basis. These historical elements add significantly to the physician's ability to provide optimal patient care.

Most clinical situations provide an adequate opportunity for a careful *review of systems*. Occasionally, patients cannot provide details of their illness, and then available resources, including family, friends, previous medical records, and emergency medical personnel, will be used to glean what information is available. A review of systems, with emphasis on estimating the patient's ability to respond to the stress of surgery, is imperative. It is sometimes tempting to attempt to summarize a lengthy review of systems with statements such as "review of systems is negative." This terminology should be avoided. It is often important to know exactly what the patient was asked, what they affirmed, and what symptoms they denied experiencing. Therefore, specific questions should be asked and specific answers documented. Areas of focus, explored more fully below, include in particular the

cardiorespiratory, renal, hematologic, nutritional, and endocrine systems. Within the nutritional review is sought information about appetite and weight change, which can impact healing. Further, information about the timing of the patient's last meal can affect the timing of urgent (but not emergent) operations. A full stomach predisposes the patient to aspiration of gastric contents during the induction of anesthesia. If the patient's disease process permits, it is generally best to allow gastric emptying to occur as much as possible prior to induction of anesthesia. This usually takes about 6 hours of strict *nil per os* status. If anesthesia must be induced emergently, the rapid sequence induction technique is used to optimize the chances for safe endotracheal intubation without aspiration.

Family history likewise should record the specific questions asked and the patient's actual responses. For example, family histories of bleeding diatheses, or bad reactions to general anesthesia, are of obvious interest to the surgical team, as would a history of myocardial infarction or malignancy in all of the patient's first-degree relatives.

Determining *allergies and drug sensitivities* is important and will influence selection of such critical interventions as perioperative antibiotics and anesthetic technique.

A *medication history* should also be taken. This history includes prescription drugs, over-the-counter agents, and herbal remedies (nutraceuticals). Many prescription drugs have important implications in perioperative patient management and are detailed in Table 1-1. Some drugs adversely interact with anesthetic agents or alter the normal physiologic response to illness, injury, or the stress of surgery. For example, patients who take β-blocking agents cannot mount the usual chronotropic response to infection or blood loss. Anticoagulants such as warfarin compounds or antiplatelet agents can carry specific risks, both if they are continued in the surgical period and if they are discontinued perioperatively. Patients and/or families should also be questioned about the use of dietary supplements and over-the-counter medications. The popularity of complementary and alternative medicines and the use of nutraceuticals have dramatically increased worldwide. Patients should be asked specifically about these, as many do not regard them as "medicines." Many of these nutraceuticals have the potential to adversely affect the administration of anesthetic agents, hypnotics, sedatives, and a variety of other medications. Some are thought to interfere with platelet function and coagulation, and others to potentiate or reduce the activity of anticoagulants and some immunosuppressants. These products have been classified as "supplements" and are not regulated by the Food and Drug Administration. As a consequence, robust scientific studies concerning their mechanism of action, herb–drug interactions, active drug content, effectiveness, and potential side effects are difficult to identify. Further, reliable information regarding these products is difficult to obtain. The sheer number of preparations available makes it difficult, if not impossible, to compile detailed information on all of them.

Common nutraceuticals are listed in Table 1-2, along with their indications for use and potential adverse side effects. The American Society of Anesthesiologists (ASA) recommends discontinuation of these supplements for 2 to 3 weeks prior to an operative procedure, but this recommendation is not based on sound scientific evidence. The hospital pharmacist or Doctor of Pharmacy is an excellent resource for questions in this area.

TABLE 1-1	Perioperative Medication Management		
Drug Type	**Comment**	**Preoperative Management**	**Postoperative Management**
Cardiac			
β-blockers	Abrupt discontinuation can increase risk of MI	With a sip of water a few hours before operation	Parenteral agent until taking p.o.
Atrial antiarrhythmics		With a sip of water a few hours before operation	IV β-blockers, diltiazem or digoxin until p.o. intake resumed
Ventricular antiarrhythmics	Monitor Mg, K, and Ca levels perioperatively	With a sip of water a few hours before operation	Parenteral amiodarone or procainamide
Nitrates	Transdermal (paste, patch) may be poorly absorbed intraoperatively	With a sip of water a few hours before operation	Intravenous (most reliable) or transdermal until p.o. intake resumed
Antihypertensives	Abrupt discontinuation of clonidine can cause rebound hypertension	With a sip of water a few hours before operation	Parenteral antihypertensives; if on clonidine, consider clonidine patch or alternative antihypertensive agents
Pulmonary			
Inhalers		No modification necessary	Can use nebulized or metered dose inhalers
Leukotriene inhibitors		With a sip of water a few hours before operation	
Diabetes			
Insulin	5% dextrose solutions should be given intravenously intra- and postoperatively in patients receiving insulin	½ dose usual long-acting agent at the usual time preoperatively	SSI until p.o. intake back to baseline
Oral agents (except metformin)		Hold AM of operation	SSI until p.o. intake back to baseline
Metformin	Can produce lactic acidosis, particularly in the setting of renal dysfunction or with administration of IV radiographic contrast agents	Hold for at least 1 day preoperatively	Monitor renal function closely. Resume metformin when renal function normalizes, usually 2–3 days postoperatively. SSI until then.
Antiplatelet agents/anticoagulants			
Aspirin, clopidogrel, ticlopidine		D/C 7 days preoperatively	Resume when diet resumed
Warfarin		Hold until INR normalizes, usually 3–5 days. If anticoagulation critical, maintain anticoagulation with heparin	Resume when diet resumed
Heparin		Discontinue 4 hr preoperatively	Resume 6–12 hr postoperatively, provided no increased risk of hemorrhage thought to exist
Osteoporosis agents			
SERMs	Associated with increased risk of DVT	Hold 1 week preoperatively for procedures with moderate to high risk DVT	
HIV agents		With a sip of water a few hours before operation	Resume when taking p.o.
Neurologic			
Antiparkinson agents			
Carbidopa/levodopa	Prolonged cessation of levodopa can lead to syndrome similar to neuroleptic malignant syndrome	With a sip of water a few hours before operation	
Seligilene	Life-threatening syndrome similar to neuroleptic malignant syndrome reported when used with meperidine	Avoid use with meperidine	Avoid use with meperidine
Antiseizure medications		With a sip of water a few hours before operation	Parenteral agents until p.o. intake resumed

TABLE 1-1	Perioperative Medication Management (continued)

Drug Type	Comment	Preoperative Management	Postoperative Management
Psychiatric			
Tricyclic antidepressants	Anticholinergic effects and conduction abnormalities can be seen		Monitor for anticholinergic side effects
Monoamine oxidase inhibitors	Life-threatening hypertension reported when used with certain sympatho-mimetics; life-threatening syndrome similar to neuroleptic malignant syndrome reported when used with meperidine	Stop 2 weeks preoperatively	
SSRIs	"Serotonin syndrome" reported when used with tramodol; some agents have associated withdrawal syndrome	With a sip of water a few hours before operation	Resume as soon as possible postoperatively
Antipsychotics	Can cause ECG abnormalities (pro-longed QT interval)		Resume as soon as possible postoperatively
Lithium	Monitor levels perioperatively		Resume when p.o. intake resumes
Benzodiazepines	Abrupt cessation can cause withdrawal		Parenterally until diet resumed
Endocrine			
Levothyroxine		Can be held for a few days if needed without adverse effect	Parenterally until diet resumed
Propylthiouracil		Preoperative β blockade for hyperthyroid patients; preoperative potassium iodide	Parenteral β blockers; resume PTU when medications can be given via NG tube
Estrogen	Can increase risk of postoperative DVT	Consider stopping for 4 weeks prior to cases with high risk of DVT	
Rheumatologic			
Methotrexate	Does not interfere with wound healing or increase wound infection rate	Continue usual regimen	Resume when taking p.o.
COX-2 inhibitors	Can impair renal function	Hold 2–3 days preoperatively	Resume when taking p.o.

SSI, sliding scale insulin; SERM, selective estrogen receptor modulator; SSRI, selective serotonin reuptake inhibitors.
From Mercado DL. Perioperative medication management. Med Clin North Am 2003;87(1):41–57.

Even in a surgical emergency, serious efforts must be made to acquire essential historical information about the patient. An emergency situation does force the physician to focus on the critical aspects of the patient's history. The mnemonic "AMPLE" history (*A*llergies, *M*edications, *P*ast medical history, *L*ast meal, *E*vents preceding the emergency) is a convenient way to remember the essential elements during a very time-pressured encounter.

PREOPERATIVE SCREENING TESTS AND CONSULTATIONS

Interpretation of Laboratory and Diagnostic Data

It is standard practice in most North American hospitals for doctors to order a battery of routine preoperative screening tests on otherwise asymptomatic patients under the mistaken belief that this practice improves patient safety, and outcome, by identifying unsuspected conditions that could contribute to perioperative morbidity and mortality. This indiscriminate practice is expensive and unwarranted. In fact, the potential harm caused by the routine screening of asymptomatic patients is greater than any benefit derived from uncovering occult abnormalities. The time and resources necessary to chase unanticipated results, the occasional performance of additional invasive (and risky) secondary procedures, and the fact that 60% of these abnormal results are ignored are arguments against unselected screening. If there is a legal liability issue surrounding preoperative screening, the latter is the most significant one. Obtaining data to establish a "baseline" is not recommended for the asymptomatic patient. Normal laboratory results obtained within 4 months of an elective operative procedure need not be repeated, since abnormalities could be predicted based on the patient's history. Preoperative screening tests are not a substitute for a comprehensive history and physical examination focused to identify comorbidities that may influence perioperative management. The need for emergency surgery, especially for patients who cannot provide historical data, obviously alters these recommendations.

Routine screening of hemoglobin concentration is performed only in individuals who are undergoing procedures that

TABLE 1-2	Nutraceuticals: Proposed Use and Adverse Effects[a]	
Product	**Use**	**Potential Side Effects**
Echinacea (*Echinacea species*)	Prevent and treat upper respiratory infections	Immunosuppression (?)
Ephedra	Sympathomimetic	Vasoconstriction, MI, CVA, herb-drug interaction with MAO-inhibitors
Feverfew (*Tanacetum parthenium*)	Anti-inflammatory, arthritis, migraine headache	Oral ulcers, abdominal pain, bleeding
Garlic (*Allium sativum*)	Cholesterol reduction, anticoagulant, ± antihypertensive, antimicrobial (?)	Irreversible antiplatelet activity (?)
		Excessive bleeding
Ginger (*Zingiber officinale*)	Digestive aide, diuretic, antiemetic, stimulant	Thromboxane synthetase inhibitor
Ginkgo (*Ginkgo Biloba*)	Anticoagulant	Increased anticoagulant effects, bleeding
Ginseng (*Panax Ginseng*)	Lowers blood sugar, inhibits platelet aggregation	Hypoglycemia, bleeding, potentiates warfarin
Glucosamine		Inhibits DNA synthesis (?)
Kava (*Piper methysticum*)	Sedation, anxiolytic	Addiction, withdrawal, increased sedative effects, extrapyramidal effects, (?) hepatitis, GI discomfort, false-negative PSA, hypertension, urinary retention
Saw Palmetto (*Serenoa repens*)	Prostatic health (BPH)	Contraindication in women
Saint John's wort (*Hypericum perforatum*)	Cerebral failure	Inhibition of neurotransmitter uptake, multiple herb–drug interactions including cyclosporin, warfarin, steroids, calcium-channel blockers, and others.
Valerian (*Valeriana officinalis*, vandal root)	Sedative	Withdrawal, enhanced sedative effects of hypnotics, sedatives, anxiolytics

[a]This table of commonly used supplements is neither all-inclusive nor comprehensive. Many of the potential adverse effects and herb–drug interactions are based on anecdotal reports or small, uncontrolled case studies.

are associated with an extensive amount of blood loss, or who may be harboring anemia unbeknownst to the treating team. Patients with a history of anemia, malignant disease, renal insufficiency, cardiac disease, diabetes mellitus, or pregnancy should have baseline determinations of serum hemoglobin concentration. Individuals who cannot provide a history or who have physical findings that suggest anemia should have preoperative baseline hemoglobin determinations. The precise definition of "extensive" blood loss will vary depending on the patient's age and comorbidities. For example, patients with known coronary artery disease should not be allowed to have a postoperative hemoglobin level below 7 g/dL. If such a patient is scheduled to undergo a breast biopsy or a hernia repair, and they are not known to be anemic, it is unlikely that the blood loss associated would precipitate an acute cardiac event. In general, major vascular or musculoskeletal operations on the extremities or operations in the chest or abdomen carry enough risk of severe (>500 mL) blood loss to justify a demonstration beforehand that the patient has sufficient oxygen-carrying capacity to withstand the stress of the planned procedure, particularly if there are significant comorbidities (e.g., cardiac failure, chronic obstructive pulmonary disease [COPD], end-stage renal disease [ESRD]). The groups of patients in whom anemia is suspected preoperatively would include patients with a history of anemia, malignant disease, renal insufficiency, cardiac disease, diabetes mellitus, or pregnancy, or patients whose cardiorespiratory review of systems suggests exertional dyspnea.

Evaluation of baseline serum electrolyte concentrations, including serum creatinine, is appropriate in individuals whose history or physical examination suggests chronic medical disease (e.g., diabetes, hypertension, cardiovascular, renal, or hepatic disease). Patients with the potential for loss of fluids

and electrolytes, including those receiving long-term diuretic therapy, and those with intractable vomiting, should also have preoperative determination of serum electrolytes. The elderly are at substantial risk for chronic dehydration, and testing is appropriate in these patients as well. Although there is no specific age that mandates automatic electrolyte screening, knowledge of the patient's medical history, medications, and systems review should guide decision making about testing.

Preoperative urinalysis is recommended only for patients who have urinary tract symptoms or a history of chronic urinary tract disease, or in those who are undergoing urologic procedures.

Screening chest radiography is rarely indicated. Despite the occasional incidental abnormality that is detected with a screening radiograph, these findings rarely receive further investigation and generally do not alter the surgical plans. Screening chest radiography in asymptomatic elderly patients is also controversial because the usefulness of this diagnostic study in this population is unclear. Chest radiography is recommended for patients who are undergoing intrathoracic procedures and for those who have signs and symptoms of active pulmonary disease.

Recommendations for screening electrocardiography are more firm. Men who are older than 40 years of age and women who are older than 50 years of age should have a baseline recording. Patients with symptomatic cardiovascular disease, hypertension, or diabetes are candidates for preoperative electrocardiography screening. Patients who are undergoing thoracic, intraperitoneal, aortic, or emergency surgery are also candidates for screening examinations. In summary, laboratory and other diagnostic screening tests should be performed only on those patients found to be at risk for specific

TABLE 1-3	Recommendations for Laboratory Testing before Elective Surgery

Test	Incidence of Abnormalities That Change Management	LR+	LR−	Indications
Hemoglobin	0.1%	3.3	0.90	Anticipated major blood loss or symptoms/history of anemia
White blood count	0.0%	0.0	1.0	Symptoms suggestive of infection, myeloproliferative disease, myelotoxic medications
Platelet count	0.0%	0.0	1.0	History of bleeding disorder/bruising, myeloproliferative disease, myelotoxic medications, splenomegaly
Prothrombin time	0.0%	0.0	1.0	History of bleeding disorder/bruising, chronic liver disease, malnutrition, recent or long-term antibiotic/warfarin use
Partial thromboplastin time	0.1%	1.7	0.86	History of bleeding diathesis, anticoagulant medication
Electrolytes	1.8%	4.3	0.80	Chronic renal insufficiency, CHF, diuretic use, other meds that affect electrolytes
Renal function tests	2.6%	3.3	0.81	Age 50, hypertension, cardiac disease, major surgery, medications that may alter renal function
Glucose	0.5%	1.6	0.85	Obesity, known diabetes or symptoms thereof
Liver function tests	0.1%			No indication, consider albumin measurement for major surgery or chronic illness
Urinalysis	1.4%	1.7	0.97	No indication
Electrocardiogram	2.6%	1.6	0.96	Men > 40, women > 50, known coronary artery disease, diabetes or hypertension
Chest x-ray	3.0%	2.5	0.72	Age > 50, known cardiac or pulmonary disease or symptoms or exam findings suggesting cardiac or pulmonary disease

LR+, Likelihood ratio that a test will be abnormal in the absence of symptoms or signs; LR−, Likelihood ratio that a test will be normal in the absence of symptoms or signs; CHF, congestive heart failure.
Adapted and used with permission from Smetana GW, Macpherson DS. The case against routine preoperative laboratory testing. Med Clin North Am 2003;87(1):7–40.

comorbidities identified during the preoperative clinical evaluation. Table 1-3 is a guide to studies that may be appropriate in the preoperative screening phase.

Specialty consultation may be required to optimize the patient's chance for a successful operation. Medical consultants should not be asked to "clear" patients for a surgical procedure; their primary value is in helping to define the degree of perioperative risk and making recommendations about how best to prepare the patient to successfully undergo his or her operation and postoperative course. Once this risk is determined, the surgical team, in conjunction with the patient or the patient's family, may discuss the advisability of a planned surgical approach to the patient's illness. Postoperative consultation should be sought when the patient has unexpected complications or does not respond to initial maneuvers that are commonly employed to address a specific problem. For example, a nephrology consultation is in order for a patient who remains oliguric despite appropriate intravascular volume repletion, particularly if the creatinine level is rising. Likewise, consultation should be obtained from specialists who have expertise in areas that the treating physician does not have. For example, a general surgeon would be well advised to obtain consultation from a cardiologist for a patient who had a postoperative myocardial infarction, no matter how benign the myocardial infarction appears.

Cardiac Evaluation

Alterations in physiology occurring in the perioperative period impose significant stress on the myocardium. The surgical stress response involves a catecholamine surge in response to the pain and anxiety associated with the operative procedure or the disease process itself. The result is an increase in the myocardial oxygen requirement. A second alteration suppresses the fibrinolytic system, predisposing the patient to thrombosis. Myocardial ischemia secondary to coronary artery disease can result in cardiac segments in which blood flow is reduced further by occlusive disease putting these segments at risk during time of additional stress. In a study of unselected patients over the age of 40, the estimated perioperative MI rate was 2.5%, and this increased with the type of procedure and selected subsets of patients. A useful approach to the consideration of cardiac risk is to consider:

1. The clinical characteristics of the patient
2. The inherent risk of the surgical procedure
3. The patient's functional capacity

Evaluation of Patients Asymptomatic for Heart Disease

All evaluations start with an assessment of baseline cardiac function. Historical aspects should include any congenital or acquired cardiac pathology or interventions including valvular and ischemic heart disease as well as a list of all drugs. Special note is taken of the patient's overall status during the physical examination. Vital signs can give important clues about the status of the cardiovascular system (i.e., tachycardia, tachypnea, postural changes in blood pressure). Jugular venous distension at 30°, slow carotid pulse upstroke, bruits, edema, and a laterally displaced point of maximum cardiac impulse all suggest some type of cardiac disease. Auscultatory findings that suggest cardiac problems include rubs, third heart sounds, and systolic murmurs.

Determining which murmurs are clinically significant and which are innocent is perplexing for most medical students. Most innocent murmurs are apical. Innocent murmurs are never associated with a palpable thrill, and there are no innocent diastolic murmurs. Maneuvers that change blood flow (i.e., Valsalva) generally do not change the character or the pitch of innocent murmurs. A patient who has hemodynamically significant aortic stenosis usually has a characteristically harsh holosystolic murmur, a slow carotid pulse upstroke, and a displaced primary myocardial impulse that is secondary to left ventricular hypertrophy. This latter finding, as well as poststenotic aortic dilation, may be seen on chest radiograph. Patients who have a history of mitral insufficiency also have an increased risk of postoperative congestive heart failure and arrhythmia.

Preoperative electrocardiogram (EKG) is appropriate in those patients with one or more risk factors (history of ischemic heart disease, history or presence of congestive heart failure, history of cerebrovascular disease, diabetes or renal impairment). Preoperative EKG is not indicated for asymptomatic patients undergoing a low-risk procedure. Although any abnormality seen on routine electrocardiography implies increased risk to the adult patient, other than acute myocardial infarction or complete heart block, abnormalities rarely require postponement of surgery, especially in asymptomatic patients.

Mild, chronic congestive heart failure is not associated with an increased occurrence of perioperative infarction. Patients with cardiomegaly on chest radiograph and even those whose clinical course is effectively managed medically do not represent high-risk groups. However, abnormal third heart sounds or signs of jugular venous distension indicate decompensation of cardiac function. These patients are in jeopardy of serious cardiac complications. The perioperative phase of the patients experience is associated with alterations in fluid and electrolyte control. Patients may be kept fasting for several days and blood loss and drains deplete fluid and electrolytes. The endocrine response to surgery will also alter flux of fluids across the various body fluid compartments. This may cause additional stress if the patient has underlying cardiac compromise.

The urgency of the required surgery may alter the risk/benefit ratio and determine how complete the preoperative cardiac evaluation will be. This segment will focus on the elective workup of a required but nonurgent procedure.

Evaluation of Patients With Known Heart Disease
The patient who is scheduled to undergo elective surgery should be questioned carefully about the nature, severity, and location of chest pain. Dates and details about infarctions, documented or suspected, should be noted, as should coronary artery bypass graft or revascularization procedures, valve replacements, and pacemaker insertions. Additional historical elements of significance include a history of dyspnea on exertion (which may signify underlying cardiac or pulmonary pathology). Other clues to the possibility of coexisting heart disease include syncope, palpitations, arrhythmia, and a history of either cerebrovascular or peripheral vascular surgery.

In the patient with previous infarction, the risk of clinical postoperative myocardial ischemia is between 5% and 10% overall, with an attendant mortality rate of 50%. This figure contrasts with a risk of <0.5% in patients with no history of infarct or clinically evident heart disease. If an elective operative procedure is performed immediately after a recent myocardial infarction, the risk of an additional acute cardiac event or death is approximately 30% within the first 3 months. The risk declines with time and reaches a plateau of approximately 5% at 6 months. If possible, elective surgery should be postponed for 6 months after a myocardial infarction.

With the exception of coronary artery bypass grafting, the patient who has unstable angina should avoid surgery, and undergo further investigation and intervention prior to an elective procedure. Although the patient with stable angina is theoretically at increased risk, no clear answer about the extent of increased postoperative risk is available for this group. In contrast, patients who have undergone coronary artery bypass have a significantly reduced danger of postoperative infarct compared with those who have angina. The risk is estimated at slightly more than 1%, with a similar mortality rate. Percutaneous angioplasty may confer myocardial protection in the postoperative period, but studies confirming the value of this procedure indicate that it is beneficial only in selected lesions. The use of various and at times multiple antiplatelet agents in the post–stent insertion phase may complicate the planned surgical procedure. Patients with any cardiac history must be evaluated carefully, and the severity of their disease must be documented. If possible, maximum myocardial performance should be achieved before any operative procedure is undertaken.

A history of diabetes increases the index of suspicion for occult cardiac pathology. Of patients with a documented history of diabetes for 5 to 10 years, 60% have diffuse vascular pathology. After 20 years, nearly all patients with diabetes have some type of vascular abnormality. In addition, the risk of mortality after a cardiac ischemic event for the patient with diabetes is higher than that for people without diabetes. Silent infarctions or ischemic events without symptoms may be discovered during investigation. Therefore, patients with diabetes, especially those with a long-standing history of the disease, should be viewed with suspicion and presumed to have some degree of cardiovascular abnormality.

Discussion and close collaboration with the anesthesia team is vital to ensure the safety and optimal management of patients in the perioperative period. Different monitoring techniques may identify instability before clinical manifestations are apparent and allow for preventative intervention in the operative and postoperative phases.

Cardiac Medications
The issue of perioperative medication and cardiac protection is not totally resolved. It is recommended that patients who are currently on β-blockers remain on them, including taking them the day of surgery. Similarly, statins should be continued as they have been shown to reduce the risk of perioperative cardiac events. If absolute postoperative hemostasis is not a requirement (as it may be in certain neurosurgical or ophthalmic procedures), then single-agent antiplatelet agents should be continued.

Previous recommendations for the antibiotic prophylaxis of endocarditis following invasive surgery have been altered within the past years. The most recent are presented by the American Heart Association (*Circulation* 2007;116:1736–1754) and currently do not support routine use of antibiotics to prevent infective endocarditis for gastrointestinal or genitourinary procedures. In selected patients undergoing respiratory system procedures, prophylaxis is recommended as well as for those having invasive dental work.

TABLE 1-4	Dripps-American Surgical Classification
Class I	Healthy patient: limited procedure
Class II	Mild to moderate systemic disturbance
Class III	Severe systemic disturbance
Class IV	Life-threatening disturbance
Class V	Not expected to survive, with or without surgery

Quantification of Surgical Risk

Based on the history, physical findings, and a few simple laboratory studies, efforts have been made to quantify surgical risk. The most commonly used system, the **Dripps-American Surgical Association Classification**, categorizes patients into five groups (Table 1-4). The system offers little guidance, however, for identifying patients who are at risk for postoperative myocardial ischemia.

The revised cardiac risk index developed by Lee (*Circulation* 1999;100:1043) is the most commonly used index of cardiac risk and attributes increased risk to:

- High-risk type of surgery
- History of ischemic heart disease
- History of congestive heart failure
- History of cerebrovascular disease
- Preoperative treatment with insulin
- Preoperative serum creatinine >2.0 mg/dL (177 μmol/L).

Based on the number of factors present, the patient is assigned to class I to IV and estimated for cardiac risk accordingly (Table 1-5). A reliable indicator of hemodynamic reserve is made by a quantitative estimate of the patient's cardiovascular functional class. A useful scale is outlined in Table 1-6.

Activity is expressed in metabolic equivalents (METs). One MET represents an oxygen consumption of 3.5 mL/kg/minute, the average for a resting 70-kg man. Achieving a heart rate of more than 100 beats/minute during cardiac stress is roughly equivalent to 4 METs.

A useful bedside/clinic assessment question is to enquire about exercise tolerance. A patient who can walk four blocks or ascend two flights of stairs without stopping or getting short of breath has reasonable exercise capacity.

The American College of Cardiology and the American Heart Association Task Forces have outlined a logical approach to the preoperative cardiac evaluation of patients

TABLE 1-6	Energy Expenditure and METs
Class	**Tasks Patient Can Perform to Completion**
I	Activity requiring >6 METs
	Carrying 24 lb up eight steps
	Carrying objects that weigh 80 lb
	Performing outdoor work (shoveling snow, spading soil)
	Participating in recreation (skiing, basketball, squash, handball, jogging/walking at 5 mph)
II	Activities requiring >4 but not >6 METs
	Having sexual intercourse without stopping
	Walking at 4 mph on level ground
	Performing outdoor work (gardening, raking, weeding)
	Participating in recreation (roller-skating, dancing fox trot)
III	Activity requiring >1 but not >4 METs
	Showering, dressing without stopping, stripping, and making bed
	Walking at 2.5 mph on level ground
	Performing outdoor work (cleaning windows)
	Participating in recreation (golfing, bowling)
IV	No activity requiring >1 MET
	Cannot carry out any of the above activities

METs, metabolic equivalents.
Source: American Heart Association, Inc. ACC/AHA 2007 guidelines on perioperative cardiovascular evaluation and care for noncardiac surgery: a report of the American College of Cardiology/American Heart Association Task Force on Practice Guidelines. Circulation 2007;116(17):e418–e499.

who are undergoing noncardiac surgery. The general recommendation is that preoperative testing should be limited to the small subset of patients who are at very high risk, when results will affect patient treatment and, most important, outcome. The algorithm developed by the Task Force on Practice Guidelines (Figure 1-1) shows a simplified five-step approach to preoperative cardiac assessment. Patients who need emergency noncardiac surgery require operative intervention without extensive preoperative testing. Postoperatively, these patients may require further cardiac evaluation. Step two identifies patients who have active cardiac conditions. Patients who are undergoing low-risk surgery (Table 1-7) may proceed with the planned procedure. A patient with a good functional capacity and no symptoms, even with a history of cardiac disease, may proceed with planned surgery. Patients with major clinical predictors (i.e., unstable coronary syndrome, decompensated congestive heart failure, significant arrhythmia, severe valvular disease) should be evaluated by noninvasive tests of myocardial perfusion. The objective of these noninvasive assessments is to identify patients who would benefit from coronary angiography and subsequent cardiac intervention before elective surgery. If the patient has only intermediate predictors or if no clinical predictors are present, then assessment for functional capacity can be estimated. Individuals who cannot meet a 4-MET demand are at increased risk for perioperative cardiac ischemia and long-term complications. Individuals who are at high risk should undergo noninvasive testing and consideration for coronary angiography. Patients who show abnormalities by noninvasive testing and

TABLE 1-5	Revised Cardiac Risk Index	
Class	**Number of Risk Factors Present**	**Percentage Rate Major Myocardial Complications**
I	0	0.4–0.5
II	1	0.9–1.03
III	2	3.6–6.6
IV	More	9.1–11.0

Source: American Heart Association, Inc. Lee TH, Marcantonio ER, Mangione CM, et al. Derivation and prospective validation of a simple index for prediction of cardiac risk of major noncardiac surgery. Circulation 1999;100:1043.

are considered candidates for coronary artery revascularization should undergo coronary angiography and subsequent intervention, as determined by the results of those studies.

Pulmonary Evaluation

The reported incidence of postoperative pulmonary complications is between 2% and 19% depending on the definition of postoperative pulmonary complications. This incidence is comparable to the incidence of postoperative cardiac complications and has a similar adverse impact on morbidity, mortality, and length of stay. The purpose of a preoperative pulmonary evaluation is to identify patients at risk for perioperative complications and long-term disability. A careful history and physical examination will usually indicate which patients are most at risk. Important elements of this history should include age, a history of smoking, presence of asthma, COPD, sleep apnea, and congestive heart failure, previous pulmonary complications during or after surgery, exercise tolerance, general health, and the type and urgency of the planned procedure. Symptoms such as coughing, wheezing, sputum production, dyspnea, snoring, and orthopnea should be noted. The physical examination should be focused on the cardiopulmonary and respiratory system. In general, there is no role for routine pulmonary function test. Specialized testing is reserved for patients who have significant risk factors or who are expected to undergo an operation that carries a relatively high intrinsic risk of pulmonary complications.

Preoperative pulmonary assessment determines not only factors that can lead to increased risk but also identification of modifiable factors that can reduce the risk of pulmonary complications. Preoperative interventions that may decrease postoperative pulmonary complications include smoking cessation, inspiratory muscle training, bronchodilator therapy, antibiotic therapy for preexisting infection, and pretreatment of asthmatic patients with steroids.

The most important and morbid postoperative pulmonary complications are atelectasis, pneumonia, respiratory

Step 1: Are there active cardiac conditions?	
Condition	**Examples**
Unstable coronary syndromes	Unstable or severe angina
	MI within 30 days
Decompensated HG (NYHA functional class IV; worsening or new-onset HF)	
Significant arrhythmias	High-grade atrioventricular block
	Mobitz II atrioventricular block
	Third-degree atrioventricular heart block
	Symptomatic ventricular arrhythmias
	Supraventricular arrhythmias (including atrial fibrillation) with uncontrolled ventricular rate (HR greater than 100 beats per minute at rest)
	Newly recognized ventricular tachycardia
	Symptomatic bradycardia
Severe valvular disease	Severe aortic stenosis (mean pressure gradient greater than 40 mm Hg, aortic valve area less than 1.0 cm², or symptomatic)
	Symptomatic mitral stenosis (progressive dyspnea on exertion, exertional presyncope, or HF)

Step 2: What is their functional capacity? MET 4 = Light housework (dusting, washing dishes); climb a flight of stairs; walk on level ground at ≥ 4 mph

Step 3: What is the risk level of the planned operation?	
Vascular (reported cardiac risk often more than 5%)	Aortic and other major vascular surgery
	Peripheral vascular surgery
Intermediate (reported cardiac risk generally 1% to 5%)	Intraperitoneal and intrathoracic surgery
	Carotid endarterectomy
	Head and neck surgery
	Orthopedic surgery
	Prostate surgery
Low (reported cardiac risk generally less than 1%)	Endoscopic procedures
	Superficial procedure
	Cataract surgery
	Breast surgery
	Ambulatory surgery

Step 4: Are there clinical risk factors? Ischemic heart disease, heart failure, diabetes mellitus, renal insufficiency, cerebrovascular disease

(continued)

FIGURE 1-1. Cardiac evaluation for noncardiac surgery based on active clinical conditions (Adapted with permission from Fletcher LA, et al., ACC/AHA 2007 Perioperative guidelines. *JACC* 2007;50(17):1707–1732.)

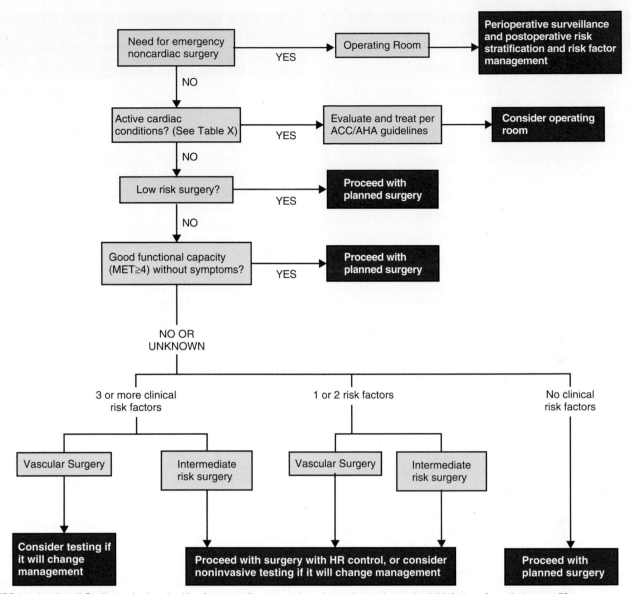

FIGURE 1-1. *(continued)* Cardiac evaluation algorithm for noncardiac surgery, based on patient and procedural risk factors, for patients ≥ age 50.

failure or prolonged mechanical ventilation, pulmonary embolism, and exacerbation of underlying chronic lung disease. Potential risk factors for postoperative pulmonary complications can be either related to the patient or the procedure and are shown in Table 1-8. While there is a significant body of scientific evidence supporting the association of most of these risk factors with postoperative pulmonary complications, the evidence for others is not as convincing.

Patient-Related Risk Factors

Patient-related risk factors include age, chronic lung disease, tobacco abuse, congestive heart failure, functional dependence, and the American Society of Anesthesiologist classification. In general, patients who have an obstruction to expiration flow for any reason are in greatest jeopardy. They may need specialized pulmonary function studies preoperatively and vigorous preoperative and postoperative pulmonary care for prophylaxis. The section on pulmonary evaluation for nonpulmonary operations describes the specific tests.

There is controversy about whether age itself is a risk factor for pulmonary complications. With increasing age, there is a progressive decline in static lung volume, maximum expiratory flow, and elastic recoil as well as a decrease in PaO_2 because of an increase in the alveolar–arterial oxygen gradient. The net effect is a loss of pulmonary reserve. The confounding factor is that many older persons also have independent risk factors for pulmonary complications. Age itself is not a contraindication to surgical intervention, but the normal changes that occur with the aging process should be kept in mind. Pulmonary disease is a risk factor and COPD increases perioperative risk for several reasons. Increased pulmonary secretions, small airway obstruction secondary to mucous plugging, inefficient clearing of secretions, and a general lack of pulmonary reserve predispose the patient to atelectasis and superimposed

TABLE 1-7	Cardiac Risk[a] Stratification for Noncardiac Surgical Procedures

Risk Stratification	Procedure Examples
Vascular (reported cardiac risk often more than 5%)	Aortic and other major vascular surgery
	Peripheral vascular surgery
Intermediate (reported cardiac risk generally 1%–5%)	Intraperitoneal and intrathoracic surgery
	Carotid endarterectomy
	Head and neck surgery
	Orthopedic surgery
	Prostate surgery
Low[b] (reported cardiac risk generally <1%)	Endoscopic procedures
	Superficial procedure
	Cataract surgery
	Breast Surgery
	Ambulatory surgery

[a]Combined incidence of cardiac death and nonfatal myocardial infarction.
[b]These procedures do not generally require further preoperative cardiac testing.

Adapted with permission from Fleisher J, et al. ACC/AHA 2007 Guidelines on Perioperative Cardiovascular Evaluation and Care for Noncardiac Surgery. J Am Col Cardiol 2007;50:1717.

TABLE 1-9	American Society of Anesthesiologists Classification and Association with Postoperative Pulmonary Complications

ASA class	Class Definition	Rates of Postoperative Pulmonary Complications by Class (%)
I	Normal healthy patient	1.2
II	Patient with mild systemic disease	5.4
III	Patient with systemic disease that is not incapacitating	11.4
IV	Patient with an incapacitating systemic disease that is a constant threat to life	10.9
V	Moribund patient who is not expected to survive for 24 hr with or without operation	NA

infection. Patients who have a history of occupational exposure to known irritants (e.g., silicone, asbestos, textile components) may have significant restrictive disease and a noticeable reduction in respiratory reserve. Also at high risk are patients who cannot cough or breathe deeply for any reason, such as those with an altered level of consciousness, neuromuscular disease, paraplegia, or weakness as a result of malnutrition.

In smokers, the relative risk of pulmonary complications is two to six times greater than that in nonsmokers. Smokers have abnormalities in mucociliary clearance, increased volume of secretions, increased carboxyhemoglobin levels, and a predisposition to atelectasis. Smokers should be asked to stop smoking at least 6 weeks before the procedure; however, compliance with this request is rare.

Functional dependence is an important predictor of postoperative pulmonary complications. Total dependence is defined as the inability to perform any activities of daily living and partial dependence is the need for equipment or devices and assistance from another person for some activities of daily life. The ASA classification, while originally designed to help in predicting perioperative mortality rates, has been proven to predict postoperative pulmonary complications (Table 1-9). Higher ASA class is associated with a substantial increase risk in complications, with patients who are higher than ASA class II having a twofold to threefold increased risk of postoperative complications compared to patients with ASA class of II or lower.

Low serum albumin level (<3.5 g/dL) has been associated with an increased risk of pulmonary complications and should be measured in all patients who may be at risk for malnutrition or in whom there is a clinical suspicion of hypoalbuminemia. Serum albumin levels should also be evaluated in patients with one or more risk factors for postoperative pulmonary complications.

Asthma used to be considered a risk factor for postoperative pulmonary complications; however, recent evidence suggests that this is not necessarily the case. Regardless, it is important that patients be compliant with prescribed antiasthma medications and good pulmonary toilet in the preoperative phase. Perioperative stress and many medications, including anesthetic agents, can provoke bronchospasm. Similarly, while intuitively it may seem that obesity and obstructive sleep apnea would also be a risk factor for pulmonary complications, current scientific evidence does not support this contention.

Procedure-Related Risk Factors

Contrary to the case of cardiac risk assessment, procedure-related risk factors are more important than patient-related factors in estimating the risk for postoperative pulmonary complications.

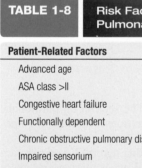

TABLE 1-8	Risk Factors for Postoperative Pulmonary Complications

Patient-Related Factors
- Advanced age
- ASA class >II
- Congestive heart failure
- Functionally dependent
- Chronic obstructive pulmonary disease
- Impaired sensorium
- Cigarette use
- Nutritional status
- Obesity
- Obstructive sleep apnea
- Cerebrovascular accident

Procedure-Related Factors
- Site of surgery (chest, upper abdomen, neurosurgery, neck, vascular)
- Duration of surgery (>3 hr)
- General anesthesia
- Emergency surgery

ASA, American Society of Anesthesiologists.

They include surgery site, duration of surgery, anesthetic technique, and type of surgery (elective vs. emergency)

Surgical Site

Patients undergoing thoracic surgery, especially if they require a lung resection, are at increased risk for pulmonary complications and are discussed separately. Among nonpulmonary operations, the risk of pulmonary complications can be stratified by the type of operation. Abdominal operations that require an upper midline incision or involve dissection in the upper abdomen are associated with a much higher pulmonary complication rate than those that are restricted to the lower abdomen. Abdominal incisions are painful and are associated with diminished functional residual capacity (FRC). These problems contribute to the higher pulmonary complication rate. Any thoracotomy incision predisposes the patient to pulmonary complications. Interestingly, the median sternotomy incision is associated with a low incidence of pulmonary complications, probably because it is associated with minimal discomfort during quiet breathing. Neurosurgical, vascular procedures and neck surgery are also associated with a higher risk of pulmonary complications.

Duration of Surgery

Prolonged surgery duration ranging from 3 to 4 hours is associated with a higher risk of postoperative pulmonary complications.

Anesthesia Technique

General anesthesia carries a greater risk of postoperative pulmonary complications than peripheral nerve conduction blocks also known as regional anesthesia. Whether spinal or epidural anesthesia is less risky is a matter of debate. General anesthesia produces an 11% reduction in FRC. Patients do not cough under anesthesia, and postoperative sedation depresses respiratory drive and inhibits coughing. The lasting effects of neuromuscular blockade can also weaken the coughing effort. Mucociliary clearance is also depressed by anesthetic agents. Anticholinergic drugs commonly thicken the patient's mucus and make it more difficult to mobilize. Tracheal intubation promotes direct colonization of the upper airway by Gram-negative organisms and sets the stage for infection. A significant portion of hospital-acquired infections is caused by iatrogenic introduction of nosocomial organisms into the tracheobronchial tree by suction catheters that are passed without attention to aseptic technique.

It is tempting to assume that regional anesthesia would obviate these problems. In fact, this assumption may be true for procedures on extremities or procedures that can be done with a very specific regional blockade (e.g., axillary block). However, spinal and epidural anesthesia are also associated with postoperative pulmonary problems. As a rule, the important factor is not the type of anesthetic agent employed, but the circumstances to which the patient is exposed (e.g., abdominal procedures, loss of periodic hyperinflation by sighing).

Pulmonary Evaluation for Nonpulmonary Operations

The pulmonary evaluation of the patient for nonpulmonary operations begins with a thorough history and physical examination as mentioned above along with an assessment of his or her functional status. Questions about activities in daily life should also be asked. For example, can the patient shovel snow (or rake the yard)? Is he or she out of breath after walking up a flight of stairs? Another important question is

whether the patient has a history of occupational exposure to known pulmonary irritants. The patient should be asked about his or her smoking history, sputum production, wheezing, and exertional dyspnea. Physical examination should begin with a general assessment of the patient's habitus. Are there signs of wasting or morbid obesity? Does the patient exhibit pursed-lip breathing? Does he or she have clubbing or cyanosis? What is the patient's respiratory pattern? Is there a prolonged expiratory phase, as in obstructive airways disease? What is the anteroposterior dimension of the chest? On auscultation, does the patient wheeze? A patient who cannot climb one flight of steps without dyspnea or blow out a match at 8 inches from the mouth without pursing the lips is a candidate for more sophisticated pulmonary function screening. Another useful bedside test is the loose cough test. A rattle heard through the stethoscope when the patient forcibly coughs is a reliable indicator of underlying pulmonary pathology and warrants investigation, beginning with a chest radiograph, with further studies ordered as appropriate to the patient's history, physical examination findings, and radiographic results.

Before the specific elements of pulmonary function tests are discussed, it is useful to review the physiologic definitions of standard lung volumes and capacities. Figure 1-2 shows a standard spirometry curve. Normal tidal ventilation is shown by A. At the end of passive tidal exhalation, the patient is said to be at FRC (shown by B in Figure 1-2). FRC is equal to the sum of expiratory reserve volume (the amount of air that can be expelled with a forced expiratory maneuver) and residual volume (the volume of air left in the lung after a forced expiration). This volume cannot be exhaled under normal circumstances. Closing volume (CV) is the volume below which the alveoli become so structurally unstable that they cannot remain open, even with the benefit of surfactant. In Figure 1-2, normal CV is shown as being slightly lower than residual volume. In a smoker, however, CV requires a much higher volume of air. Consequently, patients with lung pathology tend to have spontaneous atelectasis at much higher volumes than they would otherwise have. CV is actually greater than FRC in smokers and obese patients, whereas it is much lower than FRC in normal patients. Because FRC is the volume left in the lung after a passive tidal expiration, it is important to understand that certain lung diseases predispose the patient to atelectasis because

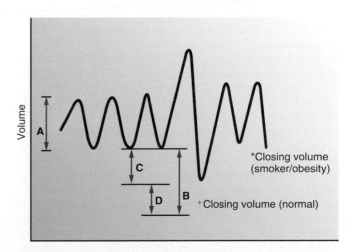

FIGURE 1-2. Spirometry. A, Tidal volume. **B,** Functional residual capacity. **C,** Expiratory reserve volume. **D,** Residual volume. ˙Closing volume for smoker/obese patient. †Closing volume for normal patient.

CV is actually greater than FRC. The most commonly used pulmonary function test (PFT) is the FEV_1. During the forced vital capacity maneuver (part of obtaining the FEV_1), the patient is evaluated for intrinsic lung disease and also for problems with the ventilatory pump that moves air into and out of the lungs.

Any patient who has significant abnormalities in respiratory function on routine history or physical examination may benefit from formal pulmonary function studies. In some patients, such information leads to a decision to postpone or modify the course of therapy. Pulmonary function studies that can potentially uncover or quantitate a condition that can be improved in the preoperative period (thereby lessening the risk of postoperative problems) are cost effective and justifiable. PFTs are often used in combination with arterial blood gas analysis to study the patient who is thought to be at high risk.

There is no evaluation strategy that precisely defines the pulmonary risk of a given patient. Although it is possible to indicate which patients are likely to fare extremely well or extremely poorly, the middle groups are difficult to stratify. At a minimum, a patient with a preoperative FEV_1 of <1 L (the amount of air that can be exhaled in 1 second during a forced expiration after the patient inhales to total lung capacity), a PaO_2 of <50 mm Hg, or a $PaCO_2$ of >45 mm Hg should have the risks of operation explained in clear terms. These risks include not only death and pneumonia, but also the possibility of long-term ventilator dependence. Because of this possibility, some patients decide against proceeding with the operation.

Pulmonary Evaluation for Pulmonary Operations

Pulmonary resections present the special problem of removal of lung tissue in a patient who is already at risk for postoperative pulmonary complications. These patients are likely to have a significant smoking history. Patients who have a greater than a 10 pack-year smoking history are at particular risk for chronic bronchitis. In general, the goal is to leave the patient with an FEV_1 of at least 800 mL postoperatively. If the predicted postoperative FEV_1 is <800 mL, the chances are significant that the patient will never wean from the ventilator postoperatively. The predicted postoperative FEV_1 is estimated by a variety of methods, ranging from simple to complex. One of the easiest ways to estimate quickly whether the postoperative FEV_1 will be low is to multiply the preoperative FEV_1 by the percentage of lung tissue that will be left after resection. For example, consider a patient with an FEV_1 of 1.8 L who is scheduled to undergo a right upper lobectomy. The percentage of pulmonary tissue to be removed is one of five total lobes (20% of the total lung tissue). This patient's predicted postoperative FEV_1 is 1.8 L—80% lung remaining postoperatively equals 1.4 L.

In the very high-risk patient who is to undergo pulmonary resection and whose predicted postoperative FEV_1 is <1 L, split perfusion radionuclide lung scanning is helpful in predicting the amount of functioning lung that will remain postoperatively. If, after careful study, the patient's predicted postoperative FEV_1 is <800 mL, the risk that the patient will not get off the ventilator is such that the patient is considered inoperable. Exercise testing is also useful in the evaluation of these patients and does not require a sophisticated pulmonary laboratory. The stair climb is a simple and reproducible method of assessing pulmonary function. The interested medical student can walk with the patient up stairs. A patient who can climb five flights of stairs can tolerate a pneumonectomy, and one who can climb three flights can usually tolerate a lobectomy. Patients with asthma and COPD should be particularly careful to be compliant with their medication regimen preoperatively.

The Patient with Renal Dysfunction

Traditionally, patients with renal dysfunction were classified under the broad categories of chronic renal failure (CRF) or acute renal failure (ARF). However, in order to standardize the definitions and better evaluate these patients, it has been recommended that the term chronic kidney disease (CKD) or acute kidney injury (AKI) be used. CKD is defined as either kidney damage or decreased kidney function for three or more months. Proteinuria or abnormalities in imaging are markers for kidney damage, and a reduction in glomerular filtration rate (GFR) is a marker for decreased kidney function. ESRD, which is a commonly used term, indicates chronic treatment by dialysis or transplantation and does not refer to a specific degree of kidney function. A GFR of <60 mL/minute/1.73 m^2 is considered the threshold for CKD. GFR can vary with age, gender, ethnicity, and body mass and is typically estimated with calculations based on serum creatinine level. Kidney failure is defined as either a GFR of <15 mL/minute/1.73 m^2 or a need for dialysis or renal transplantation. AKI encompasses the entire range of ARF from small changes in serum creatinine to loss of function requiring dialysis. AKI can be classified according to prerenal, renal, and postrenal causes. Perioperatively, the most common cause of AKI is secondary to acute tubular necrosis (ATN). The risk of AKI in surgical patients has been estimated to be approximately 1%. Factors associated with increased risk of AKI include age, past history of kidney disease, left ventricular ejection fraction of <35%, cardiac index <1.7 L/minute/m^2, hypertension, peripheral vascular disease, diabetes mellitus, emergency surgery, and type of surgery. The highest risk surgeries include coronary artery surgery, cardiac valve surgery, aortic aneurysm surgery, and liver transplant surgery.

It is estimated that approximately 15% of the general population in the United States has CKD. Surgery presents significant risks to patients with CKD or those with, or at risk of, AKI. The metabolic consequences of renal dysfunction frequently require special preparation of the patient for an elective surgical procedure. Meticulous attention to perioperative care can reduce the complication rate in patients with acute or chronic renal impairment. The extent of preoperative testing depends on the patient's comorbid conditions and should include an electrocardiogram and chest radiograph. Renal function should be assessed by accurate assessment of the fluid balance and measurement of makers of renal function including serum creatinine and blood urea nitrogen (BUN) as well as urinary electrolytes. Cardiovascular disease is the main cause of mortality in patients with CKD and therefore these patients warrant a thorough perioperative cardiovascular evaluation. Given the diverse nature of diseases that can affect kidney function, patients with kidney dysfunction requiring surgery should undergo a thorough evaluation that should include the following:

- Diagnosis (type of kidney disease)
- Comorbid conditions
- Severity of renal dysfunction as assessed by level of kidney function
- Complications related to the level of kidney function
- Risk for loss of kidney function
- Risk for cardiovascular disease

In CKD, the ability to excrete water and sodium and maintain homeostasis of the intravascular volume is impaired. Excessive preload usually does not appear, however, until renal function deteriorates to <10% of normal. Chronic volume depletion is encountered in these patients as frequently as volume overload. These patients often receive potent diuretic agents or have chronic volume contraction associated with hypertension. Maintenance of euvolemia and renal perfusion is the goal in the perioperative management of patients with CKD or AKI. For this reason, fluid management is dictated by the patient's history and disease process, not by the fact that he or she has renal impairment. For example, a patient who has ESRD and is in septic shock because of perforated sigmoid diverticulitis requires crystalloid resuscitation to correct the relative volume deficit, even though he or she is dependent on dialysis. This patient should not be fluid restricted. Invasive hemodynamic monitoring can be helpful in this patient group and allows precision in volume replacement. The ability to excrete potassium is also impaired, and patients with impaired renal function do not tolerate sudden changes in potassium level. The risk of malignant hyperkalemia is directly proportional to the serum potassium level before the last dialysis. Serum potassium levels should be <5 mEq/L before surgery. Achieving this level may require dialysis or the use of ion exchange resins. CKD is usually accompanied by chronic metabolic acidosis because excretion of fixed acids is reduced. These acids are the byproducts of metabolism and include sulfates, phosphates, and lactate. Postoperatively, the acid load can further increase as hydrogen ions are released from damaged cells in which case respiratory compensation by hyperventilation can maintain the serum pH at an acceptable level that is slightly below normal. However, if $PaCO_2$ increases even slightly, a profound exacerbation of acidosis may occur. This situation is seen in patients who cannot increase minute ventilation, who have increased dead space, or who are receiving an excessive carbohydrate caloric load.

Another electrolyte abnormality that is often seen in patients with CKD is hvypocalcemia secondary to hyperphosphatemia. Ionized calcium should be followed in these patients and supplemented as needed in the perioperative period. Oral phosphate binders and dietary restriction of phosphates may be required as well. Hypermagnesemia is also common; therefore, magnesium-containing antacids should be avoided in these patients.

Most patients with long-standing CKD are malnourished. Anorexia, which results from azotemia and the inability to handle the accumulation of nitrogenous end products, promotes depletion of both skeletal muscle and visceral protein stores. Malabsorption syndromes are common, as are overt vitamin deficiencies. Patients who receive long-term peritoneal dialysis may lose as much as 6 to 8 g protein/day, and, as a result, may have hypoalbuminemia. Anorexia and a history of weight loss suggest a catabolic state and therefore aggressive nutritional support should be provided. Patients should not be protein restricted in the perioperative phase just because they have renal failure as malnutrition significantly increases the risk of septic complications in the perioperative period.

The normochromic, normocytic anemia that is often seen in patients with CKD is usually well tolerated. The added stress and oxygen requirements that follow a surgical procedure, however, may have adverse consequences. Chronic dialysis is estimated to remove as much as 3 L blood/year, and the reduced production of erythropoietin hampers red blood cell replacement. The lifespan of red blood cells is also reduced in the uremic state. Immune responses are deficient, and, as a result, the potential for infectious complications may be enhanced. Many patients with CKD are carriers of blood-borne pathogens and also develop antibodies because of multiple transfusions, which can significantly delay typing and screening of blood products. Chronic coagulopathy secondary to heparinization during dialysis, or the coagulopathy associated with uremia, may exaggerate blood loss during surgery or in the perioperative period. A coagulation profile may help to identify intrinsic deficiencies. D-desamino arginine vasopressin (DDAVP) promotes the release of von Willebrand's multimers from endothelial cells. Thus, a dose of DDAVP may be of use preoperatively in addressing the thrombocytopathy of CKD.

Daily weighing and accurate intake and output records are essential. Exacerbation of renal failure is prevented if hypotension is avoided and medications are carefully administered. Most drugs can be nephrotoxic, and doses must be adjusted frequently based on an estimation of the degree of renal function. Angiotensin-converting enzyme inhibitors (ACEI) and angiotensin II antagonist (ARA) should be discontinued for at least 10 hours before general anesthesia to reduce the risk of postinduction hypotension. Analgesic requirements in the perioperative period are an important consideration in patients with AKI or CKD as opioids may accumulate in patients with CKD placing them at a higher risk of respiratory depression. Nonsteroidal anti-inflammatory drugs are generally not recommended because of their nephrotoxic side effects.

Patients with renal failure may require modifications in anesthetic techniques. For example, succinylcholine is generally avoided because it may promote or exacerbate hyperkalemia. Also, nondepolarizing neuromuscular blockage agents that are not renally metabolized and excreted should be selected. Cisatracurium undergoes Hoffman degradation and is often used in the anesthetic management of patients with renal failure. To minimize the risks of volume overload, electrolyte imbalances, and uremic bleeding, patients on dialysis should be dialyzed within 24 hours of surgery. Despite the formidable spectrum of potential problems faced by the surgical patient who has CKD, elective surgery can be performed safely in this patient group. Precise fluid management may be assisted in these patients with the judicious use of invasive monitoring (e.g., central venous pressure monitoring or esophageal Doppler monitoring) as the situation dictates. Electrolytes, particularly potassium, magnesium, and phosphorous, must be followed carefully. The assistance of a clinical pharmacist is indispensable in providing advice regarding how to adjust the dosage and scheduled administration of medications to these patients. Renal function is monitored by accurate assessment of the fluid balance and periodic measurements of the markers of renal function (creatinine and BUN). Renal dialysis may be needed when the patient cannot manage his or her own fluid balance, or when the detoxification or excretory function of the kidney is not performing properly. Examples of this would include volume overload with overt congestive heart failure in an anuric patient, life-threatening hyperkalemia, and intractable acidosis.

The Patient with Hepatic Dysfunction

Hepatic dysfunction was traditionally seen among patients with alcoholic hepatitis or chronic viral hepatitis. While the incidence of these conditions has not changed, the overall number of patients with hepatic dysfunction has significantly increased with the obesity epidemic. Nonalcoholic fatty liver disease has become the most common cause of chronic liver disease in the

United States. Since liver disease is common and patients with liver dysfunction are frequently asymptomatic, the preoperative assessment of all patients undergoing surgery should include a thorough history and physical examination to uncover risk factors for and evidence of liver dysfunction. The evaluation should include a careful history to identify risk factors for liver disease, including prior blood transfusions, illicit intravenous drug abuse, sexual promiscuity, a family history of jaundice or liver disease, a personal history of jaundice, excessive alcohol intake, and the use of potentially hepatotoxic medications including over-the-counter and herbal preparations. On physical examination symptoms of pruritis or fatigue or findings of palmer erythema, spider telangiectasias, abnormal hepatic contour or hepatomegaly, splenomegaly, hepatic encephalopathy, ascites, testicular atrophy or gynecomastia should be looked for. Routine testing with liver biochemical tests preoperatively for screening purposes in asymptomatic patients without risk factors or physical findings indicating liver disease is not recommended. When liver disease is suspected based on physical examination findings or liver biochemical abnormalities, additional investigations should be undertaken, and should include biochemical and serological testing for viral hepatitis, autoimmune liver disease, and metabolic disorders and radiologic evaluation with abdominal ultrasonography, magnetic resonance imaging, or computed tomography scans. Although serologic and radiologic testing is often adequate for diagnosis and perioperative risk assessment, liver biopsy remains the gold standard for the diagnosis and staging of liver disease.

Risk factors for surgery in patients with hepatic dysfunction or cirrhosis are shown in Table 1-10. The mortality of patients with liver disease depends on the degree of hepatic dysfunction, the nature of the surgical procedure, and the presence of comorbid conditions. There are several contraindications to elective surgery in patients with liver disease, as shown in Table 1-11. When these contraindications are absent, patients with liver disease should undergo a thorough

TABLE 1-11	Contraindication to Elective Surgery in Patients with Liver Disease
Acute liver failure	
Acute kidney injury	
Acute viral hepatitis	
Alcoholic hepatitis	
Cardiomyopathy	
Hypoxemia	
Severe coagulopathy (despite treatment)	

preoperative evaluation and their liver dysfunction should be optimized prior to elective surgery. Patients with advanced liver disease because of their increased perioperative risk for mortality should be managed by nonoperative measures.

In patients with cirrhosis, the Child-Pugh classification and Model for End-stage Liver Disease (MELD) score should be calculated to assist in preoperative risk assessment. The Child-Pugh class is based on the serum bilirubin and albumin levels, prothrombin time, and severity of encephalopathy and ascites (Table 1-12). In addition to predicting mortality, the Child-Pugh classification correlates with the frequency of postoperative complications, which include liver failure, worsening of encephalopathy, bleeding, infection, renal failure, hypoxia, and ascites. In general, elective surgery is well tolerated in patients with Child class A cirrhosis, is permissible with preoperative preparation in patients with Child class B cirrhosis (except those undergoing extensive liver resections or cardiac surgery), and is contraindicated in patients with Child class C cirrhosis. The MELD score is based on serum bilirubin, serum creatinine, and the international normalized ratio (INR) and is calculated by the formula:

$$\text{MELD score} = (0.957 \times \ln(\text{serum Cr}) + 0.378 \times \ln(\text{serum bilirubin}) + 1.120 \times \ln(\text{INR}) + 0.643) \times 10$$
(if hemodialysis, value for creatinine is automatically set to 4.0)

Scores range from 6 to 40, with 6 reflecting "early" disease and 40 "severe" disease. In patients undergoing laparoscopic cholecystectomy with a MELD score of <8, the mortality is 0%, while if the MELD score is >8, then the mortality is around 6%. Among patients undergoing abdominal surgery (other than laparoscopic cholecystectomy), orthopedic and cardiovascular surgery, patients with a MELD score of 7 or less have a mortality rate of 5%, patients with a MELD score of 8 to 11 have a mortality of 10% and patients with a MELD score of 12 to 15 have a mortality of 25%.

Multiple metabolic aberrations exist in the patient with hepatic dysfunction or overt cirrhosis, even before the development of ascites. The most significant change is a profound reduction in sodium excretion, frequently <5 mEq/24 hour, due to tubular reabsorption. The exact mechanism for this is unknown but is thought to be due to multiple hormonal factors. Challenging these patients with an oral sodium load further increases sodium and water retention. Many patients with hepatic dysfunction demonstrate, somewhat contrarily, intravascular volume depletion. The clinical implications of this derangement in sodium metabolism should be obvious, and

TABLE 1-10	Risk Factors for Surgery in Patients With Hepatic Dysfunction/Cirrhosis
Patient Characteristics	
Anemia	
Ascites	
Child-Pugh classification	
Encephalopathy	
Hypoalbuminemia	
Hypoxemia	
Infection	
Malnutrition	
MELD score	
Portal hypertension	
Prolonged prothrombin time (>2.5 s) that does not correct with vitamin K	
Type of Surgery	
Cardiac surgery	
Emergency surgery	
Hepatic resection	
Open abdominal surgery	

| TABLE 1-12 | Child-Pugh Classification of Cirrhosis |

Class	Albumin	Bilirubin	Ascites	Encephalopathy	Nutritional State	Mortality Rate (%)
A	>3.5	<2.0	Absent	Absent	Good	<10
B	3.0–3.5	2.0–3.0	Minimal	Minimal	Fair	40
C	<3.0	>3.0	Severe	Severe	Poor	>80

extreme diligence must be paid to fluid and electrolyte issues in the perioperative period.

Ascites increases the risk of wound dehiscence and abdominal wall hernias after abdominal surgery. Also, large-volume ascites can impair ventilation and cause respiratory compromise. Ascites can be drained at the time of surgery; however, it typically reaccumulates within days. Preoperative control of ascites with diuretics or transjugular intrahepatic portal caval shunt (TIPS) is recommended. Medical therapy for ascites includes salt restriction to 2 g/day with the combination of spironolactone and furosemide.

The underlying etiology of liver dysfunction in a significant majority of patients is alcohol; therefore, in the perioperative period, these patients are at risk for alcohol withdrawal. The alcoholic patient is protected from withdrawal symptoms by the administration of proper sedatives. The onset of mild withdrawal symptoms can occur anywhere from 1 to 5 days after alcohol is discontinued. Major symptoms generally peak at approximately 3 days, but have occurred as long as 10 days after withdrawal. These include delusions, tremors, agitation, and tachycardia. Benzodiazepines may prevent major withdrawal symptoms if they are instituted prophylactically. Table 1-13 below illustrates typical approaches to prevention of delirium tremens. Untreated delirium tremens

carries a postoperative mortality rate of as high as 50%. This rate is reduced to 10% with proper treatment. The use of intravenous ethanol, given in doses to keep serum ethanol concentrations below detectable limits, is being explored in some centers.

Patients with liver disease are at risk for increased bleeding. This impaired hemostasis can be due to decreased production of clotting factors because of hepatic synthetic dysfunction or depletion of vitamin K stores due to malnutrition or decreased intestinal absorption. Platelet abnormalities, both in number and function that can lead to bleeding tendencies, are found in patients with advanced liver disease due to portal hypertension-induced splenic sequestration and alcohol-induced bone marrow suppression.

Patients with liver disease are at significant risk for protein-energy malnutrition and patients with cholestatic liver disease are at risk for fat-soluble vitamin malabsorption. Patients with alcohol-induced liver disease are often deficient in thiamine and folate and have depleted levels of total body potassium and magnesium. These elements should be aggressively replaced to prevent abnormalities of glucose metabolism and cardiac arrhythmia. **Wernicke-Korsakoff syndrome** (i.e., ataxia, ophthalmoplegia, and confusion) may follow if thiamine is not administered prior to the administration of glucose.

| TABLE 1-13 | Examples of Medication Regimens |

Several different benzodiazepines and dosing regimens have been used and recommended. The following are examples of medications and dosing regimens.

Benzodiazepines[a]

Diazepam, 5 mg intravenously (2.5 mg/min). If the initial dose is not effective, repeat the dose in 5 to 10 min. If the second dose of 5 mg is not satisfactory, use 10 mg for the third and fourth doses every 5 to 10 min. If not effective, use 20 mg for the fifth and subsequent doses until sedation is achieved. Use 5 to 20 mg every hour as needed to maintain light somnolence.

Lorazepam, 1 to 4 mg intravenously every 5 to 15 min, or lorazepam, 1 to 40 mg intramuscularly every 30 to 60 min, until calm, then every hour as needed to maintain light somnolence.

Neuroleptics[a]

Haloperidol, 0.5 to 5 mg intravenously/intramuscularly every 30 to 60 min as needed for severe agitation. (Only to be used as adjunctive therapy with sedative–hypnotic agents.)

Ethanol Infusion[b]

I. Initiate 5% alcohol drip at 0.8 mL/kg/hr (using ideal body weight). The alcohol drip should be a continuous infusion and not discontinued or placed on hold for any diagnostic or operative procedures. The alcohol protocol is appropriate for patients admitted to a floor status level of care.

II. Measure blood alcohol content (BAC) at 6, 24, and 72 hr. If the blood alcohol level is >0.08%, hold for 2 hr and decrease rate by 50%.

III. If no symptoms of alcohol withdrawal:

after 24 hr from start, decrease rate by 50%.

after 48 hr from start, decrease rate further by 50%.

at 72 hr from start, stop and discontinue drip.

IV. If patient develops symptoms, increase rate by 50%. If symptoms continue for 6 hr, contact the resident on call.

[a]From Mayo-Smith, et al. Management of alcohol withdrawal delirium—an evidence-based practice guideline. Arch Intern Med 2004;164:1405–1412.
[b]From Dissanaike, et al. Ethanol prevents alcohol withdrawal syndrome. J Am Coll Surg 2006;203:186–191.

For a more complete discussion of surgical diseases of the liver, see Chapter 18, Liver.

The Diabetic Patient

Glycemic control is maintained by a balance between insulin and counterregulatory hormones such as glucagon, epinephrine, cortisol, and growth hormone. Surgical stress induces a neuroendocrine response with release of these counterregulatory hormones, which results in peripheral insulin resistance, increased hepatic glucose production, and impaired insulin production with the potential of hyperglycemia and even ketoacidosis in some cases. The extent of this response depends on the complexity of the surgery and the nature of postoperative complications. The task of the surgeon in managing the diabetic patient is to achieve euglycemia. It is well understood that if blood glucose levels are too low, death can quickly ensue due to starvation of glucose-dependent tissues (particularly, the brain) of their obligatory substrates. Traditionally, surgeons have erred on the side of hyperglycemia, reasoning that modest hyperglycemia is better tolerated than hypoglycemia. Recent data would suggest that it is possible, at least in the critical care environment, to achieve euglycemia safely and with better outcomes using a continuous infusion of insulin. However, the safe application of this practice to the noncritical care environment has yet to be demonstrated.

The preoperative evaluation of a diabetic patient includes assessment of metabolic control and any diabetes-associated complications including cardiovascular disease, autonomic neuropathy, and nephropathy, which could impact surgical outcomes. The surgical patient who has diabetes should be carefully questioned about the duration of the disease, insulin requirements, diet, degree of glucose control, last insulin administration, and peripheral symptoms (i.e., numbness, extremity pain). During the physical examination, special attention is given to the feet, looking for minor injuries, evidence of poor hygiene, inadequate vascular supply, ulcers, or decreased vibratory sensation. Patients who have positive findings should give meticulous care to their feet (i.e., daily washing, careful drying, application of softening lotion, protection from minor trauma, avoidance of pressure sores).

The cardiac effects of patients with diabetes were discussed previously. The incidence of cardiovascular abnormalities found on physical examination increases with the age of the patient and the duration of the diabetes. Men with diabetes may have twice the risk of cardiovascular mortality as their nondiabetic counterparts. Women have approximately four times the risk. Cardiac autonomic neuropathy may predispose patients to perioperative hypotension, so it is important to evaluate these patients for the presence of resting tachycardia, orthostatic hypotension, peripheral neuropathy and loss of normal respiratory heart rate variability.

Gastroparesis, which is also believed to be caused by autonomic neuropathy, may delay gastric emptying and increase the likelihood of aspiration. Gastroparesis is suggested if the patient gives a history of prolonged fullness after eating, or of constipation. A splash of fluid heard with the stethoscope over the stomach at a time when the stomach should be empty may suggest the presence of gastroparesis.

The risk of infection is substantially greater for the patient with diabetes. Hyperglycemia has an adverse effect on immune function, especially phagocytic activity. The reduced blood flow in patients with vascular disease, especially to the extremities, retards wound healing. Because most peripheral vascular disease in the patient with diabetes is small vessel in nature, palpable pulses are common, even in the face of tissue ischemia. Often, the extent of small vessel disease extends deep into the tissue, sparing the skin, much like a cone whose base is directed peripherally and whose apex extends in the central portion of the extremity proximally. For a patient with diabetes, ingrown toenails or minor injuries to the feet are potentially serious problems that can lead to amputation or mortality. Therefore, even minor procedures on the extremities of diabetic patients are approached with utmost caution.

Patients who require insulin to control their diabetes must have their dose adjusted to compensate for periods when food is not allowed or when the hyperglycemic response to the stress of illness, surgery, or trauma is clinically significant. Patients who have diabetes that was previously controlled by diet or oral agents may require insulin in the perioperative period. Infectious etiologies of surgical disease or postoperative infections may promote hyperglycemia and even ketoacidosis. On the other hand, overzealous administration of insulin may lead to hypoglycemia.

The perioperative management of patients with diabetes is approached as follows:

1. Insulin is available in several types and is typically classified by its length of action. Rapid-acting and short-acting insulin preparations are usually withheld when the patient stops oral intake usually at midnight the day before surgery. Intermediate-acting and long-acting insulin preparations are administered two-thirds the normal evening dose the night before surgery and half the normal morning dose the morning of surgery. Long-acting oral agents are stopped 48 to 72 hours before surgery, while short-acting agents can be withheld the night before or the day of surgery.

2. The ideal method of providing insulin in the perioperative period is debatable. Any regimen should however (1) maintain adequate glycemic control to avoid hyperglycemia or hypoglycemia; (2) prevent metabolic disturbances; (3) be easy to understand and administer. The patient should receive a continuous infusion of 5% dextrose to provide 10 g glucose/hour. Fingerstick glucose levels are monitored intraoperatively and followed postoperatively at least every 6 hours. The goal is to maintain a glucose level of between 120 and 180 mg/dL. It is generally considered preferable to have the patient at the higher end of this range because of the adverse consequences of hypoglycemia. Sliding scale use of subcutaneous insulin has been the standard method of glucose control in surgical patients. Alternatively, intravenous insulin can be used with a continuous infusion of 1 to 3 units/hour of intravenous insulin being given. This approach is particularly helpful in the brittle diabetic. In the postoperative period, close attention should be paid not only to the patient's blood sugar, but also to the patient's carbohydrate intake.

3. Diabetic ketoacidosis (DKA) can develop in patients with either type I or type II diabetes. DKA is deceptively easy to overlook because it can mimic postoperative ileus. It may present as nausea, vomiting, and abdominal distension, or in association with polyuria (which is commonly mistaken for mobilization of intraoperative fluids). For this reason, patients with type I diabetes (and many with type II diabetes) should have their urinary ketone level monitored by dipstick. This method is faster and much less costly than following serum ketone levels, and it gives a fairly accurate

picture of developing ketoacidosis. A glucose level that is <250 mg/dL does not mean that the patient is not at risk for DKA; DKA develops because of the metabolism of fuel in the absence of glucose. Hence, the development of DKA does not depend on a certain level of glucose, but on the absence of insulin.

The Adrenally Insufficient Patient

Historically, any patient who had received even small doses of glucocorticoid within the 12-month period before surgery was given preoperative glucocorticoid coverage, often in amounts well exceeding amounts produced by the hypothalamic–pituitary–adrenal (HPA) axis even in times of stress. To keep the issue of glucocorticoid replacement in some sort of perspective, it is useful to remember that patients with Cushing's syndrome produce the equivalent of 36-mg hydrocortisone/day.

Additionally, appreciation of the adverse effects of glucocorticoids has prompted a reconsideration of preoperative glucocorticoid coverage. Documented complications of glucocorticoid therapy include increased susceptibility to infection, impaired tissue healing, and abnormalities of glucose metabolism. Although high-dose glucocorticoid use was previously thought to be linked to upper gastrointestinal hemorrhage, more recent data have called this association into question.

So then, who should be considered for glucocorticoid supplementation, and how much should be given? A prednisone-equivalent dose of 20 mg/day for at least 3 weeks can be presumed to be associated with HPA axis suppression. Physical findings of a Cushingoid appearance should also raise the index of suspicion.

Present recommendations are based on the degree of surgical stress anticipated (i.e., minor, moderate, or major) and are detailed in Table 1-14. In all cases, patients should receive their morning steroid dose with a sip of water.

The role of steroids in the management of critically ill patients remains unresolved, despite recent multicenter, randomized, placebo-controlled studies. It remains difficult to conclusively demonstrate a beneficial effect of steroids in the critically ill, and the adverse effects of these agents are well described.

High-dose glucocorticoids are well known to impair wound healing. Vitamin A, 10,000 to 25,000 IU enterally for

7 to 10 days (decrease by half for parenteral use), is frequently employed to ameliorate some of the adverse effects of glucocorticoids on wound healing. Care should be taken in renally or hepatically impaired patients and supplemental Vitamin A should be of short-term use only, during the first few postoperative days, as large doses may cause Vitamin A toxicity.

The Pregnant Patient

Multiple anatomic and physiologic changes accompany a normal pregnancy, altering the presentation of many surgical diseases and mimicking others. The pregnant woman's response to these conditions can also be altered. The enlarging uterus displaces abdominal viscera and can alter the location of pain in some common intra-abdominal conditions such as appendicitis. A gravid uterus can compress the inferior vena cava and reduce venous return when the woman assumes the supine position. Pelvic venous compression produces or exacerbates hemorrhoids in over one-third of pregnant women. Lower extremity venous insufficiency and the hypercoagulable state of pregnancy itself increase the risk of venous thromboembolic events, especially if the pregnant patient is placed at bed rest.

The surgeon caring for a pregnant woman is caring, in effect, for two patients, and the mother's physiology is often preserved at the expense of reduced uterine perfusion. Some of the most significant physiologic changes during pregnancy occur to the circulatory system. Heart rate, stroke volume, and plasma volume are increased. Erythrocyte volume is also increased but not to the same degree as plasma volume, resulting in a reduction of the hematocrit. This increase in blood volume can mask blood loss or delay the classic presentation of hypovolemia, especially after injury. The appearance of normal vital signs can be deceptive and obscure fetal distress. The leukocytosis associated with a normal pregnancy reduces the utility of this laboratory test.

Respiratory rate and tidal volume are increased. This increase in minute ventilation lowers the arterial partial pressure of carbon dioxide. This occurs despite a reduction in FRC and residual volume imposed by the restriction of diaphragmatic motion secondary to the enlarging uterus. Postoperatively, the potential for atelectasis and other pulmonary complications is increased.

Most pregnant women experience reflux symptoms to some degree. Gastric acid production is increased slightly, but the primary problem is the delay in gastric emptying, the result of the action of progesterone in reducing gastric smooth muscle contractility. Nausea and vomiting are common in the first trimester, and these symptoms can be confused with gastrointestinal conditions that are surgical in nature.

It is best when possible to avoid a surgical procedure during pregnancy, but surgical emergencies must be handled when they present. If surgery is necessary, it is best performed during the second trimester, when the risk of precipitating spontaneous abortion or early labor is lowest—approximately 5% in women undergoing general anesthesia and abdominal surgery. Precipitating labor, and perhaps fetal demise, appears to be related more to the underlying pathology than the anesthesia. Laparoscopy can be performed safely as well during the second trimester, albeit with changes in trocar positioning and reducing abdominal insufflation pressure.

Appendicitis and biliary tract disease are the most common reasons for gastrointestinal surgery in the pregnant woman. Pancreatitis occurring during pregnancy is usually related to biliary tract disease. Bulk laxatives, stool softeners, and suppositories

TABLE 1-14	Stress Steroid Coverage
Magnitude of Procedure	**Steroid Replacement: Take Usual AM Steroid Dose, and:**
Minor procedures or surgery under local anesthesia (e.g., inguinal hernia repair)	No extra supplementation is necessary
Moderate surgical stress (e.g., lower extremity revascularization, total joint replacement)	50 mg hydrocortisone IV just before the procedure and 25 mg of hydrocortisone every 8 hr for 24 hr. Resume usual dose thereafter.
Major surgical stress (e.g., esophagogastrectomy, total proctocolectomy)	100 mg of hydrocortisone IV just prior to induction of anesthesia, and 50 mg every 8 hr for 24 hr. Taper dose by half per day to maintenance level.

are usually sufficient for hemorrhoids. Acute hemorrhoidal thrombosis can be drained with the use of local anesthesia. Rectal bleeding is also associated with colonic malignancy, and complaints of bleeding should not be blindly ascribed to hemorrhoids but investigated by endoscopy irrespective of gestational age.

Historically, women who were diagnosed with malignant conditions were advised to terminate the pregnancy. Fortunately, this is no longer the case. Women today share in the decision making regarding the pregnancy as well as therapeutic choices. Diagnostic delays, however, are still common in pregnant women with breast cancer. This is in part due to the normal changes that take place in the breasts of a pregnant woman. Breast masses detected in pregnant women should be investigated, and imaging is commonly employed as a first step. Mammography can be performed safely with shielding of the uterus. False-negative mammograms are unfortunately common owing to the density of the active breast tissue. Ultrasonography avoids any potential risk of ionizing radiation, but it also has an increased rate of false-negative results during pregnancy. Regardless of imaging results, biopsy should be performed on clinically suspicious masses. Core, incisional, or excisional biopsies are all appropriate choices, and can be performed under local anesthesia. Fine-needle aspiration cytology has also been shown to be accurate in the pregnant patient, but requires interpretation by a skilled pathologist.

Breast cancer in pregnant women has the same prognosis when matched for age of the patient and stage of disease, despite being predominantly estrogen receptor negative. Breast conservation surgery can be performed when appropriate and chemotherapy administered after the first trimester. Radiation therapy is held until after delivery. Continuation of the pregnancy does not appear to adversely affect outcome in women with breast cancer.

Rectal cancer is the most common colonic malignancy, and when discovered during the first half of the pregnancy should be resected. When discovered during the last half of the pregnancy, resection is generally postponed until after delivery. As in patients with breast cancer, chemotherapy is relatively safe after the first trimester, but radiation is withheld until after delivery.

One in every 14 pregnancies is complicated by injury. Every injured woman of childbearing age should be screened for pregnancy. As noted above, the changes in a woman's physiology may mask severe fetal distress. Resuscitation of the fetus requires dutiful attention to preserving the mother's blood volume and oxygenation. The classic manifestations of hemorrhagic shock signify that the fetus has been in distress for some time. Early fetal monitoring is essential in the initial assessment and resuscitation of the pregnant trauma patient. Diagnostic studies should be obtained when needed and not withheld for fear of teratogenesis. Indications for surgical exploration following maternal trauma include intraperitoneal hemorrhage, hollow visceral injury, penetrating abdominal injury, and uterine or fetal injury.

Fetal loss occurs in 15% of all women severely injured during pregnancy. Placental abruption can occur even after minor injury and is not consistently accompanied by vaginal bleeding. The presence of a hard uterus, larger than expected for gestational age, is suspicious for abruption. Disseminated intravascular coagulopathy is an ominous complication that can occur with hours of placenta abruption or amniotic fluid embolization. Because sensitization of Rh-negative women occurs with miniscule amounts of fetal Rh-positive blood, all injured Rh-negative women should be considered for Rh-immunoglobulin therapy, unless the injury is relatively minor and remote from the uterus.

The Geriatric Patient

The aging of the American population will continue for many decades to present some special challenges to surgeons. The elderly have less reserve than their younger counterparts. They are often on medications that can distort physiologic responses, for example, β-blockers. They are also often on medications that can impact the response to surgery, for example, warfarin or platelet aggregation–inhibiting agents. Their ability to negotiate everyday activities may be impaired at baseline, perhaps due to sensory impairment, difficulty in ambulation, or dementia. One of the conundrums that arises in the context of providing surgical care for an elderly patient is whether to proceed with an aggressive plan of intervention. It is always important that the patient and physician talk openly about the level of aggressiveness to be exerted on behalf of the patient. In the elderly, this issue assumes critical proportions. Repeated discussions with patients and their families should be held, beginning preoperatively and continuing in the postoperative phase. Generally, patients wish to feel that aggressive medical care will be rendered as long as there is a reasonable chance for meaningful survival. While these discussions are uncomfortable, they are as important to the patient's care as any component of the historical database. It is also important to remember that surgical care is rendered among individuals who take a personal interest in the overall well-being of the patient. Sometimes, this means that medical care focuses more on alleviating pain than on prolonging life. These discussions are best held in a quiet, comfortable place, away from distractions. It is also important to note that discussions about end-of-life issues do not constitute some sort of legal activity. There are no forms to be signed. These discussions are just like any other conversation a doctor and patient might have about the patient's care, in which the strengths and weaknesses of different approaches are compared, until the physician and patient arrive at a plan of action. The special difference, of course, is that end-of-life discussions are the patient's best chance to determine his or her destiny. These discussions should be treated with the reverence that such subject matter would naturally evoke.

OPERATIVE MANAGEMENT

Documentation

The Medical Record

The medical record is a concise, explicit document that chronologically outlines the patient's course of treatment. There are three primary purposes of the medical record. The first purpose is to record in one common and accessible location the data and thought processes that form the basis for the treatment team's understanding of the patient's status and the rationale for the treatment plans proposed for the patient. This section of the chart contains progress notes from various disciplines (Physician's; nurses; respiratory therapists; occupational, speech, and physical therapists; clinical pharmacists; clergy; nutrition support services; and so forth). It also contains data from laboratory and other diagnostic studies. The second purpose of the chart is to transmit instructions about the patient's care. This is the "orders" section. The final purpose of the chart is to provide a record of the events that occurred during the patient's care. Careful thought should be given to the information placed in the record; this information must be relevant to the course of treatment or diagnostic workup. Before notes are written, consideration should be given to the following six points:

1. Does the information pertain to patient care? Only information that pertains to the actual care of the patient should be entered into the medical record. The medical record should not be used to relay messages among consulting services. Extraneous information is inappropriate and may generate medicolegal liability. Examples include editorial comments about the appropriateness or inappropriateness of recommendations made by other Physician's. If there is genuine disagreement about the appropriate plan of management, then the reasons supporting the plan of management chosen should be documented in the chart, without editorial comment about the competency of the Physician's who have written dissenting opinions.

2. Is the information of value in documenting the treatment course? Little value is obtained in repeating factual material that has been previously documented. In teaching institutions, it is common to see history and physical examinations or progress notes recorded by students, house staff, and attending Physician's. The delivery of care in an educational environment is by necessity repetitive. Students gain important experience in writing progress notes that reflect careful and thoughtful evaluation of the patient. Students often obtain important medical information, and their notes should be carefully written. The best progress notes are those in which the assessment and plan are carefully laid out, with a clear rationale demonstrating why certain diagnostic hypotheses are being entertained, what the therapeutic options are, and why certain options are favored over others.

3. What details will be important for the future care of the patient? Operative notes are perhaps the best illustration of the importance of identifying potential needs for future care. For example, recording surgical findings is more important than noting the type of suture used to perform an anastomosis. A careful description of the abdominal organs as they are inspected and palpated may be of value if future review becomes necessary. Information about blood loss, blood and fluid replacement, and operative time is more relevant than many of the technical nuances of the operative procedure. The thought process used in diagnosing an illness or selecting a therapy is often more important than the technical details.

4. Is the information accurate? Extreme care should be taken to ensure the accuracy of information that is entered into the medical record. Confusion may occur when verbal reports of diagnostic studies written into the progress notes do not agree with formal reports, once they are typed, signed, and filed. Erroneous information can lead to disastrous results and may be more damaging than no information. Every effort should be made to maintain accuracy and consistency in the information that is recorded. In some circumstances, clinical decisions are made based on a verbal report. When this situation occurs, it is appropriate to note it (e.g., "Verbal report of positive blood culture received from the lab; plan removal of central line").

5. Are suspicions and theories clearly defined as such? An inexperienced physician may not precisely differentiate suspicions, theories, and possibilities from reality. Incorrect documentation leads to distortion of the facts in the record and misconceptions on the part of others who are peripherally involved with the patient's care. Inaccuracy is a powerful deterrent to the quality of patient care at all levels. Suspicions and theories can take on the appearance of fact if they are perpetuated over time in the medical record. Once such fallacies become embedded in the record, it can take a great deal of research within the chart to uncover the truth. Therefore, diagnostic labels should be factual rather than speculative.

6. Does the note serve the best interest of the patient, the physician, and the health care team? The medical record is kept on behalf of the patient to document the events, timing, and thinking relating to the care given during the period of hospitalization. The record is a confidential document and cannot be revealed to anyone who is not directly involved in the care of the patient, nor can it be revealed without the patient's or a responsible agent's written consent. An individual who discloses such information without this consent breaches the ethical contract between patient and physician.

Increasingly, health care providers are making the transition from a paper medical record to an electronic medical record (EMR). In 1991, the Institute of Medicine (IOM) released an influential report, "The Computer-Based Patient Record: An Essential Technology for Health Care." The IOM's vision for the EMR is of a document that (1) has a standardized format and nomenclature, (2) is easily searchable, (3) is quickly accessible to those who need to participate in the care of the patient, and (4) can be linked with databases that could improve health care in an evidence-based manner and minimize errors in the delivery of health care. In 1996, a federal law known as the Health Insurance Portability and Accountability Act (HIPAA) was passed. Compliance is required of virtually all health care providers, and failure to comply can result in civil (monetary) or criminal (imprisonment) penalties. This law specifies the ways in which medical records may be accessed, and by whom. While it was not the intent of this law to hinder medical care, it is clear that there are many reasons why great care must be taken in being certain that the medical record accurately reflects the patient's care in a manner that respects each individual's privacy. In addition to the advantages surrounding data management, a computer order entry system is considered among the most important components of a hospital's overall program to promote and ensure patient safety. The rate of EMR use has remained low, but is gradually increasing, with 25% of office-based Physician's using some EMR system as of 2005. However, only 10% of Physician's have a fully integrated EMR, with computerized order entry, computerized prescription writing, full test result reporting, and electronic progress notes. In 2009, approximately $19 billion was provided by the federal government as directed by the American Recovery and Reinvestment Act to help defray some of the large economic burden incurred by Physician's as they convert to an EMR.

The medical record can be the physician's and the patient's best ally or worst enemy. Documentation of all findings, results, rationales for diagnostic and management strategies, and explanations to the patient, particularly in terms of risks, benefits, anticipated results, and therapeutic alternatives, can protect both the patient and the physician. The art in mastering the medical record is achieving a balance between brevity and completeness.

Physician's Orders

The physician's order section of the medical record should be treated with care. Orders must be entered precisely, with the intent of being followed, not interpreted. Unfortunately, the latter is often the case because of the hasty scribblings of Physician's that may be unclear, illegible, or inaccurate, although computerized physician order entry (CPOE) is part of a robust safety program to minimize such opportunities for error. Orders should be written with sufficient detail to eliminate possible misunderstanding. There is no excuse for illegible handwriting or imprecise orders. Every aspect of the patient's life, including diet, level of activity, and access to the bathroom—even what the patient is to breathe—is the responsibility of the physician once the patient enters the hospital.

Orders include the elements listed in Table 1-15. Content and format may vary among institutions, but the principles are the same. Usually, the first orders written concern general nursing care. Identification of the physician or team that is responsible for the patient is important so that the staff knows whom to contact if problems or questions arise. Listing the working diagnosis or reason for admission gives the staff a general idea of the problem and sets the tone for the delivery of services. The frequency of vital signs is next. Any special nursing evaluations (e.g., neurologic function) are also indicated. If the physician wishes to be notified of any of these assessments (e.g., temperature >38.5°C), the staff is informed.

Diet specifications or NPO (nothing by mouth) orders are also indicated. Special diets are required by some patients (e.g., those with diabetes, those undergoing special diagnostic procedures). Too frequently, hospitalization is prolonged or expensive procedures must be repeated because of lack of attention to the details of prescribing the appropriate diet. The level of patient activity is specified as well. Such orders are generally considered routine, and some hospitals may have standard protocols. Prudent Physician's,

however, specifically write their own routine in sufficient detail to ensure that their plans are carefully followed.

Some nursing care functions must also be identified. These include special positioning, turning, pulmonary exercises, and care of wounds or drainage tubes. Foley catheters are placed to gravity drainage, nasogastric tubes to some type of suction apparatus, and wound drains to either suction or dependent drainage. The staff is informed specifically about the management of these drains or tubes. Daily care of the incision site is clearly noted. Retrograde infection from incision sites, especially with urinary catheters and wound drains, is a major contributor to morbidity. Patient positioning is extremely important in preventing pulmonary problems and preventing aspiration of the gastric contents in patients who are receiving enteral tube feedings. Other nursing instructions include the recording of fluid intake or output from urinary catheters and drains; specific instructions for tube care, stripping, or irrigation; and notification of the physician in the event of a specific occurrence (e.g., urine output <30 mL/hour, chest tube drainage >100 mL/hour).

The type and rate of intravenous fluid administration are also specified. When multiple intravenous sites are used, it is helpful to specify which fluids are to be infused at which sites.

To prevent potentially fatal medication errors, meticulous attention to detail is mandatory when writing medication orders. The notation sequence is type of drug, dosage, route of administration, and frequency. These orders should be absolutely clear and legible. If a physician is uncertain of the spelling of a drug name, he or she should consult a reference. It is important to use only standard abbreviations, and the reader is strongly encouraged to become familiar with the Official "Do Not Use" List published by the Joint Commission on the Accreditation of Healthcare Organizations (Table 1-16). Writing medications on a separate section of

TABLE 1-15	General Considerations for Writing Orders
Physician/team responsible	
Diagnosis/condition	
Immediate plans	
Vital signs/special checks/notification parameters	
Diet	
Level of activity	
Special nursing care instructions	
Positioning	
Wound care	
Tubes/drains: management and care	
Intake/output: frequency	
Intravenous fluids	
Medications: drug, dose, route, frequency	
Routine	
Special	
Laboratory orders	
Special procedures/x-ray	
Miscellaneous	

TABLE 1-16	Official "Do Not Use List" of the Joint Commission on the Accreditation of Healthcare Organizations	
Abbreviation	**Potential Problem**	**Preferred Term**
U (for unit)	Mistaken as zero, four or cc	Write "unit"
IU (for international unit)	Mistaken as IV (intravenous) or 10 (ten)	Write "international unit"
Q.D., Q.O.D. (Latin abbreviation for once daily and every other day)	Mistaken for each other. The period after the Q can be mistaken for an "I" and the "O" can be mistaken for "I"	Write "daily" and "every other day"
Trailing zero (X.0 mg), Lack of leading zero (.X mg)	Decimal point is missed	Never write a zero by itself after a decimal point (X mg), and always use a zero before a decimal point (0.X mg)
MS MSO$_4$ MgSO$_4$	Confused for one another. Can mean morphine sulfate or magnesium sulfate	Write "morphine sulfate" or "magnesium sulfate"

Source: http://www.jointcommission.org/patientsafety/donotuselist/.

the order sheet so that they are not mixed in with nonmedication orders may be advantageous; in this way, confusion and oversights are avoided. Orders for routine medications (e.g., analgesics, laxatives, sleeping pills) are written first, followed by medications for the patient's specific needs. Reviewing the medication lists daily is an excellent habit. Changes in drugs, dosage, or frequency are confusing for both the pharmacy and the nursing staff. If drugs are changed, writing an order to stop the original drug, then ordering the new one is the best approach. In most institutions, parenteral nutritional products are prepared in the pharmacy; therefore, total parenteral nutrition orders are placed with the medication orders.

Laboratory studies and special diagnostic procedures should be specified as well. Special procedures, such as radiographs, require additional thought. Request slips for these studies should specifically state the presumptive diagnosis and the reason for the test. Personal consultation with the radiologist or technician avoids confusion and prevents delays or unnecessary repetition of procedures. If those who perform the tests are aware of the reason for the testing, the results are nearly always more productive. Some procedures require special preparation of the patient; therefore, these instructions must be included in the orders. "Routine" or "daily" laboratory or radiology orders are wasteful, rarely contribute to care, and should be avoided. In the occasional situation in which serial studies are needed to follow some aspect of the patient's course, a stop time should be specified (e.g., "Please draw hematocrit q6h × 24 hour"). Laboratory and diagnostic studies should be used to confirm clinical suspicions and not as a shotgun approach to reveal a diagnosis.

The miscellaneous category in Table 1-15 is intended for other orders that may be necessary, including requests for consultation, procurement of procedural permits or old records, or admission of a patient to a special study or protocol.

The orders are only as complete as you make them. Clarity and legibility allow for efficient and appropriate delivery of services. As previously noted, computerized order entry systems are increasingly common and are widely regarded as an essential component of any program to minimize medical error.

Progress Notes

A brief *preoperative note* to summarize the workup and the pertinent physical and diagnostic studies is usually written the day before surgery. These notes serve as a checklist to ensure that the important aspects of preoperative preparation are completed. An example is shown in Table 1-17. A *night of surgery note* should be recorded to document the condition of the patient after the operation. Important information to be included in this note would be the patient's comfort level and vital signs, fluid balance, pertinent examination findings, and any critical laboratory values caregivers would need to know within the next few hours.

Daily progress notes record the patient's clinical course throughout his or her hospital stay. Noting the hospital day number, the postoperative day, or the days after injury is helpful. The format for progress notes varies among hospitals and even among services within the hospital. All notes should be dated, timed, signed, and legible. A brief, handwritten operative note should list the important elements of the operation, with consideration given to recording information that might be important in the immediate perioperative period, before the official typed report is appended to the medical record. These

TABLE 1-17	Sample Preoperative Note
Diagnosis:	Cholelithiasis
Proposed surgery:	Cholecystectomy with operative cholangiogram
History and physical:	Completed (dictated)
	Grade II/VI systolic murmur at apex
	Hypertension (controlled)
Laboratory values:	CBC: 14.5/41.5% 7,500
	Electrolytes: 140 | 4.2/26 | 101 Bun 10
	Glu 105
	CXR: NAD
	ECG: NSR-normal
	Present meds: HCTZ 50 mg qd
	Blood: type and hold (specimen in blood bank)
Operative permit:	Signed and on chart; risks, rationale, benefits, and alternatives have been explained in detail; patient understands and agrees to proceed with the surgical plans
Miscellaneous information:	
	Signature _____

CBC, complete blood count; BUN, blood urea nitrogen; GLU, glucose; CXR, chest x-ray; NAD, no appreciable disease; ECG, electrocardiogram; NSRs, normal sinus rhythm; HCTZ, hydrochlorothiazide.

important components are listed in Table 1-18. The important elements of the discharge note are listed in Table 1-19.

Event notes should be recorded whenever there is an unexpected event in the patient's course. These should briefly summarize what the problem was and the reasons for the steps taken to address the problem. *Discharge notes* should be concise and list the patient's reason for hospitalization (also referred to as the "principal diagnosis"), a brief summary of the patient's hospital course, what medications the patient is to be discharged on, what medications the patient will take after discharge, where the patient is to go after discharge, what the patient's level of activity is, and what the plan for follow-up is. It is not necessary that the discharge summary recapitulate each detail of the patient's hospitalization.

In summary, the medical record is a legal document that contains important information about the patient's hospital course and

TABLE 1-18	Operative Note	
Procedure:		
Findings:		
Surgeons:		Attending surgeon:
Estimated blood loss:		
Crystalloid replaced:		Blood products:
Anesthesia:		
Complications:		
Tubes/drains:		
Disposition:		
	Signature:	

TABLE 1-19	Discharge Note
Admission diagnosis:	Date:
Discharge diagnosis:	Date:
Operative procedure:	
Hospitalization course:	
Disposition:	
Home care instructions:	
Activity	
Diet	
Restrictions	
Wound care	
Other	
Discharge medications:	
Follow-up instructions:	
Miscellaneous:	

his or her response to diagnostic and therapeutic interventions. It is also a place where information given to the patient by the health care providers can be documented. Despite the inconvenience involved, the time and effort devoted to thoughtful record keeping returns many dividends when future review is necessary.

Tubes and Drains

Before discussing individual types of tubes and their use, it is useful to note that the size of many of these tubes is given as "French size." French size refers to the outer diameter of a catheter. Multiplying the French size by 0.33 will give the outer diameter of the catheter in millimeters.

Gastrointestinal Tract Tubes

Nasogastric tubes are usually used to evacuate the gastric contents. They are most commonly used in patients who have ileus or obstruction. The modern nasogastric tube is a sump-type tube. The sump function is achieved by bonding a smaller-diameter tube onto the larger-bore (usually 18 Fr) tube. When the main tube is placed to continuous suction, there is a small amount of air that will be drawn in by the sump tube, preventing the development of a suction lock between the main tube and the gastric wall. Therefore, sump tubes should be placed to continuous suction. You may occasionally see a nonsump tube; these should be placed to intermittent suction to break the seal that forms between the tube and the gastric wall. Nasogastric tubes may also be used to feed the patient in some cases. If feeding is the intended purpose of the tube, a soft, fine-bore tube is preferable to a stiff, large-bore tube.

Nasoenteric tubes are usually intended for feeding. These should be soft and fine bore. A word about safety is in order. Nothing should be instilled into a feeding tube of any kind (nasogastric or nasoenteric) unless the position of the tube is known. Auscultation of injected air over the epigastrium can be misleading; a tube can be intrabronchial and still transmit the sound of injected air to the epigastrium. The position of a feeding tube can only be definitively confirmed with a radiograph or by direct palpation at the time of operation. Instilling tube feeds, medications, or radiographic contrast material into an intrapulmonary (or intrapleural) tube can have lethal consequences.

Nasobiliary tubes are usually placed endoscopically, either to facilitate drainage of the biliary tree when there is an obstructing process (stone, tumor, stricture) or to facilitate drainage of bile via the biliary tract in cases of biliary fistula.

T-tubes are placed within the common bile duct for the purpose of drainage. They are kept to closed gravity drainage.

Gastrostomy tubes may be placed surgically. When placed endoscopically, they are referred to as percutaneous endoscopic gastrostomy (PEG) tubes. They may be used for drainage or for feeding.

Jejunostomy tubes can be placed surgically or endoscopically (via the stomach). When placed endoscopically, they may be placed in combination with a PEG tube. These are typically placed for long-term nutritional access.

Respiratory Tract Tubes

Chest tubes are placed into the pleural cavity to evacuate air (pneumothorax), blood (hemothorax), or fluid (effusion). They are connected to a special suction system that (1) permits a constant level of suction (usually 20 cm H_2O), (2) allows drainage of air and liquid from the pleural cavity, and (3) prevents air from entering the pleural space from the outside. This latter function is known as a "water seal." These three functions can be achieved with the use of a "three bottle system," or a proprietary manufactured chest drainage and collection system.

Endotracheal tubes for adults are cuffed to maintain a seal between the tracheal wall and the tube. These tubes are used when patients need short-term mechanical ventilation or when they cannot maintain a patent airway.

Tracheotomy tubes are placed directly into the trachea via the neck. They are used for patients who require long-term mechanical ventilation or who cannot maintain a patent airway over the long term.

Urinary Tract Tubes

Bladder catheters, commonly referred to as "Foley" catheters, are placed to straight drain.

Nephrostomy tubes are usually placed in the renal pelvis to drain urine above an area of obstruction or above a delicate ureteral anastomosis.

Tubes placed percutaneously to drain abscesses are often known as pigtail catheters. They are usually placed by interventional radiologists with the help of imaging technology.

Surgical Drains

Closed suction drains (Jackson-Pratt and Hemovac are two common types) are placed intraoperatively to evacuate actual or potential fluid collections. They are usually connected to a collapsible bulb or compressible box collection receptacle.

Sump suction drains, sometimes known as Davol drains, are very large. Although they are made of silicone, they tend to be stiff. They are placed to continuous suction and are used for situations when the drainage is expected to be thick or particulate.

Passive tubes (Penrose drains) simply maintain a pathway for fluid to follow, without suction to enhance flow. These are soft, cylindrical latex drains. Because suction is not applied to them, they are very much a two-way path for bacteria.

Wound Care

In general, surgical wounds heal either by primary intention or by secondary intention (see Chapter 7, Wounds and Wound Healing). To heal by primary intention means that the wound edges have been apposed, whether by sutures, wound clips, tapes, or dermal adhesives. To heal by secondary intention means that the wound edges have been left unapposed. Usually, there is a dressing of some sort used to collect wound fluids and help keep the wound from closing prematurely. A common situation in which healing by secondary intention would be encouraged would be in the management of an abscess. A saline-moistened cotton gauze dressing is used to gently fill the cavity. (The wound cavity should not be packed tightly because this leads to tissue ischemia.) This helps to collect drainage and to prevent the abscess cavity from sealing over. A variety of substances are used to moisten the gauze for wounds managed in this way. Some examples include 0.25% acetic acid solution, Dakin's solution (sodium hypochlorite), and povidone–iodine solutions. Each of these can be shown to inhibit fibroblast proliferation in tissue culture, and neither has any special advantage over plain, sterile saline solution.

Pain Management

It is appropriate to consider the subject of pain management in surgical patients. Physician's are often justifiably criticized for neglecting to attend to the pain of their patients as closely as they might monitor, for example, their laboratory values. Asking the patient how their pain level is should be a routine part of the review of systems taken on daily rounds, in the clinic, or in the office. For patients who cannot report pain (e.g., those in the intensive care unit, who may be mechanically ventilated and unable to speak), attention to their facial expressions and vital signs will give clues as to their level of discomfort. The nature of the patient's disease process and his or her comorbidities will determine the type of pain management strategy he or she requires. For example, many patients with thoracic or abdominal incisions are well served with epidural analgesia administered by the Anesthesia Pain Service. Where possible, intravenous patient-controlled analgesia should be used for the intense pain that accompanies the early postoperative state. Once the patient is able to take medications orally, the transition to oral pain medication is simple. In the intensive care unit, where patients may not be able to manage the patient-controlled analgesia apparatus, continuous intravenous infusions of narcotics are appropriate and should be titrated by the nurse to keep the patient comfortable without being overly sedated.

Deep Vein Thrombosis Prophylaxis

Venous thromboembolism will afflict 25% of postoperative patients if they are afforded no prophylaxis. Surgical patients are at particular risk for venous thromboembolism because they have each of Virchow's three risk factors for venous thrombosis: stasis, hypercoagulability, and endothelial injury. A variety of means have been examined in the effort to reduce the incidence of postoperative deep vein thrombosis (DVT).

Excellent evidence-based data show that surgical patients should routinely receive such prophylaxis. Low-dose unfractionated heparin is as effective in this population as low-molecular-weight heparin and is usually less expensive. Use of any heparin compound carries a small but real risk of heparin-induced thrombocytopenia (HIT). The low-molecular-weight heparins have a lower risk of associated HIT. While this thrombocytopenia is usually transient, there is a form, known as "white-clot syndrome," which can result in stroke, loss of limbs, or death. Thus, patients on routine heparin prophylaxis should have their platelet counts monitored at least every other day. If heparin is chosen, it should be given preoperatively to obtain the greatest protection. Intermittent pneumatic compression (IPC) devices produce reductions in DVT rates similar to those of unfractionated heparin and may be viewed as adjunctive. Their main liability is poor patient tolerance. The data regarding the prevention of venous thromboembolism by IPCs are not strong. Presently, the mainstay of venous thromboembolism prophylaxis in surgical patients is some form of subcutaneous heparin. The routine general surgical patient is well protected by the unfractionated heparin. Low-molecular-weight heparin is recommended for the trauma patient. Close communication with the anesthesiologists is important if epidural analgesia is being considered in a patient who might receive low-molecular-weight heparin because of the risk of spinal epidural hematoma formation.

POSTOPERATIVE COMPLICATIONS

Malignant Hyperthermia

This is a potentially fatal, hypermetabolic, autosomal dominant condition of skeletal muscle that is reported to occur in one in 14,000 children and one in 50,000 adults. Several genetic mutations are associated with malignant hyperthermia, but all result in a disruption of intracellular calcium metabolism. Problems with the ryanodine receptor (calcium-release channel) are found in over 50% of patients with this disorder, while problems with the dihydropyridine receptor are found in others. The result is a massive buildup of intracellular calcium released from the sarcoplasmic reticulum. This produces violent and sustained muscle contraction and rigidity, heat production, and acidosis. Muscle necrosis and rhabdomyolysis may occur. The clinical findings in heat stroke and neuroleptic malignant syndrome are similar, and individuals prone to malignant hyperthermia are thought to be more susceptible to these other conditions. Inhalational halogenated anesthetic agents and succinylcholine are known triggers of the syndrome as are extreme stress (heat) and vigorous exercise.

A family history of relatives who have had problems with anesthetic agents may be the only preoperative clue. Susceptible individuals may be confirmed with a muscle biopsy and stimulated contraction studies.

An abrupt rise in end-tidal carbon dioxide is the first sign. Masseter muscle rigidity is seen early in the syndrome in children, but not consistently in adults. Body temperature may climb by 1° to 2° every 5 minutes and reach extraordinary levels. Temperature elevation, on the other hand, may not present for up to 36 hours after exposure to the triggering agent. Tachycardia, cyanosis, and muscle rigidity are prominent features. Compartment syndromes may develop. Rhabdomyolysis may produce myoglobinuria. Cardiac rhythm disturbances appear to be associated with the hyperkalemia and hypercalcemia that accompany muscle necrosis. Mixed respiratory and metabolic acidosis is common, and a bleeding diathesis similar to disseminated intravascular coagulopathy has been reported.

Early recognition is the key to successful treatment. Thirty years ago, mortality rates ranged as high as 70% but today have been reduced to <5%. The first step in management is to discontinue the triggering agent. Dantrolene, a muscle relaxant that blocks calcium release from the sarcoplasmic reticulum and disrupts excitation–contraction coupling, is the only agent available for treatment. It is given by rapid intravenous push in doses of 1 mg/kg (both adults and children) and continued until symptoms subside or a maximum dose of 10 mg/kg has been reached. Dantrolene is also available in oral form, and although the absorption is slow, it is consistent. Prophylactic oral dosing is 4 to 8 mg/kg in three to four divided doses 1 to 2 days prior to elective surgery and continued for 1 to 3 days following the procedure. Patients taking oral dantrolene may notice somnolence and muscular weakness. Hyperthermia is treated by cooling blankets, but not to the point where the patient is shivering. Renal support in the form of mannitol, bicarbonate (controversial), and volume infusion is provided in the case of myoglobinuria from rhabdomyolysis. A careful search for occult compartment syndrome is made and, if found, fasciotomy is performed. Respiratory support with mechanical ventilation is frequently required to correct the respiratory component of the acidosis. Dantrolene is usually effective in managing the metabolic component of the acidosis, and bicarbonate infusion is not generally recommended. Hyperkalemia is managed in the standard fashion with exchange resins and insulin therapy if necessary. Seizure activity is treated with benzodiazepines.

Atelectasis

Despite the frequent occurrence of atelectasis—in up to 90% of patients having a general anesthetic—there is no consensus regarding its etiology, its treatment, or even its clinical significance. The definition of atelectasis varies from that of a simple collapse of the adult alveolus to one that requires clinical features of collapse or consolidation, unexplained fever (temperature >38°C), a positive chest radiograph, or evidence of infection on sputum microbiology. Alveolar unit collapse occurs with essentially all general anesthetics, regardless of the agents used.

General anesthesia results in a reduction of FRC by 400 to 500 mL in the adult. This reduction may fall below CV in many patients. The supine positioning loads the diaphragm, especially if mechanical ventilation and paralytic agents are used, compressing lung tissue in the basal segments by as much as 5%. Extrapolated to the entire lung, this represents up to 20% of all functioning alveolar units. It is easy to see that obesity multiplies this effect. Under anesthesia, patients do not sigh or cough, and mucociliary cleaning of the tracheobronchial tree is impaired. Mucous plugging of small airways may result. Absorption atelectasis, the uptake of gas from the alveoli in the face of proximal obstruction, further contributes to lung unit collapse. This is especially true if high concentrations of oxygen are used for induction or during the surgery. A loss or a change in the physical properties of surfactant may further contribute to the process. The effect is an increase in shunt fraction, that is, low ventilation to perfusion ratio, resulting in hypoxia. The postoperative period is characterized by incisional pain, somnolence from analgesic use, suppressed cough, lack of mobility, and nasopharyngeal instrumentation. These factors all contribute to perpetuation of a situation in which tidal ventilation is reduced and periodic re-expansion of collapsed alveolar units by maximum inspiratory efforts is suppressed.

Debate continues over whether atelectasis is associated with fever or whether the condition predisposes (or is the prodrome) to more serious respiratory problems such as pneumonia or the adult respiratory distress syndrome. There is experimental evidence that atelectasis alters host defenses, but the clinical significance of these findings has yet to be elucidated.

Management of postoperative atelectasis should begin preoperatively, under ideal conditions, by encouraging cessation of smoking for 8 weeks preoperatively and the institution of inspiratory exercises. Chest physiotherapy may also begin, particularly for patients with productive cough or chronic bronchitis. Re-expansion techniques (incentive spirometry) are appropriate for all patients. Some may even benefit from chest physiotherapy. The most important strategies involve adequate postoperative pain management, frequently obtained with epidural analgesia, and early mobilization. One of the advantages of minimally invasive surgery is the significant reduction in atelectasis as well as other more serious pulmonary problems. Pharmacologic interventions and diaphragmatic pacing have not enjoyed much clinical success or enthusiasm, although these interventions are still practiced in some centers.

Surgical Wound Failure

Wound healing is a complex, but predictable and highly orchestrated, series of cellular, hormonal, and molecular actions that are initiated at the time of injury. The details of wound healing are discussed in detail in Chapter 7, Wounds and Wound Healing. Acute wound healing failure involves an alteration in this process as the result of mechanical forces, infections, or aberrations of the normal biologic response of injured tissue.

Dehiscence, or acute surgical wound failure resulting in disruption of the fascial closure, is acute mechanical failure of the surgical closure. The force exerted across the wound is greater than the strength of suture material or of the fascia itself. This latter failure is generally due to ischemia of the tissue from suture material placed too tightly or becoming too tight as edema develops at the site of wounding. Poor suturing technique can also be to blame. Local infection can also lead to destruction of the fascia.

The spontaneous discharge of serous fluid from a wound is a sign heralding acute fascial dehiscence. These patients should be returned expeditiously to the operating room for examination and repair of the closure. Perhaps nothing is more dramatic, for both patient and doctor, than witnessing dehiscence of the abdominal closure and evisceration of the abdominal organs. In such a case, the exposed organs should be covered with sterile towels soaked in saline solution and the patient taken to the operating room immediately. Occasionally, a deep space infection—a subphrenic, pelvic, or interloop abscess—is associated with this problem. (See Chapter 9, Surgical Infections, for further discussion of intra-abdominal infections.)

Surgical-Site Infection

It is estimated that over 500,000 cases of surgical-site infections occur in the more than 27 million operative procedures performed yearly, representing one-quarter of all nosocomial infections. The frequency varies from hospital to hospital, surgeon to surgeon, operation to operation, and patient to patient, and is presently followed as one of a number of quality measures reported to the federal government, tracked by third-party payers and employer consortiums and available in the public domain. Surgical-site infections are the second most common nosocomial infection and will occur in 2% to 5% of all surgical patients. Emerging antibiotic-resistant organisms are a growing problem. Surgical-site infections increase the length of hospital stay and hospital costs. Furthermore, acute wound failure can have devastating consequences in the form of fascial dehiscence, pseudoaneurysm formation, anastomotic leak, fistula formation, incisional hernia, deep space infection, and mortality.

Factors contributing to surgical-site infections are discussed in Chapter 8, Surgical Infections. Signs of surgical-site infections are those associated with inflammation: redness (rubor), swelling (tumor), localized heat and erythema (calor), and increased pain at the incision site (dolor). Tachycardia may be the first sign and fever may develop only later. Spontaneous drainage from the surgical wound indicates that there has been a delay in recognition of this postoperative problem. Delay in recognition leads to destruction of the fascia and contributes to dehiscence or incisional hernias. Prompt drainage minimizes these sequelae and antibiotics play a secondary role, unless there are extenuating circumstances. Failure of the patient's tachycardia, fever, or ileus to resolve should suggest a deeper site of infection, and additional diagnostic studies may be necessary. Occasionally, the diagnosis is made by surgical exploration.

Guidelines have been developed by the Centers for Disease Control to minimize the incidence of surgical-site infections and are shown in Table 1-20.

TABLE 1-20	Center for Disease Control Surgical-Site Infections Prevention Guidelines, 1999

Recommendation	Strength of Recommendation
Do not remove hair unless it interferes with the operation	1A
If removed, remove immediately before operation with electric clippers	1A
Shower or bathe with antiseptic agent night before surgery	1B
Surgeon performs surgical scrub for 2–5 min with appropriate antiseptic	1B
After scrubbing, keep hands up and away from body; dry hands with sterile towel; don sterile gown and gloves	1B
Identify and treat all remote infections before surgery	1A
Keep hospital stay as short as possible	II
Administer antimicrobial agent only when indicated and select based on published recommendations for a specific operation and efficacy against most common pathogens	1A
Administer antimicrobial agents by IV timed to ensure bactericidal serum and tissue levels when incision made	1A
Maintain therapeutic levels during operation and, at most, a few hours after closure	1A
Before colorectal elective operations, in addition to IV antibiotics, mechanically prep the colon with cathartic agents and enemas; administer nonabsorbable oral antimicrobial agents in individual doses the day before surgery	1A
For cesarean sections in patients at high risk, administer IV antimicrobial agents immediately after cord is clamped	1A
Do not use vancomycin routinely for prophylaxis	1B

1A, Strongly recommended for implementation and supported by well-designed experimental, clinical, or epidemiologic studies;
1B, Strongly recommended for implementation and supported by some experimental, clinical, or epidemiologic studies and strong theoretical rationale;
II, Suggested for implementation and supported by suggestive clinical or epidemiologic studies or theoretical rationale.

Modified from Mangram AJ, Horan TC, Pearson MI, et al. The Hospital Infection Control Practices Advisory Committee. Guideline for prevention of surgical site infection 1999. Infect Control Hosp Epidemiol 1999;20:247–280, with permission.

Fever

An elevation in a patient's core temperature postoperatively is so common that many mistakenly consider it a normal postoperative state. Next to requests for laxatives, analgesics, and sleep aids, calls from the nursing staff regarding temperature elevation are perhaps the most common. If asked to define fever, most will offer a simple thermal definition without the important corollaries as to time of day, anatomic site of temperature determination, or the apparatus used to take the measurement. The benchmark of 37°C as normal body-temperature was established circa 1868 and has only recently been critically reviewed. To describe fever in purely thermal terms is a misleading oversimplification. The febrile response is a complex physiologic reaction to a stimulus that involves not only a cytokine-mediated rise in core temperature, but also the generation of acute-phase proteins and activation of the endocrine and immune systems (Table 1-21). The pure thermal definition of fever is further flawed because it implies a single entity when in fact it represents a pasticcio of many different temperatures, each representing a different body region and state of activity. Additionally, fever should not be confused with hyperthermia, which is a rise in body temperature not associated with a pyrogen.

The causes of fever are multiple and include noninfectious (Table 1-22) as well as infectious etiologies (Table 1-23). Some conditions have been classified as both infectious and noninfectious, for example, acalculous cholecystitis, phlebitis. The classification, obviously, depends on whether the condition is associated with bacterial infection.

The Society of Critical Care Medicine has adopted the guideline that a temperature elevation to 38.3°C is the trigger to initiate an investigation. The evaluation process begins with a review of the circumstances surrounding the patient: patient location (intensive care unit vs. ward), length of hospitalization, presence of mechanical ventilation and its

TABLE 1-21	Characteristics of the Febrile State

Endocrine and Metabolic
Increased production of glucocorticoids
Increased secretion of growth hormone
Increased secretion of aldosterone
Decreased secretion of vasopressin
Decreased levels of divalent cations (necessary for bacterial replication)
Secretion of acute-phase proteins
Autonomic
Shift in blood flow from cutaneous to deep
Increased pulse and blood pressure
Decreased sweating
Behavioral
Shivering (rigors)
Search for warmth (chills)
Anorexia
Somnolence
Malaise

Adapted from Saper CB, Breder CD. The neurologic basis of fever. N Engl J Med 1994;330(26):1880–1886, with permission.

TABLE 1-22	Noninfectious Causes of Fever
Alcohol/drug withdrawal	
Atelectasis	
Posttransfusion fever	
Drug fever	
Cerebral infarction/hemorrhage	
Brain injury	
Adrenal insufficiency	
Myocardial infarction	
Pancreatitis	
Acalculous cholecystitis	
Ischemic bowel	
Aspiration pneumonitis	
ARDS	
Subarachnoid hemorrhage	
Fat emboli	
Transplant rejection	
DVT/phlebitis	
Pulmonary emboli	
Gout/pseudogout	
IV contrast reaction	
GI bleeding	
Cirrhosis (without primary peritonitis)	
Neoplasia	
Decubitus ulcer	

Adapted from Marik PE. Fever in the ICU. Chest 2000;117(3):855–869, with permission.

duration, instrumentation (e.g., catheters, vascular lines, tubes in the nose or chest), duration of the instrumentation, medications, surgical sites and the reason for the surgical procedure (e.g., elective, emergent, trauma, gastrointestinal tract), current treatments, and diagnosis. This first step, if performed carefully and thoughtfully, will indicate the direction the doctor should take to investigate the cause of the fever. Secondly, a directed physical examination is performed to look for clues and/or confirmation of a suspected source. Table 1-23 can be used as a checklist to guide the evaluation process. Only after these two steps have been taken should consideration be given to ordering diagnostic studies. Undirected blanket ordering of laboratory tests, random cultures, and radiographs are appropriate only in very specific circumstances (e.g., patients on prolonged mechanical ventilation, those who are immunosuppressed, or those with indwelling catheters or monitoring devices). For the majority of postoperative surgical patients, a selective approach to confirmatory testing is cost-efficient, effective, and high-quality medical practice.

The most common nosocomial infectious causes of fever in the intensive care units are ventilator-associated pneumonia, sinusitis, catheter-related sepsis (primarily gram-negative), *Clostridium difficile* colitis, abdominal sepsis, and complicated wound infections. Notably absent from this list are urinary tract infections. Unless it is pyelonephritis, a urinary tract infection is rarely a cause of fever. The standard definition of a urinary

tract infection (a colony count $>10^5$ CFU/mL) does not apply to catheterized intensive care patients. Further, bacteriuria and urinary tract infection are not synonymous. Most patients with urinary catheters for more than 24 hours will have bacteria or white cells in the urine, and this should not trigger antimicrobial therapy.

Once the diagnosis is established, appropriate therapeutic steps can be taken. As mentioned previously, in a few select clinical circumstances, it is appropriate to use broad-spectrum antibiotics. Generally speaking, these situations involve critically ill patients in whom withholding antibiotic therapy for 24 to 48 hours until definitive cultures or diagnostic studies are completed could lead to disastrous consequences. Most intensivists select broad-spectrum drugs, chosen on the basis of sensitivity profiles of their own units, and then switch to more focused therapy when the cultures return.

The question arises as to whether the fever itself should be treated with antipyretics. Much divergent opinion on this issue exists, and there is little prospective scientific evidence to support either position. Fever is an adaptive response that conferred a survival advantage on warm-blooded animals. Temperature elevation enhances immune function by increasing antibody production; increasing cytokine expression; enhancing neutrophil, lymphocyte, and macrophage function; and reducing bacterial replication. Temperature elevation also confers a resistance to bacterial invasion. Still, some health care providers feel that fever is harmful and noxious and should be suppressed. The conclusions that can be drawn from the literature are summarized as follows:

- Short courses of antipyretics in approved doses carry a low risk of toxic side effects.
- The benefits of antipyretic use to the patient are uncertain, other than perhaps the analgesic effect. The loss of the immunoprotective effects of fever is concerning and potentially harmful. There are no good comparative data on this issue. The increase in metabolic demand (10% for each degree Celsius increase) associated with fever may be poorly tolerated in the elderly or debilitated, especially those with cardiac or pulmonary conditions.
- Children should not be given aspirin.
- Antipyretics do not prevent febrile seizures or raise the seizure threshold.
- Cooling blankets should not be used to treat fever (although they are used to treat hyperthermia). The patient should not be cooled to the point of inducing shivering.
- If antipyretics are used, they should be used on a scheduled basis and not as the occasion arises.
- Indomethacin and nonsteroidal anti-inflammatory drugs should not be used in patients with coronary artery disease.
- Anything that increases the cerebral metabolic rate in patients with traumatic brain injuries (e.g., fever, seizures) increases cerebral oxygen demand and cerebral blood flow. This can increase intracranial pressure.

PERIOPERATIVE SAFETY

In 2000, the IOM issued a report, *To Err is Human*, which looked at population-based studies of medical error. The report concluded that between 44,000 and 98,000 Americans die yearly in hospitals from medical mistakes. This report brought the issue of medical safety to the forefront of our national consciousness. A cross section of stakeholders

TABLE 1-23	Physical Examination Checklist for Investigating Cause of a Fever	
Anatomic Site	**Condition**	**Clue**
Head and Neck		
	Sinusitis/otitis	Nasal/oral instrumentation/facial fracture
	Meningitis	Skull fracture/instrumentation/craniotomy/CSF leak
	Parotitis/periodontal abscess; Peritonsillar/pharyngeal abscess	Elderly/periodontal disease/dehydration/oral instrumentation Immunosuppression/facial fracture
	Deep neck infection	Surgery/penetrating injury (especially digestive tract)/periodontal disease
Thorax		
	Pneumonitis/lung abscess	Intubation/mechanical ventilation/contusion/penetrating injury/aspiration
	Mediastinitis	Esophageal injury/sternotomy/neck exploration/penetrating thoracic injury
	Empyema	Hemothorax/tube thoracostomy/duration of thoracic instrumentation
	Endocarditis	Central vascular access/TPN/valvular disease (e.g., mitral valve prolapse)/periodontal disease
	Pericarditits Bronchitis/tracheitis Esophagitis	Immunosuppression/broad-spectrum antibiotics
Abdomen and Retroperitoneum		
	Intra-abdominal abscess	Previous celiotomy/splenectomy/visceral organ repair/anastomosis/ enteric contamination/bullet tract/possible missed injury
	Acalculous cholecystitis	Age/hypotension/broad-spectrum antibiotics/diabetes
	Ischemic viscera	Mesenteric injury/hypotension/pressors
	Colitis	Broad-spectrum antibiotic use/diarrhea
	Pancreatitis (necrotizing)	Hypotension/biliary stones/splenectomy/direct injury
	Urinary tract	Bladder instrumentation/comorbid urinary tract disease/urinary tract injury/diabetes
	Prostatitis	Instrumentation/duration/age
	Primary peritonitis	Hepatic failure/cirrhosis/ascites
	Pylephlebitis	Intra-abdominal process/abscess
	Occult perirectal abscess	Hematogenous malignancy/diabetes/
	Diverticular disease/appendicitis	Preexisting disease/direct injury
	TOA/endometritis	
Extremities		
	Occult compartment syndrome	Unconscious/extremity fracture/casts/hypotensive episodes/ immobilization (gluteal compartments)/ crush injury
	Phlebitis/arteritis	Duration of hospitalization/instrumentation/injury
Wounds (Surgical or Traumatic)		
	Superficial or deep abscess	Presence/contamination/time to definitive management/GI injury/diabetes/vascular disease
	Necrotizing soft tissue infection	GI injury/diabetes/immunosuppression
	Necrotizing myositis/ischemia	Occult compartment syndrome/unconsciousness
	Decubitus ulceration/abscess	Immobilization

within the health care system, from government policy developers (e.g., the Center for Medicare and Medicaid Services) to business (e.g., the Leapfrog Group), to regulators (e.g., Joint Commission on the Accreditation of Healthcare Organizations), as well as individual practitioners and their professional bodies (e.g., the American College of Surgeons), took note and began to approach the problem of patient safety from a more scientific and systems-based perspective. In 2006, the National Quality Forum published a list of "never events," which are listed in Table 1-24. The medical community has

relied heavily on Crew Resource Management strategies in designing systems to minimize error, and, if error should occur, generate useful (rather than accusatory or recriminative) discussion. Principles such as standardization of care, structured handoffs, simplification, use of forcing functions (e.g., computer order entry), avoiding reliance on memory, timeouts, and use of checklists prior to procedures have helped reduce the volume of medical error. The U.S. Department of Veterans Affairs originally developed the National Surgical Quality Improvement Program (NSQIP), which has been

TABLE 1-24	Events that Must Never Occur

Surgical Events

Surgery performed on the wrong body part

Surgery performed on the wrong patient

Wrong surgical procedure on a patient

Retention of a foreign object in a patient after surgery or other procedure

Intraoperative or immediately postoperative death in a normal healthy patient

Product or Device Events

Patient death or serious disability associated with the use of contaminated drugs, devices, or biologics provided by the health care facility

Patient death or serious disability associated with the use or function of a device in patient care in which the device is used or functions other than as intended

Patient death or serious disability associated with intravascular air embolism that occurs while being cared for in a health care facility

Patient Protection Events

Infant discharged to the wrong person

Patient death or serious disability associated with patient disappearance for more than 4 hr

Patient suicide, or attempted suicide resulting in serious disability, while being cared for in a health care facility

Care Management Events

Patient death or serious disability associated with a medication error

Patient death or serious disability associated with a hemolytic reaction due to the administration of ABO-incompatible blood or blood products (transfusion of the wrong blood type)

Maternal death or serious disability associated with labor or delivery on a low-risk pregnancy while being cared for in a health care facility

Patient death or serious disability associated with hypoglycemia, the onset of which occurs while the patient is being cared for in a health care facility

Death or serious disability (kernicterus) associated with failure to identify and treat jaundice in newborns

Stage 3 or 4 pressure ulcers acquired after admission to a health care facility

Patient death or serious disability due to spinal manipulative therapy

Environmental Events

Patient death or serious disability associated with an electric shock while being cared for in a health care facility

Any incident in which a line designated for oxygen or other gas to be delivered to a patient contains the wrong gas or is contaminated by toxic substances

Patient death or serious disability associated with a burn incurred from any source while being cared for in a health care facility

Patient death associated with a fall while being cared for in a health care facility

Patient death or serious disability associated with the use of restraints or bedrails while being cared for in a health care facility

Criminal Events

Any instance of care ordered by or provided by someone impersonating a physician, nurse, pharmacist, or other licensed health care provider

Abduction of a patient of any age

Sexual assault on a patient within or on the grounds of a health care facility

Death or significant injury of a patient or staff member resulting from a physical assault (i.e., battery) that occurs within or on the grounds of a health care facility

---

adopted by the American College of Surgeons. NSQIP provides to each surgeon risk-adjusted outcome data. This has in turn led to reductions in complication rates and in mortality. An Institute for Healthcare Improvement 100,000 Lives campaign enlisted 3,100 hospitals to implement six new proven safe practices:

- **Deploy Rapid Response Teams**…at the first sign of patient decline
- **Deliver Reliable, Evidence-Based Care for Acute Myocardial Infarction**…to prevent deaths from heart attack
- **Prevent Adverse Drug Events (ADEs)**…by implementing medication reconciliation
- **Prevent Central Line Infections**…by implementing a series of interdependent, scientifically grounded steps
- **Prevent Surgical-Site Infections**…by reliably delivering the correct perioperative antibiotics at the proper time
- **Prevent Ventilator-Associated Pneumonia**…by implementing a series of interdependent, scientifically grounded steps

Implementation of these practices has been estimated to have resulted in approximately 122,000 lives saved. Finally, current approaches to team-based care emphasize clear communication with a tone of mutual respect in an atmosphere in which it is safe to call attention to error. A cornerstone of this approach is the recognition that no one individual can possibly single-handedly possess the expertise to coordinate every aspect of a patient's care. The highly hierarchical model of health care delivery with the physician at its center is transitioning to a truly multi- and interdisciplinary model.

SAMPLE QUESTIONS

Questions

Choose the best answer for each question.

1. A 52-year-old man is in the clinic to discuss treatment of a newly diagnosed pancreatic cancer. He has no significant past medical history. He takes no medications. There is no evidence of metastatic disease, and the tumor is small and appears to be resectable by pancreaticoduodenectomy (Whipple procedure). Optimal treatment would also include adjuvant radiation therapy and chemotherapy. Informed consent for this patient is best defined as

   A. a form that can be used as a legal defense should a complication occur during the treatment of the patient's problem.

   B. a process in which the physician and patient discuss the risks and benefits of different approaches to the patient's problem.

   C. a process in which every possible complication of treatment is enumerated.

   D. a theoretical construct with little practical utility.

   E. a philosophical principle that applies to surgical procedures but not medication administration.

2. A 60-year-old woman is being evaluated for surgery to repair an abdominal aortic aneurysm under general anesthesia. She smoked a pack of cigarettes daily for 35 years, but quit 5 years ago when she had a myocardial infarction (MI) complicated by congestive heart failure. She still has occasional orthopnea. She also has hypercholesterolemia and hypertension. Which one of the following factors suggests the greatest risk for a cardiac complication following her surgery?

   A. History of cigarette smoking

   B. Congestive heart failure with orthopnea

   C. General anesthesia

   D. Hypertension

   E. Hypercholesterolemia

3. A 45-year-old man with a 25-year history of hepatitis C and cirrhosis is found to have a small hepatocellular carcinoma of the right lobe of the liver. In order to assess his risk for surgical therapy, an estimate of liver dysfunction given by the model for end stage liver disease (MELD) score is needed. Which one of the following laboratory studies is needed to calculate a MELD score for this patient?

   A. Alkaline phosphatase

   B. Serum creatinine

   C. Serum ammonia

   D. Serum albumin

   E. Serum gamma glutamyl transpeptidase (γGT)

4. Which of the following patients is at the *lowest* risk for postoperative deep vein thrombosis?

   A. An 18-year-old male with femur and lumbar fractures

   B. A 55-year-old morbidly obese female undergoing total knee replacement

   C. A 62-year-old man undergoing prostatectomy for cancer

   D. A 45-year-old woman undergoing hysterectomy and bilateral salpingo-oophorectomy and debulking for ovarian carcinoma

   E. A 38-year-old woman undergoing carpal tunnel release

5. A 28-year-old man is undergoing an operation for right inguinal hernia. The anesthesiologist notices that his end-tidal CO_2 value rises abruptly, and the patient's jaw is stiff. The patient's temperature is 41°C, his heart rate is 130 beats/minute, and his blood pressure (BP) is 130/75 mm Hg. Which of the following abnormalities would be expected if a sample of his blood were tested at this point in the operation?

   A. Hyperkalemia

   B. Hypocalcemia

   C. Alkalosis

   D. Anemia

   E. Hypoalbuminemia

Answers and Explanations

1. Answer: B

Informed consent is a process in which the physician and patient discuss the risks and benefits of different approaches to the patient's problem. This includes discussion of the most likely outcomes of treatment (including the decision to observe rather than operate). Informed consent permeates most of the discussions physicians have with their patients, although the discussions may not be labeled as such. It applies to medication choices as much as to surgical decision making, although a separate consent form is generally not obtained each time a new medication is prescribed.

2. Answer: B

General anesthesia does not itself increase risk of cardiac complications. The factors that do increase such risk include ischemic heart disease, congestive heart failure, chronic kidney disease, cerebrovascular disease, or high-risk operations such as major vascular surgery.

3. Answer: B

The MELD score formula is (0.957 × ln(Serum Creatinine) + 0.378 × ln(Serum Bilirubin) + 1.120 × ln(INR) + 0.643) × 10 (if hemodialysis, value for creatinine is automatically set to 4). Albumin is a component of the Childs-Pugh classification, but not the MELD score. Alkaline phosphatase is useful in determining biliary tract obstruction. Gamma GT is very sensitive for hepatobiliary disease and is best used to determine if an isolated elevation of alkaline phosphatase is due to liver rather than bone disease.

4. Answer: E

Patients who are immobile, who have congestive heart failure or malignancy, who undergo pelvic or joint replacement operations, or who have vertebral, pelvic, or long bone fractures are at highest risk. Carpal tunnel release does not confer increased risk of deep vein thrombosis.

5. Answer: A

This is a classic description of malignant hyperthermia. The typical electrolyte picture is that of rhabdomyolysis, with hyperkalemia, hypercalcemia, and acidosis. Malignant hyperthermia is not known to affect red cell mass or albumin levels. The patient should be given 100% oxygen, the operation should be stopped and the wound closed, and dantrolene should be administered.

2

Fluids, Electrolytes, and Acid-Base Balance

DAVID ANTONENKO, M.D. • MARY-MARGARET BRANDT, M.D. • DAVID REINES, M.D. •
HILARY SANFEY, M.D. • ARETI TILLOU, M.D.

Objectives

1. Know normal electrolyte composition of body fluids.

2. Understand the fluid compartments in the body and how they vary with age and obesity.

3. Understand and treat common electrolyte abnormalities in surgical patients.

4. Understand methods of determining normal and perioperative fluid requirements for patients.

5. Understand normal acid–base status of surgical patients and how to treat abnormal acid–base situations in surgical patients.

For most physicians, the topics of fluids and electrolytes are boring, mundane, and generally glossed over or ignored. Unfortunately, this indifference or lack of understanding regarding fluid and electrolyte management results in a host of complications. Some of these complications include increased length of stay, increased cost, wound infection, delayed wound healing, anastomotic failure, and tachyarrhythmia. There are some estimates that one in five patients develops one or more complications as a result of fluid and electrolyte management errors. Many of these complications are preventable if the physician pays as much attention to the nuances of fluids and electrolytes as to the more "exciting" aspects of surgery, such as the operating room.

Understanding and managing fluids, electrolytes, and acid–base status are critical aspects of the treatment of surgical patients. This chapter provides a brief overview of fluid, electrolyte, and acid–base balance before discussing clinical problems specific to surgery and surgical patients. It is intended to be an introduction to this subject. For more complete and comprehensive information, see the many available texts and articles in the literature, some of which are listed at the end of this chapter. A table of **normal serum laboratory values** for common electrolytes is provided in the online glossary.

NORMAL PHYSIOLOGY

Total Body Water and Compartments

Total body water (TBW) in the adult varies according to age, sex and lean body mass. Historically, and in most textbooks, this refers to the healthy, young 70-kg male who now accounts

for <1% of the population. Unfortunately, the information regarding this young male is usually applied to the other 99% of the population, which results in so many of the complications seen in surgical patients. One must extrapolate, not apply directly, this information to the care of patients.

In both males and females, TBW is directly proportional to muscle mass, which is about 70% water, and inversely related to fat, which is about 10% water. Consequently, TBW equivalent to 60% of weight only applies to the small fraction of today's population who are male, young, and physically fit. TBW may be as little as 35% of weight in the morbidly obese; the very elderly, who lose muscle as they age; or those who lose muscle rapidly because of disease or injury. TBW is estimated to be about 55% in young healthy physically fit females.

TBW is partitioned into two main compartments. In the ideal young healthy male, the intracellular fluid represents about two-thirds of TBW (40% of body weight, or about 28 L in a 70-kg man), and the extracellular fluid (ECF) one-third (20% of body weight, or about 14 L in the same individual). However, as noted previously, in those with significant reductions in lean body mass or the morbidly obese, these ratios change such that extracellular space fluid in these individuals may equal or even exceed intracellular fluid as a percentage of total body water.

There is little difference in the electrolyte composition of the two ECF subdivisions, plasma and interstitial space. In plasma (Table 2-1), sodium is the chief extracellular cation with smaller amounts of potassium, calcium, and magnesium present. The corresponding anions are chloride, bicarbonate, and smaller amounts of proteins, sulfates, and organic acids.

TABLE 2-1	Normal Plasma Values of Common Electrolytes	
Electrolytes	**Concentration**	**Units**
Cations		
Sodium	135–145	mEq/L
Potassium	3.5–5.0	mEq/L
Calcium	8.0–10.5	mg/dL
Magnesium	1.5–2.5	mEq/L
Anions		
Chloride	95–105	mEq/L
Bicarbonate	24–30	mEq/L
Phosphate	2.5–4.5	mEq/L
Sulfate	1.0	mEq/L
Organic acids	2.0	mEq/L
Albumin	3.0–5.0	g/dL
Total protein	6.0–8.4	g/dL

In the interstitial space, the ionic composition differs from plasma only with respect to its lower concentration of protein and the related minor changes in chloride and bicarbonate levels. In contrast to the extracellular compartment, the intracellular dominant cations are potassium and magnesium and the dominant anions are phosphates, sulfates, and proteins. The striking differences in intracellular and extracellular electrolyte composition are maintained by selective permeability of cellular membranes. Free diffusion of proteins, chloride, and multivalent ions is limited. Various transporter systems in the cell wall promote the movements of electrolytes across the cell membrane such that sodium remains mainly outside the cell and potassium primarily in the cell. Water is rapidly and freely diffusible among all compartments including intracellular fluid.

Movement of water from one compartment to another is passive and determined by the action of physical forces exerted across the intervening membranes. The capillary membrane that separates the interstitial and intravascular spaces, under most circumstances, is freely permeable to water, electrolytes, and solutes, but not to proteins. Consequently, the net flow of water between these two spaces is a function of the balance between fluid pressures generated on either side of the membrane and the effective **colloid osmotic pressures**. Colloid oncotic pressure is generated by the higher concentrations of nondiffusible protein in the plasma and the endothelial glycocalyx. On the other hand, the exchange of water between the intracellular and interstitial compartments is totally determined by osmotic gradients across the cell membranes. Normally, there is no gradient and no significant net water flow in either direction because the **osmolarity**, or number of osmotically active particles per liter of solution on either side of the membrane, is the same. When ECF becomes hypo-osmolar relative to normal values, water flows into the cells in which the osmolarity is higher. A new equilibrium is reached, and the osmolarity of both compartments is less than the normal 285 mOsm/L. Similarly, hyperosmolarity develops in both compartments if extracellular osmolarity is increased. In this case, osmotic equilibrium is reached by an egress of water from the cell into the extracellular space. In contrast, isotonic fluid expansion or contraction of the extracellular space, which has no effect on osmolarity, does not include such movements of water between the cells and the interstitial fluid.

Sodium

Total body sodium is estimated at 63 mEq/kg, but one-third is fixed in bone. The other two-thirds or 40 mEq/kg, most of which is extracellular, is the exchangeable fraction. Sodium and its related anions represent 97% of the osmotically active particles that are normally present in the ECF compartments. Extracellular osmolarity is estimated by the formula:

$$\text{Osmolarity} = 2 \times [\text{Na+}] + [\text{glucose (mg/dL)} \div 18] + [\text{blood urea nitrogen (BUN)} \div 2.8],$$

where $[\text{Na}^+]$ is serum sodium concentration. If the value approximates 290 ± 10 mOsmol/L, it can be reasonably assumed that extracellular osmolarity is within normal limits.

The normal adult sodium requirement is 1 to 2 mEq/kg/day, although the usual oral intake far exceeds this amount. Normal kidneys excrete sodium when intake is high and conserve it when intake is low maintaining fairly constant body sodium. Renal sodium resorption can be so efficient that nearly none is lost in the urine during maximum conservation. Assuming normal renal perfusion and membrane function, both sodium and water are filtered at the glomerulus. In the proximal tubules, large amounts of each are recovered. Ultimately, however, the determination of renal conservation or excretion of sodium or water depends on selective processes that occur at more distal tubular sites.

Sodium resorption in exchange for potassium and hydrogen ion secretion in the distal tubules is a direct effect of the adrenal cortical hormone **aldosterone**. This action helps to maintain both extracellular volume and osmolarity. Extracellular volume reduction, particularly in the intravascular space, is a potent stimulus for aldosterone release. This response is triggered by a decrease in renal perfusion, which causes the juxtaglomerular apparatus to secrete renin. Renin, in turn, cleaves angiotensinogen to produce angiotensin I, which is then converted by angiotensin-converting enzyme (ACE) to angiotensin II, a potent stimulator of aldosterone secretion. When activated by a decrease in volume, stretch receptors in the atria can also increase aldosterone secretion. The potassium level, which is usually inversely related to serum sodium concentrations, is the most sensitive stimulator of aldosterone, acting via depolarization of cells in the zona glomerulosa. Adrenocorticotropic hormone (ACTH) can also stimulate aldosterone production, but this is a minor role. The secretion of aldosterone is suppressed by extracellular volume expansion, increased sodium concentration, and decreased potassium concentration.

Antidiuretic hormone (ADH, Vasopressin) is released from the posterior pituitary gland in a diurnal fashion, peaking between 2 and 4 o'clock in the morning, and to a lesser extent in the early afternoon. The early morning peak is usually not considered in patients and as a result, unnecessary fluid infusions in response to a drop in urine output and a perceived hypovolemia are common. For example, if a patient is in the postoperative phase, has normal blood pressure and pulse pressure, and has warm extremities and full veins, increased fluid infusions in response to an early morning drop in urine output are not indicated.

There is increased ADH secretion in response to decreased blood volume; increased plasma osmolarity; and, to a lesser extent, angiotensin II and other secondary stimuli. It increases the reabsorption of water from cells in distal convoluted tubules and collecting tubules through aquaporins in the apical membrane of these cells. This effect and its modulation are important in the regulation of fluid volume and osmolarity in the body. Intracranial osmoreceptors adjacent to the anterior wall of the third ventricle and in the hypothalamic, supraoptic, and paraventricular nuclei initiate ADH secretion when plasma osmolarity rises. They also inhibit ADH secretion when plasma osmolarity decreases. The production and release of ADH also depend on the activity of volume receptors in the right and left atria. Decreased extracellular volume sensed in the right atrium and the carotid arteries leads to ADH secretion. Increased volume sensed in the left atrium leads to inhibition of ADH release. Volume-dependent responses usually override the effects of the osmoreceptor controlling system when the two are in conflict.

Potassium

In the normal young adult, total body stores of potassium are approximately 50 to 55 mEq/kg, 98% of which is intracellular at a concentration of 150 mEq/L cell water. The ECF compartment (including plasma) of the ideal 70-kg young male contains a total of 70 mEq of K^+ (present at a concentration of 3.5 to 5.0 mEq/L in 14 L of ECF). The normal adult daily potassium requirement is 0.5 to 0.8 mEq/kg/day and is directly proportional to lean body mass. The usual potassium intake averages 100 mEq/day, but 95% is excreted in the urine and 5% is lost in feces and sweat. In the kidney, most of the filtered potassium is resorbed in the proximal tubular system. Nevertheless, selective secretion or absorption in the distal tubule determines net renal excretion or conservation. Unlike its ability to conserve sodium, the kidney can only decrease potassium excretion to approximately 10 mEq/L. Potassium excretion is directly related to circulating levels of aldosterone, cellular and extracellular potassium content, and tubular urine flow rates. Acid–base disturbances also exert a significant influence.

Acid–Base Balance

Discussions in this chapter reflect the more common historical interpretation of acid–base balance and acid–base disturbances. However, a more recent interpretation of acid–base using the concept of strong ion difference is gaining support. If the student is interested multiple references to this approach to acid–base, search for the term "strong ion difference."

Acid–base balance is in effect the body's management of large amounts of endogenously produced hydrogen ion. There is a 40 to 60 mmol load of fixed nonvolatile organic acids (i.e., sulfuric, phosphoric, and lactic acids), some of which are ingested and some of which are produced by metabolic activity. In addition, 13,000 to 20,000 mmol of carbon dioxide (CO_2) constitutes the volatile acid load. Normally, the free hydrogen ion concentration of ECFs is maintained at 40 nmol/L or at a pH of 7.40 ± 0.05. Maintenance at this level is accomplished by the combined action of three mechanisms:

1. Buffering systems that are present in all body fluids and that immediately offset changes in hydrogen concentration
2. Pulmonary ventilation changes that can promptly adjust the excretion of CO_2
3. Renal tubular function, which, over time, can contribute by modulating the urinary excretion or conservation of acid or base

The bicarbonate–carbonic acid buffer system in ECF is one of the most important components. Its relation to pH is described by the Henderson-Hasselbalch equation and its modifications:

$$pH = pKa + \log [HCO3]/[H2CO3]$$
$$pH = 6.1 + \log [HCO3]/0.03 \times Paco2$$
$$7.4 = 6.1 + \log 24 \text{ mEq/L}/1.20 \text{ mEq/L}.$$

A more useful variation of these equations is:

$$[H+] = 24 \times Paco2/[HCO3].$$

CO_2 is transported in the plasma in three forms: dissolved CO_2, CO_2 bound to proteins, and free bicarbonate. If the laboratory reports CO_2 content in the serum electrolyte panel, [HCO_3^-] concentration can be roughly calculated from the serum electrolytes by subtracting 1 for the dissolved CO_2, and 1 to 2 for the bound fraction. If [$Paco_2$] and [HCO_3] are normal, then the [H^+] is 40 nmol. The value for [H_2CO_3] can be determined as the arithmetic product of a proportionality constant (0.03) and the $Paco_2$. In clinical practice, direct measurements of arterial pH and $Paco_2$ are readily available, and [HCO_3^-] can be calculated or derived from a nomogram, assuming all measurements are reliable. The pH is determined by the ratio [HCO_3^-]/[H_2CO_3], which normally is approximately 20:1. A change in either the numerator or the denominator can alter the ratio and the resulting pH value. In addition, a change of either [$H_2CO_3^-$] or $Paco_2$ can be compensated by a corresponding change in the same direction of the other, restoring the ratio to 20:1 and the pH to 7.40. Thus, pulmonary regulation of $Paco_2$ and renal tubular regulation of plasma HCO_3^- are important determinants of extracellular pH.

As effective as the [HCO_3^-]/[H_2CO_3] buffer system is, and as available as its substrates are from metabolic sources, even in combination with all other extracellular buffers it cannot maintain arterial pH at normal levels in the face of all challenges. Intracellular buffer systems play a major role. As much as 50% of fixed acid loads and 95% of hydrogen ion changes that result from excessive retention or excretion of CO_2 are buffered in the cells. The movement of hydrogen into and out of the cell involves cationic exchanges that cause reciprocal shifts of potassium. Thus, **acidosis**, in which hydrogen ions move from an area of high concentration (extracellular) to an area of low concentration (intracellular), causes potassium to move out of the cell. Alternatively, if intracellular hydrogen ions increase, potassium moves to the extracellular compartment. As a result, the potassium concentration in interstitial fluid (and serum) increases. On average, for every 0.1 change in pH, the K^+ changes inversely by about 0.3 mEq/L. **Alkalosis**, in which hydrogen ions move from an area of high concentration (intracellular) to one of low concentration (extracellular), causes the opposite movement of potassium into the cell. As a result, the extracellular potassium concentration decreases. Thus, acidosis is associated with hyperkalemia, and alkalosis is associated with hypokalemia. The usual assumption of a direct relation between serum levels and total body stores of potassium is not valid. Changes in serum potassium concentration that are induced by acid–base alterations can have significant clinical implications, particularly with regard to myocardial irritability and function. For example, if the serum potassium is measured as 3.4 mEq/L and the pH is 7.20, the true serum potassium may be as low as 2.8 mEq/L when the pH is corrected to normal.

FLUIDS AND ELECTROLYTES IN THE PERIOPERATIVE PERIOD

The three essential components that must be addressed when considering fluid and electrolyte therapy for surgical patients are:

- Maintenance
- Resuscitation
- Replacement

Maintenance involves meeting the requirements for fluid and electrolyte intake that and deficits that are present. Replacement refers to the provision for ongoing and additional losses that occur during the course of therapy. Each component must be addressed in the three phases of surgical care: that is, preoperative, intraoperative, and postoperative. With each component of therapy, comorbidities such as the presence of cardiac or renal disease and the pathophysiology of the clinical problem being treated must also be considered.

With no unusual stresses or losses and normal renal function, the fluid and electrolyte balance is maintained by the intake of adequate amounts of water, sodium, potassium, and chloride to balance daily obligatory losses. Intake is calculated to balance outputs of 12 to 15 mL/kg/day urine, 3 mL/kg/day stool water, 0 to 1.5 mL/kg/day sweat, 10 mL/kg/day combined insensible losses from the lungs and skin and an endogenous input of approximately 3 mL/kg water from the oxidation of carbohydrate and fat. These estimates apply to adults. More universal guidelines for calculating fluid and electrolyte requirements have also been devised. Probably the most accurate calculations are based on surface area, but they are cumbersome, requiring measurement of height as well as weight and a nomogram for transposing the measurements into a value for surface area. For this reason, the common practice is to determine water and electrolyte needs as a function of age and weight. Guidelines for fluid and electrolyte requirements using age and body weight are shown in Tables 2-2 and 2-3. If the entire intake is to be delivered intravenously, 5% dextrose in water is used to meet most of the water requirements because the kidney reabsorbs nearly all of the sodium and chloride that the body needs. The fluid used to replace ongoing losses or existing deficits should reflect the composition of the deficits or losses as much as possible. Usually, 0.45% or 0.9% saline can be given to provide the necessary sodium and chloride. Potassium is added in divided amounts to the various solutions. In this way, its delivery is spread out over time.

Overall estimates of daily needs must be adjusted for fever and high ambient temperatures. Insensible skin and pulmonary losses increase with elevations of body temperature (10% to 15% per °C, 8% per °F). These losses may require an additional 500 mL or more of salt-free water per day in febrile patients. Similar needs for more water because of increased pulmonary insensible losses occur in patients with tracheostomies who are breathing unhumidified air or gas mixtures, especially with hyperventilation. In a slightly different way, requirements for

TABLE 2-3	Daily Electrolyte Requirements	
Electrolyte	**mEq/kg**	**Example: 70 kg, 175 cm male**
Sodium	1.0–2.0	70–140 mEq
Potassium	0.5–0.8[a]	35–56 mEq
Chloride	1.0–2.0	70–140 mEq

[a]Potassium requirements are directly proportional to lean body mass.

both salt and water increase when ambient temperatures rise to more than 32°C (85°F). This increase is caused by hypotonic salt losses from sweating. Additional intravenous fluid replacement with 0.45% saline may be appropriate in this case. However, since the sodium loss in sweat is directly proportional to the rate of secretion and may exceed 100 mEq/L, additional sodium infusions may be required in cases where sweat rate and volume are unusually high.

As with all aspects of good surgical care, the management of fluid and electrolyte balance starts with assessment. The surgeon uses the information obtained from a thorough history and physical examination to identify current or potential problems and determine what laboratory data are needed to confirm the diagnosis. Preoperative risk assessment and management is essential. In the context of elective surgery, the standard precaution of "loading" the patient with fluids before surgery to prevent intraoperative hypotension is incorrect since it has been recently shown that the vast majority of patients admitted for elective surgery do not have hypovolemia, as was previously thought.

The initial workup could reveal underlying comorbid conditions that would have a significant impact on the patient's ability to tolerate an operation. These findings may significantly influence the fluid therapy during and after the operation. If stressful surgery is contemplated (e.g., abdominal aortic aneurysm repair, pulmonary or pancreatic resection), central venous or pulmonary arterial monitoring in the perioperative period may be required. However, systolic and mean blood pressure and heart rate have been shown in the noncritically ill patient to be as predictive, if not more predictive, of fluid needs compared with central monitoring. A history of diuretic and digitalis therapy may call attention to the possibility of hypokalemia or hyponatremia. Low preoperative serum potassium levels can fall even lower during surgery, particularly in patients who are under general anesthesia, are hyperventilated, and/or have hypocapnic respiratory alkalosis. If hyponatremia is present on admission, the margin of safety between asymptomatic and symptomatic low serum sodium concentrations is reduced, making, even relatively small, additional decreases potentially hazardous. Depending on the severity of the planned surgery, a patient with chronic pulmonary obstructive disease may need an arterial blood gas evaluation as part of the preoperative

TABLE 2-2	Daily Fluid Requirements					
	Adult, mL per Kilogram			**Child > 5 kg, mL per Kilogram**		
Per m²	**Age 25–55**	**Age 55–65**	**Age > 65**	**First 10 kg**	**Second 10 kg**	**>20 kg**
1,200 mL	35	30	25	100	50	20

workup. Similarly, BUN, serum creatinine, and electrolyte studies are indicated in a patient who has a history of chronic renal disease. With any of these disorders, any deficits and ongoing needs must be identified and addressed in the preoperative period.

Fluid, electrolyte, and acid–base imbalances must be identified and treated promptly in patients who are acutely ill. This requirement is even more important in patients who need an urgent operation. The admitting history and physical examination should clarify the extent of the deficit, and appropriate directed laboratory data should be obtained immediately. In patients who are vomiting or who have had prolonged gastric drainage, the presence of hypokalemic, hypochloremic metabolic alkalosis should be anticipated, rapidly confirmed and treated with replacement of volume, potassium, and chloride losses. In these circumstances, profound potassium depletion is present if the urine pH is acidic (this **paradoxical aciduria** is explained in more detail later). If emergency surgery is indicated, potassium replacement may be needed in 10 to 20 mEq/hour doses. If more than 10 mEq/hour is infused, the patient should be placed on a cardiac monitor.

Isotonic vascular volume depletion caused by fluid sequestered into interstitial space, either systemically as seen in sepsis or inflammatory response syndrome or locally such as with peritonitis (bacterial or chemical), intestinal obstruction, extensive soft tissue inflammation or trauma, is common. The term "third space loss" should be abandoned since the fluid sequestered in the interstitial space in areas of injury is still part of the functional ECF. Like hemorrhage, these fluid shifts to the ECF effectively reduce intravascular volumes, and must be replaced promptly. Balanced salt solutions (lactated Ringer's solution or normal saline) are normally used to replace the isotonic losses. The indications of how much to give are not always apparent. In this case, clinical observation of hemodynamic changes (i.e., tachycardia, narrowed pulse pressure, hypotension), decreasing urine output (<0.5 mL/kg/hour), and laboratory evidence of isotonic volume contraction (i.e., rising hematocrit and serum BUN: creatinine ratio >20:1, urine sodium concentrations <20 mEq/L) makes it clear that the losses are significant. With continuous monitoring as intravenous fluid is given, improvements in hemodynamic parameters and hourly urine output, to near-normal values, indicate that vascular volume has been restored to normal levels. The goal is to optimize the hemodynamics, not to maximize them. The latter has been shown to increase morbidity and mortality. To avoid clinically significant dilutional hyponatremia, care must be taken to limit the intravenous administration of hypotonic solutions (i.e., D5W, 0.45 NS, etc.) to patients who need large volumes of fluid to replace deficits in circulating blood volume.

During surgery, attention is focused on maintaining circulating volumes and adequate tissue perfusion as monitored by urine flow rates and central venous or pulmonary arterial pressures. Crystalloid solutions are used initially to replace whole blood losses, but packed red blood cells and **colloid** solutions may also be used. For patients who undergo major abdominal or thoracic surgery, Ringer's Lactate or normal saline solution should be used to replace the isotonic fluid sequestered in injured tissue. The use of hypotonic intravenous fluid should be limited to the replacement of evaporative water losses since these hypotonic fluids lead to dilutional hyponatremia. In patients who have compromised pulmonary function, arterial blood gas and pH studies are performed intraoperatively to monitor gas exchange and acid–base balance.

In the immediate postoperative period the fluid, electrolyte, and acid–base needs of the patient, for the most part, are related to monitoring and maintaining hemodynamic stability, and the adequacy of ventilation. Careful attention should be paid to the volume and electrolyte content of all fluids given to the patient. This needs to be accurately recorded in the medical record that is reviewed in the daily care of the patient. In many patients who have had relatively uncomplicated and stress-free elective surgery (i.e., inguinal herniorrhaphy, cholecystectomy) and in whom oral intake will be resumed within 48 hours, this process is accomplished simply by physical examination and serial observations of pulse rate, arterial blood pressure, respiratory frequency, and urine output, and by the administration of intravenous fluids as described for maintenance in Table 2-2. Another guideline frequently cited in the literature for estimating normal daily fluid requirements is the 4:2:1 rule, which states that for normal maintenance fluids per hour, 4 mL are given for the first 10 kg, 2 mL for the second 10 kg, and 1 mL for the remainder of the weight. This rule or the 100:50:20 rule recommended for children (as seen in Table 2-2) should not be used to estimate fluid requirements in the elderly since substantially more fluid would be infused than is actually required. The differences in fluid requirements using these different methods of calculating fluids may seem trivial at times, but the significance can be more clearly seen if as an example we apply each method to the young 70-kg male and the elderly 70-kg slightly obese male whose lean body mass is substantially reduced. The 4:2:1 rule would result in 110 mL/hour or 2,640 mL infused in 24 hours. The 100:50:20 rule used mostly in pediatrics would result in 2,500 mL in 24 hours, not much different and probably not clinically significant. However, since the elderly patient has less lean body mass, we should apply the 25 mL/kg rule (Table 2-2), which would result in only 1,750 mL required for 24 hours. In many patients, this would not seem important but if given over 3 days, the elderly patient would receive over 2 L of excess fluid and if given for 5 days he would receive almost 4 L of excess fluid. Since the elderly have decreased renal and cardiac function, this excess fluid could result in pleural effusions, pulmonary and peripheral edema (particularly if the patient is also hypoproteinemic), and even congestive heart failure. This excess fluid is *not* innocuous. It is imperative that changes in lean body mass and weight with age be considered when calculating fluid requirements.

In patients who have had more surgically stressful procedures that involve extensive dissection or resection, the fluids needed may be greater because of the fluid sequestered in the area of dissection (i.e., soft tissue injury) but must also be adjusted appropriately in patients with clinical conditions that might affect fluid balance such as known compromise of cardiac, renal, or pulmonary function. In these patients, additional monitoring with central venous or pulmonary arterial pressure, hourly urine output collected with an indwelling catheter in the bladder, and serial arterial blood gas with pH measurement may be necessary. Inadequate respiratory gas exchange may require the use of endotracheal intubation and mechanical ventilation. Infusions are needed to replace fluids that move into interstitial space in local areas of injury or systemically such as in sepsis syndrome or inflammatory response syndrome. This fluid shift can continue for 48 to 72 hours, or even longer in the elderly. In addition to daily maintenance needs, gastric, intestinal, biliary, and pancreatic drainage should be replaced. If these losses are >1,000 mL

TABLE 2-4	Composition of Normal Body Fluids[a]			
Fluid	**Na+**	**K+**	**Cl-**	**HCO3-**
Plasma	135–150	3.5–5.0	98–106	22–30
Stomach	10–150	4–12	120–160	0
Bile	120–170	3–12	80–120	30–40
Pancreas	135–150	3.5–5.0	60–100	35–110
Small intestine	80–150	2–8	70–130	20–40
Colon	50–100	10–30	80–120	25–30
Perspiration	30–50	5	30–50	0

[a]The composition of most gastrointestinal fluids and of perspiration varies according to the rate of secretion

in 24 hours, consideration should be given to replacing these deficits milliliter for milliliter with an appropriate intravenous infusion. The electrolyte content of these infusions generally can be determined by knowing the electrolyte composition of the fluid lost, as described in Table 2-4.

To determine more accurately what must be replaced, fluid samples may be analyzed for their electrolyte composition. Daily weights are used to assess fluid volume depletion or retention, recognizing that gains or losses >250 g (~0.5 lb) represent changes in body fluid content. As valuable as it is to monitor ECF status, weight gains and losses related to interstitial sequestration of fluid and their management must be considered. During replacement of these losses, weight gains do not represent hypervolemia. Rather they are caused by the replacement of needed extracellular volume to compensate for the volume that was lost or sequestered. Similarly, diuresis and associated weight loss is expected 3 or more days postoperatively when the sequestered fluid accumulations are mobilized (i.e., moved into the intravascular compartment). This excreted fluid should not be replaced. When this fluid is mobilized, intravascular volumes are likely to be high, making additional intravenous fluid infusion undesirable. On the other hand, in patients who are receiving parenteral nutrition with hyperosmolar glucose solutions, increased urine output should not be interpreted simply as appropriate excretion of excess fluids. In fact, the high urine output in these patients may be caused by osmotic diuresis that is independent of the patient's volume status. This condition requires prompt recognition and correction with intravenous fluids to avoid severe hyperosmolar volume contraction.

Several issues in perioperative management may account for the administration of excessive amounts of fluid. These include errors in the assessment of preoperative fluid deficits; dehydration, primarily derived from prolonged preoperative fasting and bowel preparation; the status of the circulation and cardiac function after general and regional anesthesia; the extent of blood loss; the desire to avoid blood transfusion; alternate reasons for a decrease in urine output; and misinterpretation of central venous pressure (CVP) or pulmonary pressures (if measured) from fluid infusion.

Administration of fluid in excess to the patient needs may cause several problems after surgery and needs to be avoided. Hypervolemia increases demands on cardiac function, due to an excessive shift to the right on the Frank-Starling myocardial performance curve, and may potentially increase postoperative cardiac morbidity. Hypervolemia also stimulates the production of atrial natruretic factor, which results in endothelial changes causing a leakage of fluid from the vascular system into the interstitium. Fluid accumulation in the lungs may predispose patients to pneumonia, respiratory failure, pleural effusions, and pulmonary edema. The excretory demands of the kidney are increased, and the resulting diuresis may lead to urinary retention mediated by the inhibitory effects of anesthetics and analgesics on bladder function. Gastrointestinal motility may be inhibited, prolonging postoperative ileus. Excess interstitial fluid may decrease tissue oxygenation with implications for wound (anastomotic) healing.

Close attention to a patient's fluid needs, particularly in the elderly or those with compromised renal or cardiac function, must continue until the patient's renal and gastrointestinal functions return to normal and all fluid, electrolyte, and nutritional requirements are being met by oral intake. At this point, with the exception of chronically ill patients, who may have ongoing needs, requirements should stabilize.

FLUID AND ELECTROLYTE DISORDERS IN A SURGICAL PATIENT

Disorders of Volume

Loss of intravascular volume is the most common cause of hypotension and low urine output in the surgical patient. The loss may be secondary to hemorrhage internally such as from traumatic injury, from gastrointestinal bleeding, or from external losses such as lacerations. Vascular volume may also decrease due to loss of plasma into the interstitial compartment due to burns, sepsis, and local or systemic inflammatory response to injury. Fluid losses from the gastrointestinal tract (e.g., vomiting, diarrhea, nasogastric suction) as well as increased evaporation of water as a result of fever or open abdominal surgery are also common.

Hypervolemia and increases in total body water above requirements (fluid overload) are usually secondary to excess replacement of fluids or to renal failure. The **majority** of surgical patients do not demonstrate early congestive heart failure even during resuscitation.

Volume Depletion

Volume depletion may be due to acute blood loss, ECF loss, or total body water reductions. An accurate history and physical examination is essential to ascertain if one or all of the deficits are present. For the most part, losses from the gastrointestinal tract are from vomiting, diarrhea, nasogastric suction, and from enteric **fistulas**, resulting in ECF volume depletion. As shown in Table 2-4, most fluids from the gastrointestinal tract are isotonic and therefore can be replaced with most common replacement fluids such as normal saline or Ringer's lactate. The intracellular compartment is affected only if osmolar concentrations change. Because of acid secretion from the stomach, gastric losses usually result in a large fluid and chloride loss and significantly less sodium loss. Since the chloride loss is also associated with hydrogen loss, patients usually become alkalotic, and their kidneys compensate for this by holding onto sodium and excreting potassium. The resulting hypochloremic, hypokalemic metabolic alkalosis needs to be treated with a higher chloride solution such as normal saline.

Isotonic depletion of functional extracellular volume also occurs with "third space losses," which are similar to serum (plasma minus some protein). These are particularly significant in burns, crush injuries, long bone fractures, peritonitis, severe pancreatitis, intestinal obstruction, pleural effusions, and large areas of soft tissue infection. Excess urinary loss of water and electrolytes can lead to volume depletion as is seen with diuretic therapy, high output renal failure, or with osmotic diuresis associated with nonelectrolyte hyperosmolar solute loading (e.g., glucose, mannitol, angiographic contrast media). Finally, there are volume depletions involving losses of water and excess of solute. These losses include excessive free water excretion associated with primary deficiencies of ADH, including diabetes insipidus. This is most commonly seen in head injury patients, but nephrogenic causes of diabetes insipidus and increased evaporative losses from burn injuries or increased sweating with evaporative losses from the skin and respiratory tract in a febrile patient can also cause this problem. These hypotonic losses create a hypernatremic hyperosmolar state in the extracellular compartment that draws water from the cell. This repletion of the extracellular space typically is seen with very high urine output, and hypotension is a late effect. Volume loss due to hemorrhage and the resulting hypotension are more fully explained in the chapter on shock.

Presentation and Diagnosis

Volume loss from the extracellular space (which holds ~40% of the total body water or 20% of total body weight in the young healthy man) is usually more rapid than loss from the intracellular space. More recent studies suggest the average blood volume of an adult is a little over 6% of body weight, not the 7% commonly quoted in many publications but is increased with living at higher altitudes to about 6.5% and to 7.5% to 8.5% in children and neonates. In order to demonstrate clinically significant physiologic changes, usually one needs to lose more than 10% to 15% of the intravascular volume. Signs of plasma volume deficits include signs of reduced tissue perfusion as seen with whole blood loss. Tables 2-5 and 2-6 demonstrate what the signs of ECF loss are in normal adults. These may be exacerbated or hidden in the older population as seen in Table 2-6. Neurologic and cardiovascular signs are more prominent with acute losses whereas tissue signs may not be evident for up to 24 hours. In acute circumstances, a clinician is more dependent on hemodynamic parameters such as change in heart rate, pulse pressure and **oliguria**, elevated hematocrit and urinary concentration in the case of interstitial fluid sequestration, or decreased hematocrit and oliguria, and urinary concentration in the case of blood loss. As renal perfusion becomes more restricted, BUN and soon creatinine rise. It is imperative that the clinician understands the difference between acute renal failure as a cause for oliguria and a rise in BUN and creatinine, and oliguria associated with fluid depletion showing a rise in BUN and creatinine. Obviously, these are opposites in treatment for one would exacerbate the problems of the other. Several methods are used to distinguish prerenal failure from renal failure. The more accurate test would be to obtain serum and urine electrolytes. A urine sodium concentration of <20 mEq/L, a BUN/creatinine ratio of 20:1, and urine **osmolality** >400 mOsm/L (in the absence of glycosuria or the excretion of other osmotically active particles) are all helpful. A more exact test is the fractional excretion of sodium (Fe_{Na})

$$Fe_{Na} = [(U_{Na} \times P_{CR})/(P_{Na} \times U_{Cr}) \times 100].$$

A FeNa of <1% is characteristic of prerenal azotemia while >2% is most common with renal injury. In acute renal failure, urine sodium usually increases to >40 mEq/L as renal tubular absorption of sodium is impaired. The BUN/creatinine ratio falls to 10 or less because creatinine starts to rise faster than BUN, and urine osmolality approaches plasma osmolality of 270 to 280 mOsm/L.

TABLE 2-5	Signs of ECF Depletion		
	10% Depletion	**20% Depletion**	**30% Depletion**
Clinical	2% weight loss	4% weight loss	6% weight loss
	Thirst	Apathy	Stupor or coma
	Mildly reduced urine output	Drowsiness	Skin cool, pale, cyanotic, with poor turgor
		Decreased skin turgor	Eyes sunken
		Dry mucous membranes	Tachycardia
		Longitudinal tongue furrowing	Pulse weak and thready
		Tachycardia	Hypotension
		Orthostatic hypotension	Urine output <15 mL/hr
		Urine output < 30 mL/hr	
Laboratory	Slightly elevated hematocrit[a]	Elevated hematocrit[a]	Greatly elevated hematocrit[a]
		Elevated WBC	
	Slightly elevated urine specific gravity	Modest elevation in BUN and creatinine	Elevated BUN/creatinine ratio (>10:1 up to 25:1)
		Elevated BUN/creatinine ratio (>10:1 up to 25:1)	Urine[b] specific gravity <1.020, urine osmolarity <500 mOsm/L, urine sodium >20 mEq/L
		Urine specific gravity ≥1.020, urine osmolarity >500 mOsm/L, urine sodium ≤10–15 mEq/L	
Comments	Findings can be overlooked on evaluation	Findings are always evident	Findings are very obvious

[a]In the absence of bleeding, hematocrit increases about 1% for every 500 mL ECF deficit.
[b]These urine findings reflect acute tubular necrosis.

TABLE 2-6	Responses to ECF Depletion in the Elderly	
System	**Signs or Symptoms in Younger Persons**	**Signs or Symptoms in Persons >65 Years Old**
Intravascular	Orthostatic hypotension	Common in healthy elderly
	Hypotension	May be masked by preexisting hypertension
	Tachycardia	Maximal heart rate decreases with age
	Reduced pulse volume	Masked by rigid vessels
	Reduced CVP or PaOP	May not reflect heart function or volume status
	Oliguria	May be less marked if preexisting renal impairment is present
	No signs of fluid overload or heart failure	Preexisting hypoproteinemia and ankle edema may be present
Interstitial	Dry skin and mucous membranes	Common in the elderly
	Dry tongue	Unreliable at any age
	Reduced tongue volume	May be useful
	Sunken eyes	A late sign at any age
	Reduced skin turgor	Unreliable in the elderly
Miscellaneous	Reduced deep tendon reflexes	May be an age-related change
	Distal anesthesia	May be an age-related change
	Drowsiness	May be caused by infection, medication, hypothyroidism, or depression
	Apathy	May be caused by infection, medication, hypothyroidism, or depression
	Anorexia	May be caused by infection, medication, hypothyroidism, or depression
	Stupor or coma	A late, nonspecific sign
	Ileus	A late, nonspecific sign

CVP, central venous pressure; PaOP, pulmonary artery opening pressure.

Treatment

The most efficacious test that a physician can do is a good history and physical examination. A measurement of postural blood pressure and pulse can be very helpful (orthostatic measurement). An increase of >10 heartbeats per minute or a decrease >15 mm Hg systolic blood pressure on a sitting patient should raise suspicion of intravascular depletion. This is more valuable in younger patients since the elderly may not be able to compensate and sudden drops in blood pressure may occur. Correction of the volume depletion requires a diagnosis that depletion is the problem, an estimate of the extent of the depletion, and an estimation of what fluid losses need to be replaced. Table 2-5 helps to describe the difference between a 10%, 20%, and 30% depletion of ECF, although these are fairly inexact findings. Hypotension usually does not occur in a young healthy adult, until there is a loss of at least 25% intravascular volume. Isotonic extracellular deficits caused by intestinal, biliary, pancreatic, or third space losses are best treated with lactated Ringer's solution or normal saline if hyperchloremia is not a problem (Table 2-7). Large volumes of Lactate-containing solution should be used with care in patients who have gastric outlet obstruction as a cause of vomiting or nasogastric secretions because these patients become hypochloremic and metabolically alkalotic. The pH of Ringer's Lactate is approximately 6.5 while the pH of normal saline is approximately 5.0. Inadequate replacement of chloride and inadequate correction of the alkalosis can exacerbate both of these problems. For replacement of nasogastric output, a solution of one-half normal saline (77 mEq/L of sodium, 77 mEq/L of chloride) with 20 to 40 mEq/L of potassium most likely will match the electrolyte losses from the vomiting. Glucose solutions should not be utilized for resuscitation or for most replacements. The addition of 50 g of glucose to a solution that is given rapidly may result in hyperglycemia and an osmotic diuresis. Glucose solutions also frequently have somewhat lower pH than solutions not containing glucose. How fast one corrects the volume is commensurate with the need and the ability of the patient to accept the fluid load that is delivered. The longer a deficit has taken to occur, the more cautious a clinician should be in replacing it. These electrolyte abnormalities will be discussed in more detail in the next section. When deficits are moderate, complete replacement should be carried out, at least over 24-hour periods. If deficits are large and consequences severe with physiologic abnormalities such as hypotension and tachycardia, and needs are more urgent; the therapeutic priority should be to correct the hemodynamic and perfusion inadequacies as rapidly and safely as possible. The rapidity of resuscitation is dependent not only on the patient's physiology and on the acuity of the physiologic changes, but also on the ability to deliver the fluid. Smaller intravenous lines, such as 20- and 22-gauge, significantly restrict the amount of fluid that can be given rapidly. Poiseuille's law states that the amount of resistance to flow through a system is dependent on the radius to the fourth power ($R = \eta L/\pi r^4$). This means that using a 16-gauge intravenous compared to a 20-gauge can more than double the amount of fluid given over for a period of time. A bolus is an amount of fluid given as fast as possible (not "999" on an infusion pump). A rapid infusion of a liter of crystalloid solution, or in case of bleeding, blood, may be necessary to achieve hemodynamic stability. In cases of ongoing massive fluid losses, the infusion of fluid must obviously exceed the egress of fluid; therefore, it is not unusual for patients to receive several liters over a rapid period of time in order to

TABLE 2-7	Composition of Commonly Used Intravenous Solutions					
	Glucose (g/L)	Na⁺ (mEq/L)	K⁺ (mEq/L)	Cl⁻ (mEq/L)	Lactateᵃ (mEq/L)	Ca⁺⁺ (mEq/L)

	Glucose (g/L)	Na⁺ (mEq/L)	K⁺ (mEq/L)	Cl⁻ (mEq/L)	Lactateᵃ (mEq/L)	Ca⁺⁺ (mEq/L)
0.9% Sodium chloride ("normal" saline)		154			154	
Lactated Ringer's solution		130	4.0	109	28	3.0
5% dextrose water	50					
5% dextrose in 0.45% sodium chloride	50	77		77		
3% sodium chloride		513		513		

ᵃConverted to bicarbonate.

stabilize the hemodynamics. Once again, one should not use a glucose-containing solution during these rapid corrections because of the iatrogenic hyperglycemic-induced osmotic diuresis, which may actually increase fluid losses. Volume losses are corrected with isotonic solutions. Ringer's Lactate is the fluid of choice for blood loss and should be given with a 3:1 ratio because there is little oncotic gradient, and the egress of the isotonic fluid from the intravascular to the extracellular space is rapid. The infusions of colloid solutions, which contain albumin, are not usually indicated in the rapid resuscitation of traumatic injury for multiple reasons. The use of normal saline is acceptable as a replacement fluid with the caveat that if one is using large amounts of normal saline, one risks hyperchloremia and worsening acidosis. Lactated Ringer's is usually the preferred solution for large-volume resuscitation.

While replacing fluid, one must be also aware that potassium abnormalities must be corrected rapidly along with abnormalities of glucose and osmolality changes. If changes are chronic and severe, too rapid correction of sodium and osmolality may result in dire neurologic consequences and swelling of the neurons (pontine demyelination).

Determinations of end points for resuscitation are still mainly clinical in nature. Weight changes are extremely difficult to document accurately in the acute stages. Measurement of fluid input and output gives some valuable data for large fluid shifts, but is not very valuable in making immediate clinical decisions. During resuscitation, repeat examination of the patient is imperative with the examination of vital signs such as pulse, blood pressure, urine output, and if possible or necessary, additional monitoring with central venous or pulmonary artery catheters. Electrolytes and serum lactate and blood pH, as well as base excess calculations, should be selectively used to help determine end points of fluid resuscitation.

If there is no acute renal failure or significant chronically compromised renal failure, then a urine output of >0.5 mL/kg/hour in adults or 1.0 mL/kg/hour in children should be achieved. This volume of urine output indicates adequate repletion of vascular volume. If the patient is showing signs of prerenal azotemia, these should resolve rapidly with repletion of the fluid.

It is often said that the dumbest kidney is smarter than the smartest doctor. Similarly, in the absence of continuing blood loss, hemoglobin may not reflect immediate losses, and replacement of blood and electrolytes is necessary to once again stabilize the vital signs mentioned above. Transfusing blood in stable patients should not be undertaken unless there is either symptomatology or the hemoglobin is <7 g/dL. However, in the acute situation, replacing blood is much more empiric, and this rule does not apply, especially in the unstable patient. A patient who is losing blood and is hemodynamically unstable usually requires blood in addition to significant amounts of crystalloid.

Prognosis

The prognosis for patients with volume depletion depends first on the underlying physiology including the duration of the loss; secondly, the amount of depletion that takes place without repletion, and the ability to stop the ongoing losses. As patients arrive in severe shock for prolonged period of time, resuscitative efforts must be extremely aggressive and may not succeed. Most patients who arrive shortly after their fluid loss or are in the hospital while they are losing fluid should be able to survive. Part of the surgeon's responsibility is to control any blood loss and to replace all losses from the gastrointestinal tract or other sites.

Volume Excess

Volume excess, for any or all fluid compartments, can occur from abnormal fluid retention, excessive or inappropriate fluid intake, or a combination of both. However the terms "fluid overload" and "volume excess" are frequently used indiscriminately and inappropriately. For example in many situations involving inflammatory response syndromes or sepsis, the patient may develop peripheral edema or pleural effusions but still have an intravascular volume deficiency. Patients who have signs of congestive heart failure may present with a gastrointestinal bleed, and they are hypovolemic even though their total body water is increased. Too often physicians equate edematous states with vascular hypervolemia, which leads to inappropriate care. The physician caring for the patient should determine as closely as possible, based on history and physical examination, the status of each fluid compartment and then detail this in the documentation (medical record). For example in the patient with sepsis syndrome, the physician might document (or at least think) "the patient has an increase in interstitial fluid causing peripheral edema but based on their heart rate and blood pressure the patient also has a vascular volume deficit." In the case of the patient with congestive heart failure and a GI bleed, the statement (or thought) should be similar, that is, "the patient has a vascular volume deficit even though she has peripheral edema." There are certainly circumstances where all compartments are increased in which case the statement (thought) could be "the patient has an increase in all fluid compartments and is particularly hypervolemic." By being more descriptive, there is less chance of misinterpretation by other physicians reading the notes and therefore less chance of error in treating the patient.

Intravenous fluid therapy with balanced salt solutions is a common iatrogenic cause of ECF expansion. Overexpansion of the extracellular compartment may occur immediately during or after surgery, during trauma resuscitation, or later when maximal hormonal responses to stress (i.e., increases in ADH and aldosterone) are operating to diminish sodium and water excretion by the kidney. Frequently, even though the interstitial fluid may increase, the vascular volume may be decreased, increased, or even normal. The risk for increased ECF is greater in any patient that has comorbidities that may contribute to ECF expansion but particularly the elderly.

Hypotonic fluid excess is usually due to inappropriate administration of salt-poor solution resulting in hyponatremia. Hypernatremic extracellular volume expansion is due to the administration of sodium loads that are not balanced by appropriate water intake. In this case, water moving out of cells in response to increased extracellular osmolarity may result in intracellular depletion of water but increased interstitial and vascular volumes. Hypertonic extracellular volume expansion can also be induced by the rapid infusion of nonelectrolyte osmotically active solutes (e.g., glucose, mannitol). In this case, hyponatremia rather than hypernatremia is present. Plasma sodium concentration decreases as a result of dilution by the solution being infused, and the sodium-free water is drawn from the cells into the extracellular space in response to the osmolar gradient created by the infused nonelectrolyte solute load. If the patient has hyperglycemia, the measured serum sodium will decrease 3 mEq/L for every 100 mg/dL increase in serum glucose above 100 mg/dL.

Presentation and Diagnosis

The clinical presentation of extracellular volume excess may range from simple weight gain, small decreases in hemoglobin and hematocrit (signifying hemodilution), modest elevation of peripheral and CVP, and dependent sacral or lower extremity edema; to extreme changes with congestive heart failure, pleural effusions, pulmonary edema, anasarca, and hepatomegaly.

Treatment

Treatment is adjusted according to the severity and rate of development of fluid compartment changes and related clinical findings. If it is determined that the patient has an increase in all fluid compartments, treatment might be as simple as fluid or sodium restriction. If symptoms are severe, the patient may need diuresis along with replacement of potassium losses. If the patient in thought to have a vascular volume deficit, then careful replacement with crystalloid or blood products may be needed, even though the patient has peripheral edema suggesting an increase in total body water. Treatment should also be specific to the organ system or systems affected and should be instituted according to appropriate guidelines for treating those diseases.

Prognosis

If properly diagnosed and treated, most patients do well. However, major morbidity and even death can occur if patients are misdiagnosed or treated inappropriately.

Disorders of Electrolyte Concentrations

As noted previously, a thorough history and physical are essential in determining the etiology and proper treatment of electrolyte imbalances. Electrolyte imbalances are rarely isolated because the body must maintain electrical neutrality; complex homeostatic and metabolic mechanisms exist to maintain the neutral state. Attempts to correct a low serum level by simple oral or parenteral replacement of an ion may not improve the patient's condition because associated abnormalities are not treated. Although electrolyte abnormalities are often corrected easily, if untreated they may be fatal. Artifactual abnormalities of serum electrolytes may result from numerous factors including improper collection or handling of blood specimens. Table 2-1 shows normal values for most electrolytes, but they may vary slightly from one laboratory to another.

Sodium

The sodium ion is the principal solute that determines ECF osmolarity and fluid volume balance in the body. An increase in extracellular sodium concentration creates an osmotic gradient that draws water out of cells. A decrease in extracellular sodium concentration does the reverse. These changes in cell volume produce the symptoms associated with abnormal serum sodium concentrations. Disorders of sodium balance are usually associated with disorders of fluid balance.

Hyponatremia

Hyponatremia results from the presence of excess body water relative to total body sodium and the failure of the kidneys to excrete the excess water. The serum sodium concentration does not always reflect true total body sodium content, or even osmolarity. For example, total body sodium may be increased in patients with chronic cardiac, hepatic, or renal disease, but hyponatremia persists because of a proportionally greater increase in water. Alternatively, total body water may be normal or decreased, but there is a proportionally greater decrease in total sodium.

Etiology Hyponatremia may be associated with decreased, increased, or normal ECF volume and each requires a different approach to correct the abnormality. The more common causes of hyponatremia are shown in Table 2-8. In surgical patients,

TABLE 2-8	Causes of Hyponatremia
Excess Water	Ingestion or infusion of excess free water (e.g., psychogenic polydipsia, or replacement of isotonic gastrointestinal and third space fluid losses with hypotonic fluid)
	Physiologic response to surgical stress, starvation, or hypovolemia (causing enhanced metabolic production of free water)
	SIADH (syndrome of inappropriate ADH secretion)
	Enhanced ADH activity
	Advanced cardiac, renal, or hepatic disease
Excess Sodium Loss	Thiazide diuretics
	Metabolic alkalosis
	Ketoacidosis
	Adrenal insufficiency
Artifactual	Hyperlipidemia
	Hyperproteinemia

ADH, antidiuretic hormone.

dilutional hyponatremia occurs most commonly when hypotonic fluids are used to replace significant isotonic gastrointestinal or third space losses. The concern in this situation is that intravascular volume may be restricted even though the patient may have decreased volumes of one or more of the body compartments, leading to more problems with fluid balance. Catabolic breakdown of body tissues, which occurs with surgical stress and caloric deprivation, metabolically generates approximately 1 mL sodium-free water for each gram of fat or muscle that is catabolized. Excretion of excess water in response to decreased serum osmolarity is impaired after surgery or other trauma due to the reabsorption of sodium and water as a result of the secretion of aldosterone and of ADH. With proper replacement of vascular volume, aldosterone secretion is blunted but ADH secretion may persist because of secondary factors such as stress that stimulate ADH secretion. Dilutional hyponatremia also occurs in patients who have advanced cardiac, renal, or hepatic disease and increased total body sodium, because these patients accumulate proportionally more water than sodium.

Artifactually very low serum sodium values are seen in the presence of severe hyperglycemia and hypertriglyceridemia, or after intravenous infusion of lipids. In the cases associated with increased lipid content, the water in the intravascular space is partially replaced so the concentration of sodium in the total sample is low, even though the concentration of sodium in plasma water may be normal, or even high.

Presentation and Diagnosis The primary clinical manifestations of hyponatremia are the signs and symptoms of central nervous system dysfunction. Osmotic forces draw water into the cells, and cerebrospinal fluid pressures increase because of cerebral and spinal cord swelling. Neurologic disturbances occur as a result. The severity of any neurological disturbance is directly related to both the degree of hyponatremia and the rapidity with which it develops. Serum sodium between 130 and 120 mEq/L may cause irritability, weakness, fatigue, increased deep-tendon reflexes, and muscle twitches if the hyponatremia developed rapidly (10 to 15 mEq/L in <48 hours, or faster), but the patient may be completely asymptomatic if it develops over time. If left untreated, severe hyponatremia may lead to seizures, coma, areflexia, and death.

In diagnosing hyponatremia, serum and urine sodium, serum and urine osmolality, and pH may be assessed. Blood tests can exclude associated electrolyte abnormalities (e.g., hyperglycemia, liver diseases, acid–base disorders). Volume status must be assessed by accurate history and physical examination.

Treatment Treatment of hyponatremia depends on the cause, severity, and nature of any associated volume abnormality. Psychogenic polydipsia is treated with water restriction. Most dilutional hyponatremia that is iatrogenically induced in the perioperative period, seen as an asymptomatic decrease in serum sodium along with modest extracellular volume expansion, is readily treated by simple fluid restriction. Thiazide diuretics cause hyponatremia by blocking the resorption of sodium and chloride in the cortical-diluting segment. However, because the resorption of salt in the ascending limb of the loop of Henle is not blocked, excretion of very concentrated urine is still possible. This concentration permits the retention of water while sodium, potassium, and chloride are depleted. The best treatment for this condition is discontinuation of the diuretic. In patients who have chronic hyponatremia, even when serum sodium concentration is very low, correction of serum sodium must be done slowly, 12 mEq/L/ day or less.

Disorders that involve total body sodium excess, in addition to disproportionate volume excess, are treated by restriction of both sodium and water.

Hyponatremia associated with volume contraction is treated with combined sodium and volume repletion, usually with normal saline or lactated Ringer's solution. The rate of repletion is dictated by the degree of volume deficit. In most cases, rapid restoration of volume and sodium is not only unnecessary but also hazardous, because it can cause rapid shifts of intracellular water and undesirable neurologic consequences.

Hypertonic saline solutions (2% or higher concentrations) are indicated *only* when hyponatremia causes life-threatening neurologic disturbances. To estimate the amount of sodium needed to correct the serum deficit, multiply the decrease in serum sodium (in milliequivalents) by total body water (in liters) as a percentage of total body weight remembering the relationship of total body water to age, sex, and body habitus:

$$mEq\ Na^+\ needed = (140 - measured\ serum\ N_a^+) \times TBW,$$

where TBW, estimated % of body water × body weight (kg).

Failure to correct total body water for age changes and body habitus could result in significant infusion of excess fluids. For example, if a patient is 75 years old but has a body mass index (BMI) of 40, they might have a total body water of as little as 40%. If the traditional formula is used with total body water of 60% body weight, the patient would receive far more sodium and water that s/he actually needs.

TBW is used because both intracellular and extracellular imbalances must be corrected. The goal is to increase the serum sodium level sufficiently to eliminate the symptoms. No more than one-half of the total calculated amount of sodium is given in the first 12 to 18 hours and at a maximum rate of 12 mEq/L of concentration per 24 hours since rapid correction of chronic hyponatremia >12mEq/L/day can cause osmotic central pontine myelinolysis. In this entity, the myelin sheaths of nerve cells in the pons are destroyed. The resulting neurologic damage is usually permanent and may be debilitating.

Over the next 24 to 48 hours, the remainder of the deficit can be corrected with normal saline. Any underlying conditions must also be treated. Responsible drugs should be discontinued, if possible. The patient usually improves for a day or so but then deteriorates, with a spectrum of neurologic findings that can include fluctuating levels of consciousness, seizures, pseudobulbar palsy, and paralysis. Some patients improve after several weeks, but others have significant permanent disability.

Prognosis Once properly treated, the prognosis of hyponatremia usually depends on the prognosis of the underlying condition. Severe neurologic symptoms may have irreversible sequelae.

Hypernatremia

Hypernatremia results from excess body sodium content relative to body water. Clinically significant hypernatremia, serum sodium >150 mEq/L, is less common than hyponatremia, but it can be just as lethal if it is allowed to progress unchecked.

Etiology Hypernatremia may result from the loss of water alone (e.g., hypothalamic abnormalities, nonreplaced insensible losses); from the loss of water and salt together (e.g., gastrointestinal losses, osmotic diuresis, excessive diuretic use, central or nephrogenic diabetes insipidus, burns, excessive sweating);

as a side effect of many drugs (e.g., alcohol, amphotericin B, colchicine, lithium, phenytoin); or from increased total body sodium without any water loss (e.g., Cushing's syndrome, hyperaldosteronism, ectopic production of ACTH, iatrogenic sodium administration, ingestion of seawater).

When body fluids become hypertonic, compensatory thirst is stimulated. Therefore, severe hypernatremia occurs only in situations in which a person cannot obtain water (e.g., infancy, disability, altered mental states).

Presentation and Diagnosis The pathophysiologic consequences of hypernatremia reflect both extracellular volume losses and cellular dehydration that result from water shifts in response to osmotic pressure. The severity of the clinical manifestation is directly related to both the degree of hypernatremia and the rapidity with which it develops. Serum sodium concentrations >160 mEq/L may be associated with signs and symptoms of dehydration, including decreased salivation and lacrimation; dry mucous membranes; dry, flushed skin; decreased tissue turgor; oliguria (except when dehydrating renal water loss is the cause); fever; and tachycardia. Signs and symptoms also include those of neuromuscular and neurologic disorders, from twitching, restlessness, and weakness, to delirium, coma, seizures, and death. Intracranial hemorrhage is a common postmortem finding in patients who die of hypernatremia; the hemorrhage is thought to result from cell shrinkage, with associated decreases in brain volume and decreased intracranial pressure, which disrupts the intracranial blood vessels. Unfortunately, many of these signs and symptoms are not very reliable in the elderly.

In addition to the history and physical, which would be the basis for diagnosing the underlying cause, measurement of serum sodium, urine sodium and urine and plasma osmolality may also help. Hematocrit may be high because of dehydration.

Treatment

The treatment of hypernatremia consists of correcting the relative or absolute water deficit, which can be estimated in several ways. The simplest accurate general rule is that for every liter of water deficit, serum sodium increases 3 mEq above the normal value of 140 mEq/L. If deficits are modest, they can be replaced orally or with intravenous 5% dextrose in water. If deficits are more severe, the TBW deficit is calculated according to the formula to estimate total body sodium. The relative water deficit (in liters) is equal to the milliequivalent change in serum $Na^+/140$. The water must be replaced slowly, with no more than one-half given over the first 12 to 24 hours. For pure water loss, 5% dextrose is infused intravenously. Therefore, if a "standard" young 70-kg patient had a serum sodium value of 150, the water deficit is calculated as follows:

$$\text{mEq change in serum } Na^+ = (\text{measured serum } Na - 140)$$
$$\times TBW \times wt \text{ in kg}$$

or

$$\text{mEq change in serum } Na^+ = (150 - 140) \times 0.6 \times 70$$
$$= 10 \times 42$$
$$= 420$$
$$\text{Water deficit in liters} = 420/140 = 3 \text{ L.}$$

In patients with associated sodium deficits, if symptoms of dehydration predominate, the vascular volume deficit is initially replaced with normal saline. If neurologic symptoms are more prominent, half-normal saline (0.45%) is used. If the sodium loss is large (e.g., diabetic hyperosmolar coma),

the volume is replaced initially with normal saline since the patient usually has a vascular volume deficit in addition to a total body water deficit. The nature of the fluid required may change as different needs become apparent. The process of reversing hypernatremia requires close monitoring. If water is replaced too rapidly, osmotic shifts can produce cellular edema. Brain cells accumulate intracellular solute slowly in response to slowly developing extracellular hypertonicity; a sudden decrease in extracellular osmolarity leads to rapid swelling of brain cells, causing serious neurologic dysfunction. As with other electrolyte disturbances, underlying problems must also be treated. *Correcting vascular volume deficit is the first priority.*

Prognosis The prognosis depends on the severity of the symptoms, the correct treatment, and the prognosis of the underlying disorder. Neurologic symptoms, once they develop, may be irreversible.

Potassium

As the principal intracellular cation, potassium is a major determinant of intracellular volume. It is a significant cofactor in cellular metabolism. Extracellular potassium plays an important role in neuromuscular function.

Hypokalemia

Hypokalemia is defined as a serum potassium <3.5 mEq/L. When total body potassium is deficient, there may also be deficiencies of magnesium and phosphorus. The exact relation between magnesium and potassium is unclear; however, many factors that cause renal potassium wasting also cause renal magnesium wasting (e.g., loop and thiazide diuretic use). The opposite is also true (e.g., potassium and magnesium sparing with amiloride). Hypophosphatemia and hypocalcemia often accompany hypokalemia. Potassium deprivation may impair calcium resorption by the kidney, resulting in a negative calcium balance. This change, in turn, alters phosphorous metabolism.

Etiology Hypokalemia may reflect potassium deficiency that results from inadequate intake, gastrointestinal tract losses, or renal losses. Hypokalemia may also reflect shifts from the extracellular to the intracellular compartment (e.g., insulin administration or alkalosis).

Gastrointestinal losses (e.g., diarrhea, vomiting, biliary or pancreatic fistulae, malabsorption and rarely villous adenoma) can be major factors in hypokalemia. The highest gastrointestinal concentrations of potassium are found in the colon and the rectum. Prolonged vomiting or nasogastric aspiration causes hypokalemia through a combination of factors. In addition to the loss of potassium in the gastric fluid, the loss of hydrogen and chloride ions produces hypochloremic hypokalemia metabolic alkalosis. The increase in extracellular pH causes movement of potassium into the cells, which makes the hypokalemia worse. As noted before, a change in pH of 0.1 units causes a reciprocal change in serum potassium of 0.3 to 0.5 mEq. As the hypokalemia worsens, in the alkalotic state, the kidneys conserve hydrogen ions by excreting potassium. Also, the high bicarbonate and low chloride concentrations in the renal tubules cause greater resorption of sodium in the distal tubule, causing additional urinary potassium loss. Finally, extracellular volume deficits stimulate aldosterone activity, which also increases renal potassium excretion. The interaction of these mechanisms, if uncorrected, produces noticeable intracellular and extracellular potassium depletion, which is not reflected in the serum level. At this point, because of the need to conserve potassium, renal tubular hydrogen ion excretion increases, urinary potassium loss decreases, and paradoxical aciduria appears (i.e., acidic urine in the presence of severe alkalosis).

Hyperglycemia, primary or secondary aldosteronism, renal tubular acidosis, elevated ACTH, licorice ingestion, acute leukemia, or corticoid excess also causes renal potassium losses. Hypokalemia is often iatrogenic, the result of treatment with thiazides, loop diuretics, or carbonic anhydrase inhibitors and inadequate replacement of potassium losses. By an unknown mechanism, magnesium deficiency decreases distal renal tubular potassium resorption. If the magnesium deficiency is not corrected, renal losses continue, and it is difficult to correct the hypokalemia.

Presentation and Diagnosis

Hypokalemia usually does not become clinically significant until serum potassium decreases to <3.0 mEq/L. In general, the severity of symptoms is proportion to the degree of deficit and the rapidity with which it develops. Additionally, the consequences of hypokalemia are exacerbated by alkalosis, hypocalcemia, and digoxin therapy. Hypokalemia may cause neuromuscular symptoms that range from skeletal muscle weakness and fatigue to paresthesias, paralysis, and rhabdomyolysis. Deep-tendon reflexes may be diminished or absent. Hypokalemia causes increased production of ammonia in the renal tubules, which may worsen hepatic encephalopathy. Other symptoms include anorexia, polyuria, and nausea and vomiting associated with paralytic ileus. Total body potassium depletion produces cellular atrophy and negative nitrogen balance. Renal tubular function is impaired, which may result in polyuria and polydipsia because of decreased concentrating ability.

Cardiac abnormalities are the most important and worrisome consequences of hypokalemia and may appear in the presence of digoxin, even with relatively mild deficits. Progressive electrocardiogram (ECG) abnormalities include low-voltage, flattened, or inverted T waves, with prominent U waves, depressed S-T segments, prolonged P-R intervals, and (at levels of ≤2.0 mEq/L) widened QRS complexes. A rapid decrease in serum potassium may lead to cardiac arrest.

If the deficiency is mild and the cause is clear from the history, serum potassium may be the only test required, with the digoxin level measured if the patient is being treated with this medication. If hypokalemia is more severe or refractory to treatment, other serum electrolytes, including calcium and magnesium, should be measured. An arterial blood gas determination can exclude acid–base disturbances, and urinary electrolytes can be used to exclude renal hyperexcretion. If the hypokalemia patient has normal blood pressure, serum bicarbonate and urine potassium should help distinguish among metabolic causes, gastrointestinal losses, dietary deficiency, and osmotic or drug-induced diuresis. If the patient is hypertensive, plasma renin and aldosterone levels may help identify the cause.

Treatment Treatment of hypokalemia involves replacing potassium and correcting the underlying cause. Whenever possible, potassium is repleted orally, with pills or liquid. Most people find the taste of potassium solutions unpleasant. Enteric-coated tablets should not be used, because they can cause small bowel ulceration. In patients with normal kidneys, the oral dose should not exceed 40 mEq/4 hour. If the intravenous route is required, the rate should not exceed 10 mEq/hour, with the dose repeated as often as necessary to increase the serum level to ≥3.5mEq/L. The patient should be on a monitor and the potassium should be infused through a central line if a rate higher than 10 mEq/hour is ordered. Too rapid intravenous administration can cause hyperkalemia and fatal cardiac arrhythmias. Generally, dextrose-containing solutions are not used, as intravenous dextrose increases endogenous insulin, which induces the movement of potassium into cells and causes the serum level to decrease further, making repletion more difficult. A serum potassium level lower than 2.9 mEq/L may reflect depletions of several hundred milliequivalents or more of the intracellular pool and thus require much more supplementation and close monitoring.

If hypokalemia is caused by hypomagnesemia, magnesium repletion will help correct it. When hypokalemia and hypocalcemia occur together they must both be treated; treatment of only one may cause the patient to become symptomatic to the other. *Prognosis* Most hypokalemia is moderate and relatively easy to correct. The prognosis depends on the severity of symptoms, correct treatment, and the prognosis of the underlying disorder.

Hyperkalemia

Hyperkalemia is a serum potassium level >5.0 mEq/L.
Etiology As in hypokalemia, the etiology of hyperkalemia is usually multifactorial. It can be caused by exogenous loading (e.g., from excessive dietary intake in a patient with renal failure or from parenteral sources, such as high-dose penicillin therapy), transfusions of many units of stored blood bank, or too vigorous correction of hypokalemia. Endogenous loading occurs whenever large amounts of intracellular potassium are released into the extracellular space (e.g., crush injuries, hemolysis, lysis and absorption of large hematomas, catabolism of fat and muscle tissue because of stress or starvation, or rapid rewarming after severe hypothermia). Hyperkalemia can also be caused by decreased renal excretion, which may result from adrenal insufficiency and impaired aldosterone activity, but most often it is caused by intrinsic renal disease. Shifts of potassium from the intracellular to the extracellular compartment also cause hyperkalemia (e.g., acute metabolic or respiratory acidosis, insulin deficiency, therapy with digitalis and related cardiotonic agents). In diabetic ketoacidosis, hyperkalemia may be seen, even with total body potassium deficit.

Numerous drugs may cause hyperkalemia. Impaired renal excretion can be caused by diuretics (e.g., spironolactone, triamterene, amiloride) and by nonsteroidal anti-inflammatory drugs (NSAIDs), β-adrenergic antagonists, and ACE inhibitors. Digitalis preparations, arginine, β-adrenergic antagonists, and some poisons, for example, can cause shifts of potassium out of the intracellular compartment, raising the serum level.

Artifactually high serum potassium results from hemolysis of the blood specimen, from obtaining a blood specimen from a vein into which potassium is being infused, and occasionally from high platelet or leukocyte counts.
Presentation and Diagnosis Although hyperkalemia causes peripheral muscle weakness that ultimately progresses to respiratory paralysis, the most important signs and symptoms are cardiac. The first ECG abnormality is peaked T waves, best seen in the precordial leads, at serum concentrations between 6.0 and 7.0 mEq/L. Further elevations produce multiple ECG abnormalities, including flattened P waves, increased P-R intervals, decreased Q-T intervals widened QRS complexes, depressed S-T segments, and complete heart block with atrial asystole. At elevations >8.0 mEq/L, more widened QRS complexes merge with T waves to produce a sine wave appearance. This change is followed by ventricular fibrillation and cardiac arrest.

Diagnosis is made by measuring the serum potassium level. It is usually relatively simple to determine the cause, but since significant hyperkalemia is uncommon if the kidneys are normal, serum BUN, creatinine, and urine output should also be measured. Anuric patients accumulate potassium, but a source must be sought in hyperkalemia in nonoliguric patients. Even in the presence of renal insufficiency, medication or excessive dietary intake is often responsible. A 12-lead ECG must be performed. If the patient is being treated with digoxin, a digoxin level should be obtained. If the patient had a crush injury, serum and urinary myoglobin should also be measured.

If spurious hyperkalemia is suspected (e.g., from a hemolyzed specimen, from blood drawn above an intravenous site), blood should be redrawn for a serum potassium level measurement or a plasma potassium level ordered. However, treatment of a very high serum potassium level should not be delayed while waiting for results.

Treatment The primary goal of the treatment of hyperkalemia is to reduce serum potassium to levels that are not life threatening. In mild hyperkalemia (<6 mEq/L), the simplest measures are to restrict potassium intake, eliminate causes such as potassium-sparing diuretics, and treat fluid volume or acid–base disorders. Potassium-wasting diuretics may be administered, and hormone deficiencies may be replaced.

For potassium levels between 6.5 and 7.5 mEq/L, 10 units insulin is administered intravenously along with 25 g glucose intravenously over 5 minutes. This therapy shifts potassium from the extracellular to the intracellular compartment and may reduce serum potassium by as much as 1 mEq/L. A similar shift may be created by administering a bicarbonate infusion or by injecting 45 mEq sodium bicarbonate intravenously over 5 minutes to induce a shift to a more metabolic state. These compartments shifts last only a few hours. Sodium polystyrene sulfonate, a cation-exchange resin, administered orally or rectally actually removes potassium form the body. Each gram of the resin binds approximately 1 mEq potassium. The oral dose is 25 g resin suspended in 50 mL 20% sorbitol solution every 4 to 6 hours. The rectal dose is 50 g in 100 to 200 mL 35% sorbitol given as a retention enema every 4 hours. Patients with potassium levels >6.5 mEq/L are monitored with continuous ECG.

Serum potassium levels >7.5 mEq/L in a patient with evidence of cardiac toxicity should be treated with an intravenous infusion of 10 to 30 mL 10% calcium gluconate given slowly over 5 minutes to reduce cardiac muscle electrical excitability temporarily while other methods are used to rid the body of potassium. Rapid infusion of calcium is dangerous and is justified only when hyperkalemia is severe. Electrocardiographic monitoring is advisable during treatment of hyperkalemia, and it is mandatory if calcium is being infused.

Hemodialysis and peritoneal dialysis also remove potassium form the body and may be necessary in patients with renal failure. They may be used along with more rapid methods to reduce serum potassium in moderate to severe hyperkalemia. In treating hyperkalemia with dehydration and acidosis in diabetic ketoacidosis, care must be taken not to allow serum potassium to decrease to hypokalemic levels.

Prognosis Hyperkalemia itself does not affect recovery from illness or surgery, and it is usually correctable. However, cardiac events caused by hyperkalemia may be fatal if the hyperkalemia and its effects are not promptly treated. The prognosis of patients with hyperkalemia is often related to the underlying cause (e.g., renal failure).

Chloride

Chloride is the major extracellular anion (Table 2-1). It is ubiquitous in the diet, absorbed in the small and large intestines, and excreted by the kidneys. Chloride balance usually parallels sodium balance, except when hypochloremia results from the loss of acidic gastric contents. Although no signs or symptoms are specific to abnormalities of chloride balance, changes in extracellular chloride content can significantly affect fluid, electrolyte, and acid–base balance and their management.

Hypochloremia

Hypochloremia is a serum chloride concentration <95 mEq/L. In severe respiratory acidosis, metabolic compensation involves renal tubular resorption of bicarbonate to decrease the extracellular acidosis that is caused by CO_2 retention and chloride depletion. As respiratory acidosis resolves and CO_2 retention decreases, renal excretion of excess bicarbonate allows the pH to return to normal. Hypochloremia impairs renal bicarbonate excretion, however, and if serum bicarbonate remains high in the presence of decreased CO_2 tension, metabolic alkalosis results and persists until the chloride deficit is corrected.

Etiology Hypochloremia classically results from the loss of acidic gastric contents, either by vomiting or by nasogastric suction. It can result from renal losses caused by diuretics, nonoliguric acute and chronic renal failure, or compensatory renal tubular resorption of bicarbonate in response to respiratory acidosis.

Presentation and Diagnosis The signs and symptoms are those of the accompanying disorder. The diagnosis is made by measuring serum chloride.

Treatment In general, hypochloremia is treated with solutions that contain sodium chloride and potassium chloride in a ratio reflecting the underlying problem and by serum electrolyte concentrations. Ammonium chloride is rarely needed and should not be used in patients with advanced liver disease or hepatic failure because it may precipitate or increase encephalopathy. It is important to correct hypochloremia along with other deficits in the treatment of hypochloremic hypokalemic metabolic alkalosis. Hydrochloric acid may rarely be used in severe refractory hypochloremic metabolic alkalosis. Extreme care must be taken with its use since even 1 to 2 mL of extravasation can produce substantial tissue necrosis.

Prognosis Hypochloremia has no specific prognostic significance. The prognosis depends on the underlying disorder.

Hyperchloremia

Hyperchloremia is a serum chloride level >115 mEq/L and is uncommon in surgical patients.

Etiology Hyperchloremia may occur in association with hypernatremia, in renal tubular acidosis, or after the administration of excess potassium chloride or ammonium chloride. It may be caused by surgical diversion of urine into segments of bowel (e.g., ileal urinary conduits, ureterosigmoidostomy). In these cases, the bowel mucosa absorbs excess chloride in exchange for bicarbonate, especially when evacuation of the urine is delayed.

Presentation and Diagnosis The signs and symptoms are those of the accompanying disorder. The diagnosis is made by measuring serum chloride.

Treatment There is no specific treatment of hyperchloremia. Treatment is directed at the underlying disorder.

Prognosis Hyperchloremia has no prognostic significance. The prognosis depends on the nature and treatment of the underlying disorder.

Calcium

Calcium is a common divalent cation, almost all of which is found in hydroxyapatite crystals in bone. On the surface of bone, bone calcium participates in exchange with ECF calcium. Of the small amount of calcium in the ECF, approximately 40% is bound to plasma protein and 10% is complexed with bicarbonates, citrate, and phosphate. Only the hormonally regulated ionized portion, the remaining 50%, is physiologically active. This small proportion is of vital importance, however, primarily because of its role in neuromuscular activity. The normal range of total serum calcium is 8.0 to 10.5 mg/dL, and that of ionized calcium is 4.75 to 5.30 mg/dL. Most bound calcium is bound to albumin, and total serum calcium is dependent on serum albumin. Total calcium values may appear artifactually subnormal in hypoalbuminemic patients unless a correction factor, such as the following, is used:

$$\text{Corrected total } Ca^{++} = [0.8 \times (4.0 - \text{patient's albumin})] + \text{total serum } Ca^{++}.$$

In this formula, 4.0 represent normal serum albumin. The proportion of calcium bound to proteins is dependent on pH; it is decreased by acidosis, with a concomitant increase in ionized calcium. The level of serum ionized calcium is a more accurate indicator of physiologic activity than total calcium.

The usual adult dietary intake of calcium is 1 g or more/day. Two-thirds of this calcium passes through the intestine and is excreted in stool, and one-third is absorbed in the small intestine, regulated by vitamin D. In normal kidneys, approximately 10% of filtered calcium reaches the distal tubules, where resorption is increased by parathyroid hormone (PTH) and metabolic alkalosis, or is decreased by hypophosphatemia and metabolic acidosis. Overall calcium homeostasis, largely regulated by PTH, is the result of intestinal absorption, renal excretion, and calcium exchange between bone and the ECF. Although severe abnormalities of calcium metabolism are uncommon in surgical patients, symptomatic abnormalities are seen.

Hypocalcemia

Hypocalcemia is defined as total serum calcium <8 mg/dL. It is seen in many conditions common to surgical patients, several of which are acute problems.

Etiology Hypocalcemia is often seen in surgical patients (Table 2-9). In acute pancreatitis, the etiology of hypocalcemia is unclear. It probably results from a combination of calcium binding in saponified tissue, PTH deficiency or dysfunction in the kidney and bone, and decreased protein-bound calcium as a result of hypoalbuminemia. Magnesium deficiency decreases PTH release and activity. Phosphate increases bone deposition of calcium, decreasing the available circulating pool. Inadequate intestinal absorption of calcium may result from inflammatory bowel disease, pancreatic exocrine dysfunction, or malabsorption syndromes. Excessive fluid losses from chronic diarrhea or pancreatic or intestinal fistulas may also seriously deplete extracellular calcium and cause other electrolyte abnormalities. Low serum calcium levels are seen with severe soft tissue infections, such as necrotizing fasciitis. Artifactual hypocalcemia is seen when serum albumin is low and total calcium, rather than ionized calcium, is measured. Vitamin D deficiency may result from synthetic failure in renal or hepatic disease, or from conversion to inactive metabolites caused by the anticonvulsants phenytoin and phenobarbital.

Another way to classify hypocalcemia is according to its relation to PTH, which may be (1) deficient or absent

TABLE 2-9	Causes of Hypocalcemia in Surgical Patients
Artifactual as a result of hypoalbuminemia	
Acute pancreatitis	
Surgically induced hypoparathyroidism (transient or permanent)	
Necrotizing fasciitis	
Inadequate intestinal absorption	
Inflammatory bowel disease	
Pancreatic exocrine dysfunction	
Mucosal malabsorptive syndromes	
Excessive fluid losses from pancreatic or intestinal fistulae	
Chronic diarrhea	
Renal insufficiency with impaired calcium resorption	
Hypomagnesemia	
Hyperphosphatemia	

(e.g., hypomagnesemia, any type of true hypoparathyroidism), (2) ineffective (e.g., vitamin D disorders, chronic renal failure, pseudohypoparathroidism), or (3) overwhelmed (e.g., hyperphosphatemia). Artifactual hypocalcemia occurs when the serum albumin is low and total calcium rather than ionized calcium is measured.

Presentation and Diagnosis The clinical manifestations of hypocalcemia reflect the role of calcium in neuromuscular activity. Early symptoms of hypocalcemia include circumoral tingling, numbness and tingling of the fingertips, and muscle cramps. Hyperactive deep-tendon reflexes develop, with a Chvostek sign (unilateral facial spasm when the facial nerve on the side is lightly tapped), tetany, and Trousseau's sign (carpopedal spasm), eventually progressing to seizures. The patient may be confused or depressed. Prolonged Q-T intervals are seen on ECG.

In acidosis, the ionized fraction of serum calcium increases at the expense of the bound fraction. Because only the ionized fraction is active, symptoms may not appear, even with low total serum calcium. With severe alkalosis, the reverse occurs, and symptoms may appear even when the measured total serum calcium is normal.

Hypocalcemia can occur after blood transfusion, as a result of citrate binding and dilution. However, evidence suggests that at moderate rates of blood transfusion, endogenous release of calcium from bone is adequate to prevent hypocalcemia. Only with massive transfusion and volume replacement at rates of 100 mL/minute or higher is there any need to give supplemental calcium.

Diagnosis is made by measuring serum calcium (the ionized portion if possible), along with serum potassium, magnesium, phosphate, and alkaline phosphatase. Other electrolyte abnormalities and acid–base disorders must be excluded. Serum albumin is measured, as well as BUN and creatinine. Measurement of urinary calcium can help assess calcium intake. It may ultimately prove necessary to measure vitamin D levels to help make the diagnosis of idiopathic hypoparathyroidism. During physical examination, a search should be made for a transverse surgical scar on the anterior neck, which would suggest previous thyroidectomy or parathyroidectomy.

Treatment Treatment of symptomatic hypocalcemia is directed at correcting the calcium deficit, normalizing the relation between ionized and protein-bound calcium by correcting acid–base disorders, and treating the underlying causes. When the need for correction is urgent (e.g., severe, highly symptomatic hypocalcemia), calcium gluconate or calcium chloride is infused. Hypocalcemia associated with chronic disorders is treated over the long term with oral calcium lactate. Vitamin D supplements may be needed; the high doses required in hypoparathyroidism may be reduced if urinary calcium loss is decreased with thiazide diuretics.

Prognosis Disorders of calcium balance can be treated with complete resolution of symptoms. Underlying disorders must also be identified and treated.

Hypercalcemia

Hypercalcemia is defined as an excessive amount of calcium in the blood, that is, total serum calcium >10.5 mg/dL.

Etiology The more common causes of hypercalcemia are shown in Table 2-10. In surgical patients, primary and secondary hyperparathyroidism and metastatic breast cancer are among the common causes. In fact, more than 90% of hypercalcemic patients who have no symptoms other than depression and fatigue have primary hyperparathyroidism. Malignancies cause hypercalcemia both by bony involvement and by the secretion of PTH-like substances that affect calcium metabolism. Malignancies that are sufficiently advanced to cause hypercalcemia are usually symptomatic. Mobilization of calcium from bone in bedridden patients can cause mild, asymptomatic hypercalcemia. The milk-alkali syndrome (e.g., hypercalcemia, alkalosis, and renal failure) results from excessive intake of calcium and absorbable antacids. Rare causes of hypercalcemia included Williams's syndrome (a constellation of congenital defects and abnormal sensitivity to vitamin D) and vitamin A intoxication, possibly by increasing bone resorption.

Presentation and Diagnosis The initial clinical manifestations of hypercalcemia are nonspecific: weakness, fatigue, anorexia, nausea, and vomiting. As serum calcium increases, severe headaches, diffuse musculoskeletal pain, polyuria, and polydipsia develop.

The combination of decreased oral intake, vomiting, and polyuria leads to hypovolemia and dehydration, which may become pronounced. The ECG shows shortened Q-T intervals and widened T waves. With normal or elevated phosphate, calcification may develop in the kidneys as well as in unusual locations (e.g., heart, skin). Pancreatitis and renal failure may develop as well. The renal failure has multiple causes, including volume depletion, nephrocalcinosis, and deposition of nephrotoxic myeloma proteins or light chains. When serum calcium increases to 15 mg/dL, and above, confusion and depression progress to somnolence, stupor, and coma. This degree of hypercalcemia results in death unless it is corrected promptly.

Diagnosis is made primarily by a careful history, including all medications, and blood tests. PTH levels are assessed, and imaging procedures are used to locate a tumor. Squamous cell carcinoma of the bronchus and hypernephromas can produce PTH-related peptide. In a patient with a known malignancy, the presence of symptomatic bone metastasis may be the initial presentation of some malignancies, such as those originating in the prostate or breast.

Treatment Initially, calcium intake is restricted, hydration status improved, and urinary calcium excretion increased. If the patient is symptomatic or calcium level is high, the patient should be hospitalized. Large volumes of intravenous normal or half-normal saline are infused. Loop diuretics enhance calcium excretion; however, their use is controversial except in patients with congestive heart failure because they may increase resorption of calcium from bone and worsen hypercalcemia. Great care must be taken during the process of vigorous hydration and diuresis, with close monitoring of volume status to avoid fluid overload and particularly hypervolemia. Meticulous assessment and replacement of electrolytes are necessary. Hypomagnesemia can develop as a result of forced diuresis. Bisphosphonates (e.g., pamidronate) are used in combination with calcitonin (which has a very rapid onset and short duration of action) to inhibit bone resorption. Gallium nitrate, which is nephrotoxic, is used in the treatment of cancer-related hypercalcemia unresponsive to hydration.

Corticosteroids are sometimes used as a long-term treatment to suppress calcium release from bone in patients with granulomatous disease, vitamin D intoxication, or hematologic malignancies. The usual dose is hydrocortisone 3 mg/kg/day. This treatment may take 1 to 2 weeks to produce an appreciable reduction in serum calcium.

The antineoplastic agent plicamycin (formerly called mithramycin), a DNA-binding antibiotic and an RNA-synthesis inhibitor, acutely reduces serum calcium by an unknown mechanism. It is given in small intravenous doses, 25 μg/kg, for 3 to 4 days. Calcium levels decrease within 48 hours and remain low for several days to weeks. Contraindications include thrombocytopenia, coagulopathy or other bleeding diatheses, and bone marrow suppression from any cause. Plicamycin has significant renal and hepatic toxicity.

Oral or intravenous phosphate supplements are sometimes used to form complexes with ionized calcium. Given intravenously, these supplements may produce a precipitous decrease in serum calcium, resulting in tetany, hypotension, and renal failure. Therefore, phosphate supplementation is generally not recommended.

TABLE 2-10	Causes of Hypercalcemia
Hyperparathyroidism	
Malignancy	
Metastatic cancer	
Lymphoma	
Leukemia	
Granulomatous disease	
Sarcoidosis	
Tuberculosis	
Fungal infection	
Excessive dietary intake	
Milk-alkali syndrome	
Vitamin A or D intoxication	
Thiazide diuretics	
Immobilization	
Endocrine abnormalities	
Thyrotoxicosis	
Adrenal insufficienc	

Prognosis If the cause of hypercalcemia is treatable and the hypercalcemia itself is treated appropriately before neurologic symptoms become severe, the patient should recover completely. Many of the causes of hypercalcemia are life threatening (e.g., metastatic cancer), and this prognosis determines the outcome more that the hypercalcemia itself.

Magnesium

Magnesium plays an important role in metabolism because it is a cofactor for many enzymes. It also affects neuromuscular function. At least one-half of the body's total magnesium is in bone. Most of the remainder is intracellular. Less than 1% is extracellular. Magnesium is the most common intracellular divalent cation, and most intracellular magnesium is bound to adenosine triphosphate. The average daily intake of magnesium is 15 to 30 mEq. Approximately 40% of the magnesium is absorbed, primarily in the jejunum and ileum, and it is excreted primarily by the kidneys. A higher percentage of intake is absorbed if body stores are deficient. The normal range of serum magnesium is 1.5 to 2.5 mg/dL. Normal kidneys conserve magnesium when intake is low, but hypomagnesemia develops if intake remains <0.3 mEq/kg/day.

Hypomagnesemia

Hypomagnesemia is common in surgical patients, particularly the elderly, who are often in a starvation state, experience gastrointestinal loss, or have absorption defects. When magnesium is deficient, losses of potassium and phosphorus, the other two major elements in cells, also occur. These elements are expelled from the cell, and the cells decrease in size to maintain normal intracellular composition. Severe hypomagnesemia also produces severe hypocalcemia by decreasing PTH secretion and by an apparent skeletal resistance and an impaired renal response.

Etiology The most common cause of hypomagnesemia is dietary deficiency combined with gastrointestinal loses (e.g., diarrhea, nasogastric suction) and deficiencies in other elements. Other causes include chronic alcoholism (especially during withdrawal), malabsorption (especially steatorrhea), acute pancreatitis, improperly constituted parenteral nutrition, and endocrine disorders. Hypomagnesemia also occurs as a side effect of many therapeutic drugs, particularly some diuretics, aminoglycosides, amphotericin, cyclosporine, cisplatinum, insulin, and pentamidine. Athletes and pregnant woman may be mildly hypomagnesemic.

Presentation and Diagnosis The effects of magnesium deficiency are not immediate. Like calcium, the body's other major divalent cation, magnesium affects neuromuscular function. Symptoms develop insidiously, first as nonspecific systemic symptoms that include nausea, vomiting, anorexia, weakness, and lethargy, then as neuromuscular symptoms that include muscle cramps, fasciculations, tetany, carpopedal spasm, paresthesias, irritability, inattention and confusion, and cardiac arrhythmias, along with other symptoms of associated hypokalemia and hypocalcemia.

Diagnosis is made by testing serum values, which may be normal, even in the presence of a deficiency in body magnesium.
Treatment Primary attention must be given to correcting the cause. If hypomagnesemia is mild and does not result from an absorptive defect, oral supplements are given. If it is moderate, then it is treated with intravenous magnesium sulfate at a rate of 50 to100 mEq/day because the equivalent oral dose can cause diarrhea. If symptoms are severe, an intravenous bolus

of 8 to 16 mEq of magnesium sulfate is administered, followed by intravenous infusion at a rate of 1 to 2 mEq/kg/day. Concomitant or resulting deficiencies in other elements must also be corrected, and adequate hydration must be maintained. If the patient is in renal failure, extra care must be taken not to overcorrect hypomagnesemia.
Prognosis Recovery from hypomagnesemia may be complete. The prognosis depends on the etiology, the severity of the deficiency and its symptoms, and the promptness of treatment.

Hypermagnesemia

Clinically significant hypermagnesemia is rare, especially if renal function is normal.
Etiology Hypermagnesemia can result from renal failure; any injury that causes rhabdomyolysis (e.g., crush injuries, severe burns); dehydration; severe metabolic acidosis; adrenal insufficiency; familial benign hypocalcuric hypercalcemia; or overdosage with magnesium salts in cathartics. In addition, in either mother or newborn, it can occur after treatment of eclampsia. It also occurs in patients with renal failure who use magnesium-containing antacids. Renal excretion is decreased in metabolic alkalosis.
Presentation and Diagnosis Symptomatic hypermagnesemia follows a progressive pattern, with increasing neuromuscular and central nervous system abnormalities as the serum level increases. Initial nausea is superseded by lethargy, weakness, hypoventilation, and decreased deep-tendon reflexcs. The condition then progresses to hypotension and bradycardia, skeletal muscle paralysis, respiratory depression, coma, and death. Diagnosis is made by testing serum values.
Treatment Mild hypermagnesemia is treated with oral hydration and by controlling magnesium intake (e.g., giving patients with renal failure nonmagnesium-containing antacids). Severe symptoms are reversed temporarily by intravenous calcium, and the magnesium excess is treated with hydration and diuretics, or hemodialysis.
Prognosis Recovery from hypermagnesemia may be complete. The prognosis depends on the etiology, the severity of the deficiency and its symptoms, and the promptness of treatment.

Phosphate

Phosphorus is a component of all body tissues, and it participates in virtually all metabolic processes. In a normal adult, approximately 85% of phosphorus is bound in bone and 15% is distributed in other tissues. Less than 1% is extracellular. The intestine, influenced by vitamin D, absorbs approximately 70% of ingested soluble phosphorus, and a higher proportion if dietary intake is low. The normal adult phosphorous requirement is 2 to 9 mg/kg/day. The amount of phosphorus excreted by normal kidneys is controlled by PTH and is proportional to the amount absorbed. The normal range of serum phosphate is 2.5 to 4.5 mg/dL. Circadian variation, mediated by the adrenal cortex, produces the highest serum levels during the afternoon and night and the lowest levels during the morning.

Hypophosphatemia

Hypophosphatemia is common in surgical patients. When phosphorus is deficient, there are also losses of potassium and magnesium, the other two major elements in cells. These elements are expelled from the cell, and the cells decrease in size to maintain normal intracellular composition.
Etiology The causes of hypophosphatemia are categorized as (1) inadequate uptake as a result of inadequate dietary intake, malabsorption, gastrointestinal losses, prolonged antacid use, improperly constituted parenteral nutrition, or vitamin D

deficiency; (2) increased renal excretion as a result of diuretic use, hypervolemia, corticoid therapy, hyperaldosteronism, **syndrome of inappropriate secretion of antidiuretic hormone** (SIADH), or hyperparathyroidism; or (3) compartmental shifts as a result of hormones, nutrients that stimulate insulin release, treatment of diabetic ketoacidosis, recovery from hypometabolic states, rapidly growing malignancies, or respiratory alkalosis. It is also seen in chronic alcoholism, in burns, and after parathyroidectomy or renal transplantation. Occasionally, hypophosphatemia is the first clue to alcohol withdrawal in a hospitalized patient.

Presentation and Diagnosis Severe phosphorous deficiency causes anorexia, dizziness, osteomalacia, severe congestive cardiomyopathy, proximal muscle weakness, visual defects, ascending paralysis, hemolytic anemia, and respiratory failure. Leukocyte and erythrocyte malfunction, rhabdomyolysis, hypercalciuria, and severe hypocalcemia are also seen. Central nervous system dysfunction occurs and can progress to seizures, coma, and death. If the hypophosphatemia is a result of vitamin D deficiency, metabolic acidosis may result from reduced renal hydrogen excretion.

Diagnosis is made by testing serum values, but total body phosphate deficiency may exist, even in the face of elevated serum values. Arterial blood gases, pH, and urine phosphate should be measured, along with serum potassium, calcium, and magnesium.

Treatment Severe hypophosphatemia should prompt an aggressive search for and treatment of cause. Phosphate salts may be given orally or intravenously. Other associated electrolyte abnormalities must also be treated. Diuretics may be withdrawn. VIPomas should be surgically removed.

Prognosis Repletion of phosphorus corrects or decreases most abnormalities. Respiratory failure may not be reversed completely, and the ultimate outcome is likely to depend on the prognosis of the underlying deficiency.

Hyperphosphatemia

Hyperphosphatemia is relatively common in adults and is seen even in the presence of total body phosphate deficiency.

Etiology The causes of hyperphosphatemia are categorized as (1) decreased renal excretion as a result of renal insufficiency or failure, hyperthyroidism, hyperparathyroidism or pseudohypoparathyroidism, or adrenal insufficiency; (2) increased intestinal absorption as a result of sarcoidosis or tuberculosis (both of which produce vitamin D), or excess phosphate or vitamin D ingestion; (3) iatrogenic, as a result of intravenous infusion of phosphate-containing fluids; or (4) shifts from the intracellular to the extracellular compartment as a result of acidotic states, tumor lysis, hemolytic anemia, thyrotoxicosis, or rhabdomyolysis.

Presentation and Diagnosis Hyperphosphatemia is associated with no symptoms, although in the presence of severe hypercalcemia, renal failure, or vitamin D intoxication, it may be accompanied by deposition of calcium phosphate in abnormal locations. It is diagnosed by testing serum values. Associated electrolyte abnormalities should also be identified and corrected.

Treatment Aluminum-based antacids decrease absorption by binding phosphate, and diuretics increase the rate of urinary phosphate excretion. Dialysis is used in patients with renal failure. It is often unnecessary to treat hyperphosphatemia, except by correcting excess intake and addressing associated problems.

Prognosis The prognosis of hyperphosphatemia depends on the cause.

Disorders of Acid–Base Balance

The management of acid–base disorders depends on prompt recognition and evaluation of the abnormalities involved. A good clinician uses the history and physical examination to determine the nature and the severity of the abnormalities (Table 2-11). Data provided by an arterial blood gas and a serum bicarbonate concentration allow a correct diagnosis to be made. Correction of the underlying disorder that has caused the acid–base disturbance is the ultimate goal. Identification of the disorder allows for initiation of treatment. Acid–base status is defined by the plasma pH and by the conditions of the acid–base pairs that determine it. Under normal conditions, the balance between these components is tightly controlled. Within 95% confidence limits, the pH of the arterial blood is between 7.35 and 7.43. This is a delicate homeostatic system that is controlled acutely (minutes) by the lungs and chronically (hours to days) by the kidneys.

Overview

The pH disorders of blood can be grouped into two broad categories, respiratory and metabolic. Respiratory acid–base disorders are disorders of $Paco_2$. Metabolic acid–base disorders are disorders of bicarbonate. An arterial blood pH that is <7.35 signifies acidemia, while pH > 7.45 signifies alkalemia. The normal limits of $Paco_2$ are 37 to 45 mm Hg. An arterial $Paco_2$ that is elevated above the normal range produces a respiratory acidosis. Respiratory alkalosis occurs if the $Paco_2$ is below the normal range.

Bicarbonate concentration normally varies between 22 and 26 mEq/L. A plasma HCO_3^- concentration that is <22 mEq/L

TABLE 2-11	Simple Disorders of Acid–Base Balance, with Examples	
Respiratory Alkalosis	**Metabolic Alkalosis**
Congestive heart failure	Chronic diarrhea
Cirrhosis	Cushing's syndrome
Fever	Hyperaldosteronism
Hypermetabolic states	Loop or thiazide diuretics
Hyperventilation	Massive blood transfusion
Pregnancy	Milk-alkali syndrome
Pulmonary embolus	Vomiting
Sepsis	
Respiratory Acidosis	**Metabolic Acidosis**
Chest cage hypofunction	Anion gap
Central nervous system depression	Acid ingestion
Chronic obstructive pulmonary disease	Advanced renal failure
Drugs	Hypotension
Morbid obesity	Ketoacidosis
Pneumothorax	Renal failure
Sleep apnea	Sepsis
Status asthmaticus	Nonanion gap
	Acute diarrhea
	Moderate renal failure
	Renal tubular acidosis

is defined as metabolic acidosis. Metabolic alkalosis is present when the bicarbonate level is above normal (26 mEq/L).

Simple acid–base disorders occur when there is a primary change either in the bicarbonate concentration or in the $Paco_2$ with an appropriate (normal) secondary change in the other parameter, as illustrated in the following equation:

$$H^+ + HCO_3^- \leftrightarrow H_2CO_3 \leftrightarrow CO_2 + H_2O.$$

Normally, the CO_2 that is produced is eliminated rapidly by the lungs.

Mixed acid–base disorders include all possible combinations. For example, a patient may develop metabolic acidosis and respiratory acidosis simultaneously. Another patient may have a combination of respiratory alkalosis and metabolic acidosis. In clinical practice, the presence of an isolated acid–base disorder is unusual. With normal kidney and lung function, compensation occurs. As a result, many disorders of acid–base are mixed. Two rules are helpful in assessing the degree to which the respiratory or bicarbonate component contributes to the change in pH.

1. A change in $Paco_2$ of 10 mm Hg is associated with a reciprocal change of 0.08 pH units. As the $Paco_2$ goes up, the pH goes down.
2. A change in HCO_3 of 10 mEq/L is associated with a direct change of 0.15 pH units. As bicarbonate goes up, pH goes up.

Acidosis

Regardless of the etiology, the consequences of acidemia can be life threatening. At pH < 7.2, there is a decrease of cardiac and peripheral vascular response to catecholamines including vasoactive drugs. As a result, cardiac function may be depressed and lethal arrhythmias may occur. In addition, potassium is transported to the extracellular space, and can rise to clinically significant levels, resulting in dysrhythmias.

Respiratory Acidosis

Respiratory acidosis is the result of retention of CO_2 because of pulmonary alveolar hypoventilation. It can be acute or chronic. Acute causes are typically respiratory depression as a result of narcotics, sedatives, muscle relaxants, or anesthetic agents. Decreased respiratory effort due to pain from surgical incisions, or trauma, altered mechanics of the chest wall due to rib fractures, can also cause hypoventilation. Pulmonary injury including contusions and lacerations of the lung, pneumonia, or pulmonary edema also result in hypoventilation due to an alteration in the ability to exchange gases at the alveolar level. Airway obstruction from a foreign body, misplaced or obstructed endotracheal tube, laryngospasm, or tracheal-bronchial injury can impair ventilation as well. Acute hypoventilation can be rapidly fatal if not identified and corrected. On the other hand, chronic respiratory acidosis is most often caused by advanced lung disease such as COPD. This results in a compensated hypoventilation and can be well tolerated.

Presentation and Diagnosis The acid–base disorder has a primary respiratory cause if the $Paco_2$ is abnormal and the $Paco_2$ and pH change in opposite directions. The clinical consequences of acute respiratory acidosis are caused by hypercapnia, and the accompanying hypoxia. Note hypoxia can be masked by increasing the available inhaled oxygen concentration. With mild acute respiratory acidosis, restlessness and agitation may be present. The patient may also be mildly hypertensive. With more severe elevations of $Paco_2$ levels, confusion, somnolence,

and ultimately coma can occur as a result of CO_2 narcosis. In combination with hypoxemia, cardiovascular dysfunction can occur, which may result in cardiac arrest and death. In patients with chronic hypoventilation and respiratory acidosis, the major threat is CO_2 narcosis. This can occur with the administration of supplemental oxygen. In chronic compensated respiratory acidosis, the stimulus to breathe is hypoxia, not hydrogen ion concentration in arterial blood. By adding oxygen, the stimulus to breathe is removed, and CO_2 narcosis ensues. Rules 1 and 2 can be used to determine whether respiratory changes are responsible for the acute acidotic state. If the change in pH is greater than explained by rule 1, there is a component of metabolic derangement present. Likewise, using Rule 2, the contribution from the change in bicarbonate can be determined.

Treatment Treatment of respiratory acidosis requires the identification and correction of the underlying cause of reduced alveolar ventilation while maintaining oxygenation. This may be as simple as administering supplemental oxygen, or by instituting mechanical ventilation or simply improving pain control since many patients have enough postoperative pain that their breathing is inhibited, resulting in decreased ventilation and subsequent hypercapnia. Acute hypercapnia should not be overcorrected. Sudden decreases in $Paco_2$ cause rapid ionic shifts between cellular and ECF, which can produce severe dysrhythmias. Abrupt decrease in $Paco_2$ below normal levels (for that patient) can cause cerebral vasoconstriction and decrease cerebral blood flow, particularly in patients with acute brain injury. The administration of bicarbonate as the *only* treatment for respiratory acidosis is inappropriate.

Metabolic Acidosis

Metabolic acidosis can be acute or chronic. One cause of metabolic acidosis is loss of bicarbonate from the extracellular space. This may be due to diarrhea, intestinal fistula, biliary fistula, or pancreatic fistula. Chronic bicarbonate losses occur with renal dysfunctions, ureterointestinal anastomosis, decreased mineralocorticoid activity, and the use of the diuretic acetazolamide, which is also a carbonic anhydrase inhibitor. In burn patients, the use of mafenide acetate, which is also a carbonic anhydrase inhibitor, can result in metabolic acidosis. Other losses of bicarbonate include ureterointestinal anastomosis and decreased mineralocorticoid activity. The second major cause of metabolic acidosis is an increased acid load. Lactic acidosis, one of the most common causes of a high anion gap metabolic acidosis, occurs with shock, whether hypovolemic, hemorrhagic, septic, or cardiogenic, and is due to the production of lactic acid as the body responds to the insult with anaerobic metabolism and/or increased accumulation in tissue of metabolites due to reduced cellular clearance. Ketoacidosis that occurs with untreated hyperglycemia is another cause for metabolic acidosis, as is ingestion of toxins, including salicylates, methanol, and other toxins. Liver failure can result in metabolic acidosis when the liver decompensates to the point where lactate and citrate that are normally produced by the body cannot be metabolized. Likewise, renal failure can cause metabolic acidosis when the kidney fails to retain bicarbonate as a result of injury to the tubules.

Presentation and Diagnosis Metabolic acidosis is the primary disorder if the pH is abnormal and the pH and the $Paco_2$ change in the same direction. Respiratory compensation occurs with both acute and chronic metabolic acidosis. Again, Rules 1 and 2 are useful in determining if the degree of compensation explains the disorder. Determination of the anion gap will help to distinguish the loss of bicarbonate from the presence of additional acids as the cause of metabolic acidosis. The anion gap is the difference between the serum sodium concentration and the sum of the bicarbonate and chloride concentrations in serum.

$$Na^+ (Cl^- + HCO_3^-).$$

Normal anion gap is approximately 12 ± 3 mEq/L. With loss of bicarbonate, the chloride increases and the anion gap remains normal. With the addition of metabolic acids, the chloride levels do not increase and bicarbonate levels fall, thus causing an anion "gap."

Treatment Identifying the underlying disorder causing metabolic acidosis and correcting it expeditiously are critical. Hypovolemia must be corrected, bleeding must be stopped, sepsis must be controlled, and/or cardiac function must be improved to improve tissue perfusion in order to satisfy cellular metabolic needs. Administration of bicarbonate without correcting the underlying problem will not return the pH to normal. In extreme life-threatening situation, such as when the patient is on vasopressors to maintain blood pressure, or when severe cardiac disturbances are present, the pH is <7.25, and the patient has fully compensated by hyperventilating, bicarbonate may be administered to raise the pH sufficiently to allow catecholamines to act at their receptors. Similarly, with diabetic ketoacidosis, treatment of the pH_a with bicarbonate is of little value without concomitant administration of insulin and intravenous fluids.

The amount of bicarbonate that may be needed to correct the total body base deficit can be calculated as:

$$mEq\ HCO_3^-\ needed = mEq/L\ HCO_3\ deficit$$
$$\times (patient\ weight\ in\ kilograms \times 0.25).$$

Rules 1 and 2 may be used to calculate the HCO_3^- deficit. It is advisable to replace no more than one-half of the calculated bicarbonate deficit in the first 3 to 4 hours, continuing with the additional bicarbonate over the next 12 to 14 hours. Too rapid or overzealous administration of intravenous bicarbonate may lead to cardiac irregularities, convulsions (which may not be evident if the patient is sedated and on a ventilator), metabolic alkalosis, hypokalemia, impairment of oxygen delivery to cells from capillaries and symptomatic hyperosmolarity as a result of the infusion of excessive amounts of sodium. It is *imperative* that the underlying cause of the acidosis be treated while replacing the bicarbonate.

Alkalosis

Regardless of the cause, a pH more than 7.45 indicates an alkalosis is present. Alkalosis has clinical features specific to the etiology, whether metabolic or respiratory.

Respiratory Alkalosis

Respiratory alkalosis is present when an increase in pH_a is related to alveolar hyperventilation and a reduced $PaCO_2$. This is common in surgical patients and may be caused by apprehension, pain that does not impede respiratory effort (usually in the young because pain in the elderly often reduces alveolar ventilation and therefore causes a respiratory acidosis), hypoxia, fever, brain injury, sepsis, and liver failure that results in elevated serum ammonia. Hypocapnia is also common in patients who are mechanically ventilated. The compensatory mechanism for respiratory alkalosis is renal excretion of bicarbonate, which is slow, or limited in surgical patients who have increased aldosterone levels resulting in sodium retention and associated limited bicarbonate excretion. Only with chronic respiratory alkalosis is there time for renal compensation.

Presentation and Diagnosis Acute respiratory alkalosis may appear similar to hypocalcemia with paresthesias, carpopedal spasm, and Chvostek's sign. Potassium, magnesium and calcium, and phosphate metabolism are all disturbed in alkalotic states. The acute hypocarbia can also cause cerebral vasoconstriction and decreased cerebral blood flow (1% to 3% for each 1 mm drop in $PaCO_2$). The decreased cerebral blood flow can be particularly dangerous in patients with acute brain injury, or atherosclerotic disease of cerebral blood vessels.

Treatment In the spontaneously breathing patient, the treatment is aimed, as in respiratory acidosis, to correct the underlying cause of the hyperventilation. In the patients who are mechanically ventilated, a decrease alveolar ventilation by changing respiratory rate or tidal volume will correct the alkalosis caused by mechanical hyperventilation. Chronic respiratory alkalosis usually is asymptomatic and does not require treatment.

Metabolic Alkalosis

Metabolic alkalosis occurs when the pH is elevated in association with an elevated serum bicarbonate level. It is one of the most common acid–base abnormalities in surgical patients. Renal and gastrointestinal losses of potassium and chloride result in hypochloremic, hypokalemic metabolic alkalosis. The infusion of excess bicarbonate can also cause metabolic alkalosis. Also, the administration of loop diuretics may result in a contraction of extracellular volume and metabolic alkalosis. Hypoventilation may allow for the accumulation of CO_2 and correction of the metabolic alkalosis. The kidneys' response to metabolic alkalosis initially results in alkaline urine as bicarbonate is excreted. With hypochloremic, hypokalemic metabolic alkalosis, the loss of electrolytes and the kidney's mechanism of saving potassium, absorbing bicarbonate instead of chloride and excreting hydrogen ion will result in paradoxical aciduria. As the kidney reabsorbs the bicarbonate ion, the compensatory mechanism fails. The correction requires replacement of chloride and potassium ions.

Presentation and Diagnosis The clinical problems associated with metabolic alkalosis are manifestations of hypochloremia, hypokalemic, and intravascular volume deficiency. This may be caused by gastrointestinal or renal losses and result in paralytic ileus, cardiac dysrhythmias, and digitalis toxicity.

Treatment The treatment of metabolic alkalosis requires replacement of electrolytes (particularly chloride and potassium) and of fluids specific to the type of loss, as well as control of ongoing losses. Once the kidney has adequate intravascular volume, and the electrolytes are replaced, the kidney will again excrete bicarbonate. Most metabolic alkalosis is chloride responsive and can be identified by measuring urinary chloride. In chloride-responsive alkalosis such as in uncorrected gastric losses, the urine chloride will be low, <10 mEq/L. The treatment is administration of chloride as a balanced salt solution, for example normal saline (0.9% NaCl). Chloride-unresponsive hypochloremic metabolic alkalosis is characterized by urinary chloride that is >20 mEq/L. This does not usually respond to chloride administration and may require glucocorticoid administration even when the electrolytes are corrected.

Conclusion

Acid–base disorders rarely occur in pure form. There are compensatory mechanisms that quickly work to maintain homeostasis. Compensatory mechanisms alone will not correct the disorder to normal. The combination of metabolic and respiratory causes of acidosis and alkalosis often intermingle

TABLE 2-12	Mixed Acid–Base Disorders			
Disorder		pH	Paco$_2$	HCO$_2$
Metabolic acidosis + respiratory acidosis		↓↓	↑	↓
Metabolic acidosis + respiratory alkalosis		✓	↓	↓
Metabolic alkalosis + respiratory acidosis		✓	↑	↑
Metabolic alkalosis + respiratory alkalosis		↑↑	↓	↑

to create mixed disorders (Table 2-12). Understanding the causes of the different acid–base disorders will allow correction of the defect. Remember the essential treatment is correction of the underlying disorder.

thePoint ✷ Go to http://thePoint.lww.com/activate and use your scratch-off code on the inside cover of this book to access bonus chapters, question bank, videos, and more.

SAMPLE QUESTIONS

Questions

Choose the best answer for each question.

1. A 35-year-old man is admitted for a sigmoid colectomy due to repeated episodes of acute diverticulitis. He weighs 140 kg, but his ideal body weight is 80 kg. Which of the following body compositions should be used as a basis for calculating basic maintenance fluids for this patient?

	Total Body Water (L)	Intracellular Water (L)	Extracellular Water (L)	Blood Volume (L)
A.	84	55	28	9.8
B.	70	55	15	8.4
C.	56	35	21	8.4
D.	54	32	22	5.4
E.	60	40	20	7.5

2. A 46-year-old man is in the intensive care unit following surgery for multiple gunshot wounds to the chest and abdomen sustained 2 days ago. He has bilateral chest tubes inserted for hemopneumothoraces. Damage control surgery including packing his liver and performing an ileostomy was done at that time. His urine output has decreased to 90 mL over the past 4 hours. His temperature is 38°C, blood pressure (BP) 110/85 mm Hg, and pulse 100/minute. What is the most likely cause for the drop in urine output?

A. Congestive heart failure

B. Hypovolemia

C. Acute renal failure

D. Diabetes insipidus

E. Sepsis

3. A 65-year-old man is seen in the emergency department with a 5-day history of nausea and vomiting. He has been drinking only water for the last 2 days. His BP is 100/75 mm Hg with a heart rate of 105/minute. He has a distended abdomen with no bowel sounds but no signs of peritonitis. A diagnosis of a bowel obstruction is made after x-rays of the abdomen reveal distended loops of small bowel. Which of the following abnormalities would you expect to find in this patient?

A. Na^+—110 mEq/L, Cl^-—90 mEq/L, K^+—2.8 mEq/L, CO_2—20 mEq/L

B. Na^+—150 mEq/L, Cl^-—120mEq/L, K^+—5.5 mEq/L, CO_2—20 mEq/L

C. Na^+—140 mEq/L, Cl^-—110 mEq/L, K^+—4.0 mEq/L, CO_2—26 mEq/L

D. Na^+—120 mEq/L, Cl^-—120 mEq/L, K^+—5.5 mEq/L, CO_2—18 mEq/L

E. Na^+—135 mEq/L, Cl^-—105 mEq/L, K^+—3.5 mEq/L, CO_2—24 mEq/L

4. A 30-year-old man is in the intensive care unit where he is being treated for injuries sustained in a motor vehicle crash. He sustains multiple orthopedic injuries and a severe head injury. On hospital day 4, vital signs are BP—120/70 mm Hg, pulse—76/minute, and respiratory rate on a ventilator of 12/minute. His urine output is 20 mL/hour. Serum sodium is 120 mEq/L, BUN is 18 mg/dL, and creatinine is 1 mg/dL. What is the most likely diagnosis?

A. Water intoxication due to inappropriate fluid infusion

B. Central diabetes insipidus

C. Lab error

D. SIADH

E. Increased aldosterone secretion due to hypovolemia

5. A 40-year-old woman is admitted with a 3-day history of diarrhea. She has a history of chronic renal insufficiency due to diabetic nephropathy. She is mildly acidotic. Serum potassium is 6.8 mEq/L. An ECG shows peaked T waves. Which of the following is the most appropriate initial treatment of the hyperkalemia?

A. Subcutaneous administration of 10 units of insulin plus 25 g of glucose over 5 minutes

B. Administration of a bicarbonate infusion or by injecting 45 mEq sodium bicarbonate intravenously over 5 minutes

C. Intravenous administration of sodium polystyrene sulfonate, a cation-exchange resin, to bind extracellular potassium

D. Transferring the patient to a center with hemodialysis and peritoneal dialysis capability

E. Rapid intravenous infusion of 50 mL of 10% calcium gluconate under continuous ECG monitoring

Answers and Explanations

1. Answver: D

The composition of the body varies with lean body mass (muscle) and the fat content. If one assumes that "ideal body weight" is related to the theoretical "young healthy male" discussed in most textbooks where total body water is 60% of weight and intracellular volume is 60% of total body water, then for 80 kg, the patient would have 48 L of total body water, 32 L of intracellular water, and 16 L of extracellular water. Since fat is only about 10% water, the extra 60 kg of fat only adds 6 L of water. Therefore in this patient, total body water would only be 54 L. Intracellular water changes little and therefore the ICF would be about 32 L and the ECF about 22 L. Vascular volume for the 80-kg weight would only be a little more than 6% of weight ($6.3 \pm 0.4\%$) or about 5 L. The additional 6 L of fat would add little to the blood volume so 5.4 L total blood volume would be a close approximation.

The clinical significance of these "estimations" relates to numerous clinical scenarios. For example, if one estimates that there is a serum sodium deficit of 10 mEq/L in this patient but assumes total body water is 60% of total weight, the patient would get 10×84 L of total body water or 840 mEq of sodium instead of 10×54 L of total body water or 540 mEq of sodium. The extra and unnecessary 300 mEq of sodium is equivalent to 2 L of normal saline.

If one calculates total body water requirements for daily maintenance using the standard "70-kg male" as a reference, then the 140-kg male would receive 35 mL/kg (Table 2-2) or about 4.9 L of fluid. However, using "ideal body weight" for the calculation and adding only about 10% for the increased fat content, the total fluid would instead be about 3 L. If the extra 1.9 L is given over 3 or 4 days and if the kidneys do not excrete this fluid due to numerous conditions such as syndrome of inappropriate antidiuretic hormone (SIADH), the patient in 3 days is up almost 6 L that may not be visible in this obese patient. This increased total body water could result in a host of effects including peripheral edema, pleural effusions, and cardiac and pulmonary dysfunction; lead to subtherapeutic drug levels (since many drugs such as antibiotics have volumes of distributions equivalent to extracellular or total body water); cause secondary complications from each of these effects and overall delay in discharge from hospital; and increase costs. In other words, a more accurate "guesstimate" using a similar thought process for patients decreases complications, reduces hospital stay, and reduces costs.

2. Answer: B

The most common cause for a drop in urine output after surgery is hypovolemia. This can be caused by inadequate fluid replacement to correct the sequestration of fluid into the site(s) of injury, continuing blood loss, and stimulation of various endocrine responses including an increase in aldosterone, which results in renal sodium retention and an increase in antidiuretic hormone (ADH), which result in reduced free water clearance in the kidney. Atrial natriuretic factor may be inhibited due to the reduction in atrial volume and distention. The patient has a narrow pulse pressure and increased heart rate consistent with a low stroke volume and perhaps reduced cardiac output. The latter could be due to a combination of an absolute hypovolemia and/or a relative hypovolemia if he is developing an abdominal compartment syndrome, which could also contribute to decreasing urine output. The patient is relatively young to have congestive heart failure. Acute renal failure would be possible but is unusual only 2 days after surgery. Diabetes insipidus would result in increased urine output. Sepsis or an inflammatory response syndrome would result in an increase in heart rate and a wider pulse pressure due to the vasodilation that occurs as a result of the release of various cytokines. In this patient, treatment would begin by performing a detailed physical exam followed by increased fluid infusion.

3. Answer: A

In a patient with a bowel obstruction who begins vomiting, the initial acid–base abnormality would be a hypochloremic, hypokalemic metabolic alkalosis due to the loss of hydrogen ion, chloride, and potassium from the stomach. The bowel will continue to secrete fluid into the small intestine, which will initially lead to hypovolemia that is compounded by the loss of gastric fluid. This results in an increase in aldosterone, which will result in increased reabsorption of sodium and chloride from the kidney, but since the vomiting results in a loss of chloride, eventually a reduction in chloride in the renal tubule will result in absorption of bicarbonate with the sodium. The resulting alkalosis may be associated with a mild respiratory acidosis to compensate for the metabolic acidosis. As the fluid sequestration in the small intestine increases, hypovolemia increases, which increases ADH and stimulates thirst. The kidneys reabsorb more water and sodium and the patient tries to drink but in this case only tolerates water. This results in an increase in water in relation to sodium in the extracellular fluid (even though both are reduced compared to the normal state) and a hyponatremia occurs. Now the patient has a hyponatremic, hypokalemic, hypochloremic metabolic acidosis, which is compensated partly by a respiratory acidosis. As the hypovolemia progresses due to the sequestration of fluid in the intestine and perhaps into the peritoneal cavity, the patient may develop a stage 2 shock state that results in a mild cellular acidosis, which eventually causes a metabolic acidemia superimposed on the metabolic alkalemia. Hence, the final presenting electrolyte and acid–base abnormality seen on the electrolytes in this patient is a hyponatremic, hypokalemic, hypochloremic metabolic acidemia. The first priority in the treatment of this condition is to correct the hypovolemia, in this case with normal saline since there is also a chloride deficit, and add potassium to the fluids since the patient has a profound potassium deficit that may be slightly masked by a lower than normal pH. (See relation between acidosis and potassium in text.) Since the patient is stable without signs of peritonitis, there is time to correct the fluid and electrolyte disorders before taking the patient to surgery. Failure to correct before surgery could result in multiple complications including a more profound hypotension and arrhythmias due to the low potassium. In general, correction of vascular volume takes precedence followed by correction of acid–base and potassium abnormalities and finally correction of any other fluid and electrolyte problems.

4. Answer: D

Although water intoxication due to inappropriate fluids is possible, in this patient it is unlikely since he has normal renal function as reflected by his BUN and creatinine. If he were given inappropriate fluids, he would diurese the extra fluid. Central diabetes insipidus usually results in a marked increase in urine (free water) output and would result in an increase in sodium concentration. Laboratory error is always possible, and if there is any question of this possibility, the electrolytes should be rechecked prior to initiating therapy. Increased aldosterone secretion would result in sodium retention and therefore would maintain serum sodium concentration. The most likely scenario is an increase in ADH, in this case due to the increase in intracranial pressure due to the head injury. Since the patient has a wide pulse pressure and normal output, he is at least euvolemic. Therefore, an increase in ADH is "inappropriate" for the situation. If, however, the patient had signs of decreased vascular volume including a narrow pulse pressure and increased heart rate, then the increased ADH secretion would be "appropriate".

5. Answer: A

Hyperkalemia <6 mEq/L or hyperkalemia without ECG abnormalities usually needs minimal intervention other than stopping any potassium infusion, deciding if this increase in potassium is due to a significant metabolic acidosis (since the potassium will increase at least 0.3 mEq/L for every 0.1 decrease in pH), checking to make sure the increased potassium was due to hemolysis of the blood sample, and monitoring the cardiac rhythm. If the patient has ECG evidence of peaked T waves, then prompt administration of 25 g of glucose plus 10 units of insulin is recommended followed by hemodialysis if necessary. If the T waves are higher than the R wave or if there is widening of the QRS complex and a decrease in the P-wave amplitude, immediate treatment is indicated with either infusion of 10 mL of 10% calcium chloride over 10 minutes or 10 mL of calcium gluconate over 3 to 5 minutes. Calcium chloride freely dissociates upon infusion resulting in 13 mEq of free calcium, whereas calcium carbonate results in only 4 mEq of free calcium. The remainder of the calcium is released as the carbonate is metabolized. Intravenous infusion of 50 mEq or more of sodium bicarbonate over 20 minutes may also be used. The amount of bicarbonate infused is proportional to the degree of acidosis but is usually not used unless the pH is <7.20. Rapid increase in potassium such as occurs with sudden renal failure or rhabdomyolysis may be lethal if not diagnosed and treated quickly.

3
Nutrition

GAIL CRESCI, PH.D., R.D. • BRUCE V. MACFADYEN, JR., M.D. • JAMES S. GREGORY, M.D. •
ALAN B. MARR, M.D. • JEREMY WARREN, M.D.

Objectives

1. Determine a patient's protein and calorie requirements by estimation, with the Mifflin-St. Jeor equation, the Penn State equation, and the Hamwi method, or with specific laboratory tests.

2. List at least four factors in a patient's medical history and physical examination that indicate malnutrition or risk for malnutrition.

3. Discuss the following objective assessments of nutritional status: anthropometric measurements, biochemical blood tests, immune function studies, and indirect calorimetry.

4. List at least four water-soluble vitamins, three fat-soluble vitamins, and four trace elements that must be added to long-term parenteral nutrition.

5. Briefly describe the metabolic changes that occur in short-term and long-term starvation.

6. Discuss the effect of starvation, injury, and infection on a patient's metabolism, and describe how nutritional support must be altered.

7. List several indications each for enteral and parenteral nutritional support.

8. Discuss the factors involved in choosing a route of nutritional support.

9. Describe the risks and benefits of enteral and parenteral nutritional support.

10. List at least four gastrointestinal, four mechanical, and four metabolic complications of enteral therapy, and describe appropriate prevention or treatment of each.

11. List four adverse sequelae of a total parenteral nutrition (TPN) catheter and four metabolic complications of TPN. Describe the appropriate treatment of each.

Surgeons care for patients who may have a compromised nutritional status and therefore an altered ability to heal properly. The nutritional challenges for patients with surgical disease include anorexia, inanition, accelerated gluconeogenesis, hyperglycemia, insulin resistance, and electrolyte and hormonal disturbances. Each of these can adversely affect both response to surgery or injury and a patient's ability to heal. The metabolic responses to stress, starvation, and sepsis include complex neuroendocrine and immunomodulatory responses that vary tremendously with the inciting event. In the ideal situation, the body's homeostatic response would result in a coordinated effort to mobilize sufficient nutrient substrates to maintain energy requirements, fight infection, and provide for essential bodily functions. In reality, these metabolic alterations often can act at odds to each other and result in a situation that places the patient at increased risk of nutritional failure. This chapter reviews metabolism and the impact of stress on nutritional status and describes methods to identify patients at nutritional risk in order to direct nutritional therapy to achieve the best possible outcomes.

OVERVIEW OF METABOLISM

Normal physiology relies on three essential substrates: carbohydrates, proteins, and lipids, which provide both an energy source and the substrates for chemical building blocks.

Ideally, energy needs should be based on direct measurement by calorimetry; however, this is labor intense and impractical in most critically ill patients. Indirect calorimetry is the measurement of respiratory gas exchange in order to make inference about cellular gas exchange, which equates to metabolic rate and substrate utilization. The measured parameters of indirect calorimetry are oxygen consumption (VO_2) and carbon dioxide production (VCO_2). From these measurements, respiratory quotient (RQ) and metabolic rate can be calculated. Indirect calorimetry is valid only when the respiratory gas exchange and the cellular gas exchange are equivalent. There are several limitations to using indirect calorimetry; therefore, predictive equations are often used to estimate resting metabolic rate (RMR). With more than 200 predictive equations available, very few have been validated against indirect calorimetry.

TABLE 3-1	Validated Predictive Equations for Estimating Energy Requirements

Acutely Ill Patients and Obese Patients—Nonventilated

Mifflin-St. Jeor Equation

Men: RMR = 5 + 10W + 6.25H − 5A

Women: RMR = 161 + 10W + 6.25H − 5A

Obese Patients (BMI > 30 kg/m²)

60%–70% of target energy requirements (as predicted by above equations)

11–14 kcal/kg/day actual body weight

22–25 kcal/kg/day ideal body weight

RMR = Resting metabolic rate in kilocalories/day

W = weight in kilograms

H = height in centimeters

A = age in years

Critically Ill Ventilated Patients

Penn State Equation

RMR via Penn State Equation (PSU)

RMR (kcal/d) = MSJ (0.96) + T_{max} (167) + V_E (31) − 6,212

Modified PSU[m] Equation for BMI ≥30 kg/m² and ≥60 yrs

RMR (kcal/d) = MSJ (0.71) + T_{max} (85) + V_E (64) − 3,085

BMR = basal metabolic rate calculated using the Mifflin-St. Jeor Equation (using actual body weight)

V_E = minute ventilation (L/min)

T_{max} = maximum daily body temperature in previous 24 hr (°C).

TABLE 3-2	Hamwi Method for IBW

1. IBW in Pounds and Inches

Men: 106 lb for the first 5 ft

    Plus 6 lb for every inch thereafter

Women: 100 lb for the first 5 ft

    Plus 5 lb for every inch thereafter

2. IBW in Kilograms and Meters

Men: 48.1 kg for each 1.52 m

    Plus 0.9 kg for every centimeter above 1.52 m

Women: 45.5 kg for each 1.52 m

    Plus 1.1 kg for every centimeter above 1.52 m

10% can be added for a large body frame size or subtracted for a small body frame size.

3. Body Mass Index (BMI)[a]

Weight (kg) ÷ height (m²)

BMI	BMI Classification	Disease Risk
<16	Protein–energy malnutrition—grade III	Very high
16–16.9	Protein–energy malnutrition—grade II	High
17–18.4	Protein–energy malnutrition—grade I	Moderate
18.5–24.9	Normal	Very low
25–29.9	Overweight	Low
30–34.9	Obesity—grade I	Moderate
35–39.9	Obesity—grade II	High
≥40	Obesity—grade III	Very high

[a]Body Mass Index Classification and Interpretation

It is known that various conditions can increase metabolic rate from 10% to 100% above basal metabolic rate (BMR) (e.g., trauma, burns, pregnancy, lactation). However, predictive equations that add an activity and/or injury factor above the RMR are not validated. The best-validated equations are listed in Table 3-1, correlating within 78% accuracy with metabolic rate measured by indirect calorimetry. Table 3-1 lists validated predictive equations for various types of patients.

RMR is more difficult to predict in the obese than in the nonobese person as lean body mass and body cell mass are very difficult to measure clinically. Obesity adversely affects patient care, particularly in the critically ill, and increases the risk of comorbidities such as insulin resistance, sepsis, infections, deep venous thrombosis, and organ failure. Achieving some degree of weight loss may increase insulin sensitivity, improve nursing care, and reduce risk of comorbidities. Therefore, providing 60% to 70% of energy requirements in this population promotes steady weight loss, while supplementing protein at a dose of 2.0 to 2.5 g/kg ideal body weight per day should approximate protein requirements and neutral nitrogen balance, allowing for adequate wound healing. Depending on the clinical condition, energy requirements for surgery patients range from 20 to 35 kcal/kg of ideal body weight per day. Ideal body weight (IBW) can be calculated using several formulas one of which is the Hamwi method, listed in Table 3-2.

Carbohydrate Requirements

Carbohydrates largely in the form of glucose supply 3.4 kcal of energy/g. Glycogen is the principal storage form of glucose.

Complex carbohydrates form important components of cell wall glycoproteins and glycolipids, as well as the carbon backbone of lipid and nonessential amino acids. In addition, the brain as well as red and white blood cells, are to a large extent, obligate glucose tissues. Approximately 120 g/day is necessary to maintain central nervous system (CNS) function. Glycogen stores are limited (180 g in a 70-kg person) and are usually exhausted within 24 hours in the unfed state. In the nonstressed state, the brain utilizes ketone bodies with progressive starvation. The maximal glucose oxidation rate is 4 to 7 mg/kg/minute, roughly equivalent to 400 to 700 g/day in a 70-kg person. In the hypermetabolic patient, a large portion of oxidized glucose is derived from amino acid substrates via gluconeogenesis yielding up to 2 to 3 mg/kg/minute of glucose. Exogenous insulin delivery can increase cellular glucose uptake in critically ill patients; however, it is relatively ineffective in improving glucose oxidation. In order to limit the diabetogenic response, glucose should comprise approximately 50% to 60% of total energy requirements, delivered at 3 to 4 mg/kg/minute. Supplemental insulin can then be used to maintain normoglycemia.

Protein Requirements

Proteins provide 4.0 kcal/g and account for 20% to 30% of the total daily caloric intake. Proteins and amino acids are essential components of all living cells and are involved in virtually all bodily functions. All protein in the body is functional. In the nonstressed state, approximately 2.5% of total body

TABLE 3-3	Select Serum Proteins: Classification and Functions				
Serum Protein	**Function**	**Half-life**	**Normal Range**	**Interpreting Results**	
Positive					
C-Reactive protein	General marker of inflammation and infection	5 hr	0.2–8 mg/dL	Synthesized by liver Rises during inflammation and infection Decreases when infection or inflammation resolves	
Negative					
Albumin	Maintains plasma oncotic pressure, carrier for amino acids, zinc, magnesium, calcium, free fatty acids, drugs	21 days	3.5–5.0 mg/dL	Routinely available Synthesized in liver; altered by liver disease Alterations occur in kidney disease with glomerular damage Elevated in dehydration Levels fall with protein-losing enteropathy; may be low in chronic, long-term unstressed malnutrition Negative acute-phase reactant, levels drop in inflammation, shock	
Prealbumin (transthyretin)	Thyroxine transport, formation of complex with RBP	2–3 days	18–38 mg/dL	Synthesized in the liver Highly sensitive to dietary deprivation and refeeding Elevated in renal dysfunction Negative acute-phase reactant	
Transferrin	Iron-binding protein	8 days	202–336 mg/dL	Decreased levels when diet deficient in protein Synthesized in liver; altered by liver disease Elevated in iron deficiency; pregnancy; chronic blood loss Low levels in chronic diseases, cirrhosis, nephritic syndrome, protein-losing enteropathy Negative acute-phase reactant	
Retinol-binding protein	Transports vitamin A; bound to prealbumin	12 hr	2–6 mg/dL	Highly sensitive to acute changes in protein malnutrition and dietary intake Elevated in renal failure Decreased in vitamin A deficiency Negative acute-phase reactant	

protein is broken down and resynthesized every 24 hours. More than half of this turnover is accounted for by the daily digestive process, hemoglobin turnover, muscle protein synthesis, and maintenance of normal immune function. During metabolic stress, proteins are broken down into amino acids and enter into the gluconeogenic pathway and used as a fuel source or form the basic structural elements of living cells. It is important to realize there is no protein storage per se and that any protein utilized for gluconeogenesis and acute-phase protein synthesis should be considered a loss of functional protein. Table 3-3 includes individual serum proteins, their half-life, normal range and function.

The amino acids glutamine and arginine deserve special attention. Glutamine is the most abundant amino acid. It comprises more than 50% of the free amino acid pool and is synthesized in most tissues of the body. Glutamine is the primary fuel source for the small intestine enterocytes. During catabolic illness, glutamine uptake by the small intestine and immunologically active cells can exceed glutamine synthesis and release from skeletal muscle, making glutamine a conditionally essential amino acid. Glutamine is a major contributor to homeostasis in the surgical population.

Arginine, like glutamine, is classified as a nonessential amino acid in unstressed conditions because the body synthesizes adequate arginine for normal maintenance of tissue metabolism, growth, and repair. Growth hormone, glucagon, prolactin, and insulin release are all increased with supplemental arginine. Arginine is also the substrate for nitric oxide

synthase, producing nitric oxide and citrulline. Nitric oxide is a ubiquitous molecule with significant roles in the maintenance of vascular tone, coagulation cascade, immunity, and GI tract function. While positive effects on wound healing are noted with arginine supplementation, arginine is controversial and not recommended in severe sepsis, as it is believed to contribute to hemodynamic instability via its conversion to nitric oxide.

Pediatric amino acid solutions have altered amino acid profiles from the adult solutions. This is because infants have a number of immature enzymatic metabolic pathways, rendering certain amino acids considered nonessential for adults essential in infants.

Lipid Requirements

Adipose tissue in the average 70-kg man contains approximately 140,000 kcal and serves as the primary energy storage source for the body. Lipids are calorie dense, supplying on average 9.0 kcal/g and generally should account for 10% to 30% of the total daily caloric load with a minimum of 2% to 4% as essential fatty acids to prevent deficiency. Essential fatty acids are required for the production of sterol-based hormones including cortisol, gluconeogenic hormones, and growth hormone, which are important in wound healing and the response to surgical stress. Lipids are the main component in cellular and subcellular membranes. Linoleic and linolenic acids are essential fatty acids that serve as precursors for prostaglandin synthesis and are essential for cell signaling.

If patients are being supported with parenteral nutrition (PN), they should be monitored for tolerance of lipid delivery because long-chain triglyceride solutions may diminish immune function, and cause hypertriglyceridemia. Complications may be minimized by infusing lipids continuously over 18 to 24 hours and at a rate not to exceed 0.1 g/kg/hour. Most patients tolerate infusions of lipids when provided as an intermittent or continuous infusion. Intravenous lipids in the US are omega-6 fatty acids, considered to be immunosuppressive. It is acceptable not to give lipids during the first week of PN. Once initiated, they can be given three times weekly to daily, depending on the nutritional needs of the patient. They may be combined with the other PN nutrients in solution as part of a total nutrient admixture (TNA) or given as a separate infusion.

There is a renewed interested in providing omega-3 fatty acid containing nutrition therapy to patients, as they are considered anti-inflammatory. Omega-3 fatty acids have been shown to be beneficial in critically ill patients as well as patients with chronic inflammatory processes. The omega-3 fatty acids eicosapentaenoic acid (EPA) and docosahexaenoic acid (DHA) displace omega-6 fatty acids from the cell membranes of immune cells, thus reducing systemic inflammation through the production of alternative biologically less inflammatory prostaglandins (prostaglandin E_3) and leukotrienes of the 5-series. EPA and DHA (fish oils) have also been shown to decrease neutrophil attachment and transepithelial migration to modulate systemic and local inflammation, and they also help to stabilize the myocardium and lower the incidence of cardiac arrhythmias. Additionally, they decrease the incidence of acute respiratory distress syndrome (ARDS), and reduce the likelihood of sepsis.

Other Requirements

Fluid and Electrolytes
Surgical patients often receive large volumes of fluid perioperatively. Typically, surgical patients are provided with intravenous fluids until oral intake is resumed and tolerated to maintain fluid balance. The goals of fluid management include maintenance of adequate hydration, tissue perfusion, and electrolyte balance. Insensible losses, measured losses (e.g., stool, urine, drainage, hemorrhage, open wounds), and alterations in fluid balance due to metabolic changes (e.g., fever, hyperthyroidism) or medical therapy (diuretics) must be carefully considered When ordering nutritional replacement, one must consider how to deliver maintenance, resuscitation, and replacement fluids and electrolytes. This can be done either separately from the nutritional requirements or combined with it. In the critically ill patient where fluid requirements can fluctuate, it is recommended to provide the nutrition regimen separately from the fluid requirements and then maximally concentrate the nutrition regimen. Once the patient becomes stable, the fluid, electrolyte, and nutrient requirements can be combined. Typical adult maintenance electrolyte needs are shown in Table 3-4. Careful monitoring of losses and serum concentrations should be used to guide adjustments to supplemental replacement.

Vitamins and Minerals
Vitamins and minerals are important for optimal postoperative recovery. Vitamin C is an antioxidant, required for the synthesis of collagen, carnitine, and neurotransmitters and for the immune-mediated and antibacterial functions of white blood

TABLE 3-4	General Daily Parenteral Electrolyte and Mineral Recommendations	
	Adults	**Infants and Children**
Sodium	50–250 mEq	2–4 mEq/kg
Potassium	30–200 mEq	2–3 mEq/kg
Chloride	50–250 mEq	2–3 mEq/kg
Phosphate	10–40 mmol	0.5–2 mmol/kg
Calcium	10–20 mEq	1–3 mEq/kg
Magnesium	10–30 mEq	0.25–0.5 mEq/kg

cells. Iron is essential to produce hemoglobin and myoglobin, which is necessary for muscle iron storage, and cytochromes, which are necessary for the oxidative production of cellular energy. Vitamin K is essential for blood-clotting mechanism. Trace element deficiencies of zinc, copper, manganese, and selenium can lead to impaired wound healing, glucose metabolism, and protein sulfination. Surgical patients who require steroid medications and who have healing wounds should receive supplemental Vitamin A to aid in collagen crosslinking. Recommended daily vitamin and trace element supplementation is shown in Table 3-4.

Other Additives
For patients receiving PN, medications that are most frequently added include additional trace elements, histamine-2 receptor blockers, vitamin K, and regular insulin, although the latter is not recommended unless glucose levels have stabilized.

Impact of Starvation and Stress
During the first 24 to 72 hours of nonstressed starvation, basal energy requirements are decreased and are supplied by liver and muscle glycogen stores. With persistent starvation and glycogen depletion, deamination of gluconeogenic amino acids, such as alanine and glutamine, accounts for an increasingly greater percent of the total glucose production to meet the preferential needs for glucose by the brain, CNS, and red blood cells. Body proteins cannot serve as a long-term source of fuel because of their structural and functional importance. Protein depletion in excess of 20% is not compatible with life. Fat mobilization with persistent starvation, likely resulting from decreased insulin levels, inhibits lipase and allows for intracellular hydrolysis of triglycerides. The liver only partially oxidizes most of the fatty acids it receives, so serum levels of acetacetate, β-hydroxybutyrate, and acetone increase. These ketone bodies, released by the liver, can be oxidized to CO_2 and H_2O by tissues such as the kidney and muscles. The brain also converts to using ketoacids as an energy source due to persistently low glucose levels. Utilization of ketone bodies as an energy source decreases hepatic gluconeogenesis and spares muscle protein. Although the brain and CNS can convert to utilizing ketoacids for fuel during nonstressed starvation, these by-products of incomplete fatty acid metabolism eventually become toxic. During unstressed starvation, there is a general decrease in energy expenditure and a change in the insulin–glucagon ratio to favor mobilization of stored fuels and minimize loss of lean body tissue.

The metabolic response to injury or infection can classically be divided into the ebb and flow phase. The ebb phase begins immediately after injury and typically lasts between 12 and 24 hours, but may last longer depending on the severity of injury and adequacy of resuscitation. The ebb phase is characterized by tissue hypoperfusion and a decrease in overall metabolism. Catecholamines are released to compensate for this, with norepinephrine being the primary mediator. Released from peripheral nerves, norepinephrine binds to β1 receptors in the heart and to alpha and β2 receptors in peripheral and splanchnic vascular beds. This results in increased cardiac contractility and heart rate and vasoconstriction in attempt to restore blood pressure, increase cardiac performance and maximize venous return.

The flow phase encompasses the catabolic and anabolic phases. It is signaled by high cardiac output with restoration of oxygen delivery and metabolic substrate. Although the duration of the flow phase depends on the severity of injury and illness, it typically peaks at 3 to 5 days and subsides by 7 to 10 days, merging with the anabolic phase over the next few weeks. During this hypermetabolic phase, although insulin levels are elevated, high levels of catecholamines, glucagon, and cortisol counteract most of its metabolic effects. This hormonal imbalance results in mobilization of amino acids and free fatty acids from peripheral muscles and adipose tissue. Some of these released substrates are used for energy production, either directly as glucose or through the liver as triglyceride. Other substrates contribute to the synthesis of proteins in the liver, where humoral mediators increase production of acute-phase reactants, and in the immune system for healing damaged tissues. The net result however is a significant loss of protein, characterized by negative nitrogen balance and decreased adipose stores, accompanied by enlarged extracellular water compartments.

Hyperglycemia is a common occurrence during hypermetabolic stress and results from the accelerated gluconeogenesis and relative insulin resistance. This can become quite exaggerated in patients with or without underlying diabetes. Glucose control (e.g., blood glucose 80 to 150 mg/dL) is important in surgical patients to limit infectious complications, other morbidities, and mortality.

ASSESSMENT OF NUTRITIONAL STATUS

Patients with poor preoperative nutritional status are more likely to have increased morbidity and mortality postoperatively. It has been estimated that approximately 30% to 50% of hospitalized patients are malnourished. Since addressing malnutrition may result in improved outcomes, nutritional assessment and intervention are necessary components of patient evaluation.

Nutrition Risk Screening and Impact on Surgical Complications

An appropriate history and physical examination remains a primary nutritional assessment tool. Criteria to consider when screening surgical patients for nutrition risk include magnitude of the proposed surgical procedure, medications, body mass index (BMI), recent weight changes, cachexia, changes in diet or appetite, and serum visceral protein levels (e.g., albumin in the outpatient setting, prealbumin in the acute care setting). Anthropometric measurements including various measures of muscle mass and circumference, and body composition have been used to evaluate nutritional status;

however, they have not been validated to accurately assess acute nutritional risk.

An accurate height and body-weight measurement should be obtained for all surgical patients to be used in calculating BMI and IBW (Table 3-2). A nutrition-focused history can reveal signs and symptoms of nutrient and vitamin deficiencies or toxicities (Table 3-5). Many medications have nutritionally related side effects or increase nutrient requirements. Recent unexplained lean body mass weight loss of 10% over 2 to 6 months or 5% in 1 month and a BMI > 30 or <18 are associated with increased postoperative complications. Albumin and total protein levels reflect long-term nutritional status and can be used as a simple marker for preoperative nutritional status in nonhypermetabolic general surgical patients. However, these levels can be affected by fluid shifts and in these cases serum transferrin or prealbumin levels may be evaluated along with acute-phase proteins (e.g., C-reactive protein [CRP]) to assist in delineation of an inflammatory process versus poor nutritional status.

Every surgical procedure carries some risk of postoperative complications. This risk correlates linearly with the magnitude and complexity of individual procedures. There is a linear increase in complications in patients undergoing elective GI surgery as preoperative albumin decreases from normal to levels below 2.0 g/dL/dL. Patients undergoing esophagectomy appear at risk if albumin drops below 3.75 g/dL/dL. Complications increase in patients undergoing gastrectomy or pancreatic surgery when preoperative albumin levels drop below 3.25 g/dL/dL. Patients undergoing elective colectomy have little increase risk unless preoperative albumin levels drop below 2.5 g/dL.

OPTIONS FOR NUTRITIONAL THERAPY

Patients unable to self-consume adequate nutrients orally (at least 60% of nutritional needs), require adjunctive nutritional therapy in the form of either enteral nutrition (EN) or PN.

Enteral Nutrition

EN supplies either whole or partially digested nutrients to the GI tract via a tube or via routine oral feeding. Table 3-6 lists the type of commonly used feeding tube access techniques for short-term and long-term enteral nutritional support. Critically ill patients best tolerate continuous infusion, with bolus or intermittent infusion being reserved for stable patients requiring long-term enteral feeding.

The GI tract not only functions to digest and absorb nutrients, fluid and electrolytes, but also is the body's largest immunologic organ serving as a protective barrier against intraluminal toxins and bacteria. Approximately 70% of the body's immunoglobulin-producing cells line the GI tract with 80% of the body's synthesized immunoglobulin being secreted here.

During severe physiologic stress, relative or absolute gut ischemia can occur, leading to mucosal compromise and disruption of the gut's barrier function and ultimate passage of bacteria and toxins into the bloodstream or mesenteric lymphoid system. Animal studies reveal that enteral rather than PN maintains gut mucosal integrity and immune responsiveness and prevents this gut-derived bacterial translocation. Enteral feeding remains the preferred route when the gut is functional. Studies suggest that providing at least 50% to 65% of goal calories may be required to prevent increases in

TABLE 3-5	Nutrient Deficiencies Revealed by Physical Examination

Suspected Nutrient Deficiency	Physical Findings
General	
Protein, calories	Loss of weight, muscle mass, or fat stores; growth retardation; poor wound healing; infections
Protein, thiamin	Edema (ankles and feet; rule out sodium and water retention, pregnancy, protein-losing enteropathy)
Obesity	Excessive adipose tissue
Iron	Anemia, fatigue
Skin	
Protein, vitamin C, zinc	Poor wound healing, pressure ulcers; cellophane appearance
Protein, thiamin	Body edema; round swollen face (moon face)
Essential fatty acids, vitamin A, pyridoxine	Xerosis (rule out environmental cause, lack of hygiene, aging, uremia, hypothyroidism), follicular hyperkeratosis, mosaic dermatitis (plaques of skin in center, peeling at periphery on shins)
Vitamin C	Slow wound healing, petechiae (especially perifollicular)
Niacin	Pigmentation; desquamation of sun exposed areas
Zinc	Delayed wound healing, acneiform rash, skin lesions, hair loss
Vitamin K or vitamin C	Excessive bleeding, petechiae, ecchymoses; small red, purple, or black hemorrhagic spots
Iron	Pallor; fatigue
Dehydration (fluid)	Poor skin turgor
Excess beta carotene	Yellow pigmentation of palms of hands with normal white sclera
Eyes	
Iron, folate, or vitamin B_{12}	Pale conjunctivae (anemia)
Vitamin A	Bitot spots, conjunctival xerosis, corneal xerosis, keratomalacia
Riboflavin, pyridoxine, niacin	Redness, fissuring in corners of eyes
Thiamin, phosphorus	Ophthalmoplegia
Hyperlipidemia	Corneal arcus, xanthelasma
Hair	
Protein	Hair lacks shine, luster; flag sign; easily plucked with no pain
Vitamin C, copper	Corkscrew hair; unemerged, coiled hairs
Protein, biotin, zinc	Sparse
Nose	
Riboflavin, niacin, pyridoxine	Seborrhea on nasolabial area, nose bridge, eyebrows, and back of ears (rule out poor hygiene)
Nails	
Iron	Koilonychia (considered normal if seen on toenails only)
Protein	Dull, lusterless with transverse ridging across nail plate
Vitamins A and C	Pale, poor blanching, irregular, mottled
Protein, calories	Bruising, bleeding
Vitamin C	Splinter hemorrhages
Lips and Mouth	
Niacin, riboflavin, pyridoxine	Cheilosis, angular scars
Riboflavin, pyridoxine, niacin, iron	Angular stomatitis
Tongue	
Riboflavin, niacin, folate, iron	Atrophic filiform papillae
Vitamin B_{12}	Glossitis
Zinc	Taste atrophy
Riboflavin	Magenta tongue
Teeth	
Excess sugar, vitamin C	Edentia, caries
Fluorosis	Mottled tooth enamel
Gums	
Vitamin C	Swollen, bleeding gums; receding

TABLE 3-5	Nutrient Deficiencies Revealed by Physical Examination (Continued)

Suspected Nutrient Deficiency	Physical Findings
Neck	
Iodine	Enlarged thyroid gland
Protein, bulimia	Enlarged parotid glands (bilateral)
Excess fluid	Venous distention, pulsations
Thorax	
Protein, calories	Decreased muscle mass and strength, shortness of breath, fatigue, decreased pulmonary function
Cardiac system	
Thiamine	Heart failure
Gastrointestinal system	
Protein, calories, zinc, vitamin C	Poor wound healing
Protein	Hepatomegaly
Urinary tract	
Dehydration	Dark, concentrated urine
Overhydration	Light colored, diluted urine
Musculoskeletal system	
Vitamin D, calcium	Rickets, osteomalacia
Vitamin D	Persistently open anterior fontanel (after age 18 months), craiotabes (softening of skull across back and sides before age 1 yr); epiphyseal enlargement (painless) at wrist, knees, and ankles; pigeon chest and Harrison sulcus (horizontal depression on lower chest border)
Protein	Emaciation, muscle wasting, swelling, pain, pale hair patches
Vitamin C	Swollen, painful joints
Thiamine	Pain in thighs, calves
Nervous system	
Protein	Psychomotor changes (listless, apathetic), mental confusion
Vitamin B_{12}, thiamine, vitamin B_6	Weakness, confusion, depressed reflexes, paresthesias, sensory loss, calf tenderness
Niacin, vitamin B_{12}	Dementia
Calcium, vitamin D, magnesium	Tetany

intestinal permeability in burn and bone-marrow transplant patients, to promote faster return of cognitive function in head injury patients, and to improve outcome from immune-modulating enteral formulations in critically ill patients.

TABLE 3-6	Methods for Gaining Enteral Feeding Access

Short-Term Access (<4 weeks)	Long-Term Access (>4 weeks)
Naso/oroenteric access	**Percutaneous feeding tube**
Spontaneous passage	Percutaneous endoscopic gastrostomy (PEG)
Active passage	Gastric/jejunal (PEG/J)
Bedside, assisted	Direct jejunal (DPEJ)
Endoscopic	**Laparoscopic**
Fluoroscopic	Gastrostomy
Operative (passed in operating room)	Jejunostomy
	Surgical
	Gastrostomy
	Jejunostomy

Current nutrition guidelines recommend that EN should be started early, within the first 24 to 48 hours of ICU and hospital admission. There is a "window of opportunity" that exists in the first 24 to 72 hours following admission or the onset of a hypermetabolic insult. Feedings started within this time frame are associated with less gut permeability and diminished activation and release of inflammatory cytokines. The impact of early EN on patient outcome appears to be a dose-dependent effect. Low rate feeding, often termed "trickle" or "trophic" feeds (10 to 30 mL/hour), may be sufficient to prevent mucosal atrophy, but may be insufficient to achieve the usual endpoints desired from EN therapy. If EN is unable to meet 100% of energy requirements after 7 to 10 days, then initiation of PN should be considered as to prevent excessive energy and protein deficits.

There are over 100 enteral formulations currently commercially available for a wide variety of clinical conditions, and they are constantly being reformulated. Enteral formulations are classified as medical foods by the Food and Drug Administration and therefore do not undergo this regulatory control. Enteral formulas can be classified as standard, elemental, or specialized. Table 3-7 provides an overview of various categories of enteral formulas and specifies the types of macronutrients and physical properties. The appropriate

TABLE 3-7 Overview of Select Enteral Formulations

Formula Category	Protein Sources	Calories From Protein (%)	Carbohydrate Sources	Calories From Carbohydrates (%)	Fat Sources	Calories From Fat (%)	Caloric Density (Calories/mL)	mL for 100% RDI	% Free Water	Osmolality (mOsmol/kg)
Oral supplements	Sodium and calcium caseinates, soy protein isolates	14–24	Corn syrup, sugar, sucrose, maltodextrin	47–64	Corn oil, canola oil, soy oil, sunflower oil, safflower oil	21–39	1.0–2.0	946–2,000	73–85	480–870
Standard tube feedings	Sodium and calcium caseinates, soy protein isolates	13–18	Corn syrup, maltodextrin Fiber: soy fiber, guar gum, oat fiber, FOS	45–57	Soy oil, corn oil, canola oil, MCT, safflower oil	29–39	1.0–2.0	830–1,890	77–85	270–500
High protein tube feedings	Sodium and calcium caseinates	22–25	Hydrolyzed cornstarch, maltodextrin, sucrose, fructose, oat fiber, soy fiber, guar gum	38–52	Canola oil, MCT, soybean oil, safflower oil	23–40	1.0–1.5	1,000–2,000	78–85	300–490
Elemental, semi-elemental	Free amino acids, soy hydrolysates, hydrolyzed whey, hydrolyzed casein, hydrolyzed soy	12–25	Hydrolyzed cornstarch, maltodextrin, sucrose, modified cornstarch	36–82	Soybean oil, safflower oil, canola oil, MCT, sunflower oil	3–39	1.0–1.5	1,150–2,000	76–86	270–650
Pulmonary	Sodium and calcium caseinates	17–20	Hydrolyzed cornstarch, corn syrup, sucrose, maltodextrin, sugar	27–40	Canola oil, soybean oil, MCT, corn oil, safflower oil, sardine oil, borage oil	40–55	1.5	933–1,420	76–79	330–650
Renal	Sodium and calcium caseinates	7–15	Corn syrup, sucrose, fructose, maltodextrin, sugar	40–58	Corn oil, safflower oil, canola oil, MCT	35–45	1.8–2.0	947–1,000	70–71	570–700
Diabetic	Sodium and calcium caseinates, beef, milk protein, soy protein isolates	16–24	Maltodextrin, hydrolyzed cornstarch, fructose, sucrose, guar gum, vegetables, fruits, soy fiber	34–40	Sunflower oil, soybean oil, canola oil, MCT, safflower oil	40–49	1.0–1.06	1,000–1,890 or NA	85	355–450
Immune modulated	Sodium and calcium caseinates, L-arginine, glutamine dipeptide, BCAA	22–32	Hydrolyzed cornstarch, maltodextrin, soy fiber	38–53	Canola oil, structured lipids; sunflower oil, fish oil, MCT	20–40	1.0–1.5	1,250–2,000	78–86	375–550
Hepatic	L-amino acids, whey	11–15	Sucrose, maltodextrin, modified cornstarch	57–77	Soybean oil, MCT, canola oil, corn oil, lecithin	12–28	1.2–1.5	N/A–1,000	76–82	560–690

MCT, medium chain triglycerides
FOS, fructooligosaccharides
BCAA, branched chain amino acids

selection and administration of enteral formula requires a thorough knowledge of physiology and pathophysiology of digestion and absorption. The physical form and quantity of each nutrient may determine the extent of absorption of and tolerance to the formula (e.g., long-chain versus medium-chain triglyceride). Disease-specific formulas have been developed for diabetes, renal failure, pulmonary, immune compromised, and hepatic disease. Although theoretically appealing, there is lack of prospective, randomized controlled clinical trials supporting the purported indications for most specialized formulas, except for the immune formulas. Initiation of immune formulas perioperatively in GI surgery and trauma patient's results in significantly decreased infections and infectious complications.

Parenteral Nutrition

PN is an intravenous infusion of a hyperosmolar solution, which contains macronutrients (dextrose, protein, lipids), micronutrients, electrolytes, and fluids. PN is given via a central venous catheter in order to accommodate the osmolarity of PN. PN was first developed to provide nutrition to those unable to take adequate nutrition via the GI tract. Diagnoses that commonly need PN include short bowel syndrome, chronic malabsorption, bowel obstruction, prolonged ileus, intractable diarrhea or vomiting, and high-output GI fistulas. PN solutions can be infused continuously over 24 hours or cycled over shorter intervals in stable patients.

PN increases the likelihood of hyperglycemia, even in nondiabetic patients. PN should not be initiated in someone whose blood glucose is ≥300 mg/dL; blood glucose should be treated and be between an acceptable range (80 to 150 mg/dL) prior to initiating PN. Dextrose can be initiated at 150 to 250 g/day depending on the patient's expected glucose tolerance and/or tolerance to prior dextrose infusions (e.g., IV dextrose). If after 24 hours glycemic control is acceptable, then the dextrose can be advanced to goal over the next 24 to 48 hours as tolerated. Capillary glucose measurements should be obtained—three to four times daily until the values are within acceptable ranges for 2 consecutive days. Regular insulin should be administered accordingly. Adding insulin to the PN solution should be delayed until the 24-hour insulin requirement is stable and even then authors are not uniform that adding insulin to PN is advisable.

Protein can be provided at the targeted patient goal. Surgical patients typically require 1.5 to 2.0 g/day of protein due to hypercatabolism and wound-healing needs. Protein may need to be adjusted for patients with renal or liver failure. However, patients with dialysis have an increased protein need as this therapy is also catabolic to the patient and therefore protein requirements are typically no different. Hepatic failure is associated with cachexia, and therefore withholding protein for these patients is not advised unless medical therapy is not successful in alleviating disease severity.

Lipids may be infused three to four times weekly or daily and for up to 24 hours, depending upon a patient's nutritional needs. Irrespective of the method of lipid delivery, either via TNA or as a separate infusion, maximal lipid infusion rates should not exceed 0.1 g/kg/hour. IV lipids in the United States are rich in omega-6 fatty acids and adverse effects associated with large infusions include immunosuppression and hyperlipidemia. Lipid-based sedation such as propofol needs to be included in the lipid infusion rate calculation. Maintenance

TABLE 3-8	Composition of Adult Parenteral Multivitamin and Micronutrient Products Available in the United States	
Nutrient	**Dose**	**Adult DRI**
Vitamins		
Vitamin A (retinol)	1 mg (3,300 USP units)	700–900 µg
Vitamin D (ergocalciferol	5 µg (200 USP units)	5–15 µg
Vitamin E (DL-α-tocopheryl acetate)	10 mg (10 USP units)	15 mg
Vitamin K (phylloquinone)	150 µg	90–120 µg
Vitamin C (ascorbic acid)	200 mg	75–90 mg
Folic acid	600 µg	400 µg
Niacinamide	40 mg	14–16 mg
Riboflavin	3.6 mg	1.1–1.3 mg
Thiamin	3 mg	1.1–1.2 mg
Vitamin B_6 (pyridoxine)	6 mg	1.3–1.7 mg
Vitamin B_{12} (cyanocobalamin)	5 µg	2.4 µg
Pantothenic acid	15 mg	5 mg
Biotin	60 µg	30 µg
Minerals		
Zinc	2.5–5 mg	8–11 mg
Copper	0.3–1.5 mg	0.9 mg
Manganese	60–180 µg	1.8–2.3 mg
Chromium	10–15 µg	20–35 µg
Selenium	20–80 µg	55 µg

of serum triglyceride levels <400 mg/dL is suggested during lipid infusion. For persistent or severe hypertriglyceridemia or for patients with an egg allergy, safflower oil or any oil high in essential fatty acids can be administered enterally if tolerated in attempt to alleviate the symptoms of essential fatty acid deficiency, which develops in approximately 10 to 14 days in the absence of essential fatty acid provision (linoleic and linolenic acids).

Most patients require daily multivitamin and mineral provision in their PN solution (Table 3-8). Some trace elements may need to be omitted in patients with liver failure (e.g., manganese). Electrolytes are added based on the individual need of each patient by evaluating their blood chemistries and medical therapies (e.g., dialysis) with guidelines provided in Table 3-4.

Peripheral Parenteral Nutrition

Peripheral parenteral nutrition (PPN) contains similar components to centrally infused PN, but macronutrients need to be provided at lower concentrations and more volume is required because the solution osmolality needs to be ≤900 mOsm/L. PPN is contraindicated in patients that cannot tolerate large volumes of fluid. PPN is indicated for only short periods (≤2 weeks) as it provides insufficient nutrients (800 to 1,200 kcal/day). Generally, decisions to use PPN are based on energy demands, anticipated duration of use, and availability of intravenous access. The use of PPN in severely malnourished is not indicated due to few suitable veins and insufficient nutrient provision. Utilization of PPN has decreased with the advent of peripherally inserted central catheters (PICC).

Parenteral Nutrition: Advantages and Disadvantages

PN offers an advantage in that a functional GI tract is not required. The parenteral route provides considerable ease in nutrient delivery, and studies show that nutritional requirements are more consistently met. The metabolic response to IV glucose differs from that of oral glucose. This is partially because the insulin-dependent hepatic uptake of glucose from the portal vein during first-pass physiology is greater when glucose is provided orally. This results in less systemic hyperglycemia and hyperinsulinemia. A meta-analysis comparing EPN and PN concluded that plasma glucose concentrations are lower during EN. Plasma glucose and insulin concentrations, glucose oxidation, carbon dioxide production, and minute ventilation increase in a linear relationship with calories administered in PN. Prolonged infusion of high rates of glucose (>4 mg/kg/minute) results in de novo lipogenesis in the majority of critically ill patients. Other known disadvantages of PN include increased infectious complications and morbidity, liver complications (e.g., biliary stasis, cholecystitis, liver fibrosis), bacteremia, and gut mucosal atrophy. Table 3-9 lists metabolic complications of PN.

Enteral Nutrition: Advantages and Disadvantages

The proposed advantages of EN in surgical and critically ill patients include attenuation of the metabolic response to stress, improved nitrogen balance, better glycemic control, increased visceral protein synthesis, increased GI anastomotic strength, and increased collagen deposition. Other benefits of EN include stimulation of the gut-associated lymphoid tissue (GALT), decreased nosocomial infections, enhanced visceral blood flow, increased variety of nutrients for delivery, and decreased risk of GI bleeding. While few studies have shown a differential effect on mortality, EN has consistently resulted in better outcomes by reducing infectious morbidity (generally pneumonia and central-line infections) in most patient populations and specifically abdominal abscess in trauma patients.

Despite the benefits of EN over PN, it may not be feasible to provide adequate nutrition via the GI tract. GI access difficulties remain, and there is difficulty in achieving nutrient goals with up to 50% of patients being intolerant to enteral feedings. Complications of EN include jejunal necrosis, aspiration, diarrhea, and respiratory compromise. In addition, the formulas themselves can induce problems related to their composition (Table 3-10).

TABLE 3-9	Metabolic Complications of PN	
Complication	**Possible Cause**	**Treatment**
Hypovolemia	Inadequate fluid provision, over diuresis	Increase free-water delivery
Hypervolemia	Excess fluid delivery, renal dysfunction, congestive heart failure, hepatic failure	Fluid restriction, diuretics, dialysis
Hypokalemia	Refeeding syndrome, inadequate potassium provision, increased losses	Increase IV potassium
Hyperkalemia	Renal dysfunction, too much potassium provision, metabolic acidosis, potassium-sparing drugs	Decrease potassium intake, potassium binders, dialysis in extreme cases
Hyponatremia	Excessive fluid provision, nephritis, adrenal insufficiency, dilutional states	Restrict fluid intake, increase sodium intake as indicated clinically
Hypernatremia	Inadequate free-water provision, excessive sodium intake, excessive water losses	Decrease sodium intake, replete free-water deficit
Hypoglycemia	Abrupt discontinuation of PN, insulin overdose	Dextrose delivery
Hyperglycemia	Rapid infusion of large dextrose load, sepsis, pancreatitis, steroids, diabetes, elderly	Insulin, decrease dextrose as indicated
Hypertriglyceridemia	Inability to clear lipid provision, sepsis, too much exogenous dextrose and insulin provision, multisystem organ failure, medications altering fat absorption, history of hyperlipidemia	Decrease lipid volume provided, increase infusion time, hold lipids up to 14 days to normalize levels
Hypocalcemia	Decreased vitamin D intake, hypoparathyroidism, citrate binding of calcium resulting from excessive blood transfusion, hypoalbuminemia	Calcium supplementation
Hypercalcemia	Renal failure, tumor lysis syndrome, bone cancer, excess vitamin D delivery, prolonged immobilization-stress hyperparathyroidism	Isotonic saline, inorganic phosphate supplementation, corticosteroids, mithramycin
Hypomagnesaemia	Refeeding syndrome, alcoholism, diuretic use, increased losses, medications, diabetic ketoacidosis, chemotherapy	Magnesium supplementation
Hypermagnesemia	Excessive magnesium provision, renal insufficiency	Decease magnesium provision
Hypophosphatemia	Refeeding syndrome, alcoholism, phosphate-binding antacids, dextrose infusion, overfeeding, secondary hyperparathyroidism, insulin therapy	Phosphate supplementation, discontinue phosphate binding antacids, avoid overfeeding, initiate dextrose delivery cautiously
Hyperphosphatemia	Renal dysfunction, excessive provision	Decrease phosphate delivery, phosphate binders
Prerenal azotemia	Dehydration, excessive protein provision, inadequate nonprotein calorie provision with mobilization of endogenous proteins	Increase fluid intake, decrease protein delivery, increase nonprotein calories
Essential fatty acid deficiency	Inadequate polyunsaturated long-chain fatty acid provision	Provide lipids

TABLE 3-10	Common Complications Associated with Enteral Feeding

Complication	Possible Causes	Corrective Measures
Mechanical		
Obstructed feeding tube	Crushed medications administered through tube	Give medications as elixir
	Formula coagulated in tube due to contact with acidic medium (gastric contents, medications)	Flush tube with water before and after each medication
	Formula viscosity excessive for feeding tube	Use less viscous formula and a pump
	Formula buildup inside tube	Flush tube with water under pressure several times per day
Metabolic		
Hyperglycemia	Metabolic stress, sepsis, trauma, Diabetes Mellitus	Treat origin of stress and provide insulin needed to maintain BG 110–150 mg/dL
		Avoid excessive carbohydrate delivery
Altered serum electrolytes	Inadequate electrolytes in formula	Change formula
	Refeeding syndrome	Monitor electrolytes closely (K^+, Mg^{2+}, PO_4) and replace as indicated
Dehydration	Osmotic diarrhea caused by rapid infusion of hyperosmolar formula	Avoid hyperosmolar formulas delivered into the small intestine
	Excessive protein, electrolytes, or both	Increase fluid provision or decrease protein and electrolytes
	Inadequate free-water provision	Ensure adequate free-water provision
Overhydration	Excessive fluid intake	Assess fluid intake; monitor daily fluid intake and output
	Rapid refeeding in malnourished patient	Monitor serum electrolytes, body weight daily; weight change >0.2 kg/day reflects decrease or increase of extracellular fluid
	Cardiac, hepatic, or renal insufficiency	Use calorically dense formula to decrease free-water provision
	Increased extracellular mass catabolism causing loss of body cell mass with subsequent potassium loss	Diuretic therapy
Gradual weight loss	Inadequate calories	Ensure patient is receiving estimated calorie requirements
	Malabsorption	Adjust nutrient delivery as indicated based upon patient monitoring
		Adjust nutrient composition or add PN if malabsorption of nutrients
Excessive weight gain	Excess calories	Rule out weight gain due to volume status
	Volume overload	Ensure patient receiving caloric needs
Visceral protein depletion	Active inflammatory process	Treat cause of inflammation
	Inadequate calories or protein	Adjust calorie and protein provision if inflammatory markers normal
Essential fatty acid deficiency	Prolonged (>10 days) lack of sufficient lipid provision (LCT)	Include at least 4% of daily caloric needs as essential fatty acids
Gastrointestinal		
Nausea and vomiting	Excessive formula volume or rate of infusion	Decrease rate of infusion or volume infused
	Hyperosmolar formula infusion (especially in small intestine)	Change to isotonic formula
	Delayed gastric emptying	Add prokinetic agent
	Improper tube location	Reposition tube if needed
	Very cold formula provided	Use polymeric formula as less offensive odor
	Smell of enteral formulas	Change to lower fat formula
		Provide formula at room temperature
Diarrhea	Too rapid infusion of formula	Decrease rate infusion rate
	Bolus feedings into small intestine	Only continuous feeds into small bowel
	Hyperosmolar formula infused	Change to isotonic formula
	Hyperosmolar medication infused	Avoid hyperosmolar medications or dilute with water prior to giving
	Altered GI anatomy or short bowel syndrome	Change to hydrolyzed, free amino acid and MCT oil-containing formula
	Malabsorption	Use lactose-free formula
	Lactose intolerance	Check stool for pathogens and treat accordingly
	GI bacterial overgrowth	Consider prebiotics and/or probiotics
	Antibiotic therapy	
Vomiting and diarrhea	Contamination	Check sanitation of formula, equipment and assure proper handling technique

(Continued)

TABLE 3-10	Common Complications Associated with Enteral Feeding (Continued)	
Complication	**Possible Causes**	**Corrective Measures**
Abdominal distention, bloating, cramping, gas	Rapid bolus or intermittent infusion with cold formula	Administer formula at room temperature
	Rapid infusion with syringe	Infuse continuously and gradually advance to goal
	Nutrient malabsorption or maldigestion	Hydrolyzed formula, MCT containing, lactose free
	Rapid administration of MCT	Administer MCT gradually as tolerated
Constipation	Lack of fiber	Add fiber formula
	Inadequate free water	Stool softener
	Fecal impaction, GI obstruction	Assure adequate free water
	Inadequate physical activity	Rectal exam, digital disimpaction
	Medications	Increase physical therapy if able, turn patient
Aspiration or gastric retention of formula	Altered gastric motility, diabetic gastroparesis, altered gag reflex, altered mental status	Postpyloric nutrient delivery with continuous infusion
		Add prokinetic agent
	Head of bed < 30 degrees	Elevate HOB > 30 degrees if possible
	Displaced feeding tube	Verify feeding tube placement and reposition as needed
	Ileus or hemodynamic instability	For prolonged intolerance, may need PN
	Medications that slow gastric emptying (opiates, anticholinergics)	Evaluate medications and change if able
	Gastric, vagotomy surgery	

Parenteral Nutrition Therapy Indications

Several organizations have developed practice guidelines to identify appropriate and inappropriate indications for PN (Table 3-11). PN should only be provided in those patients where enteral nutrient provision is not feasible for 7 or more days. PN should only be initiated in patients who are hemodynamically stable and who are able to tolerate the fluid volume, protein, carbohydrate, and IV lipid doses necessary to provide adequate nutrient requirements. Malnourished surgical patients benefit most if PN is provided for a minimum of 7 to 10 days preoperatively and then continued throughout the perioperative period.

ASSESSMENT OF NUTRITIONAL EFFECTIVENESS

Catabolism to Anabolism Switch

Nutritional support does not convert a septic catabolic patient into an anabolic state. Numerous hormonal and inflammatory factors are present that limit the effectiveness of exogenously administered nutritional substrates. Only the resolution of the underlying stress can reverse these effects. The switch from catabolism to anabolism is one of the signs that the hypermetabolic response of stress is resolving and the patient is improving. This is first noted by a shift from fluid retention to diuresis and loss of edema, followed shortly by a rise in serum proteins and an increase in protein utilization. This is reflected in a positive nitrogen balance.

Immune Competence

Malnutrition leads to a decline in immune function. Immune competence as measured by delayed cutaneous hypersensitivity (DCH) and total lymphocyte count (TLC) is reduced in uncomplicated severe malnutrition. In hospitalized patients, DCH and TLC have limited value due to other intervening factors, such as infection, uremia, cirrhosis, hepatitis, trauma, burns, hemorrhage, steroids, immunosuppressants, cimetidine, coumadin, general anesthesia, and surgery. Nonnutritional factors that affect TLC include hypoalbuminemia, metabolic stress, infection, cancer, and chronic diseases.

Nitrogen Balance Studies

Nitrogen balance studies are used to evaluate the adequacy of protein provision in order to reduce loss of muscle mass in hospitalized patients. Nitrogen is released as the result of metabolism of amino acids in proteins and is excreted in the urine as free urea. Therefore, urine urea nitrogen concentration increases with increased catabolism or metabolism of exogenous protein. In theory, by increasing exogenous protein, endogenous protein losses will decrease. Nitrogen balance studies reflect the balance between exogenous nitrogen intake and renal removal of nitrogen-containing compounds. Nitrogen balance studies are not protein turnover studies, which require labeled (stable isotope) protein methods.

Measurement of nitrogen balance studies is most accurate in patients who receive a defined nutrient intake such as those with enteral or parenteral feeding. For nitrogen balance calculations, amino acid products are generally assumed to be 16% nitrogen (6.25 g of protein = 1 g of nitrogen). Nitrogen balance is calculated by subtracting the excreted nitrogen (24-hour urine urea nitrogen [UUN] collection plus insensible losses) from the nitrogen intake provided in the nutrition therapy:

$$\text{Nitrogen balance} = (\text{grams of protein or amino acid intake}/6.25) - (\text{UUN} + 4)$$

A positive nitrogen balance in the range of 2 to 4 g of nitrogen per day, indicating an anabolic state, is desired, but often difficult to achieve. Validity of nitrogen balance is affected by severe nitrogen retention disorders (e.g., creatinine clearance <50 mL/minute, severe hepatic failure), massive diuresis, abnormal nitrogen losses through excessive diarrhea or large

TABLE 3-11	Indications and Contraindications for PN Therapy

Indications	Consensus
Nonfunctional GI tract	Obstruction, ileus
	Distal to site of possible enteral access
	Malnutrition awaiting surgery and need ≥7 days
	Prolonged ileus (≥7 days) with poor nutritional status
	Intractable vomiting or diarrhea
	For losses >500–1,000 mL/d
	Unable to maintain adequate nutritional status
	Short bowel syndrome
	Inability to absorb adequate nutrients enterally
	<60 cm small bowel may require indefinite provision
Inability to adequately utilize GI tract	Slow progression of enteral feeding
	Unable to provide at least 60% nutrient needs enterally for ≥7 days
	Enterocutaneous Fistula
	Fistula exhibits increased output with enteral feeding
	High-output fistula (>200 mL/day)
	Unable to safely gain enteral access
	Patient at nutritional risk
	Anticipated duration of need ≥7 days
Perioperative support	Preoperative
	Severely malnourished and EN not feasible
	Provide for at least 5–7 days preoperatively
	Postoperative
	If severely malnourished and initiated preoperative, begin as soon as resuscitated
	Provide if anticipate therapy to be for ≥7 days
Critical care	Unable to gain enteral access
	Resuscitated and hemodynamically stable
	Expected to remain NPO ≥ 7 days
Severe pancreatitis	If enteral feeding worsens condition
	Provide if anticipate therapy to be for ≥7 days
Contraindications	
No central venous access	Safe access not achievable
EN as alternative therapy	All means of providing EN not attempted
Well nourished, short duration	No indication of nutrition risk
	Anticipated need ≤7 days
Postoperative provision only	If not provided preoperatively
	Provide postoperatively only after 7 days of EN not being feasible
Grim prognosis when PN will be of no benefit	End-of-life issues preclude nutrition support

draining wounds or fistulas, skin exfoliation as in burns, and accuracy of protein and amino acid intake data.

Serum Proteins

Because of the flaws with nitrogen balance studies, serum transport proteins listed in Table 3-3 (e.g., transferrin, and prealbumin) have been used to potentially identify adequacy of nutrition intervention. All of these proteins have other functions separate from their use with nutrition assessment. Because of its rapid turnover and simplicity of assessment, serum prealbumin has historically been preferred over serum albumin and transferrin for nutritional assessment and monitoring of hospitalized patients. Prealbumin is mostly synthesized in the liver. During an anabolic state, it correlates with positive nitrogen balance. The use of serum proteins for nutrition assessment assumes that decreased levels are solely caused by malnutrition.

Aside from energy and protein intake affecting serum protein levels, there are also multiple nonnutritional factors that alter their serum values. The acute-phase response to injury is a systemic response to stress and inflammation. The liver reprioritizes transport protein synthesis (e.g., albumin, prealbumin) by downregulating their synthesis and upregulating the synthesis of acute-phase proteins (e.g., CRP). Transport proteins become a marker of severity of illness and inflammation, not malnutrition. Altering the nutritional plan when a prealbumin level is low and a CRP is high will not result in improved nutritional status and may result in complications of overfeeding. However, once the inflammation resolves and CRP levels decrease, then it may be reasonable to alter the nutritional plan if prealbumin levels remain low. In addition, due to the long half-life of serum albumin and its depletion with large fluid volumes, it is not an accurate marker during acute illness, but has been shown to be a good prognostic indicator of surgical outcome when evaluated in the preoperative, ambulatory care setting.

Other Biochemical Parameters

Other various laboratory assays exist that reflect a change in nutrition status, tolerance, or response to nutrition therapy. Electrolyte and micronutrients should be evaluated when deficiencies or toxicities are suspected. Hepatic, renal, and respiratory function strongly affects a patient's dietary prescription and should be included in the nutrition assessment and monitoring process. Iron levels, iron transport proteins, hemoglobin, and hematocrit with indices may determine an anemia of nutritional origin. Serum magnesium and calcium vary inversely with albumin levels. Correction of total serum levels of these elements should be made for serum albumin levels. Currently, only calcium has an accepted correction value calculated by the formula: $Ca_{(true)} = Ca_{(serum)} + 0.8(Alb_{(normal)} - Alb_{(actual)})$. Measurements of ionized calcium can also be used. In general total magnesium levels >1.5 mg/dL, even without albumin correction, rarely result in metabolic consequences.

COMPLICATIONS OF INITIATING NUTRITIONAL THERAPY

Refeeding Syndrome

Patients with significant premorbid malnutrition may not tolerate either the acute volume increase or caloric load. Proportional increases in carbohydrate-dependent electrolytes such as magnesium and phosphorus, protein-dependent electrolytes such as potassium, and volume-dependent electrolytes such as sodium should be made as the macronutrients are increased. This has been termed the refeeding syndrome. Refeeding syndrome may be defined as a constellation of fluid, micronutrient, electrolyte, and vitamin imbalances that occur within the first hours to days following nutrient infusion in a chronically starved patient. Refeeding syndrome can include hemolytic anemia, respiratory distress, paresthesias, tetany, and cardiac arrhythmias. Typical laboratory findings include hypokalemia, hypophosphatemia, and hypomagnesemia. Reported risk factors for refeeding syndrome include alcoholism, anorexia nervosa, marasmus, rapid refeeding, and excessive dextrose infusion. In these patients, dextrose should be limited initially to 100 to 150 g/day. In addition careful observation of potassium, magnesium, and phosphorous levels is necessary as they may fall rapidly with refeeding.

Transition from Parenteral to Enteral Nutrition

The goal in all patients is to transition from PN to EN, either via tube feeding or orally. Before discontinuing PN, assurance that the patient is consuming and absorbing adequate nutrients enterally is imperative. PN should be sequentially decreased as the enteral intake and tolerance improves to avoid complications of overfeeding. PN may be discontinued once the patient is tolerating approximately 60% to 75% of goal nutrients via the enteral route. For patients who are eating, PN may be reduced and discontinued over a 24- to 48-hour period. If PN is inadvertently but abruptly discontinued in patients who are not eating, all insulin should be stopped and blood glucose levels should be monitored for 30 to 120 minutes after discontinuation of PN. Based upon the blood glucose levels, appropriate therapy for hypoglycemia should be implemented. Previously, most clinicians advocated the immediate initiation of 10% dextrose in water ($D_{10}W$) if PN was abruptly discontinued, but most clinicians now find that it is unnecessary and that patient monitoring is adequate. If PN was used as a vehicle for medication or electrolyte administration, an alternate plan should be made once it is discontinued.

NUTRITIONAL CONCERNS FOR PATIENTS UNDERGOING SURGERY

Digestive Tract Surgery

The digestive tract is a very metabolically active organ involved in digestion, absorption, and metabolism of many nutrients; therefore, various surgical interventions involving the GI tract can result in malabsorption and maldigestion leading to nutritional deficiencies. Several examples of these are included in Table 3-12. Understanding where nutrients are absorbed in the intestinal tract will aid in determining which nutrient may become deficient postoperatively (Figure 3-1). Improving nutritional status preoperatively is important for optimal postoperative recovery.

Head and Neck Surgery

Head and neck cancer surgery patients usually present for surgery malnourished due to their disease state. Often, the tumor inhibits the patient's ability to chew and swallow normally. Preoperative treatment may involve radiation and/or chemotherapy to reduce tumor bulk. These therapies may

TABLE 3-12	Nutrition Consequences of Intestinal Surgery
Location	**Potential Consequence**
Proximal small intestine	Malabsorption of vitamins and minerals Calcium, magnesium, iron, Vitamins A, D
Gastric bypass	Protein–calorie malnutrition from malabsorption due to dumping, unavailability of bile acids and pancreatic enzymes due to anastomotic changes
	Bezoar formation
Distal small intestine	Malabsorption of vitamins and minerals Water soluble (folate, vitamins B_{12}, B_1, B_2, C, pyridoxine)
	Protein–calorie malnutrition due to dumping
	Fat malabsorption
	Bacterial overgrowth if ilealcecal valve resected
Colon	Fluid and electrolyte malabsorption—Potassium, sodium, chloride

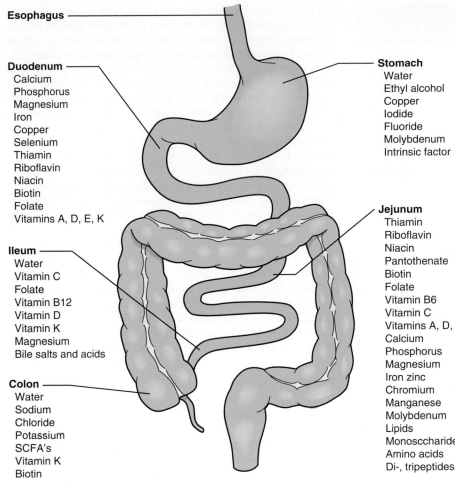

Esophagus

Duodenum
Calcium
Phosphorus
Magnesium
Iron
Copper
Selenium
Thiamin
Riboflavin
Niacin
Biotin
Folate
Vitamins A, D, E, K

Ileum
Water
Vitamin C
Folate
Vitamin B12
Vitamin D
Vitamin K
Magnesium
Bile salts and acids

Colon
Water
Sodium
Chloride
Potassium
SCFA's
Vitamin K
Biotin

Stomach
Water
Ethyl alcohol
Copper
Iodide
Fluoride
Molybdenum
Intrinsic factor

Jejunum
Thiamin
Riboflavin
Niacin
Pantothenate
Biotin
Folate
Vitamin B6
Vitamin C
Vitamins A, D, E, K
Calcium
Phosphorus
Magnesium
Iron zinc
Chromium
Manganese
Molybdenum
Lipids
Monosccharides
Amino acids
Di-, tripeptides

FIGURE 3-1. Nutrient absorption in the GI tract.

worsen the ability to swallow, so even though patients can consume some liquids and soft foods, it is often not enough to support nutritional needs. A long history of alcohol and tobacco use is commonly found among these patients, which may also affect nutrient intake. Patients typically will require nutrition therapy postoperatively as they may receive chemotherapy and/or radiation therapy, which can further delay return of adequate oral nutrient consumption. If the tumor size permits, placement of a percutaneous endoscopic gastrostomy (PEG) tube preoperatively can be performed for perioperative EN therapy. Placing a PEG, open gastrostomy, or nasoenteric feeding tube intraoperatively can be used postoperatively for EN therapy. Plans should be made as to how nutrition therapy will be provided postoperatively to avoid the use of PN if feasible.

Esophageal Surgery

There are several medical conditions that affect the esophagus and inhibit the ability to swallow. These conditions include corrosive injuries and perforation, achalasia, gastroesophageal reflux disease, and partial or full obstruction caused by cancer, strictures, or congenital abnormalities. Usually, surgical intervention is required to correct the abnormality and involves removal of a segment or the entire esophagus. The esophageal tract is then replaced with either the stomach (gastric pull-up) or the intestine (colonic/jejunal interposition). A gastric pull-up procedure results in displacement of the stomach in the thoracic cavity. This procedure results in a reduced stomach

capacity, with potential delayed gastric emptying and dumping syndrome. Another option for reestablishing esophageal continuity is by interposing a segment of colon or jejunum between the distal esophageal remnant and the stomach, or duodenum after subtotal gastrectomy. Complications following this procedure include dysphagia, strictures, and leakage at the anastomotic site. These patients may be limited to a soft or liquid diet preoperatively due to dysphagia or strictures. If the patient is unable to consume adequate nutrients orally, then a nasoenteric feeding tube may be passed if feasible. A PEG tube is not indicated if a gastric pull-up procedure is planned as the stomach is used to make the esophageal conduit; thus, a hole resulting from a gastrostomy tube would be contraindicated. Patients may require preoperative PN if the esophagus is obstructed. Intraoperatively, a jejunal feeding tube may be placed to allow for postoperative EN therapy until adequate oral intake is achieved. If enteral access is not obtained intraoperatively, then PN is indicted because patients may not resume oral intake for 7 to 10 days.

Gastric Surgery

Any gastric surgical procedure carries a chance that malnutrition can develop as a result of several postoperative consequences (Table 3-13). Dietary modifications are a key component of the medical therapy following these surgical procedures. Patients who have undergone gastric resection including the pylorus have an increased gastric emptying rate. This can result in dumping syndrome (early vs. late) caused

TABLE 3-13	Potential Nutrition Related Complications with Gastric Surgery

Procedure	Potential Complications
Vagotomy	Impairs proximal and distal motor function of the stomach
Total gastric and truncal vagotomy	Digestion and emptying of solids are retarded
	Emptying of liquids is accelerated
Total gastrectomy	Early satiety, nausea, vomiting
	Weight loss
	Inadequate bile acids and pancreatic enzymes availability due to anastomotic changes
	Malabsorption
	Protein–calorie malnutrition
	Anemia
	Dumping syndrome
	Bezoar formation
	Vitamin B_{12} deficiency
	Metabolic bone disease
Subtotal gastrectomy with vagotomy	Early satiety
	Delayed gastric emptying
	Rapid emptying of hypertonic fluids

by rapid release of a hyperosmolar load into the small bowel. This results in a constellation of symptoms: nausea, cramping, palpitations, sweating, weakness, hypotension, and diarrhea. Many patients will adapt to this after several weeks following surgery, but there are those that may need to restrict their diet indefinitely. Table 3-14 lists recommended dietary modification

for postgastrectomy patients who suffer from these symptoms. Oral supplements may be provided to increase nutrient intake, but these need to be isotonic and should not contain simple sugars. Unfortunately, many oral supplements do contain simple sugars and are hyperosmolar; therefore, they are not well tolerated postoperatively. As patients may become dehydrated due to excessive diarrhea or vomiting, they should be discouraged from drinking beverages with high simple sugar contents (e.g., Gatorade, fruit juices). The World Health Organization oral rehydration solution is the ideal beverage for these patients to consume. An ideal rehydration solution should contain water, sodium, potassium, bicarbonate, and small amounts of glucose to promote small intestinal water absorption and replenish fluid losses. PN is only indicated if enteral access is not available and the patient is malnourished and not able to tolerate adequate nutrients orally.

Anemia is a common consequence of gastric surgery. Anemia can be a result of a deficiency or malabsorption of one or more nutrients, including iron, folate, and vitamin B_{12} (Table 3-15). Total gastrectomy and some subtotal gastrectomy patients require periodic intramuscular vitamin B_{12} injections. Metabolic bone disease can also be a late complication of gastric surgery. In addition to consuming dietary calcium, patients require calcium and vitamin D supplementation.

Intestinal Surgery

If excessive lengths of intestine are removed, nutritional consequences can arise depending on the location of resection (Figure 3-1). Short bowel syndrome may occur if more than 50% of the small intestine is removed. This syndrome is characterized by severe diarrhea or steatorrhea, malabsorption, and malnutrition. Often, the patient will require long-term PN to maintain nutritional status and fluid and electrolyte balance.

TABLE 3-14	Postgastrectomy/Antidumping Diet

Principles of Diet

Postoperatively, some discomfort (gas, bloating, cramping) and diarrhea may occur. To reduce the likelihood of these symptoms, a healthy, nutritionally complete diet should be followed. Each person may react to foods differently. Foods should be reintroduced into the diet slowly.

Diet Guidelines

1. Eat small, frequent "meals" per day.
2. Limit fluids to 4 ounces (1/2 cup) at a meal. Just enough to "wash" food down.
3. Drink remaining fluids at least 30–40 min before and after meals.
4. Eat slowly and chew foods thoroughly.
5. Avoid extreme temperatures of foods.
6. Use seasonings and spices as tolerated (may want to avoid pepper, hot sauce).
7. Remain upright while eating and at least 30 min after eating.
8. Avoid simple sugars in foods and drinks.
   Examples: fruit juice, Gatorade, PowerAde, Kool-Aid, sweet tea, sucrose, honey, jelly, corn syrup, cookies, pie, doughnuts.
9. Complex carbohydrates are unlimited. Example: Bread, pasta, rice, potatoes, vegetables
10. Include a protein containing food at each meal.
11. Limit fats (<30% of total calories).
    Avoid fried foods, gravies, fat-containing sauces, mayonnaise, fatty meats (sausage, hot dogs, ribs), chips, biscuits, pancakes.
12. Milk and dairy products may not be tolerated due to lactose. Introduce these slowly in the diet if they were tolerated preoperatively. Lactose-free milk or soymilk is suggested.

TABLE 3-15	**Nutrient Deficiencies Associated with Gastric Surgery**

Deficiency	Causes

Microcytic anemia	Iron malabsorption or deficiency
	• Total and subtotal gastrectomy
	• Achlorhydria leads to insufficient
	  • cleavage of iron from food to which it's bound
	  • reduction and solubilization of ferric iron to the ferrous form
	• BII more common as primary sites of absorption bypassed
	• Reduced intake of iron-rich foods due to intolerance and reduced gastric capacity
	• Supplementation: 325 mg ferrous sulfate twice daily with coadministration of vitamin C

Macrocytic anemia	Folate, vitamin B_{12} deficiency, or anemia • Achlorhydria leads to insufficient liberation of vitamin B_{12} from protein foods it is bound • Decreased intrinsic factor leads to decreased binding of vitamin B_{12} • Reduced intake of protein-rich foods due to intolerance and reduced gastric capacity • Intramuscular vitamin B_{12} monthly injections (1,500 µg)
Metabolic bone disease	Calcium deficiency or malabsorption • BII more common than BI procedure due to bypassing the duodenum and proximal jejunum • Rapid gastric emptying can reduce absorption • Fat malabsorption can lead to insoluble calcium soap formation • Vitamin D malabsorption may accompany fat malabsorption, which can impair calcium and phosphorous metabolism • Daily supplementation: 1,500 mg calcium, 800 IU vitamin D

Pancreaticoduodenectomy

In cases of ampullary, duodenal, and pancreatic malignancy, a pancreaticoduodenectomy may be performed. This procedure is one of the most technically difficult and challenging GI surgeries and involves resecting the distal stomach, the distal common bile duct, the pancreatic head, and the duodenum. Three anastomoses must be performed: pancreatic duct to the GI tract, choledochojejunostomy, and gastrojejunostomy. The pylorus-sparing pancreaticoduodenectomy has become the preferred variation as it carries fewer postoperative nutritional consequences. Common complications following these procedures include delayed gastric emptying, dumping syndrome (if a non–pylorus-sparing procedure is performed), weight loss, diabetes mellitus, and possible malabsorption due to pancreatic exocrine insufficiency. Nutrient guidelines following these procedures are similar to those following a gastrectomy, but also may include exogenous pancreatic enzyme replacement if exocrine dysfunction is suspected.

Ileostomy and Colostomy

An ileostomy or a colostomy may be required in the varieties of intestinal lesions, obstruction, necrosis, or inflammatory bowel disease of the distal small intestine or colon or when diversion of fecal matter is necessary. These procedures involve the creation of an artificial anus on the abdominal wall by incision into the colon or ileum and bringing it out to the surface, forming a stoma. A pouch is placed externally over the stoma to collect the fecal matter. In general, patients with ostomies should eat regular diets. Foods that are gas forming or difficult to digest may be avoided to reduce undesired side effects. In the case of high-output ostomies (>800 mL/day), patients may need to avoid hypertonic, simple-sugar–containing liquids and foods, fatty foods, and foods high in insoluble fiber to reduce outputs.

LOOKING AHEAD

Nutritional assessment and support of surgical patients impacts surgical outcome. With increased pressure to decrease hospital stay and complications, nutritional status of patients is likely to become even more closely scrutinized by regulatory agencies, our hospitals, and payers. The role of PN in the achievement of full nutritional support is undergoing renewed interest and investigation, as is tailored enteral nutritional support. Prevention of complications will likely become even more important, emphasizing the role and benefit of preoperative nutritional supplementation when possible.

SAMPLE QUESTIONS

Questions

Choose the best answer for each question.

1. A 27-year-old man is in the intensive care unit 24 hours after an automobile collision. He has a left pneumothorax, multiple broken ribs, a ruptured spleen requiring splenectomy, a pelvic fracture, and bilateral femur fractures. He is intubated. He has received 6 units of PRBCs and is currently receiving IV fluids. Which one of the following best describes his metabolic response?

   A. Insulin is the major mediator of the stress response.

   B. Glycogen stores can be used for 7 days.

   C. Energy expenditure is decreased by 30%.

   D. Hepatic reprioritization of protein synthesis favors acute-phase proteins.

   E. Epinephrine and adrenocorticotropic hormone (ACTH) production are reduced.

2. A 66-year-old man is in the intensive care unit 10 days following colon resection for perforated diverticulitis. He has a history of chronic obstructive pulmonary disease (COPD) and is unable to wean from the ventilator. He has been maintained on total parenteral nutrition (TPN) and has started tube feeding. The most likely nutritional cause for failure to wean from the ventilator would be

   A. too much protein.

   B. refeeding syndrome.

   C. underfeeding.

   D. overfeeding.

   E. hyperphosphatemia.

3. A 45-year-old man was admitted to the hospital 3 days ago with nausea and vomiting due to a gastric outlet obstruction. Further studies have confirmed a gastric cancer involving the antrum of the stomach. He has a history of alcohol abuse and being homeless. The patient is thin and has temporal wasting and exposed ribs. He has an albumin of 1.9 g/dL. A nasogastric tube was placed on admission, and he was started on TPN. What is his surgical risk for perioperative complications?

   A. Moderate risk for developing surgical complications

   B. Moderate risk for developing wound complications only

   C. Low risk for developing surgical complications

   D. Cannot assess risk for surgical complications

   E. High risk for developing surgical complications

4. A 48-year-old woman is in the hospital because of nausea, vomiting, and abdominal pain. She has a history of multiple abdominal surgeries for small bowel obstruction. On admission, she was quite thin with temporal and thenar muscle wasting. Her albumin level was 1.7 g/dL. A nasogastric tube was inserted and she has been receiving TPN for 2 days. You are now called by her nurse because, in addition to nausea and abdominal pain, she's begun to feel short of breath and have tingling in her fingers. She suddenly goes into cardiac arrest. Laboratory values now show potassium—2.4 mEq/L, magnesium—1.3 mEq/L, phosphorus—1 mg/dL, and glucose—350 mg/dL. What nutritional complication may have resulted in this patient's condition?

   A. Marasmus

   B. Refeeding syndrome

   C. Overfeeding

   D. Underfeeding

   E. Kwashiorkor

5. A 46-year-old man with an enterocutaneous fistula has been maintained on TPN for several weeks. The fistula has healed and prior to removing the central line, the patient is given a unit of packed red blood cells through his central line for his chronic anemia. Two hours into his red cell infusion, a rapid response is called when the nurse discovers the patient comatose and hypotensive. What is the most likely cause of the patient's condition?

   A. Hypokalemia

   B. Transfusion reaction

   C. Hypoglycemia

   D. Air embolus

   E. Catheter-related sepsis

Answers and Explanations

1. Answer: D

The injury stress response is mediated by the counter-regulatory hormones, including ACTH, epinephrine, glucagon, and cortisol, along with the proinflammatory cytokines such as interleukins 1 and 6. Insulin is diminished during this response. The stress response results in the marked increase of energy expenditure, which is proportional to the size of the stress. Glycogen stores are rapidly depleted within 12 to 24 hours. Protein synthesis in the liver is reprioritized to produce acute phase proteins.

2. Answer: D

Patients with COPD have difficulty weaning from the ventilator secondary to CO_2 retention. Feeding with both TPN and enteral feeding is likely to provide glucose loads far in excess of 4 g/kg/day, resulting in lipogenesis. The respiratory quotient (RQ) for lipogenesis is 8.7, which signifies a high CO_2 production. This additional CO_2 could make it very difficult for a COPD patient to wean from the ventilator. (Parenteral Nutrition Advantages and Disadvantages)

3. Answer: E

Patients with a poor baseline nutritional status undergoing surgery are more likely to have increased morbidity and mortality. There is a linear increase in complications in patients undergoing elective gastrointestinal surgery as preoperative albumin decreases from normal to levels below 2 g%. Criteria to consider when screening surgical patients for nutritional risk include magnitude of the procedure, medications, recent weight changes, cachexia, changes in diet or appetite, and serum albumin. (Assessment of Nutritional Status)

4. Answer: B

Refeeding syndrome occurs when chronically starved patients lose the ability to tolerate acute changes in volume or caloric load. This results in a constellation of fluid, micronutrient, electrolyte, and vitamin imbalances within the first hours to days following nutrient infusion. These patients are typically hypokalemic, hypophosphatemic, hypomagnesemic, and hyperglycemic. This may result in symptoms, including hemolytic anemia, respiratory distress, paresthesias, tetany, and cardiac arrhythmias including sudden cardiac death. (Complications of Initiating Nutritional Therapy)

5. Answer: C

When long-term infusion of highly concentrated glucose solutions is suddenly discontinued, the increased endogenous insulin levels precipitate hypoglycemia. A blood transfusion would be more likely to elevate rather than depress potassium levels. Transfusion reactions cause fever, back pain, hemolysis, and hypotension, but not coma. The air embolus could cause both shock and unconsciousness and is unlikely to be associated with a blood transfusion. Catheter-related sepsis could induce fever and hypotension, but not coma. (Transition from Parenteral to Enteral Nutrition)

4

Surgical Bleeding: Bleeding Disorders, Hypercoagulable States, and Replacement Therapy in the Surgical Patient

HOLLIS W. MERRICK III, M.D. • KEVIN N. FOSTER, M.D. • TIMOTHY R. SHOPE, M.D. • RAVI S. SIDHU, M.D. • MARY R. SMITH, M.D. • JOHN P. SUTYAK, M.D.

Objectives

1. Using a patient's physical examination and medical history, determine the likelihood and etiology of possible bleeding disorders.

2. Name five major etiologic factors that may lead to bleeding disorders.

3. Describe the common laboratory tests that are used to assess hemostatic competence, and explain how these tests apply to the diagnosis of the conditions discussed in Objective 2.

4. Identify the acute etiologic factors that might be responsible for extensive bleeding in a patient who has received massive transfusions.

5. Name the conditions that might lead to disseminated intravascular coagulation (DIC).

6. Describe the recommended component replacement therapy for the etiologic categories named in Objective 2, as well as the definitive treatment for the underlying cause of each.

7. Describe the process of obtaining and transfusing blood, the symptoms of a transfusion reaction, and the diagnosis and appropriate management of the different types of transfusion reactions.

Bleeding may occur during surgical procedures. Although the volume of blood lost is usually not large enough to create a major problem, certain operations are invariably associated with large blood losses that may impair the normal hemostatic process. Additionally, some patients with congenital or acquired disorders of hemostasis require elective or emergency surgery. Therefore, surgeons must be prepared for significant blood losses that may have an adverse effect on patient recovery, and they must be able to manage blood loss in their patients. In addition, surgeons must be knowledgeable about common bleeding disorders and causes of hypercoagulable states, the components of blood replacement, and the problems associated with the transfusion of blood products.

THE HEMOSTATIC PROCESS

The hemostatic process involves an interaction between the blood vessel wall, platelets, and the coagulation proteins. After injury, hemostasis begins with a brief period (60 seconds) of vasoconstriction by the vessels that have muscular layers in their walls. This vasoconstriction in the region of injury only controls blood loss for a brief time and cannot offer significant control of bleeding.

The next step is mediated by **platelets**, which **adhere** to areas of vascular injury or to exposed subendothelial structures (Figure 4-1). After adhesion, the platelets extrude their contents, the most important of which is adenosine diphosphate (ADP). As a result, platelet **aggregation** occurs.

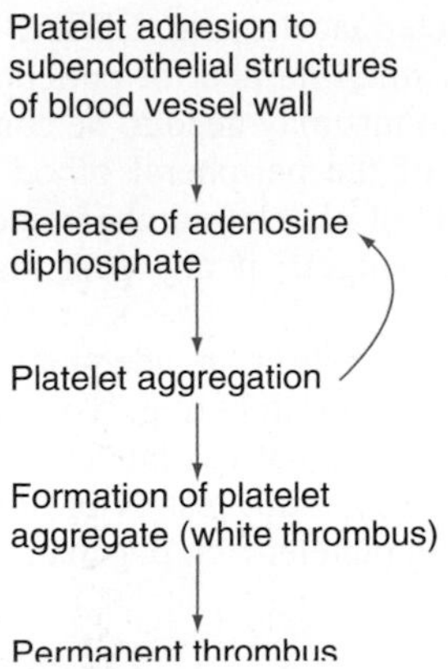

Platelet adhesion to
subendothelial structures
of blood vessel wall

↓

Release of adenosine
diphosphate

↓

Platelet aggregation

↓

Formation of platelet
aggregate (white thrombus)

↓

Permanent thrombus

FIGURE 4-1. Platelets in the control of bleeding.

This platelet-to-platelet sticking causes the initial white **thrombus**. The process from initial injury to the white (platelet) thrombus occurs independently of the coagulation pathways; hemophiliacs, for example, can generate a normal white thrombus. However, a more permanent thrombus is required for normal control of bleeding and eventual healing. This more permanent thrombus is created through the formation of **fibrin**.

The coagulation pathways use various **coagulation factors** to generate fibrin, which stabilizes the white thrombus (Figure 4-2). The **extrinsic (outside of the vessel) coagulation pathway** begins with tissue thromboplastin, which interacts with factor VII to convert factor X to factor Xa and

initiates the common pathway. The **intrinsic (inside of the vessel) coagulation pathway** requires factors XII, XI, IX, and VIII to interact and eventually convert factor X to Factor Xa. The **common coagulation pathway** involves factors X, V, II (prothrombin), and I (**fibrinogen**). The end product of coagulation is fibrin, which has a weak clot-stabilizing ability. Factor XIII (fibrin-stabilizing factor) is required to create fibrin of optimal strength (see Figure 4-2).

Bleeding may occur in the presence of a deficiency of any of the factors of the coagulation pathways, except factor XII. Additionally, although normal hemostasis requires calcium, hypocalcemia does not cause bleeding; it simply reduces effective coagulation when it is very low.

EVALUATION OF THE PATIENT

Detecting and correcting bleeding disorders before surgery is the best way to avoid major bleeding problems during and after surgery. Therefore, a careful screening for bleeding risks is an essential part of the preoperative evaluation (Table 4-1).

History

Obtaining a detailed bleeding history *is the most important step* in evaluating patients for possible bleeding problems. Patients should be asked if they have had prolonged bleeding after dental extractions, minor cuts, or previous operations; if they have prolonged or frequent menses; if they have experienced bruising after minor injury; or if they experience nosebleeds. A history of "bleeders" in the family is also important to obtain. For the individual patient, a history of bleeding

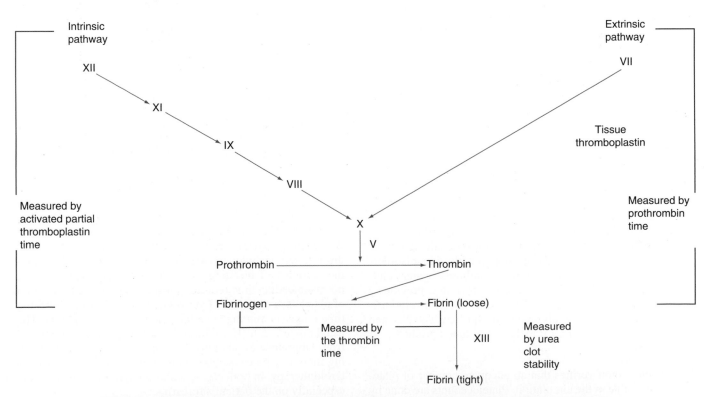

FIGURE 4-2. The coagulation pathways. Calcium and phospholipids from platelets are needed to permit the coagulation pathways to proceed at optimum rates. Activated factor XI in turn activates factor IX to become factor IXa. Factor IXa, in the presence of factor VII, platelet phospholipids, and calcium, activates factor X. The rate of this reaction is greatly increased by the presence of the platelet phospholipid. Coagulation pathways are tested as follows. Extrinsic pathway: measured by PT: monitor Coumadin therapy. Intrinsic pathway: measured by aPTT: monitor heparin therapy.

TABLE 4-1	Preoperative Evaluation for Bleeding and Clotting Disorders

Study	When Performed
History	In all patients as part of routine preoperative evaluation
Physical examination	As part of routine preoperative evaluation
Laboratory studies: PT, aPTT, platelet count, bleeding time, thrombin time	In patients with evidence of bleeding disorders or in whom excessive bleeding is anticipated because of the nature of the surgery

aPTT, activated partial thromboplastin time; PT, prothrombin time.

problems is the most important preoperative information that predicts unexpected bleeding complications. A complete history must be obtained of all medications, both prescription and over-the-counter, as these might induce or augment bleeding. Special note must be made of the presence of anticoagulant medications such as aspirin, clopidogrel (Plavix), and warfarin (Coumadin). This information is even more important than laboratory tests.

Physical Examination

The physical examination is less helpful than the history in assessing bleeding risk, because most patients with mild to moderate bleeding disorders do not have physical signs. The examiner should seek signs of blood disorders, such as splenomegaly, hepatomegaly, hemarthroses, petechiae, or ecchymoses, which can be associated with bleeding disorders. Petechiae and ecchymoses are typical of platelet disorders, whereas hematomas are more typical of abnormalities in the coagulation pathways.

Tests to Evaluate Hemostasis

Platelet count, prothrombin time (PT), and **activated partial thromboplastin time** (aPTT) should be determined in patients who provide any history suggestive of a bleeding disorder as part of the routine preoperative evaluation to exclude thrombocytopenia, a coagulation factor deficiency, or an acquired coagulation factor inhibitor. Certain other screening tests, such as bleeding time, a platelet function test on whole blood, or thrombin time, are indicated when the history or physical examination suggests a bleeding disorder. These studies should be carried out as a part of preoperative screening unless there has been a recent significant challenge to the patient's hemostatic competence. Acquired bleeding disorders (e.g., thrombocytopenia) or acquired inhibitors against clotting factors can lead to a bleeding disorder in a previously hemostatically healthy person. These tests are relatively inexpensive and may potentially avoid unexpected bleeding and the ensuing urgent need for transfusion of blood products.

Platelet Count

The platelet count verifies that an adequate number of platelets are available in the circulation. Platelet counts are done by automated methods in most institutions. However, automated counters may not be accurate at platelet counts of <40,000. Platelet counts may also be inaccurate if many red cell fragments are present or in cases of pseudothrombocytopenia due

to ethylenediaminetetraacetic acid (EDTA)-sensitive platelets, which occurs in a small number of patients. For this reason, very low platelet counts may need to be confirmed by manual methods. Review of the peripheral blood smear provides a reasonable estimate of platelet numbers and is recommended for patients before surgery if any past history of abnormal bleeding is known.

Platelets may be present in adequate numbers and yet may not function appropriately (e.g., von Willebrand disease, chronic renal failure, qualitative platelet defects). In this case, a platelet function–screening test is prolonged, and platelet aggregation done on platelet-rich plasma is abnormal.

Prothrombin Time

The PT measures the ability of the blood to form stable thrombi. It evaluates the adequacy of factors VII, X, and V; prothrombin; and fibrinogen (Figure 4-2), and both the extrinsic and common pathways. Its most common use is to monitor oral anticoagulation with warfarin (Coumadin). Today, PT is reported with the international normalized ratio (INR). The INR system overcomes the problem of variable sensitivity by standardizing the patient's PT ration using the international sensitivity index (ISI) of the particular thromboplastin. The ISI compares the locally used thromboplastin to an international standard thromboplastin. Therefore, the INR is the PT ratio that would have been obtained if the international standard had been used, and provides reliable comparisons between labs.

Mastery of the use of the INR as tool for anticoagulation therapy is important for physicians. Although most patients are adequately anticoagulated when the INR is between 2.0 and 3.0, certain patients, such as those with prosthetic heart valves, require more intensive therapy that results in an INR of up to 3.5.

Activated Partial Thromboplastin Time

The aPTT evaluates the adequacy of fibrinogen, prothrombin, and factors V, VIII, IX, X, XI, and XII in the intrinsic and common pathways (see Figure 4-2). It is the most commonly used test to monitor the effectiveness of unfractionated heparin therapy. The aPTT is normal in patients with factor VII deficiency, but it is elevated during Coumadin therapy because of reductions in factors II, IX, and X. The aPTT cannot be used to monitor most low molecular weight heparins (enoxaparin and dalteparin).

Bleeding Time

The bleeding time test is conducted by making two standard wounds (6 mm long, 1 mm deep) in the forearm of the patient with a spring-loaded lancet. The variation in the wound makes this test very technician dependent. The time from injury until the cessation of bleeding from both wounds is measured. A normal bleeding time requires adequate numbers and function of platelets and normal blood vessel walls. A normal bleeding time range (in minutes) is established by each laboratory. The usual range is 5 to 10 minutes, but small variations are found from laboratory to laboratory. A mild prolongation of bleeding time may be caused by aging skin or long-term corticosteroid therapy. In both cases, senile ecchymoses may be seen, especially on the patient's forearms.

A prolonged bleeding time is often associated with significant bleeding at surgery. Bleeding time may be prolonged by certain drugs (e.g., aspirin, or other nonsteroidal anti-inflammatory drugs [NSAIDs]). An abnormal bleeding time in a patient without a history of associated drug use indicates a potential bleeding disorder. A newly found prolonged bleeding time may be caused by any of the following disorders:

1. Thrombocytopenia
2. Abnormal platelet function because of
   a. Medication (e.g., aspirin)
   b. Dense granular disorders of platelets
3. von Willebrand disease (congenital or acquired)

Whole Blood Platelet Function Testing

Many centers no longer provide the bleeding time as a method for the evaluation of platelet function. Testing of platelet function on citrated whole blood specimens is replacing the bleeding time. The two most common instruments used are

1. PFA-100 (platelet function analyser-100). The basis of this testing instrument is *in vitro* cessation of high shear blood flow by a platelet plug, the port closure time. An initial screening is done using a collagen/epinephrine port closure time. If this time is prolonged, the collagen/ADP port closure time is evaluated. This method can identify aspirin suppression of platelet function-prolonged collagen/Epi port closure and normal collagen/ADP port closure time. Disorders of platelet function such as von Willebrand disease lead to prolongation of both port closure times.
2. VerifyNow. This instrument bases the evaluation of platelet function on platelet aggregation. The instrument can be designed to identify aspirin effect or clopidogrel effect on platelets.

Neither testing instrument has yet gained complete acceptance as a method of predicting excessive bleeding in a patient during surgery.

Thrombin Time

The thrombin time evaluates fibrinogen-to-fibrin conversion with an external source of thrombin. Prolongation of thrombin time can be caused by (1) low fibrinogen levels (hypofibrinogenemia); (2) abnormal fibrinogen (dysfibrinogenemia); (3) fibrin and fibrinogen split products; or (4) heparin (see Figure 4-2). Thrombin time is used to evaluate disseminated intravascular coagulation (DIC) and chronic liver disease.

Presurgical Evaluation of Bleeding Risk

The medical history is the most important "screening tool" in the assessment of the degree of bleeding risk in surgical patients. The age of onset of bleeding/bruising will assist in separating inherited from acquired bleeding disorders. Inherited disorders usually present in childhood if they are severe; mild inherited disorders may only manifest in adulthood, particularly at the time of surgery or other trauma. The site(s) of bleeding will provide clues concerning the underlying pathophysiology of the patient's bleeding disorder. Intracranial bleeding may be associated with disorders of platelet function (e.g., von Willebrand disease) or thrombocytopenia, while coagulation factor deficiencies usually present with intramuscular or intra-articular bleeding and less frequently gastrointestinal (GI), genitourinary (GU) or intracranial bleeding. The medication history including all prescription and over-the-counter drugs must be thoroughly clarified in patients suffering from bleeding events. The drug history must be all-inclusive even for drugs that are used sporadically. The family history warrants particular attention in addressing the pattern

of inheritance (e.g., males only as in hemophilia A or both males and females as in von Willebrand disease). The severity of bleeding in response to prior trauma, such as surgery (e.g., tonsillectomy or removal of wisdom teeth), is a very useful way to gauge the severity of the bleeding disorder: mild disorders may have very few manifestations of bleeding until challenged by significant trauma. Other significant medical disorders can magnify bleeding risk. This is particularly true of liver and kidney dysfunction.

The physical examination provides less information than the thorough history in the evaluation of patients with bleeding history or acute event. Platelet disorders, either low counts or dysfunction, will manifest similar physical findings. Petechiae, which are pinhead-sized red spots on the skin or mucous membranes that do not blanch on direct pressure, are typical of thrombocytopenia (low platelets) or thrombocytopathies (disorders of platelet function). Ecchymoses are also seen in these same disorders but usually reflect a more severe disorder and reflect significant bleeding into skin or mucous membranes. Coagulation factor deficiencies, on the other hand, present with bleeding into joints (hemarthrosis) and deep muscle bleeding (hematoma) as well as retroperitoneal bleeding. On occasion, there may be GI or GU bleeding in patients with coagulation factor deficiencies. The physical examination may not be helpful in patients with mild bleeding disorders. The site of bleeding may provide an indication of the etiology of the bleeding. Single-site bleeding is not usually due to a bleeding disorder, whereas multisite bleeding is more consistent with a bleeding disorder.

The following laboratory tests provide an adequate-enough evaluation of the patient's hemostatic competence to permit decisions to be made concerning the safety of proceeding with surgery.

- Platelet count and complete blood count (CBC)
- Platelet function testing
- aPTT
- PT
- Fibrinogen level or thrombin clotting time

CAUSES OF EXCESSIVE SURGICAL BLEEDING

Most patients are hemostatically normal before they enter the operating room. However, in some patients with large blood losses, generalized oozing is noted after a period of time. In addition, some operations (e.g., cardiopulmonary bypass, liver transplant surgery, prostate surgery, construction of portacaval shunts, trauma) are frequently associated with large blood losses. These patients develop consumption of clotting factors and platelets, causing the syndrome of consumptive coagulopathy or disseminated intravascular coagulopathy.

Preexisting Hemostatic Defects

Preexisting hemostatic defects should be suspected when a prior history of bleeding exists or when abnormal bleeding begins within the first 30 minutes of the operative period.

Congenital Bleeding Disorders

Congenital bleeding disorders, such as hemophilia and von Willebrand disease, are uncommon. Mildly affected patients may be asymptomatic. Type A hemophilia and von Willebrand disease are both characterized by deficiencies of factor VIII clotting activity (VIII), but there are differences in the

TABLE 4-2	Congenital Bleeding Disorders	
	Hemophilia A	**Von Willebrand Disease**
Incidence	25 per 100,000 in U.S.	1% of U.S. population
Pathophysiology	Reduced or absent factor VIII activity. Factor VIII molecule is present.	Reduced factor VIII activity and von Willebrand activity
Site of bleeding	Joints and intramuscular	Mucocutaneous
Inheritance	X-linked	Autosomal dominant
Patients	Only males	Males and females
Laboratory studies	Prolonged aPTT	Prolonged aPTT
	Normal PT	Normal PT
	Normal platelet function	Abnormal platelet function

TABLE 4-3	Causes of Acquired Bleeding Disorders
Advanced liver disease	
Anticoagulation therapy	
Acquired thrombocytopenia	
Platelet-inhibiting drugs	
Uremia	
Over-the-counter medications, e.g., herbal supplements	
DIC	
Primary/secondary fibrinolysis	

two disease processes (Table 4-2). Hemophilia is seen almost exclusively in males, and platelet function is normal. Von Willebrand disease affects people of both sexes. In addition to factor VIII deficiency, von Willebrand disease is associated with platelet dysfunction, which is diagnosed by decreased aggregation in response to ristocetin and is corrected by normal plasma. Von Willebrand disease is the most common inherited bleeding disorder. Although abnormal von Willebrand factor activity can be demonstrated in up to 1% of the population, the vast majority is asymptomatic with only 1 out of 10,000 showing any clinically significant signs. Von Willebrand factor has two principal functions: (1) carrier for factor VIII, preventing destruction of factor VIII in the circulation and (2) supporting platelet adhesion. Deficiency of von Willebrand activity is corrected with cryoprecipitate infusions or desmopressin (DDAVP) therapy. Cryoprecipitate is a fraction of plasma that contains von Willebrand factor, factor VIII clotting activity, and fibrinogen. DDAVP is given as an intravenous infusion or as nasal "snuff." DDAVP is a hormone that, in addition to other properties, leads to the release of von Willebrand factor from its endothelial cell storage sites. Von Willebrand disease has multiple subtypes. Von Willebrand multimer studies must be done prior to using DDAVP, as this medication must not be used in some less common types of von Willebrand disease, for example, type 2b.

Congenital platelet function disorders are uncommon and usually occur in patients who have a history of mucous membrane bleeding and easy bruising. Factor IX deficiency (e.g., Christmas disease, hemophilia B) is seen only in males and is less common (1 in 25,000 male births, about 3,300 cases in the United States) than type A hemophilia (1 in 5,000 to 10,000 male births). Type A hemophilia is treated with purified factor VIII products. Factor XI deficiency is found almost exclusively in Jewish patients.

Acquired Bleeding Disorders

Acquired bleeding disorders are more common than congenital bleeding disorders and may have a variety of causes (Table 4-3). Liver disease is a common cause of coagulation abnormalities. Inability of the liver to synthesize proteins leads to decreased levels of prothrombin and factors V, VII, and X (but not VIII), which may cause prolonged PT and aPTT. Alcohol ingestion may result in acute thrombocytopenia. Hypersplenism associated with splenomegaly may be associated with moderate thrombocytopenia due to splenic pooling of the platelets. Obstructive jaundice

may lead to clotting factor deficiencies, which can usually be corrected with parenteral vitamin K. Cirrhosis may also cause clotting factor deficiencies. These respond less well to vitamin K. However, gastrointestinal bleeding in the patient who has cirrhosis is usually caused by varices or gastritis rather than by a coagulation defect.

Anticoagulant therapy with heparin or oral anticoagulants (e.g., Coumadin) leads to acquired bleeding disorders. Coumadin causes depression of the clotting activity of four coagulation factors (II, VII, IX, and X). Because both the intrinsic and extrinsic pathways are affected by Coumadin, both PT and aPTT are prolonged. Coumadin effect can be reversed with fresh frozen plasma (FFP) in an emergency or with vitamin K. In cases of acute life-threatening hemorrhage (e.g., intracranial injury requiring emergent operation), recombinant activated factor VII has been successfully utilized to ameliorate the effects of warfarin.

Heparin prolongs both aPTT and thrombin time. Heparin (high molecular weight, or unfractionated heparin) works by increasing the speed with which antithrombin III binds to and neutralizes factors IXa, Xa, XIa, XIIa, and thrombin. Heparin effect can be reversed with protamine sulfate. A number of different low molecular weight heparins are available for use. It is important to recognize the specifics of various low molecular weight heparin preparations when selecting an agent for clinical use in specific settings. Low molecular weight heparin preparations are more difficult to reverse with protamine sulfate.

Acquired thrombocytopenia is caused by three mechanisms: (1) decreased platelet production in the bone marrow (e.g., aplastic anemia); (2) increased destruction of platelets in the peripheral blood (e.g., idiopathic thrombocytopenia purpura [ITP], DIC, heparin-induced thrombocytopenia [HIT]); (3) splenic pooling in an enlarged spleen (e.g., cirrhosis); or any combination of these three disorders (e.g., alcoholic liver cirrhosis).

Platelet function disorders are most commonly associated with medications (e.g., aspirin, clopidogrel, other NSAIDs). Unlike other NSAIDs, however, aspirin induces a defect that does not reverse; thus, patients should be instructed to avoid aspirin for 1 week before elective surgery. Clopidogrel (Plavix), used commonly for platelet-inhibiting effects, also has an irreversible effect on platelets. As with aspirin, clopidogrel should be stopped 7 to 10 days before surgery.

A second important cause of acquired platelet dysfunction is uremia. Patients who are uremic and are bleeding require dialysis before surgery to correct their platelet dysfunction.

TABLE 4-4	Mechanism of Action and Monitoring of Anticoagulants	
Mechanism of Action	**Anticoagulant**	**Laboratory Monitoring**
Xa inhibition and thrombin inhibition	Unfractionated heparin	aPTT or anti-Xa activity
Xa inhibition	Low molecular weight heparin	Anti-Xa activity
Production of inactive vitamin K–dependent clotting factors IX, X, VII, II (1972)	Warfarin	INR
Xa inhibition	Fondaparinux	Anti-Xa activity
Thrombin inhibition	Lepirudin, argatroban	aPTT

Medication-Associated Bleeding

Anticoagulants

All anticoagulants carry the risk of inducing bleeding in any patient. The most common anticoagulants that are currently in use include vitamin K antagonist (Coumadin) and heparins, both unfractionated and low molecular weight. A new class of anticoagulants, direct factor Xa inhibitors (Fondaparinux), is being used in specific settings but is likely to have expanded uses in the future. Direct thrombin inhibitors such as argatroban, bivalirudin, and lepirudin have limited indications; in particular, these drugs are used to treat patients with HIT.

Because of the increased risk of bleeding associated with all anticoagulants, great care must be taken in using these drugs (Table 4-4).

These medications must be used by knowledgeable practitioners and in settings where monitoring is available. Heparin in its unfractionated form can be monitored using the aPTT or anti-Xa activity, while low molecular weight heparins can be monitored, if needed, by only the anti-Xa activity. Anti-Xa inhibitors, such as Fondaparinux, are monitored using anti-Xa activity. Direct thrombin inhibitors, such as lepirudin, are monitored using the aPTT.

Platelet-Inhibiting Drugs

Drugs that inhibit platelet function fall into two groups. The first group consists of drugs that irreversibly inhibit platelet function. This group of drugs includes aspirin and clopidogrel (Plavix). When patients are taking these drugs and surgery is planned, the drug(s) must be stopped 7 to 10 days before planned surgery. If the surgery is required as an emergency, transfusion of platelets may be required to permit adequate hemostasis. The second group of drugs that can also alter platelet function does so by reversible inhibition of platelet function. The more commonly used drugs in this group include dipyridamole and abciximab. The platelet-inhibiting effect of these drugs disappears rapidly and usually permits surgery to proceed promptly.

Great care must be exercised in the use of anticoagulants and platelet-inhibiting agents. All medications used by the patient must be chosen with caution to ensure no adverse drug interactions occur.

Over-the-Counter Medications

Over-the-counter medications used by patients may cause bleeding. This is particularly true of herbal supplements. The following herbal supplements are known to be associated with an increased risk of bleeding, particularly in patients who are taking vitamin K antagonists: dong quai (*Angelica*), garlic, ginger, gingko biloba, ginseng, and St. John's wort. Patients often fail to advise physicians about herbal supplements because patients may not view them as medications.

Intraoperative Complications

Several common conditions contribute to bleeding during a surgical procedure. Shock may cause or aggravate consumptive coagulopathy. Massive transfusion of stored packed red blood cells may lead to bleeding. This bleeding occurs after rapid transfusion of 10 units or more of stored red blood cells over a 4- to 6-hour period. It is caused by low numbers of platelets and by dilution of the clotting factors as a result of the infusion of nonplasma fluids for volume support. For this reason, transfusion of platelets, plasma, cryoprecipitate, and calcium should be considered for patients receiving massive transfusion of red blood cells.

Acute hemolytic blood transfusion reactions may lead to DIC. When a patient is under general anesthesia, there may be no clues that incompatible blood has been infused until the onset of generalized bleeding as a result of DIC. The usual symptoms of an incompatible blood transfusion (e.g., agitation, back pain) do not occur under general anesthesia. Hemoglobinuria and oliguria provide additional clinical evidence of DIC.

Intraoperative bleeding from needle holes, vascular suture lines, or extensive tissue dissection can often be controlled through the use of local hemostatic agents. These include gelatin sponge (e.g., Gelfoam), oxidized cellulose (Surgicel), collagen sponge (Helistat), microfibrillar collagen (Avitene, Hemotene), topical thrombin (with or without topical cryoprecipitate), topical e-aminocaproic acid (EACA), and topical aprotinin.

Postoperative Bleeding

Fifty percent of postoperative bleeding is caused by inadequate hemostasis during surgery. Other causes of postoperative bleeding include a number of possible causes. Residual heparin that remains after cardiopulmonary or peripheral vascular bypass surgery can cause significant oozing or overt bleeding. Shock due to any cause that results in consumptive coagulopathy can lead to significant postoperative bleeding. Altered liver function after partial hepatectomy often is associated with bleeding. If a large portion of the liver is removed, the remaining liver may need 3 to 5 days to increase its production of clotting factors sufficiently to support hemostasis. Acquired deficiency of the vitamin K–dependent clotting factors (II, VII, IX, and X) can develop in patients who are poorly nourished and are receiving antibiotics. Supplementation with vitamin K in postoperative patients who are not able to adequately nourish themselves is essential to avoid developing these clotting factor deficiencies. Factor XIII deficiency is an uncommon disorder but must be considered as a possible cause for delayed postoperative bleeding. In this case, bleeding occurs 3 to 5 days after surgery. The diagnosis of this deficiency is confirmed by a factor XIII assay.

Disseminated Intravascular Coagulation

In any patient with postoperative bleeding, the possibility of DIC must be considered as a possible cause. This is particularly true if there is severe infection or shock. As the name DIC suggests, it is characterized by intravascular coagulation and thrombosis that is diffuse rather than localized at the site of injury. This process results in the systemic deposition of platelet–fibrin microthrombi that cause diffuse tissue injury. Some clotting factors may be consumed in sufficient amounts to eventually lead to diffuse bleeding. DIC may be acute or clinically asymptomatic and chronic. The etiology of DIC may be any of the following: (1) the release of tissue debris into the bloodstream after trauma or an obstetric catastrophe; (2) the introduction of intravascular aggregations of platelets as a result of the activation of platelets by various materials, including ADP and thrombin (which may explain the occurrence of DIC in patients with severe septicemia or immune complex disease); (3) extensive endothelial damage, which denudes the vascular wall and stimulates coagulation and platelet adhesion (as seen in patients with widespread burns or vasculitis); (4) hypotension that leads to stasis and prevents the normal circulating inhibitors of coagulation from reaching the sites of the microthrombi; (5) blockage of the reticuloendothelial system; (6) some types of operations that involve the prostate, lung, or malignant tumors; (7) severe liver disease; and (8) brain trauma or surgery may lead to DIC as the brain is rich in thromboplastin, which activates clotting if released into the circulation.

The diagnosis of DIC is established by the detection of diminished levels of coagulation factors and platelets. The following laboratory results may be useful in diagnosing DIC: (1) prolonged APTT; (2) prolonged PT; (3) hypofibrinogenemia; (4) thrombocytopenia; and (5) the presence of fibrin and fibrinogen split (FDP) products and positive D-dimers. The presence of fibrin and fibrinogen split products is caused by activation of the fibrinolytic pathway in response to activation of the clotting pathway. The D-dimer is a product of fibrin digestion by the fibrinolytic process.

The most important aspect of the treatment of DIC is to remove the precipitating factors (e.g., treating septicemia). If DIC is severe, replacement of coagulation factors is required to correct the coagulation defect. Cryoprecipitate is the best method to replace a profound fibrinogen deficit. Platelet transfusions may also be required. FFP is useful to replace other deficits that are identified, but it must be used judiciously if volume overload is a potential problem. The use of heparin to treat DIC is controversial. In rare cases, the coagulation must be inhibited with heparin or with drug therapy to prevent platelet aggregation. There is no conclusive evidence that using heparin alters the outcome of DIC. Because antithrombin III is consumed during DIC, the use of heparin as an anticoagulant may be severely compromised. Large trials are under way to evaluate the benefit of using antithrombin III concentrates and protein C concentrates as part of the treatment of DIC. Preliminary data from some trials are promising.

Bleeding Disorders Caused by Increased Fibrinolysis

Postsurgical bleeding may also be caused by disorders leading to increased fibrinolysis.

Primary fibrinolysis is a disorder that occurs when the fibrinolytic pathway is activated leading to the production of plasmin without antecedent activation of the coagulation pathways. Most commonly, primary fibrinolysis occurs after fibrinolytic therapy with drugs such as tissue plasminogen activator (tPA), which are used to lyse coronary artery or peripheral artery thromboses. Primary fibrinolysis is also seen in conjunction with surgical procedures on the prostate gland,

which is rich in urokinase. It also occurs in patients with severe liver failure. Very rare disorders of inhibitors of the fibrinolytic pathway (e.g., congenital deficiencies of α_2-antiplasmin) can also cause primary fibrinolysis. Treatment of these disorders is best accomplished by eliminating the precipitating cause such as discontinuing lytic therapy. Since the half-life of lytic agents is short (in minutes), bleeding usually stops rapidly.

If primary fibrinolysis becomes severe, EACA can be used for therapy. This drug must be used cautiously because it blocks the fibrinolytic pathway and may predispose the patient to thrombotic events.

Secondary fibrinolysis is most often seen in response to DIC. The coagulation pathway is activated, followed by the fibrinolytic pathway. Manifestations of this activation in laboratory tests include hypofibrinogenemia and the presence of fibrin split products and positive D-dimers. As the DIC is corrected, the secondary fibrinolysis resolves.

Hypercoagulable States in the Surgical Patient

Thromboembolism may occur for a number of reasons during the course of surgery and in the postoperative period (Table 4-5). Both congenital and acquired disorders can put surgical patients at risk for venous thromboembolism (VTE). The evaluation of patients for surgery must include an assessment of the degree of risk the patient has for a VTE event. Virtually all surgery carries varying degrees of risk for VTE from minimal to highly significant. A number of steps are essential in the assessment of the degree of risk in a patient.

The most important first step in the assessment of VTE risk is the medical history of the patient. The information to be obtained should address the following points. Has the patient suffered a VTE event before the age of 40 years or had an unprovoked VTE event at any age? A recurrent VTE event at any age can be a harbinger of a hypercoagulable state as can a thrombosis occurring at an unusual site (e.g., mesenteric vein thrombosis). Perhaps one of the most important points in the history is the family history, which can provide helpful clues about the risks for VTE in any patient. A significant positive family history can guide one to evaluate patients for inherited hypercoagulable risk factors.

TABLE 4-5	Differential Diagnosis of Hypercoagulable States by Site of Thrombosis
Arterial Thrombosis (e.g., Myocardial Infarction)	**Venous Thrombosis (e.g., VTE)**
Common: Antiphospholipid syndrome	Common: Factor V Leiden
Prothrombin 20210 mutation	Prothrombin 20210
HIT Syndrome	Protein C deficiency
Uncommon: Elevated PAI-1 activity	Protein S deficiency
Hyperhomocysteinemia	Antithrombin deficiency
t-PA Deficiency	Uncommon: Hyperhomocysteinemia
Anomalous coronary arteries	Factor XII deficiency
Vasculitis	Trauma
	Immobilization
	Pregnancy, oral contraceptive therapy, or hormone replacement therapy

A positive history for thrombosis associated with pregnancy, oral contraceptives, or hormone replacement therapy should alert practitioners to the possibility of an underlying hypercoagulable state. The specific complications of pregnancy that one must address in the history include recurrent fetal loss, fetal growth retardation, preeclampsia, or eclampsia. Each of these disorders can be an indicator of any underlying hypercoagulable state.

Associated disease states such as malignancy, autoimmune disorders, and chronic inflammatory state can magnify the risk for VTE, particularly if there is an underlying hypercoagulable state.

Circumstantial risk factors that add to a patient's risk for VTE include advancing age, pregnancy, immobilization, and trauma of any type including the planned surgery procedure. In addition, obesity is a significant risk factor for VTE, and as the amount of obesity in the United States continues to escalate, the risk for VTE in these patients will also. Interestingly, non-O blood group type blood does add to the patient's risk for VTE, likely due to the associated higher levels of von Willebrand factor and factor VIII.

An unexplained prolonged aPTT may herald the presence of an antiphospholipid antibody that may be associated with an increased risk for VTE in some patients. Thus the aPTT is a very useful part of the patient's preoperative evaluation.

Congenital Disorders

Congenital disorders associated with hypercoagulable states are diagnosed more frequently than in years past. They must be considered as possible risk factors for VTE in anyone with a positive family history or in patients presenting with a thrombosis at a young age (under 30 years of age). The most common cause of congenital hypercoagulable states is activated protein C resistance (APCR). The most common cause of APCR is the factor V Leiden mutation. Activated protein C binds to and neutralizes factors VIII and V, thus acting to regulate the rate at which the intrinsic and common pathways proceed. Genetically abnormal factor V (factor V Leiden) lacks the binding site for activated protein C; thus, factor V cannot be neutralized. Patients with factor V Leiden abnormality are predisposed to thromboembolic events. Additional causes of congenital hypercoagulable states include deficiencies of antithrombin III and proteins C and S. Protein C is present in the plasma in an inactive form. When thrombin is attached to thrombomodulin on the endothelial cell surface, protein C is activated. Protein S functions as a catalyst to this activation. Activated protein C has two functions: (1) as an anticoagulant (as described earlier) and (2) as an inducer of fibrinolysis. Hyperhomocysteinemia may also be associated with an increased risk of thrombosis. Some patients with hyperhomocysteinemia are found to have gene defects (e.g., MTHFR 6771). Prothrombin 20210 is an additional cause of a congenital hypercoagulable state (Table 4-6).

Acquired Hypercoagulable States

Acquired hypercoagulable states may result from a number of possible causes, which may include one or more of the following. Decreased production of naturally occurring anticoagulants, protein C and S, or antithrombin may occur in patients with significant liver disease.

Ineffective fibrinolysis secondary to reduced or defective plasminogen may also be present in patients with advanced liver disease. Very high levels of clotting factors, especially

TABLE 4-6	Initial Laboratory Evaluation of Hypercoagulable States
APCR ratio; if positive request factor V Leiden study	
Antiphospholipid antibody panel	
Antithrombin activity	
Protein C activity	
Protein S activity	
Fasting homocysteine	
Prothrombin 20210 study	
Von Willebrand activity	
Factor VIII clotting activity	

fibrinogen, von Willebrand factor, and factor VIII, which may occur in response to the stress of severe illness or trauma, have been associated with an increased incidence of VTE. Platelet counts $>1,000 \times 10^3/mm^3$ $(1,000 \times 10^9/L)$ may be seen in a small number of patients who have had a splenectomy particularly in the immediate postoperative period. Very high platelet counts are also associated with essential thrombocythemia, a myeloproliferative disorder.

The antiphospholipid antibody syndrome is an autoimmune disorder that may be associated with other autoimmune disorders or may develop in otherwise healthy people. The diagnostic criteria include a documented thrombotic event and/or pregnancy-associated morbidity and two positive antiphospholipid antibody tests done at least 12 weeks apart. Some cases of chronic DIC, as can be seen associated with malignancies, may present as a VTE.

HIT is the development of a low platelet count associated with the administration of heparin, in either its unfractionated or low molecular weight form. HIT predisposes to thrombosis. In a patient receiving heparin who develops a new or worsening thrombosis and a falling platelet count, HIT should be suspected and heparin stopped immediately. Most patients do not develop sufficient thrombocytopenia to cause bleeding. Recent (within 3 months) prior exposure to heparin may accelerate the process. The most common manifestations of HIT are arterial thrombosis causing strokes, myocardial infarctions, leg ischemia, and venous thrombosis causing deep vein thrombosis (DVT) or pulmonary embolism. The diagnosis is considered when the clinical scenario is compatible with HIT. The diagnosis is suggested with an enzyme-linked immunosorbent assay (ELISA), which detects circulating antibodies. However, this has a high false-positive rate and must be confirmed by a serotonin release assay (SRA). Since HIT predisposes to new thrombotic events, in addition to discontinuing heparin, it is necessary to anticoagulate these patients. Warfarin is contraindicated as it may cause skin gangrene (Coumadin-induced skin necrosis due to low protein C activity). Anticoagulation for a patient with confirmed or suspected HIT requires using one of the following thrombin inhibitors: argatroban, lepirudin, or danaparoid.

Management of Hypercoagulable States

Therapy for hypercoagulable states is primarily directed at (1) interfering with the coagulation pathways (with heparin, Coumadin, or both); (2) interfering with platelet function (with aspirin, clopidogrel, or other platelet-inhibiting drugs); and

(3) treating hyperhomocysteinemia (with folic acid, vitamin B$_{12}$, and other B vitamins). Therapy must be individualized both to the patient and to the site and severity of the thromboembolism. Great caution must be exercised when using warfarin in patients with protein C deficiency. These patients may develop "Coumadin-induced skin necrosis" if a long overlap period with heparin is not performed. This long overlap allows metabolism of all vitamin K–dependent proteins to reach a steady state. The duration of anticoagulation therapy requires careful consideration, and the risks and benefits of protracted anticoagulation therapy must be weighed against potential benefits.

During the perioperative period, therapy for patients with a history of thromboembolism and a documented hypercoagulable state must be planned carefully by both the surgeon and the hematologist. Low-dose heparin (5,000 international units [IUs]), subcutaneously administered, provides adequate protection from thromboembolism for short periods without compromising surgical hemostasis. Alternatively, low molecular weight heparin prophylaxis may be used. For patients with a documented hematologic risk factor for thrombosis (e.g., APCR) who have never had a thromboembolic event, prophylaxis with pneumatic compression boots or low-dose heparin is adequate. DVT prophylaxis is also covered in detail in Chapter 1, Perioperative Management of the Surgical Patient.

BLOOD REPLACEMENT THERAPY

Collection, Separation, and Storage of Blood Products

The vast majority of the blood products used in the United States are collected from volunteer donors in hospitals, community donation centers, and blood banks. Blood is typically collected from these donation centers as whole blood. The volume of a donated unit of whole blood is approximately 450 mL. This donated whole blood is initially stored in citrate–phosphate–dextrose (CPD) solution. There are few civilian indications for transfusion of whole blood. A more efficient use of donated blood is to separate whole blood into components and transfuse these individual components based on specific indications. Whole blood is separated into (1) red cells, (2) white cells, (3) platelets, and (4) plasma. Plasma is then often further separated into cryoprecipitate and specific clotting factor concentrates (for instance factor VII).

Whole blood is collected into a bag containing the anticoagulant CPD solution using a closed sterile system. A centrifuge is used to separate the platelet-rich plasma from the packed red cells into a separate container. A storage life extender (typically a crystalloid solution containing dextrose, sodium, adenine, and mannitol) is added to the packed cells, and the packed cells are frozen.

The platelet-plasma suspension is rich in platelets and has a volume of about 200 mL. Platelet concentrate is then obtained by recentrifuging the platelet-plasma suspension at a higher speed resulting in a concentration of platelets that are then resuspended in a small volume of plasma. Generally, four to six adult platelet concentrates of the same blood type are pooled together to provide an adequate dose of platelets. Many centers provide single donor pheresis platelet transfusion, which is equivalent to six platelet concentrate packs. Platelets are stored at room temperature and require continuous gentle agitation. They can be stored for a maximum of 5 days.

The platelet-poor plasma fraction is frozen and stored as FFP. It can be stored frozen for up to 12 months. Alternately, the platelet-poor plasma fraction can be further fractionated into cryoprecipitate and/or other plasma fractions or specific coagulation factors. Cryoprecipitate is rich in factor VIII and fibrinogen. It can also be stored frozen for up to 12 months.

Blood Component Therapy

Typing and Cross-Matching of Blood Components
There are over 600 known red blood cell antigens organized into 22 blood groups systems. Most of these antigens are minor and are not involved in immunologic transfusion reactions. Only two groups have immunologic relevance: the ABO and Rhesus groups. Both of these antigen groups are routinely identified for blood transfusions. An individual's ABO type is genetically determined and falls into one of four blood types depending upon the presence or absence of two antigens: A and B. Type A only has the A antigen. Type B has only the B antigen. Type AB has both antigens, and type O has neither antigen. Type O is the most common, and type AB is the least common. An individual must receive ABO-matched blood, and ABO incompatibilities are the most common cause of fatal transfusion reactions.

The Rhesus, or Rh antigen system, is also clinically important in matching blood for transfusion. There are over 50 Rh antigens, but only D antigen testing is performed. If an individual has the D antigen on the surface of red blood cells, this person is Rh positive. If an individual does not have the antigen, he/she is Rh negative.

Cross-matching is performed after A/B/Rh matching and is a process where serum from the recipient is mixed with the red blood cells from the donor. Antibodies in recipient serum to donor red cells will cause a positive crossmatch and preclude transfusion of those donor cells to this recipient.

Transfusion of Red Blood Cells
Red blood cell transfusions are available as (1) whole blood, (2) packed red blood cells, (3) washed red blood cells, (4) leukoreduced red blood cells, and (5) divided or pediatric unit red blood cells. As stated above, there are no firm current indications for transfusion of whole blood with the exception of the need for massive transfusion or need for life-saving transfusion when component therapy is not available. Washed red cells are washed with saline to remove plasma, and leukoreduced red cells are filtered to remove leukocytes. Both of these preparations are used to transfuse red cells to patients who have had hypersensitivity or nonhemolytic febrile transfusion reactions to ordinary packed red blood cells, and for transplant patients. Pediatric unit red blood cells are adult units that have been divided and concentrated into a smaller volume. The result is that a pediatric or divided unit will increase the hematocrit to the same degree in a child as in an adult when corrected for the child's weight and the volume transfused.

Transfusion of packed red cells is indicated when the red blood cell mass is decreased (as reflected in the hemoglobin concentration and/or hematocrit level) with subsequent compromise of oxygen delivery to tissues and organs. The decision to transfuse and the amount of blood to be transfused is multifactorial and must be individualized based on a number of factors including (1) the reason for anemia; (2) the degree and acuity/chronicity of anemia; (3) underlying medical conditions, particularly cardiac, pulmonary, and renal disease; (4) anticipated future transfusion requirements; and (5) hemodynamic instability.

Packed red blood cells are typically stored frozen between 1°C and 6°C. The frozen cells have a shelf life of approximately 42 days. During this period of time, there is a gradual but progressive reduction in red cell viability. Red cells stored for 5 weeks have a 70% viability. Ideally, transfused red cells survive in recipient circulation for 5 to 6 weeks. Metabolism during frozen storage causes an increase in both potassium and hydrogen ion concentration, resulting in an acidic pH level for the transfusion solution. Additionally, leukocytes and platelets within the packed red cell suspension become nonfunctional within hours of freezing. There is some evidence that transfusion of red cells stored for more than 21 days may not be as effective as transfusion of red cells stored for a shorter time.

One unit of packed red blood cells contains about 200 mL of red cells and 30 mL of plasma in a total volume of about 310 mL. The hematocrit of a typical unit of packed red blood cells is approximately 57%. Transfusion of one unit of packed red cells into an average 70-kg person can be expected to raise the hematocrit by 3% and the hemoglobin concentration by 1 g/dL.

Transfusion Triggers

Clinical experience with Jehovah's Witness and other populations who refuse blood transfusions has demonstrated the safety of relatively low hematocrits and hemoglobin concentrations. A large clinical trial demonstrated that transfusing at a hemoglobin concentration of 7 g/dL was as least as safe as transfusing at 10 g/dL. Numerous retrospective studies in a variety of patient populations have found an association between blood transfusion and poor patient outcome. Numerous other studies are in progress to define the appropriate transfusion trigger. At this point in time, arbitrary transfusion triggers cannot be justified based on numeric value alone. The decision to transfuse must be made based on individual physiologic need and clinical circumstances.

Transfusion of Fresh Frozen Plasma

FFP is the platelet-poor plasma removed from whole blood. It is typically stored frozen and thawed just prior to use. FFP contains all of the required coagulation factors in physiologic concentrations (note: the coagulation factors are not concentrated). FFP does not contain red cells, leukocytes, or platelets. FFP does not require crossmatch prior to use, but donor and recipient must be ABO compatible. Rh status is not considered.

Indications for transfusion of FFP include patients with laboratory evidence of coagulation factor deficiency (e.g., abnormally elevated PT or aPTT) with clinical bleeding or need for an invasive procedure. Coagulation factor deficiencies can result from dilutional coagulopathy following massive transfusion or resuscitation, congenital synthesis defects, anticoagulant medications such as warfarin or heparin, liver disease, malnutrition, and other acquired disorders.

Thawed FFP should be used as soon as possible and within 24 hours. One unit of FFP is approximately 225 mL in volume and can be expected to raise the level of individual coagulation factors by about 1%. The actual therapeutic effect of FFP transfusion will depend upon the several factors including absolute level of coagulation factors, synthetic capacity, and ongoing losses.

Transfusion of Platelets

Platelet transfusion is indicated for patients who have clinical coagulopathy and either an absolute thrombocytopenia or a relative thrombocytopenia due to platelet dysfunction. Platelet dysfunction often occurs as a result of medical conditions, such as renal failure, or as a result of medications such as NSAIDs and clopidogrel (Plavix). Patients with normal platelet function typically do not experience clinical bleeding until the absolute platelet count drops to 30,000 to 50,000 platelets/μL and often even lower than this. In contrast, patients with dysfunctional platelets will often manifest clinical bleeding with platelet counts in the normal range. Additional information regarding the need for platelet transfusion can be obtained from a bleeding time or whole blood platelet function testing. A bleeding time at least twice the normal limit generally indicates need for platelet transfusion.

Platelet suspensions contain some plasma and few red blood cells or leukocytes. Once received, platelets must be administered within 4 hours. The therapeutic effect of platelet transfusion depends upon the patient's pathologic state, existing platelet count, level of platelet function, weight of the patient, and number of platelet concentrates transfused. The absolute rise in platelet count is also variable. A typical transfusion of six platelets concentrates can be expected to raise the platelet count by approximately 50,000 to 100,000 platelets/μL.

Clinical Use of Recombinant factor VII

Recombinant activated factor VII (rFVIIa) was initially developed for use in hemophiliac patients. Factor VII binds to tissue factor and becomes activated. It then subsequently activates the extrinsic clotting pathway. It has a rapid onset and short duration of action. Evidence is growing that rFVIIa may also correct some factor deficiencies and clinical bleeding caused by consumptive coagulopathies, such as those associated with massive transfusions in association with trauma and surgery. Although larger trials are lacking, case reports and series have demonstrated efficacy and safety in a variety of indications and at a variety of doses. Most clinicians reserve rFVIIa for the most dire and refractory medical and surgical bleeding emergencies. Clinical trials using rFVIIa in trauma, intracranial bleeding, liver surgery, and spine surgery are ongoing.

Clinical Management of Hemophilia and von Willebrand Disease

As previously discussed, von Willebrand disease is the most common hereditary human coagulation disorder. It causes a complex coagulopathy arising from absolute or relative deficiencies of von Willebrand factor. This factor, which is produced by endothelial cells and megakaryocytes, causes platelet adhesion and formation of the platelet plug. It also forms a complex with factor VIII, facilitating its activity. Von Willebrand disease has several different pathologic subtypes. The classic syndrome is caused by a reduction in factor VIII activity. Clinical manifestations include bruising, nosebleeds, bleeding gums, menorrhagia, and muscle or joint bleeding. Most patients require no treatment. However, patients undergoing surgery or actively bleeding may require intervention. Typically, the therapeutic goal is to maintain serum levels of 25% to 50%, or 50 to 100 IU/dL, for hemostasis. Cryoprecipitate is the most reliable source of von Willebrand factor and is transfused to maintain serum activity and clinical effect. The National Institutes of Health have published a clinical guide for the treatment of von Willebrand disease (http://www.nhlbi.nih.gov/guidelines/vwd/).

Hemophilia A is a sex-linked hereditary coagulation disorder characterized by reduction in factor VIII activity. The disease affects males, and clinical manifestations include easy bruising and bleeding from minor injury. Particularly troublesome are episodes involving bleeding into joints, muscles, gastrointestinal tract, and central nervous system. Many patients with severe forms of the disease require regular transfusion of factor VIII. Additionally, patients with active bleeding, trauma, or surgery require additional transfusion. After minor surgery or trauma, 20% factor VIII activity should be maintained. For more severe trauma or surgery, 50% to 75% and even up to 90% of factor VIII activity should be maintained by transfusion. Traditionally, pooled plasma factor VIII has been transfused. More recently, recombinant factor VIII has become available.

Complications of Blood Component Therapy

Transfusion of blood and blood components is safe and efficacious when used for the correct indications. However, transfusion is not without risk. There are multiple potential side effects associated with transfusion. These can be divided into (1) metabolic derangements, (2) immunologic reactions, (3) infectious complications, (4) volume overload, and (5) pulmonary complications. There are also special considerations when transfusing large amounts of blood products over a short period of time, a massive transfusion.

Metabolic Derangements

Metabolic complications of transfusion therapy are typically seen in the context of transfusion of large amounts of blood products, or transfusion of older blood products, or both. Most common are hypocalcemia, hyperkalemia, hypokalemia, and hypothermia.

Hypocalcemia can be seen with rapid transfusion (>100 mL/minute) of citrated blood products. This can manifest as muscle tremors, ST segment prolongation, delayed T waves, ultimately decreased cardiac output, and ventricular fibrillation. This can be avoided by transfusing slowly and/or by administering calcium as intravenous supplementation. Supplementation rarely requires >1 g of intravenous calcium.

Both hyperkalemia and hypokalemia can be seen by the following mechanisms. The concentration of potassium in a unit of packed red cells is often 75 mmol/L or greater after 35 days of frozen storage. Massive rapid transfusion of >10 units of packed red cells can result in hyperkalemia. Following transfusion, the infused potassium can be rapidly taken back up into red cells resulting in hypokalemia.

Finally, rapid transfusion of multiple units of frozen blood products can result in precipitation or worsening of hypothermia. A patient receiving multiple transfusions should receive the products though a fluid warmer, and the patient's core temperature should be monitored closely.

Immunologic Transfusion Reactions

Although ABO and Rh compatibility testing and crossmatching can obviate some of the more serious transfusion reactions, minor untested and unidentified antigens and antibodies can still precipitate immunologic reactions (Table 4-7). Immunologic transfusion reactions include (1) febrile reactions, (2) acute and delayed hemolytic transfusion reactions, (3) thrombocytopenia, (4) anaphylactic shock, (5) urticaria, (6) graft versus host disease, and (7) immune suppression.

TABLE 4-7	Management of Transfusion Reactions

	Reaction	Management
Minor transfusion reaction	Fever, rash, urticaria	Observation, antihistamines
Major transfusion reaction	Fever, chills, hypotension, bleeding in previously dry areas, hemoglobinuria, decreased urine output	Immediate cessation of transfusion, send the unit of blood back to the blood bank for recrossmatch, volume expanders, pressors (mannitol, Lasix)

Febrile reactions are probably the most common immunologic transfusion reactions. These reactions typically occur as a result of antileukocyte antibodies. Symptoms and signs include fever, chills, and tachycardia. Hemodynamic instability can occur in severe cases. Patients with minor reactions can be managed expectantly, and the therapy is largely supportive. The transfusion should be stopped. Pretreatment with aspirin, antipyretics, and antihistamines can prevent future reactions. Alternately, transfusion of leukocyte-reduced red cells can also be effective.

Acute hemolytic reactions can vary in severity from minor to catastrophic. Most hemolytic reactions occur as a result of a clerical error and transfusion of ABO-mismatched blood. They can begin quickly with administration of as little as 50 mL of donor blood. Symptoms include sensation of hot or cold, flushing, chest pain, and low back pain. Signs include fever, hypotension, tachycardia, hematuria, hemoglobinuria, bleeding, and possibly acute renal failure. Successful management of hemolytic transfusion reactions rests on early diagnosis and prompt intervention. The transfusion must be immediately stopped. The remaining transfusion blood and a sample of the patient's blood are returned to the laboratory for retyping and crossmatching. Transfused and patient blood is also sent for culture to differentiate from contamination (see below). Care is primarily supportive. Hemodynamic instability is treated with volume expansion and pressors, if necessary. Some clinicians recommend administration of mannitol and/or loop diuretics such as furosemide to maintain urine output. Severe renal failure may require hemodialysis.

Graft versus host disease occurs when immunosuppressed patients receive donor leukocytes in blood component therapy. These cells are unrecognized as foreign cells by the recipient, and they mount an immune response against recipient tissues. Onset of symptoms is often delayed for weeks and includes fever, rash, liver dysfunction, and diarrhea. This can be prevented by using leukocyte-reduced red cells and/or irradiated red cells.

Transmission of Infectious Agents

Transmission of infectious agents following transfusion is rare but not zero. Blood can transmit infections caused by bacteria, viruses, and parasites.

Platelets are the most likely blood component to transmit bacterial microorganisms. Clinical manifestations include fever, chills, tachycardia, and possibly hypotension. It can be difficult to differentiate bacterial infection from other transfusion reactions. The transfusion must be stopped, the blood tested as described above, and anti-infective and supportive measures initiated.

Probably the most feared complication of transfusion of blood products is the transmission of viruses such as hepatitis B and C and the human immunodeficiency virus (HIV). Careful screening of donors and testing of blood has resulted in reduction of viral transmission to very low levels. The risk of hepatitis B transmission is about 1 in every 200,000 transfusions, and for hepatitis C, about 1 in 2 million transfusions. Likewise, the risk of HIV transmission is about 1 in 2 million transfusions.

Transfusion-Related Acute Lung Injury

Transfusion-related acute lung injury (TRALI) occurs in about 1 out of every 5,000 transfusions. It can occur with transfusion of any blood component, but is most common with transfusions that contain plasma, such as FFP or platelets. TRALI is characterized by noncardiogenic pulmonary edema following transfusion. The inciting event in TRALI is unknown, but likely immunologic. Onset of pulmonary edema and respiratory insufficiency is generally within 1 to 2 hours of beginning the transfusion, but it can happen up to 6 hours after a transfusion. Recently, a delayed TRALI syndrome has been recognized, in which onset may be delayed up to 72 hours after transfusion. Treatment of TRALI is supportive. Patients usually require intubation and mechanical ventilation. The pulmonary edema is due to pulmonary vascular mechanics and not fluid overload, so diuresis is not usually indicated. As the pathophysiology is thought to involve activation of host neutrophils by donor antibodies and cytokines, plasma-rich components such as FFP are associated with an increased risk of TRALI. Preventive efforts are focused on limiting blood donors associated with elevated anti-HLA antibodies such as multiparous women. Mortality is 5% to 10% for TRALI.

Massive Transfusion

Massive transfusion has been variously defined as the administration of >10 units of packed red blood cells in <24 hours, administration of a patient's total blood volume in <24 hours, or transfusion of more than one-half of a patient's blood volume in 1 hour. Complications of massive transfusion include dilutional coagulopathy as a result of decreased levels of clotting factors and platelets, oxygen transport abnormalities, electrolyte and acid–base derangements, hypothermia, possibly disease transmission, and development of acute respiratory distress syndrome (ARDS).

Recent studies have focused on development and implementation of massive transfusion protocols (MTPs) to simultaneously improve outcome and reduce the number of blood products transfused. One study demonstrated that transfusion of packed red blood cells, FFP, and platelets in a 1:1:1 ratio resulted in a significant decrease in 24-hour mortality in trauma patients. Other studies have confirmed these results and have also demonstrated decreased use of packed red cells, FFP, and platelets.

Key features of an effective MTP include (1) activation of protocol early in the patient's clinical course, (2) automatic delivery of red cells, FFP, and platelets in a 1:1:1 ratio, and (3) early use of rFVIIa in some studies. Proper use of an MTP should result in increased survival and decreased use of blood products.

Blood Substitutes

Blood substitutes, also known as artificial blood, can be divided into two broad categories based on intended function: volume expanders and oxygen carriers. Volume expanders are inert and are used to increase blood volume. Volume expanders may be crystalloid based, such as Lactated Ringer's solution, or colloid-based, such as hydroxyethyl starch. Volume expanders can be used to replace volume following blood loss, either as a substitute for blood if the blood loss is relatively small, or as a replacement until packed red blood cells can be transfused, in the case of larger blood loss.

Oxygen carriers are either perfluorocarbon based or hemoglobin based, depending upon the transport mechanism used. Oxygen-carrying blood substitutes are potentially useful in a number of settings and for a number of reasons including (1) easy storage and long shelf life, (2) no viral transmission, (3) potential use in battlefield and extreme scenarios, (4) immediate availability, and (5) may possibly be more cost-effective.

A recent multicenter trial of a hemoglobin-based oxygen-carrying blood substitute reported equivalent safety and efficacy to packed red cells when used in emergent trauma situations. However, the Food and Drug Administration (FDA) declined approval of this substitute due to safety concerns, and the product is not currently in production.

---

thePoint ✳ Go to http://thePoint.lww.com/activate and use your scratch-off code on the inside cover of this book to access bonus chapters, question bank, videos, and more.

SAMPLE QUESTIONS

Questions

Choose the best answer for each question.

1. A 26-year-old man is brought to the emergency department (ED) after being stabbed in the left arm in a fight. Brisk bleeding from the wound was controlled by the EMTs with a pressure bandage. Fifteen minutes later in the emergency department, the bandage is removed and only slight oozing is noted. The most likely mechanism for decreased bleeding at this time is

   A. platelet activation and aggregation.

   B. activation of the extrinsic coagulation cascade pathway.

   C. activation of prothrombin to thrombin.

   D. activation of the intrinsic coagulation cascade pathway.

   E. local peripheral vascular vasoconstriction.

2. A 55-year-old woman is scheduled for a craniotomy to remove a brain tumor. She has a history of hypertension and hypercholesterolemia, and she underwent coronary artery angioplasty with a stent placed 6 months ago. Current medications include enalapril, pravastatin, and clopidogrel. Which one of the following would most likely be prolonged?

   A. Activated partial thromboplastin time (APTT)

   B. Bleeding time

   C. Prothrombin time (PT)

   D. Thrombin time

   E. Activated clotting time (ACT)

3. A 50-year-old man is started on IV heparin for a peripheral arterial thrombosis. Three days later, it is noted that his platelet count has dropped from 200 to 35. What is the next best step in management?

   A. Discontinue heparin and administer lepirudin

   B. Continue heparin and administer argatroban

   C. Discontinue heparin and administer aspirin

   D. Discontinue heparin and administer Coumadin

   E. Continue heparin and administer a platelet transfusion

4. A patient is scheduled to undergo open abdominal aortic aneurysm repair. During preoperative testing, it is determined that his blood type is B negative. This means

   A. he has circulating antibodies to Rh antigens.

   B. he has circulating antibodies to A antigens.

   C. he has circulating antibodies to B antigens.

   D. he has no circulating antibodies to ABO antigens.

   E. his red blood cells have A antigens.

5. A 65-year-old woman with severe symptomatic anemia secondary to chronic renal disease is being transfused with packed red blood cells. A couple of minutes into the transfusion, she complains of back pain, chest pain, and shortness of breath. The most likely diagnosis is

   A. transfusion-related acute lung injury (TRALI).

   B. delayed hemolytic transfusion reaction.

   C. acute hemolytic transfusion reaction.

   D. transfusion-related volume overload.

   E. transfusion-related hyperkalemia.

Answers and Explanations

1. Answer: E

Hemostasis involves the blood vessel wall, platelets, and the coagulation cascade leading to fibrin deposition. After injury, local vasoconstriction is the first hemostatic process to occur. This is followed by platelet adherence, activation, and aggregation. Finally, the coagulation cascade leads to the deposition of fibrin.

2. Answer: B

Clopidogrel is a platelet-inhibitor medication that is often used after the placement of intravascular stents to prevent thrombosis. Like aminopsalicylic acid (ASA), clopidogrel is nonreversible; therefore, it should be stopped 7 to 10 days before surgery if normal coagulation is required. Prolonged bleeding time is associated with platelet dysfunction. The APTT (intrinsic and common pathways), PT (extrinsic and common pathway), and thrombin time (formation of fibrin from fibrinogen) evaluate specific aspects of the coagulation cascade.

3. Answer: A

Heparin-induced thrombocytopenia (HIT) is a hypercoagulable state manifest by arterial and venous thromboses. HIT occurs as a result of antibody formation to heparin–platelet complexes and results in thrombocytopenia due to intravascular platelet activation and aggregation. There is no indication for platelet transfusion. It can occur due to administration of any type of heparin. Patients must be anticoagulated with an alternative agent such as argatroban, lepirudin, or danaparoid. In this setting, starting Coumadin without starting one of these alternative agents is contraindicated as the initiation of Coumadin therapy is associated with a transient hypercoagulable state.

4. Answer: B

Multiple blood cell antigens exist; however, the ABO and Rh antigens are most clinically relevant. A person with blood type B means his red cells have the B antigen. His plasma will have antibodies to the A antigen. In patients who are Rh negative, they will not have circulating antibodies to the Rh antigens unless they have been previously exposed (e.g., during pregnancy of an Rh-negative mother with an Rh-positive fetus). Hence, in this case, although he is Rh negative, he will not have circulating Rh antibodies.

5. Answer: C

Acute hemolytic transfusion reactions are usually caused by clerical error resulting in the administration of ABO mismatched blood. Host antibodies bind to antigens in donor red blood cells resulting in hemolysis. This may result in renal failure and shock. Patients complain of shortness of breath, chest pain, and back pain. The most appropriate course of action is to stop the transfusion, provide supportive therapy, and have the blood rechecked. TRALI usually occurs after completion of transfusions. Volume overload and hyperkalemia are unlikely only minutes into a transfusion.

5
Shock: Cell Metabolic Failure in Critical Illness

KENNETH W. BURCHARD, M.D. • KAREN BRASEL, M.D., M.P.H. • JEANNETTE CAPELLA, M.D. • TIMOTHY A. PRITTS, M.D., Ph.D.

Objectives

1. Define shock, and list the two primary mechanisms that may cause cellular malfunction consistent with shock.

2. List the etiologies of these primary mechanisms that are responsible for shock.

3. List the clinical information (i.e., history, physical examination, diagnostic tests, hemodynamic parameters) that helps to determine which of the two primary mechanisms is the predominant cause of shock in an individual patient.

4. Describe the interrelation between the two primary mechanisms of shock as a cause of cellular injury.

5. Describe the general principles of management that diminish cellular injury from the primary mechanisms of shock.

Traditional descriptions of shock often use systolic hypotension (<90 mm Hg) as the defining variable. According to this criterion, classification schemes that use categories such as hypovolemic/hemorrhagic, septic, cardiogenic, and neurogenic shock are common and imply that evidence of an altered circulation is sufficient to make the diagnosis. However, certain etiologies of hypotension (i.e., neurogenic vasodilation after spinal cord injury) do not necessarily cause cellular or organ injury. In addition, cellular and organ injury may develop without hypotension reaching 90 mm Hg. Therefore, definitions of shock based on the circulatory measurement of systolic blood pressure are potentially misleading and narrow in scope.

A broader definition is that shock is a condition in which total body cellular metabolism is malfunctional. This concept dates back to 1872 when S.D. Gross described shock as "a rude unhinging of the machinery of life." When treated aggressively, this cellular metabolic dysfunction, the rude unhinging, is reversible. When allowed to continue, however, shock results in cellular death, organ damage, and the eventual death of the individual.

During the 20th century, many theories were developed to explain this cellular injury and death (i.e., disorders of circulation, disorders of the nervous system, toxemia). By 1950, two competing theories were predominant: (1) shock is secondary to inadequate oxygen delivery; (2) shock is secondary to a toxic cellular insult that can progress even when sufficient oxygen is delivered. Such conditions as severe hemorrhage and cardiac malfunction (i.e., **hypoperfusion**) were recognized throughout the century as etiologies of inadequate oxygen delivery. The recognition that the primary toxins of cellular injury are endogenous (the products of tissue injury or the consequent inflammatory response) rather than exogenous (endotoxin) emerged primarily over the last three decades. Tissue injury and the associated inflammatory response result in the production or activation of cellular molecules (i.e., cytokines, superoxide radicals, prostaglandins, adhesion molecules) that promote local cellular activation, tissue repair, and host defenses. However, sometimes this local response incites similar responses in cells that are distant from the primary insult. The result is systemic **inflammation** that can cause organ malfunction and shock.

Simultaneously, during the last two decades, experimental and clinical studies showed that these two mechanisms of cellular injury are not competitive or exclusive, but are most often additive during shock states. Simply stated, *hypoperfusion begets inflammation, and inflammation begets hypoperfusion.* The clinician must be alert to this association and must approach each patient who has the manifestations of total body cellular malfunction with the dual goals of carefully assessing circulation for oxygen delivery and the state of inflammation for cell toxicity. Restoring excellent circulation and treating severe inflammation are the primary tenets for managing the patient with shock.

This chapter describes the pathophysiology that links hypoperfusion with inflammation, provides clinical guidelines for recognizing **hypoperfusion** and **severe inflammation**, and outlines management strategies that can limit these mechanisms of cellular injury.

TABLE 5-1	Hemodynamic and Oxygen Delivery Variables	
Item	**Definition**	**Normal**
CVP	Central venous pressure; CVP = RAP; in the absence of tricuspid valve disease, CVP = RVEDP	5–15 mm Hg
LAP	Left atrial pressure; in the absence of mitral valve disease, LAP = LVEDP	5–15 mm Hg
PAOP	Pulmonary capillary occlusion pressure; PAOP = LAP, except sometimes with high PEEP levels	5–15 mm Hg
MAP	Mean arterial pressure, mm Hg; MAP = DP + 1/3 (SP − DP)	80–90 mm Hg
CI	Cardiac index; CI = CO/m² BSA	2.5–3.5 L/min/m² BSA
SI	Stroke index; SI = SV/m² BSA	35–40 mL/beat/m²
SVR	Systemic vascular resistance; SVR = (MAP − CVP) × 80/CO	1,000–1,500 dyne-s/cm⁵
PVR	Pulmonary vascular resistance; PVR = (MAP − PAOP) × 80/CO	100–400 dyne-s/cm⁵
Cao_2	Arterial oxygen content (vol%); $Cao_2 = 1.39 \times Hgb\ Sao_2 + (Pao_2 \times 0.0031)$	20 vol%
$C\bar{V}O_2V$	Mixed venous oxygen content (vol%); $C\bar{V}O_2 = 1.39 \times Hgb \times S\bar{V}O_2 + (P\bar{V}O_2 \times 0.0031)$	15 vol%
$C(a − v)\ o_2$	Arterial venous O_2 content difference; $C(a − v)o_2 = Ca\ o_2 − C\bar{V}O_2$ (vol%)	3.5–4.5 vol%
O_2D	O_2 delivery; $O_2D = CO \times Cao_2 \times 10$; 10 = factor to convert mL O_2/100 mL blood to mL O_2/L blood	900–1,200 mL/min
O_2C	O_2 consumption; $O_2C = (CaO_2 − C\bar{V}O_2) \times CO \times 10$	250 mL/min

BSA, body surface area (m2); CO, cardiac output; DP, diastolic pressure; LVEDP, left ventricular end-diastolic pressure; PaO₂, PAOP, pulmonary artery occlusion pressure; PEEP, positive end-expiratory pressure, arterial PO₂ (mm Hg); PV̄ O₂, mixed venous PO₂; RAP, right atrial pressure; RVED, right ventricular end diastolic pressure; Sao₂, arterial oxygen saturation (%); SV̄ O₂, mixed venous oxygen saturation; SP, systolic pressure; SV, stroke volume.

NORMAL PHYSIOLOGY OF CIRCULATION AND INFLAMMATION

The main function of circulation is to deliver oxygen to the capillaries. The determinants of total body oxygen delivery are listed with other commonly measured or calculated hemodynamic variables in Table 5-1. As the formula for oxygen delivery shows, the pulmonary component is limited to providing adequate arterial oxygen saturation (≥90% saturation is usually present when PaO₂ ≥ 60 mm Hg). This goal is usually readily achieved with modern respiratory therapy. Hemoglobin can be increased with the transfusion of red blood cells (RBCs), but this strategy has limited applicability (see below). Usually, the most difficult component to treat is **cardiac output**. The determinants of cardiac output are organized by both the variables that affect **ventricular function** and the variables that affect **venous return**. Depending on clinical circumstances, sometimes it is more useful to use the logic associated with alterations in ventricular physiology to enhance circulation, and sometimes it is more useful to use the logic associated with alterations in venous return physiology. This logical application of one circulatory physiology versus another ("physiologic") is described in more detail in the hypoperfusion section.

Ventricular Physiology

The major determinants of ventricular performance are listed in Table 5-2. **Preload** is the magnitude of myocardial stretch, the stimulus to muscle contraction that is described by the Frank-Starling mechanism (Figure 5-1), whereby increased stretch leads to increased contraction until the muscle is overstretched (commonly recognized clinically as congestive heart failure [CHF]; see the Hypoperfusion Section). Preload is most appropriately measured as end-diastolic volume. Because volume is not easily measured clinically, the direct proportion between ventricular volume and ventricular end-diastolic pressure

allows the measurement of pressure (typi cally measured as central venous pressure [CVP] for the right side of the heart and pulmonary capillary wedge or pulmonary artery occlusion pressure [PAOP] for the left side of the heart) to estimate volume.

Ventricular **afterload** is determined primarily by the resistance to ventricular ejection that is present in either the pulmonary (pulmonary vascular resistance) or systemic arterial tree (systemic vascular resistance). With constant preload, increased afterload diminishes ventricular ejection, and decreased afterload augments ejection (see Figure 5-1). **Contractility** is the force of contraction under conditions of a predetermined preload or afterload. Factors that may increase or decrease contractility are listed in Table 5-3. A change in contractility, like a change in afterload, results in a different cardiac function curve (see Figure 5-1).

The combined influence of increasing contractility and decreasing afterload to improve ventricular function is also shown in Figure 5-1. Heart rate is directly proportional to cardiac output (not to cardiac muscle mechanics) until rapid rates diminish ventricular filling during diastole.

Venous Return

Venous return is described by the following formula:

$$VR = (MSP − CVP)/(RV + RA/19).$$

TABLE 5-2	Determinants of Ventricular Function
Preload	
Afterload	
Contractility	
Heart rate	

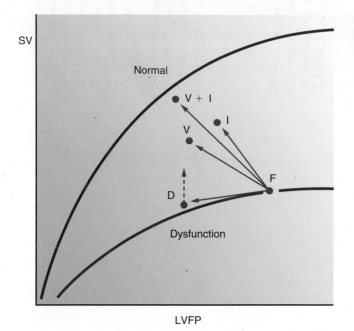

FIGURE 5-1. Expected hemodynamic response in severe left ventricular dysfunction to administration of diuretics (D), inotropic drugs (I), vasodilators (V), and a combination of vasodilators and inotropics (V + I). SV, stroke volume; LVFP, left ventricular filling pressure; F, failure.

where MSP, mean systemic pressure; CVP, central venous pressure (right atrial pressure); RV, venous resistance; and RA, arterial resistance.

This equation (including the constant, 19) was formulated by Guyton in 1973 using both calculations and empirical observation. As might be expected, alterations in arterial resistance have much less effect on venous return than alterations in venous resistance, as indicated in the formula.

MSP is not the same as mean arterial pressure. MSP is the pressure in small veins and venules. This pressure must be higher than CVP in the periphery so that blood can flow from the periphery to the thorax. Venous resistance occurs primarily in the large veins in the abdomen and thorax. Arterial resistance occurs mostly in the arterioles.

Factors that alter venous return variables are listed in Table 5-4. Surgical patients frequently have diseases or therapeutic interventions that may inhibit venous return.

Physiology of Inflammation

The normal response to tissue injury is essential for eliminating infectious organisms, wound healing, and restoring normal tissue function. The initial response to tissue damage

TABLE 5-3	Factors That Affect Myocardial Contractility
Increased	**Decreased**
Catecholamines	Catecholamine depletion and receptor malfunction
Inotropic drugs	α and β blockers
	Calcium channel blockers
Increased preload	Decreased preload
Decreased afterload	Overstretching of myocardium
	Severe inflammation and ischemia

TABLE 5-4	Factors That Alter Venous Return Variables
Increased Venous Return	
Increased MSP	
Increased vascular volume	
Increased vascular tone	
External compression	
Trendelenburg position (increased MSP in lower extremities and abdomen)	
Decreased CVP	
Negative pressure respiration	
Decreased venous resistance	
Decreased venous constriction	
Diminished Venous Return	
Decreased MSP	
Hypovolemia	
Vasodilation	
Increased CVP	
Intracardiac	
Congestive heart failure	
Cardiogenic shock	
Tricuspid regurgitation	
Right heart failure	
Extracardiac	
Positive pressure respiration	
PEEP	
Tension pneumothorax	
Cardiac tamponade	
Increased abdominal pressure	
Increased venous resistance	
Increased thoracic pressure	
Positive pressure respiration	
PEEP	
Increased abdominal pressure	
Tension pneumothorax	
Increased abdominal pressure (hours)	
Ascites	
Bowel distension	
Massive edema in the abdominal cavity	
Intraabdominal hemorrhage	
Retroperitoneal hemorrhage	
Tension pneumoperitoneum	

MSP, mean systemic pressure; CVP, central venous pressure; PEEP, positive end-expiratory pressure.

by trauma is bleeding and coagulation. This response is less likely, but not impossible, with tissue damage from ischemia or infection. Platelet activation results in the release of important chemoattractants (see Table 5-5).

Damaged blood vessels initially vasoconstrict, but this constriction is soon followed by vasodilation and increased capillary permeability secondary to the action of agents such as nitric oxide, prostaglandin E2, prostacyclin, histamine,

TABLE 5-5	Normal Inflammation
Event	**Cells Responsible**
Coagulation	Platelets
Early inflammation	Polymorphonuclear leukocytes (first few hours)
Later inflammation	Monocytes (days) macrophages
Collagen and mucopolysaccharide	Fibroblasts (maximum deposition 7–10 days)
Capillary budding	Endothelial cells (maximum 7–10 days)

TABLE 5-6	Functions of Inflammatory Cells
Cells	**Function**
Platelets	Coagulation, release PDGF, IL-1
Polymorphonuclear leukocytes	Phagocytosis, especially microbes, release IL-1, IL-8
Macrophage	Phagocytosis; stimulate fibroblast migration and growth; stimulate endothelial cell migration and growth; release FGF, PDGF, IL-1, IL-6, TNF, TFG-β, TGF-α
Fibroblast	Collagen deposition
Endothelial cells	Release of adhesion molecules
	Capillary budding

PDGF, platelet-derived growth factor; IL, interleukin; FGF, fibroblast growth factor; TNF, tumor necrosis factor; TGF, transforming growth factor.

serotonin, and kinins. When blood flow is present, this increase in vascular permeability results in the accumulation of protein-rich edema fluid (exudate).

Attracted by chemoattractants, polymorphonuclear cells (PMNs) are the first white cells to migrate to the inflammatory site (within minutes if circulation is good). White cells adhere to damaged, leaky vessels as a result of an increase in adhesion molecules, first P selectin, then E selectin, as well as intracellular adhesion molecules (ICAM-1). The adhesion molecules enhance the migration of PMNs into the interstitium. PMNs move to the site of tissue injury down the concentration gradient of attractant molecules called chemokines.

PMNs then phagocytize dead tissue and foreign objects, sometimes assisted by opsonins and preformed antibodies in the removal of bacteria. PMNs produce proteases and intracellular oxygen radicals that are critical for beneficial PMN activity. Besides proteases and oxygen radicals, PMNs can also release interleukin-1 (IL-1). IL-1 mediates temperature elevation through the thermoregulatory center and also stimulates other inflammatory activity (e.g., migration of macrophages). Another cytokine, interleukin-8 (IL-8), is a potent PMN attractant that is produced by many cell types after exposure to IL-1 and the cytokine tumor necrosis factor (TNF). The PMNs last only for a period of hours.

Within hours, tissue macrophages and circulating monocytes are also attracted by chemoattractants; they migrate into the injured area and last for days to weeks. The continuing inflammatory process is largely regulated by macrophages through mediator release, such as those listed in Table 5-6.

Fibroblast migration and angiogenesis begin next. The combined process of fibroblast proliferation and capillary budding produces granulation tissue that is friable and bleeds easily.

Fibroblasts produce collagen. This process usually accelerates 5 days after tissue damage occurs.

A summary of cellular activity in inflammation is shown in Tables 5-5 and 5-6.

As emphasized below, much of the local effect of inflammation (increased vascular permeability, nearby cellular activation, and injury) can result in the production of cytokines and other molecules that gain access to circulation. These molecules that are necessary for effective local inflammatory activity can cause distant or systemic tissue injury by the endocrine effect of these proinflammatory substances. This is particularly important as it relates to PMN and endothelial cell activation.

Effective inflammation controls infection, heals wounds, and then abates. Therefore, in addition to the proinflammatory physiology described above, there are anti-inflammatory responses that develop simultaneously to limit the action of inflammatory cells.

Such cytokines as IL-10 and IL-13 as well as the adrenal secretion of cortisol are some of the agents that serve this function.

A perfect inflammatory response, then, represents a precise balance between the proinflammatory and anti-inflammatory physiology that results in the resolution of infection and/or the healing of wounds without any deficit in either of these positive outcomes and no distant organ malfunction or failure.

HYPOPERFUSION STATES

Hypoperfusion is a decrease in total body or regional blood flow that is sufficient to result in cellular malfunction or death. Hypoperfusion is the primary mechanism that is responsible for inadequate oxygen delivery; the immediate effects of hypoperfusion on cell viability are secondary to the interruption of oxidative metabolism.

The Neurohumoral Response to Hypoperfusion

The most frequently studied models of total body hypoperfusion cause a reduction in cardiac output from loss of volume (hypovolemic hypoperfusion, i.e., hemorrhage) or loss of cardiac function (cardiogenic hypoperfusion). Either of these etiologies may result in the neurohumoral response shown in Table 5-7.

TABLE 5-7	Neurohumoral Response to Hypoperfusion
Increased	**Decreased**
Epinephrine	Insulin
Norepinephrine	Thyroxine
Dopamine	Triiodothyronine
Glucagon	Luteinizing hormone
Renin	Testosterone
Angiotensin	Estrogen
Arginine vasopressin	Follicle-stimulating hormone
ACTH	
Cortisol	
Aldosterone	
Growth hormone	

The clinically apparent effects of this neurohumoral response are tachycardia (epinephrine, norepinephrine, dopamine), vasoconstriction (norepinephrine, arginine vasopressin, angiotensin), diaphoresis (norepinephrine), oliguria with sodium and water conservation (adrenocorticotropic hormone [ACTH], cortisol, aldosterone, arginine vasopressin), and hyperglycemia (epinephrine, glucagon, cortisol, insufficient insulin). This activation of the neuroendocrine system attempts to preserve blood flow to vital organs (heart, lungs, brain) while diminishing flow to less vital organs (kidneys, gastrointestinal tract). In this way, it maintains or increases intravascular volume by limiting urine output. This response is more homeostatic under conditions of hypovolemic hypoperfusion compared with cardiogenic hypoperfusion. In the latter, tachycardia, vasoconstriction, and sodium and water retention may aggravate rather than diminish hypoperfusion by decreasing ventricular filling time, increasing afterload, and increasing myocardial stretch, respectively.

The Effects of Hypoperfusion on Inflammation

The most clearly documented association of hypoperfusion with inflammation is the effect of ischemia followed by reperfusion (**reperfusion injury**). Clinically, this effect is most obvious in patients with ischemia in isolated limbs (compartment syndrome), the brain, and the heart after cardiopulmonary bypass. However, severe systemic hypoperfusion may cause a similar response in many tissues, particularly the gastrointestinal tract.

The mechanism that is responsible for ischemia reperfusion injury appears to require both local and systemic factors. A complex interaction of oxygen free radicals, thromboxane, leukotrienes, phospholipase A2, and leukocytes participates in both regional and total body alterations in capillary permeability and organ function. Anatomic and physiologic damage to the intestine, limb, kidney, liver, and lung may occur after reperfusion, even when a specific organ (i.e., lung) was not initially hypoperfused. Because PMNs are potent producers of oxygen free radicals, these cells are central to this pathophysiology.

In the last decade, more evidence has demonstrated that hypoperfusion itself can stimulate inflammatory cell (PMN) and mediator (complement) activity, even before reperfusion.

In clinical hypoperfusion, particularly with trauma, it is difficult to separate tissue injury that is secondary only to hypoperfusion from damage from other mechanisms (e.g., a direct blow). Whatever the cause, hypoperfusion and inflammation commonly occur together.

The Effects of Hypoperfusion on Cellular Metabolism

The classic effect of hypoperfusion on cellular metabolism is anaerobic metabolism caused by an oxygen deficit. Elevated levels of lactic acid, with low pyruvate levels, characterize the glycolysis that is the primary means of adenosine triphosphate (ATP) production in anaerobic states. The reduction in ATP production that occurs secondary to the loss of mitochondrial function (2 ATP/mole production vs. 36 ATP/mole from oxidation) can result in inadequate energy to meet cellular needs, with first cell edema and subsequently cell death as a consequence.

Before cell death occurs, cell membrane function suffers from inadequate ATP production. Disordered membrane pump function allows extracellular sodium and calcium movement into cells, with water following the sodium. This sequestration of water in cells can cause a deficit in extracellular fluid, which may accentuate the fluid requirements during resuscitation.

ETIOLOGIES, DIAGNOSIS, AND MANAGEMENT OF HYPOPERFUSION STATES

The primary etiologies of hypoperfusion states in surgical patients are decreased venous return and decreased myocardial function (Table 5-8).

Decreased Venous Return: Hypovolemia

Hypovolemia (especially from hemorrhage) is the most common etiology of decreased venous return secondary to decreased MSP. Common etiologies of hypovolemia are listed in Table 5-9.

Severe hypoperfusion secondary to hypovolemia (i.e., hypovolemic shock) has been studied most frequently in experimental and clinical hemorrhage. Hemorrhagic shock not only diminishes venous return but also may cause cardiovascular alterations (Table 5-10). Cellular effects (other than lactic acidosis from anaerobic glycolysis) are listed in Table 5-11. As mentioned earlier, ischemia-induced activation of local and systemic inflammation has also been described.

The metabolic and toxic phenomena associated with hypovolemic shock, even without severe inflammation, result in loss of plasma and interstitial volume beyond what is accounted for by the primary disease process (i.e., hemorrhage, vomiting). Migration of interstitial fluid into cells and increased capillary permeability are implicated as mechanisms.

Physical Examination in Hypovolemic Hypoperfusion

Agitation, tachypnea, and peripheral vasoconstriction are common with any etiology of hypoperfusion. In the patient who has hypovolemia, vital signs and physical findings show evidence of hypoperfusion roughly in proportion to the degree of blood volume deficit. A 10% loss of blood volume (560 mL, approximately the amount donated for transfusion) produces little, if any, disturbance. A 20% loss may cause tachycardia and orthostatic hypotension. A 30% loss may produce hypotension while the patient is supine. However, a patient may

TABLE 5-8	Etiologies of Hypoperfusion
Decreased venous return	
Hypovolemia	
Pericardial tamponade	
Tension pneumothorax	
Increased abdominal pressure	
Bowel obstruction	
Tension pneumoperitoneum	
Massive bleeding	
Diagnostic laparoscopy	
Ascites	
Positive end-expiratory pressure	
Decreased myocardial function	
CHF	
Cardiogenic shock	

TABLE 5-9	Common Etiologies of Hypovolemia
Hemorrhage	
Severe inflammation or infection	
Trauma	
Pancreatitis or other causes of peritonitis	
Burns	
Vomiting or other intestinal losses	
Excessive diuresis	
Inadequate oral intake	

TABLE 5-11	Cellular Effects of Hemorrhagic Shock
Diminished transmembrane potential difference	
Increased intracellular sodium	
Decreased intracellular ATP	
Increased intracellular calcium	

be normotensive when supine, even with greater loss of blood volume (Table 5-12). As a bedside clinical measurement, blood pressure is especially useful since hypotension most commonly develops secondary to hypovolemia. Hypotension as a result of disruption of intrinsic cardiac function (cardiogenic shock) is much less common (discussed later). CHF, a distinct clinical entity from cardiogenic shock, typically results in a normal or increased blood pressure for that individual.

The neck veins are not distended unless hypovolemia is accompanied by an extracardiac increase in CVP (tension pneumothorax, pericardial tamponade, severe effort during expiration, increased abdominal pressure). An S3 gallop is not likely. And an etiology of hypovolemia may also be apparent (open wound with hemorrhage, distended abdomen, femur and pelvic fractures).

Common Laboratory Aids

Hypovolemic hypoperfusion that is severe enough to cause hypotension is associated with metabolic acidosis that is recognized either from serum electrolytes or, more precisely, arterial blood gases and blood lactic acid concentration. Elevated serum blood urea nitrogen (BUN) and creatinine levels that are indicative of renal malfunction are common. Hyperglycemia in a nondiabetic and hypothermia without environmental cooling are indicative of poor cellular metabolism.

Other tests (e.g., hemoglobin level, other serum chemistries, radiographic studies) are usually used to determine the etiology of hypovolemic hypoperfusion rather than to document the severity of the perfusion deficits.

Treatment of Hypovolemia

In the patient who has severe hypovolemic hypoperfusion, circulation must be restored simultaneously with diagnostic

and therapeutic interventions to correct the underlying cause of the hypovolemic state. When bleeding is the cause of hypovolemia, rapid and vigorous attention to the site of hemorrhage is the first principle while restoration is under way. This may be achieved by limited local efforts (e.g., pressure on a bleeding extremity) or demand operative intervention (e.g., emergency room thoracotomy, exploratory laparotomy).

The circulatory, metabolic, and toxic effects of hypovolemic hypoperfusion are best alleviated by rapid (within minutes) restoration of intravascular volume, thereby increasing MSP, venous return, and oxygen delivery. In general, two types of fluid, **crystalloid** and **colloid**, are used for volume replacement (Table 5-13).

RBC transfusion is principally indicated during active hemorrhage, and early transfusion is especially beneficial following trauma. The administration of red cells can result in increased cardiac output, increased oxygen-carrying capacity, and little, if any, leakage of red cells into the interstitium, even in the face of increased capillary permeability. The primary disadvantage of RBC transfusion is the evidence of increased mortality risk when critical care patients, who are not actively bleeding, receive red cells to maintain hemoglobin concentrations above 9 g/100 mL. Much of this risk appears to be associated with nosocomial infection and multisystem organ failure rather than infection with a transmissible disease (e.g., hepatitis C, human immunodeficiency virus). While little advantage is documented for increasing the hemoglobin to 10 g/100 mL or greater, patients with severe ischemic heart disease and poor cardiac performance may not tolerate oxygen content reductions associated with restrictive transfusion guidelines.

Potential advantages and disadvantages of various resuscitation fluids other than red cells are shown in Tables 5-14 and 5-15.

Fresh frozen plasma (FFP) should not be used primarily as a colloid. Like the transfusion of red cells following trauma, early and sufficient FFP administration appears to have a survival advantage. Ratios of 1 unit of FFP to 1.5 units of RBC or less are advocated for these circumstances. For less acute bleeding conditions, documentation of a deficiency in intrinsic or extrinsic coagulation (partial thromboplastin time > 1.5 × control, prothrombin time < 50%) should accompany the plan to use FFP.

Much more controversial than the appropriate use of FFP and RBCs are the advantages and disadvantages of the various crystalloid and colloid solutions. Most investigators agree that colloid administration results in less sodium and water administration compared with crystalloid solutions. In addition, plasma oncotic pressure is higher after the administration of colloids. Still debated is whether increased total body sodium and water gain are detrimental to organ function after resuscitation of circulation.

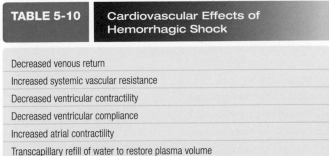

TABLE 5-10	Cardiovascular Effects of Hemorrhagic Shock
Decreased venous return	
Increased systemic vascular resistance	
Decreased ventricular contractility	
Decreased ventricular compliance	
Increased atrial contractility	
Transcapillary refill of water to restore plasma volume	
Intravascular protein replenishment from preformed extravascular protein	

TABLE 5-12	Hemodynamic Effects of Intravascular Volume Loss in Supine Subjects					
Amount (%)	Rate	Blood Pressure	Pulse	Mentation	Skin Vasoconstriction	Urine Output
≤10	5 min	NL	NL	NL	NL	NL
≤10	1 hr	NL	NL	NL	NL	NL
20	5 min	↓	↑	NL	↑	↓
20	1 hr	NL	↑	NL	NL	↓
30	5 min	↓↓	↑↑	↓	↑↑	↓↓
30	1 hr	↓	↑	↓	↑	↓
50	5 min	↓↓↓	↑↑	↓↓	↑↑↑	↓↓↓
50	1 hr	↓↓	↑↑	↓↓	↑↑	↓↓

NL, normal.

When a patient who has hypovolemia is receiving large volumes of crystalloid or colloid and is not responding well to therapy (most often seen in severe systemic inflammation, e.g., septic shock), dopamine administration is a logical adjunct. Dopamine increases left ventricular filling pressures as it increases cardiac output, probably as a result of constriction of the veins and decreased venous capacitance. This increase may occur at the expense of increasing myocardial oxygen demands. After adequate vascular volume is attained, the dopamine can usually be discontinued. Therefore, dopamine can serve as a pharmacologic surrogate for fluid administration. Since left ventricular end diastolic pressure increases with dopamine administration, left atrial pressure will increase, and the clinician should not presume that dopamine would lessen any deleterious effect that elevated left atrial pressure might exert on the lungs.

Decreased Venous Return: Pericardial Tamponade

The primary mechanism for decreased venous return during pericardial tamponade is an extracavitary increase in CVP. The etiologies of tamponade are most commonly chest trauma (penetrating and blunt) and bleeding after cardiac surgery. Acute tamponade (most often associated with chest trauma) can develop with relatively small volumes of pericardial fluid and not demonstrate classical physical findings except for hypoperfusion. Tamponade that develops less acutely is more likely to demonstrate distended neck veins, muffled heart sounds, and an increased paradoxical pulse (>15 mm Hg). In these cases, the electrocardiogram may show low voltage, the CVP is often elevated, and a chest x-ray may show an enlarging heart. However, with severe hypovolemia, the CVP may be normal despite tamponade, and may become elevated only after fluid resuscitation. An echocardiogram in both acute and subacute circumstances can show fluid surrounding the heart, with diminished ventricular volumes.

It is important to distinguish this etiology of hypoperfusion from CHF or cardiogenic shock because reducing fluid intake and administering a diuretic would reduce venous return further in tamponade. As stated, CHF usually results in normal or elevated blood pressure. Severe tamponade results in hypotension. Therefore, tamponade simulates cardiogenic shock more closely than CHF. Because cardiogenic shock requires a major insult to myocardial function (see later), hypotension with elevated CVP should increase suspicion of tamponade or a tension pneumothorax unless obvious evidence of severe myocardial malfunction is found.

Removal of the fluid surrounding the heart (pericardiocentesis/pericardial window/repair of a cardiac wound) is the most effective therapy, and it can result in a dramatic improvement in cardiac output. However, venous return also improves as a

TABLE 5-13	Fluids for Hypovolemia Resuscitation
Crystalloid	
Isotonic	
Ringer's lactate	
0.9% saline	
Hypertonic saline	
Colloid	
Red blood cells	
Fresh frozen plasma	
Albumin	
Processed human protein	
Low–molecular-weight dextran	
Hydroxyethyl starch	

TABLE 5-14	Crystalloid Solutions
Isotonic solution advantages	
Inexpensive	
Readily available	
Freely mobile across capillaries	
No increase in lung water	
Isotonic solution disadvantages	
Rapid equilibration with interstitial fluid	
Lowers serum oncotic pressure	
No oxygen-carrying capacity	
Increase in systemically perfused interstitial fluid	

TABLE 5-15	Colloid Solutions (Other than Red Cells)

Advantages
Less water administered (more resuscitation per milliliter)
Less sodium administered
Less decrease in oncotic pressure
Acid buffer (FFP)
Disadvantages
Expensive (albumin, FFP)
Transmissible disease (FFP)
Increased interstitial oncotic pressure
Depressed myocardial function (albumin: 50% reduction in left ventricular stroke work index at a pulmonary capillary occlusion pressure of 15 mm Hg)
Depressed immunologic function (albumin: decreased immunoglobulins, decreased response to tetanus toxoid)
Delayed resolution of interstitial edema
Coagulopathy: infrequent in low doses (low–molecular-weight dextran: platelet malfunction; hydroxyethyl starch: decreased factor VIII:c concentrations; albumin: decreased fibrinogen, decreased prothrombin, decreased factor VIII)

result of increasing MSP with intravenous fluid. Therefore, vigorous fluid administration should be provided despite an elevated CVP.

Decreased Venous Return: Tension Pneumothorax

Tension pneumothorax reduces venous return by producing an extracavitary increase in CVP and by increasing venous resistance in the chest. Tension pneumothorax may occur spontaneously from rupture of a bleb or, more commonly, after penetrating or blunt trauma. Physical examination shows evidence of decreased perfusion, along with decreased breath sounds and tympany over the affected thorax, tracheal deviation away from the affected thorax, and distended neck veins. Therefore, the diagnosis can be made at the bedside without radiologic assistance. However, when circulation is not severely threatened, a chest x-ray can be the principle diagnostic tool.

When circulation is threatened, treatment consists of emergently releasing the tension (e.g., placing a 14-gauge needle into the chest, placing a finger in a large penetrating injury), followed by closed thoracostomy. Administration of intravenous fluid to increase MSP is also beneficial, and neck vein distension may not be evident with severe hypovolemia.

Decreased Venous Return: Increased Abdominal Pressure

While a sudden increase in intra-abdominal pressure can result in a short-term increase in venous return (sudden decrease in venous capacitance), a prolonged (hours) increase in abdominal pressure (>25 mm Hg) diminishes venous return by increasing intrathoracic pressure, producing an extracavitary increase in CVP, and increasing venous resistance in abdominal veins. Increased abdominal pressure may be particularly detrimental to renal blood flow, but it can cause marked total body hypoperfusion despite a well-maintained mean arterial blood pressure from increased systemic vascular resistance.

Intrabdominal pressure (IAP) is increased by a variety of mechanisms (see Table 5-4). It is most easily measured with a bladder catheter: 50 to 100 mL fluid is inserted into the bladder through the fluid sampling port on a Foley catheter; the catheter is clamped distal to the sampling port; and pressure is measured by connecting the needle in the sampling port to standard hemodynamic monitoring tubing, using the pubis as the zero pressure level.

Physical examination often shows evidence of hypoperfusion along with a tensely distended abdomen and possibly distended neck veins. Such patients are usually on a ventilator, and most often the pressure needed to provide a proscribed tidal volume increases.

The most effective treatment is to relieve the pressure. However, aggressive fluid management to increase MSP may be the only option in some cases where, for instance, exploration of the abdomen is considered prohibitively risky. When hemodynamics and respiratory function are severely impaired by increased abdominal pressure, then opening the abdomen and "closing" it with a prosthetic material (synthetic or biological) or leaving it open and covered with a plastic, occlusive dressing may be the best alternative.

While intra-abdominal pressure in the 25-mm Hg range is well understood to cause marked alterations in circulatory physiology, any increase above zero is potentially detrimental to venous return, especially in patients who have a compromised circulation for other reasons in addition to the abdominal process. Therefore, some patients with an abdominal pressure <25 mm Hg will benefit from interventions to reduce this impairment to venous return. Measurement of the abdominal perfusion pressure (APP = MAP – IAP) has been advocated for patients with low systemic pressure. An APP <50 mm Hg can be used in lieu of the absolute abdominal pressure to assist in the diagnosis of the abdominal compartment syndrome.

Cardiogenic Hypoperfusion and Cardiogenic Shock

To cause cardiogenic shock, or hypotension, on a cardiac basis, cardiac function must be severely disrupted from etiologies such as those listed in Table 5-16. Hypoperfusion

TABLE 5-16	Etiologies of Cardiogenic Shock

Acute ischemia
Ventricular wall infarct
Papillary muscle infarct
Ventricular septal defect
Acute valvular disease; mitral, tricuspid, or aortic regurgitation
Arrhythmias
Rapid supraventricular
Bradycardia
Ventricular tachycardia
End-stage cardiomyopathy
Severe myocardial contusion
Severe myocarditis
Severe left ventricular outflow obstruction
Severe left ventricular inflow obstruction

of this magnitude, especially when it is secondary to myocardial infarction, is associated with a high mortality rate (~75%). Cardiogenic shock is a clinical entity distinct from CHF. In CHF, arterial blood pressure is characteristically well maintained or increases. This characteristic distinguishes cardiogenic shock (the term applied to significant reductions in systolic pressure) from CHF.

In general, the diseases listed in Table 5-16 are not subtle and do not cause gradual alterations in cardiac function. Hypotension is more often a disease of hypovolemia than a disease of severe impairment of cardiac function. When a clinician decides not to administer fluid to a hypotensive patient, he or she is actually making a diagnosis of cardiogenic shock. Cardiogenic shock is the only major circulatory deficit that can be worsened by the administration of fluid. Because cardiogenic shock is secondary to severe, usually obvious, cardiac disease, the clinician should be able to document the occurrence of a marked insult to cardiac function. Without such documentation and the associated recognition of a disease that requires aggressive monitoring and management in a critical care setting, the clinician should consider the hypotensive patient to be hypovolemic and not in cardiogenic shock.

Physical Examination

Physical examination shows hypotension, tachycardia, tachypnea, peripheral vasoconstriction, distended neck veins, agitation, and confusion. When valvular dysfunction is present, associated murmurs may be auscultated.

Laboratory Aids

Cardiogenic shock is associated with chest x-ray evidence of hydrostatic pulmonary edema, metabolic acidosis (lactic acidosis), increased CVP and PAOP, and elevated BUN and creatinine. A cardiogram often shows evidence of acute ischemia, infarct, or arrhythmias. An echocardiogram can provide information about ventricular wall motion and valve function. The cardiac index is low (<2.2 L/minute/m^2), and both systemic and pulmonary vascular resistance are high.

Treatment

As always, treatment is based on the etiology. Arrhythmias are usually the most readily treated etiology of severe cardiac impairment. Arrhythmias are diagnosed and treated as described in textbooks that cover advanced cardiac life support. When the etiology is not an arrhythmia, the same sequence of interventions used to increase cardiac output in CHF may be used for cardiogenic shock (Tables 5-17 and 5-18). However, hypotension (often <90 mm Hg systolic) makes the use of vasodilators alone less attractive. Therefore, a combination of inotropic drug support and vasodilation is frequently used. Mechanical support of the heart with an intraaortic balloon pump (IABP) increases cardiac output while reducing preload and afterload. IABP may be more successful than high-dose dobutamine in supporting patients during severe cardiac impairment. IABP may be adequate to support a patient until cardiac function improves or may be required until surgery (e.g., replacement of the aortic valve, coronary revascularization) is performed.

End Points for Resuscitation of Circulation

End points for resuscitation of circulation depend on such variables as the primary etiology of the circulatory deficit, the underlying state of the patient's circulation, and the magnitude

TABLE 5-17	Treatment of Cardiogenic Shock
Reversal of underlying disease	
Coronary artery bypass	
Valve replacement	
Rx myopathy	
Repair ventricular septal defect	
Reduce preload	
Decrease water intake	
Diuretics	
Venous dilation	
Nitroglycerin	
Calcium channel blockers	
Narcotics	
Reduce afterload	
Nitroprusside	
Antihypertensives	
Diuretics	
Narcotics	
Increase contractility	
Intravenous inotropes	
Increase arterial oxygen	
Supplemental O$_2$	
Mechanical ventilation	
Intraaortic balloon pump	

of cellular and organ malfunction recognized during the hypoperfusion insult. However, for most clinical conditions, bedside recognition of normal circulation is adequate for assessing the outcome of resuscitation. Such variables as normal (the designation of normal depends on knowledge of the patient's premorbid blood pressure) or increasing blood pressure, pulse rate of <80/minute, normal or improved mental status, urine output >0.5 mL/kg/hour, warm extremities, and resolution of metabolic acidosis usually suffice.

However, patients who have had a severe cellular insult may require more complicated hemodynamic monitoring and adjustment of circulation. Certainly, patients who are in cardiogenic shock require precise hemodynamic monitoring (i.e., pulmonary artery catheterization, echocardiogram, cardiac

TABLE 5-18	Hemodynamic Effects of Inotropic Drugs and Vasodilators

	Hemodynamic Parameters			
	Heart Rate	**Contractility**	**Preload**	**Afterload**
Dopamine	↑↑	↑	↑	↑ or NC
Dobutamine	↑	↑↑	↓	NC or ↓
Isoproterenol	↑↑	↑↑	↓	↓
Nitroprusside	±	NC	↓	↓↓
Nitroglycerin	±	NC	↓↓	↓

NC, no change.

catheterization) to make the proper diagnosis and adjust therapy. In such cases, return of the cardiac index from low (<2.2 L/minute/m^2) to normal (2.5 to 3.5 L/minute/m^2), along with normal amounts of oxygen delivery (400 mL/minute/m^2) and consumption (130 mL/minute/m^2), may allow cellular and organ function to recover. A normal cardiac index may also be adequate in patients with underlying heart disease who have a further reduction in cardiac function from noncardiac causes and then undergo resuscitation of their circulation close to baseline. Unfortunately, despite the achievement of normal cardiac index and oxygen parameters, patients with or without severe acute or chronic heart disease may continue to have cellular malfunction that progresses to organ failure and death after a severe hypoperfusion insult.

The recognition that normal circulation, oxygen delivery, and oxygen consumption may be inadequate for cellular and organ recovery after severe hypoperfusion was inferred from epidemiologic data that associated an increase in these parameters (cardiac index > 4.5 L/minute/m^2; oxygen delivery > 600 mL/minute/m^2; oxygen consumption > 170 mL/minute/m^2) with eventual survival. In patients who achieve these end points, metabolic acidosis usually resolves. This situation also portends a favorable outcome. Therefore, several investigators champion the use of fluids, inotropic drugs, and sometimes vasodilators to push for these hemodynamic end points in every critically ill patient. The results of such management remain controversial, with some studies supporting these endeavors and others finding an increase in mortality rates.

What can be used in the individual patient to determine if sufficient oxygen is being provided to the tissues? The pulmonary artery catheter (PAC) allows the measurement of mixed venous oxygen saturation (mvO$_2$ sat), measured by taking a sample from the pulmonary artery port. Healthy adults deliver hemoglobin that is close to 100% saturated with oxygen and consume about 25%. This results in an mvO$_2$ sat of 75%. When the mvO$_2$ sat measures in the 50s, most would argue that cells are demanding more oxygen than circulation is delivering. When this value is in the 70s, then oxygen delivery would appear sufficient for the demand. Values in the 60s could be interpreted either way.

Many more central venous catheters than PACs are inserted. Over the last several years, measurement of central venous oxygen saturation (cvO$_2$ sat) has been utilized to assess resuscitation end points. When measured simultaneously, most often cvO$_2$ sat is higher than mvO$_2$ sat. Therefore, cvO$_2$ sat values in the 60s are usually interpreted as indicating inadequate oxygen delivery.

As with any clinical measurement, venous oxygen saturations are subject to inaccuracies, and any value obtained should be juxtaposed with the other clinical variables described above before deciding that more therapy for circulation must be provided.

In summary, clinical evaluation is usually sufficient to recognize the "end points of resuscitation"—normal blood pressure for that individual, a slow pulse, warm extremities, good urine output, normal mental status, and resolution of metabolic acidosis (e.g., resolution of elevated lactic acid). However, many patients will continue to exhibit abnormalities in these clinical parameters even after aggressive efforts. Such patients can be more precisely evaluated with the central venous and PACs as well as echocardiographic data, recognizing that the information so obtained must not be used in isolation. Once the clinical and cellular evidence of shock has resolved (see below), then such monitoring techniques are no longer necessary.

SEVERE INFLAMMATORY STATES

As described above, inflammation is a normal response to tissue injury. Although localized inflammation in response to an insult is usually beneficial, severe tissue injury from a variety of causes (Table 5-19) can result in inflammation distant from the original disease (systemic inflammation). This inflammation may cause cellular malfunction and death in remote organs. As catalogued in the concept of the **systemic inflammatory response syndrome (SIRS)**, many disease states can cause systemic inflammation, probably as a result of the activation of cellular mediators of inflammation at remote sites.

To meet the definition of SIRS, a patient must have two or more of the following conditions: (1) temperature >38.5°C or <36°C; (2) heart rate > 90 beats/minute; (3) respiratory rate >20 breaths/minute or Paco$_2$ < 32 Torr; and (4) total leukocyte count >12,000 cells/mm, <4,000 cells/mm^3, or >10% immature forms. Many patients with systemic inflammation, but without evidence of cellular and organ malfunction (i.e., not in shock) may meet the definition of SIRS. The SIRS variables of hypothermia (<36°C) and leukopenia (<4,000 cells/mm^3) are associated with more severe inflammation, as are systolic hypotension and evidence of organ malfunction (e.g., elevated BUN and creatinine, oliguria, altered mental status, decreased arterial oxygenation, increased bilirubin, decreased platelets). These patients are in shock, even if infection is not present and the term sepsis cannot strictly be applied. Therefore, the traditional concept of septic shock is too narrow. Patients with severe systemic inflammation who exhibit these alterations are in shock. When infection is the cause of severe systemic inflammation, then septic shock can be considered the diagnosis.

Effects of Severe Inflammation on Circulation

Severe systemic inflammation is associated with alterations in both total body and regional perfusion. Mechanisms that reduce cardiac output during systemic inflammation are listed in Table 5-20.

The most common etiology of inadequate cardiac output during inflammation is decreased venous return, which results from both loss of intravascular fluid and vasodilation. Intravascular volume decreases as plasma exudes into the primary focus of inflammation (area of injury or infection). When systemic inflammation develops in response to the primary focus of inflammation, plasma may also exude into some or

TABLE 5-19	Etiologies of Systemic Inflammation (Partial List)
Infection (meets definition of sepsis)	
Trauma	
Burns	
Ischemia/reperfusion: regional or total body	
Pancreatitis	
Drug reactions	
Hemolytic transfusion reactions	

TABLE 5-20	Circulatory Disorders in Severe Inflammation: Reduced Cardiac Output

| **Hypovolemia** |
| Peripheral vasodilation |
| Increased capillary permeability, local or total body |
| Intracellular migration of fluid |
| Sequestration in gastrointestinal tract lumen |
| **Myocardial depression** |
| **Increased pulmonary vascular resistance** |
| Hypoxia |
| Platelet emboli |
| Thromboxane release |
| Serotonin release |
| White blood cell aggregation |
| **Deficits in the microcirculation** |
| Gastrointestinal tract |
| Renal |

all of the other tissues. Such exudation causes an increase in interstitial fluid, which becomes protein-rich compared with normal. In general, interstitial fluid is maintained in the extracellular space by active cellular processes that maintain cell membrane integrity and perform such functions as sodium-potassium exchange, which keeps potassium in the cell and sodium out of the cell. Severe inflammation may interfere with active cell membrane function, decrease ion-exchange capabilities, and allow more interstitial water and solutes to enter cells. Depletion of interstitial fluid is another mechanism that aggravates plasma volume loss.

Ileus is common during severe inflammation, regardless of the location of the primary focus. Ileus can cause fluid to accumulate in the lumen of the gastrointestinal tract that can be as voluminous as that sequestered during bowel obstruction.

Collectively, the exudation of plasma volume into inflammatory foci (both local and systemic), the accumulation of fluid in the gastrointestinal tract, and the migration of fluid into cells is known as the third space, to distinguish it from normal plasma and interstitial fluid spaces. The magnitude of the third space effect is roughly proportional to the magnitude of tissue injury or infection that is present. The primary effect of **third-space fluid accumulation** is to deplete plasma volume and impair venous return.

Vasodilation of the systemic veins and arterioles is characteristic of severe inflammation, and several inflammatory mediators are implicated as causative (e.g., histamine, kinins, prostacyclin, nitric oxide). Increasing the capacitance of veins decreases MSP and may decrease venous return, especially if CVP (discussed previously and in the section on venous return) does not decrease proportionally because of increased pulmonary vascular resistance.

Severe inflammation may directly depress the function of previously normal myocardial cells. Less severe inflammation may result in augmented malfunction of previously abnormal cardiac tissue. Therefore, cardiac output may be impaired and result in a physiology that is consistent with an excess, rather than a deficit, of intravascular volume (i.e., CHF, cardiogenic

shock physiology). Recognition of such **cardiogenic states** of hypoperfusion during inflammation is important for proper therapeutic intervention (see later).

Severe inflammation is associated with increased pulmonary vascular resistance. This increase in right ventricular afterload may cause dilation of the right ventricle, decreased right ventricular ejection, and impaired filling of the left ventricle. Right atrial pressure may increase and impair venous return.

In addition to the recognized effects on cardiac function and cardiac output, which can reduce total body perfusion, severe inflammation may cause deficits in the microcirculation that in turn can result in regional ischemia to organs or within organs. This ischemia will accentuate cell and organ injury. The gastrointestinal tract and kidneys appear to be particularly prone to such alterations.

Effects of Severe Inflammation on Cellular Function

Severe inflammation can result in alterations of cellular metabolism that are independent of inflammation-induced reductions in oxygen delivery, but similar to abnormalities recognized with hypoperfusion, a condition called "cytopathic hypoxia." In cytopathic hypoxia the cells behave as if there is too little oxygen because of an inflammation-induced alteration in cellular function, not because there is too little oxygen provided for cells to function properly. For instance, the elevation in lactic acid level that is associated with severe inflammation is not characteristically secondary to cellular anaerobic metabolism. Increased lactic acid production can also develop from alterations in glucose metabolism that are associated with increased pyruvate production or decreased pyruvate metabolism without mitochondrial malfunction (i.e., accelerated aerobic glycolysis). Therefore, in inflammatory states an elevated lactic acid level does not necessarily support the conclusion that a patient has inadequate oxygen delivery.

There are other physiologic disturbances that demonstrate how cells have difficulty distinguishing the insults from too little oxygen and too much inflammation. For example, the same cell-depolarizing protein molecule that appears in circulation after hypovolemic hypoperfusion is present after inflammatory insults. Such cell depolarization can result in sodium and water accumulation in the cells. Further, a decrease in serum ionized calcium is common in both hypoperfusion and inflammatory states. This decrease, shown experimentally to be associated with increased intracellular calcium, is also likely a marker for cell membrane malfunction.

Therefore, several cell function alterations—production of lactic acid, decreased cell membrane function, increased intracellular sodium and calcium—can all result from either true cellular hypoxia or as a result of inflammatory toxins, namely, cytopathic hypoxia.

DIAGNOSIS AND MANAGEMENT OF SEVERE INFLAMMATION

The clinical manifestations of severe systemic inflammation (Table 5-21) are as potentially varied as the many organs that may manifest malfunction. Most patients have hemodynamic alterations, but sometimes abnormal lung, central nervous system, hematologic, or other organ function is the primary evidence of

TABLE 5-21	Common Clinical Manifestations of Severe Inflammation
Vital signs	
Temperature elevation, hypothermia	
Tachycardia	
Tachypnea	
Hypotension with warm or cold extremities	
Change in mental status	
Respiratory insufficiency	
Ileus	
Oliguria, increased urine protein	
Elevated hemoglobin, thrombocytopenia, Leukocytosis, leukopenia	
Increased serum glucose, decreased ionized calcium	

inflammation, rather than hemodynamic changes. Therefore, a high index of suspicion of the patient at risk, augmented by evidence gathered during physical examination and selected laboratory tests, supports the diagnosis of significant inflammation.

The Patient at Risk

The first category of risk is a patient who recently acquired a disease (e.g., severe pancreatitis) or had an injury (e.g., unstable pelvic fracture with ruptured spleen) that is characterized by severe inflammation. The second category of risk is a patient who has an underlying condition (e.g., immunosuppression after liver transplantation) or who recently underwent a procedure (e.g., elective colon resection for carcinoma) that makes systemic inflammation, particularly from infection, more likely. Any patient who has had a significant episode of hypoperfusion (e.g., cardiogenic shock after an acute myocardial infarction, upper gastrointestinal hemorrhage sufficient to result in hypotension) is also at risk for systemic inflammation, either at the time of the hypoperfusion or days later.

Physical Examination

Outward Manifestations

The patient is usually restless and may have alterations in mental status ranging from delirium to coma. In fact, mental status changes may precede obvious hemodynamic or respiratory findings. These alterations sometimes lead the clinician to a misdirected evaluation (i.e., computed tomography of the brain). Such alterations in central nervous system function are rarely focal and are most consistent with a metabolic encephalopathy.

If intravascular volume is decreased, the skin is cool and possibly mottled, with vasoconstriction most often evident in both the upper and lower extremities. Capillary refill time is also decreased.

Vital Signs

Usually, severe systemic inflammation is seen as a decrease in blood pressure, an increase in heart rate, an increase in respiratory rate, and elevated temperature. Patients who have underlying cardiac disease may have hemodynamics that are more consistent with CHF (i.e., elevated blood pressure, tachycardia). Hypothermia may be present in the most severe cases.

Lung Examination

At lung examination, the lungs may be clear, even when acute respiratory distress syndrome (ARDS) is present. However, rales, rhonchi, and bronchospasm may be found. Examination findings consistent with consolidation (e.g., tubular or tubulovesicular breath sounds, egophony) may assist in locating an inflammatory process, but they are clearly not specific to systemic inflammation. The lung examination is not sufficiently specific to permit a diagnosis of systemic inflammation or other etiology of diffuse pulmonary malfunction.

Cardiovascular Examination

Hypotension and tachycardia are usually present, along with crisp heart tones. After intravascular volume is restored, the extremities are usually warm, demonstrating good capillary refill. Hypotension with warm hands and feet most often represents the response to inflammation, although anaphylaxis and a high spinal cord injury can produce similar findings. Jugular venous pressure is low by clinical examination.

As a result of plasma exudation and the other causes of plasma volume loss, the patient usually is sequestering fluid. This sequestration can be sudden or, if the patient has been monitored in a hospital setting, the positive fluid balance and an increase in weight may have been documented for several days before acute deterioration is noted.

Myocardial depression from inflammation might cause elevated jugular venous pressure, hypertension, and an S3 gallop. Myocardial depression that is severe enough to result in hypotension and a clinical picture identical to cardiogenic shock is possible. However, such myocardial malfunction is much less common than are circulatory deficiencies secondary to hypovolemia. The clinician must be careful to distinguish the fluid sequestration and positive fluid balance associated with severe inflammation (which is universal) from the same phenomena seen with cardiogenic states. Treating hypovolemia with fluid restriction and diuretics causes further circulatory embarrassment.

Fluid administration is directed at restoring and maintaining the plasma and blood volume that is threatened by the fluid sequestration associated with severe inflammation. Thus, the primary reason for fluid administration is to support circulation. Often circulation is assessed with urine output. Decreased urine output secondary to severe inflammation is most often caused by inadequate cardiac output. Therefore, it is a marker of inadequate circulation.

Laboratory Studies

Hematologic Studies

An increase in total white blood cell count, particularly young PMNs, is most common. Leukopenia denotes more severe disease and consists mostly of immature PMNs. The platelet count usually falls, and evidence of consumption of coagulation proteins, with breakdown of fibrinogen (increased prothrombin time, increased partial thromboplastin time, and increased fibrin split products or D-dimer), denotes more severe disease. Hemoglobin may increase as plasma exudes into inflammatory sites. This increase indicates hemoconcentration, and may be a useful tool in assessing intravascular volume resuscitation because plasma volume is likely to be inadequate until the hemoglobin returns to the patient's baseline value.

Lung Studies

A decrease in arterial Po_2 and Pco_2 is characteristic of severe systemic inflammation as well as many other lung disease states. The increase in physiologic shunt, which results in a decrease in arterial Po_2, is associated with stimuli that increase minute ventilation and decrease arterial Pco_2. A chest x-ray may be clear or may demonstrate loss of lung volume as well as evidence of pulmonary fluid accumulation, most often from a noncardiogenic pathophysiology (i.e., ARDS). The clinician should recognize that respiratory signs and symptoms and laboratory data during severe inflammation (shortness of breath, tachypnea, crackles, wheezing, decreased arterial Po_2, chest x-ray showing increased lung water) may be indistinguishable from those seen with CHF. In addition, he or she should recognize the dangers of misdiagnosing the effects of severe lung inflammation as CHF.

Urine Studies

Oliguria is common during severe inflammation, and is most often secondary to low intravascular volume and inadequate circulation. It gives rise to laboratory test results that are consistent with a prerenal state (e.g., elevated urine specific gravity, low urine sodium, increased urine osmolality, elevated BUN: creatinine ratio).

Serum Chemistries

An elevated blood glucose level is common during inflammation from such alterations as increased gluconeogenesis, glycogen lysis, and relative insulin resistance.

For many years, decreased total serum calcium has been recognized as associated with one particular severe inflammatory disease, pancreatitis. The amount of decrease correlates with the severity of disease. Ionized calcium is the calcium that is not bound to albumin. Therefore, it is not affected by albumin concentration that can decrease markedly during critical illness. Ionized calcium is also better correlated with parathyroid hormone release compared with total calcium.

Ionized calcium decreases with any disease that causes either severe hypoperfusion or inflammation. This decrease is not secondary to inadequate parathormone secretion. Several recent studies showed an increase in intracellular calcium during or after hypoperfusion or inflammatory states. In addition, the magnitude of the decrease correlates with the severity of disease. Although it is not specific for inflammation, ongoing severe inflammation must be considered in any patient who has decreased ionized calcium. In contrast, a normal ionized calcium level is unusual during severe inflammation or hypoperfusion. Therefore, a normal value suggests that a severe acute systemic insult is not present.

The combination of electrolyte or arterial blood gas levels that are consistent with metabolic acidosis and an elevated lactic acid level is often seen in severe inflammation. An elevated lactic acid level may develop secondary to anaerobic metabolism, suggesting hypoperfusion as the cause. However, an elevated lactic acid level can also result from metabolic alterations associated with inflammation in the presence of normal oxygen concentrations. Therefore, like ionized calcium, these abnormalities do not distinguish severe inflammation from a decrease in either regional or global perfusion. Persistent metabolic acidosis could mean that either disease is present and should prompt further diagnostic and, possibly, therapeutic efforts.

TABLE 5-22	Treatment of Severe Inflammation
Control etiology	
Infection	
Tissue injury	
Drug or transfusion reaction	
Support organ function	
Antagonize inflammatory and metabolic mediators	

Treatment

Treating the Underlying Cause

Once severe inflammation is recognized, the first principle of treatment is to determine the underlying cause and initiate appropriate therapy (Table 5-22). Infection and infection-like processes (i.e., endotoxin) are the most commonly considered etiologies of severe inflammation. However, reactions to drugs or transfusions and tissue injury without infection (i.e., early severe pancreatitis) can also cause severe systemic inflammation that is indistinguishable from that seen with the invasion of microorganisms.

While the search for the primary disease is underway and therapy is initiated, vital organ function must be supported until the primary process is under control. Unfortunately, systemic inflammation may continue despite adequate resolution of the initiating insult. In some patients, inflammation appears to become self-sustaining, as though a positive feedback system developed in one or more of the organs with systemic inflammation. For instance, ARDS initiated by an inflammatory process in the abdomen causes inflammatory cells to accumulate in the lungs. The inflammation caused by these pulmonary cells usually, but not always, subsides when the underlying illness is effectively treated. Sometimes the lung inflammation becomes subacute despite resolution of the first inflammatory focus.

As discussed later, novel therapies that focus on interrupting various steps in the inflammatory process are being studied to determine whether they can ameliorate the adverse effects of severe inflammation and improve clinical outcome. In addition, therapies designed to enhance immunologic function may prevent subsequent inflammatory insults from infection or microbiologic by-products.

Supporting Organ Function: Cardiovascular and Pulmonary

Rapid restoration of circulation during severe inflammation has been shown to reduce mortality. Support of circulation usually starts with treatment of hypovolemia. The result is usually an increase in cardiac output such that hypotension is alleviated, if not completely reversed. The temperature of the extremities also changes from cool to warm. For most patients, the combination of restoration of intravascular volume, peripheral vasodilation, and the neurohumoral response to inflammation produces a hyperdynamic (cardiac index > normal) circulatory state. Urine output and mental status usually improve. Unfortunately, pulmonary function does not characteristically improve dramatically with treatment of hypovolemia alone. Ionized calcium alterations and metabolic acidosis may or may not improve as a result of simple improvement in circulation.

RBC transfusion is reserved for patients who have ongoing hemorrhage or hemoglobin levels of <7 g/100 mL and who have abnormalities that are consistent with inadequate oxygen delivery. For patients with hemoglobin levels of more than 10 g/100 mL, simply increasing hemoglobin does not appear to significantly improve oxygen consumption.

Dopamine, usually in low concentrations (2– to 10 µg/kg/minute), is commonly administered during severe inflammation. Because dopamine, even at these low doses, tends to increase left ventricular end-diastolic pressure as cardiac output increases, this drug has a physiologic effect that is similar to fluid infusion, and is most useful when hypovolemia is the primary abnormality.

The diagnosis and treatment of a cardiogenic state usually requires more complicated monitoring than simply recording blood pressure, pulse, skin color, mental status, urine output, and electrolyte concentrations. Insertion of a PAC allows more precise measurement of cardiac filling pressures and the response to inotropic and vasodilator manipulations.

The primary advantage of PAC insertion is the ability to acquire hemodynamic data (CVP, PAOP, CI, SVR) to assist in hemodynamic diagnostic and therapeutic decision-making. Given the evidence that achieving excellent circulation is associated with improved outcome in patients who have severe hypoperfusion or inflammation, using technologic devices (which might include echocardiography) to evaluate circulation and possibly avoid continuing hypoperfusion clearly appears beneficial. This argument is not supported by data accrued during routine use of PACs, however, because critical assessment of circulation is not likely to be crucial for any common illness or surgical intervention (e.g., major vascular surgery). Likewise, it may be difficult to discern a survival advantage to using such equipment in large groups of patients in the intensive care unit. However, an individual patient may achieve a distinct advantage, especially when a therapeutic intervention that reverses hypoperfusion is documented.

The disadvantages of PAC insertion include complications related to central venous access (e.g., pneumothorax, central venous thrombosis) as well as those associated with the cardiac location (e.g., ventricular arrhythmias, damage to the tricuspid or pulmonic valves, and/or rupture of the pulmonary artery). Ventricular arrhythmias are usually not sustained, and anatomic injuries are rare. Despite the relatively low risk, PAC insertion should be used when the potential advantage, as described earlier, is considered worth the risk.

During severe inflammation, myocardial depression may be a manifestation of decreased function of the myocardial catecholamine receptors. Phosphodiesterase inhibitor drugs (e.g., amrinone), which do not require this receptor function for action, may be particularly useful inotropic agents during severe inflammation.

In a patient who is hyperdynamic, has elevated cardiac output, and has low systemic resistance states, the use of a vasoconstrictor (e.g., norepinephrine, vasopressin) may be indicated, especially when certain vessels with fixed stenoses (e.g., atherosclerotic plaques in renal, carotid, or coronary arteries) are likely to require higher mean arterial pressure for adequate perfusion. Under these circumstances, the use of such vasoconstrictors (with simultaneous documentation of no significant reduction in cardiac output) may increase mean arterial pressure and provide evidence of better organ perfusion (e.g., increased urine output).

For most patients with severe systemic inflammation from sepsis, rapid (within 6 hours of diagnosis) restoration of circulation, as defined by a cvO_2 sat >70% and normal lactic acid

concentrations, is associated with improved outcome and a decrease in inflammatory mediator concentrations. These data in humans are the most compelling evidence gathered thus far that demonstrate the association between hypoperfusion and the pathophysiology of inflammation.

Support of pulmonary function often requires mechanical ventilation using techniques related to the pulmonary disorder (i.e., Acute Respiratory Distress Network settings for ARDS). Such management is sufficient when arterial oxygen saturation is >90%.

Achieving a Balance in the Effects of Inflammation

Much experimental and clinical research has evaluated the antagonism of inflammatory and metabolic mediators in severe inflammatory states (Table 5-23). Many studies show promise, but few are emerging as "standard" therapy.

As previously stated, inflammation has beneficial effects (e.g., wound healing, defense against invasive organisms) that are important for survival during critical illness. Therefore, a successful outcome depends on a balance between the beneficial and the detrimental effects of inflammation. Therapy that

TABLE 5-23	Antagonism of Inflammatory and Metabolic Mediators
Interference with effects of endotoxin	
Clear endotoxin from circulation	
Antiendotoxin antibody	
Bind toxin to membrane	
Filter toxin out	
Interfere with binding of endotoxin to effector cells (i.e., bactericidal or permeability-increasing protein)	
Interference with the activation of pro-inflammatory cytokines	
Steroids	
Nonsteroidal anti-inflammatory agents	
Inhibition of IL-1-converting enzyme	
Interference with the activity of increased pro-inflammatory cytokines	
Anti-TNF, anti-IL-1 antibodies	
Binding of TNF and IL-1 with excess receptors	
Blocking of effector cell receptors (i.e., administration of IL-1 receptor antago nist)	
Continuous blood filtration	
Administration of anti-inflammatory cytokines	
Interference with superoxide activity	
Decrease production	
Increase scavenging	
Interference with secondary mediators	
Cyclooxygenase system	
Nitric oxide system	
Complement	
Histamine, serotonin, kinin system	
Coagulation system	
Interference with inflammatory cell activation by blocking activation receptors (i.e., inhibition of leukocyte integrin and selectin)	

IL, interleukin; TNF, tumor necrosis factor.

aggressively suppresses inflammation (i.e., pharmacologic doses of anti-inflammatory steroids) may provide short-term benefits (e.g., improvement in hemodynamic and pulmonary function), but the loss of the beneficial effects of inflammation may result in death secondary to recurrent infection or wound breakdown.

For all of the therapies listed in Table 5-23, this balance must be considered. The benefits of inflammation are primarily local (i.e., at the focus of tissue injury or infection). The detrimental effects are primarily systemic (e.g., alterations in circulation or pulmonary function). Therapies that allow local inflammation to continue while the systemic inflammation is suppressed may augment the proper inflammatory balance.

In general, these therapies are most helpful in patients who appear to have severe systemic inflammation despite usually adequate therapy for the underlying illness. For instance, consider a 65-year-old previously healthy woman who has perforated diverticulitis and undergoes a sigmoid resection with end-sigmoid colostomy. Ordinarily, fluid resuscitation, surgery, and antibiotics are sufficient to reverse the detrimental effects of this severe inflammatory illness and support the proper balance between the beneficial and detrimental effects of inflammation. However, if organ malfunction (e.g., ARDS, hyperdynamic circulation, impaired renal function) consistent with ongoing severe inflammation is still present 3 to 4 days later, then one possible explanation is that the inflammation stimulated in other organs by the perforated diverticulitis is responsible for the lack of resolution, despite therapy that is often sufficient. In other words, the detrimental and beneficial effects of severe inflammation are out of balance. Under such circumstances, therapy directed at the systemic inflammation may be warranted.

Recently, two such therapies have shown limited benefit: (1) the use of recombinant human activated protein C and (2) the use of physiologic (rather than pharmacologic) doses of hydrocortisone.

A PRACTICAL GUIDE TO THE PATIENT IN SHOCK

Once a patient is recognized to be in shock, the guiding principles are to: (1) provide an excellent circulation and (2) treat severe inflammation.

Recognize the Patient in Shock

Clearly, the first step in the evaluation and management of the patient who is in shock is to recognize that a deficit in total body cellular function is present, that is, there is a "rude unhinging." The history is the first clue to the patient who is at risk (Table 5-24). Next, bedside examination can provide

TABLE 5-24	Characteristics of the Patient Who Is at Risk for Shock
Trauma or burn	
Vascular catastrophe—ruptured aneurysm	
Acute cardiac disease	
Acute abdominal disease	
Severe extraabdominal infection	

TABLE 5-25	Bedside Examination Indicators of Shock
Hypotension	
Tachycardia	
Tachypnea	
Hyperthermia or hypothermia	
Peripheral vasoconstriction and cool extremities	
Hypotension with warm extremities	
Agitation and altered mental status	
Oliguria	

clues, but severe hypotension and marked tachycardia may not always accompany other evidence of shock (Table 5-25). Next come common laboratory data, which are frequently abnormal during shock (Table 5-26) and may provide the first clue of threatened cellular function.

Provide an Adequate Circulation

An accurate diagnosis of the state of circulation is critical.

The patient who is in cardiogenic shock requires aggressive hemodynamic monitoring as well as pharmacologic and possibly mechanical assistance of circulation (see earlier sections). This level of care clearly requires a critical care environment and physician expertise. The decision may be made to perform emergency cardiac catheterization or cardiac surgery.

The hypotensive supine adult who does not have a cardiogenic process most often has lost at least 30% of intravascular volume (~1,500 mL in a 70-kg person). Replacement with isotonic crystalloid solution requires a 3:1 ratio as the crystalloid distributes throughout the extracellular space. Therefore, 4,500 mL crystalloid solution is required to begin plasma volume restitution in this patient. Because there is no organ in the body that is improved by hypoperfusion, and because prolonged hypoperfusion induces or aggravates tissue inflammation, restitution of an adequate circulation should be accomplished rapidly (within minutes, if possible, with two large-bore intravenous lines wide open).

When decreased venous return (most often as a result of hypovolemia) is the cause of hypoperfusion, a diagnostic evaluation of the etiology of impaired venous return must occur simultaneously with restoration of circulation. Venous return can improve with fluid infusion, regardless of the underlying etiology of the decrease (e.g., hypovolemia vs. pericardial tamponade).

TABLE 5-26	Common Laboratory Abnormalities With Shock
Metabolic acidosis	
Elevated BUN and creatinine	
Leukocytosis or leukopenia	
Elevated blood glucose	
Decreased platelet count	
Decreased ionized calcium	

TABLE 5-27	Bedside Indicators of an Excellent Circulation
Normal blood pressure and pulse for the individual	
Normal mental status	
Warm extremities	
Urine output ≥0.5 mL/kg/hr	
Resolution of metabolic acidosis	

TABLE 5-28	Monitors of Circulation Status
Cardiac index	>4.5 L/min/m²
Mixed venous O₂ saturation	≥70%
Central venous O₂ saturation	70%
Oxygen delivery	>600 mL/min/m²
Oxygen consumption	>170 mL/min/m²

Ideal values indicate a good prognosis.

As described in previous sections, the circulatory parameters that indicate an excellent circulation may vary from patient to patient, but general bedside guidelines are listed in Table 5-27. More sophisticated indicators of an excellent circulation have been proposed, and may be of particular value when evidence of organ malfunction is present, despite bedside indicators that circulation is adequate (i.e., BUN and creatinine levels are increasing when the blood pressure and pulse are normal; Table 5-28).

Treat Severe Inflammation

Treating severe inflammation requires recognition that an inflammatory state is present (see discussion of severe inflammatory states). Next, the focus of severe inflammation must be localized and treated (e.g., antibiotics for pneumonia, colon resection for perforated diverticulitis). Usually, these interventions suffice. Occasionally, the other methods described in the section on severe inflammatory states are used to diminish the effects of severe inflammation.

Hypoperfusion can cause inflammation or aggravate established inflammation. Therefore, providing an excellent circulation is as much a treatment of inflammation as is the use of antibiotics or surgery. As a corollary, because inflammation can induce both total body and regional hypoperfusion, treating inflammation improves circulation.

Conclusion

Total body cellular malfunction (i.e., shock) can result from various insults that may be broadly categorized as severe hypoperfusion or severe inflammatory disturbances. Almost invariably, hypoperfusion and inflammation coexist in patients who have shock. Restoring an excellent circulation and treating severe inflammation are the keys to preserving cellular and organ function and preventing death from shock.

thePoint ✴ Go to http://thePoint.lww.com/activate and use your scratch-off code on the inside cover of this book to access bonus chapters, question bank, videos, and more.

SAMPLE CASE

A 45-year-old male alcoholic comes to the Emergency Department with a complaint of upper abdominal and back pain of 12 hours' duration. He vomits green-looking material several times. He denies hematemesis, diarrhea, bloody bowel movements, and liver disease. He is not a diabetic.

His temperature is 38.6 degrees C, his blood pressure is 90/60 mm Hg, pulse 120 bpm, respiration is 26/minute with an oxygen saturation of 92% with 4 L of nasal oxygen.

Physical examination shows an agitated middle-aged man who is pale with cyanotic fingers. His chest is clear, his neck veins are flat, his heart is without murmur or gallop. His abdomen shows epigastric distention and no scars or bulges. He has no bowel sounds. Percussion reveals tenderness in the epigastrium and palpation reveals involuntary guarding in that region. His hands and feet are cyanotic and cold.

He is disoriented to place and date.

Passage of a bladder catheter returns 100 mL of dark urine.

At the time of a recent discharge following admission for alcohol withdrawal, his hemoglobin was 13.2 g/dL. His BUN was 22 mg/dL and creatinine 0.8 mg/dL. His blood pressure at discharge was 130/70 mm Hg.

Laboratory data are:

Hgb	16.7 g/dL
WBC	16,000
Bands	35%

Platelets	96,000
Sodium	132 mEq/L
Potassium	3.2 mEq/L
Chloride	95 mEq/L
Bicarbonate	20 mEq/L
Glucose	220 mg/dL
BUN	45 mg/dL
Creatinine	1.9 mg/dL
Bilirubin	1.8 mg/dL
Alkaline phosphatase	130 mEq/L
AST	120 IU/L
Amylase	1,200 U/L

Arterial Blood Gas

pH	7.28
pCO_2	28 mm Hg
pO_2	66 mm Hg
Arterial lactic acid	6 mEq/L (normal < 2.3)
Ionized calcium	0.96 mmol/L (normal 1.12–1.22 mmol/L)
Blood alcohol	1,845 mg/L

Plain x-rays of the chest and abdomen are unrevealing. An abdominal CT scan shows a markedly enlarged, edematous pancreas, with several peripancreatic fluid collections.

DESCRIPTION OF "SURGICAL" MANAGEMENT

Severe pancreatitis provides an excellent model of the linkage between hypoperfusion and inflammation. In this case this man is suffering a "rude unhinging" as exemplified by bedside analysis (hypotension, mental status changes, cool, cyanotic extremities) and laboratory parameters (elevated lactic acid, low ionized calcium, elevated glucose). The etiology of his shock is both hypoperfusion and inflammation, but the immediately reversible component is his circulatory deficit.

As with most cases of hypotension, the primary cause of his low blood pressure is hypovolemia from loss of plasma volume. His cardiac output would be expected to be low and his systemic resistance elevated from the neurohumoral response that would override the vasodilation mechanisms of inflammation. The increase in hemoglobin by 25% provides an initial estimate of that plasma volume deficit. If he weighs 70 kg and we calculate his plasma volume as 5% body weight, then he has a plasma volume deficit of about 900 mL. Using isotonic crystalloid to replace this deficit will demand expansion of the entire extracellular space, with two thirds of that volume outside of the vascular compartment. Therefore, his initial resuscitation should consist of 3 L of warmed isotonic saline administered as rapidly as possible (two large-bore IVs) just as if he were a hypotensive blunt trauma patient.

Restoration of plasma volume is associated with better outcomes, as exemplified by studies that show increased pancreatitis mortality in patients with persistently elevated hemoglobin concentrations. Similar to the data gathered in sepsis, a principle method of limiting the severity of pancreatic inflammation and the associated shock is rapid restoration of circulation.

The surgical team must anticipate that the initial resuscitation will not immediately interrupt the inflammatory disease. The team must plan ongoing "resuscitative" fluid management to avoid recurrent episodes of shock that aggravate cellular injury. To do this the patient must be closely monitored (i.e., intensive care unit type of environment) with attention to the cellular injury risk. Admission to the regular floor with a bladder catheter as a monitoring device would be unwarranted. He should have at least CVP monitoring for both pressure and central venous saturation. An arterial pressure catheter would aid measurement of resuscitation effect from both blood pressure and blood test data. Repeat hemoglobin measurements will help discern if plasma volume is approaching his baseline. Most certainly, an increase in hemoglobin should prompt renewed efforts to expand his non-cellular blood volume.

The team should anticipate that despite rapid attention to circulation, other systemic effects of severe pancreatitis may progress from the pancreatitis itself and the systemic tissue injury that the shock engendered. For instance, worsening respiratory status would be very likely and not attributable to the fluid administration.

If hypotension persists after expansion of the plasma volume, bedside and laboratory analysis will help discern if the cardiac output is likely to still be low or that hypotension is now from the vasodilation that accompanies systemic inflammation. Better mental status, warm extremities with brisk capillary refill, good urine output, and resolution of acidosis would all support the achievement of a hyperdynamic circulation (increased cardiac output) and hypotension from a low systemic resistance. A central venous saturation >70% would also support this analysis. Under these circumstances, where hypotension is from low resistance rather than a low cardiac output, augmenting systemic resistance with a vasopressor (norepinephrine, vasopressin) will not likely prove harmful.

It is also not likely that nonsurgical physicians will recognize the similarity between pancreatitis and severe trauma and other systemic inflammatory states that produce shock. The benefit of early restoration of circulation and the magnitude of plasma volume restitution necessary for that restoration is more commonly encountered in surgical practice.

The volume of isotonic fluid provided in the first 24 hours to such a patient is another marker of the severity of the illness. Patients who sequester 10 L of fluid in 24 hours have a greater threat from their illness than patients who sequester 5 L. When the patient who sequesters more fluid exhibits more illness, the clinician should remember that pancreatitis is the illness, not the fluid. If circulation is not restored, shock will continue and death will follow. Limiting efforts to resuscitate and maintain an excellent circulation will not ameliorate the "rude unhinging."

Once circulation is satisfactory, it is possible for the inflammatory illness to continue and cause cell injury from inflammatory toxins. For pancreatitis little additional therapy is possible, except for surgery when the peri-pancreatic region becomes infected. Early surgical intervention (24 to 48 hours) is not warranted and peri-pancreatic infection usually takes several days to become evident. At that point the sterile inflammatory illness becomes "sepsis" and the principles of infection management (source control, antibiotics) are employed to limit or reverse cell injury from inflammatory toxins.

SAMPLE QUESTIONS

Questions

Choose the best answer for each question.

1. A 65-year-old man is severely injured in a dump truck rollover accident. He has sustained bilateral femur fractures, a pelvic fracture, and a pulmonary contusion. A pulmonary artery catheter is placed in order to guide you in the optimization of his hemodynamic status and guide his resuscitation. Correction of which current value will have the most dramatic impact on his oxygen delivery?

   A. Measured cardiac output of 2 L/minute
   B. Serum hemoglobin of 12 mg/dL
   C. Arterial PO_2 of 82 mm Hg
   D. Arterial oxygen saturation of 93%
   E. Pulmonary capillary occlusive pressure of 10 mm Hg

2. A 75-year-old woman with a history of congestive heart failure underwent elective sigmoid resection for severe recurrent diverticulitis. Postoperatively, she experiences shortness of breath. Physical exam and chest radiography suggest the presence of pulmonary edema. Which of the following parameters is the most accurate determinant of her left ventricular preload?

   A. Central venous pressure
   B. Pulmonary artery occlusive pressure
   C. Systemic vascular resistance
   D. Pulmonary venous pressure
   E. Left ventricular end-diastolic volume

3. A 22-year-old man is transported emergently to the hospital after sustaining a stab wound to the left chest. On initial survey, his airway is patent and he is breathing spontaneously, but he appears to be in shock. Which of the following findings best supports your working diagnosis of pericardial tamponade?

   A. Central venous pressure of 8 mm Hg
   B. Crisp S1S2 on cardiac auscultation
   C. Paradoxical pulse of 18 mm Hg
   D. Left atrial distention
   E. Increased QRS voltage on ECG

4. Two weeks following a severe motorcycle crash, a 25-year-old woman remains intubated in the surgical ICU. You are called to the bedside to evaluate a change in her condition. On evaluation, her vital signs include temperature of 39°C, heart rate of 110 beats/minute, respiratory rate of 22, blood pressure of 88/50, and arterial oxygen saturation of 96%. Her urine output has been 20 mL over the past 8 hours. On exam, she is in moderate distress and appears confused. She has crackles posteriorly in her left lung fields and her extremities are warm. A bronchoalveolar lavage is performed revealing Gram-negative rods. What is your diagnosis?

   A. Atelectasis
   B. Septic shock
   C. Systemic inflammatory response syndrome
   D. Allergic reaction to penicillin
   E. Pulmonary embolus

5. A 34-year-old woman is thrown from a horse during a trail ride and brought to the emergency department 60 minutes after the accident. She is awake but appears to be mildly confused. She complains of left chest pain that is worsened with inspiration as well as generalized abdominal pain. On exam, her airway is patent and breathing unlabored. Her pulse is 110 beats/minute. Her blood pressure is 85/62. Her breath sounds are equal bilaterally. Her neck veins are flat and her skin is cool. She is tender over her left lower ribs and left upper quadrant. You suspect that she has sustained an injury to her spleen with resultant hemorrhage. Approximately what percentage of intravascular volume loss has she experienced?

   A. 0%
   B. 10%
   C. 20%
   D. 30%
   E. 50%

Answers and Explanations

1. Answer: A

Oxygen delivery is delineated by the relationship $O_2D = (CO \times CaO_2 \times 10)$. 10 is a factor to convert mL O_2/100 mL blood to mL O_2/L blood. The key components of the relationship are CO (measured cardiac output, which in turn is defined by the relationship CO = HR × stroke volume) and arterial oxygen content (CaO_2, defined as $CaO_2 = 1.39 \times Hgb \times SaO_2 + (PaO_2 \times 0.0031)$). Of the answers listed, the most deranged from baseline is a CO of 2L/minute (average adult normal values are 4.5 L/minute for women and 5 L/minute for men), and, given the mathematical relationship of the O_2D equation, it will have the greatest impact on this value when corrected. The values given for hemoglobin (B), arterial oxygen saturation (C), and pulmonary artery occlusive pressure (E) are all near or within normal values. Even relatively dramatic changes in arterial PO_2 will have a minimal impact on O_2D given the correction factor of 0.0031 as delineated in the CaO_2 equation (answer C).

2. Answer: E

Preload is defined as the amount of myocardial stretch prior to myocardial contraction. Increased stretch leading to increased myocardial contraction is described by the Frank-Starling mechanism. Preload is most closely related to end-diastolic volume (answer E). Several other factors, including central venous pressure, pulmonary artery occlusive pressure, and pulmonary venous pressure, may also be used to estimate preload, but they are not as accurate as left ventricular end-diastolic volume for this purpose (answers A, B, and D). Systemic vascular resistance (C) is not mathematically related to preload.

3. Answer: C

As the disease process progresses, pericardial tamponade results in decreased venous return, with resultant decreased stroke volume, hypoperfusion, and shock. Clinical evidence of tamponade includes an increased paradoxical pulse (>15 mm Hg; answer C). Other signs include elevated central venous pressure (rather than normal, answer A), muffled heart sounds (rather than crisp S1S2, answer B), left atrial collapse (rather than distension, answer D), and decreased QRS voltage on ECG (answer E).

4. Answer: B

Although inflammation is a normal response to tissue injury, the patient in the above scenario is displaying evidence of a dysfunctional inflammatory response. The derangements noted are too severe for atelectasis (answer A), which is associated with slight fever and normal blood pressure. Although allergic reactions (answer D) can be associated with cardiovascular collapse, there is no history of recent medication administration given. Pulmonary embolus (answer E) may present as tachycardia and hypotension but is typically also associated with hypoxia.

To meet the definition of the systemic inflammatory response syndrome, or SIRS, a patient must have two or more of the following conditions: (1) temperature >38.5°C or <36°C; (2) heart rate >90 beats/minute; (3) respiratory rate >20 breaths/minute or $Paco_2$ < 32 Torr; and (4) total leukocyte count >12,000 cells/mm³, <4000 cells/mm³, or >10% immature forms. Although the patient in the scenario meets these criteria (answer C), the additional presence of end-organ dysfunction (hypotension, oliguria) and infection (Gram-negative rods on bronchoalveolar lavage [BAL]) make the diagnosis of septic shock more appropriate (answer B).

5. Answer: D

The patient described in the scenario has suffered a splenic injury and progressive hemorrhage over the course of the hour leading up to presentation. She is demonstrating progressive hemodynamic effects from volume loss as described in Table 5-12, including mild tachycardia and hypotension, altered mental status, and decreased skin perfusion. Blood volume loss of 0% to 10% produces little change in hemodynamics or physical exam (answers A and B). Blood loss of 20% over 1 hour results in increased pulse, but normal blood pressure, mentation, and skin palpation (answer C). Blood loss of 30% is associated with mild hypotension, tachycardia, altered mental status, skin vasoconstriction, and decreased urine output (answer D; correct answer). Loss of 50% of blood volume is associated with severe physiological derangements, including profound hypotension, severe tachycardia, obtunded mental status, and anuria (answer E).

6
Surgical Critical Care

SAMUEL A. TISHERMAN, M.D. • MELISSA BRUNSVOLD, M.D. • BRIAN J. DALEY, M.D. •
JAMES E. MORRISON, M.D. • PAUL J. SCHENARTS, M.D. • CHRISTOPHER WOHLTMANN, M.D.

Objectives

Respiratory

1. Describe the initial management of patients with acute respiratory failure.
2. Explain the differences between volume-controlled and pressure-controlled modes of ventilation.

Cardiovascular

1. Describe methods for hemodynamic monitoring.
2. Describe the hemodynamic effects of vasoactive agents, including inotropes and vasopressors.
3. List the steps involved in cardiac arrest resuscitation, including postresuscitation care.

Renal

1. Explain the difference between prerenal and renal causes of acute kidney injury.
2. List the indications for renal replacement therapy.

Liver

1. Describe the initial management of complications of liver disease, including coagulopathy, variceal bleeding, encephalopathy, and ascites.
2. List the components of the Child-Pugh classification of liver dysfunction.

Gastrointestinal (GI)

1. List the causes of intestinal ischemia.
2. Describe the physiologic changes typically seen with the abdominal compartment syndrome.

Endocrine

1. List endocrine disorders seen in critically ill patients.

Neurologic

1. List the causes of delirium in the surgical intensive care unit (SICU).
2. List the treatments for intracranial hypertension in patients with traumatic brain injury (TBI).
3. List the components of the brain death examination.

Systemic Inflammatory Response Syndrome

1. List the clinical findings found with the systemic inflammatory response syndrome.

Infectious Diseases

1. List common causes of sepsis in the surgical intensive care unit.
2. Define ventilator-associated pneumonia.

End Points of Resuscitation

1. Describe the laboratory and clinical tests that can be used to determine the adequacy of resuscitation.

Preventing Complications in the surgical intensive care unit

1. List risk factors for deep venous thrombosis in the SICU.
2. List the indications for placement of an inferior vena cava filter.

Improvements and innovations in medical care have allowed critically ill patients with very complex derangements in their physiology to benefit from medical and surgical care. In the hospitalized population in general, there is a greater complexity of care, advanced invasive monitoring, and procedures utilizing intricate technologies for diagnosis and treatment. Today's SICU integrates all these technologies along with intensive nursing, respiratory, and physician care. This setting allows scrutiny of every facet of the patient's care to result in the best outcome for that patient.

Patients who require intensive care have dysfunction of one or more of the body's organ systems, or the potential to develop such dysfunction. Early action is the key to good outcomes, whether the patient has had a TBI or hemorrhagic shock due to trauma. The SICU setting allows for early detection of abnormalities and has a system to address each and every issue.

The multiple monitoring and therapeutic interventions in the SICU require constant attention by a well-orchestrated team directed by the surgical intensivist and implemented by the nursing staff. The SICU team typically also includes respiratory therapists; pharmacists; physical, occupational, and speech therapists; dieticians; and social workers. Consultants with unique body system knowledge or competency in a unique procedure become involved as needed. The goal is for the patient to receive the right therapy at the right time, delivered by the expert in that field. One of the most important aspects of care is communication so that the multidisciplinary team, the patient, and family are all aware of the therapeutic plan.

A systematic program for care, or protocol, may be developed for many facets of care, such as ventilator weaning, burn care, etc. Each unit must adapt the protocol to meet the unique qualities of that unit. Many protocols are based on published evidence or expert consensus guidelines that link care delivered to outcome. Unfortunately, there is a dearth of data for many of the common treatments delivered today. Protocols or flow diagrams ensure that each contributory aspect is addressed and that each intervention is goal directed. Even if a therapeutic maneuver is not performed, the protocol ensures it was considered.

RESPIRATORY FAILURE

Prevention and Respiratory Monitoring

"An ounce of prevention is worth more than a pound of cure" is certainly true for surgical patients when it comes to respiratory failure, since placing a patient on mechanical ventilation has many potential complications, such as pneumonia, barotrauma, and tracheal stenosis.

In order to prevent respiratory failure, many issues must be considered. In the postoperative patient, good pulmonary "toilet," which consists of an incentive spirometer, coughing, deep breathing at least 10 times an hour, and mobilization of the patient, improves the clearance of secretions and prevents atelectasis. Mobilizing the patient allows the abdominal contents to fall toward the pelvis and increase excursion of the diaphragm. In cases of significant abdominal distension, such as bowel obstruction, a nasogastric tube can be used for decompression.

Inadequate postoperative or posttrauma pain control can result in splinting of the chest wall with poor respiratory effort. Secretions may not be cleared adequately, and pneumonia may result. Many modalities of pain control may be utilized to attain adequate pain control. Narcotics (either intravenous or oral) may be utilized, but high doses may produce respiratory depression. Nonsteroidal anti-inflammatory drugs (NSAIDs) can decrease the need for narcotics. Epidural catheters, lidocaine patches, and nerve blocks are also potential adjuncts to systemic analgesics.

Patients in the SICU should have close monitoring of their respiratory status. This begins with checking vital signs frequently, especially respiratory rate and effort. Oxygen saturation of hemoglobin is monitored by continuous pulse oximetry, allowing titration of supplemental oxygen. Carbon dioxide levels can be monitored by arterial blood gases. If a patient is having increased work of breathing, as evidenced by use of accessory muscles or abdominal breathing, the etiology for this distress must be rapidly evaluated. Astute clinicians should be able to detect respiratory deterioration by physical examination, often before the monitoring systems detect a problem.

Interventions

Respiratory failure occurs from failure of oxygenation (low PaO_2), failure of ventilation (high PCO_2), or both. During SICU evaluation, it is important to determine the cause of the respiratory failure to initiate the correct treatment. Treatment for hypoxic respiratory failure involves increasing oxygen available for transport into the pulmonary circulation (increased oxygen concentrations and mean airway pressures), and treatment for hypercarbic failure involves increasing minute ventilation. Specific ventilator strategies can target hypoxemic or hypercarbic respiratory failure.

The first intervention in patients with either respiratory distress or oxygen desaturation is usually to administer supplemental oxygen. The best way to accomplish this is with high-flow oxygen via a nonrebreather face mask. Such a mask minimizes entrainment of room air around the mask. If oxygen alone is ineffective, then positive pressure ventilation may help.

Not all patients with respiratory failure require invasive positive pressure ventilation, however. Noninvasive positive pressure ventilation can be provided via a tightly fitting face mask. The two modalities for providing this therapy are continuous positive airway pressure (CPAP), which provides a constant pressure, and bilevel positive airway pressure (BiPAP), which provides separate pressures for inspiration (IPAP) and expiration (EPAP). These modalities are best used in patients with intact mental status and reversible causes of respiratory failure (e.g., fluid overload).

If all preventive and noninvasive methods are not effective, invasive positive pressure ventilation is required. This involves intubation of the airway, usually via an oral route. Nasotracheal intubation can be used in patients who are breathing spontaneously and do not have facial trauma. Indications for intubation include inadequate oxygenation, inadequate ventilation, increased work of breathing, and inability to protect the airway from aspiration.

Prior to intubation, the appropriate equipment, such as suction, a variety of endotracheal tubes, stylets, medications, and carbon dioxide detectors, must be available. No medications should be administered until all equipment is ready. The patient's airway should be assessed (mouth opening, visualization of anatomic structures, cervical spine flexibility) so that potential difficulty with intubation can be anticipated. The most experienced person available should perform the procedure, and a backup plan must be considered. For the trauma patient with a potential cervical spine facture, in-line cervical stabilization must be maintained during intubation attempts (see Chapter 9, Trauma). The tube must be visualized passing the vocal cords and placement verified by auscultation and exhalation of carbon dioxide.

In the event that a patient cannot be intubated due to either anatomic issues or severe facial trauma, a surgical airway is necessary. Rarely, a surgical airway is the initial airway of choice. The fastest and best way to obtain a surgical airway is to perform a cricothyrotomy. A vertical incision is made over the cricoid and thyroid cartilages. A transverse incision is then made through the cricothyroid membrane. After entry into the airway is made, the tract is dilated. A no. 6 or smaller endotracheal tube is inserted until the balloon is just within the airway.

The final way to secure the airway is by tracheostomy, which can be used urgently in cases of severe laryngeal injury or in children <8 years of age. Electively, a tracheostomy is used for patients with anticipated need for a prolonged period of ventilator support to help prevent subglottic stenosis and injury to the vocal cords. Timing of tracheostomy is controversial but is based on anticipated duration of mechanical ventilation, neurologic status, underlying disease, and comorbid conditions. If needed urgently, the procedure is performed open, but if done electively, it may be done percutaneously.

Mechanical Ventilation

The primary modes of ventilation are volume control (or volume-cycled) and pressure control (or pressure-cycled). In volume control, the primary goal of the ventilator is to provide the patient with a preset tidal volume. The tidal volume is delivered regardless of the airway pressure generated by its delivery, up to a set limit to avoid barotrauma (pressure injury) to the lungs. The ventilatory modes associated with volume control are assist control (AC) and intermittent mandatory ventilation (IMV). In AC, all breaths, whether initiated by the ventilator or by the patient, provide the tidal volume set on the ventilator. The patient does little work of breathing. In IMV, machine tidal volumes are given only up to the respiratory rate set on the ventilator. Any breaths initiated above that rate will only provide a tidal volume generated by patient effort.

In pressure control mode, the airway pressure is set by the clinician. The tidal volume provided to the patient is variable and is determined by lung compliance. The goal is to allow for oxygenation without generating barotrauma, sometimes focusing on oxygenation at the expense of allowing permissive hypercarbia. The standard maximum pressure is a plateau pressure (the pressure in the lungs when a brief inspiratory pause is provided by the ventilator) of 35 cm H_2O. Inspiratory time is also controlled with this mode. For patients with severe hypoxemia, prolonging inspiratory time, even to the point of inversing the inspiratory:expiratory ratio, can help recruit alveoli and improve oxygenation. Taken to the extreme, this mode may be called airway pressure release ventilation.

Pressure support ventilation (PSV) is a form of pressure-cycled ventilation. When a patient attempts to breathe through an endotracheal tube and ventilator tubing, there is significant resistance. Positive pressure administered during inspiration helps to overcome this resistance. The positive pressure is present until inspiratory flow decreases to a certain level. PSV can be used either as a stand-alone mode of support or a supplement to IMV. Since the patient controls the respiratory rate and receives support rapidly, patients may find this mode to be more comfortable than other modes.

The pressure-cycled modes of ventilation can be combined as "bilevel" ventilation, which is a pressure-controlled mode that also allows the patient to breathe spontaneously and receive additional pressure support above controlled levels of pressure.

A final method of ventilation is high-frequency jet or oscillatory ventilation. This method is utilized to help decrease barotrauma. The tidal volumes in this method are extremely small, but the respiratory rate may be as high as 600 to 900 breaths/minute. Air is pushed in during inspiration, and expiration is passive.

The adult respiratory distress syndrome (ARDS) presents a particular ventilatory challenge. In ARDS, the patient has bilateral alveolar infiltrates without evidence of cardiac failure.

Lung compliance is significantly decreased, and the PaO_2/FiO_2 ratio is <200. Clinical trials have suggested benefit of a lung-protective ventilatory strategy using tidal volumes of 6 to 8 mL/kg to prevent barotrauma. Combinations of positive end-expiratory pressure (PEEP) and FiO_2 are adjusted to maintain adequate PaO_2 by maintaining alveolar recruitment but minimizing the toxic effects on the lungs of high levels of oxygen.

Weaning

The process of weaning from the ventilator has multiple components. The initial issue is assessing readiness to wean. The process that caused the respiratory failure must be corrected. Pain control must be adequate, but not sedating. Sedation is titrated to allow the patient to be cooperative, but not be too anxious. FiO_2 must be titrated down to <50%, and PEEP must be decreased to ≤5 cm H_2O.

Although weaning can be accomplished by progressively decreasing IMV rate or PSV level, a daily trial of spontaneous breathing on minimal ventilator support (typically pressure support of 5 cm H_2O) or a T-piece (a connector for administering oxygen through an endotracheal tube with the patient disconnected from the ventilator) tends to be more rapid. If the patient tolerates the trial with an adequate respiratory rate, tidal volume, and oxygen saturation, the patient can be extubated.

CARDIOVASCULAR FAILURE

Hemodynamic Monitoring

Arterial Catheterization

Arterial catheterization, though invasive, is relatively common in critically ill patients as it serves to allow arterial blood collection for laboratory studies as well as continuous measurement of blood pressure. Usual sites are the radial artery or the femoral artery, which has a larger size and flow. Complications of arterial catheterization are rare, but include infection, bleeding, vascular injury (pseudoaneurysm and arteriovenous fistula), distal ischemia, and thromboembolism.

Blood pressure readings from arterial catheters allow minute-to-minute monitoring. The measured pressure can be confounded by malpositioning of the transducer or dampening of the waveform by air bubbles in the tubing or excessive tubing length. Blood pressure can also be overestimated if the system is incorrectly calibrated or there is a "whip" in the waveform.

Central Venous Catheterization

Central venous catheters (CVCs) are commonly used to treat critically ill patients (Figure 6-1). Indications for central venous catheterization include the need for hemodynamic monitoring of central venous pressure (CVP) readings, administration of medications that may be irritating to peripheral vessels, and inability to obtain peripheral intravenous access. A common misconception is that large volume resuscitation requires a CVC; since these catheters typically are long, and flow rates are related not only to radius of the tube but its length, they may not provide rapid flow. The exceptions are short, large-diameter catheters, often called "introducers," as they can also be used to introduce a pulmonary artery catheter (PAC).

Complications of CVC include pneumothorax, malpositioning, infection, thrombosis, vascular injury, air embolism, and arrhythmia. Confirmation of placement in the desired location is necessary before infusing potent agents. Infections

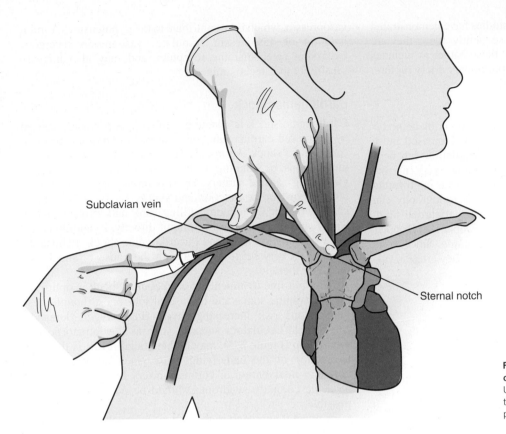

Subclavian vein

Sternal notch

FIGURE 6-1. Central venous catheterization is often accomplished via the subclavian vein. Understanding the anatomic relationships between the clavicle, subclavian vein, and the underlying pleura is important for safe cannulation.

can be decreased by careful attention to aseptic technique during placement and by using antibiotic-coated catheters. During placement, practitioners should wear a hat, mask, gown, and gloves, and use sterile drapes. Catheterization of the femoral vein carries an increased risk of infection and deep venous thrombosis compared to the subclavian or internal jugular sites. A CVC should be removed when the need for central access is over. It should not be left simply to function as an intravenous line. Air embolism can be avoided by careful control of an open CVC and by keeping patients in the head-down (Trendelenburg) position until the catheter is capped. Similarly, CVCs should be removed with the patient supine.

Pulmonary Artery Catheterization

PACs were initially developed to guide treatment in the setting of myocardial dysfunction (Figure 6-2). These catheters have at least three ports. The distal port measures pulmonary artery pressure, a proximal port measures CVP in the right atrium, and other ports can be used for infusions. The tip of the catheter has a small balloon that is inflated to facilitate passage of the catheter through the heart into the pulmonary artery. In addition, inflation of the balloon allows measurement of the pulmonary artery wedge pressure or pulmonary artery occlusion pressure, which can approximate left atrial pressure. Temperature changes at the catheter tip following injection of fluid into the catheter can be used to measure cardiac output by the thermodilution method. Mixed venous oxygen saturation, measured from a pulmonary artery blood sample, can be useful to examine the relationship between oxygen delivery and oxygen consumption by tissues.

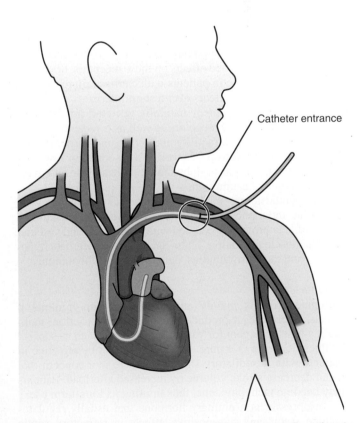

Catheter entrance

FIGURE 6-2. The pulmonary artery is cannulated using a balloon-tipped catheter placed via the internal jugular, subclavian, or femoral veins.

Despite the potential benefits, no studies have demonstrated improved outcomes with PACs. Consequently, today they are used infrequently. The risk of using these catheters includes the standard risks of CVC, as well as pulmonary artery rupture, pulmonary infarction, and endocarditis.

Other Methods of Hemodynamic Monitoring

Several newer and often less invasive methods of hemodynamic monitoring have been gaining favor. Increased pulse pressure variability during mechanical ventilation can be a simple method for identifying hypovolemia. Very narrow pulse pressures can suggest poor stroke volume as in profound hypovolemia or cardiac dysfunction. Echocardiography can provide evidence of cardiac dysfunction or pericardial fluid, as well as an estimation of volume status. Esophageal Doppler monitoring uses flow to estimate stroke volume. Since these readings are based on flow and not pressure, they are less vulnerable to changes in intrathoracic pressure.

Hemodynamic Support

Inotropes

In cardiac failure or cardiogenic shock, the contractile function of the myocardium must be supported to improve cardiac output and organ perfusion. This is commonly achieved through inotropic support with agents such as dobutamine, dopamine, epinephrine, and phosphodiesterase inhibitors. At times, vasopressors, which increase vascular tone, are also needed.

Dobutamine is a β1 agonist that increases myocardial contractility and heart rate. These effects may be at the expense of increasing myocardial oxygen consumption, which may worsen cardiac function. Because peripheral vasodilatation can occur due to mild β2 activity, dobutamine may not be the best inotrope in a patient who is hypotensive. In addition, dobutamine may lead to tachyarrhythmias, which do not improve cardiac output.

Dopamine has different effects at different doses and progressively stimulates dopaminergic, β1, and α1 receptors. Because of the combined effects on these receptors, dopamine may be a good choice in patients with cardiac failure as it can be titrated to various effects over a short interval.

Epinephrine is a potent naturally secreted adrenal hormone that stimulates β receptors as well as α receptors. It has marked effects on contractility and increasing vascular tone. Thus it is a useful inotrope, as well as a vasopressor. Epinephrine has effects similar to dobutamine on heart rate and myocardial oxygen consumption.

Phosphodiesterase inhibitors increase intracellular cyclic adenosine monophosphate (AMP). This results in increased myocardial contractility coupled with myocardial and vascular smooth muscle relaxation. These agents may exacerbate hypotension and tachyarrhythmias, but less so than dobutamine.

Vasopressors

Norepinephrine is mainly an α1 agonist with minimal β effects. Therefore, it produces potent vasoconstriction, making it a first-line agent for vasodilatory shock, such as sepsis.

Phenylephrine is a pure α1 agonist. It can be effective in patients with vasodilatory shock, but there is a concern that it can decrease stroke volume by increased afterload. Patients may become tachyphylactic, thus limiting its long-term use.

Vasopressin is a pituitary hormone that usually regulates volume status and has positive effects in refractory septic shock. Many of these patients have low levels of endogenous vasopressin, which may contribute to the hypotension. Administration of vasopressin stimulates vasopressin receptors, bypassing catecholamine receptors, and may also increase sensitivity to catecholamines.

Cardiogenic Shock

Cardiogenic shock is a state of global hypoperfusion caused by decreased cardiac function. The most common causes of cardiogenic shock are myocardial infarction, sepsis, trauma, medications, or stunning of the myocardium from cardioplegia during cardiac surgery. Dysrhythmias may also contribute to poor cardiac function and shock. Tachycardia reduces cardiac output by reducing filling time and stroke volume. Bradycardia reduces cardiac output directly. In addition, valvular dysfunction may lead to cardiogenic shock. Echocardiography is very helpful in defining the cause of shock and directing therapy.

The first-line treatment for cardiogenic shock is optimization of volume status and the use of inotropes, though these medications risk increasing myocardial oxygen demands. Mechanical circulatory support, such as the intraaortic balloon pump (Figure 6-3), may be beneficial if this is the case. Correction of the underlying cause, such as percutaneous coronary intervention or coronary artery bypass grafting for an acute coronary syndrome, should be pursued as soon as possible.

A general approach to the patient in shock is presented in Figure 6-4.

Cardiac Arrest

Sudden cardiac arrest is a frequent cause of death in the United States and is often a manifestation of coronary atherosclerosis. While cardiac arrest may occur in critically ill surgical patients with atherosclerosis, there are a variety of other reasons as well.

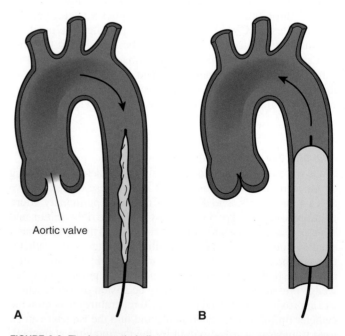

Aortic valve

A   **B**

FIGURE 6-3. The intraaortic balloon pump is placed via the femoral artery into the proximal, descending aorta. The balloon is inflated during diastole in order to increase coronary and cerebral perfusion and then deflated just before systole to decrease afterload.

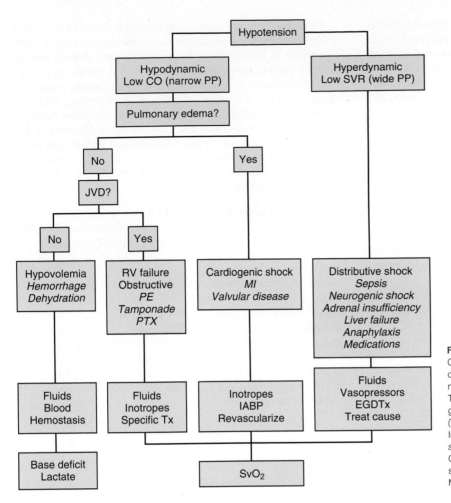

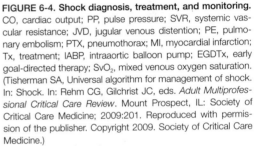

FIGURE 6-4. Shock diagnosis, treatment, and monitoring. CO, cardiac output; PP, pulse pressure; SVR, systemic vascular resistance; JVD, jugular venous distention; PE, pulmonary embolism; PTX, pneumothorax; MI, myocardial infarction; Tx, treatment; IABP, intraaortic balloon pump; EGDTx, early goal-directed therapy; SvO$_2$, mixed venous oxygen saturation. (Tisherman SA, Universal algorithm for management of shock. In: Shock. In: Rehm CG, Gilchrist JC, eds. *Adult Multiprofessional Critical Care Review.* Mount Prospect, IL: Society of Critical Care Medicine; 2009:201. Reproduced with permission of the publisher. Copyright 2009. Society of Critical Care Medicine.)

Frequently, cardiac arrest represents the end stage of acute and/or chronic illness. Less commonly, surgical patients develop sudden cardiac arrest. This may be caused by an acute myocardial infarction, pulmonary embolism (PE), acute respiratory decompensation (aspiration or mucous plugging), tension pneumothorax, or massive hemorrhage. First-line treatment for any cardiac arrest is the initiation of cardiopulmonary resuscitation (CPR). The recommendations for CPR have been developed and periodically revised by the American Heart Association based on the most up-to-date literature and expert consensus. As of the 2010 recommendations, for a suddenly unresponsive patient with abnormal or no breathing, rescuers should begin CPR. Lay rescuers should provide chest compressions only at a rate of 100 compressions per minute, while trained rescuers should also provide ventilations with a compression:ventilation ratio of 30:2. One theme throughout the recommendations is to initiate chest compressions as soon as possible and minimize any interruptions. When two providers are present and an advanced airway has been inserted (e.g., endotracheal tube, Combitube, or laryngeal mask airway), one provider should continue chest compressions at a rate of 100 compressions per minute without interruption, while the second provider delivers ventilations at a rate of 8 to 10 breaths/minute.

As soon as possible, the patient should have electrocardiographic monitoring initiated in order to assess the cardiac rhythm. If not already present, intravenous access (central or peripheral) should be established. Management at this point is dependent upon the rhythm. Ventricular fibrillation and pulseless ventricular tachycardia require defibrillation. Interruptions of chest compressions should be minimized both before and after the delivery of a shock, as well as during pulse checks. If defibrillation is unsuccessful, a vasopressor (epinephrine or vasopressin) should be administered to improve coronary perfusion pressure, followed by an antiarrhythmic (amiodarone or lidocaine).

For patients with pulseless electrical activity (PEA) or asystole, the initial treatment is a vasopressor (epinephrine or vasopressin). Atropine may be considered for asystole or PEA with a slow heart rate. More importantly, asystole and PEA are frequently caused by reversible factors. These may be remembered as the 6 H's and 4 T's: Hypovolemia, Hypoxia, Hydrogen ion (acidosis), Hypo- or Hyperkalemia, Hypoglycemia, Hypothermia, Toxins, Tamponade (cardiac), Tension pneumothorax, and Thrombosis (coronary or pulmonary). Outcome can be maximized by rapid recognition and management of these factors.

The postresuscitation care of the patient who has suffered a cardiac arrest may have a significant impact on outcome. Three main issues need to be addressed. First, the cause of the arrest needs to be determined, and any reversible pathology needs to be addressed (e.g., cardiac catheterization for acute myocardial infarction, thrombolytic therapy for massive PE). Second, the effects of the cardiac arrest on multiple organ systems, particularly the brain, should be minimized with standard SICU care. For the patient who remains comatose after normal hemodynamics have been restored, mild hypothermia (33°C to 34°C) for 12 to 24 hours has been shown to improve neurologic outcome and even survival. This can be initiated with the intravenous infusion of cold crystalloid solutions, followed by the use of ice packs or a cooling blanket, as well as new devices for therapeutic temperature management. Third, an estimate of long-term functional outcome is important. This involves serial neurologic examinations. The use of electrophysiology studies or brain magnetic resonance imaging may be helpful. To optimize long-term function, it is important for these patients to be referred for appropriate rehabilitation services once the acute medical issues have resolved.

ACUTE RENAL FAILURE

Acute renal failure, now more commonly referred to as acute kidney injury, occurs in 5% to 10% of hospitalized patients. The development of acute kidney injury results in retention of nitrogenous waste; in disturbances in fluid, electrolyte, and acid–base balance; and may also prolong the effect of the many medications that are excreted through the kidneys. Given the central regulatory function of the kidney, it is not surprising that acute kidney injury in the critical care setting is associated with a significant increase in morbidity and mortality of 150% to 300% depending upon severity of kidney injury.

The kidney is unique in its ability to regulate its own blood flow and hence regulate glomerular filtration. However, the kidney of the critically ill patient is at particular risk of hypoperfusion due to hemorrhage, hypovolemia, cardiac pump failure, and use of medications that cause vasoconstriction. The critically ill patient may also be exposed to nephrotoxic agents such as intravenous contrast, antibiotics, and antifungal agents.

Renal Monitoring

The first step in managing renal dysfunction is prevention. Primary preventative strategies include insuring adequate hydration, maintenance of perfusion pressure by keeping the mean arterial pressure >60 mm Hg, and limiting exposure to potentially nephrotoxic agents.

Early identification of renal dysfunction allows earlier treatment and results in an improved outcome. Kidney function is an excellent indicator of systemic perfusion and is relatively easy to monitor, though urine output alone is only one measure of renal function. An adult should make at least 0.5 mL/kg/hour and children 1 mL/kg/hour. Production of urine in amounts less than this should prompt immediate investigation. There are limitations to using urine output as a monitor of systemic perfusion and a measure of renal function. It is possible to have high-output renal failure, in which the kidney produces large volumes of urine but is not reabsorbing electrolytes or excreting nitrogenous waste products. In the setting of evolving or established renal failure, urine output alone may not correlate with systemic perfusion.

Due to these limitations, monitoring of urine output needs to be supplemented with other markers of renal function. Determination of serial serum concentrations of blood urea nitrogen (BUN) and creatinine are easily obtained and relatively easy to interpret. Urea is the end product of protein and amino acid catabolism. Under normal conditions, approximately 90% of nitrogen excretion is by the kidneys, depending upon glomerular filtration rate. Unfortunately, in the critical care setting, the BUN is of only limited value, as BUN is also affected by production of nitrogenous wastes, for example, by use of high-protein diets, reabsorption of hematomas, and digestion of blood from the GI tract.

Determination of serial serum creatinine levels has greater utility for measuring renal function in the critical care setting. Creatinine is formed from the nonenzymatic degradation of creatine and phosphocreatine in muscle. The tubular reabsorption of creatinine is negligible. As a result, serum creatinine is an excellent reflection of glomerular filtration. Because creatinine production reflects muscle mass, the value needs to be considered in relation to body muscle mass. Because of this limitation, the trend in serum creatinine and the calculation of creatinine clearance may be better measures for monitoring renal function. Creatinine clearance, currently the best measure of renal function, is calculated as

$$\text{Creatinine Clearance (mL/min)} = [\text{Urine Cr (mg/dL)} \times \text{Volume (mL/24 h)}]/ [\text{Serum Cr [mg/dL]} \times 1,440 \text{ (min/24 h)}]$$

Measuring the concentrating abilities of the renal tubules may be used to distinguish oliguria due to prerenal causes, such as hypovolemia, from that caused by intrinsic renal failure due to impaired tubular function. The ability to reabsorb sodium and water is compromised in cases of intrinsic renal failure, but not in cases of prerenal azotemia. The fractional excretion of sodium is the most accurate means of distinguishing prerenal from renal causes of azotemia. The fractional excretion of sodium is calculated as

$$\text{FENa} = [(\text{Urine Na} \times \text{Serum Cr})/ (\text{Urine Cr} \times \text{Serum Na})] \times 100$$

In normal individuals, the FENa is <1% to 2%. In an oliguric patient, a value of <1% suggests a prerenal cause. A value of >2% to 3% suggests compromised tubular function.

Management of Acute Kidney Injury

The first step in managing such a patient is to acquire a relevant history. This includes the patient's baseline state of health, baseline laboratory values, and recent exposure to known nephrotoxins. The hospital record, including operative notes, should be reviewed for episodes of hypotension or blood loss and for the amount and type of fluid resuscitation. The next step is to determine the source of renal dysfunction, that is, pre-, intra-, or postrenal. Pre- versus intrarenal causes can be evaluated using the FENa. Postrenal failure from ureteral or bladder obstruction can usually be determined by placement or flushing of a urinary catheter. Ultrasound imaging can rule out bilateral obstruction of the ureters and provides additional information about inflow into the kidney. The most common type of acute kidney injury in the SICU is acute tubular necrosis secondary to ischemia.

Once the cause of renal dysfunction is determined, the next step is to maximize perfusion with appropriate hydration and cautious use of vasoactive agents. An all too common mistake in surgical patients is to assume that the prerenal etiology is solely lack of hydration. While this is a very common cause, decreased cardiac output is also common and may require inotropic or vasopressor support. Another frequent error is the use of "renal dose dopamine" to improve renal function. Because dopamine at low doses increases sodium excretion, thus increasing urine output, it was originally thought to improve renal function. Unfortunately, large clinical trials have demonstrated this not to be the case. Insuring adequate oxygenation is also important when resuscitating the injured kidney.

Because of the kidney's role in eliminating many medications, the doses of certain medications need to be adjusted ("renal dosing"), and some medications need to be discontinued. In particular, medications known for their nephrotoxicity should be avoided.

Renal dysfunction can lead to platelet dysfunction and an increased risk of bleeding. Acutely, this can be treated with 1-deamino-8-D-arginine vasopressin (desmopressin) or conjugated estrogens. Renal replacement therapy (dialysis) is also effective.

Renal Replacement Therapy

Similar to patients with chronic kidney disease, disturbances in the volume and composition of body fluid are the main indications for renal replacement therapy. The most common indications are volume overload, electrolyte disturbances (typically hyperkalemia), metabolic acidosis, and severe azotemia (particularly causing pericarditis).

All forms of renal replacement therapy (also commonly known as dialysis) rely on the principle of allowing water and solute transport through a semipermeable membrane. Ultrafiltration achieves volume removal by using a pressure gradient to drive water across the membrane. Removal of solute occurs through diffusion from an area of higher concentration across the membrane to an area of lower concentration.

Types of renal replacement therapies are classified as intermittent or continuous. Examples of the former include hemodialysis, typically delivered for 3 to 4 hours several days per week. Advantages of this therapy are rapid removal of solute and volume and rapid correction of electrolytes and acidosis. The main disadvantage, however, is systemic hypotension due to rapid fluid shifts, particularly in critically ill patients. In those patients, continuous renal replacement therapy, which occurs over several days, may be better tolerated. Because this mode is continuous and gradual, control of volume removal, azotemia, electrolyte balance, and acid–base status may be easier.

Renal replacement therapy requires large-bore venous access (Figure 6-5). Acutely, nontunneled and noncuffed CVCs can be used. Typically, these are placed in the internal jugular or femoral veins, sparing the subclavian veins to prevent strictures and thrombosis that would complicate long-term access. For long-term access, tunneled and cuffed dialysis catheters can be placed to decrease risk of infection. Alternatively, an arteriovenous fistula can be surgically created directly between the vessels or using graft material, such as polytetrafluoroethylene.

A general approach to the patient with acute renal failure is illustrated in Figure 6-6.

LIVER FAILURE

Liver disease is common, often caused by alcohol abuse or viral hepatitis, although other causes need to be considered. Complications of chronic liver failure that may result in ICU admission include variceal hemorrhage, encephalopathy, spontaneous bacterial peritonitis (SBP), and hepatorenal syndrome. In addition, liver disease may be a comorbidity of patients presenting with another disease process.

Coagulopathy

Coagulopathy is present in patients with liver failure since key coagulation factors are synthesized in the liver. Correction of

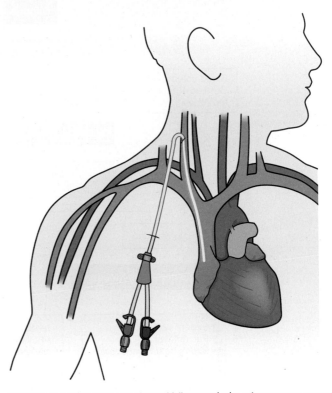

FIGURE 6-5. Patients with chronic renal failure require long-term venous access for dialysis. A dialysis catheter may be tunneled under the skin . A dialysis catheter with an adherent antibiotic-or silver-impregnated cuff can be tunneled under the skin.

coagulopathy with fresh frozen plasma (FFP) is the first line of treatment in a bleeding patient, but the effect is transient, since the production of clotting factors remains impaired. Patients with mild liver dysfunction may respond to administration of vitamin K. In some circumstances, there may be a role for recombinant activated factor VII.

Variceal Bleeding

Initial evaluation of a patient with variceal bleeding, just like that for any other patient with gastrointestinal bleeding, should proceed systematically with stabilizing the patient, first controlling the airway and breathing, then working to assess and establish adequate circulation, including transfusion of packed red blood cells. FFP and platelets may also be required to correct coagulation defects and thrombocytopenia.

While this resuscitation is undertaken, steps should be taken to control ongoing blood loss. Administration of octreotide, a synthetic analogue of somatostatin, can decrease portal blood pressure. Vasopressin also reduces portal pressure but may cause myocardial ischemia and is less effective than octreotide. After the bleeding episode has been resolved, β blockade is employed to reduce cardiac output and splanchnic blood flow to prevent recurrent bleeding.

Definitive control of hemorrhage typically requires endoscopic intervention, with either banding or sclerosis of the varices. Complications include perforation, ulceration, and stricture, as well as abdominal distention, worsening encephalopathy, recurrent bleeding, and infection.

In the face of massive uncontrolled bleeding, balloon tamponade, using the Sengstaken-Blakemore or Minnesota tube (nasogastric tube with gastric and esophageal balloons) can be a temporizing measure. Prior to insertion of the tube, it is critical

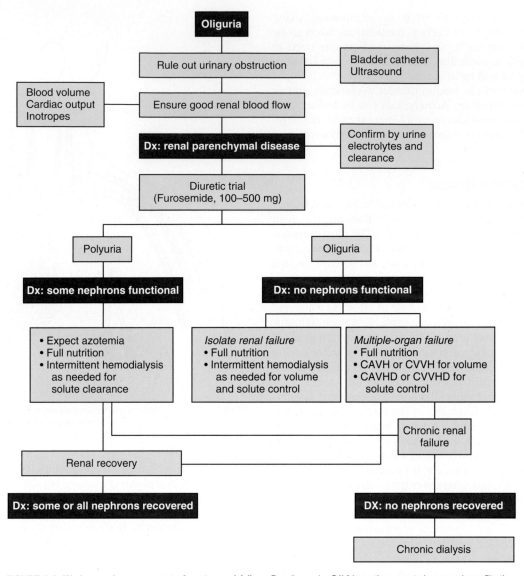

FIGURE 6-6. Workup and management of acute renal failure. Dx, diagnosis; CAVH, continuous arteriovenous hemofiltration; CVVH, continuous venovenous hemofiltration; CAVHD, continuous arteriovenous hemodiafiltration; CVVHD, continuous venovenous hemodiafiltration. (From Mulholland MW et al., eds., *Greenfield's Surgery*, 4th ed. Philadelphia: Lippincott Williams & Wilkins, 2006:208.)

to intubate the patient's airway because of the risk of aspiration. The tube is inserted like an orogastric or nasogastric tube. Gastric position is confirmed radiographically. The gastric balloon is inflated and drawn cephalad to apply internal pressure on the varices. The tube is then secured under traction, such as by fastening it to a face mask or a football helmet on the patient or attaching it to an orthopedic traction system. If there is ongoing bleeding, the esophageal balloon may be inflated. Other complications of balloon tamponade include esophageal ischemia or perforation.

If other interventions fail, a portosystemic shunt, such as the transjugular intrahepatic portosystemic shunt (TIPS), can be placed to reduce the high pressure in the varices. Surgical shunts are the final option, usually of last resort, as these are associated with high morbidity, including worsening hepatic encephalopathy. Operative portosystemic shunts most commonly involve placement of prosthetic grafts between the portal and systemic systems (e.g., mesocaval shunt) to partially decompress the portal system as in an "H-graft." Complications include shunt thrombosis, infection, and worsening encephalopathy.

Hepatic Encephalopathy

Hepatic encephalopathy is characterized by a decline in neurologic function that is associated with poor hepatic function. The severity is described in Table 6-1. The most common precipitating factor is GI bleeding. The differential diagnosis

TABLE 6-1	West Haven Criteria for Grading Hepatic Encephalopathy
Grade	**Symptoms**
1	Trivial lack of awareness, euphoria or anxiety, impaired performance of cognitive tasks
2	Lethargy or apathy, inappropriate behavior
3	Somnolence responsive to verbal stimulus, confusion and disorientation
4	Coma

for hepatic encephalopathy includes metabolic encephalopathies such as hypoglycemia, hypoxia, uremia, and electrolyte abnormalities or intracranial lesions such as hemorrhage or abscess. Toxic encephalopathy, such as alcohol intoxication, must also be excluded.

While the specific pathology of hepatic encephalopathy is not entirely understood, the prevailing theory is that it results from increased blood ammonia levels from nitrogenous substances within the gut lumen and increased stimulation of γ-aminobutyric acid (GABA) receptors. Ammonia levels do not correlate well with the level of encephalopathy. Other substances, such as aromatic amino acids, also seem to play a role. After controlling precipitating factors, treatment centers on pharmacologically reducing the production and/or absorption of ammonia from the gut. First-line therapy is generally lactulose, which acts to acidify the colon, trapping nonabsorbable ammonium in the gut lumen and causing diarrhea, further eliminating nitrogen. Drawbacks include diarrhea and abdominal distension. Reduction of urease-producing gut flora with antibiotics may also help relieve severe encephalopathy. Neomycin is an aminoglycoside traditionally used for this purpose; however, it is associated with ototoxicity and nephrotoxicity with prolonged usage. Other antimicrobial agents such as metronidazole and rifaximin are well tolerated and effective.

Ascites

Ascites is rarely the principal reason for critical care admission but is frequently associated with hemorrhage, renal failure, or hepatic encephalopathy. Refractory ascites may result in the development of abdominal compartment syndrome, causing hypotension from impaired venous return or respiratory compromise. Paracentesis (Figure 6-7) is a temporizing measure in refractory ascites.

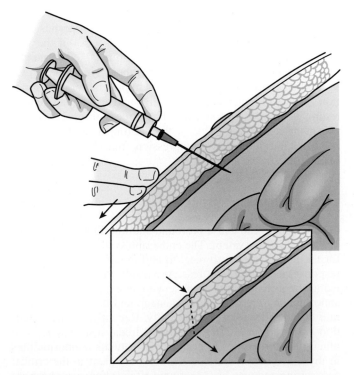

FIGURE 6-7. Paracentesis is accomplished via either a subumbilical or flank approach. Care must be taken to avoid injury to bowel. Ultrasound is frequently used.

TABLE 6-2	Child-Pugh Classification of Liver Dysfunction		
	Score		
	1	**2**	**3**
Encephalopathy grade	None	1 and 2	3 and 4
Ascites	Absent	Mild	Moderate
Bilirubin (mg/dL)	<2.0	2.0–3.0	>3.0
Albumin (g/dL)	>3.5	2.8–3.5	<2.8
International normalized ratio (INR)	<1.7	1.7–2.3	>2.3

Class is based upon the sum of the scores: Class A: 5–6; Class B: 7–9; Class C: 10–15.

Spontaneous Bacterial Peritonitis

Spontaneous bacterial peritonitis (SBP) is a spontaneous infection of ascites in the absence of a primary intra-abdominal source of infection. Infection results from translocation of intestinal bacteria. Common clinical manifestations include fever, abdominal pain, and unexplained encephalopathy, although asymptomatic presentations are not uncommon. Paracentesis is the most effective way to diagnose SBP by finding >250 neutrophils/mL of ascitic fluid, with or without a positive ascitic fluid culture. Treatment is based on the organism sensitivity, but fluoroquinolones and third-generation cephalosporins may be used empirically.

Hepatorenal Syndrome

Hepatorenal syndrome is a difficult problem characterized by the development of acute renal failure in a patient with end-stage liver disease. The pathophysiology involves reduced renal blood flow due to splanchnic vasodilation associated with portal hypertension, leading to decreased effective circulatory volume and activation of the renin–angiotensin system. Hepatorenal syndrome typically presents as a slow decline in renal function; however, new insults such as infection or bleeding can cause a precipitous drop in renal function. Medical management centers on improving splanchnic blood flow with pharmacologic intervention. The most common agents used are midodrine as a vasoconstrictor and octreotide to inhibit vasodilation. The best hope for improvement in these patients remains restoration of liver function through transplantation.

Severity of Liver Failure

The severity of liver dysfunction can be described using the Child-Pugh classification (Table 6-2; also see Chapter 18, Liver). It's important to note that typical "liver function tests," including transaminases, alkaline phosphatase, and γ-glutamyl transferase, depict injury to the hepatocytes or canaliculi, but not liver synthetic function. Measurement of bilirubin or prothrombin time (international normalized ratio) can be more useful.

Liver Transplantation

Liver transplantation is the most effective treatment for chronic liver failure, with an overall 1-year survival at 88% (see Chapter 22, Liver). Patients with liver failure should be referred for transplantation when hepatic dysfunction becomes clinically evident. The prognostic model for end-stage liver disease (MELD) score predicts liver-related mortality based on a formula involving the serum creatinine, serum bilirubin, and INR. The MELD score is used to allocate donor livers to the most appropriate patient and in some centers is replacing the Child's classification for risk assessment. It is a complex regression equation that is available online on the United Network for Organ Sharing Web site (www.unos.org/resources/meldpeldcalculator.asp) for quick calculation.

Acute Liver Failure

Acute liver failure (ALF) or fulminant hepatic failure is defined by a rapid decline in liver synthetic function combined with encephalopathy not attributable to another cause. This occurs in the setting of a previously normal liver, as in acetaminophen toxicity, or as a deterioration of compensated liver disease. When possible, the cause of ALF should be treated as a first line of therapy. Examples include antiviral therapy for hepatitis B or *N*-acetylcysteine for acetaminophen toxicity.

Supportive management of these patients focuses on the complications of ALF such as respiratory failure, hypotension, coagulopathy, GI bleeding, renal failure, sepsis, and encephalopathy. Cerebral edema is the primary cause of death in ALF. Clinical manifestations include elevated intracranial pressure (ICP), which, without intervention, progresses to eventual brainstem herniation and brain death. Management includes invasive ICP monitoring and aggressive management of elevated ICP, with a goal of maintaining ICP below 20 mm Hg. In extreme circumstances, pentobarbital-induced coma or induction of mild hypothermia has been utilized.

GASTROINTESTINAL MONITORING AND FAILURE

Gastrointestinal Function

Normal GI tract function is to ingest food, digest it, and mobilize the resulting suspension, absorb the useable constituent components, and store the waste products until a socially acceptable time arises for elimination. The quiescent gut receives about 5% of cardiac output, which can increase to 30% during a large meal. The GI tract itself is composed of rapidly dividing mucosal cells, which are susceptible to ischemia. In addition, the GI tract is filled with immunologic cells interacting with the immense mucosal surface area present in the gut for absorption. Abnormalities affecting the gut in the SICU can be divided into altered function or anatomic changes.

Although physical examination of the abdomen in critical care is difficult and often fails to secure a diagnosis, it still must be performed. What is not detected is as important as what is detected; therefore, additional testing is usually necessary. Normal GI tract function is usually expected in the SICU, even if the patient is not receiving enteral feeding. Feeding intolerance, marked by vomiting, diarrhea, and constipation, is common and may be the result of illness, injury, drugs, immobility, or a combination of any or all. Simple measures to prevent intolerance include elevating the head of the bed and assuring frequent evacuation.

Gastrointestinal Integrity

Changes in the gut anatomy fall into two major areas—loss of mucosal integrity or ischemia. Mucosa anywhere in the GI tract may be injured; the stomach and the colon are the most common locations. Gastric erosion, often called stress-related mucosal disease (SRMD), thought to be due to reduced mucosal perfusion, can lead to gastritis or ulceration. Improved hemodynamic resuscitation has reduced gastric ulceration, but there are still subsets of SICU patients at risk for SRMD who require acid prophylaxis (upper GI bleeding, prolonged ventilation [>48 hours], and coagulopathy). Prophylaxis for SRMD involves the administration of H2 antagonists, proton pump inhibitors, or cytoprotective agents. The colon can also ulcerate or blister from the toxin produced by *Clostridium difficile*.

Ischemia to the gut can occur from obstruction of splanchnic blood flow to the vessels from embolism, or from intense vasoconstriction during hypotension. Clinically, gut ischemia is marked by abdominal pain and a lactic acidosis, but, early on, abdominal tenderness and peritoneal signs may be absent. Therapy involves removing or bypassing the vascular obstruction and resecting irreversibly damaged ischemic bowel. Ischemia may also result from nonocclusive mesenteric ischemia and is the manifestation of global inadequate bowel perfusion. Treatment requires improved hemodynamics. When ischemic bowel is found, it is paramount that the surgeon insure adequate blood supply to the remaining bowel, and a repeat intraoperative evaluation is often needed to determine bowel perfusion status.

Abdominal Compartment Syndrome

Abdominal compartment syndrome is a result of elevated intraperitoneal pressures that affect not only intraperitoneal organs but extra-peritoneal organ systems as well. Intraperitoneal pressures, measured via the bladder, >25 cm of water denote abdominal hypertension and are common in obesity or postresuscitation (following injury or ischemia) victims due to generalized bowel edema. The same physical properties exist for the abdomen as with other anatomic spaces—if the volume of organs and/or fluids increases within a fixed space, the pressure will rise. Abdominal compartment syndrome is present when those elevated pressures impair pulmonary function, urinary output, and renal function and also impair venous return, leading to hypotension. Early recognition is critical; treatment is decompression of the peritoneal cavity by paracentesis, intraluminal decompression, muscle paralysis, or opening the fascia surgically.

ENDOCRINE DYSFUNCTION

Critical illness can cause profound and interlinked alterations of the endocrine system. The endocrine system is responsible for the body's ability to react to and modify the physiologic responses to trauma and stress. As a result, patients with preexisting endocrine disease or those with unrecognized endocrine abnormalities are difficult to manage and have an increased rate of complications and mortality. Recently, greater attention has been focused on acquired adrenal insufficiency and glucose abnormalities in critically ill patients. Abnormalities in thyroid function are also relatively frequent in the critical care setting and may have profound effects; however, these are often not initially considered.

Adrenal

The adrenal glands are part of the neuroendocrine axis. Production of glucocorticoids, catecholamines, mineralocorticoids, and sex hormones are all important factors in the body's ability to respond to critical illness. There is great controversy about the incidence, diagnosis, and treatment of adrenal insufficiency in the SICU. In the general population, the incidence of adrenal insufficiency is <0.1%, but it may be as high as 28% in critically ill patients. The most common cause of adrenal insufficiency is previous steroid use. However, other common causes of adrenal insufficiency in the critical care setting include infection, systemic inflammation, and sepsis. While the incidence of adrenal insufficiency in the critically ill may be underappreciated, the detrimental impact of such dysfunction is well recognized. The reported mortality of this condition may be as high as 25% but is decreased to 6% with early recognition.

Absolute or relative insufficiency of cortisol production in the critically ill patient is particularly important, given its role in the maintenance of vascular tone, endothelial integrity, vascular permeability, and total body water distribution. It also potentiates the vasoconstrictor actions of both endogenous and exogenous catecholamines.

Critically ill patients are at risk for the development of adrenal insufficiency of critical illness (AICI). The usual signs and symptoms of adrenal insufficiency such as fatigue, weight loss, nausea, abdominal pain, and hyperpigmentation of the skin are not typically apparent in this group of patients. Rather, these patients typically present with hypotension, unresponsiveness to catecholamine infusions, and/or ventilator dependence. Electrolyte abnormalities (hyponatremia, hyperkalemia) and hypoglycemia may also be present and not recognized as adrenal insufficiency.

Diagnostic criteria for adrenal insufficiency in the critically ill are not well established and are controversial. In general, a cortisol level obtained in the presence of severe endogenous stress (hypotension, shock, sepsis) evaluates the entire axis and can be considered superior to traditional adrenocorticotrophic hormone stimulation testing. Random serum cortisol levels that are <20 µg/dL may be sufficient to diagnose adrenal insufficiency in critically ill or injured patients. If the patient is in refractory shock, it may be most prudent to treat the patient empirically with hydrocortisone and then taper the daily dose over the next several days as the illness subsides. Formal testing after resolution of the critical illness will help determine if this was primary adrenal insufficiency or a secondary insufficiency requiring additional workup and treatment.

Glucose Disorders

Hyperglycemia occurs in many critically ill and injured patients. While diabetes may be the etiology in a few patients, hyperglycemia due to increased sympathetic and adrenal activity and activation of the cytokine cascade are the most common causes in the critically ill patient. Certain medications commonly used in the intensive care unit such as β-blockers, cyclosporine, catecholamines, total parenteral nutrition, and glucocorticoids promote hyperglycemia. Hyperglycemia may also be caused by decreased insulin release due to electrolyte abnormalities such as hypokalemia and stress-induced glycogenolysis and hepatic gluconeogenesis.

Regardless of the mechanism, hyperglycemia is associated with organ dysfunction in the cardiovascular, cerebrovascular, neuromuscular, and immunologic systems.

Hyperglycemia has been associated with an increased risk of in-hospital mortality, because it causes release of free fatty acids that may induce arrhythmias in ischemic hearts, volume depletion due to osmotic diuresis, and worse outcomes after head injury. Hyperglycemia impairs white blood cell functions including chemotaxis, phagocytosis, and oxidative burst pathways. As a result of white blood cell impairment, postoperative wound infections, pneumonia, urinary tract infections, and bacteremias are all increased in hyperglycemic patients.

While it is still controversial, there is accumulating evidence that tight control of the blood glucose improves outcomes in critically ill and injured patients. Too strict glucose control may be more dangerous because of episodes of hypoglycemia, so the proper range of appropriate blood glucose levels for specific subgroups of intensive care patients is still under investigation.

In patients with type I diabetes mellitus, diabetic ketoacidosis (DKA) may develop in critically ill and injured patients. These patients may present with symptoms of nausea, abdominal pain, excessive thirst, or fatigue. Patients with DKA may also present with hemodynamic instability and altered level of consciousness. Since mortality may approach 10% to 15%, rapid identification and treatment is mandatory. Laboratory data suggestive of DKA include a blood glucose level between 400 and 800 mg/dL, anion gap metabolic acidosis, and the presence of serum and urine ketones. Hyperkalemia is common despite the presence of a total body potassium deficit. Treatment consists of rapid volume replacement with normal saline infusion and correction of hyperglycemia with an insulin drip. Glucose levels should be monitored frequently, and intravenous fluid should be converted to 5% dextrose with hypotonic saline once the blood glucose is corrected to below 250 mg/dL. Hypokalemia and hypophosphatemia frequently develop during treatment and should also be corrected.

Hypoglycemia also occurs in the intensive care, most frequently during intensive blood glucose control. Hypoglycemia is associated with increased mortality as well as impaired neurologic and cognitive function. Rapid identification and treatment is necessary to prevent permanent neurologic injury.

Thyroid Disorders

The metabolic rate of all tissues is dependent upon thyroid hormones. As such, excessive or deficient levels of thyroid hormone, when unrecognized or untreated, create life-threatening problems in critically ill patients. Critical illness may alter production of thyroid hormone through regulatory changes in thyroid-stimulating hormone (TSH), peripheral metabolism, or alteration in binding proteins. The spectrum of thyroid function abnormalities seen in the SICU occurs on a continuum, ranging from thyroid storm to hypothyroidism and myxedema coma.

Thyroid storm is an example of severe hyperthyroidism, which may be precipitated by physiologically stressful events including surgery, trauma, childbirth, and critical illness. The classic symptoms are high fever (105°F to 106°F), high output cardiac failure and mental status changes. The diagnosis of thyroid storm is based on a nondetectable TSH and elevation of T3 (triiodothyronine) and T4 (thyroxine) levels. Other laboratory findings frequently include elevation of white blood cell count, calcium, blood glucose and hepatic transaminases. Because the turnaround time on these tests may be prolonged, treatment should be initiated based on clinical suspicion. As death occurs in up to 20% of patients, with the most frequent cause being cardiac failure, treatment should be directed at control of the catecholamine-induced cardiac symptoms, typically with propranolol or other β-blockers. Decreasing production and release of thyroid hormones, blocking their peripheral actions and addressing the primary cause are the mainstays of treating thyroid storm. Propylthiouracil and potassium iodide decrease the release of T3 and T4.

Hypothyroidism is also relatively common in the SICU. While rare, myxedema coma is the most severe result of hypothyroidism with mortality rates of >60%. This may be precipitated by the stress of traumatic injury, surgery, burns, and cardiovascular events. Clinical features include reduced metabolic rate, hypothermia, ileus, bradycardia, decreased cardiac contractility, hypotension, and hypoventilation. The mental status changes associated with hypothyroidism range from lethargy to coma. Laboratory workup reveals an elevated TSH, very depressed T4, hyponatremia, and low blood glucose. Characteristic electrocardiogram changes are sinus bradycardia, low-voltage QRS, flat or inverted T waves, prolonged intervals, and heart block. Treatment consists of supportive SICU care, external warming, infusing of glucose-containing intravenous fluids, and thyroxine replacement.

Sick euthyroid syndrome is a common finding in the SICU. It is not clear if this is an adaptation to critical illness or a true pathologic process. This typically is identified by an isolated decrease in T3 with normal TSH. Currently, specific therapy is not recommended.

NEUROLOGIC DYSFUNCTION

Sedation/Analgesia

ICU patients frequently require analgesia and/or sedation, particularly when they need mechanical ventilation. Typically, medications to sedate intubated patients are administered as a continuous infusion and titrated to allow evaluation of neurologic function, yet assure that the patient is comfortable and does not cause harm by inadvertently removing critical devices, such as endotracheal tubes. Excessive dosing of these medications can cause respiratory depression, hypotension, and prolonged sedation, leading to prolonged time on the ventilator or in the SICU.

For pain, a narcotic infusion is usually used. If the patient is awake, there is no reason a patient-controlled analgesia (PCA) device or enteral narcotic cannot be used. Adjuvants, such as NSAIDs or regional anesthesia, can decrease the need for narcotics. If frequent neurologic assessments are needed, short-acting narcotics, such as remifentanyl, may be used.

Sedation is usually achieved with a short-acting medication such as propofol, midazolam, or dexmedetomidine. Although a number of sedation scales have been developed, no single scale is clearly superior to the others. The important issue is choosing a drug and titrating the drug to a particular effect rather than using one agent for everyone or every malady. Usually, the goal is to have a calm, but responsive patient. Deeper levels of sedation may be required in some circumstances, such as difficulty with ventilation requiring high airway pressures, intracranial hypertension, or an open abdomen.

Because these medications are frequently administered continuously, there is a danger of accumulation of the medication, leading to delayed awakening, increased need for mechanical ventilation, and prolonged SICU stay. To decrease this risk, a daily interruption of sedation has become a standard practice. Once the patient awakens to the point of responding to commands, the infusion(s) can be restarted at half the previous rate and then slowly increased as needed. This way, the minimum effective dose is determined at least once each day.

Delirium

Delirium, defined as a state of acute or fluctuating mental status and inattention, plus disordered thinking or altered level of consciousness, is very common in surgical patients. Delirium may be further classified as hypoactive (lethargic) or hyperactive (agitated). The initial management of the patient should include assessment and reversal of any immediately life-threatening issues, including compromise of the airway, breathing, or circulation. Once these issues have been addressed, the cause for the delirium must be determined. The cause may not be evident and frequently is never clearly determined. Despite this, a rapid evaluation for reversible causes should be undertaken. Common causes for delirium in postoperative patients can be divided into patient (e.g., alcoholism, endocrine disorders), acute illness (e.g., sepsis, head trauma), complications of the acute illness (e.g., hypoxemia, hypovolemia, and electrolyte abnormalities), and iatrogenic factors (e.g., medications). Early sepsis is a frequent cause of delirium, with the delirium preceding more typical physical and laboratory findings suggestive of sepsis. Any focal neurologic findings should prompt a computed tomography (CT) scan of the head. Except for vascular, neurological, or cardiac patients, stroke is very infrequent.

The workup for a patient with delirium should include a thorough neurologic examination as well as complete physical examination, measurement of oxygen saturation, electrolytes, and complete blood count. Endocrine disorders should be entertained based on suggestive history. All medications should be reviewed for their potential neurologic side effects. Without localized focal neurologic findings, a CT scan of the head, though often warranted, is unlikely to demonstrate an abnormality.

Once reversible causes for delirium have been managed, pharmacologic therapy is appropriate, though no drugs are specifically approved for treatment of delirium. There is no clear consensus on the best medications. Drugs that can cause respiratory or cardiovascular depression, such as benzodiazepines, should generally be avoided. These drugs may also increase confusion. Typical antipsychotics, such as haloperidol, are often used. It is usually best to begin with low doses and then to evaluate the patient's response to therapy. Atypical antipsychotics may also have benefit, including risperidone and quetiapine. The greatest dangers of such medications involve cardiac arrhythmias, particularly *torsades de pointes* in patients with prolonged QT intervals. Altering environmental factors, such as light and sound, may help. Attempts to assist patients in obtaining adequate sleep at night can help.

Alcohol Withdrawal Syndrome

Patients who regularly abuse alcohol or benzodiazepines can develop tolerance such that they require higher and higher levels to attain the same effect. When they cease or reduce their intake, they are at risk for developing withdrawal. The initial signs are usually related to elevated sympathetic tone, including hypertension, tachycardia, tachypnea, fever, and diaphoresis. These symptoms can occur within hours. Alcohol withdrawal delirium usually occurs 2 to 3 days later. The most feared complication, seizures, may also occur at this stage.

Prevention is controversial. Some advocate prophylactic administration of either alcoholic drinks or benzodiazepines. Others prefer to closely monitor the patient using a protocol, and then to titrate treatment when there is evidence of withdrawal.

Management of alcohol withdrawal includes pharmacologic treatment aimed at stimulating γ-aminobutyric acid receptors (the main receptors stimulated by alcohol). Benzodiazepines or alcohol itself (enteral or intravenous) are successful in the great majority of cases. In patients refractory to these medications, the addition of a barbiturate or propofol may be helpful.

Traumatic Brain Injury

TBI involves both the primary injury to neurons and secondary injury from hypotension or hypoxemia. Therefore, the initial management of the patient with TBI, like all patients with trauma, should include an initial assessment of the ABCs (airway, breathing, and circulation). Any episodes of hypotension or hypoxemia can significantly impact outcome from TBI.

The initial neurologic evaluation of the patient with suspected TBI includes a detailed examination of motor and sensory function. Evidence of an expanding mass lesion or herniation, such as development of a dilated, nonreactive pupil, is particularly ominous. The Glasgow Coma Scale (Table 6-3; see also Chapter 9, Trauma) is particularly

TABLE 6-3	Glasgow Coma Scale

Test and Response	Points
Eye opening	
Spontaneous	4
To voice	3
To pain	2
None	1
Best verbal response	
Oriented	5
Confused	4
Inappropriate words	3
Incomprehensible sounds	2
None	1
Best motor response	
Obeys commands	6
Localizes pain	5
Withdraws from pain	4
Flexor response	3
Extensor response	2
None	1

useful for categorizing the severity of TBI and following the patient's course. The GCS score is the sum of the scores from each of the three tests (eye opening, best verbal response, and best motor response). TBI is categorized as mild (GCS score 13 to 15), moderate (GCS score 9 to 12), or severe (GCS score ≤8).

Physical examination of patients with TBI generally does not provide sufficient information to determine appropriate management. CT of the head has become a mainstay of evaluating such patients. The finding of significant extra-axial bleeding is usually an indication for craniotomy. Epidural hematomas are caused by injury to dural arteries adjacent to skull fractures. Subdural hematomas are associated with disruption of veins with rapid acceleration/deceleration of the brain. Subarachnoid bleeding is also common with TBI. In some circumstances, the pattern of subarachnoid blood should raise concern about aneurysm rupture.

Management of patients with severe TBI is usually focused on control of ICP, which can be measured with an external ventricular drain (EVD) or fiberoptic parenchymal monitors. Strategies to decrease ICP include elevation of the head of the bed, endotracheal intubation, sedation, neuromuscular blockade, and drainage of cerebrospinal fluid. Osmotic therapy with either mannitol or hypertonic saline can decrease cerebral edema and thereby decrease ICP. Additional maneuvers to decrease ICP in refractory cases, particularly with diffuse injuries, include barbiturates and hypothermia. Surgically, resection of injured brain tissue and craniectomy (temporary removal of a section of skull to allow brain swelling to occur) may help.

The SICU management of TBI usually includes maintenance of PCO_2 ~35 Torr and cerebral perfusion pressure (mean arterial pressure-ICP) >60 mm Hg. Prophylactic anticonvulsant therapy, usually with phenytoin, is continued for 7 days.

Brain Death

Brain death has been defined as the cessation of all functions of the brain. There is no national standard for how this is determined, but there are state laws and hospital protocols. There are some generally accepted common practices. Typically, a clinical examination by two different experienced clinicians is required. Before a clinical evaluation for brain death can be performed, any confounding issues must be ruled out. The patient must have a systolic blood pressure >90 mm Hg, and a temperature >32°C. Uremic or hepatic encephalopathy cannot be present. All medications that may affect brain function must have been stopped and enough time elapsed such that their affects may be eliminated.

The clinical examination for brain death includes the testing of all cranial nerves that can be evaluated. The specific examination includes testing pupil reactivity, corneal reflex, ocular vestibular reflex (cold water calorics), oculocephalic reflex (doll's eyes reflex), gag reflex, and cough reflex. There can be no response to central (supraorbital ridge pressure) painful stimulation. The vagus nerve is tested by administering atropine. Finally, apnea must be demonstrated with allowing the PCO_2 to rise to >60 Torr. The time of death is noted as the time at which the second examiner has completed his examination. Occasionally, additional studies are needed, such as cerebral angiography or nuclear medicine perfusion studies, to demonstrate no blood flow to the brain. Electroencephalography is also occasionally used.

SYSTEMIC INFLAMMATORY RESPONSE SYNDROME

A number of physiologic and laboratory parameters are commonly seen in response to injury, infection, or inflammation from virtually any cause. This normal response is collectively called the Systemic inflammatory response syndrome (SIRS). Because it is not unique and is usually the first sign of an ongoing process, it serves as a warning sign rather than a strict diagnostic tool of disease entity, itself requiring specific intervention. The presence of SIRS should lead to increased monitoring and trigger a series of diagnostic pursuits, as this may be a sign for worsening physiologic events that will require critical care interventions.

The criteria for SIRS are somewhat vague (see Table 6-4). Two criteria must be present, and there must be a plausible situation present (e.g., the normal physiology seen with exercise meets SIRS). If SIRS is present from infection or suspected infection, this is called sepsis. If sepsis has progressed to impair the normal function of an organ or body system, it is called severe sepsis. Sepsis with hypotension is septic shock.

Organ dysfunction is common in the SICU as a result of hypoperfusion or SIRS (Figure 6-8). If more than one system is affected, multiple-organ dysfunction syndrome (MODS) is present. Individual organ failure can be tabulated and scored (Table 6-5). The sum of the scores correlates with mortality. These distinctions are necessary for not only precise nomenclature but therapeutic decisions and prognosis. For each organ system that fails, mortality increases linearly up to >80% when four organs fail. The most common organ system failing

TABLE 6-4	Systemic Inflammatory Response Syndrome
Temperature	<36°C or >38°C
Heart rate	>90 beats/min
Respiratory rate	>20 breaths/min (or $PaCO_2$ < 32 mm Hg)
Leukocyte count	<4,000 or >12,000 cells/mm³ (or >10% bands)

and requiring support is the respiratory system, followed by the cardiac and renal systems.

INFECTIOUS DISEASES

Sepsis remains a leading cause of death in the intensive care unit. Patients may require SICU admission for sepsis from a variety of causes. In addition, interventions and devices utilized in the ICU place patients at additional risk for infections and sepsis.

Sepsis is the response to an infectious process and is characterized by release of multiple inflammatory mediators. Initially there is an increase in heart rate and temperature. Loss of vasomotor tone may also occur and lead to septic shock. The Society of Critical Care Medicine has generated guidelines for the treatment of sepsis as part of their Surviving Sepsis Campaign. Critical components of these guidelines include rapid identification of the septic state, aggressive

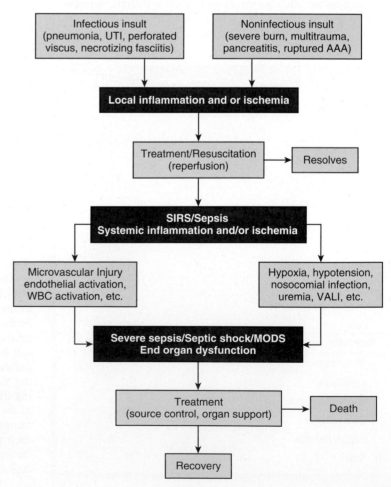

FIGURE 6-8. Pathophysiology of MODS. UTI, urinary tract infection; AAA, abdominal aortic aneurysm; SIRS, systemic inflammatory response syndrome; WBC, white blood count; VALI, ventilator-associated lung injury. (From Fischer JE, et al., eds. *Mastery of Surgery*, 5th ed. Philadelphia: Lippincott Williams & Wilkins, 2006:114.)

| TABLE 6-5 | Multiple Organ Dysfunction Score |

Organ system	Score				
	0	1	2	3	4
Respiratory (PO$_2$/FiO$_2$)	>300	226–300	151–225	76–150	≤75
Renal (serum creatinine, mg/dL)	≤1.1	1.2–2.3	2.4–3.9	4.0–5.6	>5.7
Hepatic (serum bilirubin, mg/dL)	≤1.1	1.2–3.5	3.6–7.1	7.2–14.1	>14.2
Cardiovascular (PAR)	≤10	10.1–15	15.1–20	20.1–30	>30
Hematologic (platelet count, 10^3)	>120	81–120	51–80	21–50	≤20
Neurologic (GCS)	15	13–14	10–12	7–9	≤6

PAR (pressure adjusted heart rate) = heart rate × (CVP/mean arterial pressure); GCS, Glasgow coma scale score.

Adapted from Marshall JC, Cook DJ, Christou NV, Bernard GR, Sprung CL, Sibbald WJ: Multiple organ dysfunction score: a reliable descriptor of a complex clinical outcome. Crit Care Med. 1995;23:1638–1652.

goal-directed resuscitation, source control of the septic focus, and early administration of appropriate antibiotic therapy. The initial antibiotic therapy is broad spectrum, but the spectrum should be rapidly narrowed when culture results are obtained. In cases of septic shock that are refractory to fluid resuscitation, vasopressors may be used. If vasopressor therapy is unsuccessful, vasopressin can be initiated. When these measures have failed, another consideration for the etiology of refractory septic shock is adrenal insufficiency.

A common source of sepsis in the SICU is ventilator-associated pneumonia (VAP). VAP occurs in 9% to 24% of patients with respiratory failure. Patients on the ventilator have a 3% per day risk of developing VAP. Development of pneumonia increases ICU stay and mortality. Noninvasive positive pressure ventilation and early liberation from the ventilator can decrease the likelihood of VAP.

What else can be done to prevent VAP? Good oral hygiene helps to decrease the bacterial load that may be microaspirated into the lungs. A subglottic suction catheter can remove pooled secretions and prevent biofilm formation on the endotracheal tube, though efficacy of this approach is unclear. Supine positioning increases the risk of aspiration, and as a result, the head of bed should be elevated. Patients can also be rotated to improve mobilization of pulmonary secretions. Good hand washing by healthcare workers prevents patient-to-patient cross contamination and contamination of the ventilator circuit. Malnutrition weakens the immune system, emphasizing the importance of nutritional support. Many of these interventions can be placed into a ventilator bundle or protocol to help reduce VAP in all ventilated patients.

The classic diagnosis of pneumonia is made by identifying a new infiltrate on chest radiograph, fever, leukocytosis, and increased sputum production. The ventilated SICU patient may already have an abnormal radiograph and an elevated white blood cell count and fever for other reasons. For this reason, the optimal method of diagnosis includes quantitative culture obtained by bronchoalveolar lavage (BAL) or protected telescoping catheters (nonbronchoscopic BAL), or protected specimen brush. The presence of ≥10^4 to 10^5 bacteria indicate an infection. Treatment should include early, broad-spectrum coverage. Inadequate or inappropriate coverage results in increased morbidity and mortality. The antibiotic coverage should be narrowed as soon as possible, based on final culture results.

Urinary catheters are commonly used in SICU patients. The longer these catheters are in place, the greater the risk of urinary tract infection. These catheters must be placed with meticulous sterile techniques. Care must be taken to prevent unintended removal of the catheter as it may cause trauma to the urinary tract and reinstrumentation of the tract increases the risk of infection. Each day, the necessity of a catheter should be assessed.

Antibiotics, though necessary in the SICU, can alter the flora in the colon, allowing C. difficile to flourish and become infective. Certain antibiotics, such as the quinalones and clindamycin, are more likely than are others to cause clostridial or pseudomembranous colitis. Colitis from C. difficile may result in a range of symptoms from diarrhea to toxic megacolon. Diagnosis is usually made by demonstrating the presence of the C. difficile toxin in a stool sample using a cytotoxic assay, enzyme immunoassay, or rapid polymerase chain reaction test. Treatment is by administration of oral or intravenous metronidazole or oral vancomycin.

Critically ill patients, particularly those with hypotension, peripheral vascular disease, diabetes mellitus, mechanical ventilation, and parenteral nutrition, are at risk for development of acalculous cholecystitis. Unlike cholecystitis seen in healthy patients, the etiology is not related to impaction or obstruction from gallstones. Biliary stasis and ischemia of the gallbladder wall are the causes of acalculous cholecystitis. With acalculous cholecystitis, there is a high incidence of gallbladder gangrene and perforation. Patients in the SICU may not be able to convey the typical symptoms of cholecystitis. Diagnosis can usually be made by demonstrating wall thickening, pericholecystic fluid, and tenderness with direct pressure on the gallbladder (sonographic Murphy's sign) on ultrasound. Rarely, a hepatobiliary imino-diacetic acid scan (HIDA scan) is helpful. Treatment includes broad-spectrum antibiotic coverage and fluid resuscitation. Patients who are stable enough to tolerate operation should undergo cholecystectomy. If patients are not stable enough for operation, a cholecystostomy tube should be placed.

Another cause of sepsis in the SICU is catheter-related blood stream infection (CRBSI). This is seen with any type of intravascular catheter, including dialysis catheters and peripherally or centrally inserted central lines. Risk of sepsis increases with the number of lumens and the frequency of use, as well as the use of parenteral nutrition. Femoral catheters have the highest rate of infection by site. Measures that can help prevent CRBSI include meticulous sterile technique and maximum barrier precautions at the time of insertion, use of antibiotic-impregnated catheters, and appropriate technique with each access to the catheter. The need for intravascular catheters should be assessed on a daily basis, and those not needed should be removed.

END POINTS OF RESUSCITATION

When managing patients with shock, therapy needs to be initiated as early, and as aggressively, as possible (for further discussion of shock, see Chapter 5, Shock). Once initiated, however, therapy must be titrated utilizing appropriate monitoring.

Monitoring begins with physical examination, focusing on clinical findings to estimate volume status, that is, examination of the jugular veins, mucus membranes, and skin turgor. Urine output and examination of the distal extremities (skin temperature and capillary refill) can, to some extent, estimate global perfusion.

Assuring adequate intravascular volume, that is, preload (particularly of the left ventricle), should always be the first step in resuscitation. The clinical question is whether or not the patient will respond to fluid resuscitation. Since ventricular volume cannot readily be monitored continuously, clinicians frequently rely on clinical parameters such as end organ perfusion and blood pressure.

If an appropriate clinical response is not seen, SICU clinicians can monitor pressure-related variables, such as PCWP or CVP. The relationship of the measured pressure to true ventricular preload may be influenced by many factors, including ventricular compliance (e.g., myocardial ischemia or chronic hypertension), valvular heart disease, and pulmonary vascular abnormalities. In addition, increased intrathoracic pressure, for example, from decreased lung compliance, mechanical ventilation with high pressures, increased airway resistance, or intra-abdominal hypertension, can significantly influence pressure measurements. Consequently, flow-derived variables, such as right ventricular end-diastolic volume (RVEDV), which can be estimated utilizing specialized PACs, may better estimate preload.

Another method for predicting volume responsiveness is observation of pulse pressure variability with the respiratory cycle while the patient receives mechanical ventilation. As patients become more hypovolemic, pulse pressure variability increases. Observation of respiratory variability in the pulse oximetry plethysmography can yield similar information.

Echocardiography may be the best noninvasive method of estimating ventricular filling and cardiac function, and though it is repeatable, it cannot typically be used continuously. Surgical intensivists are increasingly using echocardiography themselves.

Once the patient is adequately volume loaded, the next consideration is adequacy of cardiac output. Cardiac output can be measured using a PAC, but this is invasive and not always beneficial. Echocardiography can be more helpful. Alternative technologies for estimating cardiac output include pulse contour analysis (which can also measure stroke volume variability), esophageal Doppler ultrasound, and bioimpedance.

Adequacy of global oxygen delivery to tissues, in relation to oxygen demands, can be assessed by measuring mixed venous oxygen saturation (SvO_2). This value is used as a major resuscitation end point for cardiogenic shock and for early goal-directed therapy for sepsis. A decrease in oxygen delivery, for example, anemia, hypoxemia, or decreased cardiac output, or increased oxygen demands, for example, fever or sepsis, leads to a decrease in SvO_2. With sepsis, however, SvO_2 may be inappropriately high because of maldistribution of blood flow or cytopathic hypoxia leading to inadequate utilization of oxygen at the mitochondrial level.

Monitoring acid–base status has become a useful adjunct to hemodynamic monitoring. Inadequate oxygen delivery to tissues leads to anaerobic metabolism and lactic acidosis. Thus, measurement of either base deficit or lactate levels can reflect the level of anaerobic metabolism. Base deficit levels can be confounded by other causes of metabolic acidosis, such as alcohol intoxication, administration of normal saline resulting in hyperchloremia, or preexisting acid–base disorders. In addition, base deficit may be artificially decreased by the administration of sodium bicarbonate. Lactate can be increased in sepsis, even when global oxygen delivery is normal, because of inhibition of pyruvate dehydrogenase, cytopathic hypoxia, increased release of alanine from muscle, and decreased hepatic clearance.

Monitoring of O_2 or CO_2 in tissues that are vulnerable to global hypoperfusion (skin, muscle, GI tract) has held some promise as markers of adequate resuscitation. Near-infrared spectroscopy can be used to measure tissue oxygen, carbon dioxide, pH, oxygen saturation of hemoglobin, and tissue oxyhemoglobin coupling to cytochrome a, a3 redox. A variety of tissues can also be monitored, including muscle, stomach, bowel, and liver, but the clinical value of these measurements remains unproven.

PREVENTING COMPLICATIONS IN THE SICU

Patients in the SICU are already critically ill. Unfortunately, other complications may arise that may increase morbidity and mortality. Deep vein thrombosis (DVT), with or without the associated PE, and stress ulcers are the most common examples. Prophylactic measures are therefore taken in an effort to reduce the incidence of these complications. Recently, there has also been a national trend to focus prevention measures on infectious complications such as UTI and CRBSI. In fact, these healthcare-associated infections are thought to be so easily preventable that Medicare will no longer reimburse hospitals for the extra costs associated with their treatment. Strategies to decrease the risk of these nosocomial complications are sometimes combined into "bundles" that can readily be implemented in the SICU and can have more impact than implementing a single intervention. The compliance and impact of the bundles can be tracked.

Deep Vein Thrombosis

DVT, often within the large veins of the lower extremities and pelvis, may occur in 20% to 70% of hospitalized patients, depending upon the patient population studied and surveillance strategy. Fatal pulmonary emboli, which often occur with little warning, may occur in 0.1% to 7% of patients without prophylaxis. Risk factors for DVT include medical diseases that create the conditions described in Virchow's triad: stasis, endothelial injury to the vessel wall, and hypercoagulable state. Patients at high risk include those who are immobilized, have experienced trauma (especially pelvic or long bone fractures), are paralyzed, have cancer, or have undergone major orthopedic (hip, knee, pelvis) or abdominal/pelvic operations. Smoking, obesity, pregnancy, and the use of certain medications (birth control pills) increase the risk. The risk is also increased in patients with polycythemia and underlying hypercoagulable states.

Though often asymptomatic, common symptoms of acute DVT include leg redness, increased warmth, pain, tenderness to palpation, and leg swelling. Two extreme diagnoses related to lower extremity venous thrombosis, phlegmasia cerulea dolens, and phlegmasia alba dolens are covered in Chapter 22, Diseases of the Vascular System.

Prophylaxis for DVT includes early ambulation, compression stockings, pneumatic compression devices, and the administration of low-dose heparin (unfractionated or low molecular weight). Clinical suspicion of DVT should prompt a duplex ultrasound exam of the lower extremity. The initial treatment of DVT requires therapeutic anticoagulation with heparin or one of its derivatives, followed by oral anticoagulation with warfarin. In some patients, particularly those with a contraindication to heparin, placement of an inferior vena cava filter is indicated. Other generally accepted indications include failure of anticoagulation, a bleeding complication from the anticoagulation, or when the risk of DVT/PE is unusually high. The latter is the most controversial.

Heparin use is not without complication. Heparin-induced thrombocytopenia (HIT) may occur in 1% to 5% of patients who have been exposed to heparin. The diagnosis should be considered in patients who have received heparin and then develop a low platelet count (<150,000/m³), or a >50% decrease in platelet count from the baseline level. Twenty to fifty percent of patients with HIT may develop thrombotic complications. HIT is caused by antibodies to platelet factor 4 (PF4) and heparin. Diagnosis is made by blood testing using serologic and functional assays for heparin-dependent antibodies. Treatment requires the immediate discontinuation of all sources of heparin. If anticoagulation is still needed, alternative agents should be used including direct thrombin inhibitors (lepirudin, argatroban, bivalirudin) or heparinoids.

Stress-Related Mucosal Disease

Also known as gastric stress ulcers, SRMD has been recognized since the nineteenth century. Bleeding complications from ulcers have been noted in burn patients (Curling's ulcer) and also patients with TBI (Cushing's ulcer). Stress ulcers range in severity from insignificant superficial gastric erosions to deep ulcers with life-threatening hemorrhage. The cause is multifactorial, but is primarily related to hypoperfusion and loss of mucosal host defenses. Clinically significant bleeding may occur in 3% to 6% of patients. Mortality from bleeding may approach 50%. Patients at risk include those on mechanical ventilation, as well as those with burns, TBI, major trauma, or sepsis or those being treated with steroids. Prophylaxis for SRMD involves the administration of H2 antagonists, proton pump inhibitors, or cytoprotective agents.

ETHICS

Because of the intensity of interventions, as well as risks for mortality and long-term morbidity (which limits quality of life), ethical issues frequently arise in the SICU, particularly focused on end-of-life care. Managing the ethical issues is complicated by the fact that the surgical intensivist has rarely developed a rapport with the patient or family prior to the acute illness. In addition, the patient frequently cannot participate in these discussions. Thus, the surgical intensivist must discuss end-of-life decisions with the patients' family. As patients develop multiple organ system dysfunction or irreversible neurologic dysfunction, surgical intensivists need to address appropriate goals of care with the patient and/or family. Frequently, in alignment with the ethical principles of beneficence and nonmaleficence, the surgical intensivist should discuss changing the goals of care from trying to restore the patient to baseline function to simply making the patient comfortable and withdrawing life-sustaining therapy. Involvement by nursing staff, social services, palliative care services, and clergy is often helpful with these discussions.

CONCLUSIONS

Surgical patients frequently require critical care. The challenge for the surgical intensivist is to simultaneously diagnose the patients' conditions, while initiating appropriate therapy. Multiple organ dysfunction and the need for support of multiple organs is the norm. To complicate matters, critical care interventions carry significant risks. Not infrequently, end-of-life and other ethical issues come into play. The intensivist-led multidisciplinary critical care team must be able to manage the complexities involved in these patients in order to optimize patient outcomes.

SAMPLE QUESTIONS

Questions

Choose the best answer for each question.

1. A 68-year-old woman in the surgical intensive care unit is comatose 10 days after a motor vehicle crash during which she sustained a fractured right femur treated with an intramedullary rod within 24 hours of the injury. There were no other injuries noted on admission. She remains intubated due to hypoventilation. Vital signs are blood pressure (BP)—100/60 mm Hg and pulse—52 beats/minute. Her temperature is 35.4°C. Her chest is clear. There are no heart murmurs. Her abdomen is mildly distended but soft. There are no bowel sounds. The surgical site is healing well with no signs of infection. An electrocardiogram shows sinus rhythm with low-voltage QRS. Computed tomographic scan of her head is normal for her age. Laboratory studies show:

   Hemoglobin—8.2 g/dL
   Sodium—138 mEq/L
   Potassium—3.7 mEq/L
   Thyroid-stimulating hormone (TSH)—16.4 μU/mL
      (ref—0.5 to 5.0 μU/mL)
   T4—0.5 μg/dL (ref—5 to 12 μg/dL)

   What is the most likely diagnosis for her condition?
   A. Sick euthyroid syndrome
   B. Thyroid storm
   C. Myxedema coma
   D. Adrenal insufficiency of critical illness
   E. Graves' disease

2. A 70-year-old woman is transferred from the surgery ward to the surgical intensive care unit because of hypotension 2 days after undergoing an open low anterior resection for a sigmoid cancer. The surgery went well with minimal blood loss. The tumor was found on routine colonoscopy, and she had no symptoms and was quite healthy and active prior to surgery. Her preoperative medications were multiple vitamins and calcium supplements. Since surgery she has been receiving maintenance intravenous fluids and was stable until a few hours ago when she became hypotensive. Despite receiving boluses of normal saline and starting pressors (norepinephrine and vasopressin), she remains hypotensive. She is intubated because of lethargy and tachypnea. Her temperature is 37.4°C. Pupils are equal and reactive. Her chest is clear bilaterally. There are no heart murmurs. Her abdomen is soft and tender only near the lower midline incision. There are no localizing neurological findings. There is minimal urine output from a Foley catheter. Laboratory studies show:

   Hematocrit—33% (36% the day before)
   Sodium—129 mEq/L

   Potassium—5.1 mEq/L
   Glucose—108 mg/dL
   Arterial blood gases (ABGs) on 40% FiO$_2$–pH—7.39
   PCO$_2$—38 mm Hg
   PO$_2$—130 mm Hg
   U/A—no bacteria, negative leukocyte esterase

   What is the most likely diagnosis?
   A. Hemorrhage
   B. Anastomotic leak
   C. Pulmonary embolism
   D. Acute adrenal insufficiency
   E. Urosepsis

3. A 52-year-old man was admitted to the hospital with bilateral femur fractures and rib fractures following a motor vehicle crash. He developed a deep vein thrombosis involving the left femoral vein and was started on intravenous heparin 4 days after admission. His platelet count decreased and concern was raised for heparin-induced thrombocytopenia. Which of the following would be the best alternative anticoagulant?
   A. Clopidogrel
   B. Argatroban
   C. Warfarin
   D. Enoxaparin
   E. Aspirin

4. A 71-year-old man is admitted to the intensive care unit in septic shock secondary to pneumonia. His BP is 85/40 mm Hg and heart rate 95 beats/minute. Which of the following medications would be the most appropriate to use to treat his hypotension?
   A. Epinephrine
   B. Dobutamine
   C. Milrinone
   D. Dopamine
   E. Norepinephrine

5. A 42-year-old woman with a history of alcohol abuse is admitted to the intensive care unit with active bleeding from esophageal varices. The medication most useful for decreasing the risk of rebleeding, with the least side effects, is
   A. octreotide
   B. proton pump inhibitor
   C. beta-blocker
   D. vasopressin
   E. nitroglycerin

Answers and Explanations

1. Answer: C

While rare, myxedema coma is the most severe form of hypothyroidism. Typical features of this condition include mental status changes ranging from lethargy to coma, hypothermia, sinus bradycardia, low-voltage QRS complex on electrocardiogram (ECG), hypoventilation, and ileus. An elevated TSH and severely depressed T4 levels confirm the diagnosis. Sick euthyroid syndrome may be an adaptation to critical illness and is noteworthy for a depressed T3 level. Thyroid storm is severe hyperthyroidism and has features opposite of myxedema coma, including fever, high-output cardiac failure, and nearly nondetectable TSH with elevated T3 and T4 levels. The hallmark of adrenal insufficiency of critical illness is hypotension refractory to fluids and vasoactive medications.

2. Answer: D

Adrenal insufficiency of critical illness typically presents with hypotension refractory to fluid resuscitation and vasoactive medications. Ventilator dependence, hyponatremia, hyperkalemia, and hypoglycemia can occur but are less commonly attributed to the adrenal dysfunction. While frequently seen with chronic adrenal insufficiency, hyperpigmentation, abdominal pain, nausea, weight loss, and fatigue are not typical symptoms in the critical care setting.

3. Answer: B

In this setting, any heparin product should be stopped immediately, including low molecular weight heparin, such as enoxaparin. Use of warfarin is appropriate in the long term but will not be effective immediately. Antiplatelet therapies, such as aspirin and clopidogrel, have no proven role as substitutes for anticoagulants. The best choice is argatroban, a direct thrombin inhibitor.

4. Answer: E

Dobutamine is a beta-agonist. Milrinone is a phosphodiesterase inhibitor. Both are commonly used for the management of cardiogenic shock. Epinephrine and dopamine have mixed alpha- and beta-receptor activity. Dopamine also stimulates dopaminergic receptors. Tachycardia is a frequent side effect. Norepinephrine stimulates mainly alpha receptors, with some beta-receptor activity. Thus, it is the drug of choice for patients with distributive shock, for example, sepsis.

5. Answer: A

Although proton pump inhibitors are useful for bleeding ulcers and are usually given to patients with variceal bleeds, they do not decrease the bleeding. Beta-blockers and nitrates help prevent recurrent bleeds but are dangerous while the patient is bleeding. Vasopressin, used for years to help treat variceal bleeding, is a nonspecific vasoconstrictor and thus is risky. Octreotide can decrease rebleeding with few side effects.

7

Wounds and Wound Healing

GLENN E. TALBOY, JR., M.D. • ANNESLEY W. COPELAND, M.D. • GREGORY J. GALLINA, M.D.

Objectives

1. Define a wound, and describe the sequence and approximate time frame of the phases of wound healing.

2. Describe the three types of wound healing and the elements of each. Describe the three phases of wound healing that are distinct to each type of wound.

3. Describe the essential elements and significance of granulation tissue.

4. Describe the growth factors and cytokines involved in wound healing, their cells of origin, and their target cells.

5. Describe the clinical factors that decrease collagen synthesis and retard wound healing.

6. Describe the rationale for the uses of absorbable and nonabsorbable sutures.

7. Describe the appropriate use and toxic doses of local anesthetics.

8. Discuss the functions of a dressing.

9. Define clean, contaminated, infected, and chronic wounds, and describe the management of each type.

10. Develop a basic understanding of methods to assist in wound healing, when their use is indicated, and when it is contraindicated.

A wound, in the broadest sense, is a disruption of normal anatomic relations as a result of an injury. The injury may be intentional (e.g., elective surgical incision) or unintentional (e.g., trauma). Regardless of the cause of injury, the biochemical and physiologic processes of healing are identical, although their time course and intensity may vary. The process of wound closure is classified into three distinct types: (1) primary, (2) secondary, and (3) tertiary, based on the timing of replacement of the epithelium over the wound. Wound healing is also divided by physiologic process into three stages or phases: (1) inflammatory or substrate, (2) proliferative, and (3) maturation or remodeling. These biochemical and physiologic events are correlated with gross morphologic changes in the wound. Knowledge of these events and changes allows the physician to maximize the chances of successful healing and minimize scarring.

PHYSIOLOGY OF WOUND HEALING

Inflammation is the basic physiologic process that is common to all wounds. Clinically, inflammation is identified by the cardinal signs of redness (rubor), heat (calor), swelling (tumor), pain (dolor), and loss of function. These signs of inflammation are also seen in wound infections, which ultimately may cause wound disruption. All wounds, whether acute, chronic, or infected, have varying time courses after the primary events that lead to normal wound healing. The physiology underlying these clinical signs is a complex interaction of biochemical and cellular events.

Biochemical Aspects

Trauma activates a cascade of chemoattractants and mitogens that recruit phagocytes, fibroblasts, and endothelial cells. These chemoattractants, which include platelet-derived growth factors (PDGFs) and complement peptide (C5A), are produced during the clotting of blood by degradation of the surrounding tissue and by cells entering the wound. The initial event of clotting blood and recruitment of cells occurs in the first 1 to 2 hours after injury. The first cells that enter the wound are platelets, which come into contact with the damaged **collagen** at the time of injury. The platelets degranulate and release alpha granules that contain multiple growth factors, including PDGF and transforming growth factor-β (TGF-β).

Inflammatory cells are attracted and release a variety of cytokines and growth factors. Cytokines are soluble proteins that are secreted by a cell and influence activities of other cells. Growth factors are proteins that bind to cell receptors and initiate cellular proliferation and differentiation. Macrophages release TGF-β, macrophage-derived growth factor (MDGF), transforming growth factor-α (TGF-α), heparin-binding epidermal growth factor (HB-EGF), and basic fibroblast growth factor (bFGF). Keratinocytes also enter the wound and release TGF-β, TGF-α, and keratinocyte-derived autocrine factor (KAF). All of these cytokines and growth factors are involved in synthesis of extracellular matrix and new capillary formation. Many also act as attractants for fibroblasts and neutrophils. Table 7-1 lists growth factors and cytokines by cell of origin and their target tissues.

In addition to cytokines and growth factors, arachidonic acid is contained in the walls of cells. It is released when the

TABLE 7-1	Cytokines and Growth Factors		

Name	Cell of Origin	Target Cells/Tissue	Effect
TGF-α	Macrophages Keratinocytes	Fibroblasts, epithelial cells, and endothelial cells	Migration of target cells Extracellular matrix proteins, proliferation, and capillary formation
TGF-β	Platelet alpha granules Macrophages Fibroblasts and keratinocytes	Inflammatory cells. Fibroblasts, epithelial cells, and endothelial cells	Chemotactic for target cells Migration of target cells Extracellular matrix proteins, proliferation, and capillary formation
EGF	Platelet alpha granules	Inflammatory cells	Chemotactic for target cells
PDGF	Platelet alpha granules Fibroblasts and endothelial cells	Inflammatory cells	Chemotactic for target cells Extracellular matrix proteins, proliferation, and capillary formation
IL-1	Macrophages, monocytes, and keratinocytes		Increases collagen synthesis, activates neutrophils, increases keratinocyte migration
IL-2	T lymphocytes	Fibroblasts, inflammatory cells, and T cells	Attracts fibroblasts and inflammatory cells, activates T cells
IL-6	Fibroblasts and inflammatory cells	Fibroblasts Inflammatory cells	Fibroblast proliferation Chemotactic for inflammatory cells
IL-8	Macrophages and endothelial cells	Leukocytes	Recruitment and activation
IFN-γ	T lymphocytes	Monocytes and macrophages	Activation of target cells
TNF-α	Macrophages, monocytes, fibroblasts, mast cells, and keratinocytes	Macrophages, monocytes, endothelial cells, and neutrophils	Mediates tissue repair, endothelial cell activation, and tissue remodeling

cells are injured. The degradation of arachidonic acid into prostanoid derivatives of prostaglandins and thromboxanes causes a number of responses associated with the inflammatory response, including vasodilation, swelling, and pain.

Physiologic Aspects

At the same time that these biochemical events are developing, leukocytes are marginating, attaching to vessel walls, and migrating through the walls toward the site of injury (Figure 7-1). In addition, venules are dilating, and lymphatics are being blocked. This inflammatory response in the wound occurs for a variable period, depending on local tissue and host factors. Some of these factors are responsive to manipulation by the physician.

PHASES OF WOUND HEALING

Understanding the phases of wound healing is important in treating conditions and diseases that affect various stages of the healing cascade (e.g., diabetes mellitus, malnutrition, and chronic illnesses). The three phases of wound healing are (1) inflammatory or substrate, (2) proliferative, and (3) maturation or remodeling. The second and third phases are relatively constant, regardless of the type of wound healing. These phases begin only when the wound is covered by epithelium. Figure 7-2 shows the phases of healing, comparing cells and collagen concentrations with wound strength over time.

Substrate Phase (Inflammatory)

The substrate phase is also known as the inflammatory phase, lag phase, or exudative phase. The main cells involved in this process are polymorphonuclear leukocytes (PMNs), platelets, and macrophages. Shortly after a wound occurs, PMNs appear and remain the predominant cell for approximately 48 hours. These

leukocytes may be the origin of many inflammatory mediators, including complement and kallikrein. Small numbers of bacteria are handled by the macrophages that are present in the wound. However, if a large number of bacteria are present, especially in the neutropenic patient, clinical infection will occur. The neutrophil is not crucial for normal wound healing, but the macrophage is. Monocytes enter the wound after the PMNs, reaching maximum numbers approximately 24 hours later. They evolve into macrophages, which are the main cells involved in wound débridement. Another biochemical event associated with débridement is activation of tissue matrix metalloproteinases (TMMPs). In the absence of injury or inflammation, these degradative, proteolytic enzymes normally are quiescent, in part due to TMMP inhibitors, which also reside in normal tissue. After injury, TMMP inhibitor activity dramatically falls, and TMMP activity is stimulated. Activated TMMP enzymes, working in conjunction with leukocyte enzymes, degrade surrounding matrix proteins such as collagen and necrotic cellular macromolecules. These enzymes break down devitalized tissue structures, which is required for subsequent events in wound healing. Experimental wounds that are depleted of macrophages and monocytes show marked inhibition of fibroblast migration, proliferation, and loss of collagen production. Macrophages, which can secrete more than 100 different molecules, are an important producer of growth factors. Some of these factors are TGF-β, which stimulates the proliferation of fibroblasts, and interleukin-1 (IL-1), which is partially responsible for regulating the repair of damaged tissue. IL-1 is an important growth factor in the regulation of many processes in the inflammatory response; it may induce fever, promote hemostasis by interacting with endothelial cells, enhance fibroblast proliferation, and activate T cells.

As clot, debris, and bacteria are being removed from the wound, substrates for collagen synthesis are being arranged. In primary wound healing (discussed later), the substrate phase occurs over approximately a 4-day period. The wound is edematous and erythematous. This normal process may be difficult

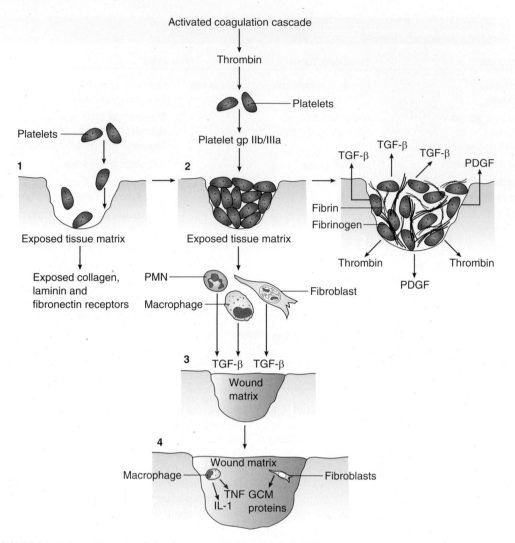

FIGURE 7-1. At tissue injury, a provisional wound matrix is established. (1) Platelets bind to exposed wound matrix receptors. (2) After wounding, the coagulation cascade is activated, generating thrombin, which activates platelet glycoprotein (Gp) IIb/IIIa and increases platelet aggregation. A provisional wound matrix is formed and is made up of platelets, fibrin, fibrinogen, and fibronectin. The activated platelets in the wound generate TGF-β, PDGF, and thrombin. (3) TGF-β is strongly chemotactic for neutrophils, macrophages, and fibroblasts, recruiting these cells into the provisional wound matrix, where they are also subsequently activated by TGF-β. (4) Increasing concentrations of TGF-β result in macrophage activation, producing increased amounts of tumor necrosis factor-α (TNF-α) and IL-1. TGF-β also stimulates fibroblast production of extracellular matrix proteins. These reactions further enhance migration of macrophages and fibroblasts into the wound, facilitating tissue repair. (Based on Greenfield LJ. *Surgery: Scientific Principles and Practice.* Baltimore, MD: Lippincott Williams & Wilkins, 2001, Fig. 5-15.)

to distinguish from early signs of wound infection. In healing by secondary or tertiary intention (discussed later), this phase continues indefinitely until the wound surface is closed by ectodermal elements (i.e., epithelium for skin, mucosa in the gut).

Proliferative Phase

The second and third phases of wound healing are relatively constant, regardless of the type of wound healing. These phases begin only when the wound is covered by epithelium. The proliferative phase is the second stage of healing. It is characterized by the production of collagen in the wound. The wound appears less edematous and inflamed than before, but the wound scar may be raised, red, and hard. The primary cell in this phase is the fibroblast, which produces collagen.

Collagen is the principal structural protein of the body. It has a complex, three-dimensional structure. Collagen synthesis begins with the production of amino acid chains in the cytoplasm of the fibroblast. These α-chains are unique in that each third amino acid is glycine. Two amino acids, hydroxyproline and hydroxylysine, are found only in collagen. These amino acids are required for hydroxylation during collagen synthesis by specific enzymes. Important cofactors involved in the hydroxylation process are ferrous ion, α-ketoglutarate, and ascorbic acid. Insufficient consumption of one of the cofactors can lead to an interruption of the proliferative phase. The absence of ascorbic acid leads to the production of defective, unhydroxylated collagen, which leads to wound breakdown. Most physicians are familiar with scurvy, which is caused by vitamin C deficiency, characterized by impaired wound healing, cutaneous sores, and a hemorrhagic gingivitis.

Maturation Phase (Remodeling)

The third, and final, phase of wound healing is the remodeling, or maturation, phase. It is characterized by the maturation of

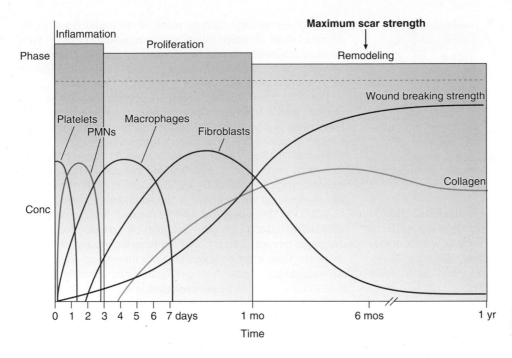

FIGURE 7-2. Phases of wound healing comparing cells and collagen concentrations with wound strength over time.

collagen by intermolecular cross-linking. The wound scar gradually flattens and becomes less prominent and more pale and supple. This phase is a time of great metabolic activity. Collagen is deposited in the wound, and existing collagen is remodeled and removed; thus, there is no net collagen gain in the wound. The maturation process clinically corresponds to the flattening of the scar. Wound maturation in an adult takes from 9 to 12 months.

CLASSIFICATION OF HEALING WOUNDS

Wounds may be classified as acute or chronic. Acute wounds include all surgical incisions as well as wounds sustained as a result of acute trauma. Acute wounds are expected to pursue the normal phases of wound healing previously described in an orderly and timely manner, culminating in full epithelialization and formation of a scar. In contrast, a chronic wound is one in which the normal wound healing process is frustrated or arrested for some reason. Examples of typical nonhealing chronic wounds include chronic venous stasis ulcers, pressure sores, and diabetic foot wounds.

Primary Intention

Acute wounds may be managed in one of several ways. The most common method is to primarily close the wound, resulting in *healing by primary intention*. The term applies to all surgical incisions and lacerations that are closed with sutures, staples, adhesive, or any technique by which the surgeon intentionally approximates the epidermal edges of a wound. It also includes tissue transfer techniques and flaps that may be used to close larger defects. The advantages of this approach to wound management are that it is easiest for the patient to manage the wound, there is a rapid return of function of the wounded part, and the final cosmetic result is superior (Figure 7-3). The one major disadvantage of primary closure of a wound is the risk of wound infection.

Secondary Intention

An alternative to primary closure of a full-thickness wound is to leave it open, or let it *heal by secondary intention* (Figure 7-4).

Classically these wounds are treated with "wet-to-dry" dressings wherein a gauze sponge is moistened with saline and used to pack the wound, covered with a dry dressing; the moist sponge dries out, and when it is removed and changed once or twice a day, gentle débridement of the wound is achieved. Granulation tissue, characterized by friable reddish "granules" of tiny capillary buds, will form in the base of the wound. Epithelial cells cannot migrate across granulation tissue, however, so healing in secondary intention occurs primarily by wound contraction. Myofibroblasts at the edges of the wound exert a centripetal force, which gradually draws the edges of the wound together. Wound contraction occurs to a greater extent in areas of the body where the surrounding tissues are redundant, such as the abdomen and buttock, and is not as pronounced in areas such as the scalp or pretibial area where the skin is taut. The disadvantages of leaving a wound open are that daily dressing changes are required until the wound is healed, which may take some time, and the final result is a cicatrix that may be unsightly. The one advantage of applying this

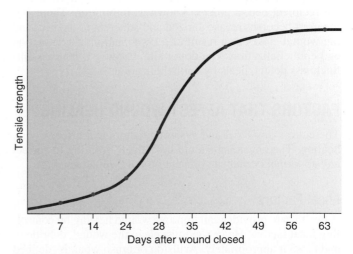
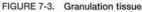

FIGURE 7-3. Granulation tissue.

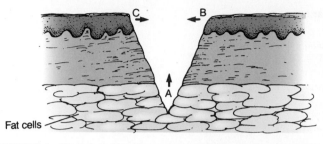

FIGURE 7-4. Wounds that heal by secondary intention. **A,** Granulation tissue forms at the base. **B,** The wound margins contract. **C,** The epithelium migrates.

method of wound management is that wound infection is virtually impossible. Thus, secondary intention is applied to wounds that are highly contaminated, such as a subcutaneous abscess after incision and drainage, or where the likelihood of wound infection is deemed too great, as in open appendectomy for perforated appendicitis.

Delayed Primary Closure

In delayed primary closure, sometimes called *healing by tertiary intention*, the wound is initially managed as a secondary intention wound, that is, left open with dressing changes. After a matter of about 5 days or so, when the wound is clean and granulation tissue is abundant, the wound edges are actively approximated. This approach is successful because granulation tissue, while not sterile, is extremely vascular and as such is highly resistant to infection. Delayed primary closure combines the advantages of primary wound closure in terms of final cosmetic result and rapid return to function while significantly reducing the risk of wound infection.

Skin Grafting

For large surface area full-thickness wounds that cannot be closed primarily, an alternative to the lengthy application of secondary intention is skin grafting. Split-thickness skin grafts consist of epidermis and a portion of the underlying dermis and are harvested using a dermatome. Before it is placed on the open wound, the graft may be meshed with a device that creates fishnet-like perforations or interstices in it. The perforations allow the graft to expand to cover an irregularly shaped wound and also prevent pooling of blood or serum underneath the graft, which would prevent take. For the first 48 hours, the grafted skin derives its nutrients by passive absorption from the recipient bed, a process known as imbibition. Thereafter the graft becomes revascularized and adherent to the bed, and the wound closes as a result of a combination of contraction and epithelialization. The donor site, because it is not a full-thickness defect, heals by epithelialization.

FACTORS THAT AFFECT WOUND HEALING

There are many local and systemic factors that affect wound healing. The physician should be actively working to correct any abnormality that can prevent or slow wound healing.

Local Factors

A health care provider can improve wound healing by controlling local factors. He or she must clean the wound, debride it, and close it appropriately. Avulsion or crush wounds (defined

below under general management of wounds) need to be debrided until all nonviable tissue is removed. Grossly contaminated wounds should be cleaned as completely as possible to remove particulate matter (foreign bodies) and should be irrigated copiously.

Bleeding must be controlled to prevent hematoma formation, which is an excellent medium for bacterial growth. Hematoma also separates wound edges, preventing the proper contact of tissues that is necessary for healing.

Radiation affects local wound healing by causing vasculitis, which leads to local hypoxia and ischemia. Hypoxia and ischemia impede healing by reducing the amount of nutrients and oxygen that are available at the wound site.

Infection decreases the rate of wound healing and detrimentally affects proper granulation tissue formation, decreases oxygen delivery, and depletes the wound of needed nutrients. Care must be taken to clean the wound adequately. All wounds have some degree of contamination; if the body is able to control bacterial proliferation in a wound, that wound will heal. The use of cleansing agents (the simplest is soap and water) can help reduce contamination. A wound that contains the highly virulent streptococci species should not be closed. Physicians should keep in mind the potential for *Clostridium tetani* in wounds with devitalized tissue and use the proper prophylaxis.

Systemic Factors

In addition to controlling local factors, the physician must address systemic issues that can affect wound healing. Nutrition is an extremely important factor in wound healing. Patients need adequate nutrition to support protein synthesis, collagen formation, and metabolic energy for wound healing. Patients need adequate vitamins and nutrients to facilitate healing; folic acid is critical to the proper formation of collagen. Adequate fat intake is required for the absorption of vitamins D, A, K, and E. Vitamin K is essential for the carboxylation of glutamate in the synthesis of clotting factors II, VII, IX, and X. Decreasing clotting factors can lead to hematoma formation and altered wound healing. Vitamin A increases the inflammatory response, increases collagen synthesis, and increases the influx of macrophages into a wound. Magnesium is required for protein synthesis, and zinc is a cofactor for RNA and DNA polymerase. Lack of any one of these vitamins or trace elements will adversely affect wound healing.

Uncontrolled diabetes mellitus results in uncontrolled hyperglycemia, impairs wound healing, and alters collagen formation. Hyperglycemia also inhibits fibroblast and endothelial cell proliferation within the wound.

Medications will also affect wound healing. For example, steroids blunt the inflammatory response, decrease the available vitamin A in the wound, and alter the deposition and remodeling of collagen.

Chronic illness (immune deficiency, cancer, uremia, liver disease, and jaundice) will predispose to infection, protein deficiency, and malnutrition, which, as noted previously, can affect wound healing.

Smoking has a systemic effect by decreasing the oxygen-carrying capacity of hemoglobin. Smoking may also decrease collagen formation within a wound. Hypoxia results in a decrease in oxygen delivery to a wound and retards healing. Every physician should encourage patients to stop smoking for general health reasons.

GENERAL MANAGEMENT OF WOUNDS

Local Anesthetics

To reduce patient discomfort when debriding or suturing wounds, local anesthesia may be required. Of the two pharmacologic classes of local anesthetics, the amide group is most commonly used and includes xylocaine, bupivacaine, mepivacaine, and prilocaine. The second pharmacologic class is the esters and includes procaine, chloroprocaine, tetracaine, and cocaine. If a patient has a known sensitivity to one family of local anesthetics, the physician may select the other. However, the ester anesthetics may not be used in individuals with sensitivity to p-aminobenzoic acid (PABA).

All local anesthetics reversibly inhibit the conduction of nerve impulses by decreasing the membrane permeability to sodium, which decreases the rate of depolarization and leads to an increase in the excitability threshold of the nerve and inhibition of the nerve impulse. Clinically, the order of loss in nerve function is pain, temperature, touch, proprioception, and skeletal muscle tone.

Solubility, protein binding, and the pH and the vascularity of the tissues determine duration of action of the local anesthetics. Another important factor is the inclusion of a vasoconstrictor, which is most commonly epinephrine. Amides are protein bound and are metabolized in the liver by ring hydroxylation, oxidative N-dealkylation, cleavage of the amide linkage, and conjugation. Esters are metabolized by pseudocholinesterase to PABA and diethylaminoethanol. Individuals with sensitivity to PABA therefore should not receive an ester local anesthetic.

The physician needs to evaluate carefully the wound size and consider whether excessive amounts of local anesthetic will be required to treat a wound. If the maximum dose will be exceeded, general anesthesia will need to be employed. For example, the toxic limit of xylocaine, a frequently used local anesthetic, is 7 mg/kg given in 1 hour. The clinician should remember that 1 mL of xylocaine 1% contains 10 mg of drug. Another way to consider this is that 50 mL of xylocaine 1% is the toxic level for a 70-kg person. Major side effects of local anesthetics include central nervous system (tinnitus, blurred vision, tremors, and depression) and cardiovascular effects (myocardial depression, atrioventricular [AV] block, and decreased cardiac output). Table 7-2 gives the name, maximum dose, onset of action, and duration of action of the more commonly used local anesthetics.

Local anesthetics containing vasoconstrictors (i.e., epinephrine) should not be used in tissues supplied by end arteries, such as the nose, digits, penis, and ear. Necrosis of this tissue can result from vasoconstriction.

TABLE 7-3	Steps in Wound Care

1. Sterile preparation and draping
2. Administration of local anesthetic
3. Hemostasis
4. Irrigation and débridement
5. Closure in layers
6. Dressing and bandage

Classification of Wounds

A **clean wound** is one that is relatively new (<12 hours) and has minimal contamination. Clean wounds are classified according to presentation and method of injury. The clean wound needs to be debrided, if necessary, and closed using the proper suture material (see below). Wound edges should be approximated without tension. Skin edges should not be overlapped, since this would result in undergrowth of the epithelial layer. Table 7-3 lists the steps in wound care.

An **avulsion** injury occurs when the skin has been violated by shearing forces and underlying tissue has been undermined and elevated, creating a flap or total loss of skin. The flap or avulsed tissue is composed of skin with or without the underlying fat and muscle. This type of wound needs thorough cleaning, débridement of necrotic tissue, and closure if appropriate. Efforts should be made to suture the "flap" of tissue down with absorbable suture and then close the wound edges. It is also helpful to place a pressure dressing over this wound to decrease fluid collection. If an open wound has been created, a full-thickness flap containing the appropriate layers of tissue or a skin graft may be required to cover the defect.

An **abrasion** is a superficial loss of epithelial elements, with portions of the dermis and deeper structures remaining intact. Usually, only cleansing of the wound is required, because the remaining epithelial cells regenerate and migrate to close the wound. Careful cleansing is critical to prevent traumatic tattoos, which can result from debris in the wound. Desiccation of an abrasion should be avoided by applying a layer of petroleum jelly or antibiotic ointment.

Puncture wounds generally do not require closure. Management consists of assessment of the damage to underlying vital structures and examination for a foreign body. Radiographs are often helpful in assessing the presence of a foreign body. This wound must be carefully followed clinically to detect any developing infection at an early stage.

TABLE 7-2	Local Anesthetics			
Type/Name	**Maximum Dose**	**Maximum Dose with Epinephrine**	**Onset of Action**	**Duration of Action**
Amides				
Xylocaine	4.5 mg/kg–350 mg	7 mg/kg–500 mg	1–5 min	60/90 min
Bupivacaine	2.5 mg/kg–175 mg	3.5 mg/kg–225 mg	5–10 min	12/18 hr
Esters				
Procaine	350 mg	600 mg	1–2 min	60 min
Chloroprocaine	11 mg/kg–800 mg	14 mg/kg–1000 mg	6–12 min	60/90 min

TABLE 7-4	Suture Material					
Suture	**Trade Names**	**Raw Material**	**Stranding**	**Type**	**Retention of Tensile Strength**	**Where Used**
Nylon	Nurolon	Synthetic	Mono/polyfilament	Nonabsorbable		Skin
Polyester	Dacron, Tevdek, Ethibond	Synthetic	Polyfilament	Nonabsorbable		Skin, mucosal areas, fascia
Silk		Natural	Polyfilament	Permanent[a]	2 yr	Below skin
Catgut		Natural	Monofilament	Absorbable	7 days	Below skin
Chromic Catgut	Chromic	Natural	Monofilament	Absorbable	14 days	Below skin
Polyglycolic acid	Vycril, Dexon	Synthetic	Polyfilament	Absorbable	14 to 30 days	Below skin
Polypropylene	Prolene	Synthetic	Monofilament	Permanent		Skin, fascia, vasculature, and tendon/bone
Polyglyconate	Maxon	Synthetic	Monofilament	Absorbable	30–60 days	Below skin, fascia, bowel, ducts
Polydioxanone	PDS	Synthetic	Monofilament	Absorbable	60 days	Below skin, fascia, bowel, ducts
Poliglecaprone	Monocryl	Synthetic	Monofilament	Absorbable	30–50 days	Subcuticular skin closure
Poly (L-lactide/glycolide)	Panacryl	Synthetic	Polyfilament	Absorbable	90 days	Bone, tendon, and fascia
Stainless steel			Mono/polyfilament	Nonabsorbable		Bone, fascia, and skin

[a]Absorbs over 2 yr but is considered permanent.

Crush injuries are often accompanied by the loss of significant amounts of tissue that may initially appear viable. Nonviable tissue must eventually be débrided, and the wound closed with either a skin graft or a myocutaneous flap.

Suture Material

Suture material, size, and type should be chosen based on the type of tissue that is being sutured (Table 7-4). Suture size is graded by a number or by a zero (0). The more zeros, the smaller the suture. Suture size number 1 is larger than 0, which in turn is larger than 2-0 (00). Suture can be as small as 9-0 or 10-0. A 3-0 or 4-0 suture is used for skin on the torso and extremities, whereas a 5-0 or 6-0 suture is appropriate for the more delicate tissues of the face and neck. A 2-0 to 4-0 suture is appropriate for closure of deeper tissues.

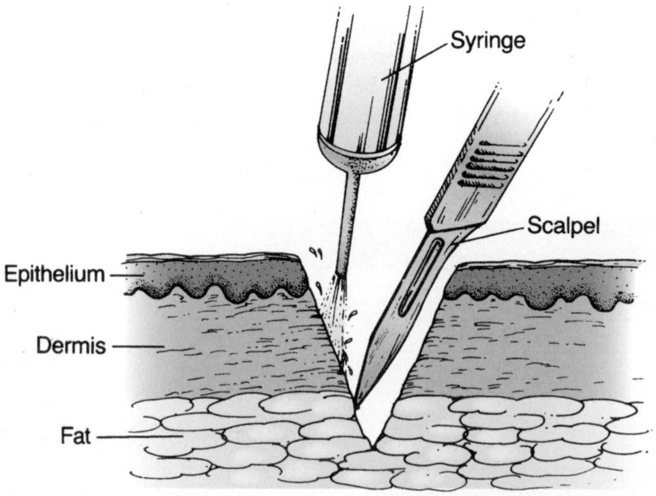

Wound Closure

It is important that the wound be prepared properly prior to closure by thorough cleaning and débridement (Figure 7-5), as discussed above. When suturing, the physician should remember several important details:

1. There should be no tension on the wound edges, because tension can lead to necrosis of the skin. If the wound will not close without excessive tension, another management plan (e.g., rotational flaps, skin graft) should be considered.
2. Sutures in the skin of the torso and extremities should be left in place for 7 to 10 days.
3. Sutures on the face and neck should be left in place for only 4 days.
4. Knots should be secure but not so tight as to strangulate the tissue.
5. Monofilament nonabsorbable suture should be used on the skin because it is less reactive.
6. Deep suture should be absorbable and placed in the tissues that have the greatest strength. For closure of muscle, it is the fascia that provides the greatest strength. For closure of the skin, the dermis provides the strength (Figure 7-6).

FIGURE 7-5. Sharp débridement and saline lavage to prepare the wound for closure.

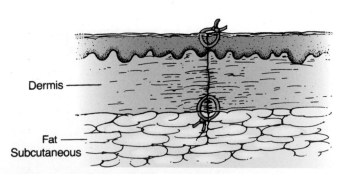

FIGURE 7-6. The dermis is approximated for strength, and the epidermis is closed to seal the wound and align the surface cells.

Dressings

A dressing is usually placed over the closed wound to protect the wound, immobilize the area, compress the area evenly, absorb any secretions, and be aesthetically acceptable. Proper wound dressing should fulfill all of these criteria without compromising adequate coverage of a wound. The dressing should provide sufficient bulk to protect the wound from trauma. The bulk provided by fluffed gauze and gauze pads allows for adequate absorption of wound secretions and helps to immobilize the area. A plaster splint or cast may provide further immobilization. An outer layer of firmly wrapped rolled gauze and a loosely but evenly applied elastic roll can provide even compression and an aesthetically acceptable appearance.

Suture Removal

Sutures used for skin closure are removed when they have done the job for which they were placed. Sterile forceps and fine scissors are the basic instruments that are used to remove sutures. The use of sterilized supplies is important for infection control. The suture is grasped with forceps and cut and then gently removed.

Figure 7-7 shows the stages of wound healing, from débridement of necrotic skin and soft tissue, to formation of a granulation bed and placement of a skin graft, to a healed wound with a combination of skin graft and advancement flap.

MANAGEMENT OF CONTAMINATED, INFECTED, AND CHRONIC WOUNDS

Contaminated Wounds

All wounds are contaminated to a greater or lesser extent. Even the wounds that are considered clean have a bacterial inoculum (see Table 7-5 for classification of wounds). Proper wound care, with débridement and adequate lavage, can markedly diminish the inoculum and result in successful primary wound healing. Exceptions to primary closure of these contaminated wounds include a very high bacterial inoculum (e.g., human bite, farm injury), a long time lapse since the initial injury, the suspected or known presence of species, and a severe crush injury. In these instances, delayed closure is the preferred management.

Keeping buried sutures to a minimum is important when closing any wound. Excessive use of buried suture provides foreign body for bacterial contamination. Monofilament skin sutures are used to reduce the possibility of wound infection. If the surgeon has doubts about the extent of contamination or the safety of the closure, delay is the judicious approach to wound management. Delay allows time for further débridement and reduction of the bacterial count to $<10^5$ bacteria/gram of tissue. Follow-up within 48 hours detects early signs of clinical infection.

Infected Wounds

Infected wounds are sometimes difficult to detect. Proper management begins with identifying the truly infected wound. Any layperson can observe **pus** exuding from a severely inflamed wound and tell that the wound is infected. On the other hand, the most experienced surgeon will have no better chance than the flip of a coin in identifying the level of bacterial contamination in a chronically granulating wound.

The number of bacteria that can be tolerated and still allow successful wound closure is the most precise definition of an infected wound. A wound is considered infected when the level of contamination is $>10^5$ organisms/gram of tissue. The proper management of the infected wound is to decrease the bacterial count to 10^5 or less organisms/gram of tissue so that the wound may be closed. Débridement is the most important technique to decrease the bacterial count. Frequent cleaning of a wound can also decrease the bacterial count. Dressing changes should be limited to twice per day to prevent adversely affecting the progression of healing within an open wound. Systemic antibiotics are of little use in local bacterial control because they do not penetrate the granulating wound bed. However, topical antibacterials (e.g., mafenide acetate, silver sulfadiazine) are effective and may be used. Because of possible corneal irritation, mafenide acetate or silver sulfadiazine should not be used on the face. Biologic dressings (e.g., allograft, amniotic membrane) also decrease the bacterial level. Successful adherence of a biologic dressing indicates a reduced bacterial count and accurately predicts success with either wound closure or autograft. Successful wound management requires diligent preoperative, intraoperative, and postoperative care as well as meticulous surgical technique. Proper handling of tissues, adequate débridement, careful placement of sutures, and bacteriologic knowledge of the wound are critical aspects in wound closure.

Chronic Wounds

Wounds that are slow to heal are classified as chronic. They include diabetic foot ulcers, venous stasis ulcers, and open wounds that have failed to close. These wounds are stalled in the inflammatory phase of healing. They have poor granulation tissue formation, altered cell cycles, and biochemical imbalances. Studies have shown that chronic wounds have elevated levels of inflammatory cytokines and TMMPs. The presence of both inhibits or slows the natural progression of healing. The increased concentration of TMMPs is enhanced by the associated decrease in protease inhibitors. In addition, there is an increase in degradation of fibronectin and other important matrix components. Chronic wounds are difficult to deal with and take time and patience. Débridement of the wound, careful cleaning, and dressing changes have been the only hope in advancing healing in a chronic wound. Negative pressure devices, recombinant growth factors, hyperbaric oxygen, and enzymatic débridement ointments are some of the methods that have been used to assist in wound healing.

Chronic wounds develop when normal healing mechanisms are not capable of repairing the tissue injury. They are a consequence of the equilibrium between the systemic and local factors favoring healing and those that oppose it being tilted toward chronicity. Malnutrition, uremia, and the hyperglycemia of diabetes are examples of systemic factors that retard healing. Edema, infection, arterial insufficiency (ischemia), fecal soiling, and pressure on the wound are examples of local factors that can impair healing. Appreciation of the role of these factors and judicious intervention to counter them often are key to successful management.

Four types of chronic wounds are generally encountered in clinical practice: pressure ulcers, venous stasis ulcers, arterial insufficiency ulcers, and diabetic neuropathic ulcers. All are more common in the elderly. Each type of ulcer reflects local factors that promote repeated bouts of trauma or injury in the wound bed, leading to prolonged or repetitive inflammatory stimulation of the wound, including promotion of leukocyte

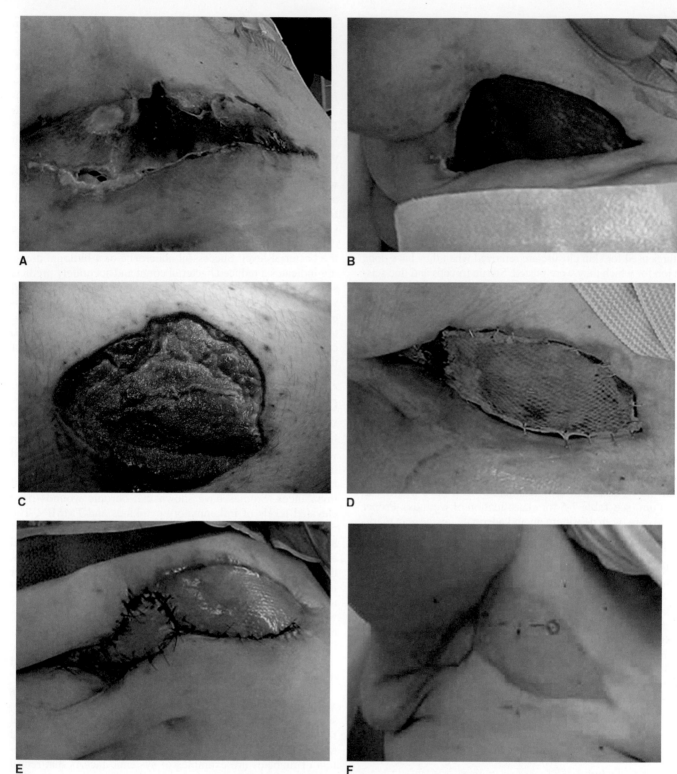

FIGURE 7-7. **A,** Example of necrotic skin and soft tissue. **B,** Wound after proper débridement of all necrotic skin and soft tissue.
C, Granulation bed. **D,** Initial placement of split-thickness skin graft. **E,** Skin graft with lateral advancement full-thickness graft.
F, Healed wound with combination of skin graft and advancement flap. Note the radiation tattoo markings.

TABLE 7-5	Wound Classification	
Wound Classification	Average Infection Rate (%)	Examples
Clean	3	Atraumatic, no gastrointestinal (GI) or genitourinary system (GU) or respiratory track (R) involvement
Clean–Contaminated	8	Minor sterile breaks, entrance into GI, GU, or R tract without significant contamination
Contaminated	15	Entrance into GI, GU, or R tract with spillage of contents, traumatic wounds with soil and particulate matter
Dirty	35	Infection within tissue, that is, abscess

activity, TMMP degradation, and, in some, repeated infection. Successful management starts with the correct diagnosis of the type of ulcer. It continues with specific steps to alleviate the continuing pathologic influences, which usually include local factors specific to the type of chronic wound, but may include systemic factors that need to be addressed.

Pressure Ulcers

Pressure ulcers develop in neurologically impaired patients or those with critical illness who are bedridden and cannot protect their skin with appropriate reflexes and spontaneous movement to relieve pressure. As many as 10% of acutely hospitalized patients develop bedsores, which progress from partial- to full-thickness injuries if not well managed. Patients with chronic spinal cord injury are at particular risk for pressure ulceration due to a loss of both sensation and motor function below the level of spinal injury. The common sites for pressure ulceration are the heel, sacrum, and ischial tuberosities (bony prominences that bear increased pressure in the bedridden or wheelchair-bound patient). Pressure ulcers can be classified and graded using the information in Table 7-6.

Pressure ulcer prevention starts with frequent turning and repositioning of the patient at risk. Particular attention to the heel is necessary, and protective devices such as foam heel pads are not as effective as floating the foot off the bed with a pillow under the calf. Rotating the patient from side to side with pillows helps to prevent pelvic ulceration. Once a pressure sore has developed, it may be necessary to use specialized pressure relief mattresses, including elaborate air-fluidized supports, to minimize pressure. Pelvic pressure ulcers often have small skin defects overlying large cavities and become severely infected from fecal soiling. Aggressive surgical débridement and drainage to control infection may be

required, and ultimately rotational skin or myocutaneous flaps are necessary to close the defect and achieve primary healing. The most common local care applied to pelvic pressure ulcers is probably saline-moistened gauze with twice-daily changing. A particularly useful new modality is the negative pressure wound vacuum device (Wound VAC—Vacuum Assisted Closure system, Kinetic Concepts, Inc., San Antonio, TX), which is a porous sponge packed into the wound connected to negative pressure. The negative pressure applied by the VAC stimulates more rapid closure of the wound, while simultaneously promoting drainage and creating a moist wound environment favorable for the ingrowth of granulation tissue.

Venous Stasis Ulcers

Venous stasis ulcers are the most common chronic wounds developing in adults (Figure 7-8). Venous insufficiency from venous valvular incompetence affects approximately 15% of adults, with typical symptoms of leg discomfort, heaviness,

TABLE 7-6	Pressure Sore Classification/Grade
Grade	Description
Grade 1	This is a nonblanching erythematous area on intact skin.
Grade 2	Partial-thickness skin loss with the involvement of the epidermis and/or the dermis. This is usually superficial and can appear as a blister or abrasion.
Grade 3	Full-thickness skin loss with necrosis of subcutaneous tissue that can extend to the fascia.
Grade 4	Full-thickness skin loss with necrosis. Destruction can involve muscle, bone, and tendons.

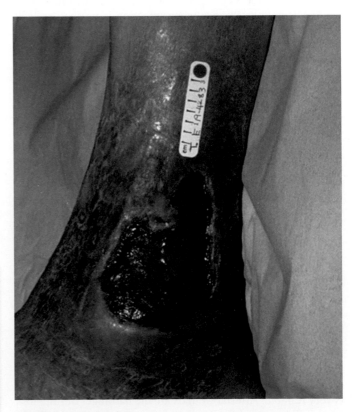

FIGURE 7-8. Venous ulcer.

and edema. Ulceration in patients with chronic venous insufficiency is relatively uncommon, with an overall incidence of 1 per 1000 per year. Venous ulcers generally are superficial wounds in the anteromedial aspect of the leg ("gaiter zone"), not involving the foot. The underlying pathophysiology is a consequence of venous hypertension transmitted to the microcirculation of the skin. Incompetent valves in the deep and superficial veins draining the lower extremity lead to the transmission of elevated pressure to the venous side of the capillaries in the skin. This effect is exacerbated when the leg is dependent and alleviated when the leg is elevated. The consequences include anatomic changes in the capillaries that slowly enlarge and become tortuous. Additionally, the increased filtration and subsequent deposition of plasma proteins and red cells alter the interstitium around the capillaries. The red cells break down in the tissue, causing deposition of hemosiderin pigment. The chronic consequence is hyperpigmentation and edema (termed *dermatofibrosis*) of the leg above the ankle. Patients with chronic venous insufficiency who develop a wound have impaired healing because of both (1) decreased skin perfusion as a consequence of elevated venous pressures in the capillaries and (2) decreased delivery of oxygen and glucose to tissues as a consequence of edema and protein deposition in the interstitium. An additional factor is the tendency of the wounds to weep fluid copiously, with maceration of the surrounding normal tissues and further skin damage.

Management of venous ulcers starts with compression, either with paste bandages (Unna boots) or with multiple-layer dry bandages (Charing Cross or dry boots). Multiple-layer dry dressings are generally more effective, because they provide more pressure and allow variation in the medications and topical devices applied directly to the wound bed. Routine management of venous ulcers starts with establishing a clean wound bed with sharp débridement of necrotic tissue, using systemic antibiotics when infection is present, as well as teaching the patient to elevate the limb as much as practical. Local care requires weekly or biweekly application of compression bandages, often with topical application of medications or devices directly to the wound, which promotes healing. Most venous wounds will heal in several months with continued compression therapy. Refractory wounds may require surgery to ablate the abnormal veins transmitting pressure to the involved skin or skin grafting.

Arterial Insufficiency Ulcers

Arterial insufficiency ulcers result from atherosclerotic obstruction of the main conduit arteries supplying the lower extremity, although other causes of occlusion such as thromboembolism may apply (Figure 7-9). Chronic arterial ulcers may resemble venous ulcers or any chronic wound, with variable appearances and degree of granulation. They tend to excite little inflammation, and may extend into deeper structures to expose bone or tendon. Typically, arterial ulcers involve the toes, which can be mummified and black (dry gangrene) or have suppuration with oozing (wet gangrene), but any part of the foot, ankle, or leg may develop ulceration or nonhealing wounds. The presence of black, infarcted skin or multiple wounds should strongly raise the suspicion for arterial disease. Pedal pulses are usually absent, but in doubtful cases diagnostic vascular ultrasound to assess the arterial circulation is very reliable. Arterial wounds are the harbinger of limb loss from infection, and the presence of an arterial wound should

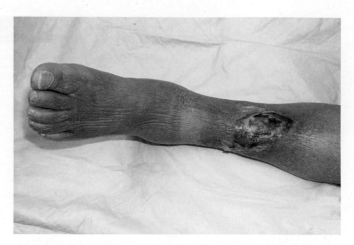

FIGURE 7-9.   Arterial ulcer.

prompt timely and aggressive intervention to salvage the limb and prevent major amputation.

Management of arterial wounds usually entails mechanical arterial interventions to improve tissue perfusion. Focal obstructions and occlusions are occasionally present and can be treated with endovascular balloon angioplasty or stenting, but most often long segments of arterial occlusion mandate bypass surgery with synthetic conduits or autologous saphenous veins. Without arterial reconstruction, approximately 25% of wounds can be healed with local care alone. It is hard to predict which wounds will respond to local care; therefore, the impetus to perform arterial surgery is high. Local care before revascularization is generally conservative: wet-to-dry gauze or antibiotic ointments are widely employed modalities. After arterial reconstruction, management options include excision of the wound and primary closure (e.g., toe amputation), or skin grafting. These interventions are occasionally successful without revascularization, but the chance for success with these minor surgical procedures depends greatly on the adequacy of arterial perfusion, and generally they should be deferred until after successful arterial reconstruction.

Diabetic Neuropathic Ulcers

Diabetic neuropathic ulcers result from a combination of factors. Diabetic patients tend to develop polyneuropathy of the long neurons supplying the foot and lower extremity. Motor neuropathy leads to atrophy of the intrinsic muscles of the foot, leading to derangements in bony architecture that depends on intrinsic muscle tone for proper alignment. The resulting deformities include Charcot's foot, which is a collapse of the midfoot with plantar subluxation of the ruined bones, and clawing of the toes with plantar subluxation of the metatarsal heads (Figure 7-10). In both cases, the change in bony architecture leads to excessive weight bearing on surfaces at risk for pressure ulceration. In addition, diabetic polyneuropathy often causes sensory deficits, and a lack of proper protective reflexes contributes to promoting the chronic wound. Elevated glucose in poorly controlled diabetes independently retards wound healing and inhibits the leukocyte response to infection; often, all measures to promote healing will fail without tight control of glucose. Arterial disease is frequently present in diabetics. Approximately 40% of diabetic neuropathic ulcers have an element of contributing arterial ischemia, which adds to the difficulty of treating these wounds. Typically, diabetic neuropathic ulcers are found at a site of increased weight bearing, such as

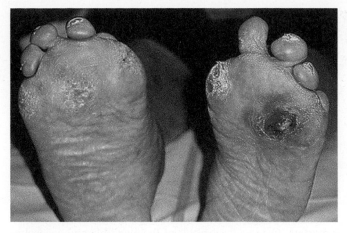

FIGURE 7-10. Charcot's foot.

a subluxed plantar surface of a metatarsal head, the heel, or on the dorsal surface of a toe that is rubbing against a shoe. Wounds typically have a fibrotic granulated bed surrounded by hypertrophic skin (callus), which identifies the exposure to excess pressure. Proper care for the diabetic wound starts with an appreciation of the burden imposed by the nonhealing wound. For each year a diabetic wound remains open, a 25% risk of limb loss is present. As a consequence, aggressive and timely intervention is mandated.

Management starts with control of infection. Wounds that penetrate into bone or joint usually require surgical débridement followed by secondary healing or, when possible, primary closure after limited amputation. Specialized shoe gear to alleviate pressure is generally indicated. The most effective means to reduce pressure on a foot wound is a wheelchair, which will remove all pressure on the foot until the wound is healed. Another option, which is often successful, is to immobilize the foot in a cast to redistribute pressure and eliminate shear. Many different types of specialized shoes with cushioned soles and pressure relief features are available, and custom-made shoes with deep toe boxes and accommodative insoles are appropriate for management of the healed foot. Minor surgical procedures to treat bony deformity such as extensor tendon tenotomy to correct clawing or Achilles tendon lengthening to correct equinus deformity may be very helpful interventions and should be considered when local care measures are not successful. Arterial surgery may be required when ischemia is a prominent factor. Local wound care to keep the granulating wound clean and free of infection can be supplemented with topical medication in lieu of moist gauze. Frequent débridement of the wound and regular shaving of surrounding calluses are important steps, as well as aggressive treatment of nail diseases.

Advanced Care for Chronic Wounds

Management of chronic wounds requires a significant investment of resources, and many novel and technically sophisticated methods for stimulating healing of wounds have been devised in recent decades. Compared to medical interventions for other diseases, wound care therapy has not been as rigorously subjected to randomized prospective trials, and there is not much clear evidence that any one of these modalities has better efficacy compared to conventional care or other advanced modalities. Nonetheless, all of these newer treatments have developed proponents and seem to have a place in the management of chronic wounds. These newer modalities include the following:

1. Intermittent negative pressure devices
2. Topical foams and occlusive bandages to promote a moist wound environment
3. Topical application of growth factors and collagen preparations to promote healing
4. Topical use of broad-spectrum antimicrobial compounds to decrease the bacterial burden of the wound
5. Topical enzyme preparations
6. Use of engineered living skin substitutes
7. Hyperbaric oxygen therapy

Negative pressure applied to the wound (as described earlier) is a method of wound healing that promotes new tissue growth, removes edema fluid, reduces TMMPs, and assists in contraction of the wound. These devices are used in wounds that are not infected and have undergone adequate débridement. It is contraindicated in wounds that have cancer growth, untreated osteomyelitis, active bleeding, or necrotic tissue.

Topical foams and occlusive bandages are devices that, when placed over an open wound, prevent loss of moisture and desiccation. The typical moist-to-dry gauze dressing change regimen that is normally adequate for acute wounds may be suboptimal for chronic wounds. With gauze-packing methods, the wound tends to become overly dry, leading to damage to the wound tissue. With topical occlusive covers, however, desiccation is prevented, and the resident proteolysis enzymes (TMMPs) can better promote autolytic débridement. Foams typically are porous and allow absorption of exudates from a wound, but do not have an adhesive backing. Other devices are impermeable or permeable membranes made of polyurethane or other synthetic polymers that allow variable flux of water vapor. Occlusive dressings that allow sufficient flux of water to prevent excessive fluid in the wound often are optimal. One risk with occlusive dressing methods is that without regular changes, bacterial overgrowth may be promoted.

Growth factor therapy with topically applied PDGF can stimulate chronic wounds to heal. It seems to be particularly useful in diabetic ulcers, where prospective, randomized, multicenter clinical trials showed complete wound healing to be almost twice as likely to occur with PDGF therapy compared to wounds treated otherwise. Venous ulcers appear to respond well to PDGF therapy. A new growth factor, keratinocyte growth factor II (KGFII), is in clinical trials with promising early results. KGFII has the unique ability to stimulate keratinocyte migration. Topical application of devitalized tissue (thin sheets of animal skin or intestinal submucosa) and purified collagen preparations are widely used to promote healing. These biologics may work to counteract excessive TMMP activity in the wound. Some evidence indicates that TMMPs are bound and inactivated by topical collagens. An alternative hypothesis for how collagen and tissue products stimulate healing is that they mimic the architecture found in healing acute wounds, and thus stimulate chronic wound cells by providing growth factors or other cues that promote normal wound healing.

Topical broad-spectrum antimicrobial preparations include 1% silver nitrate solution, which has been used for over a century to inhibit bacterial growth in burns and other chronic wounds. Other silver preparations such as Silvadene cream and films that slowly release silver into wounds are widely used. Topical iodine solutions have good antimicrobial activity, but are too cytotoxic for recurrent use. A better preparation is cadexomer iodine, a formulation of starch granules with elemental iodine, which both absorbs exudate from the wound and promotes a sterile environment. This is one of the few topical antimicrobials supported by randomized clinical trials. Specific topical antibiotics such as gentamicin and metronidazole ointment also can be useful in promoting wound healing, especially when wound cultures indicate that sensitive organisms are present. Dilute acetic acid (e.g., 0.25%) suppresses pseudomonas colonization and infection and is widely used in lieu of saline to moisten gauze when wet-to-dry gauze-packing regimens are employed.

Debriding wounds of necrotic tissue or fibrinous exudates is an important adjunct to wound management. An alternative to sharp surgical débridement is the use of ointments containing degradative enzymes such as collagenase or papain. These products can significantly expedite healing. Cross-hatching the crust or necrotic tissue covering the wound with a scalpel prior to starting topical enzyme therapy increases the efficacy. One product, a combination of papain with copper and chlorophyll (Panafil), appears to be a particularly useful adjunct for many chronic wounds, but to date, supporting randomized clinical trial data are absent.

Recent advances in tissue engineering have led to the commercial production of synthetic living skin substitutes. These are bilayers of fetal fibroblasts growing over collagen layers mimicking the dermal layer of skin. These products are increasingly employed to promote healing of burns and chronic wounds. They appear to have some ability to promote healing by providing keratinocytes to cover the wound and possibly through the elaboration of growth factors.

Hyperbaric oxygen therapy is another of the newer modalities used to stimulate wound healing. Treatment entails placing a patient in a chamber of pure oxygen at three atmospheres of pressure, with daily exposures of up to 8 weeks. Exposure to high-pressure oxygen increases tissue oxygen levels, which seems to promote healing in some refractory wounds, although other effects of high oxygen levels may be important. Osteoradionecrosis of the mandible and anaerobic soft tissue infections are particularly sensitive to hyperbaric therapy, but randomized clinical trials have shown disappointing efficacy with this therapy for chronic diabetic and arterial ulcers.

thePoint ✳ Go to http://thePoint.lww.com/activate and use your scratch-off code on the inside cover of this book to access bonus chapters, question bank, videos, and more.

SAMPLE QUESTIONS

Questions

Choose the best answer for each question.

1. A 42-year-old woman is seen in clinic 2 weeks after undergoing left partial mastectomy and sentinel lymph node biopsy for stage 1 breast cancer. Whole breast radiation is recommended. She is concerned about the effects of radiation on her incision. Which of the following statements is least accurate regarding radiation effects and wound healing?

   A. Rapidly dividing cells are the least affected by radiation therapy.

   B. Radiation effects on fibroblasts should be negligible.

   C. Radiation causes increased amounts of collagen deposition.

   D. Long-term effects of radiation are often reversible after 24 months.

   E. Wound healing is impaired postradiation secondary to venous injury.

2. A 28-year-old ultimate fighter is seen in clinic 2 weeks after undergoing splenectomy for a ruptured spleen sustained during a prize fight. He is feeling well with minimal incisional pain. There is a midline laparotomy incision that appears to be healing well without evidence of infection or other problems. He wants to know when his incision will be healed enough for him to return to professional fighting. Regarding the tensile strength of his wound,

   A. it will increase steadily over the first 6 weeks and achieve maximal strength by 12 weeks.

   B. it will achieve maximal tensile strength at the point of maximal collagen deposition.

   C. it will take a full year for the wound to regain the same tensile strength as preoperatively.

   D. wound tensile strength reaches 90% at 26 weeks and this is its plateau.

   E. collagen deposition reaches a maximum level in the first 6 weeks and is quickly degraded thereafter.

3. A 52-year-old man is in the operating room undergoing an emergent laparotomy because of a perforated ulcer. There is free intraperitoneal perforation and approximately 2 L of murky green fluid with obvious vegetable matter is suctioned from the peritoneal cavity. A Graham patch is performed to close the perforation. The abdomen is irrigated with normal saline and suctioned until all return is clear of green fluid and vegetable matter. After closing the fascia the next most appropriate step would be

   A. interrupted skin closure.

   B. closure of skin with a skin closure polymer (i.e., Dermabond).

   C. wound left open and wound care until clean and granulating and then delayed closure.

   D. closure of skin with staples.

   E. subcuticular suture skin closure.

4. A 55-year-old man is seen in clinic prior to undergoing elective repair of a large umbilical hernia. He is otherwise healthy and has had no previous surgery. He takes no medications. He does not smoke and does not drink alcohol. Except for a large reducible umbilical hernia, his physical exam is normal. Which micronutrient supplementation would not be beneficial to this patient to improve wound healing?

   A. Vitamin C

   B. Vitamin E

   C. Vitamin K

   D. Vitamin A

   E. Zinc

5. A 25-year-old man is in the hospital recovering from open surgery for perforated appendicitis performed 5 days ago. Postoperatively his wound was left open with daily debridement and local dressing changes. Today, local anesthesia is applied and the wound is closed with a nylon suture at the bedside. This represents an example of

   A. primary closure.

   B. composite graft closure.

   C. delayed primary closure.

   D. healing by secondary intent.

   E. local flap closure.

Answers and Explanations

1. Answer: D

The effects of external beam radiation often cause local tissue damage and impaired wound healing. Given the sensitivity of radiation to the various phases of the cell cycle, rapidly dividing cells are the most sensitive to radiation. Two major manifestations of impaired wound healing secondary to radiation are the result of direct injury to fibroblasts, leading to a lack of collagen, and endothelial cell injury resulting in inefficient wound healing. The effects of radiation are permanent and irreversible cell damage, as manifested by progressive fibrosis and obliterate endarteritis.

2. Answer: D

Collagen secretion is initiated by fibroblasts in the first 24 to 72 hours after injury. Peak collagen production begins by 1 week postinjury. By 3 weeks after injury, collagen synthesis and collagen deposition/degradation achieve a steady state. After 3 weeks, wound tensile strength remains <30%. As the maturation process takes place, tensile strength increases consistently until it plateaus approximately 6 months (26 weeks) after injury. This strength is generally around 90% of original tensile strength, and preinjury tensile strength will never be reached.

3. Answer: C

This is a contaminated surgical field. Wound infection in this setting can be as high as 15% of wounds, regardless of irrigating until clear. Allowing the wound to stay open with wound care until robust granulation is occurring and the wound bed is clean reduces this risk once the delayed closure is done. If the wound granulates but continues to have a high bacterial load, it can be allowed to heal by secondary intention.

4. Answer: C

Vitamins integral for wound healing are vitamin C and vitamin A. Vitamin C is required for the conversion of proline and lysine to hydroxyproline and hydroxylysine. Vitamin C deficiency or scurvy leads primarily to the failure of collagen synthesis. Vitamin E is an antioxidant, aids in immune function and fibroblast stimulation, and inhibits prostaglandin synthesis. Selenium is important for lymphocyte function and protects membranes from free radical damage. Zinc is possibly the most essential element for wound healing. Zinc deficiency leads to decreased fibroblast proliferation, decreased collagen synthesis, and likely decreased lymphocyte, cellular, and immunity. While vitamin A deficiency impairs wound healing, supplemental vitamin A benefits wound healing. Vitamin A enhances immune function, macrophage proliferation, collagen synthesis, and epithelial integrity. Supplemental vitamin A therapy can improve wound healing in patients receiving corticosteroids, cancer patients, diabetics, and patients undergoing chemotherapy. Vitamin K is involved in coagulation factor formation.

5. Answer: C

Surgical wounds can heal in several ways. An incised wound that is clean and suture closed is said to heal by primary intention. Primarily closed wounds are of a smaller volume in a clean surgical field. Often, because of bacterial common contamination or tissue loss, a wound will be left open to heal by granulation tissue formation. This is healing by secondary intent, and the wound must synthesize granulation tissue, contract at the wound periphery, and eventually cover the surface area with epithelial cells. Delayed primary closure represents a combination of the first two, consisting of the placement of sutures, allowing the wound to stay open for a few days, and then subsequent closure of the sutures. Delayed primary closure requires that the wound be free of excess bacteria. This is generally accomplished by good local wound care with irrigation and debridement if necessary during a postoperative interval. Wounds heal faster following delayed primary closure than by secondary intent.

8

Surgical Infections

R. NEAL GARRISON, M.D. • GLEN A. FRANKLIN, M.D. •
OSCAR GUILLAMONDEGUI, M.D., M.P.H. • LEWIS J. KAPLAN, M.D. • DAVID A. SPAIN, M.D.

Objectives

1. Define surgical infection and the pathogenesis that leads to wound infection following surgery.

2. Discuss the risk factors that may lead to infection following a surgical procedure.

3. Review the four classifications of surgical wounds and the frequency of infection associated with each class.

4. Describe the principles of prophylactic antibiotics and appropriate drug selection.

5. Review antibiotic resistance and its consequences on surgical infection.

6. Discuss the common causes of postoperative fever and the diagnostic steps for evaluation.

7. Define the different types of soft tissue infection.

8. Review common sites of surgical infection and the treatment options associated with each.

9. List the viral occupational hazards for surgeons and review personal protective strategies.

10. Describe surgical quality improvement measures and their impact on surgical infections.

11. Review case presentations of typical surgical infections including presentation, diagnosis, and treatment.

The term *surgical infection* encompasses a wide variety of disease states and pathogens. Frequently, this term is used to refer to those infections that occur postoperatively and that are associated with the surgical site. Commonly, this category of infection is specifically related to the wound itself and ranges from a simple cellulitis to deep wound infection with abscess. With the increasing emergence of virulent pathogens and resistant organisms, the term surgical infection is also being applied to a host of diseases that require urgent surgical evaluation and treatment. Many of these infections are community acquired requiring simple incision and drainage; however, more complex and invasive infections prompt exploration, operative drainage, and radical debridement. Many adjuncts to the surgical treatment of these infections are frequently utilized including antibiotics, repetitive irrigation, local debridement and wound care with dressing changes, and topical antimicrobial therapy.

Treatment options for the surgeon are wide and varied requiring an understanding of the etiology of the invading organism, the physiologic response of the host, and the pathophysiology of the infection. The proliferation of antibiotic use and the availability of many "big gun" broad-spectrum antibiotics have allowed the emergence of many virulent bacteria, fungi, and viruses that are resistant to standard treatment strategies. Likewise, the population is aging and contains many more persons at risk for severe infections particularly with the advent of the immunosuppression required for transplantation

and the immunosuppressive effects caused by cancer treatment with steroids and chemotherapy. In addition, trauma and injury can cause a selective immunosuppressive state creating an additional segment of the population at risk. The prevalence of these risk factors has increased over the past two decades and provided the surgeon with many new challenges and opportunities for intervention in the area of surgical infection. This chapter reviews the basic principles associated with surgical infections including the risks, sources, diagnosis, and treatment for many commonly seen diseases.

PATHOGENESIS OF INFECTION

Scheduled operative procedures, traumatic injury, and nontraumatic invasion of local tissue by bacteria can all lead to severe infections that may require surgical intervention. Following bacterial soilage of host tissues, the body initiates a well-defined process of host defense. The inflammatory response includes multiple mediators (e.g., cytokines, chemokines, kinins, histamine) released from mast cells and granulocytes that alter the local tissue response and increase capillary permeability. **Complement**, fibrinogen, and **opsonins** are concentrated in the region of bacterial invasion. Circulating neutrophils undergo diapedesis, marginating via the area of increased capillary permeability into the interstitium. Chemoattractants at the site of injury from local macrophages, platelets, and endothelial cells provide a chemical gradient for neutrophils to follow. Once the neutrophils come in contact with the bacteria, opsonins bind the foreign particle and facilitate the process of phagocytosis. The engulfed organism or foreign particle is then surrounded within the phagosome, and intracellular killing and digestion are initiated by the release of lysosomal enzymes, hydrolases, and superoxide compounds within the neutrophil. Dead phagocytic cells, fibrin, opsonic proteins, both viable and nonviable microorganisms, and bacterial products are the components of "**pus**." The microenvironment of an abscess or purulent collection is relatively hypoxic and acidotic. Thus, most cellular and enzymatic functions are inhibited. These areas are often difficult to penetrate with antibiotics and deep seeded collections frequently require operative drainage in addition to antibiotic therapy. The density and virulence of the bacterial contamination versus the efficacy and effectiveness of the host immune response determines the level and severity of infection. This relationship is represented by the schematic equation:

$$\frac{\text{Dose of bacterial contamination} \times \text{virulence}}{\text{Resistance of host}} = \text{Risk of infection}$$

There are several host factors that will affect bacterial virulence and the cellular host response, which may alter the pathogenesis of the infectious disease (Table 8-1). Retained wound hematomas provide an iron-rich environment that will potentiate bacterial growth while the hemoglobin content will inhibit the effectiveness of the neutrophil response in eradicating the microorganisms. Blood is an excellent bacterial growth agar and meticulous care must be given prior to wound closure in obtaining hemostasis. Likewise, dead tissue provides a means of bacterial growth not well penetrated by host defenses. Careful wound debridement and irrigation of all nonviable tissue is necessary for adequate healing. Foreign bodies, such as suture, drains, urinary catheters, and intravenous catheters, provide potential portals of bacterial entry and must be evaluated for their risk of infection versus benefit and necessity for patient care.

Systemic factors (e.g., shock, hypovolemia, hypoxia, comorbid disease) will also affect the host response to infection. Shock leads to tissue hypoperfusion and a metabolic acidosis that weakens host defenses mechanisms. Hypoperfusion of end-organ tissue and subsequent cellular dysfunction increases septic complications in patients who have traumatic injury or who are postoperative from elective surgery. Oxygenation is an essential metabolic component for phagocytosis and intracellular killing. Inadequate oxygen delivery (related to both hypoperfusion and inadequate oxygenation) results in acidosis at the site of bacterial contamination and will significantly increase the likelihood of subsequent infection. Patient comorbid diseases must also be considered when assessing infection risk. Diabetics have impaired neutrophil function and microcirculatory disease, while obese patients frequently have poor tissue perfusion secondary to the poor blood supply in adipose tissue. Malnutrition will increase the vulnerability of the host to infection and alcoholism impairs the host immune response. The use of systemic corticosteroids is common in many disease states. Steroid use, cancer chemotherapy, and transplant immunosuppression will all greatly increase the host risk for postoperative or surgical infection. A chronic disease that alters immune system function like acquired immunodeficiency syndrome (AIDS) also poses great infectious risk following injury or surgery.

In addition to neutrophil migration into the site of injury, the systemic inflammatory response includes multiple mediators. Tissue macrophages are stimulated to produce cytokines that have profound regulatory effects on other cellular and humoral cascades. One of the best known and characterized is tumor necrosis factor alpha (TNF-α). This factor, released primarily by macrophages, is responsible for producing a hypermetabolic state and initiating the inflammatory cascade, including stimulating the release of other proinflammatory cytokines, chemokines, and adhesion molecules. There are several well-known proinflammatory cytokines and many anti-inflammatory cytokines comprising a complex regulatory system within the host response (Table 8-2).

TABLE 8-1	Risk Factors That Increase the Incidence of Surgical Infection
Local Wound	
Wound hematoma	
Necrotic tissue	
Foreign body	
Obesity	
Contamination	
Systemic	
Advanced age	
Shock (hypoxia, acidosis)	
Diabetes mellitus	
Protein–calorie malnutrition	
Acute and chronic alcoholism	
Corticosteroid therapy	
Cancer chemotherapy	
Immunosuppression (acquired and induced)	
Remote site infection	

TABLE 8-2	Pro- and Anti-Inflammatory Cytokines
Proinflammatory Cytokines	**Basic Actions**
Interleukin 1 (IL-1)	Fever, sickness syndrome, upregulates acute phase proteins, acts synergistically with TNF-α
Interleukin 6 (IL-6)	Stimulates synthesis of acute phase proteins, B cell proliferation
Tumor necrosis factor (TNF-α)	Activates neutrophils, stimulates adhesion molecule formation, increases vascular endothelium permeability, acts synergistically with IL-1
Anti-inflammatory Cytokines	
Interleukin 4 (IL-4)	Suppresses IL-1 and TNF-α production, decreases IL-8 and adhesion molecule formation
Interleukin 10 (IL-10)	Inhibits IL-12 production, decreases proinflammatory cytokine synthesis
Interleukin 13 (IL-13)	Suppresses IL-1 and TNF-α production, decreases IL-8 and adhesion molecule formation

In summary, the interaction between the pathogen and host will determine whether contamination has no real sequelae or clinical infection occurs. Several local and systemic factors can shift the balance in favor of the bacterial invasion and determine whether or not the infection remains local or progresses to systemic. The biological response of the host will follow one of three pathways: (1) the host defenses overcome the bacterial invasion, (2) the bacteria overwhelm the host, or (3) the bacteria and host achieve a "standoff" (abscess formation) where both coexist for some time period. The primary goal of surgical therapy is to reduce the bacterial concentration (incision and drainage) and improve the local environment (debridement) to shift the balance away from bacterial invasion and reestablish the opportunity for the patient's defenses to eradicate the microorganisms.

Classification of Surgical Wounds

Surgical wounds are divided into four classifications based on the level of potential bacterial contamination (Table 8-3). This categorization system is commonly reported in documentation from the operating room and provides a fairly good risk stratification for postoperative wound infection (surgical site infection, SSI). The source of contamination from each type of wound determines the pathophysiology and often treatment options for the infection once it occurs. *Clean* wounds are the most common category and include most elective surgical procedures where the gastrointestinal (GI) tract or biliary ductal system is not violated. Most SSIs from these types of procedures are caused by gram-positive organisms frequently from the operating room environment or staff. The patient's skin is also a potential source of wound contamination. The rate of SSI should be very low in these types of procedures. *Clean–contaminated* wounds are secondary to elective opening of the GI tract or biliary system. The bacterial flora is endogenous to the patient and causes polymicrobial infections. *Contaminated* procedures include gross spillage of GI contents either prior to (perforated viscus) or during the course of the operation. The SSI rate is variable dependent on the level of spillage and virulence of the pathogen. These infections are also polymicrobial. Finally, *dirty* wounds are those with established infection prior to surgical intervention. The rates of infection are high, polymicrobial in nature, and often require multiple interventions to resolve. Typical strategies for prevention of SSI are targeted to the etiologies and sources of bacterial contamination inherent to this classification system.

Categories of Surgical Site Infection

SSIs can be divided into categories based on the level of tissue penetration. Treatment strategies can be varied, but usually involve opening of the wound with debridement and drainage. The extent of bacterial invasion into the surrounding soft tissue and/or systemic dissemination of the infection will determine the need for oral or intravenous antibiotics. Superficial and incisional SSIs involve the skin and subcutaneous tissues. These are the most common types of SSI. Clinically, they range from simple cellulitis of the wound to overt infection of the wound bed above the fascia. Treatment includes oral antibiotics (gram-positive coverage the most common) for cellulitis and reopening of the wound for those infections with incisional purulent drainage and involvement of the deeper tissues. Subcutaneous abscess formation may occur that will require incision and drainage. The true rate or incidence of this type of SSI is unknown since many are treated as outpatients and never reported to quality assurance databanks. Although more common in clean/contaminated and contaminated wounds, this type of SSI can occur in any setting a wound has been created.

Deep incisional SSIs extend into the muscle and fascia. These infections require opening of the wound and frequently surgical debridement of necrotic tissue. Wounds of the abdomen are at high risk for fascial necrosis and dehiscence. Careful observation of the wound is required and some of these wounds will require fascial debridement and reapproximation. Antibiotics are more frequently utilized than in the superficial SSI, along with continued daily local wound care. The more severe forms of these infections include necrotizing fasciitis (extension of the infection along fascial planes), systemic infection, and **sepsis**. Source control of the infection and radical debridement is necessary along with the use of intravenous broad-spectrum antibiotics.

Infections of the organ/intracavitary space following surgery are also categorized as SSI. These infections include secondary peritonitis, intra-abdominal abscess, and empyema. Often related to inadequate source control from the original bacterial contamination event, these infections require surgical intervention. Sometimes accessible by percutaneous drainage methods, the original incision does not always need to be explored. However, subfascial collections can manifest as wound drainage and be confused with deep incisional SSI as the abscess attempts to extrude itself from the deeper space between fascial sutures. In addition to drainage, deep space infections will also require intravenous antibiotics. Intra-abdominal infections can often be polymicrobial; thus broad-spectrum coverage should

TABLE 8-3	Classification of Surgical Wounds			
Wound	**Bacterial Contamination**	**Source of Contamination**	**Infection Frequency (%)**	**Examples**
Clean	Gram-positive	Operating room environment, surgical team, patient's skin	3	Inguinal hernia, thyroidectomy, mastectomy, aortic graft
Clean-contaminated	Polymicrobial	Endogenous colonization of the patient	5–15	Elective colon resection, gastric resection, gastrostomy tube, common bile duct exploration
Contaminated	Polymicrobial	Gross contamination	15–40	"Spill" during elective GI surgery, perforated ulcer
Dirty	Polymicrobial	Established infection	40–50	Drainage of intra-abdominal abscess, resection of infarcted bowel

be started with antibiotic de-escalation once final culture and sensitivity data become available. Anaerobic coverage should be considered based on the most likely source and indigenous bacterial contaminants (i.e., gastric, small intestine, colon, or pancreas). Intrathoracic infections are less frequently polymicrobial and antibiotic selection should be targeted at the most commonly occurring organisms for each patient's particular disease state. Patients with deep space infections can become quite ill very quickly with systemic extension of the infection and sepsis. Rapid diagnosis and treatment is necessary to prevent further morbidity and mortality from these infections. Computed tomography (CT) is a very helpful diagnostic tool when this type of infection is suspected clinically. Many isolated collections are amenable to percutaneous drainage techniques utilizing radiographic guidance with ultrasound and CT. Source control is paramount and ongoing contamination from infected implanted devices or anastomotic breakdown will still require operative intervention.

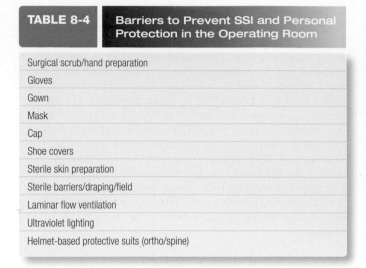

TABLE 8-4	Barriers to Prevent SSI and Personal Protection in the Operating Room
Surgical scrub/hand preparation	
Gloves	
Gown	
Mask	
Cap	
Shoe covers	
Sterile skin preparation	
Sterile barriers/draping/field	
Laminar flow ventilation	
Ultraviolet lighting	
Helmet-based protective suits (ortho/spine)	

PREVENTION OF SURGICAL INFECTIONS

Mechanical Preparation

The prevention of infection in patients undergoing elective surgical procedures or those who have been injured is paramount for quality patient care. There are numerous principles to the prevention of SSI that begin with adequate wound preparation. Most surgical infections are directly related to the patient's own endogenous flora, thus appropriate skin preparation is necessary. Body hair should be clipped not shaven to prevent skin irritation and breakdown creating a portal of bacterial entry into the wound bed. Hair removal should occur immediately before the planned procedure. Skin preparation includes the use of povidone–iodine solution or chlorhexidine-containing solutions to reduce the number of endogenous flora. Adhesive sterile plastic drapes are frequently used during vascular procedures to avoid contact of prosthetic grafts with the surrounding skin. The reduction of operative time and maintaining normothermia during the procedure has also been shown to significantly reduce the rate of SSI. Recent evidence suggests that perioperative glycemic control has positive effects as well.

Good surgical technique also plays a significant role in the reduction of postoperative infection. The complete removal of devitalized tissue and the meticulous removal of any foreign material are important in infection control. Likewise, adequate hemostasis and the lavage of any large blood clots from the wound will decrease SSI as blood is an excellent medium for bacterial growth. Finally, a reduction in wound physiologic dead space via the use of layered closures and closed suction drainage will assist in the prevention of wound infection. Ultimately, adequate tissue perfusion and oxygenation are key preventive measures. As previously discussed, the primary risk for SSI includes the classification of the surgical wound (i.e., clean versus clean contaminated vs. contaminated).

While most postoperative wound infections are related to the patient's endogenous flora, the operating room environment also contributes to the rate of infection. This environment includes the equipment, climate, ventilation, surgeon, and operating room personnel. The operating room attire and aseptic techniques utilized are designed to minimize this source of contamination. Table 8-4 lists common "barriers" to limit operating room environmental contamination of the surgical wound. Surgical scrubbing of the hands or use of antibacterial gels decreases the colony count of flora in the hands. Presumably, this will limit the inoculum of bacteria should barrier breakdown occur at any point during the procedure. Commonly used barriers include gloves, cap, gown, mask, and shoe covers. These not only protect the patient but also along with eyewear protect the surgeon and other personnel. Needle stick injuries place health care workers at risk for blood-borne pathogen infection including hepatitis B and C as well as human immunodeficiency virus (HIV). Hepatitis B carries the greatest risk of infection and seroconversion. It is estimated that as many as 800,000 needle sticks occur in health care workers each year in the United States. Preventive techniques include double gloving, no touch handling of sharps, needle and scalpel safety sheaths, and appropriate sharp disposal. Of course, the best preventive measure is awareness and careful handling of sharp instruments.

Perioperative Antibiotics

The use of perioperative **prophylactic antibiotics** relates to the magnitude of surgical intervention and the presumptive microbes to be encountered in the elective surgical setting. Adequate dosing of the antibiotic is paramount for effectiveness at the tissue level with the timing of the infusion to obtain maximal tissue and serum concentration at the point of incision and throughout the operative case considered. In general, antibiotics administered after the contaminating event are not effective in the prevention of surgical infections. The use of preoperative antibiotics has been shown to reduce the rate of SSIs by 33% to over 80%. This reduction in infections leads to decreased intensive care unit (ICU) and hospital length of stay, hospital costs, risk of readmission, and decreased mortality.

The ideal antibiotic allows maximal effect against the presumed contamination bacteria with minimal effect to the host/patient. Antibiotic effectiveness is based upon the minimum inhibitory concentration (MIC) or minimal bactericidal concentration (MBC) against bacteria. The MIC refers to the lowest concentration necessary to visibly inhibit growth under typical conditions. The MBC is the lowest concentration to eradicate 99.9% of the bacteria in a given time.

To insure adequate serum and tissue levels, initial antibiotics are given within 1 hour prior to the incision. Lengthy

TABLE 8-5 — Prophylactic Antibiotic Selection for Elective Surgery

Surgical Procedure	Approved Antibiotics
Cardiac or vascular	Cefazolin, cefuroxime or vancomycin
Hip/knee arthroplasty	Cefazolin, cefuroxime or vancomycin
Colon	Cefotetan, cefoxitin, ampicillin/sulbactam or ertapenem **OR** Cefazolin or cefuroxime + metronidazole *If β-lactam allergy:* Clindamycin + aminoglycoside or quinolone or aztreonam **OR** Metronidazole with aminoglycoside or Metronidazole + quinolone
Hysterectomy	cefotetan, cefazolin, cefoxitin, cefuroxime or Ampicillin/sulbactam *If β-lactam allergy:* Clindamycin + aminoglycoside or quinolone or aztreonam **OR** Metronidazole + aminoglycoside or Metronidazole + quinolone **OR** Clindamycin monotherapy
Special Considerations	For cardiac, orthopedic and vascular surgery, if the patient is allergic to β-lactam antibiotics, vancomycin or clindamycin are acceptable substitutes.

Current (2008) guidelines for prophylactic antibiotic selection established by The Surgical Care Improvement Program initiative of the Federal Center for Medicare and Medicaid Services.

procedures require redosing depending on the pharmacokinetics of the chosen agent. The chosen agent should be well tolerated and safe, have a long half-life and possess an antimicrobial spectrum appropriate for planned procedure. A compendium of accepted guidelines is outlined in Table 8-5. Cephalosporins with activity against the organisms likely to be encountered are typically the first line agents provided no allergy or contamination exists. The antibiotic coverage spectrum will occasionally require a second agent.

Perioperative antibiotic use requires an understanding about the type of case to be performed and the level of contamination perceived (see Table 8-3). Clean cases with little risk of contamination do not require antibiotic coverage. However, prophylaxis is utilized in clean cases where prosthetic material (i.e., mesh, vascular graft orthopedic device) is used as a means to reduce the likelihood of device infection. The risk of infection for clean cases should be <1%. For cases in which there is risk of minimal endogenous contamination, (clean contaminated) the source must be considered. Hollow viscus, such as gastric or biliary tree involvement, require the addition of gram-negative and anaerobic bacteria coverage, and the SSI risk rises by approximately threefold over clean cases. Contaminated cases involve gross spillage from bowel perforation and polymicrobial bacterial involvement. The overall risk of site infection for contaminated cases increases 5- to 10-fold over clean cases. Dirty wounds involve existing contaminated or established infection and are at the highest risk for infection to develop, reaching approximately 50% in most series. Antibiotics are considered therapeutic in these cases. Antibiotics are not a surrogate for surgical technique and attention to detail is important in the perioperative management of the patient.

Perioperative antibiotic therapy is continued in the postoperative setting only for <24 hours. For the majority of surgical cases, antibiotic infusion for more than 24 hours has been shown to increase bacterial resistance and have no further improvement on SSI rates. In certain surgical interventions, such as cardiac surgery, use may be extended to 48 hours. In colorectal surgery, extending the antibiotics for two doses postincision decreased incisional infections by up to 60%. When antibiotics are used to treat existing infection, the prophylactic agent is usually continued until specific cultures dictate a more specific agent. Should the prophylactic agent need to be extended for treatment of established infection, such as would occur with ruptured appendicitis as a clinical example, appropriate chart documentation should indicate the shift from prophylaxis to a treatment modality.

Adverse effects from prophylactic antibiotic therapy range from anaphylaxis, or severe drug reaction, to mild inflammatory allergic reactions such as a rash. The emergence of drug-resistant bacteria or development of a *Clostridium difficile* infection is unusual when the duration of use is confined to the perioperative time frame. The continued use of the antibiotic in question should be replaced with an alternate, effective medication or discontinued entirely should one of these adverse events occurs. The emergence of resistant organisms has been linked to inappropriate antibiotic utilization over time, particularly when broad-spectrum agents are continued without clear clinical evidence. Efforts to prevent development of bacterial resistance include the use of narrow-spectrum agents, high doses above the mean inhibitory concentration, and a short time course of use. In most surgical scenarios, antibiotics are an adjunct to operative therapy.

Recently, the Surgical Care Improvement Program (SCIP) was implemented as a national quality improvement initiative by the Federal Center for Medicare and Medicaid Services (CMS). The goal of this program was to utilize evidence-based standardized protocols to reduce the incidence of surgical complications 25%. The program focused on four key elements: surgical infection prevention, adverse cardiac events, prevention of thromboembolic events, and prevention of postoperative pneumonia. There are six key quality indicators related to the perioperative management of surgical patients that relate to surgical infections:

1. Prophylactic antibiotic delivery within 60 minutes prior to incision
2. Prophylactic antibiotics consistent with approved guidelines
3. Cessation of prophylaxis within 24 hours following surgery
4. Appropriate hair removal (clipping)
5. Glucose control for cardiac surgery
6. Normothermia for colorectal surgery

Data reporting and audits are hospital based and compliance is closely monitored.

ESTABLISHED INFECTION

Surgical infections can be grouped as community-acquired or hospital-acquired. Community-acquired infections are active inflammatory processes that were present before and, in many cases, are the reason the patient requires treatment.

Hospital-acquired infections occur as a consequence or during treatment and are termed *nosocomial*. All infections that occur after surgical procedures are considered nosocomial. Thus, peritonitis that occurs as the result of diverticulitis is usually a community-acquired infection, but an intraperitoneal abscess that results from a leak of a colonic anastomosis is classified as a postoperative hospital-acquired problem.

Several caveats should be considered in choosing a therapeutic antibiotic to treat established infection. Culture and antibiotic sensitivity should be obtained for all established infections and, if indicated, the antibiotic should be switched to a narrow-spectrum drug effective against the specific organisms identified (de-escalation therapy). However, because of the arbitrary testing environment of the laboratory, in vitro sensitivity does not always correlate with clinical effectiveness. Other factors that are considered when choosing an antibacterial therapeutic agent include tissue penetration, drug concentration, function of organs that either metabolize or excrete the drug, and the inherent toxicity of the agent. Because of the complexity and interaction of these variables, a clinical pharmacist is often asked to assist in choosing an appropriate therapeutic antibiotic. Regardless of the drug chosen, an ongoing daily assessment of the response of the patient to the therapy is an essential standard of care. If patient improvement is noted, that course of action should be continued but if there are little or no signs of effectiveness, both the drugs used and the site of infection being treated should be reconsidered.

Antibiotic resistance is a prominent concern in the treatment of surgical infection. Resistance means that a structural or metabolic change within the microorganism enables the bacteria to resist the antimicrobial actions of specific drugs. The development of resistance is usually mediated by either genetic material transfer via plasmid exchange from other organisms or spontaneous chromosomal mutation. Once resistance mutations for a given drug occur within the microbial population, the continued use of the antibiotic preferentially promotes the growth of the resistant organism by eliminating the sensitive microbial population. Clinical practice concerning the choice of drug and duration of therapy is of utmost importance in preventing or at least delaying the development of resistance. Systemic antibiotic therapy should be used only when there is evidence that systemic signs of infection exist. Most surgical infections require drainage and debridement as the initial therapeutic intervention and antibiotics are used as an adjunct to these mechanical treatments. With few exceptions, therapeutic antibiotics should not be used beyond 10 to 14 days because such use only encourages the emergence of resistant strains.

Nosocomial Infections

Sepsis is a leading cause of death in the ICU and it has been estimated that over 200,000 people die each year in the United States from sepsis. The mortality rate of severe sepsis associated with shock and trauma remains substantial at 25% to 50%. The treatment of nosocomial infection is largely supportive; control of the site of infection by drainage or debridement, initiate appropriate antibiotic treatment, and support failing organs.

Choosing the correct empiric antibiotic for the right indication can have a significant impact on the outcome of surgical infections. Selecting the right antibiotic is a function of knowing the medical comorbidities, the type of patient, the site of the infection being treated (pneumonia, intra-abdominal abscess, etc.), and the most likely causative organisms for that specific infection. Knowledge about the specific hospital unit's bacteria and resistance patterns encountered can be valuable in this regard.

The importance of antibiotic choice can be directly linked to outcome. For example, up to 30% of patients with catheter-related bloodstream infections have inadequate antimicrobial therapy. The mortality for these patients is more than twofold greater compared to patients with adequate antimicrobial coverage, 62% versus 28%, in large series. Very similar findings have been demonstrated for patients with ventilator-associated pneumonia (VAP). Essentially, the risk of mortality is increased by 30% to 50% if the wrong empiric antibiotic is selected or delays in starting the correct antibiotic occurs. Thus, early and appropriate diagnosis and treatment of infections should be a major priority in postoperative patients. Given the significant morbidity, mortality, and cost associated with postoperative infection, prevention whenever possible is the best treatment.

Postoperative Fever

Fever that occurs in the postoperative period can be an early indication of developing infection. The traditional six "Ws" listed in Table 8-6 provide a considered approach to help identify an etiology for the fever. Invariably, an early temperature elevation is due to lung atelectasis, which usually responds to an increase in deep breathing and cough or suction to clear secretions from the airway. Febrile responses that occur later in the postoperative course point to the surgical wound, urinary tract, intravenous catheter site phlebitis, or deep vein thrombophlebitis as potential sources. The development of deep infections or abscess is usually identified as a late occurrence. Drug fever is an unusual event that should only be considered when all other obvious causes of fever have been ruled out. A postoperative fever should stimulate a careful patient examination and chart review to identify an etiology. Antibiotic treatment should only be initiated when and if a specific infectious site and bacterial organism has been identified.

Surgical Site Infections

SSI occur in 2% of all operations and account for approximately 20% of all hospital-acquired infections leading to increased cost for treatment and an average increase in hospital length of stay by 3 to 7 days. Given the morbidity and cost associated with these infections, prevention is key as discussed in the perioperative antibiotic section of this chapter. The diagnosis of wound infection is made in the majority of cases by local examination. Erythema and purulent drainage herald an underlying infection. Local infections usually respond to simple drainage and frequent dressing changes.

TABLE 8-6	The "W's" of Postoperative Fever	
Site/Source	**Postoperative Timing (days)**	
Wind	1–2	
Water	2–3	
Wound	3–5	
Walking	5–7	
"**W**" abscess	7–10	
Wonder drugs	Anytime provided other etiologies have been ruled out	

Fascial involvement may require formal operative debridement. In all cases, bacterial cultures should be collected and antibiotics adjusted accordingly.

Hospital- and Ventilator-Associated Pneumonia

Hospital-associated pneumonia (HAP) and (VAP) occur in up to 5% of surgical patients. VAP is a serious infection occurring in surgical patients. The incidence is approximately 5% to 10% but may occur in up to 40% of seriously injured trauma or surgical patients who require prolonged mechanical ventilation as a result of the injury or from preexisting pulmonary disease. The mortality rate of VAP can be as high as 15% to 20%. Attempts at prevention have led to the development of a group of interventions that when enacted together seems to have a great impact when compared to any individual effort. There are four major components in this group: (1) elevation of the head of the bed to 30°, (2) daily sedation vacation and assessment for weaning, (3) stress ulcer prophylaxis, and (4) venous thromboembolism prevention. Adherence to these recommendations has demonstrated a significant reduction in the length of time patients require ventilator assistance, which leads to a reduction in VAP rates.

The diagnosis of VAP in surgical patients may be difficult. A clinical diagnosis based on criteria such as fever, leukocytosis, sputum Gram stain, and chest radiograph findings may only confirm the diagnosis of VAP in 60% of patients. Thus, early attempts at obtaining deep bronchial specimens and accurate cultures are needed. A quantitative bronchial aspirate of $>10^5$ organisms/mL of aspirate is diagnostic of invasive infection. Once diagnosed with VAP, the presumptive empiric antibiotic(s) must be chosen. This will largely be based on the patient's risk of having resistant organisms. In general, patients in the hospital for <7 days are at low risk and antibiotic selection should be driven by local and hospital unit experience. Patients who are immunocompromised or have been in the hospital for 10 days or greater are at high risk for infections with resistant organisms. In this setting, empiric antibiotic coverage should include methicillin-resistant *Staphylococcus aureus* (MRSA) and resistant gram-negative rods. Once the causative organism is identified by culture, empiric antibiotics should then be tailored to the narrowest possible spectrum to cover the organism(s). Frequent airway suction is an integral part of VAP therapy. Specific antibiotic treatment for 8 days is sufficient for most patients, but a lack of clear clinical signs of treatment success, such as improvement in ventilation parameters or pulmonary infiltrate, require repeat culture and antibiotic adjustment.

Urinary Tract Infections

Urinary tract infections (UTIs) are often diagnosed in surgical patients but rarely are the cause of significant physiologic consequences. However, the occurrence of UTIs does add costs to hospital care. The greatest risk factor for developing a UTI is the presence of an indwelling bladder catheter. Prevention requires aseptic placement, maintenance of the closed drainage system, and daily urethral hygiene. There has been considerable push to remove urinary catheters early in the patient's postoperative course given that there is little data to support their ongoing use in most patients. In the absence of systemic signs of infection, UTI will usually respond to a urinary antiseptic and catheter removal if possible. Urine colonization that is associated with a chronic indwelling catheter does not ordinarily require treatment. The diagnosis of postoperative UTI is considered with a quantitative bacterial culture of more than 100,000 organisms/mL urine. In surgical patients where the urinary tract has been instrumented, colony counts at or above those numbers are seen; however, in the absence of a functional or anatomic obstruction to urine flow, a postoperative fever should not be attributed to the urinary tract even with positive cultures. Surveillance for other sources of fever should be undertaken in these clinical scenarios. *Pseudomonas*, *Serratia*, and other antibiotic-resistant gram-negative organisms are the usual pathogens cultured and antibiotic therapy requires specific culture and sensitivity data. Systemic treatment is usually deferred in the absence of positive blood cultures.

Empyema

Pleural effusions are common in complicated surgical patients. Most often these are due to volume overload, sympathetic effusions (e.g., postsplenectomy) or a parapneumonic effusion. When a postoperative patient with signs of infection (fever, leukocytosis, etc.) develops a pleural effusion, the composition of the fluid should be determined by thoracentesis. A transudative effusion is due to increased hydrostatic forces and has low protein content, whereas an exudative effusion is due to increased permeability and has high protein content. Determining the fluid lactate dehydrogenase (LDH), glucose, pH, cell count, and Gram stain can help differentiate an exudate. Exudative effusions due to inflammation have a pH < 7.2, a glucose < 60 mg/dL and/or a LDH > 3× serum levels. They may be Gram stain or culture positive, although in up to one-third of patients with empyema, organisms are not identified in the fluid. In symptomatic patients or large volume effusions (>50% of hemithorax) associated with the characteristics of an exudate on thoracentesis sampling, adequate drainage of the pleural space must be accomplished. In some circumstances, repeat therapeutic thoracentesis may be sufficient, but, surgical drainage is usually required either with video-assisted thoracic surgery or for more advanced cases, thoracotomy and decortication. The diagnosis can usually be confirmed by CT scan and identification of a loculated rim-enhancing pleural collection (Figure 8-1). Antibiotics should be chosen based on the most pertinent pleural fluid and/or tracheal cultures.

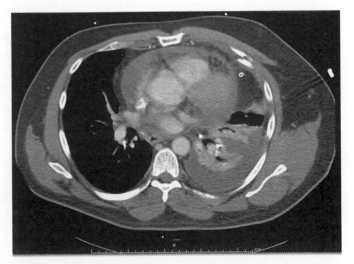

FIGURE 8-1. CT scan of chest demonstrating left pleural collection with compressed atelectatic lung consistent with empyema.

Intra-Abdominal Infections

The most common cause of intra-abdominal infections in surgical patients is perforation or leakage from a hollow viscus that leads to bacterial seeding of the peritoneal cavity. There are two responses to this: either abscess formation or generalized peritonitis. Peritonitis is further classified as primary, secondary, or tertiary. An example of primary peritonitis is spontaneous bacterial peritonitis that occurs without a breach of GI tract or peritoneal cavity (uncommon in surgical patients), is usually monomicrobial, and seen in chronic alcoholics. Secondary peritonitis is polymicrobial and occurs as a result of spillage of gut organisms from the GI tract or contamination from indwelling catheters (peritoneal catheters). Tertiary peritonitis occurs in critically ill patients and persists or recurs at least 48 hours after apparent adequate management, is polymicrobial, and reflects a failure of host defense rather than source control.

The change in the bowel lumen environment from aerobic proximal to anaerobic in the colon influences the bacterial population and thus likely causative organisms for intra-abdominal abscess or secondary peritonitis depend on the location within the GI tract leading to contamination. Infections derived from the proximal GI tract (stomach, duodenum, biliary, and proximal small bowel) contain gram-positive and gram-negative aerobic and facultative bacteria that are capable of growth under either aerobic or anaerobic conditions. Infections from the distal small bowel will be due to gram-negative aerobic and facultative bacteria. Colonic contamination produces infections with facultative and obligate anaerobic bacteria. Tertiary peritonitis generally represents a failure of treatment and therefore antibiotic resistant or unusual organisms such as MRSA, *Pseudomonas*, *Candida*, and *Enterococci* are common.

Postoperative intra-abdominal infections may be very difficult to diagnose. Physical findings may be masked by decreased consciousness or difficult to detect due to postoperative pain. The diagnosis should be considered in any patient with recent abdominal surgery or at risk for reduced splanchnic blood flow (vasopressors or prolonged shock) who demonstrates any signs of sepsis or organ dysfunction (respiratory distress, supraventricular tachycardia, renal or liver dysfunction). Broad-spectrum antibiotics should be started ASAP for any postoperative patient that demonstrates signs of systemic sepsis. Blood cultures should be obtained in any patient with signs of systemic sepsis, but the primary diagnostic test is CT with PO) and IV contrast. Usually the CT scan will suggest what type of source control is needed. Percutaneous drainage guided by ultrasound or CT is the initial intervention of choice for localized accessible abscesses. Operative source control is needed when there is (1) generalized peritonitis, (2) a source of ongoing contamination such as bowel perforation or an anastomotic leak or fistula, (3) devitalized tissue requiring debridement, or (4) failure of percutaneous drainage. In all cases of peritonitis, primary source control is an imperative step in the treatment plan. Systemic antibiotics alone will seldom be adequate therapy.

Community-Acquired Infections

Skin and Soft Tissue Infections and Tetanus Immunization

Common soft tissue infections are outlined in Table 8-7. Soft tissue infection, due to a break in the skin barrier, initially presents with spreading cellulitis. The blanching erythema of cellulitis is caused by group A *Streptococci*, which respond to penicillin therapy. Staphylococci with gross suppuration (pus) may also be the cause of cellulitis. Suppurative lesions require local incision and drainage in addition to antibiotic therapy. Increasingly, community-acquired methicillin-resistant *Staphylococcus aureus* (cMRSA) is the offending organism that has been associated with overuse of antimicrobials in the community setting.

Soft tissue infections characterized by pathogen invasion, tissue ischemia, and systemic signs of sepsis are collectively termed necrotizing soft tissue infections (NSTIs). Four types of NSTI include necrotizing cellulitis, fasciitis, myositis, and vasculitis. All are surgical emergencies requiring aggressive fluid resuscitation, broad-spectrum antimicrobial prescription and wide surgical debridement of the necrotic tissue. The most

| TABLE 8-7 | Common Soft Tissue Infections |

Infection	Etiology	Typical Organism(s)	Physical Findings	Treatment
Cellulitis	Break in skin barrier	*Streptococcus*	Warm to touch, diffuse erythema, tenderness	Systemic antibiotics and local wound care
Furuncle, carbuncle	Bacterial growth within skin glands and crypts	*Staphylococcus*	Localized induration, erythema, tenderness, swelling with purulent drainage	Incision and drainage, systemic antibiotics
Hidradenitis suppurativa	Bacterial growth within apocrine sweat glands	*Staphylococcus*	Multiple small localized subcutaneous abscesses, drainage, commonly from axilla and groin	Incision and drainage of small lesions, systemic antibiotics, large areas will require wide local excision and skin grafting
Lymphangitis	Infection within lymphatics	*Streptococcus*	Diffuse swelling and erythema of distal extremity with areas of inflamed streaks along lymphatic channels	Local wound care, systemic antibiotics, removal of any foreign body, elevation of extremity
Gangrene, NSTIs	Destruction of healthy tissue by virulent microbial enzymes	Synergistic: *Streptococcus/ Staphylococcus* Mixed aerobic/ anaerobic *Clostridium*	Necrotic skin/fascia, swelling and induration, foul smelling discharge, crepitus with subcutaneous emphysema, frequently with toxic systemic signs and symptoms of sepsis	Radical debridement/amputation of involved tissues, aggressive local wound care with frequent debridement as necessary, parenteral broad-spectrum antibiotics

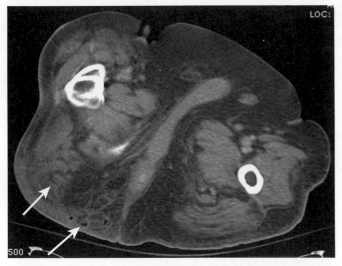

FIGURE 8-2. CT scan of pelvis demonstrating gas and fluid along fascial planes in the perineum consistent with the diagnosis of Fourier's gangrene.

characteristic finding is pain out of proportion to physical examination. Cellulitis occurs early, and bullae, skin discoloration, and crepitus develop later. The diagnosis is based on clinical exam, which is supported by laboratory (leukocytosis and hyponatremia) and CT scan findings of asymmetric tissue inflammation, fluid along fascial planes, and occult foci of gas. Fournier's gangrene is an eponym that specifically applies to NSTI of the genitalia and perineum (Figure 8-2). The vast majority of these infections are polymicrobial, but approximately 20% are monomicrobial.

Two monomicrobial NSTI deserve specific attention: Group-A *Streptococcal* infection and *Clostridial* myonecrosis. Necrotizing streptococcal gangrene rarely occurs in surgical patients. These infections are characterized by non-blanching erythema, with blisters and frank necrosis of the skin. Nonblanching erythema indicates subdermal thrombosis of the nutrient blood supply of the skin. Extensive surgical debridement of the affected area, in combination with of Wound high-dose penicillin and clindamycin, is an appropriate treatment. A Gram stain of blister fluid or tissue obtained during the debridement is useful in differentiating this infection from other necrotizing infections of the skin and skin structures.

Clostridial myonecrosis or *Clostridial* cellulitis are fulminant life-threatening infections characterized by tissue necrosis and rapidly advancing crepitus (i.e., gas gangrene). Either may occur as early as 1 day postoperatively or after tissue injury, most commonly from puncture wounds, and carries a high mortality rate. Therapy is as for other NSTI but must incorporate high-dose penicillin (esp. for *Clostridium perfringens*) as for GAS infection; clindamycin is a reasonable alternative in patients with penicillin allergy as is tigecycline, a glycylcycline related to tetracycline. Hyperbaric oxygen therapy to vastly increase local O_2 concentration, directly kill bacteria, and support WBC oxidative burst has also been successfully utilized as an adjunct for NSTI in general, and *Clostridial* myonecrosis and GAS in particular, but is not a substitute for aggressive surgical debridement. Tetanus toxoid immunization, along with adequate surgical debridement without primary wound closure, prevents *Clostridial* myonecrosis or cellulitis in most patients who are at risk. Tetanus

antitoxin is administered to patients with high-risk wounds who have an uncertain history of immunization.

Tetanus

Tetanus (lockjaw) is caused by the exotoxin produced by *Clostridium tetani*. After an incubation period of 2 days to several weeks, a prodromal symptom complex of restlessness, headache, masseter muscle stiffness, and muscular contractions in the area of the wound evolves. Violent generalized tonic muscle spasms usually follow within 24 hours, culminating in acute respiratory arrest. The keystone of management is the prevention of exotoxin production by debridement and cleansing of all wounds in which devitalized, contaminated tissue is present, coupled with an immunization program. All patients who sustain tetanus prone wounds, as described in Table 8-8 receive tetanus prophylaxis in accordance with the recommendations of the Committee on Trauma of the American College of Surgeons as outlined in Table 8-9. Patients who have not been immunized within 10 years should receive tetanus immune globulin (human). The use of systemic antibiotics for Clostridia should be considered for all tetanus-prone wounds to eliminate residual tetanus bacilli.

Breast Abscess

Breast abscess characterized by localized severe tenderness, swelling, and redness associated with a mass, is a common *Staphylococcal* soft tissue infection. Postpartum women are particularly at risk for this infection during lactation. Parenchymal breast abscesses also occur and are secondary to trauma with subsequent fat necrosis. Development of breast abscess in a nonlactating woman should alert the physician to the possibility of an underlying malignancy. Antibiotics will address the cellulitis, but urgent incision and drainage is required to treat the abscess. Typically, the abscess wall should be biopsied at the time of drainage. Since abscess walls do not have a distinct blood supply, delivery of antibiotics, white blood cells, and oxygen is quite limited. Delays in surgical intervention may result in necrosis of large amounts of breast tissue.

Perirectal Abscess

These abscesses result from infection within the crypts of the anorectal canal and present as a tender mass in the perianal area. Perirectal abscess may extend into the pelvis above the rectal sphincter and, in diabetic or immunocompromised patients, may be fatal. Perirectal abscesses are exquisitely tender and usually require a general anesthesia to be examined and to establish adequate drainage. Antibiotics coverage is usually broad-spectrum targeting both anaerobes and aerobes and is necessary for the **bacteremia** associated with drainage

TABLE 8-8	Tetanus Risk by Wound Type	
	Tetanus Prone	**Nontetanus Prone**
Age	>6 hr	<6 hr
Type	Crush	Sharp/clean
	Avulsion	
	Extensive abrasion	
	Burns or frostbite	
Contaminants (soil, saliva)	Present	Absent

TABLE 8-9	Guide to Tetanus Prophylaxis in Routine Wound Management Among Adults Aged 19–64 Years				
Characteristic	**Clean, Minor Wound**		**All Other Wounds**[a]	
History of Absorbed Tetanus Toxoid (doses)	**Tdap or Td**[b]	**TIG**	**Tdap or Td**[b]	**TIG**
Unknown or <3 doses	Yes	No	Yes	Yes
≥3 doses	No[c]	No	No[d]	No

[a]Such as, but not limited to, wounds contaminated with dirt, feces, soil, and saliva; puncture wounds; avulsions; and wounds resulting from missiles, crushing, burns, and frostbite.

[b]Tdap (tetanus, diphtheria, pertussis) is preferred to Td (tetanus, diphtheria) for adults who have never received Tdap. Td is preferred to TT (tetanus toxoid) for adults who received Tdap previously or when Tdap is not available. If TT and TIG (tetanus immune globulin) are both used, Tetanus Toxoid Adsorbed rather than tetanus toxoid for booster use only (fluid vaccine) should be used.

[c]Yes, if >10 years since the last tetanus toxoid-containing vaccine dose.

[d]Yes, if >5 years since the last tetanus toxoid-containing vaccine dose.

Adapted from CDC Morbidity and Mortality Weekly Report, Recommendations and Reports December 15, 2006/Vol. 55/No. RR-17, Preventing Tetanus, Diphtheria, and Pertussis Among Adults: Use of Tetanus Toxoid, Reduced Diphtheria Toxoid and Acellular Pertussis Vaccine, Recommendations of the Advisory Committee on Immunization Practices (ACIP).

and periabscess cellulitis. Invasive infection may result in subcutaneous tissue necrosis, which requires wide debridement for salvage. In this instance, colostomy diversion may be considered to avoid further soilage to the area, and to avoid the sequelae of fecal incontinence if the sphincter mechanism is involved in the necrosis.

Hand Infections

While generally not life threatening, hand infections may lead to severe morbidity from loss of function as a result of tissue loss, scar, and contracture (Table 8-10). **Paronychia** is a staphylococcal infection of the proximal fingernail that erupts at the sulcus of the nail border. Drainage including resection of a portion of embedded nail and hot soaks usually provide adequate therapy. A subungual abscess is the extension of a deep paronychia and is diagnosed by fluctuance beneath the nail. **Felons** are deep infections of the terminal phalanx pulp space. These infections usually occur after distal phalanx penetrating injuries and are treated by drainage. Removal of the nail is usually necessary to permit adequate drainage. Neglected infections of the fingers may result in **tenosynovitis**, an infection that extends along the digit tendon sheaths. Drainage requires opening the sheath along its entire length to prevent necrosis of the tendon.

Penetrating injury or spread from a contiguous fascial compartment may lead to infection in one of three **deep-space compartments** in the hand. A thenar space infection causes swelling and pain directly over the thenar eminence. The thumb is held in abduction to reduce pain and tendon stretch. Loss of the normal concavity as a result of tense, painful swelling of the palm is characteristic of a midpalmar space abscess. Rarely, the hypothenar space presents in a similar fashion, with swelling and painful movement of the hypothenar eminence. Urgent incision and drainage is required for these infections and empiric broad-spectrum antibiotics, later based on culture data, are generally continued for 7 to 10 days depending on the response to therapy.

Human bites of the hand are common, and the potential infectious nature should not be underestimated. Contamination of these wounds with **polymicrobial** aerobic and anaerobic oral flora contributes to invasive deep-space infections, including tenosynovitis. Copious irrigation, debridement of devitalized tissue, hand elevation, and broad-spectrum antibiotics are required to reduce the potential for infectious complications. Human bites are the only penetrating injury of the hand in which primary closure is not employed. Human oral flora includes the invasive pathogen *Eikenella corrodens*, an organism that is known to suppurate along tendon sheaths

TABLE 8-10	Common Hand Infections		
	Location	**Signs**	**Treatment**
Felon	Pulp space of digits	Swollen, indurated, tense, throbbing distal finger; point tenderness	I & D over length of phalanx along side of finger
Paronychia	Skin over mantle of nail and lateral nail folds	Swelling/induration of nail folds, point tenderness, purulent drainage	I & D at base of nail; removal of nail if infection beneath nail
Tenosynovitis	Tendon sheath	Throbbing, pain with movement, entire finger swollen, tenderness over sheath, finger held semiflexed	I & D over length of sheath and bursa; systemic antibiotics usually indicated
Fascial space	Spaces of hand/thenar regions	Tenderness of involved space, swelling over region involved, limited motion	I & D along surface lines of projection; systemic antibiotics indicated
Human bites	Point of skin penetration and underlying regions	Injury site wound, induration and swelling, purulent drainage, limited motion	Wide debridement and irrigation; systemic antibiotics and tetanus immunization indicated

I & D, incision and drainage.

leading to extensive tissue destruction. The hand and upper extremity are often injured by animal bites as well. Debridement and irrigation are required (as for human bites), but the pathogens involved are likely to be aerobic *Pasteurella* species from both dogs and cats.

Foot Infections

Foot infections result from direct injury or, more commonly, from mechanical and metabolic derangements that occur in patients with diabetes. Trauma-related infections are best prevented by adequate wound cleansing at the time of injury. Established infections should raise concern that a retained foreign body or underlying osteomyelitis is present. Plain radiography will identify the majority of retained foreign bodies in the foot, but ultrasound, CT scan, or magnetic resonance imaging may be required to localize nonradiodense objects. All foreign bodies associated with infection require localization and removal for healing to occur. Osteomyelitis diagnosed by bone destruction on plain radiographs or better characterized by bone scan requires operative debridement.

Foot infections in patients with diabetes are a common problem because of neuropathy, the resultant bone deformities, and the vascular compromise that occurs in this population, which leads to ischemic and pressure-related ulceration. Ulcers on the plantar aspect of the forefoot underneath a metatarsal head are typical for such pressure ulcers. A thorough examination of the infected foot should determine the extent of vascular and neurologic impairment. Plantar space infections may present with dorsal cellulites and all dorsal cellulitis should trigger a search for a plantar source. Osteomyelitis is a frequent component of diabetic foot infection, and any persistent or extensive infection should be evaluated for bone involvement. Cultures of involved tissue (not just surface swabs) should be obtained, followed by initial empiric broad-spectrum antibiotic therapy, debridement, and drainage. Initial therapy should cover *Pseudomonas* due to its prevalence in this patient population. Efforts should focus on limb salvage in these patients, because amputation is a frequent morbid consequence of these complex infections. Such efforts may require management of concomitant more proximal vascular disease. Antibiotics alone may be insufficient to clear infection and allow tissue healing without specific wound dressings, correction of pressure points by orthotic foot wear, or surgical debridement and arterial inflow improvement.

Biliary Tract Infections

Biliary tract infections are usually a consequence of obstruction within the biliary tree, involving either the cystic or the common bile duct. The bacteria most commonly involved include *Escherichia coli*, *Klebsiella* spp., and *Enterococcus* spp., while anaerobes are not commonly encountered. Antibiotics are utilized as an adjunct to surgical and/or endoscopic intervention for effective drainage and infection resolution. A cephalosporin such as cefazolin or cefoxitin would be the initial drug chosen in this clinical setting. Piperacillin also has a high level of secretion in bile and is frequently utilized for biliary tract infections.

Acute cholecystitis is the most common inflammatory and infectious process in the biliary tract. It begins as a nonspecific inflammatory process secondary to gall stone obstruction of the cystic duct. Entrapped bacteria convert inflammation to an invasive infectious process. Empyema of the gallbladder occurs when infected bile is undrained, leading to purulent distension. Increased endoluminal pressure combined with invasive bacterial infection into the wall may also compromise the blood supply of the gallbladder walls, resulting in ischemia, necrosis, and perforation. Prevention of these complications is best achieved by operative intervention.

Infection proximal to a common duct obstruction from stone disease (choledocholithiasis) causes ascending cholangitis. Patients present with fulminant fever, right upper quadrant abdominal pain, and jaundice (**Charcot's triad**); the addition of hypotension and altered mental status is known as **Reynold's pentad**. These patients usually manifest severe sepsis or septic shock accompanied by hemodynamic instability, which require intravenous fluid resuscitation and vasopressor management to maintain mean arterial pressure. Prompt surgical intervention to address the obstruction is imperative. The common duct must be drained by open operation (common bile duct exploration), percutaneous radiologic methods (percutaneous transhepatic catheter placement), or endoscopic means (endoscopic retrograde cholangiopancreatography with stone extraction and sphincterotomy of the ampulla of Vater). Cholecystectomy should be undertaken once the patient's septic pathology has been corrected.

Acute Peritonitis

Acute peritonitis occurs when bacteria are present within the normally sterile peritoneal cavity. However, peritonitis is variable in severity and different segments of the intestine that may perforate have different bacterial and chemical compositions and microorganism densities. Therefore, it is inappropriate to consider all of the illnesses that are classified as peritonitis as a single disease entity. Instead, peritonitis may be classified as primary, secondary, or tertiary as discussed previously. Peritonitis causes acute abdominal pain, usually accompanied by fever and leukocytosis; these findings may be absent in those with tertiary peritonitis due to host immunoincompetence.

Examination of the abdomen typically demonstrates marked tenderness with voluntary guarding as well as rebound tenderness; involuntary guarding (board-like rigidity) is characteristic of generalized peritonitis. An upright chest roentgenogram commonly shows pneumoperitoneum beneath a hemidiaphragm with acute GI perforation and small amounts of pneumoperitoneum are readily demonstrated by CT (Figure 8-3) that may not be initially apparent on plain radiography.

Perforated gastroduodenal ulcers usually present with acute onset abdominal pain with little or no antecedent history of abdominal discomfort. Approximately 80% of patients have pneumoperitoneum on an upright chest film. The perforation allows gastric acid, bile, as well as oral microflora including fungi (if the patient has achlorhydria or is on acid suppression medication) to gain access to the peritoneal space or the retroperitoneum (depending on ulcer location). If the patient is able to make acid, the peritonitis is usually a response to chemical irritation, with no bacteria culturable from the peritoneal cavity in the first 12 hours. If the perforation persists for longer than 12 hours bacterial proliferation ensues from ongoing contamination and bacterial egress into a more alkaline environment within the peritoneal space. Operative repair of the perforation is required for source control. All patients with ulcer-associated perforation should be assessed for the presence of *Helicobacter pylori* infection. Antibiotic therapy to address oral aerobes and anaerobes is generally indicated for acute perforations for <24 hours. Established infection with

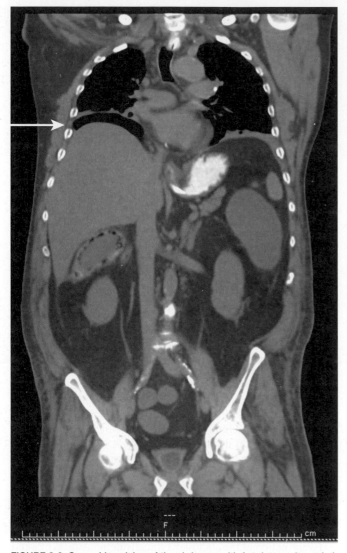

FIGURE 8-3. Coronal imagining of the abdomen with free intraperitoneal air under the right hemidiaphragm.

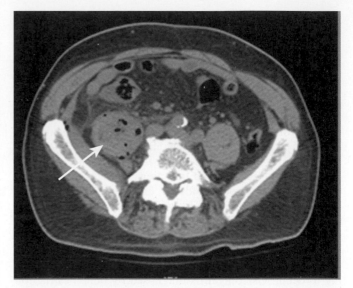

FIGURE 8-4. Localized psoas abscess following appendectomy for perforated, gangrenous appendicitis.

left > transverse > right) aerobic and anaerobic floral densities are rather high. Patients generally demonstrate peritonitis and hemodynamic instability, often presenting with septic shock. After volume resuscitation, the initiation of broad-spectrum systemic antibiotics, and often restoration of mean arterial pressure with vasopressors (norepinephrine and vasopressin) operation is generally indicated to manage the perforation, drainage of purulent collections, and debride nonviable tissue and fecal contamination within the peritoneal cavity. The etiology may be varied (ischemia, diverticulitis, perforated colon cancer, etc.) with CT scan findings including thickened bowel wall, mesenteric stranding, pneumatosis intestinalis (Figure 8-5), pericolonic collections, and pneumoperitoneum.

peritonitis and abscess indicates a need for therapeutic antibiotics whose duration exceeds 24 hours. Importantly, perforation in patients with achlorhydria (endogenous or medication induced) should prompt empiric antifungal therapy as well.

Acute appendicitis causes localized peritoneal irritation and appendiceal perforation commonly causes generalized peritonitis. In the absence of an appropriate operation, perforation may occur within 24 hours of symptom onset. Patients typically demonstrate the characteristic findings of acute, diffuse peritoneal irritation when the perforation is not contained, while a contained perforation with periappendiceal abscess formation (Figure 8-4) may induce only right lower quadrant pain and tenderness. Antibiotic therapy is directed against both aerobic (*E. coli*) and anaerobic (*Bacteroides fragilis*) enteric organisms. Treatment depends on the hemodynamic status of the patient and the presence or absence of a localized collection that is amenable to percutaneous drainage. Patients without a localized collection should undergo an emergent operation for source control. External drainage (i.e., Jackson-Pratt [JP] drain) is unnecessary and ineffective for diffuse peritoneal spillage in the absence of a localized abscess.

Colonic perforation with diffuse peritonitis creates the most virulent type of peritonitis as the colon (rectum > sigmoid >

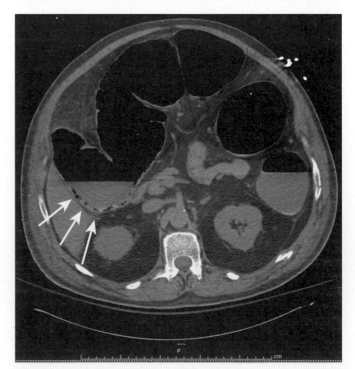

FIGURE 8-5. CT scan of abdomen with pneumatosis intestinalis visualized at the hepatic flexure of the colon.

Left and sigmoid colon perforations usually require resection of the perforated segment and diversion of the fecal stream as part of their management. Selected patients who present with a localized perforation (including mesocolonic perforation) may be initially managed without immediate operation provided the leak is adequately drained.

Peritonitis may occur from a variety of other sources besides the selected ones reviewed above. If physical findings consistent with peritonitis are present, a laparotomy prior to radiologic examination and source identification is appropriate (i.e., a typical "exploratory" laparotomy). In order to reduce patient morbidity and mortality, it is important to rapidly diagnose peritonitis and expedite operative intervention instead of awaiting radiologic studies intended to define the culpable organ system. Exploration and direct visualization will readily define the specific diagnosis and etiology and direct therapy accordingly.

Fungal Infections

Fungal infections are in general uncommon in surgical patients; however, they are increasing in frequency and severity. With the increasing utilization of broad-spectrum antibiotic coverage for many infectious etiologies, the proliferation of fungi as opportunistic pathogens has also increased in the surgical population. The patient with underlying immunosuppression, patients on chemotherapy, and older debilitated patients are also all at risk. The ubiquitous nature of fungi makes it difficult at times to differentiate colonization versus invasion. The upper GI tract and the skin are all potential sources of fungal colonization. Since they are frequently isolated from these areas in routine culture, blood or quantitative culture methodology is often required to determine true invasive infection.

Most fungal infections are self-limited and require minimal treatment (i.e., urinary tract, yeast vaginitis, dermatitis, fungal nail infections, and thrush). These infections are typically due to the *Candida* species. Common medications to treat these conditions include fluconazole, ketoconazole, miconazole, and nystatin. More severe fungal infections would include histoplasmosis, blastomycosis, cryptococcal meningitis, and aspergillosis. A more aggressive treatment regimen is needed to include intravenous antifungal agents like amphotericin B, voriconazole, caspofungin, or micafungin. The most severe forms of fungal infections require surgical debridement. Fungal burn wound and soft tissue invasive infections require rapid and radical debridement of all infected tissue. The mortality with these infections is high particularly in the immunosuppressed patient. Pulmonary manifestations of fungal disease may also require operative resection when they coalesce into a mass or abscess in lung cavities such as aspergilloma or coccidioidomycosis. Combination therapy with systemic antifungals and surgical resection are required. These infections are primarily limited to the chronically debilitated or immunosuppressed patient resulting in a high mortality despite treatment.

Viral Infections

The diagnosis and treatment of viral infections is not usually the province of the surgeon, except in cases of severely immunosuppressed patients, in whom invasive infection may mimic a bacterial etiology. However, occupational exposure of health care workers to patients who are infected with hepatitis or HIV requires an understanding of the route of transmission so that preventive measures may be undertaken.

Standard precautions including the use of personal protective equipment, reduces the likelihood of viral transmission to the health care worker. Inadvertent injury (i.e., needle-stick injury, laceration with a scalpel blade, bone fragment, or impaled object) should prompt immediate therapy including evaluation by the worker's Occupational Health Department for event reporting, source, and health care worker evaluation, and consideration for prophylactic medication administration while awaiting data. Hepatitis B, C, and HIV are the three most common viral illnesses about which the surgeon should be educated with regard to health maintenance.

The DNA virus hepatitis B is the pathogen of greatest concern for surgeons because blood or body fluid exposure is the primary route of transmission. In 5% to 10% of infected patients, a chronic carrier state develops and the individual harbors a lifetime ability to transmit the infection. Many of these chronic carriers develop cirrhosis, end-stage liver disease, or hepatocellular carcinoma. An acute infection may result in fulminant hepatic failure and death. Once hepatitis B infection is established, effective therapy is limited; however, a highly effective hepatitis B vaccine is available for individuals at risk of hepatitis B exposure. All health care workers are at risk and should undergo vaccination with follow-up antibody titers determined to ensure protection.

Hepatitis C, an RNA virus, poses a similar risk as hepatitis B because it is also transmitted by blood and body fluids. Although acute infection from hepatitis C virus is generally mild or occult, the chronic carrier state occurs in approximately 60% of patients. In these patients, chronic active hepatitis and cirrhosis typically ensue. There is an increased risk of hepatocellular carcinoma in cirrhotics who have hepatitis C. Because there is no vaccine and because over 4 million people in the United States have chronic hepatitis C, it is important that health care workers exercise standard precautions in all patient contacts. Some hepatitis C serotypes respond to early and aggressive interferon-gamma therapy following exposure; while viral eradication is possible it is the exception.

Infections secondary to the retrovirus HIV remain a focus of public concern. Although our understanding of this viral disease and its treatment continues to evolve, it is clear that blood and body fluid exposure is the primary mode of transmission. Therefore, the disease presents a potential risk to surgical care providers. With few exceptions, HIV infection appears to progress to clinical AIDS, a fatal illness. Despite the wide and continually evolving armada of antiretroviral chemotherapy that has significantly prolonged life for patients with HIV infection, prevention remains the most effective strategy when addressing HIV infection. Utilizing standard precautions to limit health care worker exposure to potentially infected blood and body fluids remains a mainstay of preventive measures throughout the hospital environment.

Multiple-Organ Dysfunction

The clinical events of acute surgical infection are most often resolved at the local site of infection with source control and systemic antibiotics. When proinflammatory products of inflammation are uncontrolled or extensive and systemic immunocompetence is compromised, an ongoing generalized septic state occurs. This generalized septic state, termed the systemic inflammatory response syndrome (SIRS), is characterized by an increase in cardiac output, reduced peripheral vascular resistance, a sustained systemic lactic acidemia, hypermetabolism, and ureagenesis.

The manifestations of SIRS, as defined by the American College of Chest Physicians, include but are not limited to a body temperature <36°C or >38°C; a heart rate > 90 beats per minute; tachypnea > 20 breaths/min or an arterial pCO_2 < 32 mmHg; a WBC count of <4,000 cells/mL or >12,000 cells/mL or the presence of >10% immature neutrophils (band forms). SIRS can be diagnosed when two or more of these criteria are present.

If left unabated, a generalized failure of individual cellular function causes dysfunction of both metabolic and vascular processes in vital organ systems. This state of hypoperfusion and hypermetabolism is termed Multiple Organ Dysfunction Syndrome (MODS). The affected vital organs fail in a sequential fashion that is a frequent precursor to death of the host. In both operative and nonoperative patients, sepsis is identified. The treatment of MODS requires assessment of all potential causes of systemic inflammation, although once it begins, the process often continues despite primary septic source control. Current management entails both organ system support (e.g., mechanical ventilation) and nutritional support to avoid metabolic and immunologic collapse. Mortality varies, but the chance of survival is diminished as the number of organ systems involved increases. When three or more organ systems, fail the mortality is >75% with renal failure having the largest impact against survival.

SUMMARY

Originally intended to refer to SSI, the term "surgical infections" has now been expanded to encompass an entire host of disease states for which evaluation by a surgeon and potential surgical intervention are necessary. SSI are in general an infrequent event from elective surgery; however, emergent procedures with gross bacterial contamination are at a much higher risk for subsequent development of postoperative infection. Many of these will require at the very least, opening of the surgical wound with daily local wound care. A small subset will require debridement and drainage with the adjunctive use of antibiotics. Careful surveillance of the wound is necessary in those patients at high risk for infection. Early identification and treatment will limit further complications related to ongoing infection. Numerous strategies targeted at prevention are being employed with protocols based on current evidence. Governmental oversight is likely to increase in the future to continue to limit SSI as a postoperative complication.

Other types of surgical infections range from cellulitis to deep organ space infections requiring a myriad of treatment techniques from oral antibiotics, incision and drainage (subcutaneous abscess), radical debridement (necrotizing fasciitis or necrotizing pancreatitis), to organ removal (i.e., appendicitis or colitis). A prompt diagnosis with rapid surgical treatment will limit morbidity and mortality in many of these diseases. Postinfections inflammatory complications (SIRS and acute respiratory distress syndrome [ARDS]) are increasing events in the ICU as critically ill patients are sustained for longer time periods. The future of surgical infections will likely involve further problems with multidrug-resistant organisms, cytokine and inflammatory modulation, and immune enhancement, although research efforts thus far have not proven to be efficacious in all these areas. The continued need for débridement and source control will provide the surgeon with a central role in the management of this varied disease.

thePoint ✳ Go to http://thePoint.lww.com/activate and use your scratch-off code on the inside cover of this book to access bonus chapters, question bank, videos, and more.

SAMPLE QUESTIONS

Questions

Choose the best answer for each question.

1. A 32-year-old man is seen in the emergency department 45 minutes after a motor vehicle collision. His only injury is a long linear laceration beginning on the left temporal forehead at the hairline and extending posteriorly for 10 cm. The edges are still bleeding briskly and the EMTs described a large amount of blood at the scene. He did not lose consciousness. His last tetanus booster was 4 years ago. Which of the following is required for tetanus prophylaxis in this patient?

   A. Tetanus immune globulin only

   B. Nothing further at this time

   C. Tetanus toxoid only

   D. Tetanus immune globulin followed by a single tetanus toxoid booster

   E. Tetanus immune globulin followed by three tetanus boosters

2. A 48-year-old man is being evaluated in the emergency department with fevers, chills, and abdominal pain for the past 24 hours. He has a history of hepatitis C infection following a blood transfusion 14 years ago for a large scalp laceration and orthopedic injuries sustained in a motor vehicle collision. He has not been to a physician for 5 years. He does not smoke or drink alcohol. He takes no medications. His temperature is 39°C and vital signs are: blood pressure (BP) 90/50 mm Hg, pulse 110/minute, and respirations 26/minute. A CT scan shows a single stone in the gallbladder that does not appear to be obstructing. The bile ducts are normal caliber and the gallbladder wall is not thickened. There is a moderate amount of fluid, mild small bowel distention, and stranding around the sigmoid colon as well as a small amount of free intraperitoneal gas around the liver. An aspirate of the peritoneal fluid shows leukocytes and mixed Gram positives and negatives on Gram stain. Laboratory values show a WBC of 19,000/mm³, total bilirubin 1.2 mg/dL, and alkaline phosphatase 40 U/L. In addition to fluid resuscitation and broad-spectrum antibiotics, what is the best step in management?

   A. Laparoscopic cholecystectomy

   B. Long-term antibiotics only

   C. Laparotomy

   D. Magnetic resonance cholangiopancreatography (MRCP)

   E. Endoscopic retrograde cholangiopancreatography (ERCP)

3. A 42-year-old woman is seen in the infectious disease clinic because of a small laceration. She is a surgeon and was assisting a surgical resident with a colon resection when she was accidentally cut with a scalpel blade during the procedure. She has received all required immunizations. Antibodies against which virus could be measured in order to assess the effectiveness of the only vaccine to prevent infection potentially transmitted from the patient to the surgeon during the operative procedure?

   A. Human immunodeficiency virus

   B. Hepatitis C

   C. Hepatitis B

   D. Cytomegalovirus

   E. Tuberculosis

4. A 30-year-old man is in the hospital recovering from splenectomy for a ruptured spleen sustained in a motor vehicle collision. He has otherwise been healthy and was not taking medications prior to the injury. A temperature of 102°F is noted on the second postoperative day. Vital signs are BP 130/80 mm Hg, pulse 100/minute, and respirations 18/minute. His pain is moderately controlled with morphine using patient-controlled analgesia (PCA). Breath sounds are diminished at both bases, more so on the left. His abdomen is mildly distended, soft and tender near the incision. The incision appears to be healing without a problem. What is the most likely cause for his fever?

   A. Atelectasis and pulmonary infection

   B. Peritonitis

   C. Urinary tract infection

   D. Suppurative thrombophlebitis

   E. Cardiac contusion

5. A 25-year-old man is seen in the emergency department because of a painful swollen forearm. Two days ago, he sustained a small laceration to his left forearm while clearing brush. It caused only minor discomfort until about 12 hours ago when the area around the laceration became more red and swollen. He has otherwise been healthy. He takes no medications. His temperature is 38°C. There is a 2-cm superficial laceration on the dorsum of his left forearm with 15-cm diameter surrounding erythema that is quite tender. The edges of the erythema were marked and 20 minutes later the erythema has extended another cm beyond the mark. The most likely causative organism is

   A. methicillin-resistant *Staphylococcus aureus*.

   B. β-Hemolytic *Streptococcus A*.

   C. *Escherichia coli*.

   D. *Streptococcus faecalis*.

   E. *Candida albicans*.

Answers and Explanations

1. Answer: B

Wounds prone to the development of tetanus include those with extensive contamination with soil, deep puncture wounds from metal objects, exposure injury complicated with frostbite, and wounds >6 hours from time of injury (Table 8-8.). Linear lacerations in general are not prone to tetanus. The extent of blood loss does not affect the need for tetanus booster administration. The patient last received tetanus toxoid <5 years ago, so nothing further is required.

2. Answer: C

This patient has secondary peritonitis. This usually involves perforation of a hollow viscus and thus involves contamination of the peritoneal cavity with multiple organisms. Gram stain and culture of the peritoneal fluid usually shows a single organism in patients with primary peritonitis and this can be treated with antibiotics without surgical intervention. In this scenario, the CT scan shows stranding around the sigmoid and fluid and evidence of free air suggestive of a diverticulitis with fecal peritonitis. Patients with underlying liver disease are prone to gallstones and are a common finding. There is no evidence of common bile duct obstruction that warrants further investigation since the alkaline phosphatase is normal.

3. Answer: C

HIV, hepatitis B, hepatitis C, and cytomegalovirus are transmitted by body fluids and blood; therefore, they pose an occupational risk to the surgeon. There is currently a highly effective vaccine for the prevention of hepatitis B in the host. No such vaccine is available for the other viral infections. Tuberculosis is not a virus but also poses a risk to health care workers.

4. Answer: A

Early postoperative fever is usually the result of atelectasis and subsequent pulmonary infection (Table 8-6). In this scenario, because of the close proximity of the left hemidiaphragm to the spleen, an infiltrate in the left lower lobe of the lung is a high probability. An adequately drained urinary tract in a young person seldom gives a high fever this early in the postoperative period. Although peritonitis from injury to a surrounding structure during the splenectomy (i.e., pancreas, stomach, or bowel) is a possibility, it is much less likely than a pulmonary source. Cardiac contusion does not elicit a febrile response.

5. Answer: B

Although cellulitis may be caused by any organism, the most likely early organism would be ß-hemolytic *Streptococcus A*. Methicillin-resistant *Staphylococcus aureus* more commonly causes local inflammation and pus formation. The other three species are rarely isolated from skin infections but more commonly are seen in infections involving the gastrointestinal tract.

9
Trauma

MATTHEW O. DOLICH, M.D. • H. SCOTT BJERKE, M.D. • JEFFREY G. CHIPMAN, M.D. •
FRED A. LUCHETTE, M.D. • LISA A. PATTERSON, M.D.

Objectives

1. Understand the concepts of the initial assessment and stabilization of the injured patient.

2. Define shock and understand the pathophysiology, etiology, and treatment of hemorrhagic shock in the traumatized patient.

3. Define the Glasgow Coma Scale (GCS) and understand its relevance in the management of traumatic brain injury.

4. Understand the concept of intracranial pressure (ICP) monitoring in traumatic brain injury.

5. Understand the various types of injuries to the spine and spinal cord, including their effects on hemodynamic status.

6. Define therapeutic interventions in traumatic brain injury.

7. Outline the mechanisms of blunt and penetrating thoracic injury, and define therapeutic interventions in patients with these injuries.

8. Understand the indications for resuscitative thoracotomy in the emergency department (ED) and the therapeutic goals of this maneuver.

9. Describe injury patterns seen in abdominal trauma.

10. Understand the concept of "damage control" surgery in the trauma setting.

11. Understand the indications for operative and nonoperative management of abdominal injuries.

12. Describe common pelvic fracture patterns and their clinical significance.

13. Understand the unique anatomy of the neck and its relationship to the diagnostic evaluation of penetrating cervical injuries.

14. Understand the concept of extremity compartment syndrome and indications for decompressive fasciotomy.

15. Understand unique issues related to trauma in elderly patients, pregnancy, and in children.

OVERVIEW AND EPIDEMIOLOGY

Trauma remains the leading cause of death in the first 44 years of life and is the fifth leading cause of mortality for all age groups. In 2006, unintentional traumatic injury resulted in over 121,000 deaths in the United States. Each year, over 43,000 deaths result from motor vehicle–related collisions, and almost 30,000 people die by firearm. More impressive is that over 2 million years of potential life are lost to unintentional injury each year in the United States, and annual trauma-related costs are estimated in excess of $400 billion. It is estimated that there are almost 20 million nonfatal injuries each year in this country alone.

In the last several decades, dramatic improvements in trauma care have resulted in increased survival rates and substantially better outcomes. Regionalization of trauma care has allowed more efficient use of limited and expensive resources. Advances in diagnostic imaging, including ultrasound and computed tomography (CT), have tremendously facilitated rapid and accurate diagnosis of traumatic injuries. Prioritization of immediately life-threatening injuries and the evolving concept of "damage control" or abbreviated surgery have further honed our ability to take care of the most severely injured patients. Trauma care has evolved into a truly multidisciplinary specialty and includes trauma surgeons, intensivists, emergency physicians, neurosurgeons, orthopedic surgeons, otolaryngologists, plastic surgeons, urologists, and physiatrists in the management of these often complex and challenging patients.

INITIAL ASSESSMENT

The initial assessment of an injured patient must quickly identify and treat immediately life-threatening injuries, then potentially life-threatening injuries, and finally life-altering injuries. The process is divided into four phases: (1) **primary survey**, (2) **resuscitation**, (3) **secondary survey**,

Exposure

The last step in the primary survey is to completely remove the patient's clothing. This allows for a complete head-to-toe examination. Additionally, it removes wet clothing that can contribute to hypothermia and may also remove any environmental toxins. Keeping the patient warm through this portion of the evaluation is critical. Hypothermia can contribute to coagulopathy and acidosis, and increases the metabolic demands of an already taxed patient.

Secondary Survey

The purpose of the secondary survey is to identify and treat additional injuries not uncovered during the primary survey. These are frequently not immediately life threatening but can cause significant morbidity and even mortality if diagnosis and treatment are delayed. The secondary survey includes a thorough physical exam, and where possible, a medical history including allergies, last meal, tetanus immunization status, and medication use.

Gastric distension is relatively common in severely injured patients. This can be exacerbated if any bag mask ventilation has occurred during the initial resuscitation. For this reason, gastric decompression with a nasogastric tube is indicated. The orogastric route should be used in patients who are intubated, those with basilar skull fractures (see head trauma section), or those with extensive facial fractures. A urinary catheter is a useful adjunct and is frequently inserted during the secondary survey. Urine production, which decreases in shock states, can be followed as an assessment of the adequacy of volume resuscitation. Bladder catheter placement should be avoided if there is blood at the penile meatus or evidence of a widened symphysis pubis for fear of a urethral transection. In these circumstances, retrograde urethrography should be performed prior to bladder catheterization to assess the integrity of the urethra and prevent false passage of the catheter. In the event of urethral disruption, suprapubic catheterization may be performed under local anesthesia with ultrasound guidance. During the secondary survey, standard monitoring includes continuous electrocardiography and pulse oximetry.

Adjunctive Studies

The results of the primary and secondary survey determine what further diagnostic studies are obtained. CT can detect many internal injuries but should be limited to hemodynamically normal patients. Abdominal ultrasound can identify the presence of intra-abdominal fluid, which in the traumatized patient is indicative of internal injuries that warrant further evaluation. Ultrasonography is now frequently performed early in the initial evaluation steps. Plain radiographs of the chest, cervical spine, and pelvis can be obtained by portable x-ray machines and also provide valuable diagnostic data.

Definitive Care

With the primary and secondary surveys complete, including the needed adjunctive studies, the definitive care plan can be created for the patient. Subsequent sections of this chapter will discuss the issues with specific injuries in more detail. The definitive care phase may also include transfer to a higher level of care for more severely injured patients.

HEAD INJURY

Head injury is the most common cause of trauma-related mortality and is responsible for approximately one-half of all traumatic deaths. Additionally, it is the leading cause of long-term disability. Injuries to the head can involve all cranial structures: skin and soft tissues, bone, and brain. Frequently, injuries to one structure are associated with injuries to others. Although primary injury to the brain (incurred at the moment of impact) is difficult to treat, propagation of the injury (secondary injury) can be prevented or limited with proper treatment. Secondary injury occurs when the injury response to the primary injury damages adjacent brain tissues resulting in a larger area of tissue damage.

Anatomy and Physiology

The anatomy of the head contributes to the patterns of injury seen in head trauma. The skin, subcutaneous tissue, and galea aponeurotica are frequently involved. Injuries to these structures include lacerations, contusions, hematomas, and even combinations thereof. The blood vessels in the soft tissues are held securely by the subcutaneous connective tissue and are prevented from retracting when severed. This characteristic can cause significant hemorrhage, especially in children. Additionally, muscles attached to the galea aponeurotica pull in opposite directions, which tends to hold wounds open and increases the propensity for ongoing bleeding.

Inside the skull, the dura mater is a thick, dense fibrous layer that encloses the brain and spinal cord. It forms the dural venous sinuses, diaphragm sellae, falx cerebri, falx cerebelli, and tentorium cerebelli. Cerebral venous blood flows into the dural sinuses through bridging veins, which can be torn and result in a subdural hemorrhage. The meningeal artery lies between the skull and the dura. Fractures of the temporal and parietal bones of the cranial vault can lacerate these arteries and cause an epidural hematoma. The vascular pia directly covers the brain. Injuries to the blood vessels of the pia as well as the underlying brain can cause subarachnoid hemorrhage or cerebral contusion.

The skull and vertebral column function as a rigid, bony case surrounding the brain and spinal cord. Within the rigid case are three components, brain tissue, cerebrospinal fluid (CSF), and blood. This rigid case has implications for head injuries, as any change in pressure within the calvarium can alter blood flow or compress the brain and adjacent structures. Because the volume of the cranium is fixed, in order to maintain a constant intracranial pressure (ICP), as the volume occupied by one of the three components increases the volume of the other two must decrease. This becomes of particular concern when ICP becomes high enough that it impedes **cerebral blood flow** (CBF) and the brain becomes ischemic.

Besides ICP, CBF is affected by cerebral vascular resistance (CVR) and cerebral perfusion pressure (CPP). CPP is the difference between the mean arterial pressure (MAP) and ICP. As seen in other systems in the body, flow (Q) = change in pressure (ΔP)/resistance (r). In this case CBF = CPP/CVR.

Under normal circumstances, CBF remains constant over a wide range of CPP by alterations in the resistance of the vascular system (CVR). This is known as autoregulation. However, autoregulation is frequently impaired or lost after brain injury. Normal ICP is usually <10 mm Hg. When ICP exceeds 20 mm Hg the brain is at risk for ischemia. As ICP rises, the body attempts to maintain CPP by increasing the systemic blood pressure (MAP). This early response to increased ICP is known as the **Cushing reflex**. In addition to an increased MAP, this reflex is associated with bradycardia and a decreased respiratory rate. Continued increases in ICP usually result in herniation syndromes and brain death.

The tentorium cerebelli is a stiff and unyielding membrane dividing the brain hemispheres from the cerebellum. The brain stem also passes through this tentorium. Any increased pressure above it will push the brain past the tentorium and compress adjacent structures such as the oculomotor nerve. When this happens the ipsilateral pupil becomes dilated and immobile (fixed). As herniation progresses, the corticospinal (pyramidal) tract in the cerebral peduncle can be compressed causing contralateral spastic weakness and a positive Babinski sign. As mentioned, the Cushing reflex can be seen with increasing ICP, which further compresses the brain against the tentorium and causes dysfunction of the cardiorespiratory centers that reside in the medulla. The associated hypotension and bradycardia that follow usually signal impending brain death.

Clinical Evaluation

The neurologic exam begins in the initial evaluation of the trauma patient and when possible includes pertinent details about the injury. Specific information should be sought regarding loss of consciousness, seizure activity, level of alertness post injury, and extremity motor function. A complete neurologic examination is performed that focuses on the level of consciousness, pupillary function, sensation, and the presence of lateralizing extremity weakness. The neurologic evaluation is repeated during the initial evaluation and throughout hospitalization to detect any progressive deterioration of neurologic function. Hypertension, bradycardia, and a slow respiratory rate are generally indicative of a Cushing reflex in response to increased ICP after severe traumatic brain injury. It should be noted that hypotension in a patient with a head injury indicates blood loss until proven otherwise and should not be solely attributed to the head injury.

The GCS is a widely accepted and reproducible method to quantify a patient's level of consciousness (Table 9-1 above). It assigns scores for eye opening (E), verbal response (V), and motor response (M). The sum total of the E, V, and M scores is the GCS score. A neurologically normal person has a GCS score of 15. Coma is defined as GCS score ≤ 8. The lowest score possible is 3. The GCS score can generally be determined during the disability step of the primary survey to indicate the severity of head injury. It is also a prognostic indicator of outcome. A score of 3 to 4 is associated with a probability of mortality or a vegetative state of approximately 97%. A score of 5 to 6 corresponds with a probability of death of approximately 65%, and a score of 7 or 8 has a mortality rate of approximately 28%. It is important to note that multiple factors unrelated to head injury may affect the GCS score, such as sedatives, shock, alcohol consumption, and recreational drug use.

Other signs for head injury can be detected during the secondary survey. Scalp lacerations may be obvious but may also be hidden in the hair. Bony step-offs, indicative of skull fractures, may be palpated. Periorbital ecchymoses (raccoon eyes), perimastoid ecchymosis (Battle's sign), hemotympanum, and leakage of CSF from the nose (rhinorrhea) or ear (otorrhea) are all signs of a basilar skull fracture.

The best method for initial evaluation of head injury is a noncontrast head CT. With modern CT scanners, scans of the head are rapid and simple. The CT scan may show bleeding inside or outside of the brain, brain swelling, midline shift, hydrocephalus, and skull fractures. Although recognizing a skull fracture is important, diagnosing the underlying brain injury is more consequential. Brain injuries can occur with or without skull fractures and vice versa. Cervical spine injuries are found in as many as 15% of patients with head injury and for this reason cervical spine radiographs should be evaluated in all patients with significant head injuries.

Specific Injuries

Some specific injuries to the head deserve further discussion. The scalp is extremely vascular, and as mentioned above, can bleed significantly when lacerated. Direct pressure is often sufficient to control the bleeding, but occasionally skin clips or sutures may need to be placed to stop hemorrhage until definitive control is achieved.

Fractures to the cranium imply large forces and are usually associated with underlying brain injuries. When not displaced they usually are observed. Occasionally, when a fracture is displaced or involves a sinus cavity, surgery is required to elevate the bone or clean out the sinus cavity.

An epidural hematoma occurs when the middle meningeal artery is lacerated, often by a fracture of the overlying bone. Blood collects between the bone and the dura mater. The dura is normally tightly adhered to the skull and as a result the collecting hematoma progressively separates the dura from the skull creating a lens-shaped or convex hematoma that can be seen on CT scan (Figure 9-2). Epidural hematomas have a typical clinical presentation that includes brief loss of consciousness at the time of the injury followed by a normal

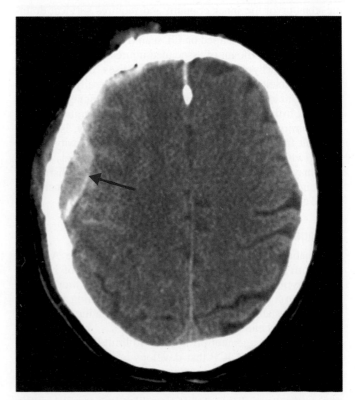

FIGURE 9-2. Epidural hematoma. A convex or lens-shaped collection of blood is typical.

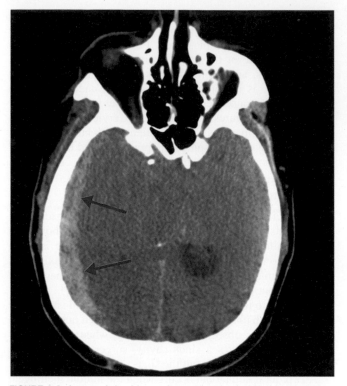

FIGURE 9-3. Acute subdural hemorrhage. High-density blood is present in a crescentic or concave shape along the right cerebral hemisphere.

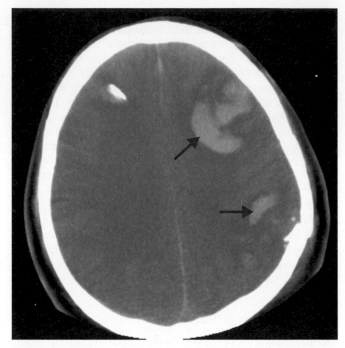

FIGURE 9-4. Traumatic subarachnoid hemorrhage with intraparenchymal cerebral contusions. Multiple foci of acute hemorrhage are noted within the left cerebral hemisphere.

mental status that progressively deteriorates over time as the hematoma expands. Without prompt diagnosis and treatment, the outcome can be devastating.

Subdural hematomas occur when blood collects between the dura mater and the brain. In this injury, the hematoma follows the contour of the inner cranium and requires surgical drainage if of sufficient size. Typically, subdural hematomas appear concave or crescent shaped on CT scan (Figure 9-3). Prognosis depends on the amount of associated injured brain tissue.

Intraparenchymal contusions or bruises occur deep in the brain itself (Figure 9-4). Treatment generally is to limit the amount of adjacent brain tissue that is damaged by the resultant inflammatory response to the original injury. Diffuse axonal injury (DAI), also known as shear injury, is thought to result from differential movement of lower density axonal tissue (white matter) in relation to higher density gray matter. This may result in tiny punctate hemorrhages and disruption of brain tissue without large extra-axial or intraparenchymal blood collections on CT.

Management of Head Injuries

The management of head injury begins with the ABCDE algorithm of the primary survey. The presence of hypoxia and/or hypotension increases the morbidity and mortality of head trauma making it imperative for the treating physician to rapidly establish respiratory and hemodynamic stability in patients with head injuries.

Another management principle is to limit as much as possible the amount of ICP that develops in response to injury. Because space within the cranium is fixed, any increase in pressure will either compress the brain itself or impede blood flow to the brain. Lack of sufficient blood flow will result in ischemic conditions and result in secondary brain injury.

There are several methods to measure ICP. The ventricular catheter method consists of placing a catheter into the lateral ventricle of the brain through a hole drilled into the skull. The catheter is connected to a transducer that allows continuous ICP monitoring as well as withdrawal of CSF as indicated to reduce ICP. A second method places a pressure monitor within the subarachnoid space through a hole drilled into the skull. This method is used when there is no need for ventricular drainage or when the ventricles cannot be cannulated. Other techniques involve placement of a fiberoptic transducer into the epidural space, subdural space, or lateral ventricle as well as the use of probes that detect tissue oxygen levels in the brain tissue, often in combination with pressure monitoring.

Besides removing CSF from a catheter placed in the ventricles, interventions to limit ICP include patient position, sedation, hyperventilation, intravenous fluid limitation, and diuretics. Keeping the head elevated and in neutral position facilitates venous drainage by gravity and helps to decrease ICP. Sedation reduces posturing and combative behavior as well as the metabolic demand of brain tissue. Moderate hyperventilation to a $PaCO_2$ of 30 to 35 mm Hg lowers ICP in most cases without causing cerebral ischemia. However, this effect is frequently short-lived and is accomplished by decreasing CBF. Therefore, hyperventilation should be considered as a temporizing measure only, while preparations are made for more definitive treatment.

Intravenous fluids are administered judiciously to ensure filling pressures that preserve adequate cardiac output. This goal can be accomplished by monitoring CVP, pulmonary capillary wedge pressure, and urine output. Mannitol is a free-radical scavenger and osmotic diuretic that effectively reduces brain swelling and lowers ICP. Caution must be used when administering mannitol to patients with multiple injuries as the diuretic effect of the drug may cause hypotension in patients with occult hemorrhage. Hypovolemia is best avoided in patients with multiple injuries, who may already have volume deficits, because hypotension increases both secondary brain injury and mortality. Hypertonic saline solutions may be administered intravenously to decrease brain swelling and maintain euvolemia. Patients with head injuries should be closely observed for seizures and treated appropriately with anticonvulsants and antiepileptic medications when seizures occur.

Operative management of traumatic brain injuries continues to evolve. Epidural hematomas, due to their arterial nature, are generally treated by surgical evacuation when large or associated with decreasing mental status. Prognosis is generally good when treatment is prompt. Subdural hematomas may be treated surgically when they result in significant mass effect, but the prognosis is more guarded and outcome is based on the amount of underlying brain injury. Subarachnoid hemorrhages and DAI are most commonly treated without operation due to risk of injuring overlying intact brain. Prognosis is variable and is dependent on the grade of injury. Recovery can take months or years.

Finally, even when head injuries are isolated, the body as a whole must be supported. Enteral nutrition is an important adjunct once the initial resuscitation of a brain-injured patient has concluded, and should be initiated early. The best possible outcomes from head injury are achieved with attention to limiting ICP while supporting the metabolic demands of the whole body.

INJURIES OF THE SPINE AND SPINAL CORD

Patients with blunt force trauma may sustain injury to the vertebral column with or without neurological compromise. Therefore, spinal immobilization is warranted to protect the patient from further injury until the spine can be clinically or radiographically cleared. Injuries may be characterized as fractures, dislocations, ligamentous injuries, or spinal cord injury. Injuries may be further characterized as stable or unstable. The flexible and relatively exposed cervical spine is the most frequent site of vertebral injury accounting for approximately half of all spine trauma. The most common site for cervical fracture or subluxation is the C5 level. Injuries can occur with flexion, extension, and rotation as well as axial loading injuries (e.g., diving accident). Head injuries are commonly associated with cervical spine fractures, therefore a patient with a traumatic brain injury should be suspected of having a cervical spine injury until proven otherwise. Approximately 5% to 30% of patients with cervical fractures will have a second noncontiguous fracture elsewhere in the spine.

The spinal canal starts out wide in the upper cervical spine and narrows further down the vertebral column, making neurological compromise and injury more likely in the lower cervical and thoracic regions. The thoracic spine is far less mobile, and has the added support of the thoracic rib cage. The thoracolumbar junction accounts for approximately 15% of all spine injuries due to the transition from the relatively inflexible thoracic spine to the more flexible and stronger lumbar spine. The spinal cord typically ends at the level of the first lumbar vertebra in adults, and the cauda equina is less likely to sustain injury associated with fracture.

Damage caused by spinal cord injury is thought to consist of a primary and secondary mechanism of injury. The primary mechanism results from the acute compression, laceration, or contusion of the spinal cord. The secondary mechanism is a delayed injury caused by a variety of biochemical processes leading to ischemia. It is crucial to prevent secondary injury to

TABLE 9-3 Segmental Motor Innervation by the Spinal Cord

Motor Function	Muscle Groups	Spinal Cord Segments
Shoulder extension	Deltoid	C5
Elbow flexion	Biceps brachii, brachialis	C5, C6
Wrist extension	Extensor carpi radialis longus and brevis	C6, C7
Elbow extension	Triceps brachii	C7, C8
Finger flexion	Flexor digitorum profundus and superficialis	C8
Finger abduction/adduction	Interossei	C8, T1
Thigh adduction	Adductor longus and brevis	L2, L3
Knee extension	Quadriceps	L3, L4
Ankle dorsiflexion	Tibialis anterior	L4, L5
First toe extension	Extensor hallucis longus	L5, S1
Ankle plantar flexion	Gastrocnemius; soleus	S1, S2

the spinal cord by treating hypoxia and hypotension, which can worsen ischemia. Ischemia is believed to be a major contributing factor for poor outcome in spinal cord injury, and several of the tenets of cerebral perfusion have been extended to provide spinal cord perfusion after traumatic injury.

A spinal cord injury is commonly described as either complete or incomplete. The complete injury will have no motor or sensory function below the level of injury. Physical examination should include inspection and palpation of the entire spine. Identifying the dermatomal level of sensory loss or dysfunction will help to make a quick assessment of the level of injury. Key sensory dermatomes include C5 over the deltoid, T4 at the level of the nipple, and T10 at the level of the umbilicus. Similarly, reflexes should be tested and motor function should be assessed for movement and strength of muscle groups and symmetry between each side. Extremity muscle groups are innervated by identifiable spinal segments making it possible to identify the level of spinal cord injury (Table 9-3).

With loss of the thoracic innervation to the intercostal muscles with an upper cervical spinal cord injury, the patient will exhibit abdominal breathing, inability to take a deep breath, and progressive respiratory compromise. Early decision to intubate the patient to assist with ventilation is often necessary and should be made in the primary survey with a complete cervical spinal cord injury. The loss of sensation with quadriplegia makes the rest of the physical exam difficult, as the patient will not be able to feel pain from other injuries distal to the cord injury. The diaphragm is innervated by C3, C4, and C5, so that an injury higher than this that involves the cord will quickly lead to apnea and death (Figure 9-5).

High thoracic or cervical cord injuries can also cause disruption of the sympathetic chain leading to neurogenic shock. Due to sympathetic vasomotor impairment to the heart, the patient can exhibit bradycardia, or lack of a tachycardia response. Due to loss of peripheral sympathetic vascular tone, vasodilatation will occur which can precipitate hypotension. The classic presentation is a patient who is hypotensive and bradycardic with warm, flaccid extremities. The normal vasomotor response is for peripheral vasoconstriction leading

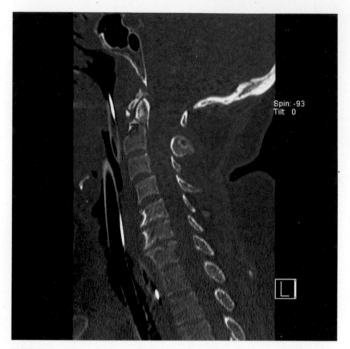

FIGURE 9-5. High cervical spinal cord injury resulting from unstable C2 odontoid fracture (*arrow*). The patient presented with apnea and hypotension from neurogenic shock.

to cool extremities in the face of hypotension related to blood loss. Initial treatment of neurogenic shock is volume resuscitation, as patients may also have concomitant hemorrhage from other injuries. Judicious use of vasopressors is warranted in a small subset of patients to prevent excessive fluid resuscitation, once hemorrhage has been satisfactorily excluded.

Incomplete spinal cord injuries occur when there are neurological findings of sensation or voluntary motor function below the level of injury. There may be a discrepancy between the level of bony injury and the level of neurologic impairment due to the spinal nerve roots exiting the spinal cord at a higher level than they exit the bony vertebral canal. This discrepancy increases with more distal location in the vertebral column. Incomplete spinal cord injuries have a better prognosis for recovery. Other forms of incomplete injury include central cord syndrome, anterior cord syndrome, and Brown-Séquard (cord hemitransection) syndrome. The most common of these is the central cord syndrome where the patient will exhibit weakness in the arms more than the legs. This typically follows a hyperextension injury of the cervical spine when there is preexisting narrowing of the vertebral canal from osteoarthritis. Sensory loss is variable. True Brown-Séquard syndromes are rare and frequently occur after penetrating injuries such as gunshot or stab wounds.

The spinal cord can be injured without a fracture of the vertebral column by either blunt or penetrating mechanisms of injury. When blunt force mechanism yields a neurological deficit without evidence of a fracture, this is termed SCIWORA: Spinal Cord Injury Without Radiological Abnormality, a nomenclature devised before the advent of magnetic resonance imaging (MRI). SCIWORA may or may not be associated with ligamentous disruption. It can occur in children where the vertebral column is flexible and the spinal cord may be stretched and injured with no evidence of injury to the vertebral column. More commonly it occurs in the elderly, where degenerative changes can lead to spinal stenosis. Even

minor head trauma can lead to significant spinal cord injury when there is severe stenosis of the spinal canal. If radiological imaging shows no evidence of a fracture, MRI gives better imaging of ligamentous structures and spinal cord.

Radiologic imaging of the spine has evolved significantly over the past two decades. Despite significant advances in imaging techniques, there is no foolproof study that completely excludes spinal injury. Plain films of the cervical spine (lateral, odontoid, and anteroposterior views) require that all seven cervical vertebrae are adequately visualized. This may be difficult due to large body habitus, degenerative bony changes, or the inability to open the mouth fully for the odontoid view. CT scan has replaced plain films in many trauma centers due to superior imaging quality and ability for three-dimensional reconstruction. The risk of scanning the neck for occult cervical injury, however, must be considered in the child or young adult. There is significantly higher radiation dosage with CT scans and a known association of head and neck radiation with the future development of thyroid cancer. MRI is a better modality for delineating soft tissue abnormalities such as ligamentous injury, spinal cord contusion, epidural hematomas, or herniated disks.

The awake patient with blunt force mechanism and neck pain may have paraspinal muscle spasm from cervical muscle strain (whiplash), or from a more serious ligamentous injury. Flexion-extension views of the cervical spine are an option to distinguish between the two. After negative C-spine x-rays or CT scanning, these views involve voluntary patient movement with imaging in flexion and extension under physician supervision, looking for bony movement that signifies instability. If the patient is unwilling or cannot move more than the 30° needed for the films, the collar is maintained for a period of a week or more and reassessed.

The spine may be clinically cleared without radiological imaging in selected patients. If a patient is alert and cooperative, is not intoxicated, has no spine pain or tenderness, and no neurological deficits, the likelihood of significant spine injury is extremely low. The presence of drugs or alcohol, altered mental status due to traumatic brain injury, or severe distracting pain from other injuries can inhibit the ability to clinically assess for vertebral injury. In these circumstances, caution is best and radiographic imaging of the spine should be obtained.

Treatment of spinal cord injury is one of the most challenging facets of trauma surgery. Spinal cord injuries have devastating effects that are long lasting, and treatment options are unfortunately limited. Despite early promising studies, there is no conclusive evidence that early high-dose intravenous steroid administration provides significant neurological benefit. Early treatment centers on maintaining spinal cord perfusion, avoiding secondary injury, and stabilization of the vertebral column. Later management is multidisciplinary and involves aggressive rehabilitation programs, rigorous physical therapy, pulmonary care, pressure ulcer prevention, and emotional support. There is currently much interest in stem cell therapy as a potential treatment for spinal cord injury.

THORACIC INJURY

Thoracic trauma accounts for approximately 25% of trauma-related deaths and follows traumatic brain injury as the second most common cause of death after traumatic injury. Certain types of thoracic injury may be rapidly fatal if not promptly diagnosed and treated; however, a number of thoracic injuries may be treated by relatively simple maneuvers such as establishment of a definitive airway or tube thoracostomy. It is estimated that approximately 15% of thoracic injuries require operative intervention. The principles of Advanced Trauma Life Support provide a stepwise framework for first diagnosing injuries that are immediately life threatening, followed by those that potentially may cause later morbidity and mortality if diagnosis is significantly delayed.

Immediately Life-Threatening Injuries Detected During Primary Survey

Tension pneumothorax is an immediately life threatening injury that results when gas builds up under pressure within the pleural space after blunt or penetrating thoracic trauma. In this setting, respiratory gases may escape from the injured lung during each respiratory cycle, or may be entrained into the pleural cavity from the outside during inspiration. If there is no route for egress of built up pressure, a tension pneumothorax results, and the ipsilateral lung collapses rapidly. Continued pressure increase displaces the mediastinal structures into the contralateral hemithorax, diminishing venous return to the heart and causing cardiovascular collapse. Death ensues rapidly if the pneumothorax is not relieved. Tension pneumothorax should be diagnosed during the initial assessment by physical examination. The affected side is hyperresonant, with diminished or absent breath sounds. The trachea is shifted to the side *opposite* the side having diminished breath sounds. Hypotension is often present, and jugular venous distension is noted secondary to superior vena caval obstruction from mediastinal shift. When tension pneumothorax is suspected, diagnosis should not be delayed by obtaining a chest x-ray, as even a brief delay in treatment may have disastrous consequences. Frequent reevaluation is necessary to detect if a simple pneumothorax develops a tension component, as young healthy patients may compensate hemodynamically during the early phases of the process. Once the diagnosis is suspected, tension pneumothorax should be treated by prompt needle thoracostomy. This is accomplished by inserting an intravenous catheter, under sterile conditions, into the affected hemithorax in the second intercostal space along the midclavicular line. This maneuver releases the tension component and allows the mediastinal structures to resume their normal anatomical positions. Needle thoracostomy is then followed by formal chest tube thoracostomy and pleural drainage as definitive management.

Open pneumothorax generally occurs in the setting of penetrating thoracic trauma when the chest wall wound remains patent. This allows the lung to collapse completely and creates a sucking chest wound. Respiratory failure may occur as work of breathing increases, since air flow via the wound may prevent generation of adequate negative inspiratory force to bring air into the lungs. Open pneumothorax should be promptly treated in the emergency department (ED) by placing a dressing over the chest wound and securing it to the skin with tape on three sides. This creates a one-way valve that allows egress of accumulated pleural gas during exhalation, but prevents inflow from the atmosphere during inhalation. In effect, this maneuver converts an open pneumothorax into a simple pneumothorax, which generally will not cause acute respiratory failure. Upon completion of the three-sided dressing, a chest tube thoracostomy should be performed to completely reexpand the lung. Operative surgical debridement and closure of the thoracic wound may be required.

Cardiac tamponade is an immediately life-threatening event that may occur in the setting of penetrating or blunt precordial injury. The most common scenario is a stab wound to the sternal region, with resultant cardiac injury. Blood escaping from the heart accumulates within the pericardial sac, resulting in cardiac compression and shock. This occurs because the pericardium is quite fibrous and nondistensible, providing little accommodation for blood leaking from the injured heart. The clinical picture of muffled heart sounds, jugular venous distension, and hypotension (Beck's triad) in a patient with a penetrating precordial injury should create a high suspicion for cardiac injury with tamponade. Other physical findings include Kussmaul's sign (increasing jugular venous distension with inspiration), and pulsus paradoxus (drop in systolic blood pressure ≥10 mm Hg during inspiration). However, these findings are quite variable, and their absence does not preclude the diagnosis of cardiac injury. Diagnosis is confirmed by bedside focused assessment with sonography in trauma (FAST), which reveals pericardial effusion (Figure 9-6). Treatment of cardiac tamponade is based on volume resuscitation to increase cardiac output, and immediate surgical decompression to release the tamponade and repair the underlying cardiac injury. In patients with cardiac tamponade who deteriorate or experience cardiac arrest in the resuscitation area, prompt ED resuscitative thoracotomy should be performed, as this maneuver may be life saving. Pericardiocentesis, or catheter aspiration of the pericardial space, should be considered in environments where resuscitative thoracotomy is not an option due to lack of experienced personnel or equipment.

Massive hemothorax is defined as the rapid loss of ≥1,500 mL of blood into the thoracic cavity, or ongoing thoracic blood loss of ≥200 mL/hour of blood over 4 to 6 hours. Clinical diagnosis is made by the presence of diminished breath sounds and dullness to percussion; plain chest x-ray may confirm the presence of retained blood or clotted hemothorax. Treatment involves tube thoracostomy and volume resuscitation to restore euvolemia, followed by operative thoracotomy

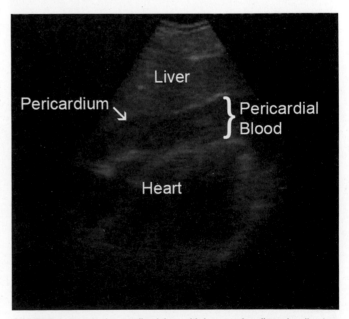

FIGURE 9-6. Penetrating cardiac injury with hemopericardium visualized on bedside ultrasound. Note the large amount of blood outside the heart within the pericardial sac.

for control of hemorrhage. Autotransfusion of shed blood may be a useful adjunct to decrease utilization of banked blood products. Massive hemothorax may occur from chest wall bleeding from intercostal muscles, pulmonary parenchyma, hilar structures, great vessels, or the heart.

Flail chest occurs when two or more adjacent ribs are segmentally fractured in two or more places. This creates an unstable segment of the chest wall that moves paradoxically out of phase with the respiratory cycle. Although the paradoxical motion of the chest wall may be dramatic on physical examination, this is not usually the cause of pulmonary failure. Rather, a flail chest typically involves a major impact to the chest, resulting in a significant **pulmonary contusion**. It is the underlying pulmonary contusion, coupled with the pain of multiple fracture ribs, that compromises respiratory status in these patients. Treatment involves aggressive pain control measures and pulmonary toilet, as well as tube thoracostomy for pneumothorax or hemothorax (which commonly coexist with flail chest). Intubation with mechanical ventilation is utilized in patients who develop pulmonary failure. Intravenous fluids should be administered judiciously, as aggressive hydration is associated with third spacing of fluid into the injured lung and worsening gas exchange. Operative stabilization of the flail segment is a newer technique that may be associated with improved pulmonary outcomes and cosmesis, but prospective studies are lacking.

Potentially Severe Injuries Detected During Secondary Survey

Simple pneumothorax occurs when gas enters the pleural space, causing collapse of the ipsilateral lung. Pleural gas may be introduced from the atmosphere in a penetrating injury, or it may emanate from injury to the lung parenchyma or tracheobronchial tree. Physical examination typically reveals diminished breath sounds on the affected side, though this finding is variable in the often loud environment of the trauma resuscitation area. Hyperresonance to percussion is often noted. Diagnosis is made by plain radiography of the chest, although bedside ultrasound may be diagnostic as well. Post-traumatic pneumothorax visible on plain radiography of the chest should be treated by chest tube placement for reexpansion of the lung.

Hemothorax results when blood or clot accumulates within the pleural space. The source of hemorrhage may be from the pulmonary parenchyma, great vessels, mediastinal structures, or chest wall. Intercostal vessels lacerated after blunt or penetrating injury may bleed significantly. On physical examination, decreased breath sounds and dullness to percussion are typical findings. Chest x-ray will confirm the diagnosis in stable patients, and treatment involves placement of a large bore (36 French) chest tube to drain the pleural space (Figure 9-7). Postprocedure x-rays should be obtained to confirm satisfactory evacuation of the hemothorax. Retained or clotted hemothorax should be treated by early thoracoscopic evacuation in the operating room, as the risk of infection (empyema) or trapped lung increases over time.

Blunt aortic injury (BAI) is a relatively uncommon but potentially lethal injury that is associated with high-speed decelerations such as motor vehicle collisions and falls from heights. The mechanism is believed to be the result of a shearing force of the relatively mobile aortic arch moving differentially in relation to the retropleural descending aorta. Direct compression of the aorta may play a role as well. Full thickness aortic rupture results in rapid exsanguination and death in the moments following injury. In survivors, the rupture is typically contained by the adventitial layers of the aorta or the mediastinal pleura. Intimal flaps or pseudoaneurysms may develop as well. BAI typically occurs in the descending thoracic aorta, just distal to the takeoff of the left subclavian artery. Chest x-ray findings suggestive of BAI include mediastinal widening, apical capping, loss of normal aortic

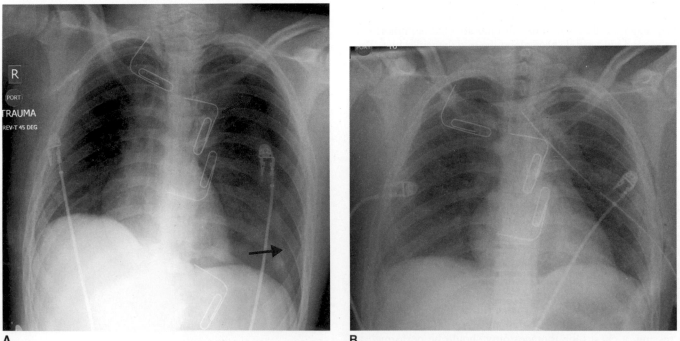

FIGURE 9-7. Left pneumothorax after penetrating chest injury. A, Lung markings are absent along the periphery of the left hemithorax. **B,** After insertion of a left chest tube, the lung has reexpanded.

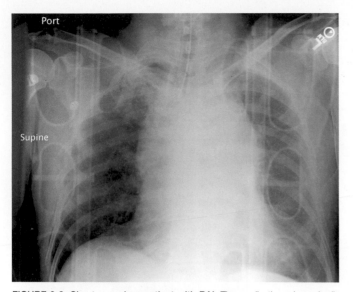

FIGURE 9-8. Chest x-ray in a patient with BAI. The mediastinum is markedly widened, the aortic contour is abnormal, a left apical cap is present, the trachea is deviated toward the right, upper rib fractures are present, and a left hemothorax is noted.

contour, depression of the left mainstem bronchus, loss of the paratracheal stripe, obliteration of the aortopulmonary window, nasogastric tube deviation, left hemothorax, and fractures of the first or second ribs (Figure 9-8). However, absence of these findings does not entirely exclude aortic injury, and patients with concerning mechanism of injury should undergo contrast-enhanced chest CT to assess the aorta (Figure 9-9). Left untreated, a significant number of aortic injuries will go on to free rupture and death. Standard treatment has been operative repair via a left thoracotomy incision. This is commonly performed with partial cardiopulmonary bypass to decrease the risk of postoperative paraplegia, which is a devastating complication of this procedure. Paraplegia results from decreased perfusion of the anterior spinal cord during aortic cross-clamping. Minimally invasive repairs using endovascular stent-grafting techniques are replacing open repair at a number of trauma centers due to the morbidity of standard open repair and the excellent results with endovascular grafts (TEVAR). Occasionally, aortic repair must be delayed

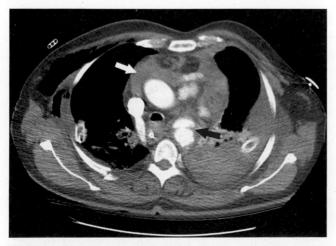

FIGURE 9-9. Chest CT in a patient with BAI. Blood is present within the mediastinum (*white arrow*), and a pseudoaneurysm of the descending aorta is depicted by the *black arrow*.

due to severity of other injuries or additional comorbidities. In such cases, careful medical management with aggressive blood pressure control is necessary to decrease the risk of free aortic rupture.

Rib fractures are one of the most common injuries of the chest, and may be sustained as a result of motor vehicle collisions, falls, assaults, and sports-related trauma. Rib fractures may be diagnosed on physical examination by noting point tenderness, and may or may not be seen on plain radiographs of the chest. CT of the chest is quite sensitive for rib fractures but is seldom, if ever, indicated to make the diagnosis. The location of rib fractures is important, as associated injuries are common. As mentioned previously, upper rib fractures may be associated with aortic or great vessel injury. Midthoracic rib fractures may be associated with pulmonary contusion or hemopneumothorax. Lower rib fractures have an association with diaphragmatic or intra-abdominal injury. Management of rib fractures primarily involves provision of adequate analgesia, as they are quite painful when untreated. Otherwise healthy young patients with one or two rib fractures may be safely managed with oral narcotic analgesics and discharged from the ED. Older patients, or those with multiple rib fractures, generally require inpatient admission. Intravenous patient-controlled analgesia (PCA) and thoracic epidural catheterization are options for aggressive pain control. The goal of treatment is to avoid splinting from pain, which impairs secretion clearance, and may result in atelectasis and pneumonia. Elderly patients with multiple rib fractures fare worse than their younger counterparts, and treating physicians should have a low threshold for ICU admission. Early intubation with mechanical ventilation is required more frequently in elderly patients with multiple rib fractures, due to decreased cardiopulmonary reserve.

Emergency Department Thoracotomy

In patients with severe traumatic injuries and hemorrhagic shock or pericardial tamponade, standard techniques using closed chest cardiopulmonary resuscitation (CPR) and volume resuscitation may be inadequate to restore perfusion. In selected cases, resuscitative left thoracotomy in the ED may be beneficial and should be considered as a potentially life-saving maneuver. ED thoracotomy allows several goals to be accomplished, including pericardiotomy for release of cardiac tamponade, open cardiac massage (which is superior to closed chest compression in establishing perfusion, particularly in hypovolemia), aortic cross-clamping to direct blood flow to the heart and brain while diminishing abdominal blood loss, intracardiac administration of resuscitative drugs, direct compression of intrathoracic hemorrhage, and potential relief of air embolism. This procedure should be considered in penetrating trauma victims who lose vital signs shortly prior to arrival or in the emergency department. Patients with pericardial tamponade who are too unstable for transport to the operating room are candidates for ED thoracotomy as well. Patients with prolonged cardiac arrest, massive blunt trauma with prehospital cardiac arrest, or pulseless electrical activity have essentially no hope for survival and should not undergo ED thoracotomy. ED thoracotomy should not be performed unless a surgeon capable of managing complex truncal injuries is available, as the patient will require immediate transfer to the operating room if vital signs are restored.

ABDOMINAL INJURY

Background

The development of trauma and emergency medical systems (EMS) over the last several decades has improved outcome from abdominal trauma. However, these systems continue to develop and improve. In 2009, during the annual running of the bulls celebration in Pamplona, Spain, four runners were gored by bulls with a 25% fatality rate even with immediate transport to the operating theater. However, structured EMS and trauma systems do significantly improve outcomes. In 1978, West and Trunkey compared trauma-related mortality in two California counties. At the time, San Francisco County had an organized trauma system with a regional trauma center while Orange County did not and transported patients to the nearest hospital. The study showed the lack of an organized trauma system or trauma center in Orange County in 1978 resulted in 10 preventable deaths from internal abdominal hemorrhage. Today, with structured trauma systems and destination criteria for trauma centers, as well as verification and designation by the American College of Surgeons and many state health departments, mortality figures for blunt abdominal trauma have equalized across the country.

Historically, abdominal trauma has been divided into two groups, penetrating and blunt. Penetrating trauma includes everything from low-energy and low-velocity stab wounds and impalement to high-energy and high-velocity gunshot wounds from military style assault weapons. Blunt trauma includes falls, assaults, crush injuries, industrial injuries and motor vehicle crashes. A combination of the two types is being seen more frequently with the proliferation of explosive devices, both in wartime and as acts of terrorism. While British and Israeli surgeons have significant historical and current experience with this type of traumatic injury, it is only recently that American surgeons treating casualties in the Afghan and Iraqi conflicts have been exposed to this third classification of abdominal injury.

From a triage perspective, unexplained hypotension in an injured patient requires immediate consideration of intra-abdominal injury. Intra-abdominal hemorrhage is a life-threatening problem and represents a significant dimension of the "C" for circulation in the primary survey: Rapid diagnosis and treatment of intra-abdominal hemorrhage is critical, as operative intervention is often required.

Anatomical Considerations

From a surgical perspective, the abdominal cavity is more than just the container for the solid and hollow abdominal viscera. It is a mobile "black box" that comprises more than 70% of the torso. In nonpregnant patients, the diaphragm can extend as high as the nipple level with the abdominal viscera in the chest. The lower limits of the abdominal cavity are the upper thigh at the groin crease and the perineum (Figure 9-10). The abdomen is divided into anatomical subunits to help facilitate the diagnostic workup of traumatic injuries. The "anterior abdomen" is defined as extending from the nipple line superiorly to the groin creases inferiorly and laterally to the anterior axillary line. The region between the anterior and posterior axillary lines is defined as the flank, and the area between the posterior axillary lines is defined as the back. Injuries to any of these areas can involve the internal abdominal

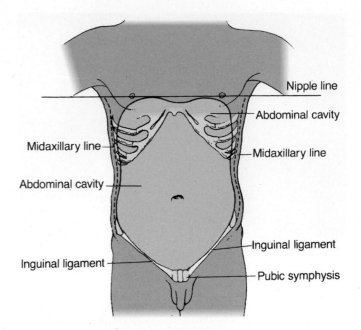

FIGURE 9-10. Surface landmarks of the abdominal cavity.

organs or vasculature resulting in hemorrhage and risk of death. The abdominal contents are partially protected by the rigid bony rib cage, the pelvis, and the lumbar spine as well as the abdominal wall musculature. Another anatomical consideration is the relative position of the hollow and solid viscera in the peritoneal cavity itself. The pancreas, kidneys, bladder, aorta, inferior vena cava, duodenum, and portions of the colon and rectum are retroperitoneal in position. The location of these organs affects injury patterns observed in both blunt and penetrating trauma.

In addition to position, the volume and size of an organ will determine its risk of injury in penetrating trauma. Penetrating trauma in the third trimester of pregnancy frequently affects the uterus and fetus. Penetrating abdominal trauma in young males most frequently injures small bowel and mesentery. In rapid deceleration, which may be incurred during a motor vehicle crash, the spleen and liver will move faster than small bowel and colon resulting in a higher chance of injury in these situations.

Initial Evaluation

The history and mechanism of a traumatic injury are extremely important in aiding determination of the relative risk and location of significant organ injury. This is frequently provided by prehospital personnel, so it is important in the initial resuscitation to allow paramedics time to provide this report. This can be safely done in 30 to 60 seconds with very little morbidity to the patient, and critical information regarding injury mechanism, restraint use, loss of consciousness, and hemodynamic status may be gleaned. After this report, the primary survey takes precedence. During the initial evaluation and resuscitation, additional insights into the presence of possible abdominal injury may be found. A blunt rupture of the diaphragm may be clinically suspected by the presence of respiratory distress, a scaphoid abdomen and bowel sounds in the chest.

The abdominal exam starts with exposure of the torso and extremities. Visual examination of the exposed abdomen, flanks, and back provide important information. Visual

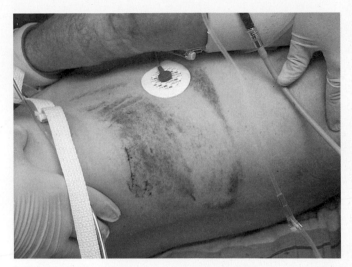

FIGURE 9-11. Blunt torso trauma with extensive contusion of the flank, associated with severe intra-abdominal injuries.

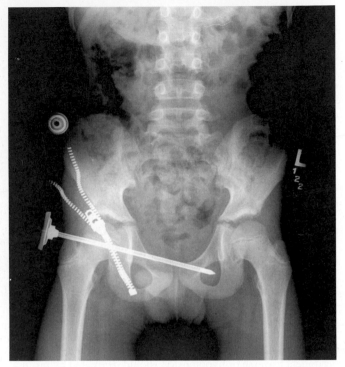

FIGURE 9-12. Penetrating trauma with impaled foreign body. Plain x-ray revealed trajectory concerning for peritoneal penetration and pelvic organ injury.

documentation of old scars, bruising, puncture wounds, lacerations, asymmetry, and distension all provide insight into what may be injured underneath the abdominal wall. It is important to remember that complete visualization of the flank and back are part of the abdominal exam in trauma, especially in cases of penetrating trauma (Figure 9-11).

There is general agreement that the palpation portion of the abdominal exam in trauma patients may be unreliable. This is, in part, due to the altered mental status created by alcohol, recreational drug use, head injury, or shock seen frequently in trauma patients. This does not mean it should not be done however. Palpation may reveal focal or diffuse tenderness, signs of peritoneal irritation, distension due to intra-abdominal hemorrhage, and fascial and muscular defects in the abdominal wall. Lateral and anteroposterior compression of the pelvis should be performed, looking for pelvic bony instability in any victim of blunt or explosive trauma. As a reminder, all of these conditions can be present but may not be initially noted on the first exam or by the first examiner for numerous reasons. Secondary and tertiary abdominal exams should be performed to minimize the risk of missed injury. Digital rectal examination should be performed in cases of penetrating abdominal trauma, and when pelvic fracture is suspected.

Adjunctive Diagnostic Tools

If there is no evidence of urethral injury or prostatic elevation on rectal exam, the insertion of an indwelling Foley urinary catheter will help guide fluid resuscitation and reveal hematuria from renal or bladder injuries. A supine abdominal x-ray of the abdomen and pelvis is often useful to determine the presence and location of bullets or other foreign bodies in hemodynamically stable patients with penetrating trauma, as these x-rays may aid in operative planning (Figure 9-12). **Diagnostic peritoneal lavage** (DPL) has historically been a rapid and reliable way of determining if intra-abdominal bleeding is present and causing hypotension in the blunt trauma patient. This procedure, which involves insertion of a catheter into the peritoneal cavity under local anesthesia, is an extremely sensitive test for intraperitoneal hemorrhage. Due to its invasive nature, however, DPL has been replaced in many situations by FAST. FAST evaluates for free fluid in the abdomen or pericardium using ultrasonographic views of the

right and left upper quadrants, heart, and pelvis (Figure 9-13). At many trauma centers, FAST is considered an extension of the bedside abdominal examination. It has been proven accurate under many conditions, and may be reliably performed by surgeons and emergency physicians, as well as radiologists.

CT of the abdomen has dramatically changed the evaluation of abdominal trauma. Continual advancement in the technology since its inception has made it the gold standard of diagnosis of abdominal injury in the trauma patient. It is usually performed in hemodynamically stable blunt trauma patients but also has utility in select penetrating trauma situations, which will be discussed later. The sensitivity and specificity of contrast-enhanced CT is unsurpassed when compared to other modalities. Newer multidetector scanners not only provide

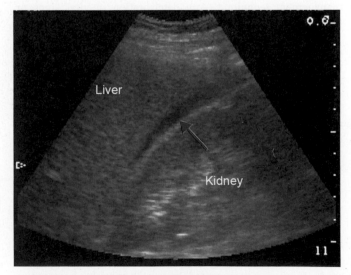

FIGURE 9-13. Positive FAST examination. Hypoechoic (dark) blood is noted in Morison's pouch between the liver and right kidney.

more detail but also are much quicker than older devices. CT angiography can be obtained less invasively and more rapidly than conventional angiography, yet with similar diagnostic accuracy. Many European trauma centers are now performing total body scans in severely injured patients and note fewer missed injuries when this technique is used. Other authors have advocated restraint, however, due to increased radiation exposure and the risk of subsequent radiation-induced malignancy developing decades after exposure.

Operative Care

A hypotensive victim of blunt abdominal trauma who does not respond to volume resuscitation or who responds transiently is considered to have an intra-abdominal source of bleeding until proven otherwise under most circumstances. On rare occasions, a spinal cord or neurologic injury will cause hypotension but in trauma patients this is more frequently due to uncontrolled intra-abdominal hemorrhage. This situation requires rapid transfer to the operating room for surgical correction of the cause of bleeding. In blunt trauma, injuries to the spleen or liver are the most frequent causes of exsanguinating hemorrhage.

The algorithm for penetrating trauma is similar but not identical. Gunshot wounds of the abdomen with clear evidence of peritoneal traverse or hypotension should be treated by prompt exploratory laparotomy, as the incidence of visceral injury is extremely high. Bullets may not travel in a straight line and one should never assume that two external gunshot wounds connect in a direct line. CT of right upper quadrant abdominal gunshot wounds in hemodynamically stable patients has been used successfully to screen for observation versus operative intervention, but the gold standard remains operative exploration. Additionally, stable patients with tangential gunshot wounds and low suspicion for peritoneal violation may be assessed by CT. In these patients CT allows visualization of the bullet tract in relation to the peritoneal cavity and abdominal viscera, thus minimizing the risk of nontherapeutic operative exploration. Low-velocity injury to the abdomen from knives or ice picks can be screened by local wound exploration but any penetration of the peritoneum mandates further evaluation or observation. In stable patients with knife wounds of the anterior abdomen and no signs of peritoneal irritation, careful observation with serial examinations over a 12- to 24-hour period is a legitimate management technique. Any deterioration in vital signs or abdominal examination mandates urgent operative exploration.

Penetrating flank wounds and back wounds from firearms are managed like abdominal wounds but CT plays a larger role in accurate diagnosis in stable patients. Penetrating trauma to these regions incurs retroperitoneal organ injury more frequently, and CT with IV, oral, and rectal contrast (also known as triple contrast CT) helps screen stable patients who may not need operative intervention. Common sense always dictates that any hypotensive patient with a penetrating wound in the abdomen, flank, or back undergo emergent exploratory laparotomy to diagnose and repair injury.

INJURY TO SPECIFIC ORGANS

Liver

Blunt liver injuries are graded from I to VI in severity, with grade I injuries represented by small capsular hematomas or parenchymal lacerations, and grade VI injuries resulting

TABLE 9-4		Liver Injury Scale
Grade[a]		**Injury Description**
I	Hematoma	Subcapsular, nonexpanding, <10% surface area
	Laceration	Capsular tear, nonbleeding, <1 cm depth
II	Hematoma	Subcapsular, nonexpanding, 10%–50% surface area
		Intraparenchymal, nonexpanding, <10 cm diameter
	Laceration	Capsular tear, active bleeding; 1–3 cm parenchymal depth, <10 cm in length
III	Hematoma	Subcapsular, >50% surface area or expanding; ruptured subcapsular hematoma with active bleeding; intraparenchymal hematoma >10 cm or expanding
	Laceration	>3 cm parenchymal depth
IV	Hematoma	Ruptured intraparenchymal hematoma with active bleeding
	Laceration	Parenchymal disruption involving 25%–75% of hepatic lobe or 1–3 segments within a single lobe
V	Laceration	Parenchymal disruption involving >75% of hepatic lobe or >3 segments within a single lobe.
	Vascular	Juxtahepatic venous injuries (i.e., retrohepatic vena cava/central major hepatic veins
VI	Vascular	Hepatic avulsion

[a]Advance one grade for multiple injuries up to grade III.

from hepatic avulsion (Table 9-4). Most liver injuries are self-limiting in nature. They bleed acutely but most stop without operative intervention. CT scanning is the diagnostic modality of choice, providing anatomic detail and accurate grading of injury (Figure 9-14). Evidence of ongoing bleeding such as contrast extravasation on CT can be managed in the interventional radiology suite with selective angioembolization of bleeding hepatic arterial branches. The hepatic artery only supplies 20% to 25% of the blood flow to the liver, so hepatic necrosis is a rare complication of this treatment. Higher-grade liver injuries, including those involving the hepatic veins or

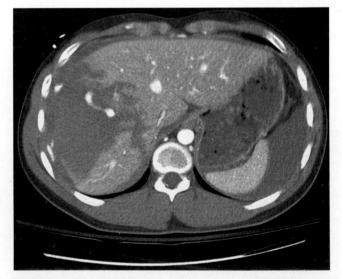

FIGURE 9-14. CT scan of the abdomen in a patient with blunt abdominal trauma and extensive hepatic injury.

retrohepatic vena cava, may result in massive hemorrhage requiring urgent operative intervention and damage control surgical techniques, as outlined in a subsequent section.

Gallbladder

The gallbladder is rarely injured in either blunt or penetrating trauma. Gallbladder injuries are best treated by cholecystectomy and are generally not repaired.

Spleen

The spleen is frequently injured in blunt abdominal trauma, especially deceleration injuries in adults or direct impact in children (e.g., bicycle handlebar or assault). Injuries are graded I to VI with higher grades more likely to require intervention (Table 9-5). Splenic salvage is the goal but must be balanced with the risk of bleeding and death in each patient. CT scan is diagnostic and facilitates planning of nonoperative management (Figure 9-15). Most low-grade splenic injuries can be managed nonoperatively by careful observation and serial monitoring of hemoglobin and hematocrit. Recurrent hemorrhage or development of peritonitis signals failure of nonoperative management and should be followed by expeditious laparotomy. Splenic injury with active bleeding and hypotension upon presentation generally requires operative management. Surgical options include total splenectomy or splenorrhaphy. The most common cause of postsplenectomy bleeding is an unligated short gastric vessel or a surgical knot that slips after resuscitation and normalization of blood volume. This can be minimized by examining the greater curvature of the stomach with a systolic pressure of at least 100 mm Hg in the operating room. Hemodynamically stable patients with IV contrast extravasation noted on CT may benefit from angioembolization of the bleeding splenic artery branches as a technique for splenic salvage (Figure 9-16). Splenectomized patients should undergo postoperative vaccination for encapsulated organisms such as pneumococcus and meningococcus to minimize the rare but

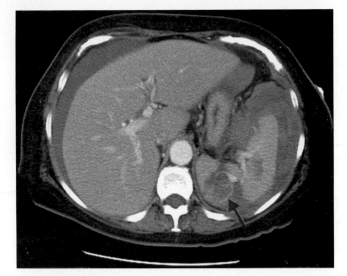

FIGURE 9-15. Splenic injury, as demonstrated by CT of the abdomen. Diffuse hemoperitoneum is present.

potentially fatal complication of overwhelming postsplenectomy infection.

Pancreas

Injury to the pancreas is relatively uncommon due to its protected retroperitoneal location. In severe blunt trauma, the body of the pancreas may be compressed against the vertebral column, resulting in transection. This usually requires operative distal pancreatectomy. Major injuries of the pancreatic head can present challenging operative dilemmas. Initial management is usually performed in a damage control setting and consists of hemorrhage control and drainage of the injury. Small injuries of the pancreas not involving the main pancreatic duct may be managed nonoperatively. Stab wounds to the back can injure pancreatic parenchyma and ducts. Evaluation

TABLE 9-5	Splenic Injury Scale	
Grade[a]		**Injury Description**
I	Hematoma	Subcapsular, nonexpanding, <10% surface area
	Laceration	Capsular tear, nonbleeding, <1 cm depth
II	Hematoma	Subcapsular, nonexpanding, 10%–50% surface area
		Intraparenchymal, nonexpanding, <5 cm diameter
	Laceration	Capsular tear, active bleeding; 1–3 cm parenchymal depth that does not involve a trabecular vessel
III	Hematoma	Subcapsular, >50% surface area or expanding; ruptured subcapsular hematoma with active bleeding; intraparenchymal hematoma >5 cm or expanding
	Laceration	>3 cm parenchymal depth or involving trabecular vessels
IV	Hematoma	Ruptured intraparenchymal hematoma with active bleeding
	Laceration	Laceration involving segmental or hilar vessels producing major devascularization (>25% of spleen)
V	Laceration	Completely shattered spleen
	Vascular	Hilar vascular injury which devascularizes spleen

[a]Advance one grade for multiple injuries up to grade III.

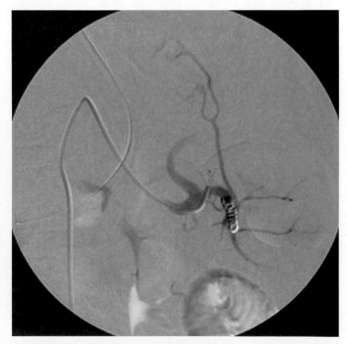

FIGURE 9-16. Angiographic embolization of splenic hemorrhage after blunt abdominal trauma. Metallic coils have been placed within the splenic artery.

includes CT scanning and endoscopic retrograde cholangio-pancreatography (ERCP).

Stomach

In blunt trauma, the full stomach may rupture, requiring urgent repair. Penetrating trauma requires operative repair as well. Gastric injury frequently coexists with diaphragmatic injury, discussed below. Bloody nasogastric aspirate in the emergency department should raise suspicion for gastric injury, though gastritis or ingested blood from maxillofacial injuries may cause this finding as well.

Diaphragm

Blunt rupture of the diaphragm usually starts at the gastroesophageal (GE) junction outward into the tendinous portion of the central diaphragm. Occasionally, blunt injury may result in complete avulsion of the posterior muscular insertion (Figure 9-17). Standard repair is done with interrupted or running permanent suture to minimize the risk of recurrence or further tearing due to its constant mobility with respiratory efforts. Care should be taken to avoid branches of the phrenic nerve when possible.

Low velocity penetrating injury to the diaphragm can occur without pneumothorax or evidence of peritoneal injury. Left sided diaphragmatic injuries are particularly concerning, due to the risk of development of diaphragmatic hernia and visceral incarceration. In addition, left sided diaphragmatic wounds are commonly associated with injuries of the stomach, colon, spleen, and small intestine. Unfortunately, injuries of the diaphragm are not readily diagnosed by FAST or CT. For these reasons, there should be a low threshold for laparoscopic or thoracoscopic evaluation of patients with left sided penetrating thoracoabdominal injuries. Small injuries of the right diaphragm may be managed without surgical repair, as the liver is protective against significant herniation in most cases.

Kidneys

The kidneys are relatively protected from injury due to their high retroperitoneal location, and encasement within Gerota's fascia. Blunt injury rarely requires operative intervention unless there is ureteral injury or calyceal leak of urine. Nephrectomy may be necessary in cases of massive destruction or complex hilar injury. Penetrating injuries are self-limiting under most circumstances unless renal artery or vein is involved. Foley catheter drainage should be maintained for 7 to 10 days, or until hematuria resolves.

Small Intestine and Mesentery

Blunt perforation of the small intestine may occur as the result of compression and resultant blowout, or by avulsion of the bowel from its mesenteric blood supply (Figure 9-18). Contusion to bowel wall may not perforate immediately, and concern for bowel injury mandates observation and serial abdominal exams if suspected. An abdominal "seatbelt sign" increases risk of this injury. Mesenteric tears with hemorrhage from arcade vessels can occur in deceleration injury and should be suspected when CT shows hemoperitoneum but no liver or spleen injury. The small bowel and mesentery are frequently injured by penetrating trauma from knife and gunshot wounds. Repair is generally straightforward and involves one layer closure with absorbable or nonabsorbable suture. Stapled repair or resection with anastomosis is appropriate as well.

Colon

Low-velocity knife injury or bullet injury to the large intestine can often be repaired primarily. More extensive wounds, including those that devascularize a segment of colon, may be successfully managed by resection with primary reanastomosis. Colostomy is seldom required in colonic trauma, with the notable exception of rectal injuries. Injuries to the rectum below the peritoneal reflection are best managed by fecal diversion to avoid perineal sepsis and allow the injury to heal. In addition, patients with colonic trauma and multiple other injuries or profound shock may be considered candidates for temporary diverting colostomy due to their increased risk for anastomotic breakdown.

Damage Control

In serious injury with shock and hypotension, it may not be possible or advantageous to attempt to repair all wounds at

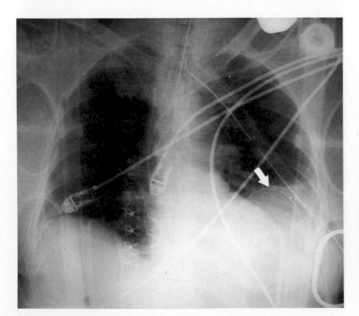

FIGURE 9-17. **Blunt rupture of the left diaphragm.** The nasogastric tube is visualized in the left hemithorax (*arrow*).

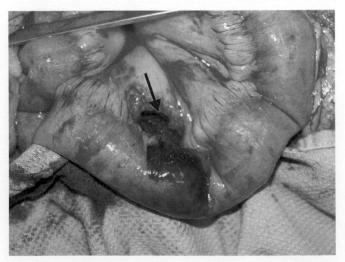

FIGURE 9-18. **Blunt abdominal trauma with avulsion injury of the small intestine from its mesentery.**

the initial operation. These patients are prone to developing a "lethal triad" of hypothermia, acidosis, and coagulopathy, which is worsened by prolonged operation and is almost universally fatal if the process is unable to be halted. Damage control technique is performed to control immediate life-threatening hemorrhage by packing of the abdominal space with laparotomy pads, or by direct ligation or repair of bleeding sites, and organ removal (i.e., splenectomy). Injured sections of small bowel or colon may be resected but not anastomosed to minimize time in the operating room. Thus, the fundamental tenets of damage control surgery are control of massive hemorrhage and control of enteric contamination of the peritoneal cavity, while attempting to minimize hypothermia, acidosis, and coagulopathy. Damage control procedures usually take 60 to 90 minutes and the patient is then transferred to the intensive care unit for resuscitation, rewarming, and correction of coagulopathy. Once stabilized, the patient is returned to the operating room for removal of hemostatic packing, restoration of gastrointestinal continuity, and definitive repair of other injuries. This step usually occurs in 12 to 36 hours after the initial abbreviated laparotomy.

Abdominal Compartment Syndrome

Aggressive crystalloid volume resuscitation and severe hemorrhagic shock will sometimes result in retroperitoneal and intra-abdominal swelling and intra-abdominal pressures above 30 mm Hg. This rise in abdominal pressure can compromise blood flow to the abdominal viscera, producing ischemia and eventual necrosis if left uncorrected. Upward displacement of the diaphragm causes pulmonary failure and increased airway pressures. Untreated abdominal compartment syndrome results in multiple organ dysfunction syndrome (MODS) and is commonly fatal. This situation may also occur in the setting of pelvic fracture or retroperitoneal hemorrhage. The clinical triad of increased airway pressures, decreased urine output, and elevated abdominal pressure constitutes abdominal compartment syndrome. Diagnosis is accomplished by measuring the pressure within the decompressed urinary bladder, as the dome of the bladder acts as a passive diaphragm and transmits the pressure within the peritoneal cavity. Treatment is achieved by opening the abdominal cavity via a laparotomy incision. This allows prompt decompression and relieves cephalad pressure on the diaphragm and thoracic cavity. Renal perfusion is restored, and urinary output promptly increases. The abdominal cavity and fascia can often be closed after swelling of the viscera has subsided but occasionally prolonged wound care, skin grafting, or complex closure techniques are required (Figure 9-19).

PELVIC FRACTURES

The bony pelvis is made up of the ilium, ischium, pubis, and sacrum, which are connected by strong ligamentous attachments. Isolated fractures to the pelvis can occur, such as to the pubic ramus or to the acetabular joint with hip dislocation. These injuries typically do not cause instability to the pelvic ring, and are rarely associated with life-threatening hemorrhage. Significant force is typically required to break the large bones of the pelvis, such as in motor vehicle collisions, pedestrian-vehicle collisions, and falls from great heights. For the more severe pelvic fractures, the fracture patterns are typically classified by mechanism of injury: Anterior–posterior (AP)

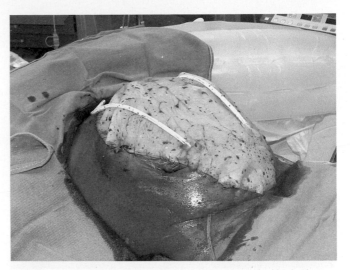

FIGURE 9-19. Abdominal compartment syndrome treated with plastic temporary abdominal closure.

compression, lateral compression (LC), or vertical shear. Of the three forces of transmitted energy, the LC mechanism (Figure 9-20) is the most common and the most stable as it is less likely to lead to ligamentous disruption at the sacroiliac joint. The AP compression fracture pattern (Figure 9-21) is also known as the open book pelvic fracture. The symphysis pubis is disrupted and the iliac wings open leading to variable amounts of sacroiliac ligamentous disruption. The appearance of the pelvis on initial radiologic imaging does not necessarily indicate the full extent of the distraction of the pelvic bones that occurred on initial impact. The least common pelvic ring disruption but most unstable is the vertical shear injury pattern, which is caused by a severe upward force that may disrupt the hemipelvis from the spine, or create a fracture of the iliac wing (Figure 9-22). This fracture pattern is often associated with other serious abdominal, pelvic, or vascular injuries.

Pelvic fractures may be suspected based on history and physical findings. If the patient is conscious, pain is usually present, particularly with movement. There may be bruising to the lower abdomen, hips, buttocks, or lower back. The bony pelvis should be manually palpated gently to illicit tenderness, deformity (such as a widened symphysis pubis), or movement

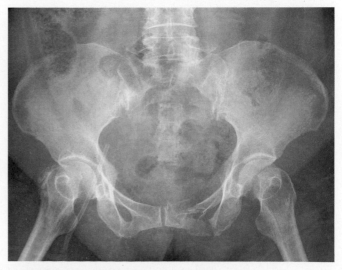

FIGURE 9-20. Pubic rami fractures from LC injury.

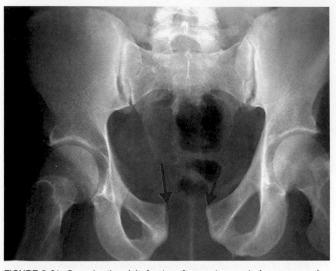

FIGURE 9-21. Open book pelvic fracture from anteroposterior compression injury.

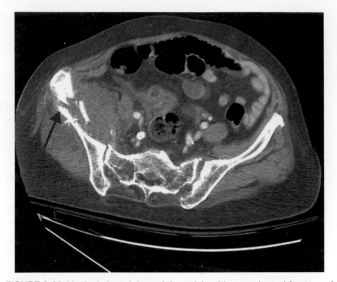

FIGURE 9-22. Vertical shear injury of the pelvis with comminuted fracture of the right iliac wing.

with gentle compression. Careful examination should include inspection for open wounds in the perineum, which would signify an open pelvic fracture. The lower extremities should be examined for alignment, length discrepancy, and pelvic pain with movement. In symptomatic patients, a plain x-ray of the pelvis is indicated to identify an unstable pelvic fracture or other pelvic abnormality, such as a hip dislocation prior to movement of the patient. CT scan of the pelvis offers a means of evaluating the bony pelvis, as well as the internal pelvic structures. Hematomas associated with pelvic fractures can range from small to quite large. Visible extravasation of intravenous contrast in a pelvic hematoma associated with an unstable pelvis is a sign of ongoing hemorrhage. Additional radiologic studies may be indicated to evaluate the genitourinary tract and exclude associated injuries.

Hemorrhage associated with a pelvic fracture can be from the bony surface, presacral venous plexus, or in approximately 10% of patients, an arterial source. Due to the severe mechanism associated with pelvic ring disruption, rapid assessment of the patient should be done to rule out other sources of blood loss, such as intrathoracic, intraperitoneal, retroperitoneal, long bone fractures, or external losses. Pelvic bleeding from the bone or small veins can be minimized by stabilizing the pelvis by one of several means: wrapping a sheet tightly around the pelvis, a pelvic binder, or pelvic external fixator. These methods work best for AP compression injuries to restore the alignment of the pelvic bones and offer some stability so that the patient can be moved in the course of their early treatment. Ongoing bleeding from an arterial source requires intervention. A critical decision is necessary in the hypotensive patient with a major disruption of the pelvis. DPL still has a role in determining whether the life-threatening hemorrhage is intraperitoneal or pelvic, as there are very different treatment options for each. As a general rule, surgical exploration is not the best option for pelvic bleeding as the small pelvic arterial branches are difficult to find in a large pelvic hematoma, and surgical exploration tends to release tamponaded venous bleeding. If the patient is taken to surgery for other injuries, such as a ruptured spleen, a pelvic hematoma can be packed off with laparotomy pads, offering a means of direct pressure internally. Care must be taken not to displace the pelvic ring further outward. Pelvic blood flow and

collaterals are extensive and angiography is both diagnostic in delineating the source of the bleeding as well as therapeutic, in that bleeding arterial vessels may be selectively embolized. Movement of the unstable pelvic bones can disrupt the pelvic arterial supply, which is based on branches of the internal iliac artery. Definitive arterial hemorrhage control is best obtained with angiographic embolization. CT scan of the pelvis in the stable patient offers a means of directing the angiographer to the most likely area of arterial injury.

Lower genitourinary injuries can occur with pelvic fractures due to the close proximity of the bladder to the pubic bones; they are usually suspected due to hematuria. The bladder may be injured by both penetrating and blunt trauma. Blunt mechanisms lead to two types of bladder injury, intraperitoneal and extraperitoneal. Extraperitoneal bladder injury is usually associated with pelvic fractures, where a bone fragment, typically the pubic bone, perforates the nearby bladder. The diagnosis is made by a cystogram demonstrating extravasation below the peritoneal reflection. Treatment is bladder decompression with a Foley urinary catheter until the laceration heals (typically 7 to 10 days). The bladder can also rupture intraperitoneally, which occurs with blunt force to the lower abdominal wall with a distended bladder. This injury may or may not be associated with pelvic fractures. Diagnosis can be made by cystogram or CT scan showing urine contrast extravasation into the peritoneal cavity. Intraperitoneal bladder injury requires surgical exploration and repair. The male urethra is also at risk of injury with disruption of the symphysis pubis. The female urethra, being shorter and straighter, is rarely injured. Typical signs associated with urethral injury are scrotal hematoma, blood at the urethral meatus, and a high-riding or nonpalpable prostate gland on rectal exam. A retrograde urethrogram should be done to evaluate for injury prior to passage of a Foley catheter in these cases. The location of injury, as evidenced by contrast extravasation on urethrogram is usually at the prostatic urethra. Blind passage of a catheter in a patient with a partial urethral tear can lead to worsening of the injury or complete transection. Inability to pass a catheter or identification of a urethral injury will require urologic consultation for definitive management. The urethra can also be injured directly with penetrating trauma or blunt force mechanisms such as straddle injuries. Bilateral pubic rami fractures can also occur with a straddle mechanism and have a common association with extraperitoneal bladder injury.

PENETRATING NECK TRAUMA

The neck is a highly complex anatomic region with critical vascular, neurologic, and aerodigestive structures concentrated within a very small area. Penetrating injuries to this region of the body are often the result of knife and gunshot wounds. Any wound that violates the platysma muscle carries a risk of injury to the great vessels, trachea, esophagus, and spinal cord, and therefore requires further assessment. For purposes of clinical evaluation and management of penetrating wounds, the anterior neck (from the midline to the anterior border of the sternocleidomastoid muscle) is divided into three zones as illustrated in Figure 9-23. Zone I extends from the sternal notch to the inferior border of the cricoid cartilage. Zone II is the area from the cricoid cartilage to angle the mandible. Zone III includes the area of the distal neck, which is from the angle of the mandible to the base of the skull.

The management of penetrating injuries has largely evolved from military experience. During World War I, nonoperative management was the standard approach but had an associated high mortality due to missed injury. During World War II, the military's policy for management of these highly fatal wounds was mandatory surgical exploration, which resulted in a significant reduction in mortality. This experience led to broad acceptance of mandatory exploration for all zone II penetrating wounds in civilian practice. During the next two decades, numerous studies reported a high rate of negative or nontherapeutic neck exploration with this policy. A number of authors

began to advocate returning to a policy of selective management guided by hard signs and symptoms of injury to the vital structures to reduce the rate of nontherapeutic exploration.

Initial evaluation of patients with penetrating neck wounds is determined by the physical examination and physiologic status. Shock or hard signs of injury to any of the vital structures in any of the three zones mandates immediate operative exploration and repair. In the hemodynamically stable patient, a more selective approach is taken for injuries to both zone I and zone III due to the difficulty in examining and operatively exposing structures in these areas. Injuries in zone I will typically require a median sternotomy for adequate exposure and repair of vascular injuries of the thoracic inlet. Similarly, operative exposure to zone III might necessitate disarticulation of the mandible, an osteotomy of the angle of the mandible, or resection of the styloid process to optimally manage a high internal carotid vascular injury at the base of the skull.

Controversy continues to center around hemodynamically stable patients with an injury located in zone II and no signs or symptoms suggestive of a major injury to a vital structure. Traditional evaluation includes angiography, bronchoscopy, and esophagoscopy in conjunction with esophagography. Other strategies are then directed at specific identified entries.

There is a growing body of literature to support the use of contrast-enhanced CT for evaluation of penetrating neck injury. Several prospective studies evaluating the use of CT angiography in penetrating neck trauma have demonstrated a sensitivity approaching 100% and a negative predictive value over 90%. One of the recognized limitations of the use of CT in the evaluation of penetrating neck trauma is its difficulty in

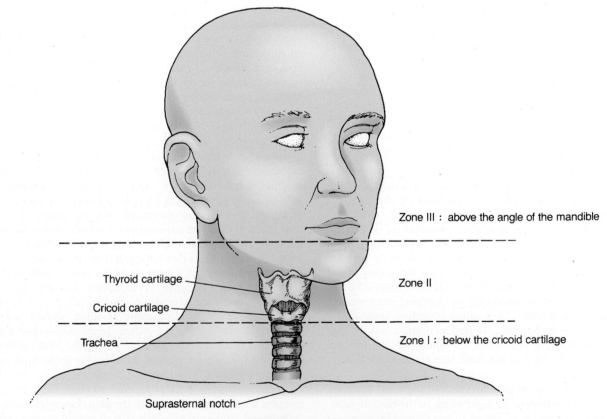

FIGURE 9-23. Zones of the neck.

detecting the trajectory of knife wounds. Specifically, small pharyngoesophageal wounds are difficult to detect with CT scan. Despite these limitations, the literature supports an increasing role for the use of CT in evaluating stable patients with a penetrating wound to any zone of the anterior neck. This imaging technique is an acceptable method to determine trajectory and thereby triage patients to the operating room, for further diagnostic studies, or observation with serial examination.

Aerodigestive Tract Injury

Aerodigestive tract injuries are seen in 10% of penetrating trauma to the neck. Optimal airway management is paramount. The translaryngeal endotracheal approach remains the best option, particularly when performed by skilled practitioners. The need for a surgical airway (cricothyroidotomy) should always be considered in any patient who might have a difficult airway. Tracheostomy should only be considered when there is a suspicion for a laryngotracheal separation after a careful translaryngeal endotracheal intubation has failed.

The preferred method of evaluating for an injury to the larynx and trachea involves a combination of direct laryngoscopy and bronchoscopy. Concomitant injuries are frequent; therefore diagnostic evaluation of possible arterial and esophageal injuries is imperative. Laryngeal injuries are classified as supraglottic, glottic, and subglottic. Supraglottic injuries typically result in a depression of the superior notch of the thyroid cartilage associated with a vertical fracture of the thyroid cartilage. Disruption of the thyroid cartilage results in a glottic injury. An injury to the subglottic region usually involves the lower thyroid and cricoid cartilage. Early definitive repair for any laryngeal injury should be the goal due to the higher incidence of stricture formation with delayed repair. Tracheal wounds should be repaired in one layer with absorbable suture. When there is an associated esophageal or arterial injury, the risk of fistulization between the two repairs is reduced by interposing a vascularized pedicle of omohyoid or sternocleidomastoid muscle. Operative management of cervical esophageal injuries requires meticulous debridement, a two layer closure of the wound, and closed suction drainage. Injuries limited to the hypopharyngeal region can be safely managed conservatively including a nasogastric tube for feeding and an empiric course of parenteral antibiotics.

Vascular Injury

When a carotid artery injury is found, several therapeutic options exist. The approach is dictated by the patient's hemodynamic status and neurologic assessment, as well as the institutional resources available. Observation or expectant management is advocated for patients who are comatose. Simple ligation of the artery is an option for those patients presenting with exsanguination or when a temporary shunt cannot be placed. The carotid artery should be repaired when the patient has an intact neurologic or changing examination. Repair may be performed by a direct operative approach or via interventional techniques. Angiointervention may be particularly applicable in high zone III injuries to the internal carotid artery at the base of the skull, due to the surgical inaccessibility of this area.

Injuries to the internal jugular vein are the most common vascular injuries with penetrating trauma. In the hemodynamically unstable patient, any venous injury should be managed by simple ligation. Otherwise, an injury to the internal jugular vein should be repaired by lateral venorrhaphy or patch venoplasty. Despite the method of repair, subsequent thrombosis is common. Massive air embolism is a rare but highly fatal complication associated with major venous injuries. A high index of suspicion needs to be maintained to diagnose this complication.

Spinal Cord Injury

Approximately 10% of penetrating neck trauma victims have an associated spinal cord or brachial plexus injury. Injuries to the spinal cord above the fourth cervical vertebrae are associated with a high mortality rate. There is no evidence to support the use of steroids in the management of penetrating spinal cord injuries.

EXTREMITY TRAUMA

Extremity injuries are quite common in blunt and penetrating trauma and may range in severity from trivial to life threatening. During the primary survey, potentially lethal injuries such as major vascular injuries, open fractures, crush injuries, and near amputations should be identified and addressed. History obtained from prehospital personnel may imply significant blood loss at the scene or in transit, and may help expedite resuscitative measures. Exsanguinating hemorrhage from major vascular injury should be treated initially with direct pressure, rather than tourniquets. Secondary survey includes a detailed neurovascular examination of each extremity, with careful evaluation of peripheral pulses, capillary refill time, skin temperature, sensation, motor function, and range of motion. Palpation may elicit tenderness suggestive of fracture or soft tissue injury. Deformity typically is associated with fractures, dislocations, or both.

Vascular injuries can be obvious or occult. The obvious or "hard signs" of acute vascular injury include pulsatile bleeding, an expanding hematoma, bruit, and an extremity that is pale, cool, and pulseless, with paresthesias or paralysis. Hard signs are an indication for operative exploration, and the general time frame for revascularization is within 6 hours. Physical findings that may be suggestive, but not diagnostic for vascular injury, are termed "soft signs." These are nonexpanding hematoma, diminished but present pulses, or absent but returning pulse. Doppler ultrasound provides a useful adjunct to physical examination of the vascular system, and allows calculation of the ankle–brachial index (ABI). The ABI is calculated measuring the systolic blood pressure (by Doppler probe) in an injured lower extremity, then dividing this number by the higher of the systolic readings from the left and right brachial arteries. Normally, this ratio is ≥1; values <0.9 are suggestive of arterial vascular injury or occlusion. In this setting, further diagnostic evaluation with arteriography or CT angiography is usually indicated.

Radiographic imaging is indicated for any extremity deformity, bony tenderness, or joint swelling as part of the secondary survey. Radiographic imaging should not lead to delay in transferring the patient to an appropriate trauma center. If a fracture is identified, typically the joints above and below the fracture are imaged as well, due to the high risk of associated injuries. Fractures are characterized by bony location, comminution, angulation, and whether they are closed or open with communication to the skin. Open fractures lead to bacterial contamination and risk of complications such as wound infection, osteomyelitis, poor bone healing, and poor functional outcome.

While a detailed discussion of extremity fractures falls outside the scope of this chapter, certain basic principles may be universally applied. Splinting of fractures is an important technique that should occur during the secondary survey, or shortly thereafter. Fracture splinting improves pain control, minimizes secondary soft tissue damage, and diminishes bleeding from the soft tissues and bone edges. While reduction of fractures and dislocations is usually accomplished by an orthopedic surgeon, a variety of splints are available for application by nonorthopedic surgeons. These may be simple cardboard or plaster constructs that can be easily applied prior to transport for diagnostic studies. It is important to note that femur fractures may be associated with significant blood loss into the soft tissues of the thigh, and should be addressed with appropriate resuscitative measures, including transfusion of blood as necessary. Patients with bilateral femur fractures may present with shock, even in the absence of other injuries. Neurovascular status should be reassessed before and after manipulation of the injured extremity. Open or compound fractures are potentially limb-threatening injuries that should be treated by a skilled orthopedic surgeon. Treatment involves prompt operative debridement of devitalized tissue, copious irrigation to remove dirt and other contaminants, fracture reduction, and administration of broad-spectrum intravenous antibiotics. As in other aspects of trauma surgery, a philosophy of damage control or "less is more" has been adopted in patients who are critically ill or who have multiple injuries. Initial management focuses on resuscitation, removal of devitalized tissue, and fracture realignment, rather than definitive operative fixation. External fixators may be applied as a temporizing measure and obviate the need for prolonged procedures or placing hardware in a contaminated field.

Dislocations should be splinted in place for transport. Reduction of the dislocation should be done as soon as possible by an experienced person after radiographic imaging to prevent complications, such as avascular necrosis of the femoral head with hip dislocation. Moderate sedation and intravenous analgesia may be required for reduction of certain dislocations. X-ray imaging is indicated prior to reduction to rule out an associated fracture that might impede reduction. Prolonged dislocation can cause traction injury to nearby nerves and vessels.

Compartment syndrome may occur after blunt or penetrating trauma. In this entity, injury results in muscular swelling and hemorrhage. When this swelling occurs in an unyielding fascial compartment, interstitial pressure rises. In the initial phases, this increase in pressure may diminish venous capillary outflow and worsen cellular injury, resulting in further swelling and interstitial fluid accumulation. Thus begins a vicious cycle, and intracompartmental pressures may continue to rise, eventually choking off arterial inflow. If left uncorrected, compartment syndrome may result in permanent nerve injury or muscle necrosis that may necessitate amputation. The muscular damage associated with compartment syndrome may be associated with myoglobinuria and rhabdomyolysis. Early signs of compartment syndrome include pain, paresthesias, and diminished sensation. The affected compartment is typically swollen and tense. Diminished pulses or capillary refill are late findings and are often associated with irreversible ischemia. Diagnosis is typically made by history and physical examination findings. Direct measurement of compartmental pressures may be accomplished with commercially available devices in cases where diagnostic uncertainty exists. In brain-injured or comatose patients, assessment of physical findings may be more difficult and direct measurement of compartmental pressures should be performed more liberally in this subset. Treatment is prompt operative fasciotomy of the involved compartments. Fasciotomy allows the injured muscle to swell without concomitant increases in pressure. Perfusion is maintained, and secondary damage is minimized. Compartment syndrome may occur in any extremity, but is most commonly associated with crush injuries of the calf, with or without bony fractures.

Myoglobinuria and rhabdomyolysis may occur after significant muscular injury or in the setting of compartment syndrome. Pigment molecules released from damaged muscle cells are directly nephrotoxic and form precipitates in the acidic milieu of the renal tubules. Treatment involves aggressive hydration with isotonic intravenous fluids. Alkalinization of the urine with intravenous sodium bicarbonate and osmotic diuresis with mannitol are adjunctive measures that are of unclear benefit. Debridement of all necrotic tissue is mandatory.

TRAUMA IN PREGNANCY

The leading causes of injury among pregnant women are transportation related, falls, and assault. Motor vehicle collision is the most common mechanism resulting in fetal death, followed by firearms, and then falls. Pregnant women between 15 and 19 years of age are at greatest risk for trauma-related fetal demise.

Young pregnant women also sustain injuries as a result of being assaulted. It is estimated that 10% to 30% of women are physically abused during pregnancy, and of these, 5% are severe enough to result in fetal death. Thus, it is mandatory for all members of the health care team to be versed in recognizing the signs and symptoms of physical abuse. This is a unique opportunity for health care providers to intervene and protect both the mother and fetus.

There are specific anatomic and physiologic changes that occur during pregnancy that may alter the maternal cardiovascular response to injury. At 10 weeks of gestation, the maternal plasma volume begins to expand and increases to 145% of the pregravid volume by full term. Total body sodium increases by 950 mEq, which increases total body water by 6 to 8 L at full term. This hypervolemia of pregnancy frequently masks signs of shock until a loss of 35% of the maternal blood volume occurs. Pregnancy also is associated with increased levels of factors VII, VIII, IX, X, XII, and fibrinogen with a reduction in fibrinolytic activity. This results in a hypercoagulable state, which increases the risk for thromboembolic events.

Cardiac output increases 25% by the end of the first trimester and continues to increase to approximately 6.2 L/min at full term. It is important to recognize that as the uterus enlarges, it compresses the inferior vena cava when the patient is supine. This will decrease venous return and cardiac preload with a resultant decrease in cardiac output.

With hypotension, the patient may experience dizziness, pallor, tachycardia, sweating, and nausea. Turning the mother onto her left side while maintaining spine precautions will displace the gravid uterus from the vena cava with a resultant increase in venous return and cardiac output.

The maternal respiratory system also undergoes changes to address the increased oxygen requirements of pregnancy. The enlarging uterus displaces the diaphragm up to 4 cm cephalad and enlarges the chest diameter by 2 cm. These changes must be considered when performing a tube thoracostomy or thoracentesis.

Gastrointestinal motility, intestinal secretion, and absorption of nutrients are reduced as serum levels of progesterone and estrogen rise throughout the pregnancy. During the latter half of the pregnancy, the angle of the gastroesophageal junction is altered, which displaces the lower esophageal sphincter into the mediastinum. These alterations also reduce the competency of the lower esophageal sphincter, which thereby increases the potential for aspiration as early as the first trimester of gestation. Thus, early insertion of a nasogastric tube will reduce the risk for aspiration.

The priorities for treatment of the injured pregnant patient are the same as those for the nonpregnant patient. Prevention of hypotension when the patient is supine is accomplished by repositioning in order to displace the uterus off the vena cava and aorta. This can be accomplished by three simple maneuvers. Placing the patient in the left lateral decubitus position, the right lateral decubitus position or the knee–chest position when supine. Alternatively, the uterus can be manually displaced to the patient's left side. Since the physiologic hypervolemia of pregnancy may mask the early signs of shock, early crystalloid resuscitation should be initiated even in the normotensive patient. The secondary survey should include a prenatal history and associated comorbid factors. Prior history of preterm labor, placenta previa, and placental abruption are risk factors for recurrence of these conditions. A urine pregnancy test should be obtained in all injured women of childbearing age, and early obstetrical consultation is recommended.

Fetal age can be rapidly estimated by measuring the fundal height on abdominal examination. Abdominal examination may reveal evidence of uterine rupture, as fetal parts may be palpable in this circumstance. A speculum examination should be performed followed by the bimanual examination only if there is no evidence of vaginal bleeding. The examination focuses on the following: vaginal blood, ruptured amniotic membranes, active contractions, a bulging perineum, and an abnormal fetal heart rate or rhythm. If the amniotic sac has ruptured, the umbilical cord can prolapse and result in compression of the umbilical vessels. Drainage of cloudy white or green fluid from the cervical os is indicative of ruptured membranes. This is an obstetrical emergency requiring urgent cesarean section. Bloody amniotic fluid is indicative of either placental abruption or placenta previa. The bulging perineum is caused by pressure from a presenting fetal part. When this occurs during the first trimester, there is a great risk of spontaneous abortion.

Rh typing is essential in the pregnant trauma patient. The Rh antigen is well developed by 6 weeks of gestation, and as little as 0.001 mL of fetal blood can cause sensitization of the Rh negative mother. Therefore, all Rh negative women should receive Rho (D) immune globulin, unless the injury is minor and remote from the uterus. The severity of fetal–maternal hemorrhage may be established by the Kleihauer-Betke test, which involves a peripheral blood smear taken from the mother. It has been suggested that a single dose of Rho (D) immune globulin, administered within 72 hours of injury, is sufficient to provide immune protection in most cases, as most fetal–maternal hemorrhages are <30 mL of blood. Although concern exists for fetal exposure to ionizing radiation, the general rule is to obtain all radiographic tests that would otherwise be indicated for the safety of the mother. This practice is based on the concept that delay in diagnosis and treatment of maternal injury correlates with poor fetal outcome.

In cases of severe trauma in late term pregnancy, perimortem cesarean section may be performed in the ED. This maneuver may be considered in cases of impending or actual maternal cardiac arrest; fetal survival has been reported when performed <4 minutes after loss of maternal vital signs.

PEDIATRIC TRAUMA

Pediatric trauma is the number one cause of death of children, as well as the number one cause of permanent disability in patients under 14 years of age. Although the principles of trauma care are the same for children as with adults, optimal treatment of the injured child requires special knowledge, careful management, and attention to the unique physiology and psychology of the growing child or adolescent. In children over 1 year and under 14 years of age, motor vehicle collisions cause 47% of all pediatric deaths related to injury. Drowning is the second most frequent cause of injury-related death in children, followed by thermal injury.

Although the resuscitation priorities (ABCDE algorithm) are the same for children as for adults, anatomic and physiologic differences require modifications to the approach. Assessment of the child's airway is the first step. Most children do not have preexisting pulmonary disease; thus a room air oxygen saturation >90% generally indicates effective gas exchange. If oxygenation is difficult, then an injury to the lung, a pneumothorax, or aspiration should be considered. In the injured child, hyperventilation is common after traumatic brain injury or shock. With either condition, intubation and mechanical ventilation is appropriate. The injured child who is combative because of hypoxia or emotional distress may also need to be intubated to facilitate further diagnostic testing. Endotracheal intubation in most settings is best managed with a protocol for rapid sequence intubation. The tube diameter can be approximated by either the width of the fingernail or the diameter of the child's fifth finger. An uncuffed orotracheal tube should be used in children <8 years of age since the cricoid ring, which is the narrowest part of the airway, will stabilize the tube. In situations where orotracheal intubation is impossible, needle cricothyroidotomy is preferred in children under 10 years of age in order to avoid injury to the delicate cricoid cartilage with a surgical incision. This may be performed percutaneously with a 14-gauge or 16-gauge intravenous angiocatheter. Nasotracheal intubation is generally not used in small children. A chest x-ray should be obtained to confirm the correct position of the endotracheal tube since a right main stem bronchus intubation is a common complication. The Broselow Pediatric Resuscitation Measuring Tape has become the standard for determining height, weight, and the appropriate size for resuscitative equipment and medication dosing in children. This device is placed on the bed next to the child, and the height measurement allows estimation of weight for dosing of medications and other therapeutic maneuvers.

The ideal initial sites for vascular access in children are the peripheral veins in the upper extremities, especially the antecubital fossa. Insertion of a percutaneous femoral venous catheter is the next best choice for emergency venous access in the pediatric patient. This should be done using the Seldinger technique and avoids the need for a surgical cutdown procedure. Intraosseous access is a very useful technique when intravenous access is difficult because of severe hypovolemia. Contraindications include proximal fractures and sites of infection. The most common site for intraosseous cannulation is the anteromedial surface of the proximal tibia, 2 to 4 cm distal to the tibial tuberosity. The needle should be angled 45° in the cephalad direction. Care should be taken to avoid the region of the growth plate and or joint space.

Age-specific hypotension is an indication for volume resuscitation of the injured child. Cardiovascular compensation by tachycardia and vasoconstriction will maintain blood pressure in the child who has had significant blood loss. Therefore, a normal blood pressure does not connote a normal circulating blood volume. A child's blood volume is approximately 8% of body weight, or 80 ml/kg. Clinical signs of decreased organ perfusion in conjunction with altered mentation are the classic findings in pediatric hemorrhagic shock. Initial resuscitation is begun with 20 mL/kg of an isotonic crystalloid solution, such as 0.9% normal saline, or lactated Ringer's solution. If there is no improvement in perfusion after a second bolus of crystalloid, then a 10 mL/kg bolus of either crossmatched or O negative packed red blood cells should be administered.

Hypothermia is a common occurrence in the pediatric trauma patient and may occur at any time of the year, including summer. The response to hypothermia includes catecholamine release, with an increase in oxygen consumption and metabolic acidosis. Hypothermia and acidosis may then contribute to posttraumatic coagulopathy. The rate of cooling and subsequent hypothermia can be reduced by warming the room (>37°C), using warmed intravenous fluids and blood (39°C), heated air warming blankets, and external warmed blankets during the initial resuscitation of an injured child.

The physical examination is the crucial first step in diagnosis since it will direct all other methods of assessment. The initial physical exam also allows the clinician a baseline for comparison with subsequent serial physical examinations. The initial imaging studies include plain radiographs of the chest, pelvis, and cervical spine. As in adults, FAST includes views of the pericardium, right and left upper quadrants, and the pelvis to detect blood. CT imaging of the head, chest, abdomen, and pelvis are the accepted diagnostic radiologic studies of choice in the majority of hemodynamically stable children suspected of having a potentially life-threatening injury. The hemodynamically stable injured child with suspected intra-abdominal injury should have a CT scan performed prior to instituting operative or nonoperative management unless an absolute indication for operation (such as diffuse peritonitis or hemoperitoneum with refractory shock) is present. In a child, the comparatively thin abdominal wall musculature and flexible rib cage provide relatively little protection from blunt injury. Thus, a high index of suspicion is necessary when evaluating children with visible bruising or contusion of the abdominal wall, such as in the setting of seatbelt-related trauma or bicycle handlebar injury. In children, the great majority of solid organ injuries can be managed without surgical intervention. As in adults, hollow viscus perforation should be managed by prompt surgical repair.

TRAUMA IN THE ELDERLY

The elderly population is the fastest growing age group in the United States and will comprise an increasingly important proportion of trauma victims. Injury is the ninth leading cause of death for citizens 65 years of age and older. Within this group, 42% reported some type of long-lasting condition or a disability. Of those aged 65 to 74, a third reported at least one disability; that number climbs to 72% in people 85 years of age and older.

Elderly trauma patients have higher injury-related mortality when compared to younger trauma patients. Much of this is due to altered physiology in all organs with aging and also the increased incidence of comorbid conditions in the elderly population. The prevalence of preexisting conditions increases with age and can be as high as 80% in those over 95 years. Differentiating the changes that derive from aging versus changes that are due to chronic disease is often difficult.

The most frequent comorbidities in the elderly involve the cardiovascular system. These diseases compromise the older trauma patient's ability to respond to hypovolemia. Rather than mounting a tachycardia and increase cardiac output, there is an increase in systemic vascular resistance resulting in a falsely reassuring blood pressure. In fact, a normal blood pressure in an elderly trauma victim frequently corresponds to profound shock when perfusion is assessed using systemic markers such as serum lactic acid level and base deficit. Cardiac physiology is also altered by antiarrhythmic and antihypertensive medications.

Aging also affects pulmonary reserve. There is a decrease in the alveolar surface area that reduces the surface tension and thus negatively effects gas exchange and forced expiratory flow. Gross anatomic changes in the thorax of the elderly include the development of kyphosis, which results in a reduction of the transverse thoracic diameter. The loss of bone density is associated with an increased rigidity of the chest wall. Chest wall compliance decreases with age, increasing work of breathing. In the elderly female, osteoporosis increases the risk for rib fractures and severe underlying pulmonary contusions. Age has been shown to be the strongest predictor of outcome and is directly proportional to mortality in patients with multiple rib fractures.

In the geriatric patient, the initial GCS score may be less reliable and more reflective of chronic disease of the central nervous system or systemic disease. A significant traumatic brain injury can result from apparently minor trauma due to the changes with aging of the meninges and a reduction in cortical brain volume. Thus, any elderly patient with a change in mental status should prompt a thorough evaluation for traumatic brain injury, including a noncontrast CT scan of the head. Additionally, many elderly patients take blood thinning drugs such as warfarin, aspirin, or other antiplatelet agents. Otherwise minor head injuries may become devastating intracranial hemorrhages in the anticoagulated patient, and prompt correction of coagulopathy with plasma or banked platelets is indicated.

Renal function begins to deteriorate at the age of 40. The number of functioning nephrons decreases by 10% per decade while the remaining functional units hypertrophy. Glomerular filtration rate (GFR) begins to decrease at 50, declining by 0.75 to 1 mL/minute/year.

Traumatic injury in the elderly is more likely to produce bowel and mesenteric infarction. The diagnosis is more difficult because the clinical examination of the abdomen may be less reliable in the geriatric population. Gastrointestinal tract traumatic wounds in the geriatric population are associated with a three- to fourfold increase in mortality compared to younger cohorts.

Cell-mediated immunity is diminished with a decrease in peripheral T-cell count and function. The antibody response to stimuli is depressed, and this places the elderly at increased risk for infection. With severe trauma they may be more prone to the development of the MODS.

Normal thermoregulatory mechanisms become less responsive with aging. Cutaneous vasoconstriction and shivering are less effective, placing the elderly at increased risk for development of hypothermia in cold environments, and after significant volume loss. Efforts to prevent hypothermia must be started immediately upon admission.

Common injury mechanisms in the geriatric population include falls, motor vehicle collisions, automobile versus pedestrian collisions, assaults, and burns. Motor vehicle collision victims over the age of 85 have a fatality rate that is seven to nine times higher than that of younger adults. Adult pedestrian injuries are more common in lower socioeconomic groups who are more likely to travel by walking. The slower pace and restricted mobility associated with aging result in the elderly pedestrian requiring longer times to cross a street, which places them at higher risk for being struck by oncoming vehicles. Violence, which is frequently viewed as a problem for the young, is an increasingly recognized cause of injury in the elderly. In the United States, 5% of all homicides are committed against people age 65 and older. The overall incidence of abuse in elderly patients is estimated to be 2% to 10%. Thus, abuse is a growing health concern in the geriatric population and should always be considered when caring for the older trauma patient. Substance abuse should be considered in elderly trauma patients, prompting screening for ethanol and recreational drugs. Consideration of causes of altered mental status should include brain injury, stroke, delirium, dementia, or intoxication. Elderly trauma patients who abuse ethanol, like their younger colleagues, are prone to delirium tremens during hospitalization.

thePoint ✳ Go to http://thePoint.lww.com/activate and use your scratch-off code on the inside cover of this book to access bonus chapters, question bank, videos, and more.

SAMPLE QUESTIONS

Questions

Choose the best answer for each question.

1. A 22-year-old man is in the emergency department after a high-speed motor vehicle collision. He complains of back pain. He is alert and oriented and is breathing normally. His oxygen saturation is normal and hemodynamically stable. There are ecchymoses on the left chest. Chest x-ray shows fractures of the left first and second ribs. The aortic knob is not clearly visible, and the mediastinum measures 10 cm. Further evaluation should include which of the following?
   A. Contrast-enhanced chest CT
   B. Repeat chest x-ray
   C. Diagnostic thoracoscopy
   D. Pericardial window
   E. Diagnostic mediastinoscopy

2. A 30-year-old man is brought to the emergency department after crashing his motorcycle at high speed into a concrete divider. He sustains severe trauma to the mid face and mandible and is lethargic upon arrival. He has copious amounts of bloody airway secretions and pulse oximetry reveals oxygen saturation levels of 82% to 85%. Two unsuccessful attempts have been made to place an orotracheal tube. The next step should be
   A. bag-valve mask ventilation.
   B. nasotracheal intubation.
   C. resuscitative thoracotomy.
   D. surgical cricothyroidotomy.
   E. bronchoscopy.

3. A 53-year-old man sustains a severe traumatic brain injury after an assault. His GCS score is 6, and an intracranial pressure monitor is inserted. Vital signs are heart rate—92 beats/minute, blood pressure (BP)—152/88 mm Hg, mean arterial pressure—109 mm Hg, and respiratory rate—16/minute. His intracranial pressure is 32 mm Hg. The patient's cerebral perfusion pressure is
   A. 120 mm Hg.
   B. 77 mm Hg.
   C. 60 mm Hg.
   D. 56 mm Hg.
   E. 32 mm Hg.

4. A 25-year-old woman is brought to the emergency department after involvement in a low-speed motor vehicle collision. She complains of feeling light-headed and states that she is 33 weeks pregnant. Vital signs are heart rate—90 beats/minute and BP—82/44 mm Hg. Abdominal examination reveals a gravid uterus but no tenderness. Chest x-ray is unremarkable, and FAST reveals no intraperitoneal fluid. A viable intrauterine pregnancy is noted, and fetal heart tones are observed. The next step in management should be
   A. cesarean section.
   B. induction of labor with vaginal delivery.
   C. left lateral tilt positioning.
   D. diagnostic peritoneal lavage.
   E. MRI of the abdomen and pelvis.

5. A 22-year-old man is brought to the emergency department after falling from a 10-foot ladder, landing on his left side. He has multiple left-sided rib fractures and a pneumothorax requiring a chest tube. Physical examination of the abdomen is unremarkable. He remains hemodynamically stable throughout the primary and secondary surveys and undergoes contrast-enhanced CT scanning of the abdomen and pelvis. CT scan reveals a grade II laceration of the spleen, with no evidence of active contrast extravasation. The next appropriate step in management is
   A. exploratory laparotomy with splenectomy.
   B. exploratory laparotomy with splenorrhaphy.
   C. splenic angioembolization.
   D. video-assisted thoracoscopy with evacuation of hemothorax.
   E. observation with serial abdominal examinations.

Answers and Explanations

1. Answer: A

The high-speed deceleration mechanism and chest x-ray findings are highly concerning for blunt aortic injury (BAI), which is most efficiently diagnosed by contrast-enhanced chest CT. Repeat chest x-ray would likely reveal the same findings but would not establish the diagnosis. Thoracoscopy is useful for evaluating the pleural space, lungs, and diaphragm, but not the aorta and great vessels. Pericardial window may be utilized to diagnose hemopericardium in suspected penetrating cardiac trauma, but not aortic injury. Mediastinoscopy is used for evaluating lymph node status in lung cancer staging but has no role in trauma. (Taken from Thoracic Injury: Potentially Severe Injuries Detected During Secondary Survey).

2. Answer: D

In the primary survey, obtaining a patent airway is of paramount importance. The patient in this scenario has an unstable airway and poor systemic oxygenation, making the establishment of a definitive airway an urgent matter. Since orotracheal intubation attempts have failed, the next step is to perform a cricothyroidotomy. Bag-valve mask ventilation is unlikely to be successful in this circumstance and does not provide a definitive airway. Nasotracheal intubation is contraindicated in severe facial trauma as false passage into the cranium may occur. Resuscitative thoracotomy may restore circulation but does not provide an airway. Bronchoscopy may be utilized after establishment of an airway to clear blood or secretions. (Taken from Primary Survey: Airway).

3. Answer: B

Cerebral perfusion pressure (CPP) is calculated by subtracting the intracranial pressure (ICP) from the mean arterial pressure (MAP). (Taken from Head Injury: Anatomy and Physiology).

4. Answer: C

In the supine position, the gravid uterus compresses the inferior vena cava (IVC), resulting in decreased venous return to the heart and hypotension. Visibly pregnant trauma patients should be placed in the left lateral tilt position (while maintaining spinal precautions) to displace the gravid uterus from the IVC. Induction of labor and cesarean section would not be indicated in the absence of fetal distress. Diagnostic peritoneal lavage (DPL) is relatively contraindicated in pregnancy, as uterine or fetal injury may occur. MRI is not utilized in the acute evaluation of abdominal trauma.

5. Answer: E

Most low-grade splenic injuries can be managed nonoperatively. The key factor is hemodynamic stability of the patient. In this patient, splenectomy and splenorrhaphy would represent unnecessary surgical options, and interventional techniques such as angioembolization should be reserved for cases of high-grade splenic injury with active extravasation of intravenous contrast. Thoracoscopy is indicated for evacuation of residual hemothorax or diagnosis of penetrating diaphragmatic injury. (Taken from Abdominal Injury: Injury to Specific Organs: Spleen).

10
Burns

JEFFREY R. SAFFLE, M.D. • MELINDA BANISTER, M.D. • MICHAEL CAHALANE, M.D. •
JONG O. LEE, M.D. • TINA L. PALMIERI, M.D.

Objectives

1. List the classification of burns by depth of injury, and indicate the anatomic and pathophysiologic differences between these injuries.

2. List the initial steps in acute care of the burn-injured patient.

3. List three types of inhalation injury and describe their pathophysiology.

4. Differentiate the pathophysiology of chemical and electrical burns from that of thermal burns.

5. List the general indications for referral of a patient to a burn center.

6. Define burn shock and outline its treatment.

7. List the advantages and disadvantages of fascial and tangential excision of burn wounds.

8. List five important general areas of care for the burn patient.

9. Discuss the principles in management of minor first- and second-degree burns that may be seen in a primary care physician's office.

10. Identify additional therapeutic principles in the diagnosis and management of chemical and electrical burns.

Major burns hold a unique position in the public imagination as the most horrifying of all injuries, a perception that is all too often correct. To patients, acute burns are the "ultimate agony," while their long-term consequences present enormous psychological, social, and physical challenges to meaningful recovery. To the treatment team, burns are long-term, labor-intensive injuries that involve every facet of surgical care. Major burns are often used as paradigms for the most severe physiologic derangements that accompany trauma.

Burns are a major public health problem as well. In the United States, about 450,000 patients sought medical attention for burns in 2007. Over 3,700 people die every year of burn-related injuries, primarily from house fires, and about 40,000 patients are hospitalized. This chapter presents basic burn pathophysiology and practical guidelines for treatment of acute burns.

A *note on illustrations*: Burns are uniquely *visual* injuries, and the ability to assess burns by sight is an essential skill both for planning initial burn care and for making decisions about such things as the need for surgery, the presence of infection, and the extent of scarring. Clinicians who cannot assess burn extent and depth accurately often make significant errors in burn evaluation and treatment. For that reason, familiarity with the appearance of burn injuries is an important objective of this chapter. To aid the reader, we have developed a set of color illustrations to better illustrate these wounds. Because of the large number of illustrations, only two appear in the text (Figures 10-1 and 10-18).

The rest are to be found in the Appendix at the end of the book. All are cited in numerical order. We strongly encourage students to view the Appendix and become familiar with the appearance of different types of burn wounds.

PATHOPHYSIOLOGY OF BURN INJURY

The skin can be injured by a variety of agents, including direct heat from flames or scalding liquids, contact with hot objects or corrosive chemicals, and electrical current. Burns are classified according to the depth of injury. Figure 10-1 shows these injuries in relation to the structures of the skin, knowledge of which will help the reader understand the physiologic effects of burns of various depths, and the findings seen on examination.

Epidermal burns ("first-degree burns") involve only the epidermis. Within minutes of injury, dermal capillaries dilate, so that these burns present as red, moderately painful areas that blanch with direct pressure, indicating the continued presence of dermal perfusion. Blistering is absent from true epidermal injuries, and the initial erythema usually resolves within a few hours. Epidermal burn injuries are limited in their physiologic effects, and even extensive burns usually require only supportive care, which consists of pain control (oral analgesics), adequate oral fluids, and application of a soothing topical compound such as neomycin sulfate ointment to prevent infection. Healing occurs within a few days as the

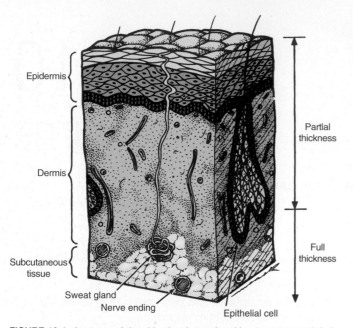

FIGURE 10-1. Anatomy of the skin showing major skin structures and their relation to partial- and full-thickness burns. Epithelial cells make up the lining of hair follicles and sweat glands, and these structures penetrate deeply into—sometimes through—the dermis. Even very deep partial-thickness burns can heal if these "epidermal appendages" survive. Dermal capillaries and nerve endings also reside in the deep dermis and survive most partial-thickness burns.

injured epidermis peels off, revealing new skin beneath. Because scarring occurs in the dermis, epidermal burns do not form scar tissue. Sunburns are often limited to the epidermis, although deeper injuries can result. Figure 10-2 shows a patient with primarily epidermal, and some superficial dermal burns.

Partial-thickness burns ("second-degree burns") extend into but not through the dermis. These injuries vary greatly in both appearance and significance, depending on their exact depth. Superficial partial-thickness burns (Figures 10-3 and 10-4) typically present with reddened skin that forms distended blisters comprised of epidermis and filled with proteinaceous fluid that escapes from damaged capillaries. The underlying dermis is moist, blanches on direct pressure, and is usually very painful, since cutaneous nerves, which reside in the deeper dermis, are intact

Deep partial-thickness injuries look very different from more superficial burns. Coagulation necrosis of the upper dermis often gives these wounds a dry, thickened texture. Erythema is often absent, and these wounds may be a variety of colors but are most often waxy white. Because epidermal appendages penetrate far into—sometimes through—the dermis, even a very deep dermal burn can heal if followed long enough. These wounds also vary in the amount of pain they produce; very deep wounds cause destruction of many dermal nerve endings and are less painful than more superficial injuries. Such wounds heal badly, however, because damaged dermis does not regenerate; instead, it is replaced by scar tissue which is often rigid, tender, and friable. For this reason, many deep dermal burns are best treated with excision of the burned tissue and skin grafting. The variable appearance of deep partial-thickness burns is illustrated by Figures 10-5 to 10-9.

During the first 24 to 48 hours postburn, burn wounds develop a coating of dead tissue, coagulated serum, and debris

called **eschar**. The exact depth of partial-thickness burns is often difficult to judge, particularly after eschar forms (see Figure 10-9). Appearance of the wound changes dramatically as eschar develops and again as it separates during wound healing. Superficial partial-thickness burns should demonstrate eschar separation within 10 to 14 days, revealing punctate areas of new epidermal growth called skin "buds," which develop from the epidermal linings of hair follicles and sweat glands (Figure 10-10). Burns of "indeterminate" depth—those that have some features of both partial- and full-thickness injuries—can often be treated conservatively for 10 to 14 days; wounds that remain unhealed should undergo grafting. Figure 10-11 illustrates such a burn. Figure 10-12 shows a burn of mixed depth on initial presentation.

Full-thickness burns ("third-degree burns") occur when all layers of the skin are destroyed. These wounds are usually covered with dry, avascular coagulum, which is relatively insensate due to destruction of nerve endings. The wound surface may be almost any color, from waxy white in the case of chemical burns, to a completely black, charred surface from flame injury. Full-thickness scald burns are often a dark red color, but the surface is dry and does not blanch with pressure. In addition, as dermal proteins are coagulated, they contract, often forming a tight, tourniquet-like constriction, which can cause circulatory compromise in the extremities. Very small, full-thickness burns can heal by contraction, but larger injuries require skin grafting because even the deepest epidermal appendages are destroyed. Figures 10-13 and 10-14 illustrate the appearance of full-thickness burns, which can be very dramatic. An additional category of burn injury, termed "fourth-degree" burns, is sometimes used to describe injuries that extend to bone.

PATHOPHYSIOLOGY OF INHALATION INJURY

Inhalation injury is a unique complication of injury from flames and smoke that is an important facet of burn treatment. Although inhalation injury is often less apparent than other manifestations of burn injury on initial presentation, it can cause severe morbidity and mortality that may overshadow those of cutaneous burns. Inhalation injury typically occurs when the patient is exposed to the toxins contained in smoke. These injuries most commonly occur during a fire in an enclosed space, so detailed information regarding the location of the patient during the fire is a critical point in the history. The treatment of inhalation injury is largely supportive. Endotracheal intubation to secure the swelling airway is mandatory. Ventilator support with positive end expiratory pressure (PEEP) is most helpful in combating the airway collapse.

Inhalation injury can present in three different ways in burn patients. First, patients exposed to large amounts of toxic smoke frequently present with *carbon monoxide (CO) poisoning*. CO poisoning is a common cause of immediate death in patients injured in building fires, and often accounts for the majority of deaths in mass casualty incidents. CO is produced from *incomplete* combustion of normal household items such as wood and cotton. CO competitively binds to oxygen receptors on the hemoglobin molecule to produce carboxyhemoglobin (COHb), which cannot transport oxygen. The tissue delivery of oxygen consequently decreases and severe hypoxia ensues. Oxygen-enriched tissues, such as the heart and brain, are the most vulnerable. At low levels,

TABLE 10-1	Signs and Symptoms at Various Concentrations of COHb

COHb Concentration (%)	Symptoms
0–10	None (normal value may range up to 10% in smokers)
10–20	Tightness over forehead, mild headache, dilation of cutaneous blood vessels
20–30	Headache and throbbing in the temples
30–40	Severe headache, weakness, dizziness, dimness of vision, nausea, vomiting, and collapse
40–50	As above; syncope, increased pulse, and respiratory rate
50–60	Syncope, tachycardia, tachypnea, coma, intermittent seizures, Cheyne-Stokes respirations
60–70	Coma, intermittent seizures, depressed cardiac and respiratory function, possible death
70–80	Bradycardia, slow respirations, death within hours
80–90	Death within an hour
90–100	Death within minutes

Reproduced from: Einhorn IN, National Institute of Environmental Health Sciences, and Schulte JH, Heldref Publications; and Herndon DN, Total Burn Care. 3rd ed. Philadelphia, PA: Saunders Elsevier, 2007:250.

CO poisoning is initially asymptomatic, but as the COHb level rises, symptoms increase. CO poisoning is particularly deadly because of its tendency to impair mental function. The patient will initially experience headache, progressing to dizziness, weakness, and syncope. In the later stages coma, seizures, and death result (see Table 10-1). CO poisoning should be strongly suspected in any patient who presents with altered mental status following exposure to smoke. Remember that pulse oximetry is not accurate in detecting CO poisoning; an arterial blood gas with direct measurement of hemoglobin saturation must be obtained to detect CO toxicity.

Treatment of CO poisoning should consist of ventilation with 100% oxygen, and must begin as soon as possible, ideally before the patient reaches the hospital. Endotracheal intubation may be needed both to protect the impaired airway and for adequate delivery of such high levels of oxygen. If a more rapid decrease in COHb concentration is deemed necessary (usually because of acute neurologic symptoms), hyperbaric oxygen therapy (HBO) may be used. HBO works by providing higher concentrations of oxygen to compete with CO for hemoglobin binding. Oxygen administered at three atmospheres of pressure produces a PaO_2 as high as 1,500 mm Hg. This provides a significant amount of dissolved oxygen for immediate use, and reduces the half-life of COHb from about 80 minutes at one atmosphere of pressure down to about 20 minutes. Appropriate equipment and personnel are required to perform hyperbaric therapy, and its use must be prioritized with other important aspects of care for acutely burned patients, including fluid resuscitation.

Burn patients may also present with *upper airway injury*. Unlike other forms of inhalation injury, which are chemical injuries, upper airway injury is produced by heat. Flash burns and explosions may produce instantaneous deep burns of the face and oropharynx, which lead to rapid, life-threatening airway edema. Remember that swelling occurs progressively over the 24 hours following injury, and that facial/airway edema can come on very precipitously. Remember also that massive facial swelling can accompany scald or chemical burns even in the absence of flames or smoke. Figure 10-15 illustrates this process. Assessment of airway patency and swelling is an important component of the initial evaluation of every burn patient (see below). Early endotracheal intubation is essential to support the airway during acute care of these patients.

Patients who inhale significant quantities of smoke can suffer *lower airway injuries*, the so-called "true" inhalation injury. Cotton, wood, and paper are the most abundant fuels burned during a house/building fire. Large amounts of CO, formaldehyde, formic acid, and hydrochloric acid are produced from the incomplete combustion of these materials. Inhalation of toxic compounds causes severe damage to the mucosal cells of the airway. Cyanide toxicity has also been reported as an infrequent cause of death following smoke inhalation. As the dead/damaged cells slough, they produce plugging, segmental collapse, and bronchiectasis. Pneumonia can occur in multiple lung segments in these patients. However, this cascade of events often takes several days to develop; symptoms may be completely absent for the first 24 to 48 hours of care, so a high index of suspicion is critical for the detection and timely treatment of these injuries. Performance of fiberoptic bronchoscopy is an important part of initial evaluation of patients trapped in enclosed spaces. Figure 10-16 shows typical bronchoscopic findings of carbonaceous debris and mucosal sloughing in a patient with inhalation injury.

INITIAL CARE OF THE BURN PATIENT

Burn patients should be considered victims of multiple trauma and many of the same treatment priorities and algorithms apply to their care as to other trauma patients. It will be assumed that the reader is familiar with the principles of Advanced Trauma Life Support outlined in Chapter 9, Trauma; this chapter on burns focuses on aspects of care that are unique to burn injuries.

Stop the Burning Process

A unique problem of burn trauma is the tendency for burns to continue producing tissue damage for minutes to hours after the initial burn has occurred. This process can further injure the patient as well as endanger medical personnel. For example, placing an oxygen mask on a victim of flame injury runs the risk of reigniting smoldering clothing. It is thus critically important to stop the burning process before proceeding with any other measures. Flame burns should be extinguished completely by dousing with water, smothering, or rolling patients on the ground. Hot liquids—especially viscous liquids like tar or plastics—can remain hot enough to burn for some time; they should be cooled immediately with cool water or moist compresses. Once cooled, such compounds can then be left in place on the patient if necessary. Caustic chemicals must be diluted immediately and completely with copious amounts of water. In recent years, widespread concern over possible acts of terrorism and mass casualty incidents involving toxic chemicals has heightened awareness of the need to decontaminate patients thoroughly both to protect the care team and to spare victims further harm.

Victims of electrocution can themselves conduct current to rescue workers. Such patients cannot be approached until the source of current is shut off.

Primary Survey

The primary survey is a quick examination designed to detect and treat immediately life-threatening conditions, beginning with evaluation of *Airway, Breathing, and Circulation* (The "ABCs"). In performing the primary survey in burn victims, special attention should be paid to the possible existence of smoke *inhalation injury*, which is a major source of both immediate and long-term morbidity and mortality. As discussed previously, inhalation injury should be suspected whenever the patient has been exposed to smoke. All three types of inhalation injury—CO poisoning, upper airway swelling, and lower airway obstruction and hypoxemia—may be present simultaneously, or any of the three may occur alone. Even in the absence of smoke exposure, patients with severe facial burns can develop massive swelling that can lead to obstruction of the supraglottic airway. Remember again that edema is progressive, and signs of airway compromise may be absent until several hours following injury; patients should be followed and reexamined regularly for this. Also during the primary survey, the examiner should note evidence of circulatory compromise in extremities caused by severe edema and constricting burn wounds. See Chapter 9 for a more detailed review of the signs and symptoms of vascular compromise accompanying trauma to the extremities.

Resuscitation

Initial resuscitation of burn victims is similar to that of other patients. If injuries appear to be major, two large-bore lines placed *intravenously* should be secured. A Foley catheter should be placed to aid in resuscitation and blood drawn for laboratory studies. Formal calculation of fluid requirements should not be performed until after the secondary survey is completed. The performance of fluid resuscitation is an important ongoing part of the definitive treatment of burn injuries, and will be discussed in detail below.

Secondary Survey

All too often, the presence of a dramatic burn wound distracts the examiner from detecting other, more urgent injuries. In addition, the swelling, discoloration, and pain that accompany burns can obscure underlying abdominal tenderness, extremity fractures, or cyanosis. For these reasons, it is imperative that a comprehensive, head-to-toe exam of every burn patient be conducted. Only after completing the secondary survey should burns be debrided by removing blistered skin and washing the burn wound thoroughly. The location, extent, and depth of burn wounds should be documented. Two mechanisms exist for doing this. One, the "Rule of Nines" is performed by dividing the body into its component parts, and assigning 9% of the total body surface area (TBSA) to each part. This is illustrated in Figure 10-17. As an alternative, many providers use the Lund and Browder chart (Figure 10-18). A completed Lund and Browder chart is illustrated in Figure 10-19. A useful computerized mechanism for doing this is available at www.sagediagram.com. These charts are used to calculate the total burn size, expressed as *percent total body surface area* (%TBSA). Only partial-thickness ("second-degree") and full-thickness ("third-degree") burn wounds should be included in this estimate of total burn size. An easy way to estimate small burns is to remember that the palm of the patient's hand (with fingers) is approximately one percent of their body surface area. This estimate of burn size is used to guide fluid resuscitation, nutrition, and other aspects of

care. Wounds should not be dressed with antibiotic creams or ointments, or wrapped with dressings, until a secondary assessment has been completed, and the burn has been evaluated.

Burn Center Referral

Over the past 50 years, specialized burn facilities have been developed to care for patients with serious burns. The American Burn Association and the American College of Surgeons have defined criteria for **burn centers**, similar to those developed for Trauma Centers. These criteria require that institutions maintain significant multidisciplinary expertise in all phases of burn treatment, and commit space, resources, and personnel to the care of patients with burns. In addition, specific guidelines for referral of patients to burn centers have been developed; these are contained in Table 10-2. The guidelines are not absolute, but are widely used as standards for treatment. As a more general rule, surgeons who do not work in burn centers should treat only patients with burns they are experienced in treating, and consider consultation with a burn center for *any* questions regarding patient management.

DEFINITIVE CARE OF BURN INJURIES

Following initial assessment, burn patients require treatment for a number of physiologic consequences of injury. Support for several different problems may be required simultaneously, although the importance and magnitude of these problems change at different times postburn. To help in organizing treatment priorities and protocols, many physicians divide burn care into three periods: *Resuscitation, Wound Closure, and Rehabilitation*. It should be emphasized, however, that these distinctions are somewhat artificial, that many aspects of care overlap these periods and that careful attention to the individual patient's needs is essential at all stages of treatment.

Resuscitation Period

This period lasts for the first 24 to 48 hours following injury. Once an acutely burned patient has been evaluated and stabilized as described previously, fluid resuscitation is the most important goal of initial treatment. Burn injury produces loss of capillary integrity, which results in edema formation. With large (≥15% to 20% TBSA) injuries, capillary leakage becomes systemic, producing total body edema, and severely depleting circulating volume, a phenomenon known as *burn shock*. All patients with burns of 10% to 15% TBSA or greater require formal fluid resuscitation. These fluid losses can exceed those of any other injury or disease; truly remarkable amounts of fluid may be required for successful resuscitation of patients with very large injuries.

A host of algorithms have been developed for burn resuscitation, but most successful regimens share several basic concepts. These are illustrated in Table 10-3, by the **Consensus formula**, a widely utilized, simple, and relatively generous resuscitation formula.

This formula calls for isotonic crystalloid fluid (lactated Ringer's solution) to be given at an initial rate determined from burn size and body weight. Because even experts disagree on the optimal quantity of fluid to be used, the formula provides a range of choices (from 2 to 4 mL of lactated Ringer's solution per kilogram body weight for every percent TBSA that is burned). Edema formation occurs throughout the first 24 hours postburn, but is most pronounced during the first 8 hours, so half the total fluid is given during that

BURN ESTIMATE AND DIAGRAM
AGE vs AREA

Area	Birth 1 yr.	1-4 yr.	5-9 yr.	10-14 yr.	15 yr.	Adult	2°	3°	Total	Donor Areas
Head	19	17	13	11	9	7				
Neck	2	2	2	2	2	2				
Ant. Trunk	13	13	13	13	13	13				
Post. Trunk	13	13	13	13	13	13				
R. Buttock	2½	2½	2½	2½	2½	2½				
L. Buttock	2½	2½	2½	2½	2½	2½				
Genitalia	1	1	1	1	1	1				
R. U. Arm	4	4	4	4	4	4				
L. U. Arm	4	4	4	4	4	4				
R. L. Arm	3	3	3	3	3	3				
L. L. Arm	3	3	3	3	3	3				
R. Hand	2½	2½	2½	2½	2½	2½				
L. Hand	2½	2½	2½	2½	2½	2½				
R. Thigh	5½	6½	8	8½	9	9½				
L. Thigh	5½	6½	8	8½	9	9½				
R. Leg	5	5	5½	6	6½	7				
L. Leg	5	5	5½	6	6½	7				
R. Foot	3½	3½	3½	3½	3½	3½				
L. Foot	3½	3½	3½	3½	3½	3½				
						TOTAL				

Cause of Burn_____

Date of Burn_____

Time of Burn_____

Age_____

Sex_____

Weight_____

BURN DIAGRAM

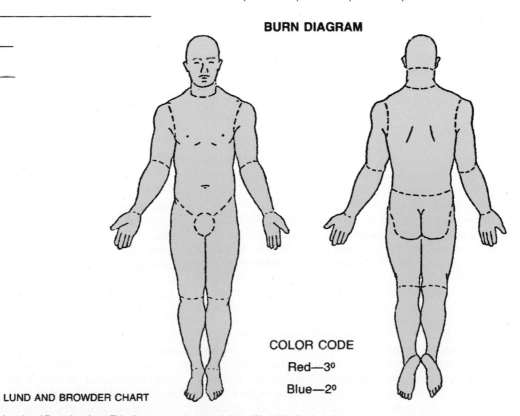

COLOR CODE

Red—3°

Blue—2°

LUND AND BROWDER CHART

FIGURE 10-18.   **Lund and Browder chart.** This diagram was developed during World War II to help document and estimate the extent of burn injuries. Following initial debridement, the examiner should draw the burn injuries on the figure, calculate how much of each body area is burned, and then add all areas to produce a total burn size. Inexperienced providers tend to overestimate burn size, and underestimate depth. We hope that the figures included with this chapter will help readers evaluate burn wounds more accurately.

TABLE 10-2	Criteria for Referral to a Burn Center

1. Partial-thickness burns >10% total body surface area (%TBSA)

2. Burns the involve the face, hand, feet, genitalia, perineum, or major joints

3. Third-degree burns in any age group

4. Electrical burns, including lightning injury

5. Chemical burns

6. Inhalation Injury

7. Burn injury in patients with preexisting medical disorders that could complicate management, prolong recovery, or affect mortality

8. Any patient with burns and concomitant trauma (such as fractures) in which the burn injury poses the greatest risk of morbidity or mortality. In such cases, if the trauma poses the greater immediate risk, the patient's condition may be stabilized initially in a trauma center before transfer to a burn center. Physician judgment will be necessary in such situations and should be in concert with the regional medical control plan and triage protocols.

9. Burned children in hospitals without qualified personnel or equipment for the care of children

10. Burn injury in patients who will require special social, emotional, or rehabilitative intervention

Referral Criteria, Advanced Burn Life Support Provider Manual. Chicago, IL: American Burn Association, 2005:76. Used with permission.

period. However, because inhalation injury, multiple trauma, and other factors can influence an individual's fluid requirements, regimens like the Consensus formula really only tell you where to *begin* resuscitation, which should thereafter be guided by frequent and repeated evaluation of the patient. Maintenance of adequate urine output (≥30 mL/hr in adults; 1 to 2 mL/kg/hr in children) is used as an indicator of appropriate fluid intake, and an important goal of treatment. The infusion rate is adjusted according to urine output and gradually decreased until a maintenance rate is reached. Vital signs, hematocrit, and other laboratory tests should be carefully monitored as well.

Fluid resuscitation does not stop fluid leakage into the interstitium; it is intended only to keep up with ongoing losses, which decrease over time. As resuscitation proceeds, therefore, so does tissue swelling. Fluid accumulating beneath the constricted eschar of a deep burn increases tissue hydrostatic pressure, sometimes to the point that circulation is compromised. Frequent evaluation of extremity pulses, sensory and motor function, and pain is essential to diagnose the progressive ischemia of a **compartment syndrome**. The treatment of this problem is **escharotomy**, an incision made through the rigid, leathery eschar to relieve the compression produced by ongoing edema, and thus restore distal circulation. Figures 10-20 and 10-21 illustrate escharotomies of the upper extremity. Compression by edema can also affect the chest and abdomen, resulting in respiratory compromise and even arrest. Escharotomies can be performed on the torso and should provide immediate relief (see Figure 10-22). Because escharotomies are always made through burn wounds, they are repaired during burn wound excision and skin grafting, and usually leave no additional scars.

However, escharotomies do not always provide adequate relief of edema-related pressure. When burns of the extremity are particularly deep, incisions through the underlying muscle fascia ("fasciotomies") may be required to produce adequate decompression. This is commonly required for high-voltage electrical injuries (see Figure 10-23). In addition, massive fluid accumulation within the tissues of the abdomen can produce an abdominal compartment syndrome and require laparotomy to relieve this compression (Figure 10-24).

Respiratory Support

Resuscitation of the patient with moderate to severe inhalation injury usually requires modifications. An inhalation injury is essentially a burn to the inside of the lungs, and the Consensus formula must be adjusted appropriately. Upon positive bronchoscopic diagnosis of inhalation injury, the %TBSA used for calculating resuscitation may be considered to increase by 20% to 30%, though the amount of fluid given should still be adjusted according to patient response. Ventilatory support and close monitoring of systemic arterial pressure, lactic acid, and urine output must be used to help titrate the amount of fluids the patient is receiving. Development of adult respiratory distress syndrome (ARDS) is very common with a severe inhalation injury. Overresuscitation with intravenous fluids can worsen the ARDS and should be avoided if at all possible. ARDS is diagnosed by a "ground-glass" appearance on chest radiograph coupled with the clinical syndrome of worsening respiratory failure. Aggressive modes of ventilator support are necessary to combat hypoxemia in patients with ARDS. Conventional ventilator settings must have adequate PEEP and low tidal volumes to minimize barotrauma. Newer ventilator modes, such as airway pressure release ventilation (APRV) and pressure regulated volume control (PRVC), are useful in the ARDS setting as they decrease barotrauma with constant airway pressure and lower tidal volumes. The APRV and PRVC modes keep the alveoli pressurized at all times, except for a very short expiration, maintaining them in an open state. These advances in ventilator management have decreased the incidence of pneumonia and chronic respiratory failure substantially. The treatment team must remain vigilant with respiratory care and positioning of the patient in order to decrease the risk of pneumonia from inhalation injuries. ARDS secondary to inhalation injury can progress to chronic respiratory failure; these patients may require tracheostomy and long-term ventilator support.

Wound Coverage Period

This phase of treatment begins immediately following fluid resuscitation, and lasts for days to weeks until the burn wound either heals primarily or is successfully replaced with skin grafts. This period comprises most of the patient's hospital care and is the period of most intensive treatment. Patients who attain successful wound closure usually survive, though they may face prolonged rehabilitation following this period of care.

Excision and Skin Grafting

Deeply burned skin is a great liability to the patient. Not only does burn eschar serve as a site for infection, but the loss of skin integrity causes increased evaporative fluid losses, severe pain, and an intense inflammatory response that can escalate, leading to multiple organ failure and death. If followed conservatively, deep eschar will eventually separate spontaneously, but this can take weeks, during which the patient is exposed to ongoing stress and risk of infection. For these reasons, most burn centers now employ **early excision**, in which burned skin is cut off the underlying tissue.

TABLE 10-3	Principles of Fluid Resuscitation for Burns: The Consensus Formula

Principles

A. Resuscitation should consist primarily of isotonic crystalloid solution because it is inexpensive, readily available, and can be given in large quantities without harmful side effects.

B. Because injured capillaries are porous to proteins for the first several hours after injury, colloid-containing fluids are not used initially.

C. Resuscitation requirements are proportional to burn size and patient's body weight.

D. Edema formation is most rapid during the first hours after injury, but continues for at least 24 hr. Therefore, half the calculated fluid is given in the first 8 hr following the burn.

E. Formulas only tell you where to BEGIN resuscitation, which must then be guided by patient response: urine output, vital signs, and mental status.

Practice: The Consensus Formula

A. The Formula: 2–4 mL lactated Ringer's × body weight (Kg) × %TBSA burns = total fluid for the first 24 hr.

B. For the first 8 hours after injury, give half the total calculation.

C. Second and third 8 hr after injury, give one-fourth the total calculation.

Example

A. A 220-lb (100 kg) man is burned while filling the gas tank on his boat. He is wearing a swimming suit, and is burned over all of both legs, his chest, and both arms. Calculated burn size is 65% TBSA.

B. Calculated fluid requirements: The Consensus formula offers a range of options, from 2 to 4 mL/Kg/%TBSA. Therefore, calculations range between the following:

Minimum: 2 mL × 100 kg × 65%TBSA = 13,000 mL in 24 hr

= 6,500 in first 8 hr = 812 mL/hr

= 3,250 mL in each of the second and third 8 hr = 406 mL/hr

Maximum: 4 mL × 100 kg × 65% TBSA = 26,000 mL in 24 hr

= 13,000 mL in first 8 hr = 1,625 mL/hr

= 6,500 mL in each of the second and third 8 hr = 812 mL/hr

C. Adjust according to patient response

1. You select an initial rate of 812 mL/hr, based on a calculation of 2 mL/kg/%TBSA. After 6 hr, the patient has received 4,872 mL of lactated Ringers. Urine output, which was initially good, has fallen to 20 mL in the past hour. Heart rate is 132, BP is 106/50.

2. At this point you should increase the fluid rate, typically by about 10%–20%. All indications point to inadequate resuscitation.

3. You increase fluids by 20%, to 974 mL/hr. Two hours later urine output again drops, to 15 mL/hr. Heart rate is 128, BP is 98/52.

4. You should again increase fluids. Most experts would NOT consider use of a diuretic at this point in time. Individual fluid requirements vary significantly, and this man appears to need more than the minimum requirements. Even if you had selected an initial rate of 1,625 mL/hr, your response to decreasing urine output should be the same—to increase fluids.

5. Three hours later, urine output has increased to 95 mL/hr. Heart rate has dropped to 90, BP is 135/85.

6. You should now begin to decrease fluids by 10%–15% per hour, with continued attention to urine output and vital signs. Fluid resuscitation is a dynamic process and requires continuous attention to detail.

Two techniques are used: **fascial** and **tangential excision**. In fascial excision, the scalpel or cautery is used to excise the entire skin and subcutaneous tissue, usually to the level of the underlying fascia. This procedure is easy to perform, relatively bloodless, and permits good skin graft "take." Fascial excision is disfiguring, however, and removal of subcutaneous fat leads to joint stiffness and poor mobility. Examples of fascial excision are shown in Figures 10-25 and 10-26. For the past two decades, the technique of "layered" or tangential excision has gained popularity. In this technique, sequential thin slices of skin are removed with a dermatome until viable tissue is encountered. This technique requires skill and produces significant bleeding. However, the cosmetic and functional results of grafting this type of wound are often superior to those of fascial excision. Tangential excision of deep partial-thickness burns permits salvaging intact dermal elements, which improves the results of skin grafting (Figure 10-27). Most surgeons wait until fluid resuscitation has been completed before beginning excisional therapy in order to permit stabilization of cardiovascular function and intravascular volume, which can be further compromised by surgical blood loss. Limited burns of mixed or indeterminate depth can be followed for 10 to 14 days before the decision to proceed with surgery must be made.

Skin grafting is usually performed at the same time as excision. At present, permanent coverage of an excised wound can only be achieved with the patient's own skin, termed **autograft**. Autografting can be performed using **full-thickness** or **split-thickness** skin grafts. Full-thickness grafts are obtained by excising an ellipse of skin from the groin or flank, which is closed with sutures. Split-thickness grafts are obtained by using a dermatome to harvest intact skin at the level of the superficial dermis, typically 0.004 to 0.015 inches in depth. This yields a graft with sufficient dermis for secure coverage of the excised burn, while leaving a wound superficial enough to heal spontaneously in 7 to 14 days. Figure 10-27 shows the performance of tangential excision and split-thickness skin grafting of a burned hand. In treating very large burns, the urgency to remove eschar often requires that excision be performed even if no donor sites are available for grafting. Although the best functional and cosmetic results are obtained when sheet grafts are placed (as shown in Figure 10-27), when insufficient autograft is available, several techniques can be used to obtain wound coverage. First, skin can be expanded by meshing or cutting multiple small slits in the skin. Many skin grafts are meshed to facilitate application and graft "take." These grafts leave a permanent mesh pattern in the skin, but produce durable coverage (Figure 10-28). Widely meshed autografts will cover larger areas, though the interstices of the mesh are prone to desiccation. For that reason, widely meshed autografts are usually covered with one of several skin substitutes, which can also be used alone to attain temporary closure of burn wounds awaiting autografting. Figure 10-29 illustrates this process. The most widely used skin substitute is cadaver **allograft** skin obtained from tissue banks. Other skin substitutes include freeze-dried pigskin, human amniotic membrane, and various synthetic materials. In recent years, considerable research has been devoted to development of a man-made "artificial dermis," which could be taken off the shelf and used to cover large burn wounds. Some of these products are used routinely, particularly in reconstructive surgery, but they still require coverage with thin autografts. Finally, it is possible to grow a patient's own epidermal cells in culture. These cultured epidermal allografts (CEAs) are expensive, fragile, and easily lost due to infection. Nonetheless, they have proved life saving in some patients with massive burns.

Infection Control

Immediately after burning, the skin surface is virtually sterile for 24 to 48 hours, before gradually becoming repopulated with bacteria. Burn eschar—especially the thick, avascular eschar of deep burns—is an ideal culture medium for bacteria, which will rapidly multiply on such a surface. These bacteria may colonize burn eschar harmlessly, or, by penetrating through the burn wound, invade intact tissues and overwhelm local defenses, producing invasive infection, termed **burn wound sepsis**. Infection is also exacerbated by the immunosuppression that accompanies severe burn injury. Burn wound sepsis is often fatal, and has until recently been the most common cause of death in hospitalized burn victims. With modern methods of wound management, however, it is now an infrequent occurrence in burn centers.

Much of the increased survival from burns achieved in the past 50 years is due to improved understanding and treatment of burn wound infections. Beginning in the 1940s, systemic antibiotics like penicillin, as well as some topical agents, were used to control microbial contamination of burn wounds. The first widely used topical antimicrobial, silver nitrate solution, proved particularly effective in controlling infections caused by *Staphylococcus* and *Streptococcus* species. A variety of Gram-negative infections then began to predominate as causes of burn wound infection. The development in the 1960s of two powerful topical agents, mafenide acetate (Sulfamylon), and **silver sulfadiazine** (such as Silvadene, Thermazene, and SSD), helped control many gram-negative bacteria, which were then replaced by resistant *Pseudomonas* as a leading cause of infection (Figure 10-30). More recently, a host of powerful systemic antibiotics, and numerous other topical agents, have helped control *Pseudomonas* infections. This success has been followed by—and to some extent, caused—the emergence of multiply resistant bacteria (such

as methicillin-resistant *S. aureus* [MRSA], *Acinetobacter*, vancomycin-resistant *Enterococcus* [VRE]), as well as fungi and other exotic organisms, as important clinical pathogens in burn victims. This problem is magnified by the development in many burn centers of entrenched, endemic microbial populations, which have proven very difficult to eradicate. Thus, as the medical community has developed evermore powerful antimicrobials for burn care, we have seen the microbial fauna adapt, and continue to present new and unforeseen problems.

The most effective technique in the battle against burn wound infection is early burn excision and skin grafting, discussed previously. It also remains true that meticulous wound care is an essential part of burn treatment during the repair phase. Beginning immediately postburn, wounds must be washed regularly, and carefully debrided of old topical creams and ointments, dried serum, and bits of loose eschar. Topical antimicrobials are only effective for a few hours, and most experts agree that their replacement, as well as regular and thorough debridement, should be performed at least twice daily. There are some new products that adhere to wounds and release antibiotics (usually silver) slowly; their use should be supervised by an experienced clinician since infection developing beneath these products can be particularly difficult to diagnose and treat. This is also true for freshly grafted burn wounds and skin graft donor sites.

As prevention and treatment of burn wound infection has become more successful, other problems have gained prominence as causes of morbidity and mortality in burn victims. In particular, pneumonia has emerged as the most common, and often the most troublesome, infection seen in burn patients. As outlined previously, smoke inhalation causes chemical injury to the small airways of the lung, leading to bronchiectasis and mucous plugging, which permit the development of infections and render them difficult to clear. Pneumonia, in turn, often serves as a stimulus for systemic inflammation and infection, leading to the development of multiple organ failure. A host of other infectious complications can occur in burn victims as well. Septic thrombophlebitis can occur in veins cannulated for vascular access. When this involves central veins, systemic sepsis, endocarditis, and death can result. Localized infections can also develop in exposed bone or cartilage, the urinary tract, salivary glands, gallbladder, and other areas. All of these complications, happily, are now seen extremely infrequently in burn treatment.

Nutritional Support

As part of the hormonal response to burn trauma, metabolic rate rises dramatically, and can exceed twice normal for prolonged periods, with a corresponding increase in nitrogen excretion. This is the most severe metabolic response seen with any type of illness or injury, and the resulting catabolism can result in a fatal degree of inanition within a few weeks. In such patients, protein malnutrition causes both wasting of respiratory muscles and immune compromise, with resulting pulmonary infection and death. For this reason, burn patients require aggressive nutritional support and close monitoring throughout the wound closure phase of treatment, and sometimes longer. Enteral feeding is clearly superior to intravenous nutrition in burn victims; patients with large injuries should undergo placement of enteral feeding tubes as soon as possible, and infusion of a high-protein liquid diet until they can demonstrate adequate oral intake. A variety of formulas has been used to predict the caloric requirements of burn patients. None is entirely satisfactory, due in large part to the wide variation seen among individuals and the fluctuations in energy expenditure that occur during the postburn course. Many experts recommend the routine measurement of energy expenditure using indirect calorimetry and of protein utilization by determining nitrogen balance at least weekly. The technique of indirect calorimetry calculates the energy requirements of an individual by measuring the oxygen consumed during normal breathing.

In recent years, improved understanding of the role of nutrition in trauma management has led to development of "customized" nutritional products aimed at the specific needs of burn and trauma patient. At present, the advantages of such products remain to be proven; provision of a basic high-protein diet (1.5 to 2.0 g protein/kg body weight daily), in quantities sufficient to satisfy caloric requirements, remains the most important principle in nutritional management of such patients.

The Rehabilitation Phase

Once burns are closed, major emphasis is shifted to rehabilitation. Providers should remember the adage that *rehabilitation begins at the time of injury*, so it is incorrect for rehabilitation to wait for wound closure. As burn wounds heal they contract, due to the presence of myofibroblasts that begin to accumulate within wounds shortly after injury, and continue to proliferate within scar. If unopposed, burn scar contractures can immobilize extremities completely, and produce significant disfigurement (Figure 10-31). Much of the therapy provided during burn rehabilitation is aimed at preventing and correcting contractures. This therapy is more effective if begun quickly, while scar tissue is still pliable, and before it can "set" into significant contractures. Scar tissue remains inflamed and continues to remodel and reshape itself for at least a year following injury. Burn patients are usually followed for at least that long. In addition to motion and stretching exercises, tight-fitting garments are frequently used to retard the growth of hypertrophic scars. These custom-made garments are worn until scar tissue softens and erythema fades. Figure 10-32 shows a custom-made clear facemask used for the same purpose. The process of recovering completely from a major burn is long and labor-intensive, but the vast majority of burn victims can return to active and useful lives with appropriate therapy. The vast majority of patients return to work or school, even following burns of 70% TBSA or greater.

Reconstructive surgery may be needed to correct particularly difficult contractures, resurface areas of unstable wound coverage, or improve cosmesis. This surgery is usually postponed until burn scars mature and soften. However, many reconstructive procedures can be avoided by early and continued application of physical therapy and other rehabilitative techniques.

SPECIAL PROBLEMS IN BURN CARE

Comprehensive care of burn patients often involves a number of issues that either are not regularly encountered in other surgical practices, or present themselves in unique ways. These include the unique features of electrical and chemical injuries, the care of patients with minor burns, problems with pain control and itching, and the increasing trend for burn centers to treat other nonburn conditions. These are reviewed here.

Chemical and Electrical Burns

Both chemical and electrical injuries can present unique problems in diagnosis and treatment. The degree of tissue damage produced by chemicals is determined by the nature of the agent, its concentration, and the duration of skin contact. Three classes of chemicals commonly produce skin injuries. *Alkalis* dissolve and combine with the proteins of the tissues to form alkaline proteinates, which contain hydroxide ions. These ions induce further chemical reactions, penetrating deeper into the tissue. *Acids* induce protein breakdown by hydrolysis, which results in an eschar that does not penetrate as deeply as the alkalis. These agents also induce thermal injury by heat generation with contact of the skin, further causing tissue damage. *Organic compounds* such as petroleum products, phenols, and others injure tissue by their fat solvent action, which dissolves cell membranes. All three types of agents also pose the risk of systemic absorption and toxicity to both patients and providers. Figures 10-33 and 10-34 show examples of chemical injuries.

A careful history should be obtained to identify the responsible chemical. Prompt treatment is imperative in minimizing tissue damage. Providers should wear protective gear and detoxify the patient completely before other care is delivered. All clothing should be removed, and any dry powders should be brushed off the skin. All chemicals should then be thoroughly irrigated with copious volume of water. Hot chemicals such as tar can be left in place once cooled completely. If the chemical composition is known, monitoring of the irrigated solution pH will give a good indication of irrigation effectiveness and completion. The local poison control center may provide important information on specific chemical injuries, their severity, and possible adjunctive treatment, but initial detoxification—with appropriate protection of personnel—should always be instituted as quickly as possible.

Patients may have metabolic disturbances from pH abnormalities or from specific chemical toxicities (such as organophosphates). An arterial blood gas, electrolytes, and hepatic enzymes should be obtained. If the patient's condition deteriorates—such as obvious progression of the wound and/or progressive metabolic deterioration—urgent surgery may be needed to remove the wound entirely. Resuscitation should be guided by body surface area (BSA) involved. Depth of injury can be difficult to determine with chemical injuries: some may be more superficial than they appear, particularly in the case of acids, while alkaline injuries may penetrate beyond that which is apparent on exam and will require more fluid for effective resuscitation volume. Once initial care and resuscitation is completed, chemical wounds are managed the same as other burn injuries.

Electrical injuries occur when current enters a part of the body, such as the hand, and proceeds through tissues with the lowest resistance, generally nerves, blood vessels, and muscles, to exit through ground. Electrical injuries are classified as low-voltage (<1,000 V) and high-voltage (>1,000 V) injuries. Low-voltage injury, which typically results from household (120 V) current, is generally limited to the area surrounding the injury. The skin has high resistance to electrical current, and many low-voltage injuries produce only small cutaneous burns. However with high-voltage injuries, typically from industrial current contact, the skin involvement may be limited but associated underlying soft tissue damage may be extensive. Current travels preferentially beneath the skin, as deeper tissues have less resistance; tissues having the highest resistance generate the most heat. Deep tissues appear to retain heat so that the tissues next to bones, especially between two bones often sustain more severe injury than more superficial tissue. In fact, superficial muscle may appear uninjured while deeper muscle near bones may be damaged. Thus the true extent of tissue damage with high-voltage injury may be impossible to determine on initial inspection. Figures 10-23 and 10-35 illustrate high-voltage electrical injuries.

Electrical injuries can cause a variety of wounds. Current flow through tissues, as described above, can result in deep tissue damage. In addition, current passing from its source to ground can generate an electrical arc or "flash" injury. Flame injuries can also result from ignition of clothing without actual current flow through the patient. Electrical injury may also be associated with falls, and can produce blunt trauma from tetanic muscle contractions. Lightning injuries are a type of very high voltage direct current injuries. The blast associated with lightning strikes can produce significant trauma, including ruptured eardrums. Late complications include development of cataracts and peripheral neuropathy.

In assessing a victim of electrical injury, the first step is to be sure that no potential for continued electrical damage exists. Current sources must be disconnected before the patient can be approached. Electrical injury can result in dysrhythmia, and many patients die from electrically induced ventricular fibrillation or cardiac standstill, so immediate attention to resuscitation is essential. All victims of electric shock should have an electrocardiogram (ECG) obtained; victims of high-voltage injury (and low-voltage injuries associated with abnormal ECG findings) should be monitored on telemetry for at least 24 hours. Because of the potential for multiple trauma from falls and muscle tetany, patients should be immobilized and treated as multiple-trauma victims. Victims of high-voltage injury should be referred to a burn center, and require formal resuscitation. These injuries often result in muscle damage and rhabdomyolysis; if untreated, this will lead to compartment syndromes and renal failure. Pigmented urine with myoglobin will appear tea colored. This is illustrated in Figure 10-36. Intravenous fluid should be given to maintain adequate urine output, which should be 100 mL/hour or greater until the urine is clear or myoglobinuria is resolved. Using bicarbonate to alkalinize urine and mannitol as an osmotic diuresis to enhance renal clearance of myoglobin have not been proven in prospective studies. Therefore use of these adjunct treatments should be individualized according to practitioners' experience.

When compartment syndrome is suspected or myoglobinuria does not improve with resuscitation, emergent operation for fasciotomy or exploration of muscles and debridement of necrotic muscle may be needed. Early amputation of an affected limb may be required in severe cases. Figure 10-23 illustrates such a case.

Care of Outpatient and Minor Burns

Although burn centers concentrate on the care of patients with major injuries, many burn wounds are small, and can be managed on an outpatient basis. More than a half million emergency department visits annually are related to burns, and over 75% are limited injuries (less than 10% TBSA). Even such small burns, however, can be important injuries, with significant associated pain, potential for infection, and disability. The overarching goals of treatment are to relieve pain, prevent infection, and encourage optimal healing with the least amount of scar formation.

Burns that involve small areas of injury can often be treated in a primary care or emergency department setting. Any burn patient with evidence of inhalation injury, circumferential burns, burns to the face, hands, or perineum, or significant comorbidities is best referred to a burn center. Minor burns in children or in the elderly are less than 5% TBSA. The size of burns is often overestimated, and the use of standardized tools such as the Lund-Browder chart (Figure 10-18) is helpful in deciding on the most appropriate location and method of treatment.

As with major burns, treatment begins with removal of the offending agent and cooling the injury. It has been shown that ice water or ice cubes increase necrosis in experimental burns but that tap water at 12 to 25°C is effective at reducing damage and providing initial pain relief. However, cooling should be applied only for a short time, as complications such as frostbite and hypothermia can result from prolonged cooling. After patient assessment and calculation of the burn depth and size, a decision is made regarding treatment in the outpatient setting, hospital admission, or burn unit transfer. Criteria for referral of burn injuries to specialized centers for care are contained in Table 10-2.

Epidermal burns without blistering do not require topical care. Treatment of superficial partial thickness injuries should begin by thoroughly washing the wound. Although controversy exists regarding the treatment of blisters, they can often be left intact. However, once they rupture, blisters should be debrided to facilitate cleansing of the wound. Once washed and debrided, burns can be covered with a variety of topical agents, including antibiotic creams (silver sulfadiazine, mafenide acetate) or ointments (neomycin sulfate, bacitracin). Commercial products containing aloe vera have also been used with success. Historically, silver nitrate and silver sulfadiazine have been used to inhibit bacterial growth in burns. Because these substances are inactivated in a burn wound environment, they require frequent reapplication. Although evidence for the direct benefits of such topical care for minor burns is lacking, it is unquestionably true that dressing these wounds relieves discomfort and provides psychological benefit to the patient. Encouraging frequent washing and reapplication of topical compounds may be their most important benefit. More recently, a variety of other silver-containing dressings (silver imbedded in hydrofibers or on polyethylene mesh, and nanocrystalline silver) have been developed for burn care. These dressings can be left on wounds for longer periods, lengthening the time between dressing changes, which reduces pain and the incidence of infection compared to traditional silver preparations. They are also cost-effective, considering the need for fewer dressing changes.

Oral antibiotics are not required for uninfected burns. Topical antibiotics and absorptive dressings are useful for most contaminated burns. Burns should be inspected daily to assess for infection and changes that become evident rapidly when infection occurs.

Deep partial-thickness burns or third-degree burns are covered initially with an antibiotic ointment and dressed. Depending on local expertise and size of the burn, they should be considered for local excision and grafting. Because these wounds heal by contraction and generate considerable scar formation, all but the smallest burns should be excised. The depth of the burn may be difficult to determine initially so frequent examination is required. Burns can deepen during the first few days because of infection or desiccation. As described previously, small burns should heal within a few weeks; burns taking longer than 3 weeks will likely form hypertrophic scars and provide an unstable epithelium. For this reason, early excision is optimal.

Treatment of Itching and Pain

Morbidity from burns extends beyond the acute phase of treatment. The pain and anxiety associated with burn injury is a significant problem. Control of pain is essential to quality patient care. Pain (the "fifth vital sign") should be assessed whenever other vital signs are taken and treated promptly and effectively. A variety of standard scales are available to quantify pain by both patients and providers.

Analgesics are most effective for acute burn pain when given on a scheduled basis, before pain can escalate. The intravenous route is preferred during the resuscitation phase; intramuscular injections should be avoided due to highly unpredictable absorption and plasma levels, and the pain of the injections themselves. Once resuscitation is completed, oral or enteral medications can be used to supplement injections as needed. Dose, route, and type of medication should be evaluated frequently to make sure pain is satisfactorily controlled.

The most commonly used analgesics for controlling acute burn pain are opioids. Morphine is most widely used. Fentanyl is shorter acting and avoids oversedation following a procedure. Oral formulations of both agents are available in addition to intravenous preparations. In addition to opioid analgesics, anesthetic agents such as ketamine and nitrous oxide can be used to provide short-term relief of pain and anxiety during procedures. For outpatient treatment, combinations of hydrocodone or oxycodone with acetaminophen are often sufficient. Nonsteroidal anti-inflammatory drugs (NSAIDs) can be used for the relief of mild to moderate pain or as adjuncts to hydrocodone/oxycodone.

Anxiety is prevalent in burn patients and can exacerbate pain. Lorazepam, diazepam, and midazolam are the main anxiolytics used in the treatment of burn-related anxiety and are often used in combination with opiate analgesics; alpha2-adrenergic agonists such as clonidine and dexmedetomidine can also have excellent sedative, analgesic, and anxiolytic effects and have been used in burn patients with good results. Table 10-4 lists a number of medications commonly used for analgesia and sedation in burn centers. It should be noted that many of these agents should be used only in an inpatient, monitored setting.

Medications by themselves often do not control pain and anxiety completely. A variety of nonpharmacological therapies have been tried to alleviate pain associated with burn injury. Other valuable adjuncts include cognitive techniques such as breathing exercises, reinforcement of positive behavior, the use of age-appropriate imagery, and behavioral rehearsal. Another approach to pain control is distraction. Distracting patients' attention using music therapy, movies, and games can help them to better tolerate pain. Computerized "virtual reality" systems can immerse patients' attention in a computer-generated world and engage them in multisensory interactions with that world, including touch, sight, and

TABLE 10-4	List of Analgesia and Sedatives Typically Used in Adult Burn Treatment	
Agent	**Recommended Dosages**	**Comment**
Opiates		
Morphine sulfate	0.03–0.1 mg/kg IV	Morphine, fentanyl, and hydromorphone (Dilaudid) are the most widely used acute analgesics. All three agents can be used with patient-controlled analgesia (PCA) devices for effective pain control. Oral preparations of these and other narcotics are preferred for long-term and outpatient use, but remember to use equi-analgesic doses when transitioning from intravenous to oral agents.
Fentanyl	50–100 µg IV, 0.5–1 µg/kg IV	
Hydromorphone	1–2 mg IV, 0.02 mg/kg IV	
Oxycodone	5–10 mg PO q 4–6 hr	These two widely used oral analgesics are less powerful than morphine and fentanyl, but share the same risks of respiratory depression and dependency. They are often used in the rehabilitative phase of burn care and for outpatients. A long-acting form of oxycodone is available.
Hydrocodone	5–10 mg PO q 4–6 hr	
Benzodiazepines		
Midazolam	0.03–0.1 mg/kg IV	These are widely used benzodiazepines for sedation and relief of anxiety. They are not good analgesics, however, so other medications should be used to provide adequate pain control.
Lorazepam	1–4 mg IV, 0.04–0.08 mg/kg IV	
Diazepam	2–10 mg IV, 0.04–0.3 mg/kg IV	
Other Agents		
Propofol	0.5–1 mg/kg IV	Frequently used for short-term sedation for procedures, and for sedation of mechanically ventilated patients. Airway support is required for use.
Ketamine	0.5–1 mg/kg IV	Can be given intramuscularly for short procedures in the outpatient setting. Associated with emergence problems, including delirium and nightmares. Can be used at a very low dose continuous infusion (0.1 mg/kg/hr).
Dexmedetomidine	0.3–0.7 mcg/kg/hr IV	Increasingly popular both for short-term sedation and more prolonged sedation of ventilated patients.
Clonidine	0.1–0.3 mg q 6–12 hr PO	Also available as a sustained-release patch. Should not be used as a single agent for pain control.

sound providing profound relief of pain and anxiety. Studies have shown a significant reduction in pain in burn patients during dressing changes and rehabilitative therapies using virtual reality systems. Augmented virtual reality involves a virtual image being overlaid onto the physical world instead of immersion into an artificial virtual world to focus patient perception away from a noxious stimulus. Hypnosis can reduce pain and can be used as an effective nonpharmacological approach to burn pain. Hypnosis uses a combination of relaxation, imagery, and cognitive-based approach.

In addition to pain, itching can be a severe, prolonged problem in burn patients. In a study from one outpatient burn clinic, 50% of the patients recalled moderate to severe pruritus. This often interfered with sleep and with quality of life in general. At times, it causes wound breakdown because of scratching. Pruritus occurred in 32% of the cases with burns smaller than 2% TBSA, almost as frequent as pruritus in major burns. Although pruritus recedes with time, it can last for up to 12 years after the burn. Treatment is often not effective, with only 36% of patients in that study reporting benefit. Topical drugs (tricyclic histamine receptor blockers, doxepin) as well as gabapentin, dapsone, ondansetron, and H1/H2 blocker combination therapy have been employed. Simple cooling, transcutaneous electrical nerve stimulation (TENS), and massage have also been useful.

Burn Unit Treatment of Other Injuries

As burn units have evolved into centers for multidisciplinary expertise, they have often been used to treat other conditions that require critical care, specialized wound management, physical therapy, and rehabilitation. Among the conditions often referred to burn centers are the major exfoliative skin disorders and necrotizing soft tissue infections (NSTIs).

Skin Disorders

Toxic epidermal necrolysis (TEN) and Stevens-Johnson Syndrome (SJS) are rare, life-threatening exfoliative disorders involving the skin. They are caused by cell-mediated immune reactions resulting in destruction of basal epithelial cells by CD8 positive cells and macrophages in the superficial dermis. T cells then migrate into the epidermis, causing keratinocyte injury and epidermal necrolysis, analogous to the graft-versus-host disease that occurs in bone marrow transplant recipients. The disorders are distinguished primarily by the extent of cutaneous involvement: TEN is defined as >30% BSA desquamation, while SJS has less than 10% BSA involvement. Patients with 10% to 29% BSA involvement have an SJS/TEN "overlap." Because TEN is the most severe form of this disorder, it is most frequently referred to burn centers for care.

Drug exposure causes 80% of all TEN cases. Dilantin and sulfonamide antibiotics are involved in 40% of all cases; however, other agents, such as nonsteroidal anti-inflammatory agents, other antibiotics, upper respiratory tract infections, and viral illness have also been implicated. High-risk groups include patients with seizure disorders, metastatic cancer (particularly brain metastases), urinary tract infections, allogenic bone marrow transplants, and human immunodeficiency virus (HIV) infections.

A viral-like prodromal phase consisting of fever and malaise is frequently reported shortly after exposure to the inciting agent. Following this, a macular rash develops that spreads, often becoming confluent. The syndrome may involve any mucosal surface, including the oropharynx, eyes, gastrointestinal tract, and tracheobronchial tree. Patients have evidence of epidermal necrosis with large areas of epidermal detachment on physical examination. Nikolsky's sign, the separation of the epidermis with moderate digital pressure, is a common physical finding. This is illustrated in Figure 10-37.

TEN and SJS treatment begins with immediate discontinuation of the inciting agent. Skin biopsy at the edge of the blistered area and adjacent uninvolved skin should be performed to distinguish TEN/SJS from infectious (staphylococcal scalded skin syndrome, viral exanthem) or immunologic disorders. Once diagnosis is confirmed, wound management is a critical component of treatment, as secondary skin infections are the major cause of death. Because TEN involves separation of the dermal–epidermal junction, it is similar to a partial thickness burn wound, which can heal without operative intervention provided that appropriate supportive therapy is given. Debridement of devitalized tissue and use of appropriate temporary wound coverage is vital. A wide range of regimens for temporary wound coverage have been proposed, including xenograft, biosynthetic wound dressings, allograft, Xeroform gauze, 0.5% silver nitrate soaks, and antimicrobial wound dressings. Figure 10-38 illustrates this. Sulfa-containing topical agents are generally avoided, because of their involvement in the etiology of TEN. To date, there are no clinical trials that prove the superiority of any given regimen. What does appear to make a difference is protocol-driven care by an experienced burn center. This includes fluid therapy, ventilator support when needed, aggressive nutrition, and physical therapy. Ocular involvement is frequent, and as many as half of the survivors have severe long-term sequelae. Ophthalmologic consultation should be obtained early in the course of the disease in order to diagnose and treat pseudomembranous or membranous conjunctivitis.

A number of systemic therapies for SJS/TENS have been proposed as well. Although systemic steroids decrease the inflammatory response, they have not improved survival in TEN/SJS after the development of desquamation. The use of immunoglobulin was recommended due to its inhibition of CD95 in an experimental model. However, clinical studies have not demonstrated benefit of immunoglobulin administration.

Mortality from TEN ranges from 20% to 75%. A multicenter review of 199 patients treated in U.S. burn centers reported mortality of 32%. Mortality risk from TEN has been associated with multiple factors, including: age more than 40 years, presence of malignancy, greater than 10% TBSA of sloughed epidermis, elevations in blood urea nitrogen level and serum glucose, acidosis (serum bicarbonate less than 20 mEq/L), and heart rate more than 120 beats/minute. Mortality is due primarily to sepsis, multisystem organ failure, and cardiopulmonary complications. Long-term sequelae include abnormal pigmentation, loss of nail plates, phimosis in men, vaginal synechiae in women, dysphagia, conjunctival scarring, lacrimal duct damage with decreased tear production, ectropion, and symblepharon (adhesion of the eyelid to the eyeball). Close follow-up and referral to appropriate specialists is needed to optimize long-term outcomes.

Soft Tissue Surgical Infections

The term "necrotizing soft tissue infections" encompasses a variety of severe infections of the skin, subcutaneous tissue, and muscle that require immediate surgical excision.

The continued use of other terms such as "necrotizing fasciitis," "Fournier's gangrene," and "Meleney's gangrene" has led to substantial confusion in the literature. Regardless of terminology, these infections share several characteristics: most are rapidly progressive, produce severe toxicity, and lead to necrosis of involved tissues, which may spread rapidly. These infections are discussed in more detail in Chapter 8, Wounds and Wound Healing, but are mentioned here because their appropriate treatment often results in large wounds that burn centers are well equipped to treat. Like burn victims, such patients often require aggressive fluid resuscitation, meticulous wound care and surgery, critical care support, and prolonged rehabilitation. Some examples of these injuries are included in Figures 10-39 and 10-40.

the**Point** ✳ Go to http://thePoint.lww.com/activate and use your scratch-off code on the inside cover of this book to access these illustrations, bonus chapters, question bank, and more.

SAMPLE QUESTIONS

Questions

Choose the best answer for each question.

1. A 63-year-old man with chronic obstructive pulmonary disease (COPD) caught his home on fire while smoking in bed. He was trapped in the house for an unknown time period before firefighters extricated him. He presents to the Emergency Center with severe facial blistering, singed nasal hairs, black intraoral mucosa, a swollen tongue, and carbonaceous sputum. His pulse oximetry reads 85% on room air, and he is obtunded. What is the next best step in management?

   A. Administer racemic epinephrine and steroids.

   B. Draw an arterial blood gas for carboxyhemoglobin levels.

   C. Secure his airway by endotracheal intubation.

   D. Place him on 10 L oxygen by humidified facemask.

   E. Transfer him to the hyperbaric oxygen chamber.

2. A 25-year-old man suffers burns to 40% total body surface area (TBSA) in an explosion at a natural gas drilling site. He requires emergent intubation and fluid resuscitation. During his first week of hospitalization, he undergoes a major operative procedure for excision and skin grafting. By the end of the third week in the hospital, his weight (which originally increased with resuscitation) has come back down, and he weighs 12 pounds less than before the injury. What is the most likely cause for his weight loss?

   A. Decreased nitrogen excretion and resulting catabolism

   B. Increased nitrogen excretion and resulting catabolism

   C. Protein malnutrition with respiratory muscle building

   D. Immune system building with increased risk of pneumonia and bacteremia

   E. Indirect calorimetry readings to support positive nitrogen balance

3. A 27-year-old man is sprayed with concentrated sulfuric acid while working in an oil refinery, sustaining burns to his face, hands, and forearms. He is brought immediately to the emergency room. On initial exam, he is awake and in pain. His clothes are soaked with acid. In addition to providing appropriate protection for all health care workers, the first step in management should be to

   A. debride his burns and complete a Lund and Browder chart.

   B. immediately place the patient in a decontamination shower.

   C. perform a secondary survey.

   D. begin fluid resuscitation.

   E. contact the local burn center for referral.

4. A 6-year-old girl was burned in a house fire and unable to escape. She was found unconscious by firefighters, who intubated her at the scene. On arrival in the burn center, she is found to have carbonaceous sputum, elevated carboxyhemoglobin levels, and burns to 30% TBSA. You should inform her parents that inhalation injury significantly increases the mortality rate of patients with major burns *mostly* due to

   A. increased metabolic rate and protein–calorie malnutrition.

   B. persistent pulmonary infection and eventual development of multiple organ failure.

   C. hypoxia.

   D. airway obstruction.

   E. increased fluid requirements for resuscitation.

5. A 19-year-old man is seen in the emergency department 20 minutes after a high-speed head-on collision with a tree, in which his car caught fire. He was not wearing a seat belt and was ejected from the vehicle. In the emergency department, he is alert, but he does not remember what happened. He admits to drinking a few beers earlier. Blood pressure is 75/40 mm Hg and heart rate 140. His airway is patent. Breath sounds are equal bilaterally. Arterial blood gases reveal a PaO_2 of 140, SaO_2 of 98%, $PaCO_2$ of 34, and pH of 7.33. He has burns to 15% TBSA, involving his anterior trunk and legs. His abdomen is covered with burns but appears distended; tenderness is hard to determine because of painful burn wounds. What is the most likely cause of his hypotension?

   A. Smoke inhalation injury

   B. Burn shock

   C. Intra-abdominal hemorrhage

   D. Ethanol intoxication

   E. Closed head injury

Answers and Explanations

1. Answer: C

This man presents with every manifestation of inhalation injury, which is the most frequent cause of death in victims of structural fires. Oxygen therapy is essential, but this man likely does not have an adequate airway. Securing his airway is the first principle of treatment. Section: Initial Care of the Burn Patient. Subsection: Primary Survey.

2. Answer: B

In response to the increased metabolic demands of a major burn, skeletal muscle is broken down to provide an available energy substrate. This results in increased nitrogen excretion, and loss of lean body mass, which can exceed a half pound per day. Cardiac muscle and respiratory muscles are not immune from these effects, and as muscle wasting continues, both heart failure and respiratory failure can occur. Loss of as little as 15% lean body mass can lead to a fatal degree of inanition within a few weeks of injury. Section: Definitive Care of Burn Injuries. Subsection: Nutritional Support.

3. Answer: B

The patient illustrates the danger that health care workers face when dealing with hazardous material spills. Unwary physicians and nurses who attempt to help this man could suffer serious burns from the acid on his clothing, which is continuing to burn the patient as well. This chemical must be neutralized before a primary survey can be conducted safely. All of the other answers are appropriate steps in treatment but should not be performed until after the patient is decontaminated. Section: Special Problems in Burn Care. Subsection: Chemical and Electrical Burns.

4. Answer: B

Though inhalation injury can produce immediate death from carbon monoxide poisoning and hypoxia, patients who survive the initial event should survive this problem. Similarly, airway obstruction is usually a treatable problem with limited time course. Pneumonia is the most worrisome complication of smoke inhalation, because it is often persistent/recurrent, and difficult to treat. Persistent infection—including pneumonia—often leads to development of the multiple organ failure syndrome, which is usually fatal. Section: Pathophysiology of Burn Injury. Subsection: Pathophysiology of Inhalation Injury.

5. Answer: C

This patient illustrates the importance of the secondary survey in victims of burn injury. This man's burns are too limited in extent to cause severe shock, especially so soon after injury. Smoke inhalation is doubtful, especially with good blood gases. There is no evidence for ethanol intoxication or closed head injury. Unless a second injury (i.e., abdominal trauma) is *considered*, it will not be diagnosed. Section: Initial Care of the Burn Patient. Subsection: Secondary Survey.

11
Abdominal Wall, Including Hernia

LEIGH NEUMAYER, M.D., M.S. • DALE A. DANGLEBEN, M.D. • SHANNON FRASER, M.D., M.SC. •
JONATHAN GEFEN, M.D. • JOHN MAA, M.D. • BARRY D. MANN, M.D.

Objectives

1. Know the relations of the layers of the abdominal wall and their pertinent reflections into the groin.

2. Define indirect inguinal hernia, direct inguinal hernia, and femoral hernia.

3. List the factors that predispose to the development of inguinal hernias.

4. Define and discuss the relative frequency of indirect, direct, and femoral hernias by age and gender.

5. Define incarcerated hernia, strangulated hernia, Richter's hernia, and sliding inguinal hernia.

6. Outline the principles of management for patients with groin hernias, including observation, surgical treatments (ante-

rior, posterior, open, and laparoscopic) for repair, and the indications for their use.

7. List the factors that predispose to the development of incisional hernias.

8. Discuss the appropriate use of prosthetic materials in hernia repair.

9. Discuss the embryology of an umbilical hernia.

10. Describe the advantages and disadvantages of open compared to laparoscopic incisional hernia repair.

11. Advise a patient on the best approach to incisional hernia management based on specific consideration of the patient's past medical and past surgical history.

The abdominal wall is of obvious importance in keeping our insides inside. Knowledge of its anatomy is vital to plan transgressions for access to the enclosed viscera and to understand the common clinical problem of abdominal wall (including groin) **hernias.** Hernias are one of the most common clinical problems addressed by surgeons, with more than 700,000 groin hernia repairs performed annually. This chapter emphasizes anatomy and embryologic development because only with that knowledge can the surgeon plan structural changes to correct symptomatic defects. The chapter reviews the pertinent anatomy and discusses the most common **hernias** and their management.

ANATOMY OF THE ABDOMINAL WALL

Surface Relations

The abdominal wall has few anatomic landmarks. Only the costal margins, anterior superior iliac spines, and umbilicus break the otherwise flat plane. Where anatomy failed, verbiage was substituted. Hypochondriacal (below the ribs), periumbilical (around the umbilicus), and epigastric (upon the stomach) are examples of colorful, but imprecise, terms. Other attempts were made to define abdominal regions by drawing imaginary lines across the abdominal wall. Thus, the abdomen was halved, trisected, and even divided into as

many as nine imaginary compartments in attempts to provide reliable topographic characteristics. The most useful of these is the creation of simple vertical and horizontal lines through the umbilicus, dividing the abdomen into four imaginary quadrants (Figure 11-1). In this format, the right upper quadrant covers such disease-prone intra-abdominal organs as the gallbladder, duodenum, right pleura, and liver. The left upper quadrant covers the spleen, stomach, left pleura, and tail of the pancreas. The left lower quadrant lies over the sigmoid colon, left ureter, and the left ovary in a woman. The right lower quadrant overlies the right ureter, cecum, Meckel's diverticulum, right ovary, and that common cause of right lower quadrant pain, the appendix.

Cutaneous Nerves

Cutaneous nerves arising from the intercostal nerves (T7–L1) supply the sensation and motor function of the anterior abdominal wall. At each level, posterior rami supply the paraspinal muscles and sensation to the back and flank (see Figure 11-2, Right). The anterior ramus running between the transversus abdominis and the internal oblique, gives rise to the lateral cutaneous nerve, which traverses the internal and external oblique muscles at about the mid-axillary line. It then branches into anterior and posterior divisions. The anterior primary ramus continues its course beyond the lateral

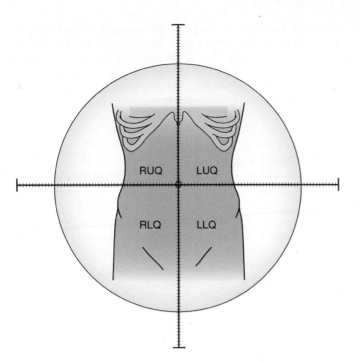

FIGURE 11-1. View of the anterior abdominal wall defining the descriptive sectors of anatomy. RUQ, right upper quadrant; LUQ, left upper quadrant; RLQ, right lower quadrant; LLQ, left lower quadrant.

cutaneous branch; anteriorly it pierces the rectus sheath, supplies the rectus muscle, and proceeds anteriorly to the midline and paramedian skin. These nerves supply the anterior and posterior abdominal walls in a dermatome-like fashion, with a relatively transverse distribution in the upper abdomen and a more oblique pattern in the groin (Figure 11-2, Left). The result of this rich cutaneous innervation is a series of dermatome-related clues to intra-abdominal diagnoses. For example, visceral afferent fibers from the appendix fol-

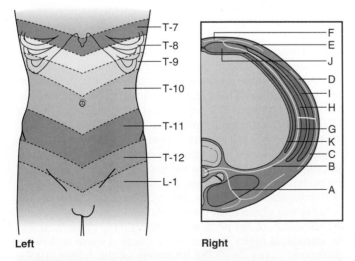

Left   **Right**

FIGURE 11-2. Left, Cutaneous nerve distribution to the anterior abdominal wall. Right, Schema of the cutaneous nerves. A, Posterior primary division. B, Anterior primary division. C, Posterior division of the lateral cutaneous nerve. D, Anterior division of the lateral cutaneous nerve. E, Lateral division of the anterior cutaneous nerve. F, Medial division of the anterior cutaneous nerve. G, Transversus abdominis muscle. H, Internal oblique muscle. I, External oblique muscle. J, Rectus abdominis muscle. K, Peritoneum.

low the same nerve distribution as the small intestine, back to their T10 origins. Therefore, early in its course, appendicitis causes central abdominal pain in the T10 dermatome distribution. Later in the course of the disease, if the inflammatory process from the appendix involves the anterior peritoneum beneath the right lower quadrant of the abdomen, this irritation is sensed by somatic afferent fibers of the T12 nerve route. It is referred back in the appropriate lower cutaneous distribution as hyperesthesia. The disease is often well described by abdominal pain findings alone. Despite this apparent degree of segmentation, considerable overlap of cutaneous nerves exists. Because of this overlap, the sacrifice of any single cutaneous nerve usually does not result in a permanent sensory loss. This safety factor is less pronounced in the lower sensory nerves (ilioinguinal and iliohypogastric). The ilioinguinal and iliohypogastric nerves both arise variably from the first lumbar nerve. The ilioinguinal nerve pierces the internal oblique muscle just superior and lateral to the internal inguinal (abdominal) ring and then runs with the spermatic cord. The ilioinguinal nerve innervates the base of the penis (or mons pubis), the scrotum (or labia majora), and the medial thigh, and is the nerve that is most frequently injured during open inguinal hernia repair. The iliohypogastric nerve is usually encountered just under the external oblique fascia, superior to the cord structures, often lying near the tendinous portion of the internal oblique muscle, and innervates the suprapubic skin. The genital branch of the genitofemoral nerve travels with the spermatic cord. Injury to these nerves can leave permanent numbness in the groin, scrotum, and anterior thigh. Entrapment of these nerves in scar tissue or sutures can result in chronic (lasting longer than 6 months) neuropathic pain for the patient. The incidence of chronic pain after inguinal hernia repair appears to be between 6% and 13%.

The abdominal wall dermatome pattern also explains why incisions that cross the oblique orientation of the nerves often result in muscle denervation and a postoperative bulge or hernia in the abdominal wall. Experienced surgeons have learned to make either midline incisions or an oblique incision in the direction of the nerve fibers to avoid this denervation.

Layers of the Abdominal Wall

A brief review of the seven individual layers that make up the abdominal wall is helpful before discussing of the role of these layers in surgical disease or their use in designing surgical repairs. The following discussion describes the anatomy of the seven individual layers, with particular attention to the origins and reflections of fascial continuity for each. The most notable reflection occurs in the groin, where all of the layers of the abdominal wall are reflected into the scrotum, much as the layers of a shirt, jacket, and overcoat are reflected off the chest wall and onto a sleeve, while maintaining constant relation to each other.

Skin

As elsewhere, Langer's lines of cleavage are present in the skin of the abdominal wall. The course of fibrous bundles and the disposition of elastin fibers in the corium produce these lines of skin tension. Across the anterior abdominal wall, these lines are oriented transversely. In the lower abdomen, like the cutaneous nerves, Langer's lines assume a slightly more oblique pattern as they course into the groins. The skin, its cleavage lines, and its superficial cutaneous innervation all are continuous onto the scrotum in the male and the labia in the female.

Subcutaneous Tissue

The subcutaneous tissue of the abdominal wall has two layers. The more superficial and fatty of the two is Camper's fascia. The deeper, more fibrous, denser layer is Scarpa's fascia. There is considerable disagreement about the precise definition and fascial connection of these two adipose layers. In general, they can be incised in any plane, with little adverse effect. Scarpa's fascia continues into the perineum as the superficial perineal fascia of Colles of the penis and the tunica dartos of the scrotum. It is from this continuity that infections and urinary extravasations proceed upwards from the perineum and the abdominal wall. The major functioning muscles of the abdominal wall are broad, flat, constricting layers. In general, these layers overlap throughout their course and join symmetrically in the midline.

External Oblique Muscle

The most superficial of these is the external abdominal oblique muscle. This muscle arises broadly from the lower eight ribs and interdigitates with the serratus anterior muscle and latissimus dorsi. In the flank, it forms a thick, broad muscle, the fibers of which run obliquely downward. However, as it courses over the anterior aspect of the abdominal wall, the fibers of its **aponeurosis** run essentially transversely. High in the abdomen, this aponeurosis fuses with the anterior half of the aponeurosis of the internal oblique muscle at the lateral margin of the rectus abdominis muscle to form the anterior rectus sheath (Figure 11-3). Lower in the abdomen, this fusion occurs near the midline.

In the groin, the aponeurotic fibers of the external oblique muscle angle downward, taking the direction of your fingers if they are placed comfortably in your jean pockets. Further laterally, this aponeurosis rolls on itself to form the inguinal (Poupart) ligament. This ligament is a free margin suspended between the anterior superior iliac spine and the pubic tubercle, with no muscular origins or insertions. Medially, the fibers of the inguinal ligament rotate and attach onto the most medial portion of **Cooper's ligament** as the lacunar ligament, which forms the medial boundary of the femoral hernia. The external spermatic fascia of the spermatic cord

is derived from the external oblique aponeurosis as the cord passes between the crura of the superficial ring. The fascia lata of the thigh is attached to the inguinal ligament. Finally, near the medial attachment of the external oblique aponeurosis onto the pubic tubercle, the aponeurosis divides, forming a triangular orifice known as the superficial or external inguinal ring through which the spermatic cord and testicle descend.

Internal Oblique Muscle

The internal oblique muscle arises broadly from the iliac crest, lumbodorsal fascia, and from the lateral part of the inguinal ligament. Its fibers are directed obliquely upward in the high flank, transversely in the midflank, and slightly downward in the low flank. Like the external oblique muscle, the internal oblique forms a broad aponeurosis that fuses into the midline and contributes to the anterior rectus sheath throughout the abdomen as well as the posterior rectus sheath in the upper abdomen (see Figure 11-3). The internal oblique muscle fibers arising from the abdominis inguinal ligament join with similar fibers of the internal oblique to form the conjoint tendon, which is inserted into the pubic crest behind the external inguinal ring.

Transversus Muscle

The transversus abdominis muscle, the deepest of the three muscular layers, has similar origins and attachments to the internal oblique, arising from the lower six ribs, the thoracolumbar fascia, the iliac crest, and the lateral part of the inguinal ligament. It fuses medially to form the rectus sheaths and the linea alba.

Transversalis Fascia

The transversalis fascia is a thin stratum of connective tissue lying between the internal surface of transversus abdominis and the extraperitoneal fat. With the descent of the testicle, the transversalis fascia establishes continuity with the internal spermatic fascia of the spermatic cord.

Peritoneum

The peritoneum is a serous membrane that lines the entire peritoneal cavity and invests the intra-abdominal structures. Details of the intra-abdominal reflections of the peritoneum and the formation of the greater and lesser peritoneal sacs are discussed in Chapter 13, Stomach and Duodenum; Chapter 14, Small Intestine and Appendix; and Chapter 15, Colon, Rectum, and Anus. The peritoneum is best described as the exquisitely sensitive final lining layer of the anterior abdominal wall. With the descent of the testicle in utero, a portion of the peritoneum is also pulled into the scrotum (Figure 11-4). With complete development, this peritoneal remnant remains as the tunica vaginalis of the testicle. In normal development, the remainder of the peritoneal connection is obliterated and the peritoneal cavity is once again a sealed space within the abdominal cavity (with the exception of the fallopian tube orifices). If this obliteration process is not completed, the result is varying degrees of persistence of an open communication between the peritoneal cavity and the tunica vaginalis. These varying degrees of patency result in an indirect hernia, a communicating or a noncommunicating hydrocele, or a mere persistent patency of the processus vaginalis, inviting herniation.

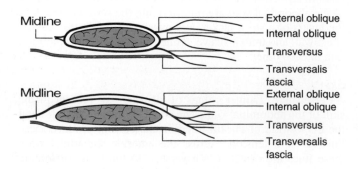

FIGURE 11-3. Cross section showing midline fascial relations above (top) and below (bottom) the semicircular line of Douglas.

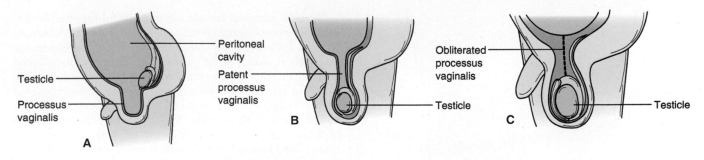

FIGURE 11-4. Peritoneal accompaniment of testicular descent. A, Before descent. **B,** Full patency of the processus vaginalis after descent. **C,** Patent remnant or noncommunicating hydrocele.

Midline Structures

All of the layers of the abdominal wall are continuous across the anterior midline. The skin, subcutaneous tissues, transversalis fascia, and peritoneum are simple continuations, but the fusions and attachments of the abdominal muscles, umbilicus, and umbilical cord remnants deserve special attention.

To understand these midline structures, the relationships between the sheaths and locations of the rectus abdominis muscles must be appreciated. The rectus abdominis muscle consists of narrow, thick bands of muscle that parallel the midline from the costal cartilages to the pubic symphysis and pubic crest. Each muscle is divided along its course by a variable number of tendinous intersections that essentially divide the muscle into a series of interconnected muscles. Above the umbilicus, the recti are separated by a dense fascial line where the aponeuroses of the abdominal muscle all come together. This fibrous line is called the linea alba. The formation of the linea alba and of the rectus sheaths is of some anatomic interest and surgical importance (see Figure 11-3). Approximately midway between the umbilicus and the symphysis pubis is an anatomic landmark, the semicircular line of Douglas (arcuate line). Above this line, the external oblique aponeurosis and the anterior leaf of the internal oblique aponeurosis and the central oblique aponeurosis fuse to form the anterior rectus sheath, and the posterior leaf of the internal oblique aponeurosis and the aponeurosis of the transversus abdominis fuse to form the posterior rectus sheath. Below the semicircular line, all three aponeuroses cross anterior to the rectus muscle, leaving only the peritoneum and the transversalis fascia between the rectus muscles and the abdominal contents. Below the semicircular line, the exact point of fusion of the aponeurotic layers to form the rectus sheath is variable. The external oblique usually joins far medially. The internal oblique and transversus fuse near the lateral edge of the rectus muscle.

Umbilicus

By the start of the second trimester, the omphalomesenteric duct disappears, the gut rotates and reenters the peritoneal cavity, and the body walls form, with the exception of a ring of variable size in the middle of the abdomen. Through this ring pass the umbilical arteries, left umbilical vein, and the allantois (a tubular diverticulum of the embryonic hindgut). At birth, these three atrophy into fibrous cords. With healing of the transected cord, the force of retraction of those vessels modifies the formation of the umbilical ring scar. These forces result in weak portions of the scar, usually at the superior portion of the umbilical defect, where later umbilical herniations can develop.

Remnants of this physiologic closure yield structures that are of occasional surgical interest. The left umbilical vein persists as the ligamentum teres of the liver, coursing in the falciform ligament from the umbilicus to the hepatic margin. Although it physiologically closes and fibroses after birth, this vessel is frequently available for cannulation in the newborn (and even occasionally in the adult) for venous access. Remnants of the omphalomesenteric duct may persist as either vitelline duct cysts, cutaneous fistulas to the umbilicus, or a Meckel's diverticulum. Finally, failure of allantois closure may result in urachal cysts or total urachal fistula, with urinary soiling at the umbilicus.

ABDOMINAL INCISIONS

Access to the abdominal cavity is obtained by surgical incisions. The ideal incision provides adequate access to the intra-abdominal organ under investigation, reestablishes the strength and form of the abdominal wall postoperatively, and leaves a cosmetically acceptable surgical scar. The following are the commonly used surgical incisions (Figure 11-5).

Midline vertical incisions are the most widely used. They are directed through the fused aponeurotic midline (linea alba), anywhere from the xiphoid to the pubic tubercle. This incision has multiple advantages, including the speed at which it can be made (no vascular structures cross the midline), its ability to provide access to all portions of the abdomen, and the fact that it can be extended easily. Consider, for example, that you explore a patient with "free air" suspecting to find a perforated duodenal ulcer. You open the upper midline to find that there is feculent intra-abdominal fluid and the cause of the free air is perforated sigmoid diverticulitis. It is easy to extend the midline incision inferiorly to gain proper exposure to the sigmoid colon. It is the incision of choice in trauma or when lack of a preoperative diagnosis requires exposure of all portions of the abdomen.

Transverse incisions are preferred by some surgeons as being more "physiologic" and are often the incisions of choice in pediatric surgery. The skin incisions are made along Langer's lines, resulting in better cosmetic scars. More importantly, they are made in line with the direction of muscle tension, so postoperative coughing or exercise tends to close the incision rather than open it (as occurs in vertical incisions). As a result, the incidence of wound dehiscence and late herniation is theoretically minimized. Transection of the rectus

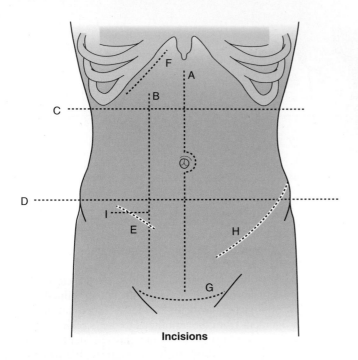

Incisions

FIGURE 11-5. Common incisions across the anterior abdominal wall. **A**, Midline incision. **B**, Paramedian incision. **C** and **D**, Two of the multiple planes of transverse incisions. **E**, McBurney incision. **F**, Subcostal incision. **G**, Pfannenstiel incision. **H**, Kidney transplant incision. **I**, Rocky-Davis incision.

abdominis muscle is not a significant problem as it heals without difficulty and functionally becomes just one more tendinous inscription.

Retroperitoneal incisions are increasingly being used for access to the aorta and vessels, kidneys, and the anterior spine. In the lower quadrants, a hockey stick skin incision is used to access the iliac vessels and bladder for kidney transplantation.

Paramedian incisions have fallen into disrepute in recent years. They add very little to the exposure provided through a midline vertical incision. In addition, they have several disadvantages: (1) they are time consuming to create and close; (2) they may denervate medial portions of the rectus muscle and overlying skin; and (3) because of their inherent weakness, they are the most prone to herniation or disruption. The farther lateral a paramedian incision is fashioned, the more detrimental it is.

Subcostal incisions (also known as Kocher incisions) are advocated because they improve visibility for certain diseases in the upper abdomen. Although they combine some of the better features of the previous incisions, they also have the disadvantages of both. Lines of muscular pull, cutaneous and muscle innervation, and skin tension are all traversed, as with a vertical incision, whereas the possibility of extension in the case of misdiagnosis is compromised. A subcostal incision can be extended across the midline bilaterally for liver transplants and exposure of the pancreas (called a "chevron" incision).

The *Pfannenstiel* incision is commonly used for obstetric, gynecological, and occasional urologic procedures. It is a transverse skin incision just above the pubic bone. The rectus fascia is divided in the midline vertically, and offers enhanced exposure and visibility. It also affords excellent cosmesis as it is well hidden by undergarments.

Specific incisions are occasionally useful for specific diseases. The best example is the right lower quadrant McBurney incision for approach to the appendix. When a preoperative diagnosis is made, all of the benefits of this well-designed surgical incision can be realized. The transverse skin incision is in line with Langer's lines, and none of the cutaneous nerves, including the ilioinguinal and iliohypogastric, are disturbed. The precise location of McBurney's point, two-thirds of the distance from the umbilicus to the anterior iliac spine, allows the placement of a small incision immediately over the diseased organ. The muscle layers are divided bluntly in line with their direction of pull, so herniation and disruption are rare. Once the procedure has been completed, the peritoneum is closed, and then some claim that no further approximation of muscle or fascia is necessary, although most would reapproximate all layers. Another incision utilized for appendectomy is the Rocky-Davis (Figure 11-5, I). This incision is transverse at the skin and then splits the muscle in an oblique direction.

HERNIAS OF THE ABDOMINAL WALL

A hernia is the protrusion of any organ, structure, or portion thereof through its normal anatomic confines. In the abdominal wall, a hernia is the protrusion of all or part of any intraabdominal structure through any congenital, acquired, or iatrogenic defect. Whenever a hernia originates through a relatively small aperture, there is a risk of **incarceration**, which occurs when the contents of a hernia become entrapped and cannot be reduced back into the abdominal cavity. Incarceration of a hernia is the most common cause of bowel obstruction in people who have not had previous abdominal surgery. It is the second most common cause of small bowel obstruction, after postoperative bands and adhesions (see Chapter 14, Small Intestine and Appendix, and Chapter 15, Colon, Rectum, and Anus). This entrapment can become so severe that the blood supply to or from the bowel is compromised (**strangulation**). The result is bowel necrosis, which may progress to intestinal **perforation**. Strangulation should be suspected when there is erythema of the overlying skin, tachycardia, fever or elevated white blood cell count; this represents a true surgical emergency. Omentum or loops of bowel can remain incarcerated within the hernia for months or years without proceeding to strangulation; in general, chronic incarcerations are not painful nor do they cause an acute bowel obstruction. Acute incarcerations, on the other hand, are more troublesome, since they are more likely to result in strangulation. When a patient presents with an acute incarceration, one should attempt reduction and proceed with surgery urgently (or emergently if reduction is not possible).

Inguinal Hernias

Indirect Inguinal Hernia
Anatomy and Pathophysiology

An indirect inguinal hernia occurs when bowel, omentum, or another intra-abdominal organ protrudes through the internal inguinal ring descending within the continuous peritoneal coverage of a patent processus vaginalis, which is anteromedial to the spermatic cord (Figure 11-6). As the epigastric vessels lie medial to the point that the processus vaginalis protrudes,

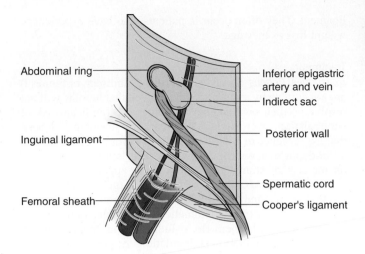

FIGURE 11-6. Indirect inguinal hernia. The posterior inguinal wall is intact. A hernia develops in the patent processus vaginalis (sac) on the anteromedial aspect of the cord. (In this figure and in Figures 11-7 and 11-8, the external oblique and internal oblique layers are not shown because they have no role in the development or repair of inguinal hernias.)

TABLE 11-1	Approximate Relative Incidence of Hernia Type		
	Direct	**Indirect**	**Femoral**
Men	40%	50%	10%
Women	Rare	70%	30%
Children	Rare	All	Rare

an indirect hernia is often defined anatomically as a hernia "lateral to the epigastric vessels." A more fundamental definition of an indirect inguinal hernia, however, is to understand that it is a congenital lesion; if the processus vaginalis does not remain patent, an **indirect hernia** cannot develop. Patency of the processus vaginalis is necessary, but not sufficient, for development of an indirect hernia. Indeed 20% of male cadaver specimens retain some degree of processus vaginalis patency. The patient's history often yields the more immediate reason for development of a hernia, usually an episode of vigorously increasing intra-abdominal pressures: for example, lifting a heavy object or coughing vigorously, which opens up the processus vaginalis and allows the organ to protrude.

A patent processus vaginalis leads to three matters of pathology in the groin, depending on the lowest point where the processus vaginalis has sealed. (1) As previously discussed, a patent processus vaginalis allows intra-abdominal contents (usually bowel and omentum) to protrude into the patent indirect sac and into the inguinal canal. (2) A communicating hydrocele is also the result of a patent processus vaginalis, but differs from the indirect hernia in that serous peritoneal fluid instead of bowel travels into the groin to whatever level the patency exists. Because there is free communication between the tunica vaginalis and the peritoneal cavity, the fluid collection is greater after standing and less after recumbency, and it worsens significantly by the formation of ascites within the abdominal cavity. (3) A noncommunicating hydrocele occurs when a small portion of the processus vaginalis adjacent to the testicle is not obliterated, but the remainder of the processus vaginalis between it and the peritoneal cavity is obliterated (Figure 11-4). This results in a fluid-filled sac (hydrocele) in the scrotum that is unchanged by position or pressure.

Clinical Presentation

Indirect hernias usually cause a bulge in the groin, typically as a result of increased abdominal pressure. In babies and young children, virtually all inguinal hernias are indirect. A 20-year-old workman hoisting a refrigerator has adequate cause for making a previously undetected patent processus develop into

a hernia. On the other hand, a 60-year-old man presenting with the new onset of a hernia should raise questions as to why this congenital lesion would appear at this late date. Often, chronic coughing from lung disease, straining at micturition due to prostatism, or straining at defecation as a result of a sigmoid obstruction may predispose to development of an inguinal hernia. When obtaining a history from this patient, a thorough review of systems should be undertaken, looking for new symptoms such as cough or constipation. These symptoms should be investigated further; in the absence of related symptoms, most believe that extensive investigation of these organ systems at the time of hernia diagnosis is not warranted. However, a rectal exam including palpation of the prostate and testing the stool for blood are considered standard in the workup of a man over age 50 presenting with a new hernia, and a routine screening colonoscopy should also be recommended if it has not previously been done. Indirect hernias are the most common hernias in both sexes and all age groups (Table 11-1). They occur more commonly on the right because of delayed descent of that testicle.

Direct Inguinal Hernia
Anatomy and Pathophysiology

In contradistinction to the indirect hernia, the direct inguinal hernia bulges directly through the posterior inguinal wall (Figure 11-7). Unlike indirect hernias whose origin is lateral to the inferior epigastric vessels, **direct hernias** bulge medial to the inferior epigastric vessels and are not associated with a patent processus vaginalis. The portion of the posterior inguinal wall through which a direct hernia occurs is referred to as **Hesselbach's triangle.** Its classic boundaries are the

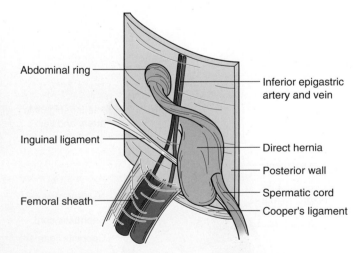

FIGURE 11-7. Direct inguinal hernia. The abdominal ring is intact. A hernia defect is a diffuse bulge in the posterior inguinal wall medial to the inferior epigastric vessels.

linea semilunaris muscle medially, inferior epigastric vessels superolaterally, and inguinal ligament inferiorly. Direct hernias tend not to protrude with the cord into the scrotum and are generally believed to be acquired lesions. Because they are acquired lesions, they are more common in older men. They occur over time as a result of pressure and tension on the fascial layers.

Clinical Presentation

Just like an indirect hernia, a direct inguinal hernia causes a bulge in the groin, ranging from very small-necked pedunculated herniations of preperitoneal fat (diverticular direct hernias) to large, bulging protrusions that destroy the entire posterior inguinal wall. Direct inguinal hernias are usually broad based and are, therefore, much less likely to incarcerate or strangulate.

Femoral Hernia
Anatomy and Pathophysiology

A third category of herniation in the groin is the **femoral hernia.** Like the direct hernia, it is an acquired lesion. Its etiology lies in a short medial attachment of the transversus abdominis muscle onto Cooper's ligament, which results in an enlarged femoral ring that predisposes to herniation (Figure 11-8). This hernia passes into the femoral canal, which is defined by the lacunar ligament medially and the femoral vein laterally. This should not be confused with the femoral triangle, which is defined superiorly by the inguinal ligament, medially by the adductor longus muscle, and laterally by the sartorius muscle, and is an important landmark during angioplasty when seeking to identify the femoral artery.

Clinical Presentation

On physical examination, femoral hernias cause bulges much lower in the groin than other hernias (below the inguinal ring and onto the anteromedial thigh). Despite maximal dilation from repeated protrusion, the femoral hernia ring is limited by rigid structures (the inguinal ligament, its lacunar attachments, and Cooper's ligament). Therefore, this hernia is very susceptible to incarceration and strangulation. Femoral hernias are often mistaken for lipomas or enlarged lymph nodes in the groin because they present as a mass inferior to the inguinal

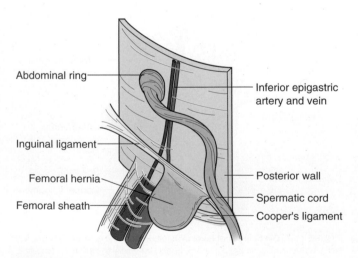

Abdominal ring
Inferior epigastric artery and vein
Inguinal ligament
Femoral hernia
Posterior wall
Femoral sheath
Spermatic cord
Cooper's ligament

FIGURE 11-8. Femoral hernia. The defect is through the femoral canal, but otherwise involves similar structures and insertions as a direct inguinal hernia.

ligament. They often occur in patients who have experienced weight loss as they age.

Treatment

Nonsurgical Options Groin hernias (direct, indirect, or femoral) are not curable by medical therapy. Given that hernias will not resolve on their own and have a perceived significant risk of strangulation, over the last 200 years the teaching has been that the presence of a hernia is indication for repair. Although an in-depth review of the literature reveals a paucity of data on the risk of strangulation, it actually appears to be quite low (well below 0.1%). Recently, two large studies (one in North America and one in England) compared observation to open mesh repair of asymptomatic or minimally symptomatic inguinal hernias in men. Both studies found an exceedingly low rate of incarceration/strangulation. Approximately one-quarter of men had progression of pain and discomfort over 4 years and subsequently underwent repair. There were no adverse consequences of postponing hernia repair until the hernia was symptomatic. Given the known risk of chronic pain in 6% to 13% of patients undergoing hernia repair and the truly negligible risk of acute strangulation, one can consider observation alone in an asymptomatic patient (it is hard to make "asymptomatic" better). Importantly, both studies excluded patients with femoral hernias because femoral hernias are thought to more likely become incarcerated; many patients with femoral hernias initially present with an acute incarceration.

When an incarceration is encountered, a few gentle manual attempts at reduction (i.e., returning the entrapped organ to the confines of the abdominal cavity) are warranted. The patient should be placed in the Trendelenburg position (head-down) and given some pain medication for relaxation if necessary. Gentle steady pressure should be applied to the incarcerated hernia. The pressure should be applied in a cephalad, lateral, and slightly dorsal direction, along the course of the spermatic cord through the inguinal canal. Although these attempts are successful in only 60% to 70% of cases and are associated with some risk to the entrapped structure, they are justified by the potential benefits of patient comfort, relief of obstruction, and prevention of strangulation, and by the diagnostic information obtained. If an incarcerated hernia is successfully reduced, repair should be undertaken in an urgent fashion. At a minimum, the patient should be admitted to the hospital for observation for 12 to 24 hours and offered elective repair before discharge.

For the occasional patient with severe comorbidities that would make any operation exceedingly high risk, palliation is sometimes sought with the use of a truss that may be used for indirect and direct hernias but not for femoral hernias. A truss is a fist-sized ball of leather, rubber, or fabric that is positioned by the patient over the protruding hernia bulge and strapped in place by a variety of belts and straps. With excellent anesthetic and surgical options, the use of a truss is unusual in the current environment.

Surgical Options for Inguinal Hernias The surgical repair of hernias is conceptually simple: (1) reduce any protruding abdominal viscus or organ to the abdominal cavity; (2) create a new, tension-free inguinal floor; (3) recreate a snug abdominal (internal) ring. Additionally, for indirect hernias, obliteration of the processus vaginalis (hernia sac) by either reduction back into the abdominal cavity or ligation at a point high against the abdominal wall prevents recurrence; for femoral hernias, the femoral space must also be obliterated or covered with tissue or mesh (plug technique).

There are many options for repair of groin hernias. There are two basic approaches: anterior (from the front, usually through a groin incision) and posterior (from the back, either through a large lower transverse abdominal incision or laparoscopically). Some repairs are tissue based, (using only the patient's own tissue); but currently most involve also placement of some type of prosthetic to replace or bolster the abdominal wall. The mesh can be placed anteriorly (outside or in between the layers of the groin) or posteriorly (inside, either preperitoneally or intraperitoneally). The physiologic principle for placing the mesh posteriorly (no matter which approach) is that when intra-abdominal pressure increases as it does with coughing or straining, the mesh is pushed up against the abdominal wall and is buttressed by the muscle instead of being pushed away from the abdominal wall.

Repair of Inguinal Hernias

Femoral hernias can be repaired through either an inguinal, thigh, laparoscopic, or abdominal approach, and a combination of approaches may be required if an incarcerated femoral hernia cannot be reduced. In some cases, dividing the iliopubic tract may facilitate reduction of the hernia. The key principle is to close the femoral canal, which can be achieved by the McVay repair and suturing to the Cooper ligament from an inguinal approach, or by a hernia plug when approaching the hernia inferiorly from a thigh incision.

Anterior Mesh Repairs

Lichtenstein Repair (Open) The Lichtenstein (tension free) repair consists of placing a piece of mesh (currently recommended to be at least 3×6 inches in size) to repair the hernia. A slit is cut in the mesh to accommodate the spermatic cord. The mesh is sewn with a nonabsorbable running suture to the inguinal ligament, starting 2 cm medial to the pubic tubercle. Two interrupted sutures are used to tack the mesh superiorly and superolaterally. A third interrupted suture is used to recreate the abdominal ring, suturing the inferior edge of each mesh tail to the inguinal ligament just lateral to the level of the abdominal ring. At least 6 cm of mesh tail are then tucked up underneath the external oblique fascia laterally. The recurrence rate is typically quoted at 1% to 6%.

Mesh-Plug Repair (Open) This repair uses a plug that looks a bit like a badminton birdie. The plug is placed in the defect (tip of the umbrella goes in first) and sewn in place. The plug can be used with or without an onlay piece of mesh similar to the Lichtenstein repair. Some surgeons consider the placement of a plug appropriate for all inguinal hernia repairs; some surgeons condemn its use entirely, considering it an unnecessary "wad" of foreign body; other surgeons use it selectively when a larger hernia has resulted in a virtual "blow out" of the inguinal floor.

Prolene Hernia System (PHS, Open) Recently, there has been increasing use of the PHS. This repair is also a tension free repair that covers the entire myopectineal orifice (MPO, for direct, indirect, and femoral hernias). The preperitoneal space is accessed and dissected out exposing the myopectineal orifice, the mesh consist of two leaflets of polypropylene, with a connector in between. The lower leaflet is deployed in the preperitoneal space, with the onlay portion covering the entire inguinal floor. This repair utilizes the standard anterior approach but it includes a preperitoneal component. This system, like the laparoscopic mesh repairs, was developed to take advantage of preperitoneal mesh placement, without the large incision needed for a traditional preperitoneal repair (Stoppa repair discussed below).

Preperitoneal Repairs

Stoppa Repair (Open) The Stoppa or preperitoneal repair places a very large piece of mesh in the preperitoneal space. The access to this space is through a transverse incision above the groin. This is the same repair as the extraperitoneal laparoscopic repair, aside from the access (through a larger incision for the open repair, compared to several small incisions for the laparoscopic repair).

Kugel Repair (Open) This repair uses a piece of mesh that has been reinforced around the edges so that it will open and stay open once in place. The preperitoneal space is accessed through a small incision in the groin over the abdominal ring. The preperitoneal space is dissected using blunt finger dissection. The oval piece of reinforced mesh is then placed into this space. It does not require suturing because the pressure of the abdominal contents holds it in place against the posterior lower abdominal wall.

Laparoscopic Repairs

Totally Extraperitoneal Repair (Laparoscopic) The totally extraperitoneal (TEP) repair is a laparoscopic repair wherein the entire repair is done without entering the peritoneal cavity. The preperitoneal space is accessed by opening the anterior rectus fascia just to one side of midline (usually the side to be repaired). The muscle is retracted laterally, and sliding a finger inferiorly along the posterior aspect of the rectus gives access to the preperitoneal space. The space is further developed using a balloon that is inflated in the space. A laparoscope camera is then placed through this incision. Trocars are placed through two other incisions; these then serve as working ports. Laparoscopic instruments are used to reduce the hernia sac back into the preperitoneal space, and then a large piece of mesh is placed and tacked with metal clips to prevent slippage. The repair of a direct hernia is technically easier than an indirect hernia, as the reduction of the intestinal contents in a large indirect hernia sac can be quite challenging. Sometimes ligation of the indirect hernia sac is required, and an inadvertent injury to small bowel or colon contained within during this maneuver can be catastrophic.

Transabdominal Preperitoneal Repair (Laparoscopic) The transabdominal preperitoneal (TAPP) repair is similar to the TEP except that the access to the preperitoneal space is gained by incising the peritoneum after placing a laparoscope into the peritoneal space. The peritoneum is reflected down and the hernia sac is reduced. The mesh is placed and tacked in the same locations, and then the peritoneum is brought back up over the mesh to minimize contact of the intestines with the tacks and mesh material.

Note that for the laparoscopic approaches the tacks are not placed laterally. The cutaneous nerve of thigh and the femoral branch of genitofemoral nerve run laterally. This lateral area is usually referred to as the "triangle of pain." This is an area bounded by the spermatic cord medially and the lateral portion of the iliopubic tract (the thickened inferior margin of the transversalis fascia seen as a fibrous band running parallel and posterior (deep) to the inguinal ligament, contributing to the posterior wall of the inguinal canal as it bridges the external iliac–femoral vessels in the subinguinal space, passing from the anterior superior iliac spine to the lacunar ligament). Another area where tacking the mesh should be avoided is the so-called triangle of doom. Its borders consist of the vas deferens medially, the spermatic vessels laterally, and the iliac vessels inferiorly. Venturing into this area with a surgical tacker could result in significant hemorrhage and thus "doom" the patient and surgeon.

Classic Tissue Repairs

The following section is presented only for the sake of completeness. Most classic repairs are no longer performed. All are open repairs.

Marcy Repair The Marcy repair is popular in very small or early indirect hernias. Because these hernias represent only a dilation of the abdominal ring, the Marcy repair simply snugs up that aperture by sewing the transversus aponeurosis on the lateral side of the ring to the transversus aponeurosis on the medial side of the ring until that layer is snug around the cord.

Bassini Repair The Bassini repair is a more superficial repair in which margins of transversus and internal oblique muscles are anchored inferiorly to the inguinal ligament with nonabsorbable interrupted suture. It was the most widely used traditional method for repair of hernias, and associated with a 10% recurrence rate.

McVay (Cooper's Ligament) Repair The McVay procedure is an anatomic repair, like the Marcy operation, that is used for larger indirect hernias and direct hernias and femoral hernias. The principle of this repair is that when the posterior inguinal wall is destroyed by the hernia, the surgical repair of that wall should be as close as possible to the original anatomy. The strong transversus aponeurosis is sewn to Cooper's ligament, along that tendon's natural insertions and the anterior femoral sheath.

Halsted Repair The Halsted repair is similar to a McVay repair except that the external oblique fascia is closed underneath the spermatic cord. It is important to know this when reoperating on these patients from an anterior approach. The cord will be in the subcutaneous tissue, literally unprotected by the external oblique fascia.

Shouldice Repair The Shouldice repair incorporates a series of four running suture lines that approximate and imbricate the transversus aponeurosis to several lateral structures. In a sense, this procedure combines a deep repair similar to McVay's with a superficial repair similar to Bassini's. The Shouldice Clinic in Canada specializes in this repair. Their results in terms of recurrence and chronic pain are as good as or better than results from open mesh and laparoscopic repairs reported in multicenter trials. This is an example of the expertise found at a highly specialized center leading to excellent results.

Reviews and Special Situations

In 2002, the Cochrane Group reviewed the literature regarding nonmesh (generally tension producing) and mesh repairs. This review of 20 randomized trials concluded that the use of mesh repair is associated with a 50% to 75% reduction in the risk of recurrence when compared to nonmesh repairs. There is also some evidence of quicker return to work and of lower rates of persisting pain among patients undergoing mesh repairs. In 2003, the Cochrane Group reviewed studies evaluating laparoscopic compared to open groin hernia repair. There were insufficient data to recommend one over the other, although the data suggest that pain is less and return to work is faster among patients undergoing laparoscopic repair. Particular advantages of the laparoscopic approach are the ability to perform simultaneous repairs when inguinal hernia is bilateral,

and to reduce the difficulty of operating through scar with the added risk of nerve injury when repairing a recurrent inguinal hernia after a previous open repair. However, operation times were longer and there appeared to be a higher risk of serious (visceral or vascular injury) complications with laparoscopic repairs. A previous retropubic radical prostatectomy precludes access to the hernia from the laparoscopic approach. The laparoscopic repair requires general anesthesia, whereas most open repairs can be performed under local, regional, or spinal anesthesia. A large trial published in 2004 evaluated laparoscopic versus open tension-free repair of groin hernias in nearly 2,200 adult men. In this trial, laparoscopic repairs were associated with a 10% recurrence rate while open repairs had a 4% recurrence rate. Further analyses from this large trial showed small differences in pain in the early postoperative period, and return to activities at 4 days in the laparoscopic group (compared to 5 days in the open group), consistent with other trials. The current recommendations for inguinal hernia repair following the findings of the Cochrane review are: in adult men, hernias should be repaired with mesh, whether the approach is laparoscopic or open, although open repair appears to be associated with a lower recurrence rate and fewer life-threatening complications.

Groin Hernias in Women Because groin hernias are much less common in women, there are no randomized trials of sufficient size from which to make recommendations. However, we can make some recommendations using data available from the Swedish hernia registry. In a study of nearly 7,000 groin hernia repairs in women, the recurrence rate was the lowest in women who had a laparoscopic repair, in large part due to the increased incidence of femoral hernias in women that might have been missed during an open repair. A laparoscopic approach allows identification and treatment of all defects.

Groin Hernias in Children In children with inguinal hernias, the hernia is repaired by high ligation (elimination) of the sac without muscle/fascia repair. A laparoscopic exploration of the contralateral groin to exclude a bilateral hernia can be performed through the ipsilateral hernia sac using a needlescope. Hernia repairs in children should have a very low recurrence rate.

Cut-Out Exercise

The authors of this chapter recognize that inguinal anatomy is complicated, and in spite of these procedures often being performed by an attending with a junior resident, the successful repair of hernias is based on an understanding of complex anatomy.

The cut-out exercise included in this chapter (Figure 11-9) simplifies the three-dimensional aspects of inguinal anatomy, which are important as surgical considerations and should illustrate the concept of primary repair for the student. It allows the student to practice using simulation. A student can cut out a mesh and place it under the cord as in the basic Lichtenstein repair. All terms and concepts used within the exercise are compatible with the information delivered in this chapter.

We recommend that you carefully remove the page from this textbook containing the exercise, take the pretest, and then fold and cut the page as directed. Taking the posttest will determine whether you have improved your understanding of hernia repair principles. (The correct answers are listed on the obverse side of the "Penrose Drain.") We believe that working through this exercise, particularly before scrubbing on a hernia repair, will be of great benefit.

THE HERNIA TEACHER

BARRY D. MANN, MD
Anne Seidman
Medical College of Pennsylvania
and Hahnemann University

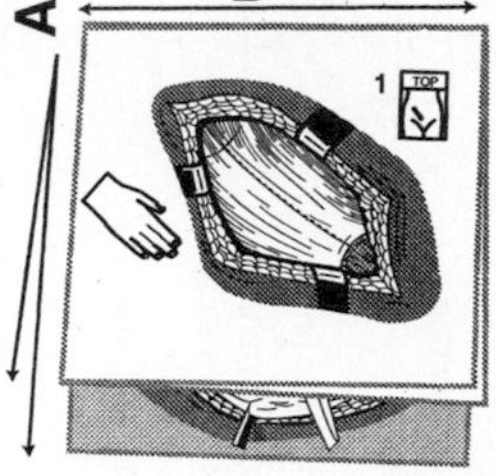

First take Pretest below.
Then fold along fold A
Fold along fold B
Cut along dotted lines C & D until "Stop Cut".

To perform a right inguinal hernia repair,
turn to Frame **1** and follow directions.

Circle T or F	Pre-test	Post-test
1. The fibers of the "conjoined tendon" separate to form the external (superficial) ring.	T F	T F
2. The cremasteric fibers invest the structures of the spermatic cord.	T F	T F
3. The illioinguinal nerve innervates the lateral thigh.	T F	T F
4. A direct sac is more closely adherent to the spermatic vessels than an indirect sac.	T F	T F
5. A finger placed through an indirect hernia sac should slip into the peritoneal cavity.	T F	T F
6. High ligation of a direct hernia sac is required for proper hernia repair.	T F	T F
7. A synthetic mesh sutured in place underneath the cord yields a satistactory hernia repair.	T F	T F
8. The origin of an indirect hernia is medial to the epigastric vessels.	T F	T F
9. The inguinal ligament is actually an extension of the external oblique aponeurosis.	T F	T F
10.Cooper's lig. is part of the "conjoined tendon".	T F	T F

FOLD B

stop cut C

8

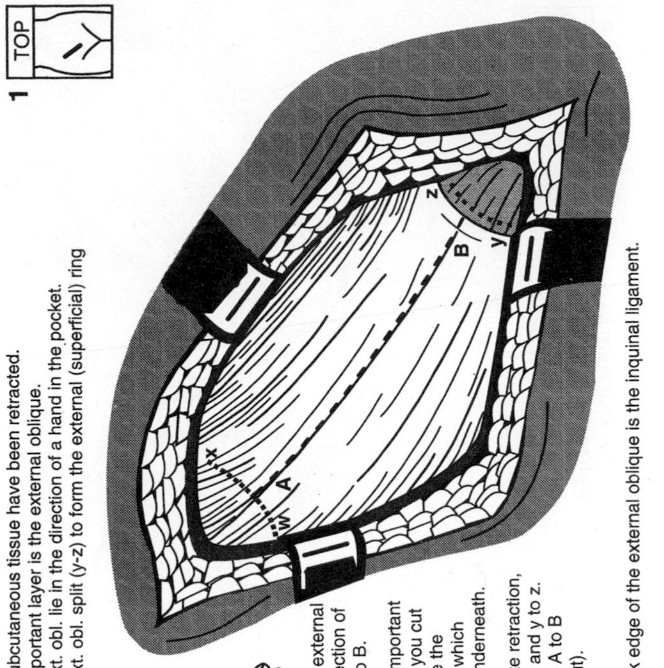

Note:
a) Skin and subcutaneous tissue have been retracted.
b) The first important layer is the external oblique.
c) Fibers of ext. obl. lie in the direction of a hand in the pocket.
d) Fibers of ext. obl. split (y–z) to form the external (superficial) ring.

Step 1 Incise the external oblique in the direction of its fibers from A to B.

*In actuality, it is important to lift upwards as you cut so as not to injure the illioinguinal nerve which may lie directly underneath.

Step 2 To facilitate retraction, incise from w to x and y to z. (In actual surgery A to B will be the only cut).

Note:
e) The rolled back edge of the external oblique is the inquinal ligament.

TOP **1**

FOLD A

k) In this drawing, your finger has replaced the penrose drain You are now teasing away the cremasteric fibers with a scissors.
When this maneuver is complete (Frame 5), you will have "skeletonized" the cord revealing ① the vessels to the testicle,
② the vas deferens (white), and ③ an indirect sac if one is present.
Turn to Frame 5, orient to **TOP** and identify these items.

TOP **4**

(TEST ANS: F,T,F,F,T,F,T,F,T,F)

Note: The origin of an indirect sac lies lateral to the inferior epigastric vessels seen underneath (in Frame 7)
Turn to Frame,**6** and orient to TOP

Step 5 Mobilize the indirect sac which lies antero-medial to the cord by incising dotted line from **G** to **H**

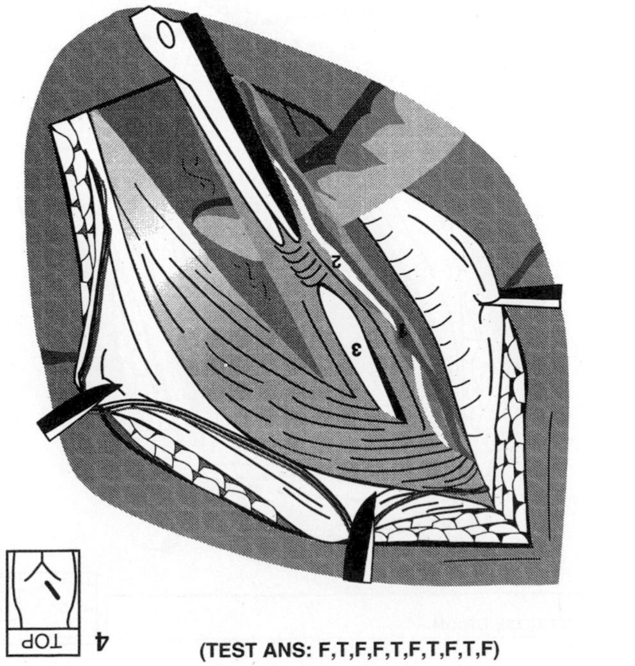

l) The Penrose drain now retracts the vessels and vas deferens (white)

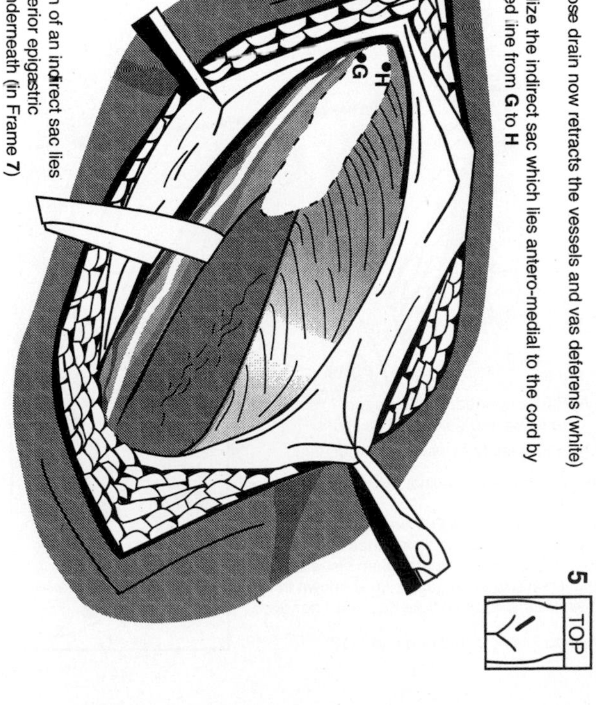

stop cut D

TOP **5**

A

FIGURE 11-9. The Hernia Teacher Cut-Out Exercise. *(Continued next page)*

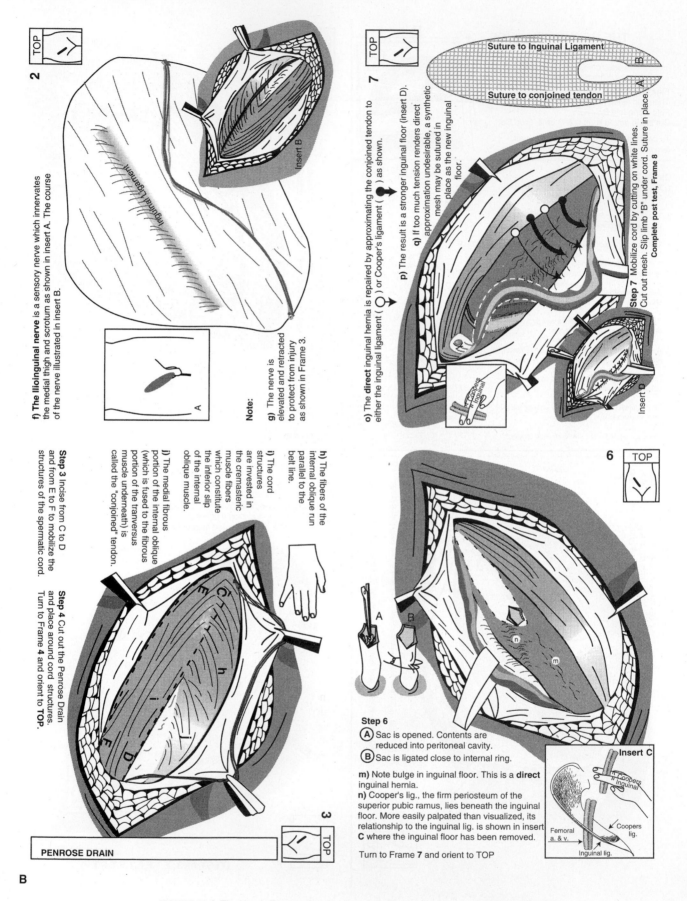

2

f) The Ilioinguinal nerve is a sensory nerve which innervates the medial thigh and scrotum as shown in insert A. The course of the nerve illustrated in insert B.

Insert B

Inguinal Ligament

A

Note:

g) The nerve is elevated and retracted to protect from injury as shown in Frame 3.

h) The fibers of the internal oblique run parallel to the belt line.

i) The cord structures are invested in the cremasteric muscle fibers which constitute the inferior slip of the internal oblique muscle.

j) The medial fibrous portion of the internal oblique (which is fused to the fibrous portion of the tranversus muscle underneath) is called the "conjoined" tendon.

Step 3 Incise from C to D and from E to F to mobilize the structures of the spermatic cord.

Step 4 Cut out the Penrose Drain and place around cord structures. Turn to Frame **4** and orient to **TOP**.

3

PENROSE DRAIN

B

Step 6
(A) Sac is opened. Contents are reduced into peritoneal cavity.
(B) Sac is ligated close to internal ring.

m) Note bulge in inguinal floor. This is a **direct** inguinal hernia.
n) Cooper's lig., the firm periosteum of the superior pubic ramus, lies beneath the inguinal floor. More easily palpated than visualized, its relationship to the inguinal lig. is shown in insert **C** where the inguinal floor has been removed.

Turn to Frame **7** and orient to TOP

6

Insert C

Femoral a. & v.   Coopers lig.

Inguinal lig.

7

Suture to Inguinal Ligament

Suture to conjoined tendon

A B
B

o) The **direct** inguinal hernia is repaired by approximating the conjoined tendon to either the inguinal ligament ( ) or Cooper's ligament ( ) as shown.

p) The result is a stronger inguinal floor (insert D).

q) If too much tension renders direct approximation undesirable, a synthetic mesh may be sutured in place as the new inguinal floor.

Step 7 Mobilize cord by cutting on white lines. Cut out mesh. Slip limb "B" under cord. Suture in place. **Complete post test, Frame 8**

Insert D

FIGURE 11-9. The Hernia Teacher Cut-Out Exercise. *(Continued from previous page)*

Complications After Groin Hernia Repair

A seroma or hematoma presents as a focal, firm swelling in the region of the hernia within 2 or 3 days after the procedure. Though this is generally a complication that is managed by reassurance that the swelling will resolve in a few weeks, it can cause great alarm, with particular concern that the hernia repair has failed. The patient should be warned of this possibility.

Later complications of hernia repair include infection of the wound or the implanted mesh. Whereas infection in inguinal hernia repair is unusual, any superficial infection must be treated aggressively in order to avoid chronic mesh infection. A persistent infection is likely to involve the prosthetic mesh, and may require reoperation for removal of involved foreign material.

A rare complication of hernia repair is ischemic orchitis, which results from injury to the testicular vessels in the spermatic cord during hernia dissection. It can be prevented by both identifying the cord structures during repair and not removing the testes from the scrotum, which can devascularize it. Ischemic orchitis can lead to testicular atrophy or severe chronic testicular pain that is relieved only by orchiectomy. Injury or fibrosis of the vas deferens can impair fertility and can lead to complete infertility in the rare case that the contralateral testicle is nonfunctional.

Nerve injury leading to numbness or neuralgia is a serious complication in inguinal hernia repair. Chronic pain (lasting more than 3 months) has been reported in up to 15% of patients undergoing groin hernia repair, therefore, the risk of this complication should be included when obtaining informed consent for the procedure. Chronic pain can result from entrapment of the ilioinguinal, iliohypogastric, or genitofemoral nerve. Care should be taken to avoid catching a nerve in a suture during the repair. Nerve entrapment may also occur due to the subsequent development of scar tissue or fibrosis. Randomized trials have been conducted to determine the best management of the nerves during herniorrhaphy. Deliberate division of the nerves results in no difference in pain or numbness. The best results are obtained when the nerves are identified and preserved (not incorporated in the repair). In rare cases, the neuropathic pain can be severe and debilitating. Various remedies have been tried to eliminate the pain of entrapped nerves with varying degrees of success. These treatments have included oral analgesics, acupuncture, local injections with bupivacaine, triamcinolone, and/or ketorolac, reoperation with division of the nerves, complete neurectomy, and removal of mesh implants.

Recurrent Hernia

The ultimate measure of success of an inguinal hernia repair is a low rate of hernia recurrence. Traditionally, a recurrence rate of 10% was accepted, until a rate of recurrence as low as 1% was reported by Lichtenstein. Recent multicenter randomized trials report recurrence rates ranging from 4% to 10%. Watchful waiting is acceptable treatment for a recurrent hernia, though patients may be motivated to seek definitive treatment for the condition for which they originally sought surgical intervention. Failure to diagnose multiple hernias at the time of initial operation (i.e., missing an indirect hernia sac during repair of a direct hernia, or missing a femoral hernia), failure to close an enlarged internal ring, and excessive tension on the repair are the leading causes of recurrent hernia. A postoperative hematoma or undue tension may cause mesh to become dislodged from the pubic tubercle medially, which is the most frequent cause of recurrence of a direct hernia. After failed anterior repair, a laparoscopic posterior repair (either TAPP or TEP) is the preferred surgical approach to a recurrent hernia. A laparoscopic approach provides the advantages of operating through unscarred tissue planes, a low incidence of mesh and wound infection, a lower risk of injury to the spermatic cord structures and nerves, and the ability to assess for additional hernias.

Other Abdominal Wall Hernias

Anatomy and Pathophysiology

Other abdominal wall hernias include umbilical hernias, omphalocele, and gastroschisis. An umbilical hernia, by far the most common, is also of least significance and threat to the patient. It is the small (usually <1 cm) defect in the abdominal wall that results from incomplete umbilical closure. Small portions of omentum, bowel, or other intra-abdominal organs may protrude through this fascial defect. In adults, even if umbilical closure occurred, the umbilical scar is subject to stretching and a defect that can enlarge and produce a hernia. The other two types of abdominal wall herniation are much more severe, affect only the newborn, and, fortunately, are very uncommon. An omphalocele occurs when, after incomplete closure of the abdominal wall by the time of birth, a portion of the abdominal contents herniates into the base of the umbilical cord. Unlike the simple umbilical hernia, which is covered by skin, in omphalocele, the abdominal contents are separated from the outside world by only a thin membrane of peritoneum and the amnion. Gastroschisis is an even more severe failure of abdominal wall development. It causes a full-thickness abdominal wall defect lateral to the umbilicus. The hernia of gastroschisis is into the amniotic cavity, so there is no sac. There is no covering of any kind over the intestinal contents, which protrude from the lateral edge of the umbilicus. (See Chapter 3, Pediatric Surgery, in Lawrence et al. eds., *Essentials of Surgical Specialties*, 3rd ed.)

Clinical Presentation

Because the developmental process of the abdominal wall continues into extrauterine life, small protrusions of this type are very common in infants. Unless incarceration occurs, they are best ignored until the preschool years (age 4) as most resolve spontaneously. Despite their innocuous nature in infancy, however, umbilical hernias are some threat in adults, and operative repair is recommended in an adult. The rigid surrounding walls of the linea alba predispose the patient to incarceration and strangulation of protruded organs. Omphaloceles and gastroschisis are perinatal emergencies that require immediate surgical attention. (See Chapter 3, Pediatric Surgery, in Lawrence et al. eds., *Essentials of Surgical Specialties,* 3rd ed.)

An umbilical hernia in a cirrhotic patient presents special considerations. Ascites should be controlled initially by medical therapy such as diuresis, peritoneovenous shunt, or transjugular intrahepatic portosystemic shunt (TIPS), since the rate of complications and hernia recurrence are increased in the presence of ascites. Repair of minimally symptomatic umbilical hernias should be deferred and treated simultaneously during liver transplantation. Careful discussion with the patient of both the risks of future hernia incarceration and strangulation as well as the increased mortality of surgical intervention in cirrhotics should be undertaken before making the final decision to operate.

Treatment

The treatment of umbilical hernia is as straightforward in concept as that of groin hernia: (1) reduce the abdominal contents and (2) establish the continuity of the abdominal wall. Commonly used folk remedies (e.g., stuffing cotton balls into the umbilicus, taping coins over it to prevent protrusion) only delay developmental closure or complicate the hernia with necrosis of the overlying skin. Surgical procedures for a simple umbilical hernia are as straightforward in execution as they are in concept. In children and in adults with defects <1.5 cm in diameter, a primary repair (placing sutures to close the defect) is generally recommended. For defects larger than 1.5 cm, a mesh repair is recommended, since the recurrence rate for mesh repairs when the defect is larger is about half that of nonmesh repairs.

By necessity, surgical therapy for omphalocele and gastroschisis is intricate and complex, including bowel resection and the formation of extra-anatomic compartments fashioned with prosthetic materials. Despite these efforts, the mortality rate for these lesions remains high. (See Chapter 3, Pediatric Surgery, in Lawrence et al. eds., *Essentials of Surgical Specialties,* 3rd ed.)

Incisional (Ventral) Hernias

Anatomy and Pathophysiology

Incisional hernias can develop through any prior fascial incision and occur with an incidence of 10% after previous laparotomy. Deep wound infection is the most common cause of incisional hernias, although other factors such as poor surgical technique, or poor wound healing due to cirrhosis, malnutrition, malignancy, immunosuppression, and steroid dependence, may play a role. Factors that increase intra-abdominal pressure such as obesity, chronic obstructive pulmonary disease (COPD), or constipation as well as some cancers (colon and prostate) are also thought to increase the risk of incisional hernias. The risk of recurrence increases with each additional repair. Incisional hernias are usually diagnosed by visualization of a bulge with an associated palpable fascial defect. In obese patients, abdominal computed tomography (CT) scan may be needed for diagnosis. The patient may complain of the bulge, pain, or discomfort at the site. The patient can also present with a bowel obstruction if the hernia becomes acutely incarcerated. The risk of incarceration and strangulation is higher with smaller defects. If an incisional hernia is not repaired early, the defect may enlarge with time and an operation may become more complex. Some patients develop extremely large incisional hernias, often after multiple abdominal operations. Their defects can result in a "loss of the abdominal domain." These defects present a challenge to repair.

Treatment

The fascial defect of small incisional hernias may be successfully reapproximated with sutures, but most incisional hernias will require repair with mesh, which can be performed via either an open or a laparoscopic approach. Obese patients may benefit from preoperative weight loss, and smoking cessation may be beneficial for patients who smoke.

Whether a repair is performed open or laparoscopically, key principles are the same: (1) avoid injury to intra-abdominal structures, (2) create a tension-free repair, and (3) overlap mesh onto fascia by 3 to 5 cm to prevent recurrence. Mesh can be placed either intra-abdominally, preperitoneally (between peritoneum and muscle), or on top of the fascial layers. The mesh is often secured around the periphery with tacking sutures placed through stab incisions in the skin. These tacking sutures may be brought through all layers of the abdominal wall, through the mesh, then back through mesh and abdominal wall and tied (Figure 11-10). Stab incisions are closed with surgical adhesive tape strips (Steri-Strips).

Component separation using autogenous tissues is an alternative to mesh repair of incisional hernias. There are several variations, but most involve making relaxing incisions through one or two fascial layers of the lateral abdominal wall. This allows approximation of the midline fascia medially. Defects <5 cm wide in the upper and lower abdomen and 10 cm wide in the midabdomen are amenable to closure with component separation. Larger defects will require mesh because there is a limit to the distance the muscles and fascia can be mobilized without causing a defect elsewhere.

Repairs of incisional hernias with mesh are associated with a recurrence rate of about 10% to 20%, most often attributable to excessive tension on the fascial closure. The risk of recurrence increases with each subsequent repair. An infection of a mesh can be quite challenging to manage and ultimately may require removal of the previously implanted mesh.

Other Hernias

Pantaloon Hernia

The **pantaloon hernia** is the simultaneous occurrence of a direct and an indirect hernia. The pantaloon hernia causes two

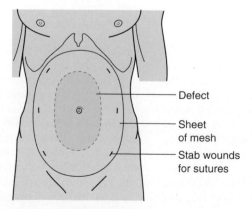

FIGURE 11-10. Incisional hernia repair. The mesh is secured around the periphery with tacking sutures placed through stab incisions in the skin and is brought through all layers of the abdominal wall, through the mesh, and then back through the mesh and abdominal wall. The sutures are then tied.

Defect

Sheet of mesh

Stab wounds for sutures

Suture
Skin
Muscle/fascia
Mesh
Peritoneum

Skin
Muscle/fascia
Mesh
Peritoneum

bulges that would be seen intraoperatively, straddling the inferior epigastric vessels.

Sliding Hernia

A **sliding hernia** is any hernia in which a portion of the wall of the protruding peritoneal sac is made up of some intra-abdominal organ (usually sigmoid on the left, cecum on the right). As the sac expands, the organ is drawn out, into the hernia. There are few physical exam signs to distinguish these from other inguinal hernias, through the presence of an incompletely reducible hernia or the finding of colon in the scrotum on barium enema is most suggestive. Its repair involves the careful return of the organ to the abdominal cavity and avoidance of an inadvertent entry into the bowel or bladder, followed by the traditional sequence of obliteration of the sac and closure of the fascial defect.

Richter's Hernia

Richter's hernia is the name given to a hernia at any site through which only a portion of the circumference of small bowel incarcerates or strangulates. Because the entire lumen is not compromised, symptoms of bowel obstruction can be partial or absent.

Spigelian Hernia

Spigelian hernias are rare herniations through the semilunar line, which is the lateral margin of the rectus muscle, at or just below the junction with the semicircular line of Douglas. Unlike groin hernias, these hernias lie cephalad to the inferior epigastric vessels. The tight aponeurotic defect predisposes them to incarceration. The patient should be offered surgical repair, typically via the open approach; the placement of mesh is typically not required.

Grynfelt's Hernia

Grynfelt's hernia is a wide-mouthed hernia that protrudes through the superior lumbar triangle, which is bounded by the sacrospinalis muscle, the internal oblique muscle, and the inferior margin of the 12th rib. Diagnosis is hampered by the protrusion of these hernias under the latissimus dorsi muscle.

Petit's Hernia

Petit's hernia protrudes through the inferior lumbar triangle, which is bounded by the lateral margin of the latissimus dorsi, the medial margin of the external oblique, and the iliac crest. Like the superior lumbar hernia, these hernias are broad, bulging hernias that usually do not incarcerate.

Littre's Hernia

Any groin hernia that contains a Meckel's diverticulum is Littre's hernia. This type of hernia is usually incarcerated or strangulated at presentation, and may require a laparotomy for intestinal resection.

Amyand's Hernia

Any groin hernia that contains the appendix is an Amyand's hernia. If appendicitis develops it can present a confusing clinical picture.

Obturator Hernia

Obturator hernias are deceptive hernias, often of Richter's type, that protrude through the obturator canal. They are much more common in women and usually occur in the seventh and eighth decades. An obturator hernia is classically diagnosed by the symptoms of intermittent bowel obstruction and paresthesias on the anteromedial aspect of the thigh as a result of compression of the obturator nerve (Howship-Romberg sign). The hernia can sometimes be palpated as a mass on rectal exam. The mortality rate is high (up to 40%), and urgent surgical intervention via laparotomy is warranted.

Hesselbach's Hernia

Like a femoral hernia, Hesselbach's hernia protrudes onto the thigh beneath the inguinal ligament, but courses lateral to the femoral vessels.

Epigastric Hernia

An epigastric hernia, which is due to congenital or acquired weakness of the midline linea alba, protrudes through the crossing midline fibers above the umbilicus. It is more common in men than in women, and 20% of epigastric hernias are multiple. Surgical repair is recommended, and the hernias often can be closed primarily. Recurrences are frequently the result of failure to recognize multiple small defects.

Diastasis Recti

Diastasis recti is not a hernia; it is a midline fascial weakness, not a fascial defect. It should be distinguished from an epigastric hernia. It occurs when the rectus muscles separate in the upper midline, making a wide linea alba, and is often associated with rapid weight change. When the patient contracts the recti (for instance, when trying to sit up), this widening can be mistaken for a hernia because it does cause a bulge, often cosmetically bothersome to the patient. Diastasis is not a true hernia (no fascial defect), so reassurance of the patient is the best treatment.

thePoint ✳ Go to http://thePoint.lww.com/activate and use your scratch-off code on the inside cover of this book to access bonus chapters, question bank, videos, and more.

SAMPLE QUESTIONS

Questions

Choose the best answer for each question.

1. A 46-year-old man comes to your office 6 months after an open inguinal hernia repair complaining of pain, which has never resolved after his surgery. On further questioning, he complains of radicular pain into the testicle, which worsens with sitting for longer than 10 minutes. On exam, he is hyperesthetic overlying his scar and has numbness over the ipsilateral scrotum and medial thigh. All else is normal. Injury to which nerve is the most likely cause for his pain?

   A. Femoral nerve

   B. Hypogastric nerve

   C. Lateral femoral cutaneous nerve

   D. Ilioinguinal nerve

   E. Vagus nerve

2. A 40-year-old man comes to clinic because of a large incisional hernia. One year ago, he underwent a splenectomy for a ruptured spleen following a motor vehicle crash. There is a large hernia in the epigastrium in the central portion of a long midline incision. A laparoscopic incisional hernia repair is recommended to the patient. Which of the following should be included in the discussion with the patient while obtaining informed consent?

   A. Risk of conversion from a laparoscopic procedure to a hand-assist procedure

   B. Whether the patient has insurance coverage

   C. The type of sutures used for mesh fixation

   D. The manufacturer of the prosthetic material

   E. The hernia recurrence rate

3. A 28-year-old man comes to clinic because of an inguinal hernia. He works as a stonemason and first noticed the hernia when he developed a painful bulge while lifting a bag of cement. He has otherwise been healthy and takes no medications. An open inguinal hernia repair with mesh has been recommended. During a discussion of the anticipated risks, which of the following represents the most common complication?

   A. Recurrence

   B. Urinary retention

   C. Reduced fertility

   D. Chronic pain

   E. Ischemic orchitis

4. A 62-year-old man is in the operating room undergoing an open left inguinal hernia repair. A large indirect sliding hernia is found, and during the dissection, the sigmoid colon is inadvertently injured. The colotomy is easily repaired with sutures. Which of the following hernia repairs should be used in this situation?

   A. Bassini repair

   B. Halsted repair

   C. Marcy repair

   D. Cooper's repair

   E. Lichtenstein repair

5. A 32-year-old man comes to the emergency department with an acutely incarcerated inguinal hernia. With sedation, the hernia is reduced and he feels better. Eighteen hours later, he complains of increasing abdominal pain and has diffuse tenderness on examination. He most likely had which of the following?

   A. Diastasis recti

   B. Petit's hernia

   C. Epigastric hernia

   D. Amyand's hernia

   E. Richter's hernia

Answers and Explanations

1. Answer: D

Because of its path alongside the spermatic cord, lying on top of the internal oblique muscle, the ilioinguinal nerve is susceptible to entrapment by most anterior repair techniques. The symptoms described by this patient are most consistent with the distribution of sensory innervation of the ilioinguinal nerve.

2. Answer: E

In general, informed consent for a hernia repair should include the most common risks, which would include recurrence, chronic pain, urinary retention, and possible numbness of the area. If one needed to convert from a laparoscopic repair, the conversion would be to open, not hand assisted. While insurance coverage may be an issue for payment for the hospital, it is not part of informed consent, nor are the types and manufacturers of the materials used for the repair.

3. Answer: D

Recurrence after open inguinal hernia repair is reported to be between 1% and 6%. Urinary retention is observed in approximately 10% of patients—particularly older men—and patients should be able to urinate before discharge home. Chronic neuropathic pain from nerve entrapment is observed in 6% to 13% of patients. Impaired fertility and ischemic orchitis from injury to the vas deferens and spermatic vessels, respectively, are rare complications (<5%).

4. Answer: A

An unexpected injury to the colon during an open hernia repair will change the wound classification to a contaminated procedure and significantly increase the risk of wound infection. Thus, mesh placement with a Lichtenstein repair should be avoided. Performing the more traditional Bassini repair that involves suturing Poupart's ligament to the conjoint tendon will be associated with a higher risk of hernia recurrence but avoids significant wound complications. The Halsted repair is a largely historical procedure, which left the spermatic cord in the subcutaneous tissues. A Cooper repair (also known as a McVay repair) is more difficult to perform than a Bassini repair and would not offer additional benefit in the repair of a sliding hernia, while the Marcy repair would be insufficient to offer any meaningful prevention of recurrence of a sliding hernia.

5. Answer: E

A Richter's hernia involves only a portion of the circumference of a bowel wall and typically is recognized with bowel incarceration or strangulation (sometimes after reduction of the hernia, causing an acute abdomen when the bowel perforates). Diastasis recti is a fascial weakness, not a true fascial defect, and does not require surgical intervention. Petit's hernia is a broad, bulging hernia that usually does not incarcerate. Amyand's hernia contains the appendix and sometimes can present with findings of appendicitis. Epigastric hernias typically are small and often contain preperitoneal fat only. They are often recognized early by the patient in the event that the hernia becomes incarcerated, and strangulation is unlikely to ensue.

12
Esophagus

CARLOS M. LI, M.D. • JAMES A. McCOY, M.D., PH.D. • HWEI-KANG HSU, M.D.

Objectives

1. Describe the general anatomy of the esophagus with respect to location, adjacent structures, and areas of narrowing.

2. Describe the arterial and venous anatomy and innervation of the esophagus.

3. Describe the histological layers of the esophageal wall.

4. Describe the swallowing mechanism in physiological terms.

5. Describe the imaging and functional studies used for the workup of esophageal disease.

6. Describe the anatomic and physiologic factors that predispose to reflux esophagitis.

7. Describe the symptoms of reflux esophagitis, and discuss the diagnostic procedures needed to confirm the diagnosis.

8. List the indications for operative management of esophageal reflux. Discuss the physiologic basis for the antireflux procedure used.

9. List the two major cell types of esophageal cancers.

10. List the known etiologic factors for esophageal cancers.

11. List the symptoms that suggest esophageal cancer.

12. Outline a plan for diagnostic and staging evaluation of a patient with suspected esophageal cancer.

13. Describe the surgical procedures to resect esophageal cancer.

14. Describe the etiology and presentation of traumatic perforation of the esophagus and the physical findings that occur early and late after this type of injury.

15. Describe the workup, management, and surgical management of esophageal perforation.

16. Describe esophageal hiatal hernia with regard to anatomic type and the relative need for treatment.

17. Describe the pathophysiology, diagnostic workup, (including the radiologic and manometric characteristics) and management of achalasia.

18. List the common esophageal diverticula in terms of their location, symptoms, and pathogenesis.

The esophagus connects the oropharynx to the stomach. The complex anatomy and physiology of the esophagus belie its simple function as a conduit for passage of oral contents into the stomach. Regardless of the medical specialty chosen, the future physician will likely encounter a clinical situation where knowledge of esophageal diseases will prove useful. Although this chapter covers various topics on esophageal disease, the medical student should focus on the workup and management of three commonly encountered esophageal diseases. They include gastroesophageal reflux disease (GERD), esophageal carcinoma, and esophageal perforation.

ANATOMY

General Anatomy

The esophagus, a muscular alimentary tube of approximately 25 cm length, connects the pharynx to the stomach. The esophagus starts at the level of the cricoid cartilage (level of the sixth cervical vertebra) and ends just below the diaphragm (level of the eleventh thoracic vertebra). It can be subdivided into four segments, the cervical esophagus (3 to 5 cm long), the proximal and middle thoracic esophagus (18 to 22 cm long), and the distal abdominal esophagus (3 to 6 cm long). For endoscopic mapping purposes, the esophagus starts at around 15 cm from the incisors and ends at about 40 cm from the incisors. It traverses the thorax in the posterior mediastinum. Structures closely associated with the esophagus include the trachea and left atrium (both anterior to the esophagus) and the descending thoracic aorta (the aorta travels along the left of the esophagus and then swings posterior to the esophagus as it passes through the diaphragm) (Figure 12-1). Because the aorta runs along the left side of the esophagus, most surgical approaches to the esophagus are performed through a right thoracotomy (Figure 12-2).

Three anatomic areas of esophageal narrowing are of clinical significance, since ingested foreign bodies often lodge there and food impaction can occur there. They include the proximal esophagus at the level of cricopharyngeus muscle, the midesophageal at the level of the aortic arch, and a distal narrowing at the level of the diaphragm (Figure 12-3). There are two functional sphincters in the esophagus, an **upper esophageal sphincter** (UES), at the level of the cricopharyngeus

CT Scan Cross-Section

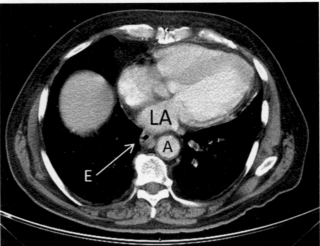

E: esophagus
A: aorta
LA: left atrium

B

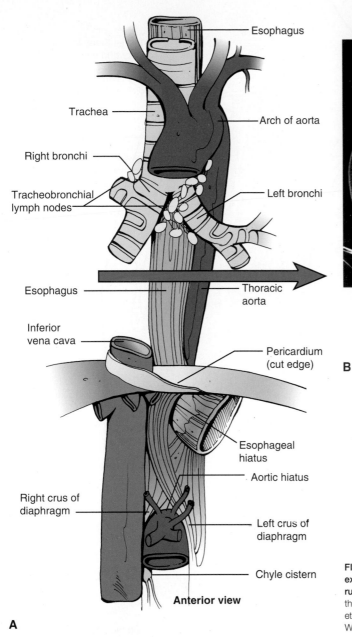

Anterior view

A

FIGURE 12-1. **A,** Anterior view with the lung and the heart removed to expose the posterior mediastinum where the esophagus and the aorta run. **B,** CT scan shows cross-sectional cut at the shown level with the aorta on the left and the heart anterior of the esophagus. (**A,** Reprinted from Fischer JE, et al. *Fischer's Mastery of Surgery*, 6th ed. Philadelphia, PA: Lippincott Williams & Wilkins, 2012:793, with permission.)

muscle, and a **lower esophageal sphincter** (LES), between the esophagus and stomach.

Arterial Supply

The cervical esophagus is supplied by the inferior thyroid artery from the thyrocervical trunk artery. The thoracic esophagus is supplied by the bronchial arteries and smaller esophageal arteries from the thoracic aorta. The distal esophagus is supplied by branches of the left gastric artery (Figure 12-4).

Venous Drainage

The cervical esophagus drains mainly through the inferior thyroid vein. The thoracic esophagus drains mainly through the azygos vein and hemiazygos vein. The distal esophagus is drained through the coronary and left gastric vein, which drain into the portal venous system (Figure 12-5). In liver cirrhosis

with portal vein hypertension, the lower esophageal venous plexus provides collateral drainage from the portal venous system to the azygos veins, leading to esophageal varices.

Lymphatic Drainage

Lymphatics from the cervical esophagus drain into the deep cervical (jugular) lymph nodes. The thoracic esophagus drains into lymph nodes found in the posterior mediastinum, such as the paratracheal and pulmonary hilar lymph nodes. The distal esophagus drains into the celiac, left gastric, and parahiatal lymph nodes (Figure 12-6). Initial lymph node spread is determined by the location of the esophageal carcinoma.

Innervation

Innervation of the esophagus is based on the autonomic nervous system with sympathetic and parasympathetic fibers

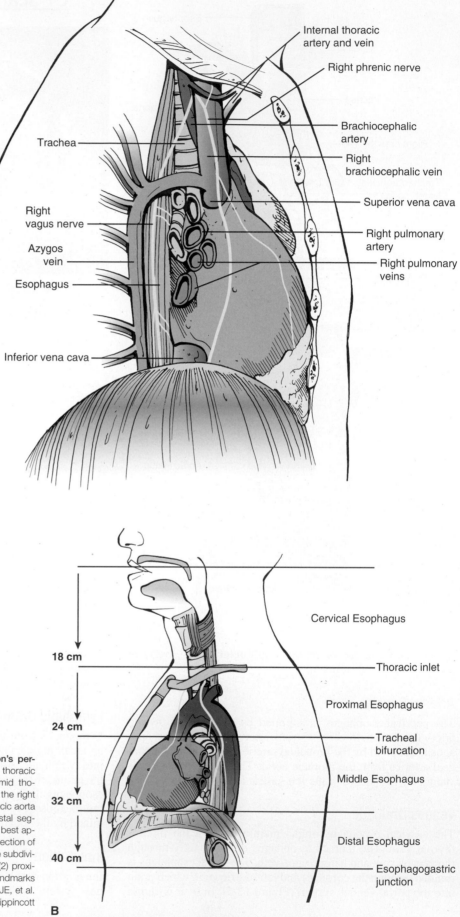

FIGURE 12-2. Esophageal anatomy from a surgeon's perspective. A, Through a right thoracotomy, most of the thoracic esophagus is accessible. As a result, proximal and mid thoracic esophageal lesions are best approached through the right chest. **B,** From a left thoracotomy, the descending thoracic aorta obstructs access to the esophagus, except for the distal segment. As a result, distal thoracic esophageal lesions are best approached through the left chest, especially if en-bloc resection of a distal esophageal lesion is planned. Also shown are the subdivision of the esophagus into four segments (1) cervical, (2) proximal, (3) middle, and (4) distal esophagus, and their landmarks and distance from the incisors. (Reprinted from Fischer JE, et al. *Fischer's Mastery of Surgery*, 6th ed. Philadelphia, PA: Lippincott Williams & Wilkins, 2012:794, with permission.)

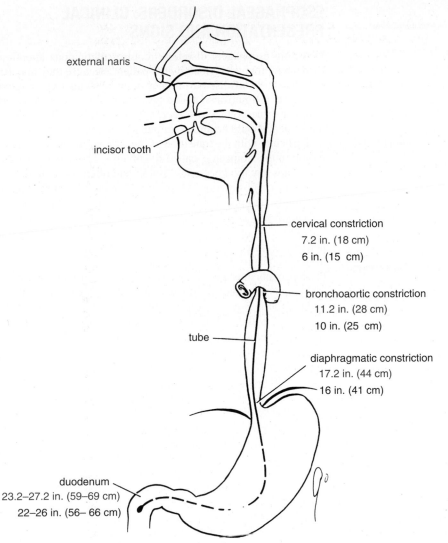

external naris

incisor tooth

cervical constriction
7.2 in. (18 cm)
6 in. (15 cm)

bronchoaortic constriction
11.2 in. (28 cm)
10 in. (25 cm)

tube

diaphragmatic constriction
17.2 in. (44 cm)
16 in. (41 cm)

duodenum
23.2–27.2 in. (59–69 cm)
22–26 in. (56–66 cm)

FIGURE 12-3. Shown are three areas of normally occurring esophageal constriction where foreign bodies and food impaction have a tendency to become **lodged.** (Reprinted from Snell R. *Clinical Anatomy*, 4th ed. Philadelphia, PA: Lippincott Williams & Wilkins, 2003, with permission.)

exerting opposing effects. The proximal esophagus receives its nerve fibers through the recurrent laryngeal nerves of the vagus nerve and cervical sympathetic chain. Damage to the recurrent nerve not only disrupts the vocal cords but also the swallowing mechanism of the upper esophagus increasing the risk of aspiration. The mid- and distal esophagus receives autonomic innervations from the vagus and thoracic sympathetic chain. An intramural nerve plexus of sympathetic and parasympathetic fibers is located in the muscularis propria, between the circular and longitudinal muscle layers (myenteric plexus). The myenteric plexus controls peristaltic activity of the esophagus and, when damaged, can lead to achalasia (failure of esophageal muscle relaxation). Afferent visceral pain fibers of the esophagus travel via sympathetic fibers to the upper thoracic spinal cord, sharing a similar pathway with cardiac sensory fibers. As a result, pain from the heart (angina) can resemble esophageal pain (spasm, acid reflux). The motor innervation of the esophagus is supplied through the vagus.

Histology

The esophageal wall consists of four main layers. They include (1) mucosa (containing a layer of superficial and deep mucosa),

(2) submucosa, (3) muscularis propria (the muscularis propria is made up of two layers, an inner circular layer and an outer longitudinal layer), and (4) adventitia (paraesophageal tissue). The esophagus does not have a serosal layer, unlike most of the gastrointestinal (GI) tract. On endoscopic ultrasound (EUS) imaging, the esophagus is seen as five discrete boundaries, correlating to the mucosa (seen as two layers) (1) superficial mucosa and (2) deep mucosa, (3) submucosa, (4) muscularis propria, and (5) adventitia (paraesophageal tissue) (Figure 12-7). The muscularis propria layer of the esophagus transitions from striated muscle fibers (proximal 1/3) to smooth muscle fibers type (distal 2/3). The esophageal mucosa is lined by a layer of nonkeratinizing, stratified squamous epithelium. In GERD, there is abnormal reflux of gastric contents into the distal esophagus, leading to abnormal transformation of normal squamous epithelial cells into intestinal columnar cells (**Barrett's esophagus**) (Figure 12-8).

PHYSIOLOGY

At rest, most of the esophagus is in a relaxed state except for the upper and LESs where resting pressures are high (15 to

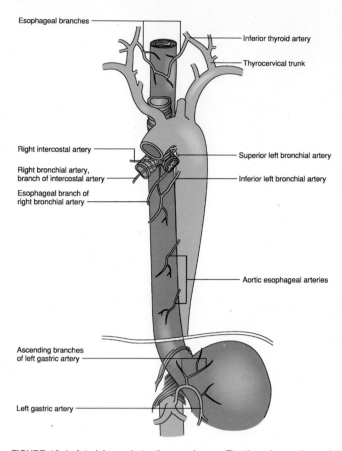

FIGURE 12-4. Arterial supply to the esophagus. The thoracic esophagus is supplied by multiple small branches arising from the descending thoracic aorta. Because of the small size of these arterial vessels, blunt and "blind" dissection of the esophagus is possible without the risk for severe bleeding. (Reprinted from Mulholland W, et al. *Greenfield's Surgery*, 4th ed. Philadelphia, PA: Lippincott Williams & Wilkins, 2006, with permission).

30 mm Hg). The resting high pressures of the sphincter help prevent reflux and regurgitation of digestive material back up the esophagus. The swallowing mechanism is voluntarily initiated from the nucleus ambiguous (located in the medulla). When the swallowing mechanism is initiated, there is temporary relaxation of the UES, allowing the food to enter the upper esophagus. The bolus is propelled down the esophagus by a primary peristaltic wave. The LES relaxes in anticipation of the food bolus, allowing the food to enter the stomach.

After passage of the bolus, the LES returns to its normal high resting pressure, preventing reflux of stomach contents. Normally, swallowing a bolus of food causes a primary peristaltic wave. Secondary peristaltic waves are not part of the normal swallowing mechanism but occur with esophageal dilatation or irritation, or if there is obstruction that prevents bolus progression. It is believed to represent a "backup" clearing process of residual material in the esophagus after the swallowing process. Tertiary waves are abnormal, nonpropulsive "fibrillation" of the esophagus thought to be correlated with anxious emotional states of the patient. Figure 12-9 shows the typical peristaltic activity initiated by the swallow mechanism and the method of intraluminal manometry to record this process.

ESOPHAGEAL DISORDERS: CLINICAL PRESENTATION AND SIGNS

Detecting esophageal disorders requires meticulous attention to the symptoms described by the patient, because they may be manifestations of disease in other organ systems (e.g., angina pectoris or asthma) or signs of a systemic problem (e.g., collagen vascular or neurologic disorders). To better assess the patient, the student should become familiar with several terms.

Difficulty with the transition of ingested substances from the mouth to the stomach is called **dysphagia**. The patient usually complains that food becomes "stuck" and often is able to define the point of obstruction. Dysphagia occurs with both liquids and solids, and pain is usually not a component of the process. **Odynophagia** is painful swallowing. It can be due to esophageal infection (e.g., *Candida* esophagitis, Cytomegalovirus, or herpesvirus infection), a foreign body in the esophagus, or injury to the esophagus. **Globus hystericus** is a "lump in the throat"; these patients must be evaluated carefully because the sensation may represent a mass lesion and not a psychological symptom.

Heartburn is also known as **pyrosis** or **water brash**. It is associated with GERD, achalasia, and esophageal **strictures.** In exploring the diagnosis of GERD, it is best to allow patients to describe their symptom complex in their own words. Heartburn that spontaneously disappears over a period of months without therapy may be a sign of a severe disease process (e.g., esophageal stricture or carcinoma).

Regurgitation is the passive return of ingested material into the oropharynx. **Vomiting** is the active return of stomach contents to the oropharynx.

Recurrent episodes of bronchitis or pneumonia, particularly in the very young and the elderly, may be signs of recurrent aspiration of esophageal or gastric contents because of esophageal obstruction, congenital malformation, diverticula, or esophageal motility disorders. Esophageal disease must also be considered in the differential diagnosis of anemia and bleeding. Ulcerative esophagitis is the most common cause of esophageal bleeding and usually causes occult blood in the stool.

Hiccup, or **singultus**, is a sign of diaphragmatic irritation and may indicate a diaphragmatic **hernia**, acute gastric dilation, or subendocardial myocardial infarction.

Esophageal disease may cause signs and symptoms that are often indistinguishable from those of angina pectoris. Some historical features may help to differentiate between the two disease processes. Symptoms related to the esophagus are typically aggravated by changes in body position, particularly bending over. The symptoms are relieved by belching and only marginally relieved by nitroglycerin. Nitroglycerin relieves the symptoms of diffuse esophageal spasm. Usually, other symptoms related to the esophagus can be elicited from the patient. In any case, cardiac and esophageal evaluation must proceed simultaneously since myocardial ischemia and esophagitis are both common diseases.

DIAGNOSTIC EVALUATION OF THE ESOPHAGUS

Barium Esophagography

In most cases, a contrast esophagram is the first study obtained for the workup of esophageal dysphagia, regurgitation, or heartburn.

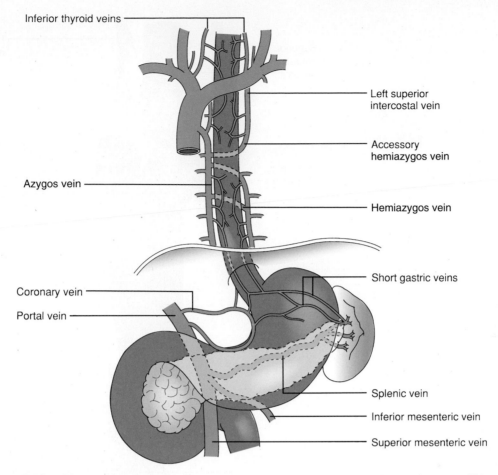

FIGURE 12-5. Venous drainage of the esophagus. Most of the drainage occurs through the azygos vein system, which communicates with the portal venous system via the coronary and short gastric veins. In portal vein hypertension, these collaterals enlarge and can lead to esophageal varices. (Reprinted from Mulholland MW, et al. *Greenfield's Surgery*, 4th ed. Philadelphia, PA: Lippincott Williams & Wilkins, 2006, with permission.)

The patient swallows barium, while monitored with real-time video, to assess esophageal motility and to look for hiatal hernia, diverticula, or obstruction. When a hiatal hernia is suspected, video recording is performed in various positions to increase intra-abdominal pressures, maximizing the yield for identifying the presence of the hernia. Barium study also provides good visualization of any esophageal structural disease. Because of its general availability and usefulness in identifying motility and structural disorders, the esophagram is the preferred initial study.

Esophageal Manometry

Esophageal manometry allows for direct, simultaneous measurement of intraluminal pressures at multiple levels. Manometry study is used to assess the function of both upper and LESs, and it also identifies contraction abnormalities in esophageal motility disorders. Esophageal manometry study is performed by nasally inserting a tube containing multiple levels of water-filled or solid-state pressure transducers into the esophageal lumen. Peristaltic wave activity and sphincter function are studied by measuring intraluminal pressure along the esophagus during "wet" swallows with water (Figure 12-9). With esophageal manometry, detailed information on LES abnormalities is obtained (including function and anatomy of the physiological LES). Manometric study is indicated in the workup of achalasia, esophageal spasm, and GERD.

Esophageal pH Monitoring

The monitoring of distal esophageal pH is useful in the workup for GERD. This is performed in a 24-hour outpatient study, where a pH probe sensor is inserted via nasal catheter to the level just above the LES. The patient is then encouraged to go through a "normal day," with routine meals and activities, while distal esophageal pH is monitored continuously (Figure 12-10). Wireless technology has made pH probe transducers (inserted endoscopically) more tolerable for patients. Because of the greater comfort, the pH probe can be left in longer (allowing for studies of up to 48 to 72 hours), increasing the yield for detecting acid reflux. A different pH probe is used for identifying bile acid (nonacidic) reflux. Proton pump inhibitors (PPIs) and H2 blockers are discontinued for several days before a pH study for GERD is performed.

The 24-hour pH study is used to collect six measures of abnormal pH (<4) exposure in the distal esophagus. They include (1) percentage total time with pH < 4, (2) percentage upright time with pH < 4, (3) percentage supine time with pH < 4.0, (4) number of episodes pH < 4, (5) number of episodes more than 5 minutes with pH < 4, and (6) longest episode (in minutes) with pH < 4. The patient's results are compared to that of normal subjects, and a composite score is calculated based on the "normal" mean and the standard deviation values of these measures. This composite score is commonly known as

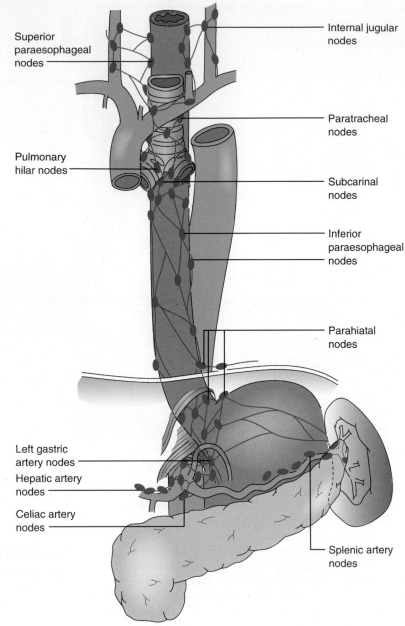

FIGURE 12-6. Lymphatic drainage of the esophagus. Lymphatic drainage and tumor spread from distal esophageal cancer occur to the inferior paraesophageal and celiac lymph nodes, while the proximal/midesophageal cancers spread to superior paraesophageal, paratracheal, and internal jugular lymph nodes. (Reprinted from Mulholland MW, et al. *Greenfield's Surgery.* 4th ed. Philadelphia, PA: Lippincott Williams & Wilkins, 2006, with permission).

the DeMeester score. The DeMeester score obtained is believed to be very specific in identifying the patient who would benefit from antireflux surgery.

Imaging Studies

Compared to other available studies, computed tomography (CT) and magnetic resonance imaging (MRI) provide limited additional information when assessing for esophageal disease. Esophagram, endoscopy, and EUS provide superior local structural evaluation of the esophagus. However, CT and MRI can provide useful assessment of distant metastasis in esophageal carcinoma, especially when combined with positron emission tomography (PET) scanning (an important step in the staging of esophageal cancer). CT and MRI can provide some information regarding disease involvement of surrounding structures, such as the aorta, trachea, and the lymph nodes. It should be emphasized that apparent involve-

ment of these structures on CT scan does not alone exclude surgical respectability, as it is difficult to differentiate between inflammatory changes from direct carcinomatous invasion. The CT scan is useful in the workup of suspected esophageal perforation.

Upper Endoscopy

Direct endoscopic examination of the esophagus is mandatory for all esophageal disease. It has a role in the diagnosis and treatment of various esophageal diseases. Endoscopy allows for direct visualization of any pathology, and it provides access for biopsies. Through endoscopy, the physician can perform dilatations of strictures and inject pharmacologic agents to treat varices and LES disorders. More recently, techniques have been described for limited surgical procedures, such as the stapling of esophageal diverticula. When esophageal diverticular disease is suspected, or in severe caustic

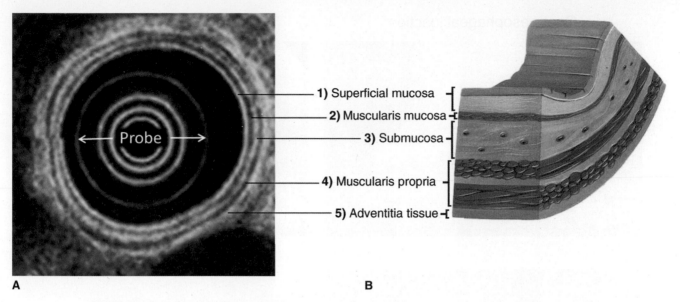

FIGURE 12-7. **A,** Endoscopic ultrasound (EUS) of the esophagus. **B,** The five histologic layers of the esophagus correlating with those seen on the ultrasound. EUS provides an accurate picture of the depth of tumor wall invasion, an important step in staging esophageal cancers.

esophageal injury, endoscopy is performed with caution, as there is increased risk for perforation. In GERD, endoscopic examination is used to evaluate the extent of mucosal injury, and for monitoring the presence of atypical histologic changes in Barrett's esophagitis.

Endoscopic Ultrasound

Endoscopic ultrasound (EUS) of the esophagus is used to obtain detailed imaging of esophageal wall and adjacent lymph node pathology. To perform EUS, an ultrasound probe is introduced endoscopically to the area of interest. Detailed imaging of the esophageal wall is seen as five discrete layers, and any adjacent lymph nodes can also be visualized for guided biopsy. EUS is used in the staging workup of esophageal cancer. With EUS, tumor depth and invasion can be evaluated for T staging, and abnormal lymph nodes can be located for fine needle aspiration N staging (Figure 12-11). EUS is also useful in guiding fine needle aspirations of suspicious lymph nodes adjacent to the esophagus, helping with N staging. EUS is also useful in identifying other intramural lesions, such as leiomyomas.

ESOPHAGEAL DISEASES

GERD and esophageal carcinoma are the most frequently encountered esophageal diseases. A thorough fund of knowledge in these two esophageal entities forms the essential basis for this chapter. In addition, esophageal perforation is commonly referred to the surgeon as an emergency consultation, and a thorough understanding on the workup and management of it will complete the basic foundation for managing esophageal disease. Because of their significance, these three esophageal disorders are presented first, while other less commonly encountered diseases are added at the end for completeness. The common surgical procedures of the esophagus are described within each of these clinical scenarios, but the surgical approach and techniques can be applied to most any esophageal pathology.

Gastroesophageal Reflux Disease

Gastroesophageal reflux is the backward flow of gastric contents into the distal esophagus, past the LES. Occasional reflux of gastric contents into the distal esophagus is seen as a "physiologically normal" process, which makes the distinction between "normal" and "pathologic" GERD difficult to define. In 2006, a Global Evidence-Based Consensus group formulated the definition of GERD as "a condition which develops when the reflux of stomach contents cause troublesome symptoms and/or complications." GERD is caused by an incompetent LES. Poor LES function is commonly caused by prolapse of the abdominal segment of the esophagus and stomach into the chest, as in a hiatal hernia. Other causes of LES incompetence are increased intra-abdominal or gastric pressures from gastric obstruction, food- or drug-induced LES relaxation, and abnormal esophageal peristaltic activity. While GERD is frequently associated with a hiatal hernia, not all patients with GERD have a hiatal hernia (numbers vary between 50% and 90%), and not all patients with hiatal hernia have GERD (numbers vary between 13% and 84%).

The symptoms of GERD include heartburn, regurgitation, and dysphagia. The most common complaint is dyspepsia after heavy, greasy meals and is described as a burning or pressure-like discomfort in the epigastrium. The symptoms of GERD can be confused with angina pain because of the common sensory pathway of the esophageal and cardiac sympathetic nerves. Not infrequently, the diagnosis of coronary artery disease is delayed because the symptom of chest pain is attributed to GERD. Antacid therapy often improves the symptoms of GERD. The symptoms of GERD can be induced by having the patient lie supine or lean over (as in tying their shoes). Consumption of caffeine and alcohol frequently exacerbates the symptoms due to their effect on LES competence. GERD should be in the differential diagnosis of cryptic recurrent aspiration pneumonias, especially in the elderly and disabled patient.

Late complications of GERD include stricture of the distal esophagus (Schatzki's ring) and intestinal metaplasia of the distal esophageal mucosa (Barrett's esophagus). The concern

Gastroesophageal junction   Endoscopy

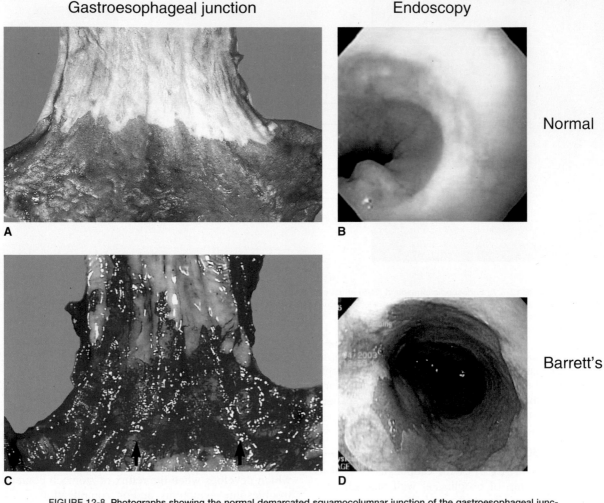

Normal

Barrett's

FIGURE 12-8. Photographs showing the normal demarcated squamocolumnar junction of the gastroesophageal junction as compared to the abnormal Barrett's columnar cell esophagitis (seen in GERD). **A** and **B,** The anatomic and endoscopic appearance of a normal demarcated squamocolumnar junction. **C** and **D,** Barrett's esophagus, where "tongues" of abnormal pink columnar cells are seen invading into the whitish normal squamous tissue zone. (**A** and **C,** Reprinted from Mills SC. *Histology for Pathologists,* 3rd ed. Philadelphia, PA: Lippincott, Williams & Wilkins, 2007, with permission. **B,** Reprinted from Fischer JE, et al. *Fischer's Mastery of Surgery,* 6th ed. Philadelphia, PA: Lippincott Williams & Wilkins, 2012:796, with permission. **D,** Reprinted from Mulholland MW, et al. *Greenfield's Surgery.* 4th ed. Philadelphia, PA: Lippincott Williams & Wilkins, 2006, with permission.)

of Barrett's esophagus is its predisposition to the development of high-grade dysplasia leading to malignant transformation of the distal esophagus. Current recommendations for managing patients with Barrett's esophagus associated with low-grade dysplasia include routine follow-up endoscopy every 6–12 months with 4-quadrant biopsies every 1–2 cm of involved esophagus.

Diagnosis
Aggressive workup for GERD is usually reserved to when surgical intervention is being considered, or if late complication of GERD is present, such as stricture or Barrett's esophagitis. The workup for GERD should include (1) barium swallow, (2) esophageal manometry, (3) 24-hour esophageal pH study, and (4) upper endoscopy. Positive barium study can demonstrate reflux in the presence of a hiatal hernia, a distal stricture, or shortened esophagus. Esophageal manometry is used to assess the function of the LES and can identify other esophageal motility issues. Esophageal pH study is used to confirm abnormal acid exposure of the distal esophagus. Endoscopy is useful in visualizing inflammatory changes in the distal

esophageal and to assess for intestinal metaplasia and atypia from Barrett's disease. Confirmation of these aggressive diagnostic studies will help ensure that surgical intervention is appropriate and likely to be successful.

Medical Treatment
Currently, the initial therapies for GERD should include behavioral modifications and the use of PPIs. Behavioral modifications include changes in eating habits, appropriate postural behavior, and avoidance of triggering agents (Table 12-1). PPIs have been found to successfully control symptoms in the majority of patients with GERD (>90% success). For patients who fail or cannot comply with nonoperative management, surgical intervention remains a reasonable option. The development of "less invasive" laparoscopic procedures for GERD has decreased the threshold for surgical intervention.

Surgical Treatment
Surgery is mainly reserved for patients with GERD who have failed conservative management, cannot continue PPIs, or

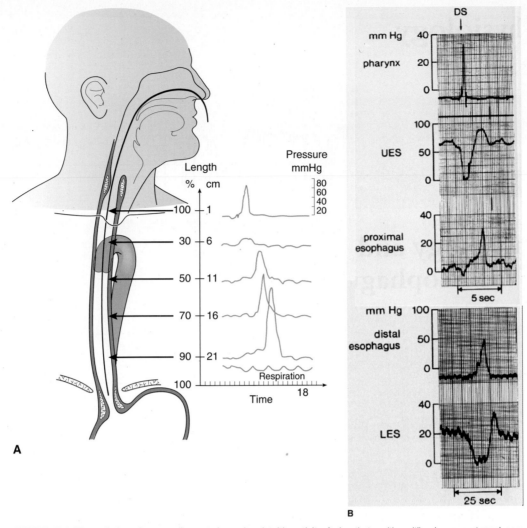

FIGURE 12-9. The technique for recording esophageal peristaltic activity. A, A catheter with multilevel pressure transducers is inserted into the esophagus to temporally measure intraluminal pressures during swallows. **B,** Actual recordings of esophageal activity at different levels during dry swallow (DS). Note that the upper (UES) and lower (LES) esophageal sphincters have a resting tone between 50 and 20 mm Hg, which relaxes during a swallow and then rebounds back up after passage of the bolus to prevent reflux. (**A,** reprinted from Mulholland MW, et al. *Greenfield's Surgery,* 4th ed. Philadelphia, PA: Lippincott Williams & Wilkins, 2006, with permission. **B,** Reprinted from Shields TW, et al. *General Thoracic Surgery,* 7th ed. Philadelphia, PA: Lippincott Williams & Wilkins, 2009:1692,1694, with permission.)

develop a complication from GERD. In the pediatric population, aspiration pneumonitis is a common indication for recommending an antireflux procedure. Predictors of successful response to surgery include (1) a positive pH test, (2) presence of typical reflux symptoms, and (3) symptomatic relief with PPIs. There is no definitive evidence that successful surgical intervention reverses or prevents the progression of Barrett's esophagus, and continued surveillance for malignancy is recommended.

The principles of antireflux surgery include (1) restoration of an intra-abdominal segment of esophagus, (2) reconstruction of the esophageal hiatus in the diaphragm, and (3) reinforcement of the LES, usually with a **fundoplication**. The purpose of the fundoplication wrap is to accentuate or recreate the gastroesophageal flap mechanism, (where distension of the stomach fundus leads to external compression of the LES, reinforcing its closure) (Figure 12-12). Numerous antireflux procedures have been described; they include the Nissen, Belsey, Hill, Dor, and Toupet procedures. These procedures can be categorized into complete or partial stomach wraps,

and transabdominal versus thoracic surgical approaches (Table 12-2).

Currently, the Nissen fundoplication is the most commonly performed antireflux procedure. It is usually performed through a transabdominal approach and consists of a complete (360°) fundoplication wrap, while the other procedures are considered partial wraps (Figure 12-13).

Some surgeons believe there is less postoperative dysphagia and gas bloat after a partial wrap, while other surgeons believe there is a lower recurrence rate of GERD after a complete wrap. In the end, if the principles of antireflux surgery are followed, (restoration of the intra-abdominal esophageal segment, repair of esophageal hiatus, and reinforcement of the LES) similar excellent results have been reported for the various antireflux procedures (success rate of >90%). Mortality should be <1%. Newer surgical approaches are based on these same principles and differ mainly on the current trend for a "minimally" invasive laparoscopic approach for performing the surgery.

The Collis gastroplasty procedure is used in combination with a fundoplication when there is esophageal shortening

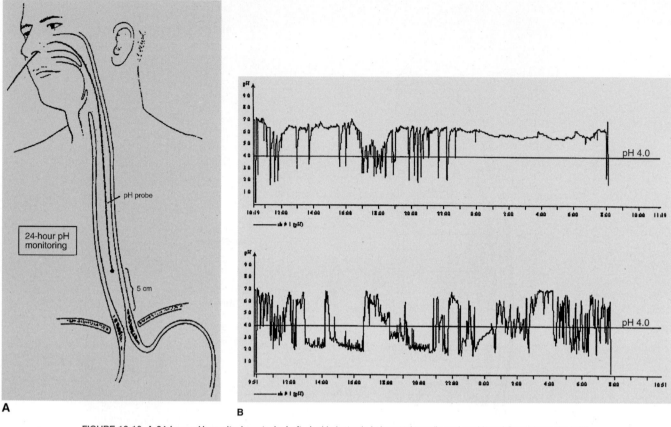

A

B

FIGURE 12-10. A 24-hour pH monitoring study. **Left**, A pH electrode is inserted nasally and positioned 5 cm above the LES. **Right**, pH tracings in patients with abnormal acid reflux. In the upper tracing, short episodes of pH < 4.0 (*line*) suggest defective lower esophageal function. In the lower tracing, the episodes of pH < 4.0 (*line*) are prolonged, suggesting poor esophageal clearance of acid reflux. (Reprinted from Shields TW, et al. *General Thoracic Surgery*, 7th ed. Philadelphia, PA: Lippincott Williams & Wilkins, 2009:1713, 1709, with permission.)

from chronic severe GERD. In the Collis gastroplasty procedure, a segment of "distal" esophagus is reconstructed from the stomach. This results in the lengthening and creation of a "neo" intra-abdominal esophagus (Figure 12-14).

Esophageal Carcinoma

Between 1987 and 2007, the incidence and mortality rate for esophageal cancer have remained constant despite significant shifts in histological type in the United States. Incidence per

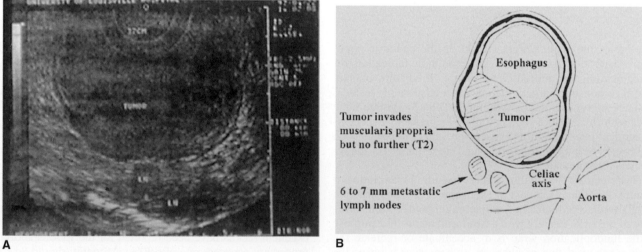

A

B

FIGURE 12-11. Endoscopic ultrasound (EUS) is the most accurate means to determine the depth of tumor invasion in the esophageal wall. **A**, Example of an actual ultrasound image of esophageal tumor. **B**, Correlating schematic drawing. Tumor depth invasion (T staging) has strong prognostic implications in the treatment and outcome of esophageal cancer (see Table 12-3 for staging details). EUS is also valuable in identifying and guiding fine-needle aspiration of suspicious paraesophageal lymph nodes. (Reprinted from Shields TW, et al. *General Thoracic Surgery*, 7th ed. Philadelphia, PA: Lippincott Williams & Wilkins, 2009:1713, 1999, with permission.)

TABLE 12-1	Behavioral Modifications for Treating GERD			
	Modification	**LES Competency**	**Gastric Pressure and Emptying**	**Mucosal Irritant**
Dietary behavior	Eat small meals		+	
Dietary content	Avoid lying down after meals		+	
	Avoid acidic foods			+
	Avoid fatty meals	+	+	
	Avoid caffeine, chocolate	+		
Postural modification	Elevate the head of the bed		+	
Social habits	Avoid smoking	+		+
	Avoid alcohol	+	+	+
Medications	Avoid anticholinergics, calcium, β-blockers, xanthines, and aspirin	+	+	+
Obesity	Lose weight		+	

year has remained around 4 to 5 per 100,000, with mortality rate being similar at 4 to 5 per 100,000. Overall survival for patients diagnosed with esophageal cancer remains dismal at around 20% for 5 years, mainly due to advanced disease at the time of diagnosis. Two histological types of esophageal cancer are seen, squamous cell carcinoma (SCC) and adenocarcinoma. Although both types of esophageal carcinoma carry a poor prognosis and are managed similarly, their etiology, epidemiology, and anatomic characteristics are different enough to warrant distinction between the two.

Until recently, SCC was the most common type of esophageal cancer seen in North America and Europe (recently,

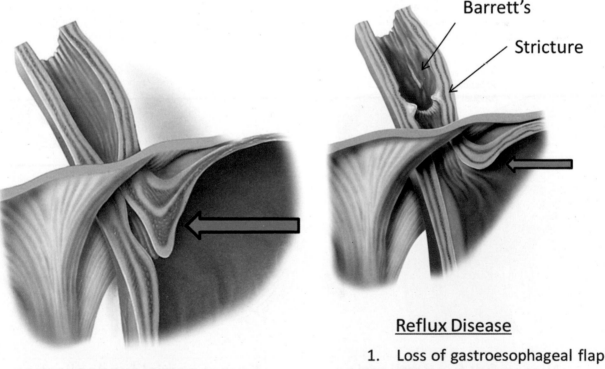

Barrett's

Stricture

Reflux Disease

1. **Loss of gastroesophageal flap**
2. **LES incompetence**
3. **Loss of intra-abdominal esophagus**

Normal

A

B

FIGURE 12-12. **The gastroesophageal junction in normal and reflux disease states.** Normally, the gastroesophageal flap (*large arrow*) is formed by overlap of the stomach fundus on the distal esophagus, aiding the competency of the LES by external compression when the stomach distends after a meal. With reflux disease, there is associated loss of this flap mechanism (*small arrow*), LES incompetence, and migration of the intra-abdominal esophagus into the thorax. Antireflux procedures attempt to restore these physiological principles. Complications from chronic reflux disease include Barrett's esophagus and stricture. (Reprinted from iDAMS.lww, asset (A) 9965ef.tif and (B) 9965E_HR.eps provided by Anatomical Chart Co.)

TABLE 12-2	Antireflux Procedures	
Procedure	**Degree of Stomach Wrap**	**Surgical Approach**
Nissen	360	Abdominal or thoracic
Belsey-Mark	240	Thoracic
Toupet-Dor	180	Abdominal
Hill	0[a]	Abdominal

[a]*Although the Hill procedure does not attempt to wrap the stomach around the distal esophagus, it still follows the key principle of reinforcing the LES by accentuating the gastroesophageal flap valve.*

adenocarcinoma has surpassed SCC in prevalence). There is a higher incidence of SCC seen in African Americans and males (near 4:1 ratio). SCC is seen mainly in the mid- to proximal segment of the esophagus but can also involve the distal segment. There has been a strong association between alcohol and tobacco consumption with SCC. Other factors believed to increase risk for SCC include high dietary intake of nitrosamine, dietary deficiencies in vitamins and minerals (including Plummer-Vinson syndrome), genetic predisposition (tylosis), achalasia, and history of caustic injury to the esophagus.

Adenocarcinoma has surpassed SCC as the most common esophageal cancer type encountered in North America and Europe. Its incidence in the western world has increased fourfold over the past two decades. Prevalence of adenocarcinoma is higher in Whites than in African Americans. It involves the distal esophagus and is associated with Barrett's esophagus from GERD. Although the association between adenocarcinoma and Barrett's disease is not disputed, the role for PPI and antireflux procedures as a means to slow or reverse Barrett's disease (thereby decreasing the risk for developing adenocarcinoma) remains controversial.

Diagnosis

Due to the increased prevalence of adenocarcinoma in the West, the clinical presentation and history for esophageal carcinoma have changed. Both types of esophageal cancer usually present with dysphagia to solid food and weight loss, but with adenocarcinoma, there is frequently associated history of reflux disease. On presentation, the patients with adenocarcinoma are usually healthier, with less advanced disease, especially if they have been undergoing surveillance endoscopy of Barrett's disease. Patients with SCC usually present with more advanced disease, greater weight loss, and history of smoking and alcohol abuse.

Workup for esophageal cancer is mainly for confirming the diagnosis and staging of the cancer. Initial diagnostic study is frequently the barium swallow to evaluate the cause of dysphagia. Barium swallow is the first study performed and will typically demonstrate stricture with irregular filling defect (Figure 12-15).

CT scan can be useful in defining the extent of the tumor and abnormal-appearing lymph nodes. However, CT scan alone is not enough to prove tumor invasion of adjacent structures, since distinction between local inflammatory reaction and tumor invasion is not possible. Endoscopic evaluation is mandatory for histologic confirmation of esophageal cancer. In patients with Barrett's dysplasia, endoscopic surveillance with routine biopsies helps identify early malignant changes. Endoscopic ultrasound is performed to define depth of tumor

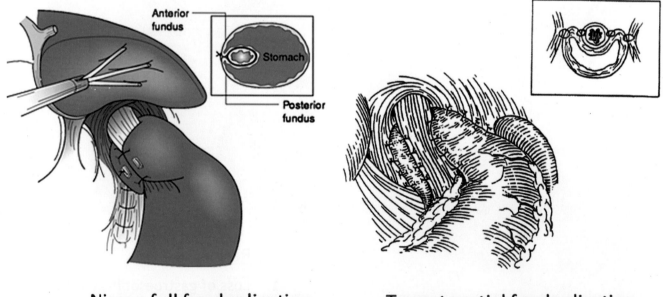

Nissen full fundoplication

A

Toupet partial fundoplication

B

FIGURE 12-13. Two examples of fundoplication procedures. **A**, The Nissan fundoplication procedure is a full 360° wrap. **B**, The Toupet fundoplication is a partial 180° wrap. Note that in the Nissen, the esophageal hiatus is also tightened, while in the Toupet, anchoring sutures are placed from the fundoplication to the crus of the esophageal hiatus. This prevents slippage of the fundoplication into the chest, where the fundoplication would cease to be effective. In all fundoplication procedures, the gastroesophageal flap is recreated where a portion of the fundus overlaps the distal esophagus to provide external compression support of competency for the distal esophagus. (**A**, Reprinted from Mulholland MW, et al. *Greenfield's Surgery*, 4th ed. Philadelphia, PA: Lippincott Williams & Wilkins, 2006. **B**, Reprinted from Kaiser LR, et al. *Mastery of Cardiothoracic Surgery*, 2nd ed. Philadelphia, PA: Lippincott Williams & Wilkins, 2007:125, with permission).

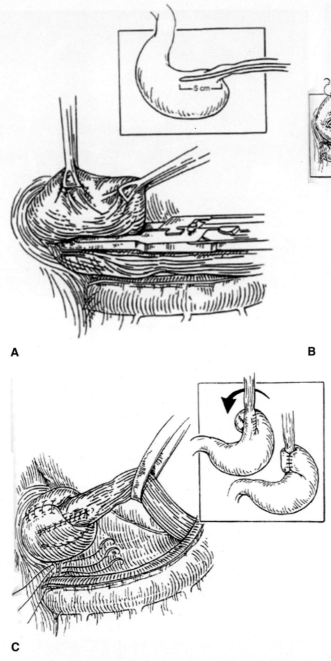

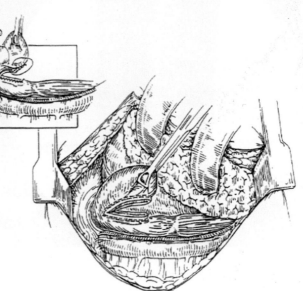

FIGURE 12-14. When the esophagus is shortened and retracted into the chest from chronic GERD, the Collis gastroplasty procedure is used to recreate a distal "esophageal" tube from the stomach. A and B, The shortened esophagus is lengthened 5 cm by stapling the fundus into a tube of "neo" esophagus. **C,** The gastroplasty is combined with a fundoplication to prevent reflux. (Reprinted from Kaiser LR, et al. *Mastery of Cardiothoracic Surgery*. 2nd ed. Philadelphia, PA: Lippincott Williams & Wilkins, 2007:128,129, with permission).

invasion and in assisting with localizing adjacent suspicious lymph nodes for fine needle aspiration. In tumors involving the proximal and midesophagus, bronchoscopy is performed to rule out tracheobronchial involvement. The combination of CT scan and PET scan is helpful in identifying distant metastasis. Other than lymph nodes, the distant organs most commonly involved with metastatic disease are the liver and the lungs.

Staging

Once diagnostic studies are completed, the esophageal cancer can be staged using the current 2009 TNM staging definitions (American Joint Committee on Cancer) (Table 12-3). In the most recent update on esophageal cancer staging, squamous cell and adenocarcinoma are graded differently, with tumor location used only for the staging of squamous cell cancer. Remembering the TNM criteria for each stage is difficult,

but a useful guideline to remember is the distinction between early (≤ Stage IIa) from more advanced stages of esophageal cancer. For Stages IIa or earlier, there is limited local tumor invasion and no lymph node involvement, with no metastasis. A more detailed description of early stage esophageal cancer is shown in Table 12-4.

The distinction between early stages (I and IIa) and more advanced stages (IIb and IV) is useful, as current 5-year survival is 50% or greater for the early stages as compared to <30% for advanced stages.

Surgical Treatment

Surgical resection remains the best chance for cure of esophageal cancer. Despite significant improvements in surgical morbidity and mortality, long-term outcome after attempted curative resection remains poor, with most series reporting an overall 5-year survival rate of 20%. Only in the early stages

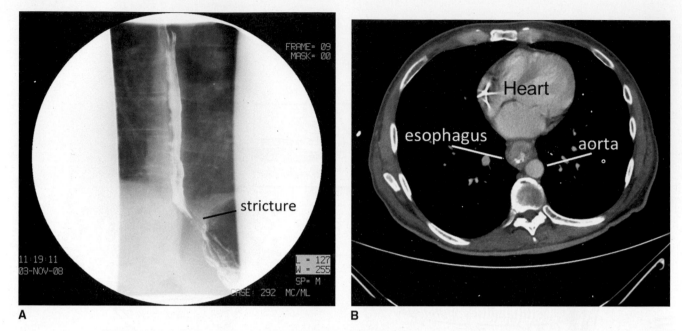

FIGURE 12-15. **A,** Barium swallow and **B,** corresponding CT scan cut demonstrating a distal esophageal cancer.

(contained tumor with no lymph node involvement, or tumors that show complete regression [0] after preoperative chemoradiation) has there been significant long-term survival of >50%.

Surgical treatment of esophageal carcinoma is based upon the principle of complete local resection of the tumor with reconstruction of the alimentary tract by using another segment of the GI tract. Variations on the procedure depend upon what segment of the GI tract is used for esophageal reconstruction and the surgical approach used for resecting the tumor.

Esophageal Substitutes

Esophageal substitutes that have been used for reconstruction include stomach, colon, and jejunum. Which of these is used depends upon availability, location of the resected esophageal segment, and surgeon preference. Surgeons who have an interest in performing esophagectomies should be familiar with more than one technique, as options may be limited by the clinical history (prior gastrectomy, vascular disease, etc.).

The stomach is the most frequently used conduit in esophagectomies. The advantage of using the stomach includes its rich vascular supply, ease of surgical mobilization as a vascularized pedicle, and the need to create two less GI anastomosis. When used as a conduit, the left gastric and the short gastric arteries are divided, allowing the fundus to be mobilized into the chest or neck. The stomach is then left with blood flow coming from the right gastric and gastroduodenal arteries. Because the vagus is divided during esophageal resection, a pyloromyotomy is often performed to facilitate gastric emptying. The drawbacks of using the stomach as a conduit include the risk of ischemia in the fundus because of dependent collateral flow and postoperative gastroesophageal

| TABLE 12-3 | American Joint Committee on Cancer Esophageal Cancer TNM Definitions |

T (Tumor Depth)		N (Regional Nodes)		M (Metastasis)		G (Histologic Grading)		Location (Squamous Cancer)	
T0	No visible tumor	N0	No nodes	M0	No metastasis	G1	Well differentiated	Upper Thoracic	20–25 cm
Tis	High-grade dysplasia	N1	1–2 nodes	M1	Distant metastasis	G2	Moderately differentiated	Middle Thoracic	>25–30 cm
T1	Lamina propria or submucosa	N2	3–6 nodes			G3	Poorly differentiated	Lower Thoracic	>30–40 cm
T2	Muscularis propria	N3	≥7 nodes			G4	Undifferentiated	Esophagogastric junction	
T3	Adventitia	—	—	—	—	—	—	—	—
T4a	Pleura, pericardium, diaphragm (resectable)	—	—	—	—	—	—	—	—
T4b	Aorta, vertebrae, trachea (unresectable)	—	—	—	—	—	—	—	—

American Joint Committee on Cancer, 2009.

TABLE 12-4	Criteria for Early Stage (≤ IIa) of Esophageal Cancer

	T	N	M	G	Location
Adenocarcinoma stage ≤ IIa	≤ T2	N0	M0	Any	Not applicable
Squamous cell carcinoma stage ≤ IIa	T1	N0	M0	Any	Any
	T2-3	N0	M0	G1	Any
	T2-3	N0	M0	G2-3	Lower

reflux symptoms after destruction of the LES mechanisms. Reflux appears to be more common when an intrathoracic gastroesophageal anastomosis is used, as compared to a cervical anastomosis.

The left colon can also be used as an esophageal substitute, and it is the next most frequently used after the stomach. Some surgeons prefer using the left colon to the stomach due to its longer available length, favorable vascular anatomy, and close size match with the esophagus. The left colon is used in an isoperistaltic fashion, with a vascular pedicle dependent upon the left colic artery branch of the inferior mesenteric artery. As compared to the stomach, the colon has the advantage of a longer and more relaxed reach to the cervical esophagus. The colon is also more resistant to acid reflux. The disadvantages of using colon include the need to perform two additional anastomoses and the greater technical experience needed in assessing and mobilizing the colon vasculature. Preoperative colonoscopy and visceral angiography is required to verify absence of pathology and adequate blood supply to the colon. There are two ways of routing the colon interposition graft. The preferred route is through the resected esophageal space in the posterior mediastinum. An alternative route is through the retrosternum, which is used if the posterior mediastinal space is not available due to extensive disease or scarring, or if the diseased esophagus cannot be safely removed. The retrosternal route is not optimal because of a more circuitous route, increasing the risk of obstruction due to kinking of the conduit, especially at the thoracic inlet.

The jejunum is rarely used as an esophageal substitute. It is occasionally used as a free graft, especially when a short segment of the cervical esophagus is resected. The jejuna-free graft is placed as an interposition graft between the esophageal ends, with its vascular supply reconstructed through microvascular anastomosis of the jejunal vessels to the neck vessels. A pedicled jejunal graft for extensive esophageal reconstruction is difficult to create due to its unfavorable vascular anatomy. Jejunal reconstruction via a Roux-en-Y connection (see stomach chapter for description) can be used when total gastrectomy is combined with distal esophagectomy.

Surgical Procedures

Surgical resection of the esophagus can be performed by either a thoracotomy or a transhiatal approach. Both frequently require a concomitant incision through either an abdominal incision or a cervical incision, or both. Each technique has its proponents, claiming advantages in operative mortality, postoperative morbidity, and cancer survival. The thoracotomy approach for esophageal resection has been the historical standard, with proponents claiming a cleaner and visually direct resection of the tumor. However, because a thoracotomy is often associated with a higher morbidity than an abdominal incision, the transhiatal approach was introduced. This approach, which avoids a thoracotomy, may provide significant advantages in certain clinical scenarios, such as in some patients with poor pulmonary function, or those who have had previous major thoracic procedures. A transhiatal esophagectomy is performed via a cervical and abdominal incision, with the esophagus and the tumor removed partly by blunt, blind hand dissection. The main advantage of this technique is avoidance of a thoracotomy incision. The argument against transhiatal esophagectomy is the risk of limited access to uncontrolled bleeding and the limited resection of large tumors involving surrounding esophageal tissue. Although there have been multiple retrospective studies supporting either the thoracotomy or transhiatal surgical approach (with respect to cancer survival and perioperative complications), the surgeon should be familiar with both surgical techniques. Tumor location, clinical history, or patient functional status may enhance the theoretical advantages of one approach over the other.

Three main surgical approaches have been described in performing a thoracotomy. The most common approach is via the right thorax combined with an abdominal incision (Ivor Lewis). In an Ivor-Lewis approach, the gastroesophageal anastomosis is located in the right chest (Figure 12-16). For tumors involving the proximal and midesophagus, a three-incision (abdominal, right thoracotomy, and cervical) approach has been described (McKeown). The McKeown procedure is similar to the Ivor Lewis, other than the addition of the third cervical incision and a cervical gastroesophageal anastomosis. The potential advantages of the McKeown include wider surgical margins due to more extensive proximal resection of the esophagus and construction of a cervical anastomosis, where the consequences of a possible anastomotic leak are less severe than an intrathoracic anastomotic leak. For a distal esophageal tumor extending into the stomach with extensive local disease, a left thoracoabdominal incision has been advocated by some, through which an extensive "en-bloc" resection can be performed with the theoretical benefit of a cleaner oncological resection.

To avoid the morbidity of performing a thoracotomy, a transhiatal approach for esophageal resection has been proposed. The operation consists of two incisions: an abdominal incision and a cervical incision. The stomach and lower esophagus are mobilized via the abdomen, and a cervical incision is used to mobilize the upper esophagus. Part of the removal of the midesophagus is performed by a blunt, blind hand dissection (Figure 12-17). The fundus of the stomach is mobilized to the neck for a cervical anastomosis. Arguments for a transhiatal approach include avoidance of a painful thoracotomy incision, decreased lung trauma from mechanical retraction, and avoidance of an intrathoracic anastomosis. Concerns on using the transhiatal approach include a limited resection of large tumors (especially those involving the midesophagus), greater potential for local tumor spillage from blunt dissection, and the greater stretch of the stomach to reach the neck. The extra distance required for the stomach to reach the neck can contribute to an increased risk for anastomotic failure due to tension and ischemia. The transhiatal approach seems to be ideally suited for local limited disease involving the distal esophagus, as commonly seen with malignant transformation of Barrett's disease.

Again, it should be emphasized that despite strong proponents for each of the above-mentioned approaches, there is no definitive study demonstrating a clear advantage of one technique over the other. Understanding of the theoretical benefit and drawbacks of each technique, and familiarity of

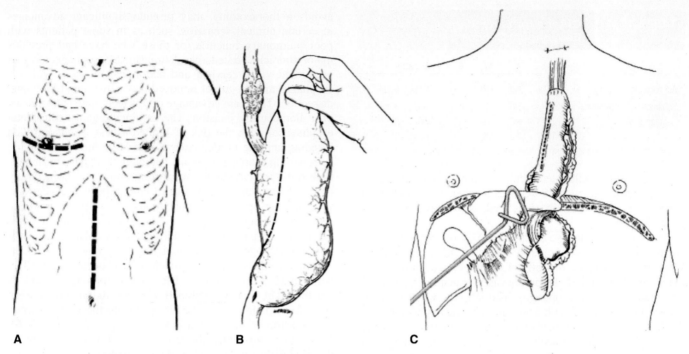

A **B** **C**

FIGURE 12-16. A, In the Ivor-Lewis approach for esophageal resection, two separate incisions are made. B, The initial abdominal incision is used to mobilize the esophageal replacement conduit (usually the stomach) into the right chest. C, A second incision is made into the right chest, to complete the resection of the distal esophagus and to reestablish GI continuity by anastomosing the stomach to the proximal esophagus. (Reprinted from Kaiser LR, et al. *Mastery of Cardiothoracic Surgery*, 2nd ed. Philadelphia, PA: Lippincott Williams & Wilkins, 2007:145,143,161, with permission).

using more than one surgical approach, would allow the surgeon to map a treatment course best serving the individual patient.

More recently, the advent of laparoscopic techniques for esophageal resection has started to provide an alternative approach to patients with resectable esophageal cancer. The laparoscopic equivalent of the thoracotomy and transhiatal esophagectomies has been described with similar long-term cancer survival outcomes, but with decreased surgical morbidity due to less invasive incisions. There is a long learning curve, and currently only limited centers have the expertise to perform successful laparoscopic esophagectomy.

Neoadjuvant Therapy

Because of the dismal prognosis in advanced esophageal cancer, the role for neoadjuvant (preoperative) therapy has been intensively pursued. Because most esophageal cancer presents at an advanced stage, the goal of neoadjuvant therapy is to "down stage" the tumor and improve cancer survival after surgical resection. Multiple prospective randomized trials have been conducted, with many studies showing improved cancer survival with neoadjuvant chemoradiation and surgery, as opposed to surgery alone. Most neoadjuvant chemoradiation therapy protocols include a course of 5-fluorouracil and cisplatinum with 45 Gy radiation over 6 to 7 weeks, followed by surgical resection a month after completion of treatment. Not all studies demonstrated improved survival, and the cost of increased perioperative mortality and morbidity must be weighed in. The greatest survival benefit occurs in the patient who demonstrates a complete response to neoadjuvant therapy (with no residual tumor found in the resected specimen).

In summary, use of neoadjuvant chemotherapy remains controversial, and its use is dependent on the institution or physician. The benefit of some survival improvement with neoadjuvant therapy must be balanced against the treatment cost, the increased perioperative morbidity, and the delay in surgical intervention to complete chemoradiation therapy.

Palliative Management

Palliative interventions for patients with terminal esophageal carcinoma are directed toward relief of severe dysphagia and obstruction. With advances in endoscopic approaches such as stents, laser coring, and phototherapy, surgical intervention is rarely indicated for palliation. Chemoradiation remains an effective means of palliation, and its effect is more durable. However, the benefit of palliative chemoradiation does not occur immediately and takes several weeks before the patient sees any improvement. Most endoscopic palliative interventions can provide immediate relief, but there is a higher risk of complications due to perforation, and their effects may not be long lasting.

Dilatation

Immediate improvement of dysphagia can be obtained using dilators or balloon expansion. These techniques of dilatation are relatively simple and readily available in most hospitals, but their effect is usually of short duration. The main risk is that of perforation.

Stents

Endoscopically placed expandable metal stents have replaced the old plastic, rigid tubes for treating obstructing lesions. They can provide immediate relief but require expertise in sizing and placing of the stent. Recurrence of obstructive symptoms can occur within a few months, requiring reintervention. Complications include stent migration, food

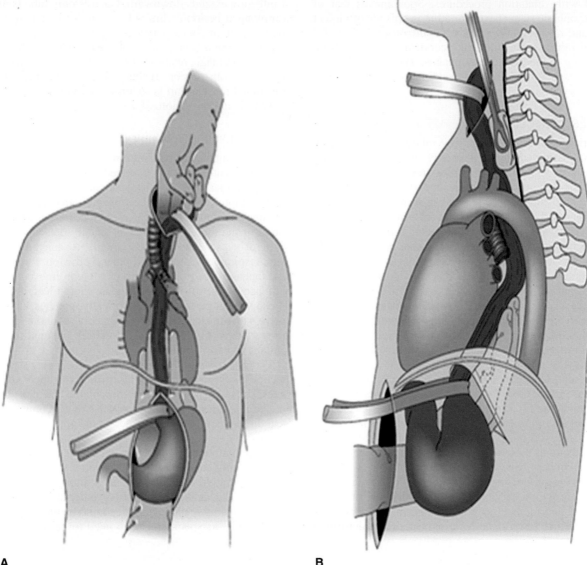

A   **B**

FIGURE 12-17. A and B, In a transhiatal esophagectomy, partial blunt dissection is performed by hand through a cervical and abdominal incision. Temporary hemodynamic instability by the compression of the heart during hand dissection of the thoracic esophagus can occur. Usually, the stomach is brought up to the neck where a gastroesophageal anastomosis is created. (Reprinted after Orringer MB. Surgical options for esophageal resection and reconstruction with stomach. In: Baue AF. Geha AS, Hammond GI, eds. *Glem's Thoracic and Cardiovascular Surgery*, 5th ed. Norwalk, CT: Appleton & Lange, 1991:799, with permission.)

impaction, and perforation. Stents are used for mid- and distal esophageal tumors and can be associated with significant reflux when placed in the distal esophagus.

Laser and Photodynamic Therapy

Endoscopically guided laser "coring" of obstructing tumors can be effective but carries a high risk of perforation. Photodynamic therapy consists of using photosensitizing agents followed by local light therapy to ablate the tumor. Because of limited depth of penetration by the laser light, risk of perforation is decreased, but the extent of tumor debulking is therefore limited.

Radiation and Chemoradiation

Chemoradiation therapy can be very effective and durable in decreasing tumor mass and improving dysphagia. Compared to the other palliative modalities, there is less limitation from tumor location and size or the availability of endoscopic expertise. The limiting factor of chemoradiation is the lag

period of weeks to achieve effect and systemic debilitation from chemotherapy.

Ideally, centers treating patients with advanced esophageal cancer should have expertise in multiple options of palliation, as it is likely that the patients will need more than one approach for their disease. Ultimately, the goal of palliation is to provide a "comfortable" quality of life in the limited time available for the patient. Any aggressive palliative intervention must be weighed against potential for major complications and need for acute hospitalization.

ESOPHAGEAL PERFORATION

Traumatic injury to the esophagus is a frequently encountered surgical emergency seen in thoracic surgery. Currently, esophageal perforation commonly results from instrumentation of a diseased esophagus and is especially associated with dilatation procedures. Spontaneous tear of the distal esophagus can also occur after an episode of violent vomiting and retching (**Boerhaave's syndrome**). It is useful to separate injury occurring at the cervical esophagus from that occurring at the thoracic esophagus. The etiology, prognosis, and management differ, depending on the location of the perforation.

Cervical Esophageal Injury

The majority of cervical esophagus injuries are caused by endoscopic instrumentation, especially at the level of the cricopharyngeal sphincter. Penetrating trauma to the neck is another common cause of cervical esophageal injury, as it is more vulnerable due to its locality when compared to the thoracic esophagus. The immediate concern of cervical esophageal injury is sepsis. The ability for infection from a cervical esophageal injury to rapidly extend into the posterior mediastinum (posterior descending mediastinitis) is a classically described entity. The retrovisceral space is located posterior to the esophagus and anterior to the prevertebral fascia. Due to the retrovisceral space, which connects the paracervical esophageal space to the posterior mediastinum, infection can rapidly descend from the neck into the mediastinum (Figure 12-18).

Initial symptoms of cervical esophageal injury include pain with swallowing and neck flexion. Tenderness and crepitus may be present. On plain x-ray films, air may be seen in the retrovisceral space, possibly extending into a pneumomediastinum. Indication for surgical intervention in suspected cervical esophageal injury can be based on history, clinical exam, and simple x-rays. A positive barium esophagram study is not mandatory, as up to 20% of these studies may be negative.

Treatment of cervical esophageal injury consists of intravenous antibiotics, surgical debridement, and drainage. Surgical approach is through a cervical incision on the side of injury. Drainage and debridement of the retrovisceral space are performed, extending down to the superior posterior mediastinum if infection extends downward. Gastrostomy tube is placed if a prolonged period of limited oral intake is anticipated. Primary repair of the esophageal injury is attempted, but not required as most cervical esophageal injuries will heal with adequate drainage, restricted oral intake, and absence of distal esophageal obstruction. If there is associated tracheal injury, a pedicled muscle flap is incorporated into the procedure to prevent fistula formation.

Thoracic Esophageal Injury

Thoracic esophageal perforation is most commonly caused by instrumentation of a diseased esophagus, usually after attempted dilatation of a distal esophageal obstruction. Spontaneous rupture of the distal esophagus can occur after violent retching and emesis (Boerhaave's syndrome). Major perforation of the thoracic esophagus usually presents with acute signs of sepsis, and it is commonly associated with chest pain, respiratory distress, and pleural effusion. Recent history of esophageal instrumentation or violent emesis, associated with acute onset of clinical distress, should lead to suspicion of esophageal perforation. Historically, patients with a Boerhaave's tear present in a more clinically dramatic fashion and have a worse prognosis due to greater contamination from spillage of gastric contents.

Workup starts with plain x-rays, which may demonstrate pneumomediastinum and pleural effusion. An upper GI swallow and CT scan are helpful in determining the extent of injury and infection. Assessment for the presence of concomitant esophageal disease is needed to help determine optimal surgical management.

Treatment options include expectant medical management or surgical intervention. Much has been mentioned on nonoperative management with antibiotics, nasogastric drainage, and distal tube feeds or parental nutrition. However, nonoperative management should be the exception, and not the rule, as specific criteria need to be met for medical

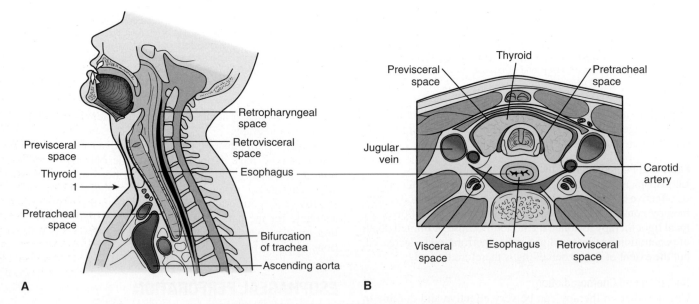

FIGURE 12-18. The retropharyngeal space and the retrovisceral space are a plane of loose connective tissue running behind the pharynx and esophagus, anterior to the vertebral bodies. This tissue plane is a potential space connecting the posterior pharynx and esophagus down into the posterior mediastinum **(A)**. Because it consists of loose connective tissue, infections arising from the pharynx or cervical esophagus can travel quickly down into the posterior mediastinum (posterior descending mediastinitis). The numeral (1) represents the level of cross-sectional view illustrated in **(B)**.

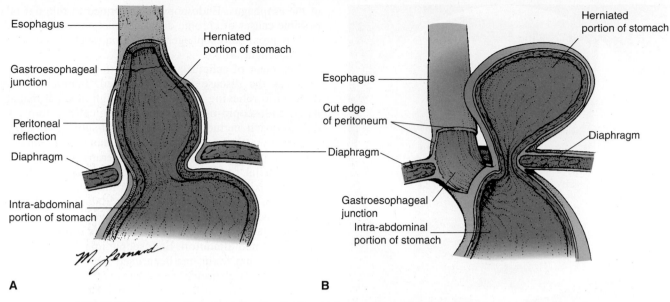

FIGURE 12-19. Type I and type II hiatal hernias. A, In type I (often associated with GERD), the gastroesophageal junction and proximal stomach slide into the chest due to weakening of the esophageal hiatus. **B**, In type II, the gastroesophageal junction remains anchored in the abdomen, and a weakening in the phrenoesophageal ligament allows the stomach or other intra-abdominal viscera to roll up into the chest. (Reprinted from Smeltzer SC, Bare BG. *Brunner & Suddarth's Textbook of Medical-Surgical Nursing*, 9th ed. Philadelphia, PA: Lippincott Williams & Wilkins, 2000, with permission.)

management of esophageal perforation. They include a limited perforation with drainage of contrast back into the esophagus, with no clinical signs of infection and no pleural effusion.

Surgical principles for managing esophageal perforation include good debridement of infected tissues, two-layer repair of the mucosa, and muscularis layer with reinforcement using a pedicled intercostal flap. Any concomitant esophageal disease needs to be identified and addressed, as any residual obstruction or pathology can affect the success of the surgical repair. This includes concomitant myotomy for LES disease and dilatation of fibrotic stricture, and in some cases, esophagectomy may be required for obstructing esophageal carcinoma. In the presence of terminal esophageal cancer, T-tube drainage via the perforation or intraluminal stenting may be alternatives to consider. Surgical esophageal exclusion has been used in managing significant esophageal injury when the patient is too ill to tolerate an extended surgical procedure for repair. Esophageal exclusion is achieved by stapling off the injured segment, cervical drainage by a spit fistula, gastrostomy tube, and local debridement. Spontaneous recanalization across the staple line can occur, or reconstruction with colon or jejunum can be offered after recovery.

HIATAL HERNIAS

There are four types of hiatal hernias described. The most common type is the sliding hiatal hernia (type I), which is frequently associated with GERD. In type I, the gastroesophageal junction slides in and out of the chest through the esophageal hiatus. In the other three types of hiatal hernias, there is a component of prolapse by the stomach or other abdominal organs into the chest.

In type II (paraesophageal) hernia, there is isolated stomach prolapsed through a weakened phrenoesophageal ligament, but preservation of the gastroesophageal junction in the abdomen. Type III hernia is a combination of sliding and paraesophageal hernia, and type IV involves herniation of other organs including the colon and spleen (Figure 12-19).

Plain chest radiography can demonstrate the presence of air-fluid level in the mediastinum or left chest consistent with herniation of the stomach. Contrast upper GI with swallow is considered the gold standard for identifying the presence of advanced hiatal hernias. CT scan can provide further detail on the anatomy of the hernia.

Asymptomatic type I hiatal hernia can be observed, as there is no risk for **incarceration**. Surgical intervention for type I hernia is determined by the symptoms of gastroesophageal reflex, and operative approaches are similar to the ones described in the above section of GERD. Frequently the esophagus is shortened in advanced type I hernias, and a Collis gastroplasty is needed to reconstruct the distal esophagus in addition to a fundoplication procedure.

Management of asymptomatic type II hernia is controversial. Because of the potential for acute **strangulation** and ischemia, some physicians believe that elective repair should be recommended for asymptomatic paraesophageal hernias. However, the incidence of acute incarceration and infarction is considered rare, and close observation with patient education seems a reasonable alternative to prophylactic surgery. When surgical repair is indicated due to symptoms (postprandial pain, dyspnea), it consists of hernia reduction, reconstruction of the diaphragmatic defect, fundoplication, and anchoring of the stomach with a gastrostomy tube or gastropexy.

ESOPHAGEAL MOTILITY DISORDERS

Achalasia

The most common motility disorder affecting the esophagus is achalasia, which translates as "failure to relax." The primary abnormality is believed to be a degenerative disease

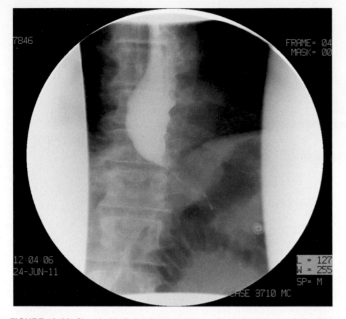

FIGURE 12-20. Classic bird's beak appearance of achalasia seen during barium swallow due to proximal esophageal dilatation associated with failure of the distal esophageal sphincter to relax.

of the myenteric (Auerbach's) neural plexus, which leads to denervation of the esophagus with resultant failure of relaxation of the LES upon swallowing. As the disease progresses, there is deterioration of the normal peristaltic activity of the esophageal body. The patient starts to develop symptoms of dysphagia to both solids and liquids and frequently complains of regurgitation. Characteristic adaptations seen in dysphagia from achalasia include changes in swallowing motions resembling a bird, with neck extension and multiple swallowing attempts. Diagnosis is confirmed by barium swallow (bird's beak sign) and manometric studies (Figure 12-20).

On manometric studies, there is failure of the LES to relax with swallowing, combined with weak peristaltic contractions

of the esophagus. Endoscopy is performed to rule out other possible causes of chronic distal obstruction, which can also lead to proximal esophageal dilatation, such as carcinoma (pseudoachalasia).

Treatment of achalasia is limited to palliative interventions, as the disease cannot be cured. Interventions are directed to relieving LES spasm through medical management, endoscopic intervention, or surgical myotomy. Initial approach includes the use of oral/sublingual nitrates and calcium channel blockers to promote LES relaxation prior to meals. Initially, medical therapy is helpful, but the beneficial response does not last, as patients develop tachyphylaxis to the drugs. Current mainstay of treatment for achalasia is endoscopic balloon dilatation of the LES. These sessions tend to be quite effective, with duration of the effect lasting for up to a few years, and usually responding to repeated dilatation. Endoscopic injection of the LES with botulinum toxin has been used with limited success. Patients who are surgical candidates and have failed endoscopic dilatation can be referred for a Heller myotomy of the LES (Figure 12-21).

The myotomy can be performed through a transthoracic or transabdominal incision. Studies have been done to demonstrate the advantage of one approach over the other, but ultimately surgeon preference and clinical history are major determinants of surgical technique. Many surgeons emphasize the importance of extending the myotomy into the proximal segment of the stomach. There is debate as to whether a concomitant fundoplication is needed to prevent gastroesophageal reflex after making the LES incompetent. Currently, a laparoscopic approach for the myotomy provides better patient comfort and the advantage of better visualization of the myotomy, possibly improving long-term outcomes.

Hypermotility Diseases

Hypermotility diseases of the esophagus include diffuse esophageal spasm and nutcracker esophagus. Symptoms are dysphagia and chest pain, and diagnosis is based on manometric

FIGURE 12-21. Heller myotomy for the treatment of achalasia, in which the distal esophageal sphincter is divided down to the mucosa. Some surgeons combine a fundoplication procedure to minimize reflux, although there is some controversy with a risk for causing residual distal obstruction. (Reprinted from Kaiser LR, et al. *Mastery of Cardiothoracic Surgery*, 2nd ed. Philadelphia, PA: Lippincott Williams & Wilkins, 2007:166, with permission).

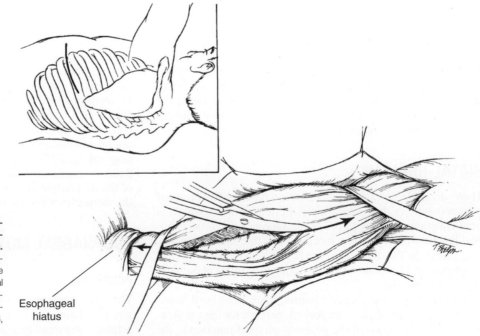

Esophageal hiatus

studies. Management is usually limited to medical treatment with nitrates and calcium channel blockers. Rarely, for diffuse esophageal spasm, an extended **esophageal myotomy** from the aortic arch level to the stomach is performed.

Esophageal Diverticula

An esophageal diverticulum is an outpouching from the wall and is classified as either pulsion or traction diverticula. Pulsion diverticula are more common and are associated with esophageal motility dysfunction. They are usually located in the proximal or distal esophagus. Because they lack a full muscle layer, pulsion diverticula are considered to be false diverticula. Traction diverticula are usually located in the midesophagus and develop from local lymph node inflammatory reaction causing traction on the esophageal wall. They are not associated with esophageal dysmotility and are true diverticula in that all layers of the esophageal wall are involved in the diverticula.

Pulsion Diverticula

Zenker's Diverticula

Zenker's diverticula are classified as pulsion diverticula and occur in the cervical esophagus. They are associated with cricopharyngeal muscle dysfunction, with failure to relax on swallowing causing proximal obstruction. Anatomically, they occur posteriorly, in the transition area of weakness between the hypopharynx and the esophagus, just above the cricopharyngeus muscle. Patients are typically elderly and may have some swallowing disorders associated with previous transient ischemic attacks or strokes. Patients with symptomatic Zenker's have regurgitation of recently swallowed food or pills, dysphagia, choking, or halitosis. Diagnosis is confirmed by barium swallow (Figure 12-22).

Endoscopy is not necessary for diagnosis but, if performed, should be done with caution as perforation can occur. Patients with symptoms are treated by myotomy of the cricopharyngeal muscle and diverticulectomy or diverticulopexy (inversion and fixation of the diverticulum to promote drainage by gravity). Newer endoscopic approaches have been described where the cricopharyngeus muscle is divided with an endoscopic stapler creating an esophagodiverticulostomy.

Midesophageal and Epiphrenic Diverticula

Epiphrenic diverticula occur in the distal third of the esophagus and are generally associated with dysfunction of the LES. Pulsion diverticula can also occur in the midesophagus and are also associated with esophageal dysmotility, such as diffuse spasm or achalasia. Epiphrenic diverticula can be caused from complications of GERD such as stricture. Symptoms of these diverticula are similar to other esophageal diverticula including dysphagia, regurgitation of undigested food, and occult aspiration. When symptomatic, they are referred for surgical intervention. Workup includes barium swallow, and in these diverticula, manometric studies to identify esophageal dysmotility pathology is needed. Surgical approach for epiphrenic diverticula is usually through a left thoracotomy, with diverticulum resection and repair, followed by stricture dilatation or an extensive distal myectomy to prevent recurrence.

Traction Diverticula

Traction diverticula are commonly associated with inflammatory paratracheal lymph node disease associated with tuberculosis or histoplasmosis. Usually they are asymptomatic and are left alone. The complication of fistula formation to the trachea or adjacent blood vessel can occur, which will lead to respiratory and bleeding symptoms. Surgical treatment consists of excision of the diverticula and repair of the adjacent structure. Frequently, an interposition flap of tissue is used to prevent recurrence and promote healing.

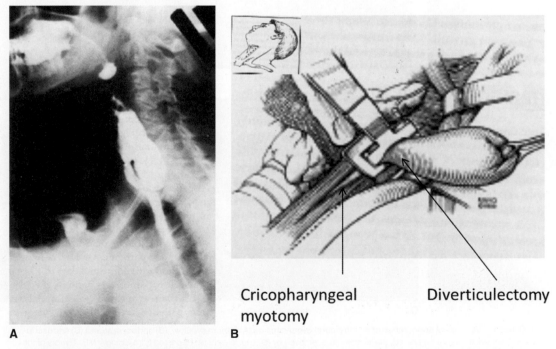

A **B**

FIGURE 12-22. A, Barium swallow shows a Zenker's diverticulum. B, Surgical treatment consists of a cricopharyngeal myotomy to relieve obstruction and usually a diverticulectomy. (Reprinted from Shields TW, et al. *General Thoracic Surgery*, 7th ed. Philadelphia, PA: Lippincott Williams & Wilkins, 2009:1963,1965, with permission.)

BENIGN ESOPHAGEAL LESIONS

Benign esophageal lesions are uncommon and are categorized by location in the esophageal wall. They commonly present with dysphagia. The most common benign neoplasm is the leiomyoma, which is located in the muscularis layer. The second most common benign mass is an esophageal cyst, which is located in the outermost adventitial layer, partially involving the muscularis layer. The granular cell tumor and fibrovascular polyp are the most common mucosal/submucosal lesions. Most of these lesions occur in the mid- to distal esophagus and commonly present with dysphagia. Barium swallow demonstrates a smooth well-defined mass occupying the lumen of the esophagus. Diagnostic workup includes direct endoscopic visualization and endoscopic ultrasound (Figure 12-23).

Asymptomatic masses can be observed, since there is minimal risk for malignant transformation of these lesions. Fine needle aspiration or biopsies should be avoided as these rarely provide adequate differentiation between a benign leiomyoma and a malignant leiomyosarcoma. Additionally, invasive manipulation of a cyst can result in iatrogenic infection requiring immediate surgical resection. When symptomatic, leiomyoma can be surgically removed by enucleation of the lesion with reapproximation of the muscle layer. Resection can be approached via standard thoracotomy, video-assisted thoracoscopic approach, or endoscopic approach (for smaller lesions). As expected, prognosis is excellent with good results and no recurrence.

FOREIGN BODY INGESTION

Foreign body ingestion is common in toddlers and mentally ill adults. The history must be confirmed with appropriate imaging studies. Most foreign body ingestion in adults is due to food impaction (poorly chewed meat or bones). The majority of impaction occurs at the level of cricopharyngeus muscle. Once past the cervical esophagus, most objects are able to pass into the stomach, and if held up at the lower esophagus, it is usually due to abnormal esophageal motility or stricture. Diagnosis is based on plain x-ray of the neck and chest. This should include lateral views of the neck to rule out cervical or mediastinal emphysema. Barium study is contraindicated as there is high risk for aspiration, and contrast delineation does not add to management of these patients. CT scan of the neck and chest can provide useful additional information. Underlying esophageal disease should be considered (e.g., foreign body lodged on an acid-induced structure), especially if impaction occurs in the distal esophagus.

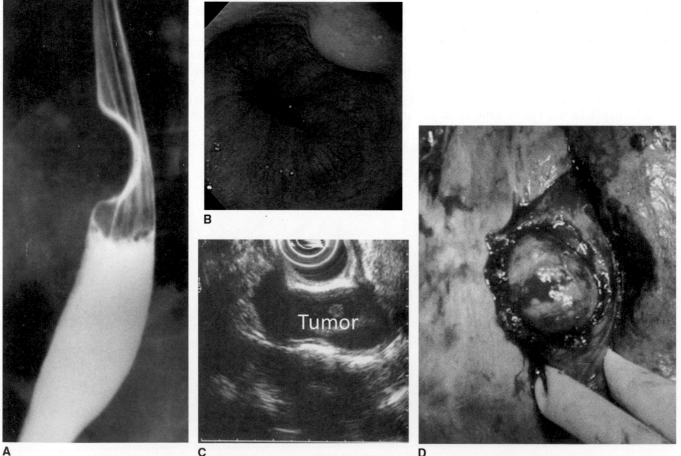

FIGURE 12-23. Typical appearance of an intramural leiomyoma on (A) barium swallow, (B) endoscopy, and (C) endoscopic ultrasound. If surgery is pursued, the leiomyoma is removed by **(D)** enucleation. (**A,** Reprinted from Orringer MB, Tumors of the esophagus. In: Sabiston DC Jr, ed. *Textbook of Surgery*, 13th ed. Philadelphia, PA: WB Saunders, 1986:736, with permission. **B,** Courtesy of Dr. Michael Kochman, Hospital of the University of Pennsylvania, Philadelphia. **C** and **D,** Reprinted from Shields TW, et al. *General Thoracic Surgery*, 7th ed. Philadelphia, PA: Lippincott Williams & Wilkins, 2009:1978,1980, with permission.)

Once the diagnosis is confirmed, the patient is best treated with gentle extraction using a rigid esophagoscope under general anesthesia. In rare instances where endoscopic removal is not possible, or there is associated perforation, open surgical removal may be necessary. Perforation of the esophagus is the most serious complication to rule out in a patient after extraction of the foreign body. A contrast study to exclude esophageal perforation should be performed before the patient is discharged. If perforation of the esophagus is identified, management is as described above in the section on esophageal perforation.

INGESTION OF CAUSTIC MATERIALS

Ingestion of caustic materials, either accidentally (as by children) or intentionally (as by an adult in a suicide attempt), is a medical emergency. Compared to ingestion of acid products, ingestion of alkaline products (e.g., Drano, Liquid Plumr) results in greater full-thickness esophageal injury. Ingestion of acidic material often leads to more superficial injury. The long-term complication from ingestion of caustic material is stricture formation.

Evaluation

The most important aspect of treatment is the early identification of the etiologic agent (e.g., acid, alkaline, specific toxin), because each agent requires a different approach. Second, careful physical examination of the oropharyngeal cavity is required to estimate the severity of injury, and the physician should be prepared for emergent fiberoptic endotracheal intubation, as these patients may develop rapid upper airway edema. Flexible endoscopy is urgently performed to assess the extent of injury and should be performed early (within 48 hours) to minimize the risk of perforation. Injury severity is graded by degree of depth, from first-degree burns being superficial to third-degree burns being transmural. The risk of perforation and stricture formation increases with the depth of injury.

Treatment

Induced vomiting and neutralization of caustic substances are not suggested because they are potentially harmful and ineffective. Airway maintenance is the first priority, followed

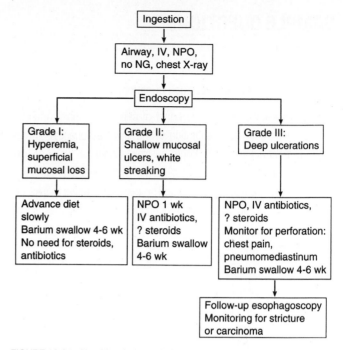

FIGURE 12-24. Algorithm for caustic ingestion. IV, intravenous; NG, nasogastric tube; NPO, nothing by mouth.

by maintenance of esophageal patency. During initial endoscopic evaluation, if second- or third-degree burns are identified, percutaneous gastrostomy should be performed for nutritional intake and future access for string-guided retrograde dilatation to prevent stricture formation. The use of antibiotics as adjuvant therapy is controversial. Steroids have not been proven effective in preventing stricture formation. Other than stricture formation, long-term complications include the increased risk for developing squamous cell cancer of the esophagus. Surgical resection, if indicated due to perforation or refractory stricture formation, is challenging due to extensive scarring in the tissues surrounding the esophagus. Surgical resection frequently requires the use of colon interposition as the stomach is frequently damaged. If scarring is deemed too intense to preclude safe esophageal resection, a substernal route for colonic interposition is performed. Figure 12-24 shows an algorithm for caustic ingestion.

SAMPLE QUESTIONS

Questions

Choose the best answer for each question.

1. A 50-year-old man has the onset of chest pain shortly after he undergoes pneumatic dilatation of the lower esophageal sphincter to treat achalasia. An upper gastrointestinal (GI) water-soluble contrast study shows free extravasation of the contrast material at the level of the distal esophagus. The decision is made to take the patient to the operating room for immediate repair. The best surgical incision to use is a(n)

   A. median sternotomy.

   B. right thoracotomy.

   C. left thoracotomy.

   D. abdominal incision.

   E. left thoracoabdominal incision.

2. A 50-year-old woman comes to the clinic because of severe heartburn and regurgitation after meals and on lying down. She has been on long-term proton pump inhibitors with good relief of symptoms but now wants to have antireflux surgery. Her body mass index (BMI) is 32.4. The preoperative study most useful in predicting symptomatic relief from antireflux surgery is a(n)

   A. contrast barium swallow.

   B. CT scan of the chest and abdomen.

   C. upper endoscopy.

   D. esophageal manometry study.

   E. 24-hour pH monitoring study.

3. A 43-year-old woman is being considered for antireflux surgery. She has a long history of reflux symptoms that are now only partially controlled with lifestyle changes and a proton pump inhibitor. Upper endoscopy showed a small hiatal hernia and a short segment of intestinal metaplasia, but no evidence of dysplasia.

She wants to know the possible advantage of the Toupet (partial) fundoplication as compared to the Nissen (full) fundoplication. The theoretical advantage for the Toupet fundoplication procedure is

   A. decreased morbidity and mortality when compared to the Nissen procedure.

   B. better long-term relief from gastroesophageal reflux disease (GERD).

   C. decreased postoperative symptoms of dysphagia and gas bloat.

   D. prevention of malignant progression of Barrett's disease.

   E. avoidance of a thoracotomy incision.

4. A 74-year-old man has a recent diagnosis of adenocarcinoma of the distal esophagus. He has a long history of reflux and Barrett's esophagus, and a recent upper endoscopy and biopsies confirmed the diagnosis. A staging workup is planned. What is the best study for assessing T (tumor invasion depth)?

   A. Barium swallow

   B. CT scan with oral and intravenous contrast

   C. Upper endoscopy with rebiopsy

   D. Positron emission tomography (PET) scan

   E. Endoscopic ultrasound

5. A frail 85-year-old man underwent upper endoscopy with dilation and biopsy of a distal esophageal stricture. Concerned about a perforation, the endoscopist obtained a water-soluble contrast upper GI study that confirmed a perforation. Nonsurgical management is acceptable if

   A. the patient has a new left pleural effusion.

   B. the patient has an obstructing carcinoma.

   C. the patient develops pain.

   D. the perforation is over 24 hours old.

   E. the upper GI study shows leak of contrast, which drains back into the esophagus.

Answers and Explanations

1. Answer: C

The best exposure of the distal thoracic esophagus is through a left thoracotomy. Anatomically, the upper and middle thoracic esophagus runs along the right side of the aorta, but the distal esophagus swings anterior and then to the left of the aorta to exit into the abdomen. The esophagus is not accessible through a median sternotomy because it lies in the posterior mediastinum with the heart lying anterior to it. A right thoracotomy is used to expose the proximal and middle thoracic esophagus. A left thoracoabdominal incision is a large morbid incision and is not necessary for the repair of the perforation and to perform a myotomy.

2. Answer: E

Evidence of abnormal acid reflux obtained from a positive 24-hour pH study is the best indicator for likely benefit of an antireflux procedure in gastroesophageal reflux disease (GERD). The other studies offered above can provide additional information on GERD but are not as sensitive in identifying potential surgical candidates for antireflux procedure. A barium swallow can identify a hiatal hernia, associated strictures, or shortened esophagus. A CT scan provides very little additional information but may demonstrate the presence of a hiatal hernia. Upper endoscopy is useful in identifying and monitoring progression of Barrett's disease. Manometric study, when abnormal, is useful in identifying motility dysfunction, which may affect surgical outcome.

3. Answer: C

Because the Toupet procedure is a partial fundoplication, there is less risk for developing dysphagia or from having difficulty burping as compared to a full encircling fundoplication. Both the Toupet and Nissen procedures can be performed laparoscopically with minimal morbidity and mortality. Because the Nissen is a full fundoplication, many proponents argue that it provides better protection from recurrent reflux. No antireflux procedure has been conclusively shown to prevent or reverse Barrett's disease, and continued periodic endoscopic monitoring is recommended. Both the Toupet and Nissen procedures are usually performed through an abdominal incision.

4. Answer: E

The endoscopic ultrasound is the best way to assess the depth of tumor invasion (T stage) and is also useful in identifying adjacent abnormal lymph node for fine needle aspiration (N stage). A barium swallow is a good initial study in the workup of dysphagia and helps locate the level of the lesion. A CT scan may show gross invasion of adjacent structures but cannot differentiate tumor depth. Upper endoscopy is used to obtain biopsies to confirm carcinoma, but depth of invasion cannot be determined from the biopsy specimen. A PET scan is used to identify distant metastasis but does not have the resolution to determine tumor depth.

5. Answer: E

Conservative management is acceptable if contrast study shows a contained leak that drains back into the esophageal lumen. A new left pleural effusion is indicative of a more severe leak, which should not be managed conservatively. Obstructing lesions cannot be ignored, as any obstruction will exacerbate the leak. Pain is indicative of excessive leak of GI contents into the mediastinum and pleura, which cannot be managed conservatively. Duration of perforation should not dictate whether surgical intervention is or is not pursued.

13
Stomach and Duodenum

JOHN T. PAIGE, M.D. • TIMOTHY M. FARRELL, M.D. • DANIEL B. JONES, M.D. •
SAAD SHEBRAIN, M.D. • KIMBERLEY E. STEELE, M.D.

Objectives

1. Describe the clinical significance of aspects of gastric and duodenal anatomy in the pathophysiology and therapy of peptic ulcer disease (PUD).

2. Review the physiology of gastric acid secretion and its role in the development and treatment of gastric and duodenal ulcer disease.

3. Understand how the physiology of vitamin B_{12} absorption can lead to deficiency after certain gastric operations.

4. Compare and contrast the pathophysiology, evaluation, and treatment of gastric and duodenal ulcer disease.

5. Discuss the presentation, classification, and treatment of adenocarcinoma of the stomach.

6. List the diagnostic options for identifying the location and etiology of benign ulcer disease.

7. Describe the common operations performed for the treatment of complicated ulcer disease and discuss their complications.

8. Identify the clinical and biochemical features of Zollinger-Ellison syndrome (gastrinoma) that aid in differentiating it from benign ulcer disease and discuss therapeutic options in its treatment.

9. Review the classification, pathophysiology, and therapy of obesity.

10. Describe the advantages and disadvantages of common procedures performed for the treatment of severe obesity and list their complications.

ANATOMY

Stomach

The stomach is a gastrointestinal (GI) capacitance organ usually located in the left hypochondrium and epigastrium, interposed between the esophagus and duodenum. There are anatomic relationships with the diaphragm superiorly, the spleen and liver laterally, the pancreas posteriorly, and the greater omentum inferiorly. Normally, the stomach can expand to accommodate a liter or more of ingested food, which it prepares for digestion and absorption.

The gastroesophageal (GE) junction is defined histologically by a mucosal change from squamous to columnar epithelium, and functionally by a high-pressure zone known as the lower esophageal sphincter (LES). In healthy individuals, the LES is intraperitoneal, >2 cm long, and has a resting pressure above 6 mm Hg. A hypotonic LES or hiatal hernia may contribute to gastroesophageal reflux disease (GERD). With swallowing, a coordinated relaxation of the LES occurs to facilitate entry of food into the stomach. Impaired LES relaxation and esophageal aperistalsis define the condition called **achalasia**.

The gastroduodenal junction is marked histologically by a definite mucosal change from gastric epithelium to intestinal epithelium (striated columnar cells with interspersed goblet cells) and functionally by a discreet 1 to 3 cm long smooth muscle valve known as the pylorus. The pylorus prevents reflux of duodenal contents into the stomach and, in association with the antral pump, controls gastric emptying. After ingestion of a meal, particles larger than 3 to 5 mm are retained in the stomach until the final "cleansing" wave of peristalsis occurs several hours later.

The stomach is divided into three distinct regions based on histologic and physiologic differences. The most proximal portion, the *fundus*, plays a crucial role in capacitance by undergoing receptive relaxation. As food traverses the pharynx and esophagus, vagal stimulation causes relaxation of the fundus, limiting increases in the intragastric pressure as food is stored. The fundus is the site of the autonomic pacemaker that is responsible for initiating gastric motor activity. The middle portion of the stomach, the *corpus*, contains most of the acid-producing parietal cells, as well as pepsinogen-producing chief cells and enterochromaffin-like (ECL) cells. The corpus is important for hydrochloric acid (HCl) secretion, storage of gastric contents, and peristaltic grinding against the pylorus. The most distal region, the *antrum*, contains G cells, which produce gastrin, but not the parietal cells. For this reason, a surgeon performing an **antrectomy** for ulcer disease must be certain to extend the resection to the proximal duodenum, since *retained antrum* in this now isolated, non–acid containing segment will hypersecrete gastrin causing recurrent ulcers

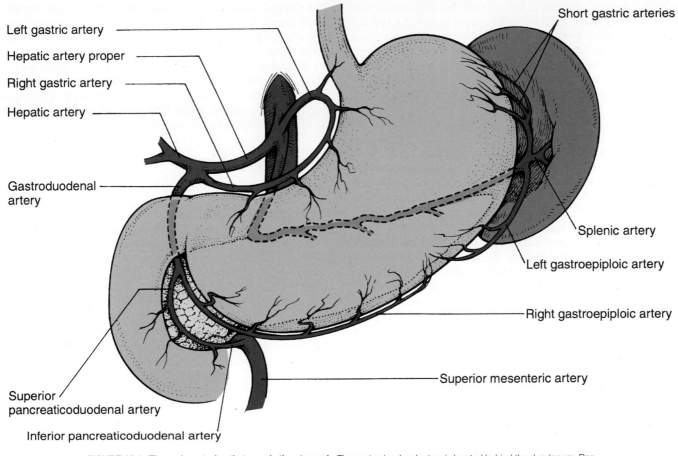

FIGURE 13-1. The major arteries that supply the stomach. The gastroduodenal artery is located behind the duodenum. Posterior penetrating duodenal ulcers may erode into this artery and cause hemorrhage.

in the remaining proximal stomach or at the anastomosis to small bowel (marginal ulcer). Finally, mucus-secreting goblet cells are found throughout the entire stomach.

The wall of the stomach has four layers: the mucosa, submucosa, muscularis, and serosa. The mucosa is arranged in a coarse rugal pattern and has a complex glandular structure. It is separated from the submucosa by the muscularis mucosa. Its abundant blood supply arises from the rich vascular network of the submucosa. The muscularis surrounds the submucosa in three layers of smooth muscle: the outermost longitudinal, the middle circular, and the innermost oblique. The gastric pacemaker in the fundus is located in the circular muscle layer. The serosa overlies the muscularis and is the outermost covering.

The arterial blood supply to the stomach includes the right and left gastric arteries, the right and left gastroepiploic arteries, the short gastric arteries, and the gastroduodenal artery (Figure 13-1). Because of this abundant blood supply, unintended surgical devascularization of the stomach rarely occurs. Sympathetic innervation parallels arterial flow.

Parasympathetic innervation via the vagus nerves contributes to HCl production by the parietal cell mass and motor activity of the stomach. As the vagus nerves traverse the mediastinum, the left trunk rotates so that it enters the abdomen anterior to the esophagus (Figure 13-2), whereas the right trunk rotates so that it enters posterior to the esophagus. The right vagus gives off a posterior branch to the celiac plexus, from which nerves pass to the midgut (pancreas, small intestine, and proximal colon), and, sometimes, a small branch that travels behind

the esophagus to innervate the stomach, known as the criminal nerve of Grassi. When not properly identified and divided during a parietal cell or truncal vagotomy, this nerve will continue

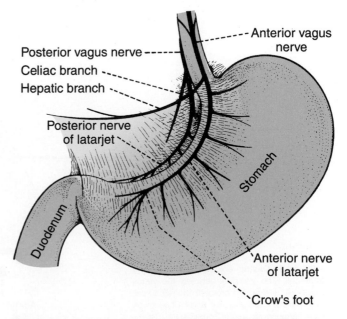

FIGURE 13-2. Branches of the vagus nerve innervate the stomach, pylorus, and duodenum. If the distal nerve of Latarjet is denervated, the pylorus does not relax in response to normal stimuli.

to stimulate acid secretion in the stomach, leading to recurrent peptic ulcer disease (PUD). The left vagus gives off a hepatic branch that passes through the gastrohepatic ligament and innervates the gallbladder, biliary tract, and liver. Below these branches, both vagus nerves continue down the lesser curvature and give off side branches that innervate the stomach and terminal branches that innervate the pylorus (crow's foot).

Duodenum

The duodenum is a "C-shaped," mostly retroperitoneal, 25- to 30-cm tube connecting the stomach to the jejunum. Anatomically, it is divided into four regions: the duodenal bulb (first part), the descending duodenum (second part), the transverse duodenum (third part), and the ascending duodenum (fourth part). The *duodenal bulb* receives chyme from the stomach via the pylorus. The *descending duodenum* receives enzymes from the pancreas and bile from the liver via the ampulla of Vater at the posteromedial aspect. In addition, the accessory pancreatic duct empties through the nearby lesser duodenal papilla. The *transverse duodenum* crosses the midline from right to left, and the *ascending duodenum* becomes the jejunum at the ligament of Treitz, where the small bowel becomes an intraperitoneal organ. The descending duodenum contains the intestinal pacemaker. Brunner's glands throughout the duodenum are the sites of mucus secretion, protecting the duodenal mucosa from gastric acid injury.

The duodenum is also an endocrine organ, with secretion of secretin and cholecystokinin (CCK) in response to the arrival of gastric acid and ingested fats. These hormones signal the hepatobiliary system to deliver bile and the pancreas to deliver bicarbonate and digestive enzymes such as trypsin, lipase, and amylase.

The blood supply to the duodenum comes primarily from the gastroduodenal artery and the superior mesenteric artery, although other smaller vessels are contributors (Figure 13-1).

The gastroduodenal artery is the first branch of the hepatic artery proper. It courses immediately posterior to the duodenal bulb and divides into the superior pancreaticoduodenal arcades. A **duodenal ulcer** that penetrates through the posterior wall of the duodenal bulb does so in the vicinity of the gastroduodenal artery. If the vessel wall is exposed to the digestive enzymes and acid, erosion and massive bleeding may occur. The superior mesenteric artery arises from the descending aorta and supplies the inferior pancreaticoduodenal arcades.

PHYSIOLOGY

Hydrochloric Acid Secretion

Gastric acid secretion is a complex, highly regulated process in which multiple specialized gastric and duodenal cells play an essential role. A well-developed mucosal defensive mechanism is also present in the stomach to protect it from caustic injury. The parietal cell rests at the heart of this elaborate system.

Gastric acid is secreted under basal and stimulated conditions. The basal acid secretion occurs in a circadian rhythm with highest levels occurring during the night and lower levels during the morning hours. When stimulated, the parietal cell undergoes morphologic and functional changes. The former includes fusion of many cytoplasmic tubulovesicles, on which proton pumps are expressed, with the canalicular membrane moving the proton pumps to a position in which they can actively exchange H^+ for K^+. The H^+, K^+, –ATPase is responsible for creating the concentrated acid environment within the lumen of the stomach (Figure 13-3). It accomplishes this task by actively secreting hydrogen ion against a 1,000,000:1 concentration gradient. Gastric acid secretion is an active process that requires a high amount of energy provided by adenosine triphosphate (ATP). Chloride ion is transported into the lumen in conjunction with this process. Water and bicarbonate

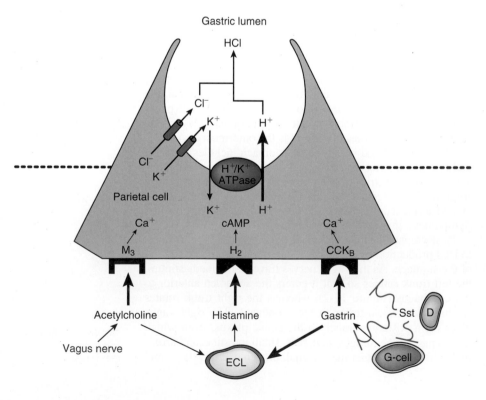

FIGURE 13-3. Gastric acid secretion by the parietal cell. The interplay between the vagus nerve, G cell, and enterochromaffin-like (ECL) cell leads to parietal cell stimulation and HCl secretion via three hormonal receptors. Somatostatin (Sst) release inhibits this acid secretion. M_3, muscarinic 3; H_2, histamine 2; CCK_B, cholecystokinin B; D, D-cell; ATP, adenosine triphosphate; cAMP, cyclic adenosine monophosphate.

are by-products of this reaction, and they passively diffuse into the plasma and extracellular space. When stimulated, 60% to 70% of proton pumps in the parietal cell become active. The proton pumps are recycled back to the inactive state in cytoplasmic vesicles once parietal cell activation ceases. Direct blockage of this fundamental step inhibits gastric acid production. Proton pump inhibitors (PPIs), developed by the pharmaceutical industry, work in this manner. They have dramatically altered the therapy of duodenal ulcer and gastric reflux disease.

The parietal cell membrane has three important receptors involved in HCl secretion: a cholecystokinin B (CCK_B) **gastrin** receptor, a muscarinic 3 (M_3) acetylcholine (Ach) receptor, and a histamine 2 (H_2) receptor (Figure 13-3). Activation of gastrin and M3 receptors leads to activation of the protein kinase C/phosphoinositide pathway, while activation of H_2 receptors by histamine leads to activation of the adenylate cyclase pathway with an increase in cyclic adenosine monophosphate (cAMP). Each pathway regulates a series of kinase cascades that control the pump mechanism. These receptors engage in a synergism in which simultaneous activation of two or more of them by the appropriate ligand augments acid secretion. Conversely, when any one of these sites is blocked, the other sites become less responsive to stimulation. Thus, when vagal innervation is interrupted, the parietal cell response to gastrin becomes blunted.

Mechanisms of Acid Stimulation

The capacity of the stomach to secrete HCl is almost linearly related to parietal cell mass. Gastric acid secretion by the parietal cell mass occurs in a sequential order divided into three general phases: cephalic, gastric, and intestinal. Each phase has distinct mechanisms of activation.

Cephalic Phase

This initial phase is mediated by the central nervous system (CNS) and stimulated by the sight, smell, or thought of food that activate afferent neural pathways to the CNS. Efferent activity proceeds from the hypothalamus to the stomach via the vagus nerve. Ach release by the vagus has three actions:

1. Directly: Ach stimulates the parietal cell directly by binding to its M_3 receptor. Activation of this receptor leads to an intracellular cascade resulting in the release of HCl.
2. Indirectly: Ach stimulates acid secretion by activating antral cells that produce gastrin-releasing protein (GRP). GRP then promotes gastrin secretion from antral G cells.
3. Ach can stimulate the ECL cells to release histamine, which subsequently stimulates gastric acid secretion through H_2-receptor stimulation.

In addition to food's visual and olfactory stimulation of acid release, its actual physical presence in the mouth activates the vagal pathway. Surgical division of the vagal nerves supplying the parietal cell mass blunts this parasympathetic response, decreasing acid secretion. In addition, anticholinergic blockade of the M_3 receptor can inhibit the response. Such anticholinergic agents, however, are not nearly as effective as other acid inhibitors now available, have multiple side effects, and are not used clinically.

Gastric Phase

The gastric phase is activated once the food enters the stomach. Stretch receptors within the stomach activate intragastric parasympathetic reflex pathways that promote further Ach release. In addition, chemical and stretch receptors within the antrum detect alkalinization, antral distension, and the presence of amino acids. In response, the G cells release gastrin. The gastrin enters the venous circulation and exerts both a direct and indirect effect:

1. Directly: Some gastrin binds the CCK_B receptors on the parietal cells, promoting HCl secretion. This direct mechanism of action is the weaker of the two.
2. Indirectly: Gastrin promotes acid secretion mainly via the ECL cells. Here, gastrin activates receptors, causing histamine release from the ECL cells. The histamine then binds the H_2 receptors on the parietal cells, stimulating acid release.

Gastrin is the most potent stimulus for acid secretion in humans. It exhibits marked heterogeneity, being processed into multiple fragments from the initial preprogastrin produced by the G cells. Three main forms include 14-, 17-, and 34-amino acid species. Of these, the 17-amino-acid gastrin is the most biologically active in stimulating acid secretion. It has a short half-life of only 2 to 3 minutes, and, like all fragments, is neutralized in the small intestine and kidney.

Certain foods can also stimulate acid secretion. Both alcohol and caffeine act directly on the mucosa to increase HCl release. Proteins also seem to promote acid secretion indirectly via their breakdown products (amino acids) as described above.

Intestinal Phase

The intestinal phase of gastric acid production occurs with the arrival of the products of digestion in the small intestine. Although knowledge regarding this phase is somewhat limited, it is associated with substantial elevations in various serum peptides. Some of them, like enterooxyntin, stimulate gastric acid output. Other peptides are inhibitory (see the section on mechanisms of acid suppression and mucosal protection below). The parietal cell H_2 receptor may play an important role in this phase of acid secretion.

Mechanisms of Acid Suppression and Mucosal Protection

When stimulated, the parietal cell mass in the stomach can drop the pH to as low as 1.0. In this acidic environment, pepsinogen is activated to pepsin and begins to hydrolyze proteins into peptones and amino acids. Unchecked, this process would lead to severe caustic injury and autodigestion of the stomach. Fortunately, several mechanisms exist to suppress acid secretion and protect the gastric mucosal lining.

Endocrine-Mediated Acid Suppression

The release of acidic chyme into the duodenum stimulates the secretion of numerous gut inhibiting hormones (so-called enterogastrones: secretin, somatostatin, vasoactive intestinal peptide (VIP), gastric inhibitory polypeptide (GIP), neurotensin) that help suppress gastric acid production. **Secretin**, a 27-amino-acid peptide released by duodenal S cells, plays an important role in this suppression. Its secretion is stimulated by luminal acidity, biliary salts, and fatty acids. In turn, secretin inhibits gastrin release, gastric acid secretion, and gastric motility. **Somatostatin**, a tetradecapeptide, is another important mediator. Its secretion is stimulated by a drop in gastric pH and acts directly on the parietal cells to inhibit acid secretion. In addition, it inhibits gastrin release when gastric luminal pH drops to <1.5. Finally, somatostatin reduces histamine release from ECL cells. CCK and GIP, both released by cells in the duodenum, also act to suppress gastric acid production. Thus, an enterogastric feedback mechanism exists in which duodenal peptides help suppress acid production in the stomach once food enters the intestines.

Gastric Mucosal Protection

Within the stomach is a sophisticated, highly efficient barrier system that protects the gastric mucosal lining from caustic injury and digestion. The first barrier is a mucus-bicarbonate layer produced by the gastric epithelial cells. The mucus is a mucopolysaccharide that attaches to the luminal surface of the gastric mucosa, creating a protective mucous gel barrier that impedes diffusion of ions and molecules such as pepsin into the cells. The bicarbonate is secreted in exchange for chloride ions. The amount of bicarbonate produced by the stomach can only neutralize a small portion of the maximum acid output. The gastric lining, however, is preserved because the gel-like mucosal barrier traps the secreted bicarbonate. Any back-diffusion of hydrogen ions into it, therefore, leads to their rapid neutralization and clearance. As a result, even though the pH in the stomach may drop to as low as 1.0, the pH at the luminal surface of the mucosal cells rarely falls below 7.0. When this mechanism is not functioning adequately, as seen in *Helicobacter pylori* infection, damage to the mucosa can occur, and **gastritis** or **gastric ulcers** can result. Bicarbonate secretion is stimulated by calcium, prostaglandins, cholinergic input, and luminal acidification.

The second barrier is prostaglandins that play an important role in gastric epithelial defense/repair by stimulating mucus-bicarbonate secretion by epithelial cells, inhibiting HCl secretion by parietal cell and improving gastric mucosal blood flow.

Vitamin B₁₂ (Cobalamin) Absorption

Vitamin B_{12} is a water-soluble vitamin with a key role in the normal functioning of the nervous system and in the formation of blood cells. The stomach and duodenum play an important role in vitamin B_{12} (cobalamin) absorption. To be properly absorbed in the terminal ileum, vitamin B_{12} must be complexed to intrinsic factor (IF). This glycoprotein is produced by the parietal cells in the stomach and binds to vitamin B_{12} after pancreatic proteases have isolated it in the proximal small bowel. Failure of any step in this sequence can result in vitamin B_{12} deficiency with the subsequent development of megaloblastic anemia, irreversible sensory neuropathy, and dementia.

The Schilling test is an effective means of determining the cause of vitamin B_{12} deficiency, which could be either pernicious anemia or small intestinal bacterial overgrowth. In the first part of the test, a patient is given an oral dose of radiolabeled cobalamin followed by an intramuscular injection of unlabeled vitamin. The excretion of cobalamin in the urine is then determined by collecting a 24-hour urine sample. An abnormal value corresponds to less than 10% excretion of vitamin. Abnormal results are followed by a repeat Schilling test using radiolabeled cobalamin bound to IF. Urinary excretion in this case will be normal if IF deficiency, as seen in pernicious anemia, is responsible for the poor vitamin B_{12} absorption. It will remain abnormal in cases of bacterial overgrowth or ileal disease causing the vitamin deficiency. Finally, the Schilling test can also be administered using radiolabeled cobalamin bound to proteins in scrambled eggs. An abnormal result in this situation would suggest failure of the vitamin to dissociate from the ingested food, as occurs in patients with achlorhydria.

Duodenal Bicarbonate Secretion

Like the stomach, the duodenum has several mechanisms of mucosal protection. Mucus is produced by Brunner's glands, helping to create a protective barrier over the mucosa. In addition, the duodenal cells secrete sodium bicarbonate via a transmucosal electrical gradient. This production is up to six times greater than that of the stomach. As a result, the sodium bicarbonate can neutralize all of the hydrogen ions that are normally presented to the duodenal bulb. Additional bicarbonate comes from the pancreas. It, however, only neutralizes a small amount of the total acid load.

Duodenal bicarbonate is stimulated locally by mucosal irritation. Pancreatic bicarbonate is released in response to secretin stimulation. It increases the volume of pancreatic secretions of bicarbonate and water. The cells of origin of these secretions are the centroacinar cells.

BENIGN GASTRIC DISEASE

Gastric Ulcer Disease

PUD includes benign ulcers of the stomach and duodenum. In most cases, gastric and duodenal ulcers have similar pathophysiology, clinical presentation, medical therapies, and surgical indications. There are, however, certain considerations with respect to gastric ulcers, such as the risk of underlying malignancy, which must be remembered during evaluation and management. This chapter, therefore, discusses each entity in separate sections to emphasize such differences. Because much overlap does exist, however, similarities will be covered in the sections on duodenal ulcer disease.

In recent decades, improved understanding of the etiologic role of *H. pylori* and nonsteroidal anti-inflammatory drugs (NSAIDs) has shifted PUD treatment algorithms dramatically away from surgery. These agents have been shown to promote ulcer formation by altering the balance between the protective and potentially harmful components of the gastric environment. *H. pylori* infection causes a chronic active gastritis, with dysregulation of gastrin and acid secretion. NSAIDs inhibit cyclooxygenase 1 (cox-1), which is essential for prostaglandin synthesis, thereby altering local blood flow, mucus production, and bicarbonate secretion in the stomach. In such cases, acid and pepsin activity overcome gastric mucosal defensive mechanisms, exposing the lining of the stomach to damage. Taken together, *H. pylori* infection and NSAID use, either alone or in combination, are thought to be the etiology of most benign gastric ulcer disease worldwide. Tobacco use is also an important risk factor. Although alcohol is a strong promoter of acid secretion, its role in ulcerogenesis remains uncertain.

Classification

Before the current understanding of PUD etiology, a classification scheme for gastric ulcers was developed, based on anatomic location and usual pathophysiology, to better direct application of acid suppressive and resective procedures. Type I gastric ulcers (most frequent) occur along the lesser curvature of the stomach in the zone above the antrum. Type II gastric ulcers arise in combination with duodenal ulcers. Type III gastric ulcers develop in the prepyloric region. Type IV gastric ulcers (least frequent) occur high on the lesser curve near the GE junction. Types I and IV are associated with normal or low acid output; types II and III are associated with gastric acid hypersecretion, like duodenal ulcers.

The characteristics and behavior of *H. pylori* likely explain the patterns behind the above-noted classification scheme for gastric ulcers. These small, curved, microaerophilic, gram-negative rods are spread from person to person via gastrooral or fecal-oral transmission, and can colonize the antrum of the stomach, causing local mucosal inflammation. In patients with a high gastric acid output, this colonization can extend distally into the duodenal bulb if the duodenal mucosa undergoes gastric metaplasia. In patients with a low gastric acid output, the colonization spreads more proximally into the cardia, with particularly dense activity at the transition zone between the antrum and the cardia. Such observations help explain why type I and type IV gastric ulcers are associated with low acid output, why type II ulcers are associated with duodenal ulcers, and why type II and type III ulcers are associated with acid hypersecretion.

NSAID-induced ulcers fall outside the above classification system. They can occur anywhere in the stomach, and respond differently to treatment. Consequently, some authors have proposed an additional type V classification for gastric ulcerations due to NSAIDs.

Clinical Presentation and Evaluation

The clinical presentation of benign gastric ulcers depends on the severity of the disease process. In uncomplicated gastric ulcers, patients typically complain of a characteristic gnawing epigastric pain that can radiate to the back. Often, since this pain is associated with ingestion of food, patients develop anorexia and weight loss. In cases of complicated gastric ulcers, patients may or may not have these antecedent symptoms prior to perforation or bleeding. Up to 10% of NSAID-induced ulcers present with a complication without warning. The presentation, evaluation, and initial treatment of complicated gastric ulcers follow the description for complicated duodenal ulcers presented later in this chapter.

Evaluation of a patient suspected of having an uncomplicated gastric ulcer begins with a thorough history and physical examination. In addition to determining the duration and character of symptoms, risk factors are sought. In particular, the patient should be questioned regarding current tobacco or NSAID use, prior PUD, or history of *H. pylori* infection. Physical examination should focus on searching for signs of a malignant process.

Esophagogastroduodenoscopy (EGD) confirms the presence of an ulcer. This study involves the passage of a fiberoptic scope from the mouth into the esophagus, stomach, and duodenum. The mucosa is examined in detail. Photographs may be taken for documentation and for comparison in subsequent evaluations of healing. Because of the 2% to 4% risk of underlying malignancy, all gastric ulcers require multiple biopsies at the time of endoscopy to establish the presence or absence of carcinoma. Endoscopic features suggestive of malignancy include a bunched-up ulcer border or large (>3 cm) ulcer size. Biopsy specimens should include samples incorporating the margin of the ulcer. Cytology and brushings are also helpful as an adjunct to biopsy. Despite such guidelines, false-negative results are still possible due to the small sample size of the biopsy specimens. The presence of achlorhydria in a patient with gastric ulceration is also suggestive of a malignant process. Finally, all patients with gastric ulcers, like those with duodenal ulcers, require testing to determine the presence or absence of *H. pylori* infection. Samples can be obtained for this purpose at endoscopy.

A less invasive diagnostic modality, which is still occasionally used, is barium upper GI contrast study. The patient is required to drink a specified amount of barium, after which multiple x-rays are taken as the contrast passes through the

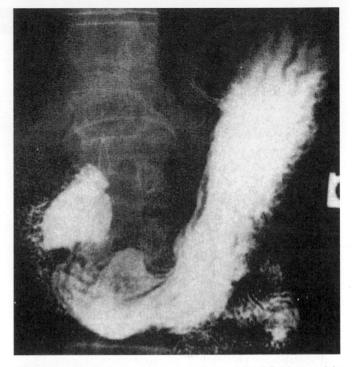

FIGURE 13-4. Moderate-sized ulcer seen on lesser curve of distal stomach in this barium upper GI study.

stomach and into the duodenum. A small crater is typically seen extending outward from the stomach (Figure 13-4). The disadvantage of this test is that biopsies of the ulcer are not possible, which may lead to eventual endoscopy anyway.

Medical Treatment

First-line therapy for uncomplicated gastric ulcer disease is medical and follows guidelines similar to those for uncomplicated duodenal ulcer disease. In brief, this regimen includes cessation of all potential ulcerogenic agents (tobacco, NSAIDs, aspirin, steroids, alcohol), treatment of *H. pylori* infection with appropriate antibiotics, and acid suppression therapy (Table 13-1).

Additional options for gastric ulcer treatment include the administration of cytoprotective agents such as sucralfate and misoprostol. Sucralfate is an aluminum salt containing sulfated sucrose. On ingestion, the sucrose polymerizes, coating the gastric ulcer with a protective barrier that prevents further injury. Misoprostol is a prostaglandin E1 analogue that promotes gastric mucosal protection by enhancing the defensive mechanisms of the gastric lining. Even with the best medical therapy, refractory and recurrent gastric ulcer disease often may occur.

Repeat endoscopy is mandatory after initiating medical treatment of a gastric ulcer. After 6 weeks, the ulcer should show substantial (>50%) healing. While another course of medical therapy followed by endoscopy may be applied, failure of a gastric ulcer to heal completely with adequate medical therapy and follow-up is highly suggestive of an underlying malignant process. As such, multiple biopsy specimens of the margin of the ulcer should be taken at each EGD. Careful histologic review of these specimens is important. Even so, despite the best efforts of pathologists, false negative results do occur. Other tests such as cross-sectional imaging and endoscopic ultrasound may be applied to further characterize a lesion. Still, even in the absence of definitive diagnosis, failure of ulcer healing is an indication for elective operation unless a compelling reason exists to preclude a given patient as an operative candidate.

TABLE 13-1	Useful Medications Related to PUD		
Medication	**Action/Class**	**Indication**	**Dosage**
Clarithromycin	Antibiotic	*H. pylori* infection	500 mg po BID (triple therapy)
Amoxicillin	Antibiotic	*H. pylori* infection	1 g po BID (triple therapy)
Metronidazole	Antibiotic	*H. pylori* infection	400 mg po BID (triple therapy)
			400 mg po TID (quadruple therapy)
Tetracycline	Antibiotic	*H. pylori* infection	500 mg po daily (quadruple therapy)
Bismuth	Antacid	*H. pylori* infection	120 mg po daily (quadruple therapy)
Omeprazole	Proton pump inhibitor	*H. pylori* infection/ulcer healing	20 mg po BID (triple and quadruple therapy)
			80 mg IV bolus then 8 mg/hr × 72 hours (bleeding ulcer)
			20 mg po/IV daily prophylaxis

Surgical Treatment

Standard operative therapy for nonhealing, obstructing or refractory gastric ulcers includes excision, because of the possibility of malignancy. For ulcer types I, II, and III, a generous antrectomy (50% gastrectomy) is most commonly performed, and GI continuity is restored to either the proximal duodenum (**Billroth I** reconstruction, Figure 13-5), a loop of proximal jejunum (**Billroth II** reconstruction, Figure 13-6), or a transposed limb of jejunum isolated from biliopancreatic secretions (Roux-en-Y reconstruction, Figure 13-7). All of these reconstructions carry risk of marginal ulcers on the intestinal side of the gastroenteric anastomosis. Roux-en-Y reconstruction, in particular, may be associated with impaired gastric emptying and intestinal transit. Patients with type II and type III ulcers often receive truncal vagotomies in addition to antrectomy to further decrease gastric acid secretion. Type IV ulcers, given their proximal location, may require near total gastrectomy with Roux-en-Y reconstruction, though local excision is also an option. Every resected gastric ulcer

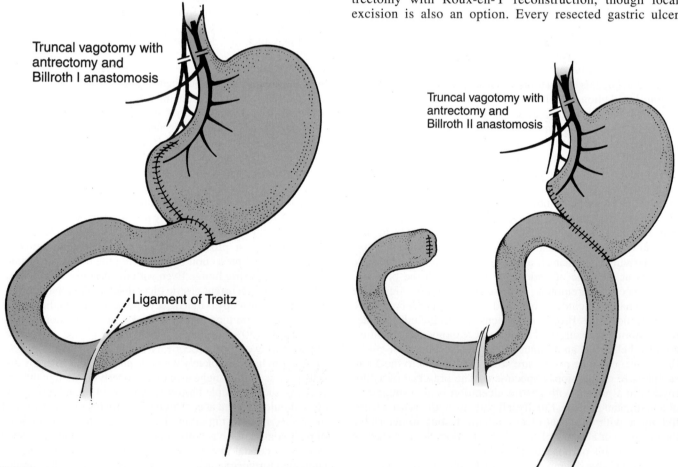

Truncal vagotomy with antrectomy and Billroth I anastomosis

Ligament of Treitz

Truncal vagotomy with antrectomy and Billroth II anastomosis

FIGURE 13-5. An antrectomy removes the distal portion of the stomach, where gastrin is produced. In addition, it removes the pylorus, thus allowing gastric emptying after vagotomy. In a Billroth I reconstruction, the duodenum is anastomosed to the stomach in continuity.

FIGURE 13-6. In a Billroth II reconstruction, the duodenum is not attached to the stomach; the stomach is anastomosed to a proximal loop of jejunum. This procedure is particularly useful when the duodenum is extensively scarred.

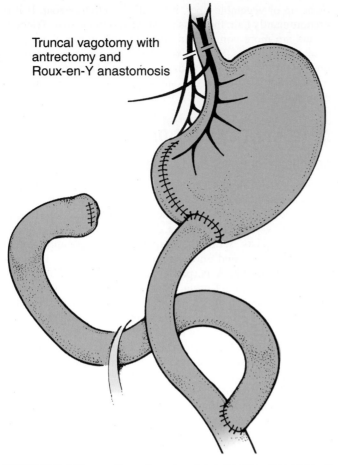

Truncal vagotomy with
antrectomy and
Roux-en-Y anastomosis

FIGURE 13-7. A Roux-en-Y anastomosis reduces the reflux of small bowel contents into the stomach. Peristalsis in the small bowel carries food and fluid away from the stomach. This procedure is particularly useful when a patient has a history of alkaline reflux gastritis.

must undergo careful histologic review to verify that a gastric carcinoma is not hidden in the depths of the crater. For this reason, complete excision of the ulcer is always required. If a gastric carcinoma is present, appropriate evaluation and adjunctive treatment should be instituted. The recurrence rate after surgical treatment of a gastric ulcer is very low.

In the case of an emergent operation for a perforated pyloric channel ulcer that was previously unrecognized, many surgeons will choose to treat by oversew and omental patch without resection, since the patient is often acutely ill, evaluation and treatment for *H. pylori* infection or NSAID injury have not yet been implemented, and the risk of malignancy is low. In this strategy, follow-up endoscopy is required to confirm complete healing.

Acute Gastritis

Acute gastritis produces an inflammation of the stomach mucosa that may be associated with erosions and hemorrhage. Presenting symptoms vary, and may include nausea, vomiting, hematemesis, melena, or hematochezia. *H. pylori* infection, NSAID or aspirin use, bile reflux, alcohol ingestion, irradiation, and local trauma can all contribute to this inflammatory response. Treatment involves acid suppression, removal of the noxious agent, occasional gastric decompression, and nutritional support.

Stress Gastritis

Stress gastritis is another important cause of acute inflammation. It typically occurs in patients suffering from severe physiologic stress, and, if not properly recognized and treated, can lead to significant morbidity and mortality. Patients develop mucosal erosions beginning in the proximal stomach and progressing rapidly throughout the rest of the organ. Classic presentations include ulcer formation in major burn victims (Curling's ulcer) and patients with CNS injury (Cushing's ulcer). This form of gastritis may also occur in other critically ill patients, such as those with severe trauma or organ failure. Medical prophylaxis using PPIs, H_2-receptor blockers, sucralfate, or misoprostol has been advised in intensive care patients. Prophylaxis should be started early in critical illness, since stress gastritis typically develops within 48 hours of the onset of physiologic stress.

Once stress gastritis is present, aggressive acid suppression is essential. Intraluminal pH should not decrease below 4.0. Treatment includes intravenous administration of PPIs or H_2 blockers. Alternatively, antacids can be directly delivered into the stomach via a nasogastric tube. Sucralfate and misoprostol remain helpful adjuncts.

Hemorrhage is the most common complication of stress gastritis, and it may be life threatening. Patients may present with blood per rectum or in nasogastric aspirate, or with a drop in blood count or unexplained hemodynamic instability. Immediate treatment should focus on initial fluid resuscitation and stabilization. Upper endoscopy confirms the diagnosis, and may be facilitated by preprocedure gastric lavage to clear the stomach of clots. Isolated sites of bleeding may be treated with electrocautery, heater probe, injection of vasoconstrictive agents, or laser therapy. Acid suppression is optimized, and preparations are made with the blood bank for immediate or subsequent transfusion as clinical parameters mandate. Serial blood counts are followed to confirm resolution of the bleed.

In cases of persistent bleeding, more aggressive interventions are required. Selective visceral angiography (typically of the left gastric artery) with embolization is one such option, and operative therapy is another. Of the several possible surgical interventions, oversewing of the bleeding erosions, with possible vagotomy and pyloroplasty (see Complicated Duodenal Ulcer Disease), is an expeditious, conservative procedure that controls hemorrhage in approximately 50% of patients. If bleeding recurs, total gastrectomy may be indicated.

Hypertrophic Gastritis (Menetrier's Disease)

Hypertrophic gastritis, also known as Menetrier's disease, is a rare disorder of the lining of the stomach characterized by massive hypertrophy of the gastric rugae. The exact etiology of the disease is unknown, but it is believed to be autoimmune in character. In particular, tumor necrosis factor (TNF)-β overexpression is believed to be implicated. Thickening of the mucosal folds occurs as a result of hyperplasia of the mucus-secreting cells in the corpus and fundus. Patients may present with epigastric pain, nausea, vomiting, occult hemorrhage, anorexia, weight loss, and diarrhea. Progression of disease is associated with a protein-losing gastropathy that may lead to hypoproteinemia and peripheral edema. Diagnosis is most often made by upper endoscopy with mucosal biopsy, although a full thickness surgical biopsy is sometimes required.

Treatment is typically nonoperative. Acid suppression therapy with PPIs, H$_2$-receptor antagonists, or antacids should be initiated. A high-protein diet and careful monitoring of nutritional status is essential. Anticholinergic medications are sometimes useful to decrease protein loss from the gastropathy. In rare instances, total gastrectomy may be required. Menetrier's disease is a risk factor for the development of adenocarcinoma of the stomach.

Mallory-Weiss Syndrome

An upper GI hemorrhage secondary to linear tearing of the mucosa at the GE junction is a well-described phenomenon known as Mallory-Weiss syndrome. Typically, these tears form after episodes in which a strong Valsalva maneuver causes mechanical stress on the mucosa in this region. Retching (often from acute alcohol intoxication), heavy lifting, childbirth, vomiting, blunt abdominal trauma, and seizures have all been associated with the syndrome. Patients typically present with hematemesis, melena, or hematochezia after such an antecedent history. Evaluation focuses on hemodynamic assessment and verification of a tear as the bleeding source. A nasogastric tube is placed, and gastric lavage is performed. The presence of blood should prompt endoscopic evaluation. The tears are best visualized on retroflexion of the flexible endoscope. Nuclear scintigraphy or selective angiography can also provide a diagnosis if endoscopy is unavailable. Laboratory investigations should include determination of coagulation parameters and serial blood counts. A blood sample is sent for type and crossmatch.

Initial therapy involves fluid resuscitation and stabilization. Acid suppression is then instituted with either PPIs or H$_2$-receptor blockers. Most bleeding will stop without further intervention; however, if bleeding persists, endoscopy is repeated, and the tear is treated with electrocautery, heater probe, or injection therapy. Selective angiography with embolization may also be therapeutic. Surgery is a last resort. The presence of subserosal staining along the lesser curve at the time of exploration is pathognomonic. Gastrotomy with oversewing of all tears is undertaken. Rebleeding after any of the above interventions typically occurs within 24 hours.

Gastric Polyps

Gastric polyps are rare, but they have been seen more frequently with increased utilization of diagnostic upper GI endoscopy. These polyps may be hyperplastic or adenomatous in nature. Hyperplastic polyps are more common and are typically benign, although rare cancerous transformation has been reported. Adenomatous polyps have a higher risk of malignant degeneration, especially those >1.5 cm. When a gastric polyp is diagnosed, the physician should consider the possibility of other polyps within the GI tract and polyposis syndromes.

One example is Peutz-Jeghers syndrome. This condition is marked by the presence of multiple benign polyps in the small intestine and sometimes other portions of the GI tract, and melanin spots on the lips and buccal mucosa. Peutz-Jeghers syndrome is an autosomal dominant trait that has a high degree of penetrance. In these patients, conservative therapy is indicated because the tumors are hamartomas and are infrequently malignant.

Bezoar

The accumulation of a large mass of indigestible fiber within the stomach is known as a **bezoar**. If the material is made up of vegetable fiber, it is called a phytobezoar. If it is predominantly hair, the mass is called a trichobezoar. Trichobezoars are more common in children and among inmates of mental institutions. Patients with large bezoars can sometimes present with gastric outlet obstruction. Although most bezoars may be broken up using the endoscope, some require surgical gastrotomy for removal.

MALIGNANT GASTRIC DISEASE

Adenocarcinoma of the Stomach

Almost 95% of stomach cancers are adenocarcinomas. Worldwide, adenocarcinoma remains a leading cause of cancer-related death. Its overall incidence, however, has been steadily declining over the last 50 years. Additionally, marked regional variability exists. While the frequency of adenocarcinoma in the United States and Europe remains relatively low, it is considerably higher in Asia, particularly Japan and China. High rates are also seen in Russia, Chile, and Finland. Environmental factors, especially diet, are thought to account for this discrepancy, since émigrés from these high-risk areas who settle in the United States have a lower incidence of disease.

Important risk factors for gastric adenocarcinoma include *H. pylori* infection, pernicious anemia, achlorhydria, and chronic gastritis. A history of caustic injury from lye ingestion also increases the risk of malignant degeneration. Finally, the presence of adenomatous polyps in the stomach is considered a risk factor.

Classification of Gastric Adenocarcinoma

Adenocarcinoma of the stomach can be divided into various classification schemes related to its clinical and histologic appearance. In the United States, cancers are often categorized into ulcerative, polypoid, scirrhous, and superficial spreading subtypes based on their endoscopic appearance. Of these, ulcerative carcinomas are by far the most frequent. Even though some differences in prognosis do exist between certain subtypes, the usefulness of this classification system is somewhat limited.

Two distinct histologic types of gastric adenocarcinoma exist: intestinal and diffuse. The intestinal type is well differentiated with glandular elements. It is more common in regions with a high incidence of disease. Typically, it occurs in older patients and spreads hematogenously. The diffuse type is poorly differentiated with characteristic signet ring cells. It occurs in younger patients and has an association with blood type A. It spreads via the lymphatics and local extension.

Linitis plastica is the term used to describe the complete infiltration of the stomach with carcinoma. In this situation, the stomach can look like a leather bottle. Patients with this variant of gastric cancer have a particularly poor prognosis.

Clinical Presentation and Evaluation

The clinical presentation of gastric adenocarcinoma depends on its stage. Early cancers are usually asymptomatic. As a result, in the United States they often go unrecognized until later in their progression. In Japan, these early cancers are more frequently diagnosed because of an aggressive endoscopic screening protocol. The low incidence of gastric carcinoma in the United States, however, makes the cost of such a program prohibitive.

More advanced disease leads to the development of symptoms. Patients can complain of vague epigastric pain similar to that produced by gastric ulceration. Often, it can be present for an extended period of time. Unexplained weight loss is another early complaint. As the disease progresses, patients begin to have more specific symptoms. Dysphagia, hematemesis, melena, nausea, or vomiting develops. Patients may also present with new onset iron deficiency anemia or guaiac-positive stools.

The initial evaluation for a patient suspected of having gastric carcinoma begins with a thorough history and physical examination. Risk factors are determined, and the patient is queried regarding lack of energy and unintentional weight loss. Physical examination should focus on signs of advanced disease. An enlarged left supraclavicular lymph node (Virchow's node) or a palpable umbilical node (**Sister Mary Joseph's node**) indicates distant lymphatic spread. Additionally, a palpable rectal ridge (Blumer's shelf) or the presence of ascites suggests peritoneal dissemination. All these findings are ominous signs and worrisome for extensive disease. On abdominal exam, the presence of an epigastric mass may indicate a locally advanced tumor.

Diagnostic workup and clinical staging should follow the National Comprehensive Cancer Network (NCCN) consensus guidelines. Upper endoscopy is essential to characterize the location and extent of disease. Additionally, multiple biopsies of the lesion are required to obtain a histologic diagnosis. Often, endoscopic ultrasound is undertaken to determine the depth of tumor invasion, an important aspect of staging. Metastatic spread to the lungs, liver, and ovaries (Krukenberg's tumor) does occur. Imaging studies to rule out such involvement are therefore necessary. A chest radiograph and computed tomography (CT) of the abdomen and pelvis are adequate screening modalities. Although the role of positron emission tomography (PET) as a primary imaging modality has not been established, it has been demonstrated to be useful for detecting advanced disease and should be considered during clinical staging. Laboratory investigations include a complete blood cell count, electrolytes, creatinine level, and liver function tests. Upper GI series are not necessary and can miss some cancers, especially the superficial spreading subtype.

Because gastric carcinoma can spread intra-abdominally, metastasis to the peritoneum and the omentum do occur. Such lesions are difficult to identify using conventional CT. As a result, laparoscopy has become a key component of staging. Patients who do not have any evidence of metastatic disease on initial workup now undergo laparoscopic staging. During this procedure, the abdomen is carefully explored for evidence of peritoneal, hepatic, or omental disease. Any suspicious lesions are biopsied. Abdominal washings are typically taken as well, and the local extent of tumor determined. The presence of metastatic disease precludes curative resection and can help avoid an unnecessary laparotomy.

Treatment

Complete surgical resection in an attempt to cure gastric adenocarcinoma should only be undertaken in the presence of localized disease. Considerable debate exists regarding the extent of such a resection. For most distal lesions, many surgeons favor a radical subtotal gastrectomy. In this procedure, approximately 85% of the stomach is removed, including the omentum. The proximal portion of the resected specimen is then immediately examined by the pathologist (i.e., frozen section) to verify that it is free of tumor involvement. Only after such verification is GI continuity restored by means of a Roux-en-Y gastrojejunostomy. Total gastrectomy is reserved for either large distal lesions or more proximal tumors. Splenectomy or pancreatectomy may also need to be included in the operative procedure. They should, however, be avoided unless absolutely necessary.

Another controversial topic is the extent of lymph node dissection at the time of resection. The Japanese favor a radical lymphadenectomy. In the United States, a less extensive dissection is undertaken. Comparisons between the two approaches in Japan point toward improved survival in those patients having the radical lymph node removal. These results have not been duplicated in Western countries. In fact, the more extensive dissections seem to cause higher morbidity without a survival benefit. The reason for such a discrepancy is poorly understood.

Current NCCN guidelines recommend perioperative (pre- and postoperative) chemotherapy using epirubicin, cisplatin, and 5-fluorouracil for potentially resectable lesions that clinically appear to invade beyond the lamina propria or have positive nodes. Chemoradiation therapy is also an option. Less invasive lesions (i.e., those only invading the submucosa) can be excised without preoperative chemoradiotherapy. Postoperative chemoradiotherapy using 5-fluorouracil with or without leucovorin is recommended after surgical resection except in cases where the tumor only invades the mucosa. Another exception is in patients who received preoperative epirubicin, cisplatin, and 5-fluorouracil. These patients should receive this same regimen in the postoperative period.

As mentioned earlier, the best cure rates are reported in Japan, where there is a high percentage of the superficial spreading type. Even with this type of tumor, the 5-year survival rate is <50%. In most studies from English-speaking countries, curative resection is associated with a 5-year survival rate of less than 10%. Pathologic staging of the resected specimen is the best predictor of survival (Figure 13-8). The case for early diagnosis is made in studies that evaluated the 5-year survival rate in patients who had an incidental carcinoma found during stomach surgery for supposed benign disease. Some studies report that the 5-year survival rate in this highly selected cohort approaches 75%.

Patients with metastatic disease cannot be cured. Palliative therapy should focus on quality of life. Because the morbidity and mortality associated with palliative surgery can be high, it should be undertaken with caution. In selected patients with good preoperative status, it may be beneficial. The resection should include the lesion, with an adequate cephalic margin, and the entire stomach distal to the tumor. Clear indications for palliative surgical intervention include proximal or distal tumor obstruction and bleeding. Endoscopic stent placement and laser therapy are also palliative options. Chemotherapy and radiation offer little help but are employed on occasion.

Gastric Lymphoma

The stomach is the primary source of almost two-thirds of all GI lymphomas. Patients with gastric lymphoma tend to be older, and the non-Hodgkin's variant predominates. Patients typically present with symptoms similar to those seen in gastric adenocarcinoma. Upper abdominal pain, unexplained weight loss, fatigue, and bleeding are all encountered. Diagnosis can often be made with tissue biopsies during upper

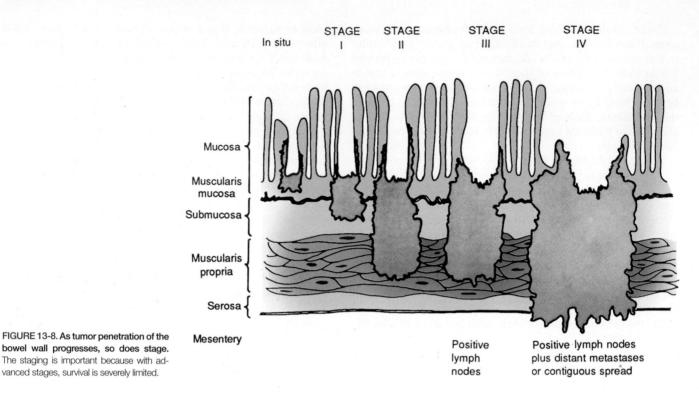

FIGURE 13-8. As tumor penetration of the bowel wall progresses, so does stage. The staging is important because with advanced stages, survival is severely limited.

endoscopy. Sometimes, however, the presence of lymphoma is only determined at the time of surgical exploration. If the diagnosis is made preoperatively, the workup should follow that undertaken for any lymphoma to determine its stage. Chest radiography, abdominal CT, and bone marrow biopsy all should be undertaken.

The treatment of primary gastric lymphoma is somewhat controversial. Some specialists advocate chemotherapy alone, citing high 5-year survival rates in early stage disease. Such treatment, however, does run the risk of causing gastric perforation or hemorrhage, necessitating surgical intervention. Other physicians believe that operative resection of grossly involved tissue is the best option. Such treatment can be followed with chemotherapy or radiation treatment. When the lesion is confined to the stomach, the 5-year survival of such a resection can approach 75%.

Gastrointestinal Stromal Tumor

Formerly known as leiomyomas and leiomyosarcomas, gastrointestinal stromal tumors (GISTs) are submucosal growths of the GI tract arising from a variety of cell types. The stomach is the most common site for these masses. GISTs can be either benign or malignant, but, unless direct invasion is present, differentiation between the two is often difficult. Large tumor size (>6 cm) and tumor necrosis suggest malignancy. Typically, such a determination is made only after the pathologist has counted the number of mitotic figures under high-powered field. The finding of more than 10 such figures per 50 fields is considered evidence of malignancy.

The clinical presentation of GISTs is similar to other gastric tumors. Many patients are asymptomatic. Nonspecific abdominal pain can occur. Bleeding and obstruction can be manifestations. Finally, some patients present with an abdominal mass. Evaluation typically involves upper endoscopy, which reveals a submucosal mass. Central ulceration may be present. Biopsy is usually nondiagnostic. Endoscopic ultrasound may

be employed. Abdominal CT should be performed to determine the tumor size, presence of invasion, and evidence of metastasis. The liver is the most common site for disseminated disease.

Treatment of a stomach GIST involves local excision. A margin of 2 to 3 cm should be included in the resection specimen. Enucleation is avoided because of the risk of malignancy in the tumor. Likewise, the tumor capsule should not be disrupted to avoid spillage. Depending on the extent of the tumor, a more extensive gastric resection may be needed. Patient survival following resection depends on the presence of malignancy. The prognosis for a benign lesion is excellent. Malignant GIST, however, can be quite aggressive. In such cases, chemotherapy using imatinib mesylate has been effective.

BENIGN DUODENAL DISEASE

Uncomplicated Duodenal Ulcer Disease

In the United States, PUD accounts for billions of dollars in health care expenditures. Nearly 500,000 new cases are diagnosed annually. As a result, the number of adult Americans having active disease remains relatively constant at approximately 2 million. Duodenal ulcers constitute the majority of this disease burden. They typically form in the duodenal bulb. *H. pylori* and NSAIDs are important ulcerogenic agents. An association with tobacco also exists. In contrast to gastric ulcers, duodenal ulcers rarely harbor any underlying malignancy. Their workup and treatment, therefore, differ somewhat from the evaluation and therapy of gastric ulcers.

Most duodenal ulcer disease is uncomplicated. Dramatic changes in the understanding and treatment of this disorder have occurred over the last two decades. The identification of *H. pylori* as a potential ulcerogenic agent and the development of effective acid suppression medications are now recognized as seminal events in the evolution of care. In the process, the treatment of PUD shifted from the domain of the surgeon to that of the internist.

Clinical Presentation and Evaluation

The clinical presentation of uncomplicated duodenal ulceration has features similar to that of uncomplicated gastric ulcer disease. Patients often complain of a burning epigastric abdominal pain that is gnawing in character. It may radiate to the back, especially if the ulcer is located in the posterior aspect of the duodenal bulb. Certain aspects of presentation, however, are different from uncomplicated gastric ulceration. The pain typically occurs 1 to 3 hours after food ingestion and is accentuated by fasting. It may awaken patients from sleep. Relief from pain typically occurs after use of over-the-counter acid suppressants. Food intake can also improve pain. In such a situation, a recent history of weight gain may be noted.

A thorough history and physical examination remain important components of the initial evaluation of the patient suspected of having uncomplicated duodenal ulceration. In addition to characterizing the nature of the pain, risk factors are determined. They include a history of PUD, prior *H. pylori* infection, NSAID ingestion, or tobacco use. Physical exam focuses on the abdomen. Mild epigastric tenderness on palpation may be present. Finally, signs of occult blood loss are sought. Pallor, orthostasis, and guaiac-positive stools are significant findings.

Traditional Diagnostic Testing

Classically, the diagnosis of uncomplicated duodenal ulcer disease was made by means of an upper GI contrast study using barium (upper GI series). Although it is now infrequently used for making such a diagnosis, an understanding of its mechanics is helpful. In this examination, barium and air are swallowed. The esophagus, stomach, and duodenum are then observed fluoroscopically. Finally, radiographs are made for permanent documentation. During the procedure, care is taken to observe swallowing mechanics, peristaltic activity, gastric distensibility, and pyloric function; the mucosal pattern is noted; evidence of organ displacement is sought, and the pyloric sphincter size and shape are determined.

The upper GI series is still a widely available, inexpensive, and safe exam. Unfortunately, it tends to miss many acute lesions of the duodenum. In such cases, ancillary findings such as duodenal spasm, deformity, or mucosal swelling may suggest the diagnosis. Even so, it is no longer a useful primary diagnostic modality for PUD given current practice patterns.

Gastric acid analysis is another classic evaluative study for uncomplicated duodenal ulcer disease. In this test, a nasogastric tube is placed into the stomach for collection of gastric aspirates. Samples are obtained over a 1-hour period before and after the administration of an intravenous acid secretagogue, usually pentagastrin. Most patients with uncomplicated duodenal ulceration have a high (>4.0 mEq/hour) basal acid output. Over two-thirds have an elevated stimulated acid output.

Gastric acid analysis is particularly useful in identifying the rare patient who develops duodenal ulceration due to an occult gastrinoma (see the discussion under Zollinger-Ellison Syndrome below). In such an individual, the basal acid output may be 10 times the upper limit of normal. The parietal cell mass is often maximally stimulated by elevated baseline serum gastrin levels. Accordingly, the stimulated acid output increases only minimally compared to basal output values. Due to evolutions in the care of both PUD and gastrinoma, however, gastric acid analysis has also fallen into disuse.

Current Diagnostic Testing

Today, the diagnosis of uncomplicated duodenal ulceration is often made empirically. In the patient with typical signs and symptoms, noninvasive testing for the presence of *H. pylori* infection is undertaken. Both quantitative and qualitative serologic antibody testing exists. These studies have the advantage of low cost and wide availability. Their accuracy, however, depends on the probability of infection. In developed countries, they are particularly useful at identifying active *H. pylori* infection among younger patients, because of its low incidence. The presence of antibody in older individuals, however, is a less reliable indicator of active disease, since it can persist for years after the infection has been successfully eradicated.

Other useful noninvasive diagnostic studies are the urease tests. They identify the presence of *H. pylori* infection by indirectly detecting the organisms urease activity. Urease hydrolyzes urea into ammonia and carbon dioxide. The increased carbon dioxide can be detected in either the blood or breath of the patient. PPIs and bismuth compounds must be withheld several weeks prior to such testing to prevent false-negative results. The main advantage of the urease tests is that they identify only active disease. They are also useful in documenting successful eradication of the bacteria.

A final noninvasive study is the fecal antigen test, which identifies the presence of *H. pylori* using antibodies. Like the urease tests, it is positive only during an active infection. Again, care must be taken when interpreting results in patients on PPIs and bismuth compounds. It is helpful in verifying eradication of the bacteria after therapy.

Upper endoscopy is the diagnostic modality of choice and should be employed in patients with characteristic symptoms. In such cases, endoscopy provides a means of direct visualization and characterization of the ulceration. Additionally, it can also identify concomitant disease or suggest an alternative diagnosis. Finally, it provides a means of obtaining biopsies. Rarely, samples are taken from a mass associated with the duodenal ulceration. More typically, gastric tissue is obtained to test for the presence of *H. pylori*. Since this infection is typically confined to the distal stomach in duodenal ulcer disease, these samples should be taken from the antrum. Both tissue culturing and histologic review can detect the organism. These methods are, however, time consuming and expensive. An alternative method is the rapid urease test. A tissue biopsy (usually antral) is placed on a pH-sensitive indicator containing a large amount of urea. In the presence of *H. pylori*, the urease produces ammonia and carbon dioxide, altering the media pH and producing a color change (CLO [*Corynebacterium*-like organism] test). Like its noninvasive counterparts, it is positive only during active infection. Because these studies are inexpensive and quick, they have become a popular means of bedside screening for the presence of *H. pylori* after routine endoscopy. Finally, they are useful in verifying complete eradication of infection after appropriate therapy.

Treatment

The treatment of uncomplicated duodenal ulcer disease is nonoperative. It is aimed at promoting ulcer healing and preventing its recurrence. Such goals are best achieved by the removal of all ulcerogenic agents and the institution of acid suppression therapy. To this end, tobacco and NSAID (including aspirin) use should be discontinued indefinitely. Additionally, *H. pylori* infection must be eradicated. Unfortunately, this organism is tenacious, and antibiotic resistance is growing. As a result, two or more antibiotics are required to treat adequately any infection. Currently, antibiotic therapy is combined with acid suppression using PPIs or H_2-receptor antagonists.

Recommendations are similar to those in the Maastricht-2 2000 consensus report. First-line therapy involves a minimum of 7 days of treatment involving acid suppression with dual antibiotic therapy using clarithromycin and amoxicillin or clarithromycin and metronidazole. Second-line regimens include repeating first-line treatment interchanging amoxicillin and metronidazole or instituting traditional quadruple therapy. This regimen consists of an acid-suppression drug, bismuth, metronidazole, and tetracycline for a minimum of 7 days (14, classically). Due to increasing antibiotic resistance, patients should undergo some form of testing for the presence of *H. pylori* after treatment. Eradication of *H. pylori* leads to more rapid healing of duodenal ulcers, resolution of gastritis, and lower recurrence rates for both duodenal and gastric ulcers.

Acid-suppression therapy should be continued until the ulcer is healed. If the etiology of the ulcer is apparent, PPIs or H_2-receptor antagonists can usually be discontinued after a relatively short time interval. If the etiology of the ulcer is unclear, they should be continued until its cause is determined and treated.

Complicated Peptic Ulcer Disease

Complicated PUD has four main manifestations: perforation, hemorrhage, gastric outlet obstruction, and intractability. As a result, the presentation, evaluation, and initial treatment of complicated duodenal ulcer disease and complicated gastric ulcer disease are the same. Differences in care can arise at the time of surgical intervention.

Clinical Presentation and Evaluation

The type of complication determines the clinical presentation and evaluation. Patients with perforated ulcers present with acute onset of severe epigastric pain. Often, they are able to report the exact time of day that the symptoms began. Physical examination usually reveals tachycardia and evidence of a rigid (surgical) abdomen resulting from diffuse chemical peritonitis. Occasionally, however, a more localized peritonitis may develop as gastric acid drains into the right paracolic gutter. In such cases, the patient presents with right lower quadrant rebound tenderness very similar to that seen in acute appendicitis. Evaluation should include an upright chest radiograph. Evidence of free intraperitoneal air (**pneumoperitoneum**) outlining the diaphragm or liver is diagnostic of a perforated intra-abdominal viscus (Figure 13-9). Patients should also have a complete blood count and basic metabolic panel drawn.

A patient presenting with a bleeding ulcer will report hematemesis, melena, or blood per rectum. Massive bleeding can occur, and some patients may exhibit signs of early or late shock. Physical examination may reveal hypotension, tachycardia, pallor, mental status changes, and active bleeding. In such cases, volume resuscitation with crystalloid or whole blood should be immediately instituted. Evaluation of any GI hemorrhage should focus on determining the site of bleeding. A nasogastric tube is placed, and gastric lavage performed. The presence of blood suggests an upper GI source. Endoscopy is confirmatory. Additionally, it allows characterization of the ulcer and determination of *H. pylori* status. Patients with bleeding ulcers should have serial hematocrits followed and coagulation parameters determined. Finally, blood type and crossmatch should be ready at all times.

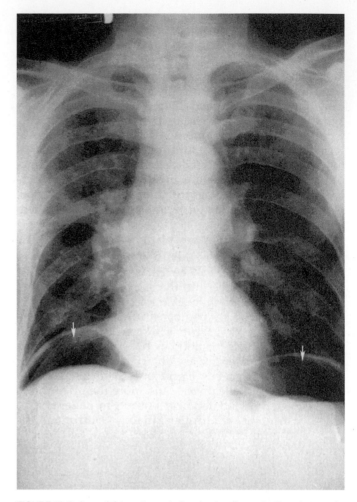

FIGURE 13-9. An upright posteroanterior chest radiograph often shows subdiaphragmatic air (*white arrows*) in patients with a perforated ulcer.

Patients with gastric outlet obstruction resulting from chronic ulcer scarring will complain of inability to tolerate oral intake. In particular, they may report projectile vomiting of food shortly after eating, much like infants with pyloric stenosis (see Chapter 3, Pediatric Surgery, in Lawrence et al. eds., *Essentials of Surgical Specialties*. 3rd ed.). A history of weight loss is common. These patients often delay seeking medical attention. As a result, they suffer from varying degrees of dehydration. Physical examination may reveal upper abdominal fullness, decreased skin turgor, dry mucus membranes, or epigastric peristaltic waves. Evaluation should focus on assessing the extent of metabolic derangement. Electrolyte and creatinine levels are informative. Often, these patients develop a hypokalemic, hypochloremic metabolic alkalosis. In severe cases, they will have evidence of paradoxical aciduria as the distal renal tubules sacrifice hydrogen ions for potassium (see Chapter 3, Fluids and Electrolytes).

Finally, patients with intractable ulcers will have symptoms of persistent disease after adequate nonoperative therapy. Often, these individuals will have undergone multiple treatments for ulceration without relief or healing. Additionally, they may develop recurrence of disease after an apparently successful initial therapy. Fortunately, such patients are becoming less frequent. Physical examination in these patients mirrors findings seen in uncomplicated PUD. Intractability should alert the clinician to the possibility of rarer causes of ulceration (see the section on Zollinger-Ellison syndrome below). Evaluation should be directed accordingly.

Treatment

The treatment of complicated PUD typically involves an initial stabilization phase. During this period, the patient is resuscitated and nonoperative therapies are instituted. Depending on a patient's complication and response to treatment, this phase can be definitive. Otherwise, the patient will require operative intervention. At the time of surgery, two objectives should be met. First, the complication should be properly treated. Second, a definitive antisecretory procedure should be performed. In this way, ulcer recurrence is minimized. Antisecretory procedures are discussed more fully under the intractability section below.

Perforation

A perforated ulcer is a surgical emergency. Patients should be prepared for the operating room with fluid resuscitation and nasogastric decompression. At the time of surgical exploration, the site of perforation is identified. Typically, this is an ulcer located on the anterior aspect of the duodenal bulb. Because of potent PPIs and success in treating *H. pylori*, definitive acid-reducing surgery is much less commonly performed today during acute surgical treatment of a perforation. More commonly, oversewing the ulcer with buttressing with a tag of omentum (Graham patch) is performed followed by intensive treatment with PPIs and antibiotics to eradicate *H. pylori*. Both open and laparoscopic repair of simple perforated duodenal ulcers have been described.

Complex perforated duodenal ulcers can be therapeutic challenges. Large, friable ulcers are difficult to close. In such circumstances, more extensive procedures are required. They focus on patching the opening or excluding it from the flow of GI contents. Adequate drainage of the duodenal region is essential.

In rare cases, patients with a perforated ulcer may be treated nonoperatively. Typically, the patient is a clinically stable elderly individual with multiple medical problems who presents relatively late (12 or more hours) after the onset of symptoms. Because of the high operative risk, these patients are treated with nasogastric decompression, volume resuscitation, nothing by mouth, and serial abdominal exams with blood laboratories. If the perforation has sealed off, they will improve and avoid operation. Surgical intervention, however, is indicated if any clinical deterioration occurs.

Hemorrhage

In patients who have upper GI hemorrhage, initial stabilization is necessary. At least two large-bore intravenous lines are inserted. Volume resuscitation then follows Advanced Trauma Life Support (ATLS) guidelines: 2 L of crystalloid is followed by whole blood. The stomach is decompressed using a nasogastric tube. High-dose PPI therapy is instituted. Finally, any coagulation abnormalities are corrected.

Hemorrhage is initially treated by upper endoscopy. Options include electrocautery, heater probe, or injection therapy. Using such techniques, most cases of bleeding can be successfully stopped. Endoscopic signs worrisome for risk of rebleeding include active hemorrhage at the time of endoscopy, a visible vessel in the ulcer crater, and fresh clot on the ulcer. Endoscopy may be repeated if rebleeding occurs. Angiography and selective embolization is sometimes employed in patients who have a very high operative risk.

Surgical intervention is reserved for refractory bleeding. In general, a transfusion requirement of six or more units of blood over the first 12 hours is an indication for surgery. Elderly patients or those who are hemodynamically unstable may require earlier operative therapy. Younger, more stable patients can be resuscitated longer. At the time of laparotomy, the bleeding artery is ligated. In the case of a posterior duodenal ulcer, duodenotomy with three-point U-stitch fixation of the ulcer bed is necessary. In a type IV gastric ulcer, left gastric artery ligation may be necessary.

Gastric Outlet Obstruction

In patients with gastric outlet obstruction, the stomach is decompressed with a nasogastric tube for 5 or 6 days, or until it returns to near-normal size. During this time, the patient is allowed nothing by mouth. Nutrition and fluids are administered intravenously. Because most patients are hypochloremic and alkalotic, initial resuscitation should be with normal saline crystalloid solution. Malnutrition is ameliorated by total parenteral nutrition. Careful monitoring for electrolyte abnormalities is undertaken.

Most cases of gastric outlet obstruction require operative intervention because of the cicatricial scarring around the site of the ulcer. Such procedures require either removal of the obstruction or its bypass. Typically, antrectomy can be performed with appropriate reconstruction. If this cannot be done, a gastroenterostomy to drain the stomach must be created. An acid-reducing procedure is also necessary.

In some cases, the gastric outlet obstruction develops due to mucosal edema rather than scarring. The prolonged nasogastric decompression helps decrease the swelling and provides resolution of the obstruction. Endoscopy, however, is still required to characterize the extent of scarring, biopsy any suspicious lesions, and screen for *H. pylori*. Occasionally, an operation can be avoided.

Intractability

Patients with ulcers unresponsive to conventional medical management have intractable disease. They may require surgical intervention to decrease acid secretion. The surgeon can alter such secretion through interruption of the vagal neural pathway with or without removal of the gastrin-producing cells in the antrum.

The most straightforward approach to vagal interruption is by means of a truncal vagotomy. In this procedure, all vagal trunks at or above the esophageal hiatus of the diaphragm are completely transected. As a result, the entire parietal cell mass is denervated. Unfortunately, truncal vagotomy also denervates the antral pump, the pyloric sphincter mechanism, and most of the abdominal viscera. Gastric motility is disrupted, and a gastric drainage procedure is required to facilitate gastric emptying. Otherwise, gastric antral dilation occurs, stimulating gastrin release. The most common complementary drainage procedure is pyloroplasty, which is performed by incising the pylorus horizontally and closing it vertically (Figure 13-10). Various modifications of pyloroplasty have been proposed, and most are known by eponyms. If pyloroplasty is not possible, gastroenterostomy is an alternative. Many surgeons add distal gastrectomy (**antrectomy**) to the truncal vagotomy (Figure 13-5). Antrectomy augments the effect of vagotomy by removing the bulk of the gastrin-producing cells (G cells). In this way, both the cephalic phase and the gastric phase of acid stimulation are interrupted. Truncal vagotomy with antrectomy

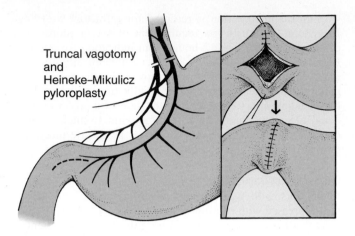

FIGURE 13-10. When the trunk of the vagus nerve is divided, a pyloroplasty is also performed to allow gastric emptying. This pyloroplasty is the most common type performed.

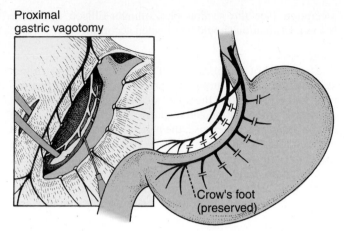

FIGURE 13-12. A proximal gastric vagotomy (highly selective vagotomy) denervates the acid-producing parietal cells without interfering with the antral pump or pylorus.

is associated with a lower recurrence rate than truncal vagotomy with pyloroplasty (1.5% vs. 10%).

Selective vagotomy provides total denervation of the stomach, from above the crus of the diaphragm down to and including the pylorus (Figure 13-11). This procedure spares the parasympathetic innervation of the abdominal viscera. Like truncal vagotomy, however, it denervates the antral pump and pylorus, necessitating some type of drainage procedure. Most surgeons employ pyloroplasty. Advocates of this type of vagotomy claim that it more completely denervates the stomach compared to a truncal vagotomy. They also emphasize that the parasympathetic innervation to other abdominal organs (liver, gallbladder, pancreas, small intestine, and proximal colon) is spared. Finally, proponents note the similar frequency of postgastrectomy syndromes (see section on postgastrectomy syndromes below) between the two forms of vagotomy.

The most recent approach to vagal interruption to gain popularity is **proximal gastric vagotomy** (Figure 13-12). It is also known as parietal cell vagotomy or highly selective vagotomy. In this procedure, the vagus nerve is identified as it courses along the lesser curvature of the stomach. The branches innervating the parietal cell mass are then individually divided. Near the level of the antrum, the nerves forming

the "crow's foot" are preserved. This maneuver maintains the normal innervation and functioning of the antral pump and pyloric sphincter mechanisms, obviating the need for a drainage procedure. Patients with gastric outlet obstruction as a result of PUD are not candidates for this procedure. Proximal gastric vagotomy has the lowest incidence of postgastrectomy syndromes. The ulcer recurrence rate is 10% to 15%, but the morbidity and mortality rates are relatively low. Patients with ulcer recurrence after proximal gastric vagotomy can now be relatively easily managed with antisecretory medications.

The decision about which procedure to perform on an individual patient is complicated. It is based on the age of the patient, the likelihood of ulcer recurrence, the severity of symptoms, and the patient's sex and weight. The procedures that have the highest cure rate (i.e., truncal vagotomy and antrectomy) also have the highest incidence of postgastrectomy side effects, such as **dumping syndrome** (Table 13-2).

Likewise, procedures with the lowest cure rate have the lowest incidence of side effects. Therefore, the surgeon's responsibility is to select the procedure for each patient that is likely to be effective in treating the ulcer diathesis while minimizing the likelihood of side effects. It is possible to predict which patients are at high risk for postgastrectomy complications; young, thin women are particularly vulnerable. In these patients, it may be advantageous to avoid performing truncal vagotomy, especially with the availability of proximal gastric vagotomy, which is an excellent alternative.

Duodenal Polyps

Duodenal polyps typically arise as a part of an inherited familial disorder. One of the more well known of these genetic conditions is familial adenomatous polyposis. Patients having this autosomal dominant syndrome develop multiple adenomatous polyps in the colon and gastroduodenal region. Because of the possibility of malignant degeneration of these polyps, close monitoring is required. Most patients require early prophylactic removal of the colon. All patients need routine endoscopic surveillance of the stomach and duodenum with removal of any polyps. The presence of cancer or villous adenoma in a duodenal polyp requires surgical excision. Another important condition is Peutz-Jeghers syndrome (see section on gastric polyps above).

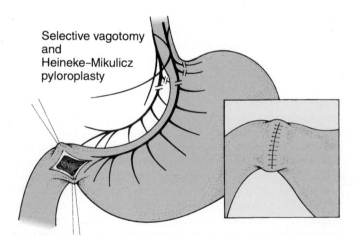

FIGURE 13-11. Because a selective vagotomy denervates the pylorus, a pyloroplasty is performed to allow gastric emptying.

| TABLE 13-2 | Relative Incidence of Recurrence and Operative Mortality Rate Expressed as Percentages |||||||||

| | Recurrence Rate (%) | Operative Mortality Rate (%) | Dumping | | Afferent Loop Syndrome | Blind Loop Syndrome | Alkaline Reflux Gastritis | Metabolic Sequelae |
			Early	Late				
Vagotomy/pyloroplasty	5–10	1–2	2+	2+	0	0	1+	1+
Vagotomy/antrectomy Billroth I	1–2	1–4	2+	2+	0	0	1+	1+
Vagotomy/antrectomy Billroth II	1–3	1–4	3+	3+	2+	2+	2+	2+
Selective vagotomy	5–10	1–2	2+	2+	0	0	0	1+
Proximal gastric vagotomy	10–15	1	0	0	0	0	0	0
Total gastrectomy	0	2–5	3+	2+	0	0	0	2+

These numbers are averages taken from the larger series published in the literature. The relative incidences of the postgastrectomy syndromes are expressed on a scale of 0 to 4+, with 0 indicating relative absence of symptoms and 4+ indicating frequent profound symptoms.

MALIGNANT DUODENAL DISEASE

Zollinger-Ellison Syndrome

Although very rare, **Zollinger-Ellison syndrome** is perhaps the most well-known endocrine tumor disorder. It is the direct result of a gastrin-producing neoplasm (gastrinoma). The resultant hypergastrinemia causes near maximal stimulation of the parietal cell mass. HCl is constantly secreted, leading to the well-described clinical manifestations of the syndrome. Over two-thirds of these tumors are located in the gastrinoma triangle, an anatomic triangle whose apices include the junction of the cystic duct with the common bile duct, the junction of the second and third portion of the duodenum, and the neck of the pancreas.

Gastrinomas can occur sporadically or as part of an inherited familial disorder. A strong association exists with the multiple endocrine neoplasia type 1 (MEN-1) syndrome. This disorder is characterized by the clinical constellation of pituitary adenomas, hyperparathyroidism, and pancreatic islet cell tumors (of which gastrinomas are the most common). Approximately 60% of all gastrinomas are malignant. Unfortunately, about half of the patients with the malignant variant of the disease die within 5 years of diagnosis. Because of its slow growth pattern, however, long-term survival up to 15 years is seen in some patients.

Clinical Presentation and Evaluation

A high degree of suspicion is necessary to identify patients with Zollinger-Ellison syndrome. Often, the diagnosis is suggested by unusual clinical presentations. One such manifestation is the patient complaining of ulcer-like symptoms with concomitant chronic or severe diarrhea. Additionally, patients may present with extremely virulent ulcer diathesis. In such cases, they will have multiple duodenal ulcers or ulceration in atypical locations (jejunum or ileum). Finally, patients may report a personal or family history of refractory PUD or endocrine disease.

Evaluation begins with a thorough history and physical examination focused on establishing the presence of any of the above-mentioned associations. In particular, a personal or family history of MEN-1 diseases is sought. Diagnosis rests on establishing the presence of hypergastrinemia with hypersecretion of acid. A fasting serum gastrin level is therefore necessary. Care, however, must be taken to make sure that the patient has discontinued any PPIs for at least 1 week prior

to testing. PPI use increases gastrin levels. The presence of elevated gastrin levels above 1,000 pg/mL is often considered diagnostic. Abnormal values <1,000 pg/mL should prompt further confirmatory testing. The investigation of choice is the secretin stimulation test. In addition to being safe, it has a high specificity and sensitivity. Fasting serum gastrin levels are obtained at 2, 5, 10, 15, 30, 45, and 60 minutes after the intravenous infusion of secretin. An elevation in the baseline gastrin value is seen in patients with Zollinger-Ellison syndrome. For most laboratories, this increase must be ≥200 pg/mL. The presence of acid hypersecretion is established by measuring the gastric pH. A value of 2.5 or less is considered positive. Gastric acid analysis can also be performed.

Once the diagnosis of Zollinger-Ellison syndrome has been established, further evaluation should focus on tumor localization and clinical staging. Commonly used imaging modalities include CT, magnetic resonance imaging, and ultrasonography. Somatostatin receptor scintigraphy and endoscopic ultrasound are also popular. These neoplasms are often quite small and, as a result, their preoperative localization can be quite difficult. A thorough search should be undertaken, however, because knowing the site of the primary tumor helps with operative planning. The liver is the most common site for metastatic disease.

Finally, all patients with newly diagnosed Zollinger-Ellison syndrome should undergo some form of screening for MEN-1 syndrome. Although genetic testing is available, it requires thorough pretest counseling. A more straightforward screen is to obtain a serum calcium level. If it is elevated, a parathyroid hormone level should be determined. The presence of hyperparathyroidism is highly suggestive of concomitant MEN-1 (see Chapter 20, Surgical Endocrinology).

Treatment

Traditional therapy for Zollinger-Ellison syndrome involved total gastrectomy with esophageal anastomosis in an effort to treat the often-virulent ulcer diathesis. Although this procedure provided absolute protection from recurrent ulcer disease, it was associated with a high mortality. Additionally, significant aberrations in metabolism could occur. Pernicious anemia, malnutrition, and weight loss were all encountered. Fortunately, advances in the surgical and medical treatment of the disorder have made total gastrectomy a very rare intervention.

Because of these same advances, however, some controversy exists regarding current therapeutic interventions. Most experts now agree that patients with Zollinger-Ellison syndrome should be placed on high-dose PPIs to lower the production of HCl. By doing so, they help prevent ulcer diathesis and improve the hypersecretory diarrhea. H_2-receptor antagonists have become second-line agents. Surgical exploration is indicated in patients having sporadic gastrinoma without metastasis. At the time of laparotomy, a proximal gastric vagotomy is performed to decrease acid secretion. In addition, a thorough search is made for the tumor. If it is found, it is resected. Cure is possible with successful removal of the neoplasm.

The role of surgery in patients having gastrinoma in association with MEN-1 is more controversial. If hyperparathyroidism is present, a parathyroidectomy is indicated because it helps attenuate gastrin release. Because cure is rarer in patients with MEN-1, some experts do not recommend surgical exploration in patients without metastasis. Other specialists contend it is helpful, especially in the hands of experienced surgeons.

The presence of metastatic disease decreases survival. Some experts recommend surgical debulking. Other options include chemotherapy and hepatic embolization. Hormonal manipulation using long-acting synthetic analogues of somatostatin (octreotide) can also be effective. Octreotide suppresses the elevated gastrin concentrations and may help in slowing tumor growth. All patients with metastatic disease, as well as those whose tumors could not be found at surgical exploration, require continued PPI therapy.

Adenocarcinoma of the Duodenum

The duodenum is the most common site for adenocarcinoma in the small bowel. Approximately two-thirds of these lesions are located in the second part of the duodenum, usually in the periampullary region. Fortunately, it is a rare disease because patients typically present late in its course. Symptoms can range from nonspecific abdominal pain with weight loss to those of intestinal or gastric outlet obstruction. Some patients will present with melena or hematochezia due to ulceration of the lesion. Physical examination often is unremarkable. Diagnosis is often made by means of upper endoscopy with tissue biopsy. CT is helpful to determine evidence of local invasion or metastatic spread.

Surgical excision is indicated in resectable disease. Pancreaticoduodenectomy is typically performed if the tumor is present in the first or second portion of the duodenum. An extended small bowel resection with duodenojejunostomy is an option if tumor is limited to the third or fourth portion of the duodenum. Patients with unresectable disease or evidence of metastasis at the time of exploration should have a diverting gastroenterostomy. Postoperative radiation therapy may be helpful. In patients with positive lymph nodes, prognosis is very poor, with 5-year survivals below 15%.

Duodenal Lymphoma

Lymphoma of the duodenum is also relatively rare; most small bowel primaries occur in the ileum. The clinical presentation is similar to that for duodenal adenocarcinoma. Abdominal pain, weight loss, and fatigue are common. Complications include perforation, bleeding, or obstruction. Endoscopy may be helpful in diagnosing duodenal lymphomas. CT assists in determining disease extent. If the diagnosis is made prior to surgical exploration, complete clinical staging is performed, following guidelines similar to those for gastric lymphoma. Wide surgical excision with staging should be performed if disease appears resectable. Adjuvant chemotherapy can be

employed postoperatively. Patients with disseminated disease receive chemotherapy and local radiation.

POSTGASTRECTOMY COMPLICATIONS

Postgastrectomy Syndromes

The innervated intact stomach is a careful guardian of the GI tract. When the stomach is denervated, and especially when the pyloric mechanism is ablated, the exquisite control of gastric emptying is abolished. This change, in association with the anastomotic characteristics of many reconstructions, is the reason for most common postgastrectomy syndromes. Several reconstructions produce a defunctionalized limb of intestine or place the duodenum or jejunum at risk for obstruction or bacterial overgrowth. Others allow easy ingress of bile and duodenal secretions into the gastric pouch. These aberrations in normal anatomy produce the various postgastrectomy syndromes.

In the evaluation of a patient with a complicated postoperative course, an upper GI series may be performed. This series is used to document the extent of gastric resection and type of reconstruction, to determine the cause of vomiting (if present), and to assess gastric emptying and motility. Gastric emptying can also be defined more physiologically by administering a radionuclide labeled meal followed by sequential imaging. Clues to the diagnosis can also be acquired by examination with an endoscope, which allows direct visualization and biopsy.

Early Dumping Syndrome

Early dumping syndrome is characterized by a select set of symptoms that occur after the ingestion of food of high osmolarity. This type of meal may contain a large quantity of simple and complex sugars (e.g., milk products). Approximately 15 minutes after the meal is ingested, the patient has anxiety, weakness, tachycardia, diaphoresis, and, frequently, palpitations (i.e., vasomotor symptoms). The patient may also describe feelings of extreme weakness and a desire to lie down. Crampy abdominal pain may also be present. Often borborygmi are heard, and diarrhea is not uncommon. Gradually, the symptoms clear.

The patient with early dumping has uncontrolled emptying of hypertonic fluid into the small intestine. Fluid moves rapidly from the intravascular space into the intraluminal space, producing acute intravascular volume depletion. As the simple sugars are absorbed and as dilution of the hypertonic solution occurs, symptoms gradually abate. Intravascular volume is replenished as fluid shifts from the intracellular space and is absorbed from the intestinal lumen. Fluid shifts, however, do not explain all of the symptoms associated with early dumping. The release of several hormonal substances, including serotonin, neurotensin, histamine, glucagon, VIP, kinins, and others, is believed to contribute to the symptom complex. The use of a somatostatin analogue to block these hormonal substances may be of benefit to some patients.

This problem is best treated by avoiding hypertonic liquid meals, altering the volume of each meal, and ingesting some fat with each meal to slow gastric emptying. Liquids are ingested either before the meal or at least 30 minutes after the meal. Frequent small meals (i.e., 6 per day) are also encouraged. Although beta-blockers (e.g., 10 to 20 mg propranolol hydrochloride) taken 20 minutes before a meal were in the past recommended by some authors, their use has been superseded by somatostatin in treating early dumping. Often, it is begun after a trial of acarbose (see Late Dumping Syndrome below). In some patients with Billroth I or II anastomoses and recalcitrant symptoms, surgical construction of a Roux-en-Y gastrojejunostomy may be necessary. This procedure works by delaying gastric emptying.

Late Dumping Syndrome

As in early dumping, the patient suddenly has anxiety, diaphoresis, tachycardia, palpitations, weakness, fatigue, and a desire to lie down. In late dumping, the symptoms usually begin within 3 hours after the meal. This variant of dumping is not associated with borborygmi or diarrhea. The physiologic explanation for late dumping involves rapid changes in serum glucose and insulin levels. After the meal, a large bolus of glucose-containing chyme is presented to the mucosa of the small intestine. Glucose is absorbed much more rapidly than when the intact pylorus is present to meter gastric emptying. Extremely high serum glucose levels may occur shortly after the meal and may elicit a profound outpouring of insulin. The insulin response exceeds what is necessary to clear the glucose from the blood, and subsequently, hypoglycemia results. The symptoms in late dumping are the direct result of rapid fluctuations in serum glucose levels.

Nonoperative therapy for this syndrome includes the ingestion of a small snack 2 hours after meals. Crackers and peanut butter make an excellent supplement to abort or ameliorate the symptoms. Acarbose, an α-glycosidase hydrolase inhibitor, is now employed to treat symptoms of late dumping syndrome. Typically it is started after dietary modification fails. If symptoms cannot be controlled by nonoperative management, then either conversion of the previous procedure to a Billroth I (if not already present) or construction of a Roux-en-Y gastrojejunostomy is considered. Surgical intervention is considered only in patients who do not respond to aggressive nonoperative therapy. Table 13-3 summarizes the differences between early and late dumping syndromes.

Postvagotomy Diarrhea

Almost half the patients who undergo truncal vagotomy experience a change in bowel habits (i.e., increased frequency, more liquid consistency). In most cases, the symptoms improve or disappear with time. However, a small percentage of patients (<1%) have severe diarrhea that does not relent with time.

These patients may experience diarrhea that is explosive in onset, is not related to meals, and occurs without warning. Causes of postvagotomy diarrhea include enhanced intestinal motility (vagal denervation), rapid gastric emptying, bile malabsorption and bacterial overgrowth.

In most patients with postvagotomy diarrhea, fluid intake is restricted and the intake of foods that are low in fluid content is increased. Antidiarrheal/antimotility agents such as codeine, diphenoxylate hydrochloride, or loperamide may be of benefit. Cholestyramine, which binds bile salts, or somatostatin analogues may also be used. Antibiotics may be considered for bacterial overgrowth. If the postvagotomy diarrhea is severe or is refractory to medical management, a reversed 10-cm segment of jejunum is inserted 100 cm distal to the ligament of Treitz. This procedure delays small bowel transit time, but has many inherent problems.

Afferent Loop Obstruction

Afferent loop obstruction occurs only after gastrectomy with a Billroth II reconstruction. It is usually associated with a kink in the afferent limb adjacent to the anastomosis. Pancreatic and biliary secretions are trapped in the afferent limb, where they cause distension. Symptoms usually include severe cramping abdominal pain that occurs immediately after the ingestion of a meal. Patients often characterize the pain as crushing. Within 45 minutes, the patient feels an abdominal rush that is associated with increased pain, followed by nausea and vomiting of a dark brown, bitter-tasting material that has the consistency of motor oil. These symptoms result from the spontaneous, forceful decompression of the obstructed limb. Classically, no food is present. The symptoms resolve with vomiting. These patients often have profound weight loss because they stop eating to prevent the pain. The best treatment is exploration of the abdomen and conversion of the Billroth II anastomosis to either a Roux-en-Y gastrojejunostomy or a Billroth I gastroduodenostomy.

Blind Loop Syndrome

Blind loop syndrome is more common after a Billroth II procedure than after a Roux-en-Y procedure. It also occurs in patients who underwent bypass of the small intestine secondary to radiation injury or morbid obesity (e.g., ileojejunal bypass). Blind loop syndrome is associated with bacterial overgrowth in the limb of intestine that is excluded from the flow of chyme. This excluded limb of intestine harbors bacteria that proliferate and interfere with folate and vitamin B_{12} metabolism. A deficiency of vitamin B_{12} leads to megaloblastic anemia. The bacterial overgrowth may cause deconjugation of bile salts and lead to steatorrhea. Patients often have diarrhea, weight loss, and weakness, and they are often anemic. A Schilling test using cobalamin bound to IF is often abnormal. Treatment consists of orally administered, broad-spectrum antibiotics that cover both aerobic and anaerobic bacteria (e.g., tetracycline). After successful therapy, a repeat Schilling test will be normal. Unfortunately, regrowth of bacteria can occur. As a result, antibiotic therapy is often only a temporizing step. Many of these patients require conversion to a Billroth I gastroduodenostomy.

Alkaline Reflux Gastritis

Alkaline reflux gastritis is seen in patients in whom duodenal, pancreatic, and biliary contents reflux into the denervated stomach. These patients have weakness, weight loss, persistent nausea, and epigastric abdominal pain that often radiates to the back. In addition, they are often anemic. Upper endoscopy

TABLE 13-3	Comparison of Early Versus Late Dumping Pathophysiology	
	Early Dumping	**Late Dumping**
Presentation	15–30 min after a hyperosmolar meal	1–3 hr following a hyperosmolar meal
Symptoms	Abdominal: nausea, vomiting, diarrhea, abdominal cramps, Vasomotor: sweating, weakness, palpitations, dizziness	Vasomotor: sweating, weakness, palpitations, difficulty concentrating, hunger
Etiology	Rapid emptying of hyperosmolar contents into the small bowel causing osmotic shifts and release of vasoactive substances	Rapid change in serum glucose and insulin levels resulting in rapid decline in blood sugar levels (hypoglycemia)

will reveal an edematous, bile-stained gastric epithelium that is atrophic and erythematous. Mucosal biopsies should be taken away from the anastomosis. They demonstrate inflammatory changes with a characteristic corkscrew appearance of submucosal blood vessels. Nuclear scintigraphy will often demonstrate delayed gastric emptying.

Although a variety of medical regimens have been proposed to treat alkaline reflux gastritis (e.g., oral ingestion of cholestyramine, antacids, H_2 blockers, or metoclopramide), none is uniformly satisfactory. Surgical correction consists of diverting the duodenal contents away from the stomach with a long-limb Roux-en-Y gastrojejunostomy. The minimum distance between the gastrojejunostomy and the entry point of the biliopancreatic limb draining the digestive juices into the intestine is *40 cm* (18 inches). Such a reconstruction is effective therapy in most patients.

Marginal and Recurrent Ulcer Disease

Marginal ulcers develop on the jejunal side of a gastrojejunostomy anastomosis. They are thought to occur secondary to ischemia but smoking has also been implicated. Patients may present with abdominal pain during eating as well as nausea and vomiting. Upper endoscopy reveals an ulcer on the jejunal side no more than 2 cm distal to the anastomosis. Conservative management is attempted first. It includes discontinuing tobacco use and initiation of a PPI. In severe cases, patients may need to be made NPO and total parental nutrition is started in order to promote healing through bowel rest and nutritional supplementation. If the ulcer is recalcitrant to medical management, surgical revision of the anastomosis is required.

Recurrent ulcer disease following surgical intervention in benign PUD is most commonly due to incomplete vagotomy. Often, the posterior vagal trunk or a branch of the right posterior nerve (criminal nerve of Grassi) is left intact. Each operation has its accepted recurrence rate. Truncal vagotomy and antrectomy has one of the lowest rates at around 2%. Proximal gastric vagotomy has the highest at approximately 12%. Traditionally, confirmation of an incomplete vagotomy was made by means of the Hollander test, in which gastric acid output was measured after creating an insulin-induced hypoglycemia in the patient. This rather dangerous diagnostic procedure was abandoned and replaced by one in which gastric acid output was determined after sham feeding. Currently, upper endoscopy is used to help confirm persistent vagal innervation to the stomach. Congo red is used to demonstrate areas of pH drop in the gastric mucosa after the administration of an acid secretagogue (pentagastrin). Such regions have intact vagal innervation. Treatment options include long-term PPIs versus reoperative vagotomy.

For patients with recurrent ulceration and verified complete vagotomy, a more thorough evaluation is required. In particular, a search for an endocrine etiology should be initiated. A family history of MEN-1 should be sought. Calcium and parathyroid hormone levels should be obtained to look for hyperparathyroidism. Gastrin levels should be drawn to rule out the presence of a gastrinoma. Therapy should follow guidelines described in the Zollinger-Ellison syndrome section.

Gastric Atony

Many gastric reconstructions result in the denervation of the stomach and ablation of the pylorus. As a result, gastric motility is altered. Rapid emptying of liquids is common and can result in both early and late dumping syndrome (see above). Additionally, delayed emptying of solids due to gastric atony can occur. This phenomenon is poorly understood. Over half of all patients with a Roux-en-Y gastrojejunostomy demonstrate substantial delays in gastric emptying on ^{99m}Tc-labeled egg albumin scintigraphy. Only about half of these patients with delayed emptying, however, exhibit any symptoms. Frequently, such symptoms will improve with time and not require intervention. Conservative management includes small meals throughout the course of the day and avoidance of tobacco and alcohol. If medication is required, promotility agents such as metoclopramide or erythromycin may be beneficial.

Metabolic Disturbances

Although a variety of metabolic abnormalities are identified after gastric resection, anemias are the most common. Vitamin B_{12} or folate deficiency from decreased absorption can lead to megaloblastic anemia in up to 20% of patients. Treatment involves appropriate supplementation. Iron deficiency secondary to altered absorption or chronic blood loss can produce a microcytic anemia in as many as 50%. Iron replacement therapy is often required. In the case of chronic bleeding, the source (often reflux gastritis) must be identified and treated.

Altered bowel function is common following gastric reconstructions. Approximately one in four patients has frequent, loose stools postoperatively (see Table 13-4 for medications to treat postgastrectomy syndromes). The increased intestinal transit can have detrimental side effects. If rapid enough, steatorrhea can develop. Calcium and magnesium can chelate to the intestinal fats, leading to decreased absorption with resultant osteomalacia. Supplemental calcium as well as bisphosphonates can prevent such bone loss.

TABLE 13-4	Useful Medications Related to Postgastrectomy Syndromes

Medication	Action	Indication	Dosage
Acarbose	Alpha-glucosidase hydrolase inhibitor	Late dumping syndrome	50–100 mg po TID
Cholestyramine	Bile salt binding agent	Postvagotomy diarrhea; alkaline reflux gastritis	1 packet daily to start
Somatostatin	Secretory inhibitor	Postvagotomy diarrhea; dumping syndrome	Long-acting form—20 mg IM monthly
Metoclopramide	Promotility agent	Gastric atony	10 mg po 30 minutes before each meal and at bedtime
Sucralfate	GI protectant	Marginal ulcer; alkaline reflux gastritis	1 g po QID
Diphenoxylate hydrochloride	Antidiarrheal agent	Postvagotomy diarrhea	5 mg po QID
Loperamide	Antidiarrheal agent	Postvagotomy diarrhea	4 mg followed by 2 mg po after each unformed stool; not to exceed 16 mg/day.

SURGICAL TREATMENT OF OBESITY

Obesity

With well over half the U.S. population overweight and nearly one-third obese, weight and its effect on health have become important topics of research and concern. Obesity is now a well-recognized risk factor for a multitude of comorbid conditions responsible for early mortality and billions of dollars in health care expenditures. Because of a dearth of effective nonoperative therapies, bariatric surgery has become a mainstay of treatment for the severely obese. As a result, it has experienced a rapid rise in use over the last decade.

Obesity is the result of an imbalance in energy homeostasis. A positive caloric accumulation leads to the storage of excess energy as fat. This positive balance can be due to either increased energy intake or decreased energy expenditure. A mere 10 kcal/day (one saltine cracker) of extra energy can result in a 1-lb weight gain over the course of a year. Both genetic and environmental influences are responsible for the development of obesity. For example, energy intake may increase secondary to altered appetite regulation, a genetic influence, or as a result of greater food availability, an environmental cause. Likewise, energy expenditure can be decreased due to a genetically determined low body metabolism or from an environmentally related sedentary lifestyle. Such a plethora of potential sources for weight gain emphasizes the multifactorial nature of obesity. An understanding of the classification, evaluation, and treatment of obese patients is essential for providing quality care to this often-marginalized group of people.

Physiology of Appetite Regulation

Appetite regulation has become an area of intense research over the last decade, increasing our understanding of energy homeostasis. The hypothalamus, stomach, and adipocyte all play important roles in this complex process (Figure 13-13). Food intake is triggered by the release of the hormone ghrelin from gastric oxyntic cells. This compound stimulates the release of neuropeptides in the "hunger center" of the hypothalamus, increasing caloric consumption. To signal adequate caloric load, the adipocyte releases the hormone leptin, which activates the "satiety center" of the hypothalamus. In this manner, food intake is decreased.

The stomach, adipocyte, and hypothalamus, therefore, constitute an intricate hormonal axis that helps to control energy homeostasis via regulation of appetite. Defects within this axis can lead to energy imbalance with important metabolic consequences. For example, leptin-receptor deficiency results in loss of the satiety signal and the development of obesity. It is one of the few disorders for which exogenous leptin administration is potentially curative. Likewise, ghrelin overproduction is thought to contribute to the hyperphagia and obesity seen in patients with Prader-Willi syndrome.

Classification of Obesity

By definition, obesity is an excess of total body fat. By contrast, overweight is an excess of body weight. An individual can therefore be overweight but not have excess body fat. Obesity can occur in the setting of increased (hypermuscular), normal, or decreased (sarcopenic) lean body mass. Multiple techniques exist to measure total body fat. Each, however, has its drawbacks, making none ideal. Hydrostatic weighing, in which an individual is immersed in water, is very accurate, but

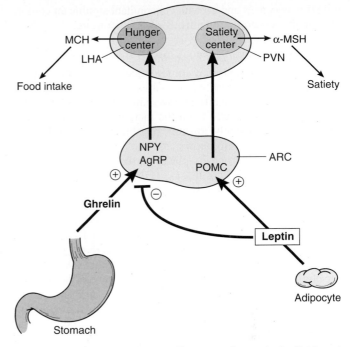

FIGURE 13-13. Hormonal axis controlling energy homeostasis. Ghrelin and leptin activate first-order neurons in the arcuate nucleus (ARC) of the hypothalamus, leading to stimulation of the hunger and satiety centers. NPY, neuropeptide Y; AgRP, agouti-related protein; POMC, propiomelanocortin; LHA, lateral hypothalamic area; PVN, paraventricular nucleus; MCH, melanin-concentrating hormone; and α-MSH, α-melanocyte-stimulating hormone.

costly and cumbersome. Anthropometry comparing skinfold thickness is easier, but very operator dependent. Bioelectrical impedance analysis provides a useful indirect measurement by determination of resting energy expenditure. It, however, requires overnight fasting.

Given the difficulties with determining total body fat, the body mass index (BMI) has become a useful surrogate marker. It is calculated by dividing an individual's weight in kilograms by the square of his or her height in meters:

$$BMI = weight \ (kg)/\left[height(m)\right]^2$$

Using the BMI, a person can be classified into various weight categories reflecting total body fat (Table 13-5). Even though very helpful, the BMI can occasionally overestimate (as in body builders) or underestimate (as in the elderly) total body fat. The classification system based on BMI provides the basis by which individuals are treated for overweight and obesity. Surgical intervention is reserved for two groups of people: those having

TABLE 13-5	Weight Classification and Risk of Illness Based on BMI	
BMI Range	**Weight Classification**	**Risk of Illness**
<18.5	Underweight	Increased
18.5–24.9	Ideal weight	Normal
25.0–29.9	Overweight	Increased
30.0–39.9	Obese	High/very high
40.0 or greater	Severely obese	Extremely high

Adapted with permission from Bessesen DH, Kushner R. Evaluation and Management of Obesity. Philadelphia, PA: Hanley and Belfus, Inc., 2002.

a BMI between 35 and 40 with concomitant significant comorbid conditions and those with a BMI of 40 or more.

Clinical Presentation and Evaluation

Severely obese patients may come to medical attention because of poor quality of life, problems with self-image, or to prevent or reduce medical conditions associated with obesity. These *comorbidities* may stem from the metabolic changes related to excess fat, namely insulin resistance, atherosclerosis, dyslipidemia, vein thrombosis, and cholelithiasis, or from the physical strains that obesity places on the body, namely sleep apnea, degenerative joint disease (DJD), GERD, and urinary stress incontinence. Additionally, some disorders have a combined metabolic and physical etiology, such as hypertension, infertility, psychosocial illnesses, and heart failure.

According to a 1991 National Institutes of Health (NIH) consensus conference on GI surgery for severe obesity, adult patients are candidates for surgery if they meet BMI criteria for clinically severe obesity, have failed attempts at diet and exercise, are motivated and well informed, and are free of significant psychological disease. In addition, the expected benefits of an operation must outweigh the risks. Since then, many data have validated these candidacy criteria, and others are emerging in support of extending indications for bariatric surgery to include carefully selected patients with BMI below 35 kg/m^2 or age <18 years.

There are no absolute contraindications to bariatric surgery. Relative contraindications include severe heart failure, unstable coronary artery disease, end-stage lung disease, active cancer diagnosis or treatment, cirrhosis with portal hypertension, uncontrolled drug or alcohol dependency, and severely impaired intellectual capacity.

Preoperative preparation is similar for all bariatric procedures. The components include determining a patient's indications for surgery, identifying issues that may interfere with the success of the surgery, and assessing and treating comorbid diseases. The typical assessment includes psychological testing, nutrition evaluation, and medical assessment.

Patients referred for bariatric surgery are more likely than the overall population to have psychopathology such as somatization, social phobia, obsessive–compulsive disorder, substance abuse, binge-eating disorder, posttraumatic stress disorder, generalized anxiety disorder, and depression. Most bariatric programs therefore require psychological evaluation before allowing a bariatric procedure. An extensive assessment performed by a mental health professional will allow appropriate therapy for poorly controlled psychological conditions, and will identify any history of physical or mental abuse that might interfere with postsurgical recovery and adaptation.

Preoperative nutritional counseling should include assessment of actual and required caloric intake, screening for detrimental eating habits, and education regarding required postoperative dietary changes. Sometimes, a preoperative very-low-calorie diet (VLCD) is implemented to reduce liver volume to improve access for a minimally invasive bariatric approach. In association, a fitness evaluation is useful to determine baseline level of function and to provide education and resources about a postoperative exercise program.

Medical assessment includes a thorough history and a physical examination with systematic review to rule out treatable endocrine causes of obesity, and to identify comorbidities that may complicate the surgery. Routine studies include baseline nutritional measures, as well as cardiovascular assessment by electrocardiogram and possible stress test to identify occult coronary artery disease. Respiratory evaluation may include chest x-ray, blood gas, and pulmonary function tests, with specific attention to the possibility of obesity hypoventilatory syndrome (daytime hypercapnia). Medical conditions need to be optimized using a multidisciplinary approach prior to surgical intervention.

Treatment

Managing overweight and obese patients requires a variety of skills of various health care practitioners (physicians, nutritionists, registered dieticians, psychologists, and exercise physiologists) working as a team to help patients learn to make the changes they need to make over the long term. In 1998, the NIH developed guidelines on the Identification, Evaluation, and Treatment of Overweight and Obesity based on BMI for appropriate weight loss interventions (Table 13-6). These criteria help health care workers in determining the best weight loss approach for a person of any given size. Treatment for overweight and obese people falls into three broad categories: behavior modification (diet and exercise), pharmacotherapy, and surgical intervention. All three therapies are able to induce a degree of weight loss. Only bariatric surgery, however, has been successful in helping people lose a significant amount of weight and keep it off.

Behavior Modification

The 1998 NIH guidelines recommend behavior modification for any patient who is obese and for those individuals who are overweight with comorbid conditions. Two main forms of modification exist: reduction in energy intake (diet) and augmentation in energy expenditure (exercise). Dietary modification is an effective means of inducing weight loss. There are two forms; the most common one is the low-calorie diet (LCD), which aims for an energy deficit ranging from 500 to 1,000 kcal/day. For women, this negative energy balance is reached on 1,000 to 1,200 kcal/day. For men, it requires an intake of 1,200 to 1,500 kcal/day. Following such guidelines, patients will lose about 0.45 to 0.90 kg/week. The goal of such therapy is a 10% weight loss over 6 months. The second form is a VLCD, which limits energy intake to less than 800 kcal/day. It often consists of high-protein liquid meals supplemented with essential vitamins, minerals, fatty acids, and electrolytes. Short-term weight loss can be dramatic, with some individuals losing up to 20 kg in as little as 3 months. The long-term weight loss from VLCDs, however, is not different from that produced by LCDs. VLCDs should not be used routinely for

TABLE 13-6	National Institutes of Health Guidelines for Treatment of Overweight and Obesity		
BMI Range	**Behavior Modification**	**Pharmacotherapy**	**Surgery**
25.0–26.9	Yes[a]	No	No
27.0–29.9	Yes[a]	Yes[a]	No
30.0–34.9	Yes	Yes	No
35.0–39.9	Yes	Yes	Yes[a]
40 or more	Yes	Yes	Yes

[a]Comorbidities present.

BMI, body mass index.

Adapted from 1998 National Institutes of Health clinical guidelines.

weight loss therapy because they require special monitoring due to increased risk of complications (hyperuricemia, gout, cardiac complications, and cholelithiasis). As a result, they are not recommended as therapies in the 1998 NIH guidelines.

VLCDs fall into two categories: those that primarily restrict fat intake and those that primarily restrict carbohydrate intake. Both diets produce weight loss that is insufficient to affect any major change in health status. A description of each type of diet follows.

Reduced Carbohydrate Diets: These diets are based on the belief that increased carbohydrate consumption is responsible for weight gain. They therefore focus on severely limiting carbohydrate intake in an attempt to lose weight. Even though these diets can cause a decrease in weight, it is often due to diuresis from depletion of glycogen stores. Furthermore, ketogenesis resulting from the low availability of carbohydrates leads to appetite suppression. Weight, therefore, is often regained when the diet is abandoned and carbohydrates reintroduced. Finally, to keep carbohydrate intake low, protein and fat content are increased. The high fat exposes the individual to the risk of atherosclerotic changes and their sequelae. The high protein is potentially detrimental to renal function, especially in borderline cases. Care should be taken, therefore, in pursuing these reduced carbohydrate programs.

Reduced Fat Diets: Since fat is the most energy-dense macronutrient (having 9 kcal/g), its reduction is useful in decreasing total energy consumption. In fact, both reduced carbohydrate and reduced fat diets are really only effective in the setting of decreased caloric intake. A reduced fat diet provides the additional benefit of decreasing atherosclerotic risk. It is therefore the recommended approach in promoting weight loss.

Physical Activity: Unlike decreasing energy intake, increasing energy expenditure is much less effective in causing weight loss. It results in minimal reductions, both alone and in combination with dietary restriction. Typical recommendations suggest increasing activity to reach an energy expenditure of 1,000 kcal/wk. Such an energy deficit can be obtained in a single day of dietary restriction, showing why increased activity does not lead to significant weight loss. It is, however, very effective in preventing weight regain after successful loss because of its role in long-term weight maintenance.

Energy expenditure comes from three main sources. The basal metabolic rate (BMR) produces the most energy. It is defined as the amount of energy required to keep sodium and potassium where they belong, to keep the body warm, to pump blood, to breathe, and to perform other basic functions. A small contribution comes from the thermic effect (TEF) of the digestion of food. Physical activity produces the rest. Of the three, physical activity is modifiable. It can be increased by adjusting lifestyle habits, such as taking stairs instead of an elevator, or engaging in structured exercise. The latter is the most useful in reaching recommended energy expenditure goals. For example, walking two miles a day for 5 days a week will produce an expenditure of 1,000 kcal/wk.

Although often effective over the short term, behavior modification fails to result in many long-term successes. Maintaining a dietary restriction or structured exercise protocol can be difficult, and people often lapse. The lost weight is regained with additional pounds. Unfortunately, only a small fraction of individuals who lose weight by behavior modification are able to keep it off.

Pharmacotherapy

Pharmacotherapy can enhance weight loss in selected obese patients and should be used only as a part of comprehensive weight management program that includes behavior therapy, diet, and physical activity. However, effective use of weight loss medications requires long-term therapy and monitoring. Trials showed that initial responders tend to continue to respond whereas initial nonresponders are less likely to respond even with increased dosages. The 1998 NIH guidelines recommend pharmacotherapy for obese individuals. Additionally, anyone with a BMI of 27 to 30 and concomitant comorbid conditions can be considered for drug treatment. There are a large number of antiobesity drugs in different stages of development. Currently, only one long-term weight reduction agents is U.S. Food and Drug Administration (FDA) approved, sibutramine and orlistat. The association of fenfluramine and dexfenfluramine with cardiopulmonary complications (valvular disease with aortic insufficiency and pulmonary hypertension) resulted in their rapid removal from the market in 1997. More recently, sibutramine's association with an increased risk of cardiovascular events (myocardial infarction and stroke) has led to its removal in 2010.

Orlistat is a potent pancreatic lipase inhibitor. It promotes weight loss by reducing intestinal fat absorption by roughly 30%. The higher the fat content of the ingested food, the more effective is the drug. Side effects include steatorrhea, fecal leakage, bloating, and increased flatulence. Long-term use results in about a 10% weight loss. Initial dosing is 120 mg three times a day. Multivitamins are sometimes given in conjunction with orlistat to ensure against a theoretical reduction in the absorption of fat-soluble vitamins. Weight regain is common after its cessation.

Developments in the basic sciences suggest targeting the regulatory signals and pathways with different new drugs that have different mechanisms of action. Most of this work is still undergoing investigation. Included in the list are recombinant leptin, drugs acting on neuropeptide Y receptor subtypes responsible for feeding effects, CCK agonists, β3-adrenergic receptor agonists, and drugs targeting uncoupling protein 3 in human skeletal muscles. Also on the list are endocannabinoid system blockers, which have a weight-loss effect. They are used in many countries but not in the United States.

Surgical Intervention

Surgery remains the only proven modality effective in inducing and maintaining weight loss and in reducing lifetime obesity-related morbidities and mortality. It is reserved, however, for severe cases, given the inherent risks of operative intervention. In 1991, an NIH Consensus Development Conference established criteria by which patients should be considered for operative treatment of obesity (Table 13-7). These guidelines have served as the basis for subsequent societal and organizational recommendations related to weight loss surgery. In addition to the previously mentioned BMI thresholds reiterated in the 1998 NIH guidelines, potential surgical candidates must have failed at nonoperative attempts at weight loss. They also must be psychologically stable and willing to follow postoperative

TABLE 13-7	Indication for Bariatric Surgery for Morbid Obesity
Individuals with a BMI of 40 kg/m² or greater	
Individuals with a BMI of 35–40 kg/m² with significant obesity-related comorbidity.	

TABLE 13-8	Types of Weight Reduction Surgery

Restrictive Procedures

Adjustable gastric banding (AGB)

Vertical banded gastroplasty (VBG)

Sleeve gastrectomy (SG)

Malabsorptive Procedures

Biliopancreatic diversion (BPD)

Biliopancreatic diversion with duodenal switch (BPD/DS)

Combination of Malabsorption and Restriction

Roux-en-Y gastric bypass (RYGBP)

diet instructions. Finally, they must not have any medical (i.e., endocrine) cause for their obesity. Operative therapy should be pursued only after these criteria have been met.

Bariatric procedures induce weight loss by decreasing energy intake. Three mechanisms are responsible for this decrease (Table 13-8). Restrictive operations limit food intake by forcing the patient to eat smaller portions. Adjustable gastric banding (AGB), sleeve gastrectomy (SG), and vertical banded gastroplasty (VBG) are the most common examples of such interventions. Malabsorptive operations alter food processing by limiting its absorption in the intestines. Biliopancreatic diversion (BPD) with or without duodenal switch (BPD/DS) is the most popular of these procedures. Among combined restrictive and malabsorptive operations, the Roux-en-Y gastric bypass (RNYGB) is the most common procedure. In general, restrictive procedures are less extensive than malabsorptive ones, but they result in less overall weight loss and cure of comorbid conditions. Malabsorptive procedures, on the other hand, have better weight loss but increased risk of problems with malnutrition. Both types of operations can be performed by either an open or laparoscopic approach. Laparoscopic procedures decrease the rate of wound infection and incisional hernia formation. Recent work has also demonstrated that, for RNYGB, the laparoscopic approach has a lower overall morbidity and in-house mortality compared to the open approach.

Currently, the four most common bariatric operations in the United States are RNYGB, AGB, SG, and BPD/DS.

RNYGB is currently the most common operative intervention for severe obesity in the United States. Important features include the creation of a small proximal gastric pouch with a Roux-en-Y gastrojejunostomy (Figure 13-14). The pouch is typically created by transecting the stomach. The Roux limb measures from 75 to 150 cm in length. Weight loss averages from 75% to 85% excess body weight (EBW) within a couple of years. Nutritional problems tend to be less severe than BPD or BPD/DS. Long-term weight loss of 60% EBW at up to 15 years is documented.

AGB has increased in popularity in recent years. The advent of laparoscopic variations of AGB has contributed to this trend. Key aspects of this procedure include creation of a proximal gastric pouch using an inflatable band and placement of an access port (Figure 13-15). A pars flaccida technique is used to create a posterior gastric tunnel from the lesser curve to the angle of His. The band is then positioned and secured by imbricating its anterior aspect. The distal fundus is sutured to the proximal gastric pouch. The port is placed on the abdominal muscle fascia. Adjustments of the band are made by instilling sterile solution percutaneously via the access

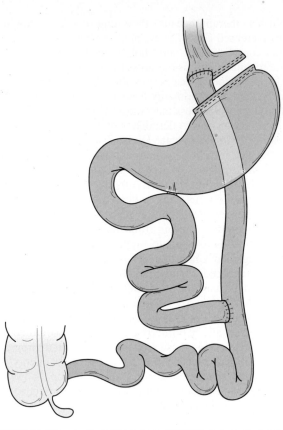

FIGURE 13-14. Roux-en-Y gastric bypass (RNYGB). In a gastric bypass, the stomach is transected unevenly, creating a small proximal pouch. A Roux-en-Y gastrojejunostomy is then created. Weight loss occurs due to decreased food intake as well as some malabsorption. Gastric bypass is currently the most common bariatric procedure performed in the United States.

port. If adjustments are not done under fluoroscopic guidance, incremental increases in the band size are undertaken to avoid overfilling it. Patients with the adjustable band lose from 45% to 55% EBW over the first few years. Long-term U.S. data is limited, since FDA approval occurred only in 2001. However, long-term results (12 year follow-up) from the United Kingdom have shown that laparoscopic AGB can achieve effective, safe, and stable long-term weight loss with low complication rates.

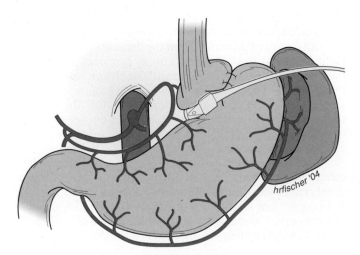

FIGURE 13-15. Adjustable gastric banding (AGB).. An inflatable band is placed around the proximal portion of the stomach, creating a small pouch and restricting food intake. The stoma size into the distal stomach can be adjusted by inflating or deflating the band.

SG is a restrictive procedure, in which the surgeon removes approximately 85% of the stomach laparoscopically so that the stomach takes the shape of a tube or "sleeve" (see stomach in Figure 13-16). This procedure is not reversible. Unlike many other forms of bariatric surgery, the pylorus and stomach innervation remain intact. SG results in excellent weight loss and comorbidity reduction that exceeds, or is comparable to, that of other accepted bariatric procedures. Long-term data are limited, but the 3- and 5-year follow-up data have demonstrated the durability of the SG procedure.

BPD and BPD/DS are more complex procedures. BPD is basically a subtotal gastrectomy with a very distal Roux-en-Y reconstruction. BPD/DS involves SG, duodenal transection with duodenojejunostomy creation, and very distal jejunoileostomy (Figure 13-16). Both operations can result in 70% to 90% EBW loss within the first few years, but nutritional problems can be severe. Given their complexity and issues with malnutrition, the BPD and BPD/DS have not enjoyed the same popularity as other bariatric procedures in the United States.

Historically, VBG was one of the most commonly performed bariatric procedures in the United States. The critical aspects of performing a VBG include the creation of a proximal gastric pouch by stomach partitioning and the reinforcement of the stoma with banding. Partitioning is usually via gastric stapling, and polypropylene is a popular banding material. Patients typically lose between 30% and 50% EBW within the first couple of years. Weight regain, however, can occur due to staple line breakdown. Addition-

ally, revisional operations can be frequent. Such results have led to the abandonment of VGB as a first-line bariatric procedure.

Complications of Bariatric Operations

Given the dramatic increase in bariatric surgical procedures, patients with a history of bariatric surgery are increasingly being seen by surgical and nonsurgical practitioners alike. Knowledge of the common complications of bariatric surgery is essential in the evaluation and treatment of such patients. Such complications can be classified as early, that is, occurring perioperatively or before the patient is discharged from the hospital, or late, that is, occurring after the patient has been discharged (Table 13-9). Late complications may occur within weeks of surgery, or may take years to develop. Furthermore, each type of bariatric procedure has its own unique complications, in addition to the complications common to all surgical procedures, such as bleeding and infection.

Early Complications

Anastomotic Leak

Anastomotic leak occurs in up to 5% of patients undergoing gastric bypass or BPD/DS. While intraoperative testing of the anastomosis may reduce this risk, it remains one of the most common complications. The gastrojejunostomy is most likely to be the site of leakage. Classic signs and symptoms of peritonitis may not be present or may be difficult to recognize in the obese patient. Abdominal pain, unexplained tachycardia, tachypnea, and hypoxia should raise suspicion of a leak. Abnormal output from a drain placed at the anastomosis at the time of surgery is also highly suggestive. Imaging with an upper GI series or abdominal CT with oral contrast should be performed promptly. Conservative management with percutaneous drainage and parenteral nutrition may be attempted in the hemodynamically stable patient. If this is unsuccessful, or if the patient is clinically unstable, immediate operative exploration, drainage, and repair (if possible) is performed.

Deep Vein Thrombosis and Pulmonary Embolus

Bariatric patients are at increased risk for deep vein thrombosis (DVT) and pulmonary embolus (PE) for several reasons.

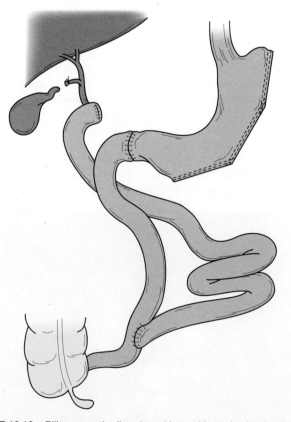

FIGURE 13-16. Biliopancreatic diversion with or without duodenal switch (BPD/DS). In a BPD/DS, the stomach is reduced in size, the gallbladder is removed, the proximal duodenum is divided and reanastomosed to more distal small bowel, and a short common channel is created via a jejunoileostomy. Weight loss is predominantly secondary to malabsorption, and complications related to malnutrition are more frequent in this procedure.

TABLE 13-9	Comparison of Early Versus Late Complications for the Three Most Common Bariatric Procedures

Early Complications	Late Complications
Anastomotic leak[a]	Nutritional disturbances[a,b,c]
Deep venous thrombosis and pulmonary emboli[a,b,c]	Marginal ulcers and anastomotic strictures[a]
Bleeding[a,b,c]	Internal hernia[a]
Infection[a,b,c]	Afferent limb syndrome[a]
Splenic or visceral injury[a,b,c]	Cholelithiasis[a,c]
	Band slippage[b]
	Esophageal dilatation[b,c]
	Band erosion[b]

[a]Roux-en-Y gastric bypass
[b]Adjustable gastric band
[c]Sleeve gastrectomy

Adipose tissue itself causes metabolic changes that increase thrombogenesis. Obese patients are often less mobile, especially after surgery. Increased adipose tissue in the lower extremities compresses the veins and impairs venous outflow. Finally, venous stasis from general anesthesia and the prothrombotic, proinflammatory postsurgical state combine to render bariatric patients particularly susceptible to developing venous thrombosis. Aggressive prophylaxis is important to help minimize risk. Combination therapy including low molecular weight heparin, sequential compression devices, and early ambulation is recommended.

DVT typically presents as painful, unilateral swelling of a lower extremity. Diagnosis is made using duplex ultrasound of the affected extremity. However, given the limited sensitivity of ultrasound in obese patients, treatment is often instituted in the absence of a clearly positive study, if the clinical presentation is sufficiently suggestive. Either enoxaparin or unfractionated heparin may be used for initial treatment, followed by oral anticoagulation with warfarin for 6 months.

PE can manifest as hypoxia, tachypnea, tachycardia, dyspnea, or chest pain. The severity of the presentation can range from mild symptoms to cardiovascular collapse. Diagnosis is usually made by helical CT. As with DVT, therapy consists of immediate institution of anticoagulation using enoxaparin or unfractionated heparin, followed by long-term warfarin anticoagulation. Therapy should be started presumptively if CT scanning cannot be obtained immediately. Patients deemed to be at unusually high risk of PE due to history of DVT/PE, extreme obesity (BMI > 60), or chronic venous stasis should be considered for placement of a vena cava filter prior to surgery.

Late Complications
Nutritional Disturbances

Not surprisingly, the therapeutic nutrient restriction imposed by bariatric surgery may also lead to significant nutritional deficiencies. Such disturbances are more likely to occur in patients undergoing malabsorptive procedures, such as RNYGB, than in restrictive procedures, such as gastric banding. Bariatric surgical patients are instructed to consume extra protein (60 to 80 g) on a daily basis to ensure that the metabolic demands of the body are met, but patients who do not adhere to the regimen may develop protein energy malnutrition. Additionally, various vitamin and mineral deficiencies can occur. Of these, iron, vitamin B_{12}, folic acid, thiamine, calcium, and vitamin D deficiency are the most important. Iron deficiency is the most common, and develops in up to 50% of gastric bypass patients. The gastric pouch produces only a very small amount of acid and therefore absorbs less iron. Also, the duodenum, a major location for iron and calcium absorption, is bypassed. Patients with preexisting iron deficiency, and menstruating women, should take 65 mg of elemental iron daily, plus vitamin C, which improves absorption. Vitamin B_{12} deficiency is the next most common, and can produce neurologic symptoms and megaloblastic anemia. In gastric bypass, the distal stomach is isolated from the food stream, preventing IF from combining with vitamin B_{12} to permit absorption in the ileum. For this reason, gastric bypass patients are routinely administered intramuscular or sublingual vitamin B_{12}. Thiamine deficiency often presents with neuropathic symptoms, and daily thiamine supplementation, usually in the form of a multivitamin, is recommended. Calcium absorption is also decreased in bypass patients, and routine calcium and vitamin D supplementation is necessary to avoid osteoporosis and osteomalacia.

Because of the potential to develop serious nutritional disturbances, bariatric patients require lifelong follow-up. Such care usually involves yearly office visits to review adherence to dietary recommendations and measurement of vitamins B_{12}, A, D, and E, thiamine, folate, calcium, and prealbumin.

Marginal Ulcer

An ulcer occurring on the jejunal side of the gastrojejunostomy is termed a marginal ulcer. Such ulcers are thought to be caused by impaired perfusion of the jejunal mucosa due to interruption of the blood supply by the staple line at the anastomosis. Smoking and the use of NSAIDs or steroids such as prednisone may also contribute. Marginal ulcers may occur as early as several weeks, or as late as 1 year postoperatively. Patients present with abdominal pain, upper GI bleeding, nausea, and vomiting. Patients may lose weight due to fear of eating, as food may worsen the symptoms. Diagnosis is made with upper endoscopy, and treatment consists of protection of the GI mucosa with PPIs and sucralfate. Total bowel rest with parenteral nutrition is sometimes necessary. If the ulcer is recalcitrant to conservative management revision of the gastrojejunostomy may be necessary.

Stricture

Healing of the gastrojejunostomy may be complicated by the development of a stricture. This complication usually occurs within 6 months of the surgery. Patients typically complain of progressive intolerance of solids and liquids, with postprandial abdominal pain and vomiting. Upper endoscopy is the diagnostic procedure of choice. If a stricture is present, pneumatic balloon dilation can be performed to open the anastomosis. The endoscope should be able to enter into the Roux limb after dilation. Multiple dilatations are sometimes necessary.

Internal Hernia

Reconfiguration of the small intestine in gastric bypass necessitates the creation of openings in the mesentery. These defects may permit herniation of colon or small bowel, with resultant partial or complete obstruction. The presenting symptoms are those of intestinal obstruction, namely, postprandial abdominal pain, nausea, and vomiting. Because the herniation may occur intermittently, symptoms may come and go. Furthermore, upper GI series and abdominal CT may be normal in a large percentage of cases, and diagnostic laparoscopy may be necessary to diagnose and repair the defect (Figure 13-17).

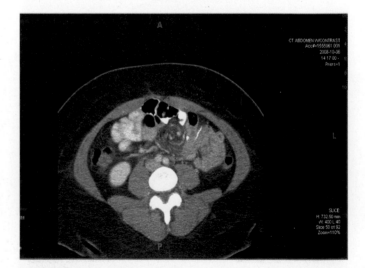

FIGURE 13-17. CT scan demonstrating an internal hernia following gastric bypass. Note the swirling of the mesenteric fat.

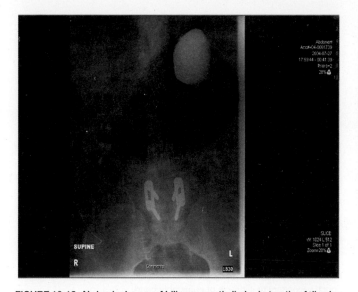

FIGURE 13-18. Abdominal x-ray of biliopancreatic limb obstruction following gastric bypass. Note the distended stomach remnant.

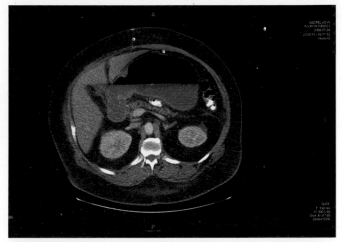

FIGURE 13-19. Abdominal CT of biliopancreatic limb obstruction after gastric bypass. Note the distended gastric remnant filled with air and fluid.

Biliopancreatic Limb Obstruction

Obstruction of the biliopancreatic limb, that is, the blind gastric pouch, duodenum, and proximal jejunum, may occur due to inflammation at the jejunojejunostomy. This complication, which typically occurs within 1 month postoperatively, results in the accumulation of bile and pancreatic secretions in the afferent limb and gastric remnant. Patients complain of abdominal pain, nausea, and nonbilious vomiting. Decompression can be accomplished through the placement of a percutaneous gastrostomy tube, which is then removed after the inflammation subsides and the jejunojejunostomy reopens (Figures 13-18 and 13-19).

Cholelithiasis

About a third of obese patients will develop cholelithiasis during the rapid weight loss following gastric bypass surgery. The risk is lower with restrictive procedures. This statistic has led to the routine administration of ursodeoxycholic acid, 300 mg twice daily, for 6 months postoperatively. This medication decreases the risk of developing cholelithiasis to around 2%. Side effects include diarrhea, dyspepsia, and abdominal pain. While screening for gallstones with ultrasound is not routinely suggested for all patients, most surgeons will perform cholecystectomy at the time of initial operation if patients have known preexisting cholelithiasis or symptoms of biliary colic.

For a list of useful medications related to bariatric surgery complications, see Table 13-10.

Adjustable Gastric Band Complications

Gastric band complications include band slippage and erosion. Slippage of the band, which usually occurs as a late complication, results in movement of the distal stomach through the band with formation of an enlarged proximal pouch. Food can become lodged in this region, causing nausea and vomiting. Additionally, patients may develop reflux symptoms. In severe cases, gastric outlet obstruction occurs and the stomach can become strangulated. Overtightening of the gastric band can lead to dilation of the distal esophagus. Diagnosis of these complications is obtained with upper GI radiographs, which can show proximal dilation, poor movement of contrast, and improper orientation of the band (Figures 13-20 and 13-21). Initial treatment includes complete deflation of the band. Occasionally, the prolapse or dilation will resolve, and the band can be slowly reinflated. Operative reduction of a prolapse with band repositioning or replacement is often necessary (Figure 13-22).

TABLE 13-10	Useful Medications Related to Bariatric Surgery Complications		
Medication	**Action**	**Indication**	**Dosage**
Heparin	Antithrombin III inhibitor	DVT/PE	Heparin nomogram used in most hospitals for therapy 5,000 units subQ TID for prophylaxis
Low molecular weight heparin/enoxaparin	Antithrombin III inhibitor	DVT/PE	1 mg/kg subQ BID for therapy 40 mg subQ daily or BID for prophylaxis
Warfarin	Vitamin K-dependent protein inhibitor	DVT/PE	Dosage varies depending on patient factors. International Normalized Ratio (INR) goal of 2–3
Ursodeoxycholic acid	Gallstone formation inhibitor	Gallstones	300 mg po BID for prophylaxis

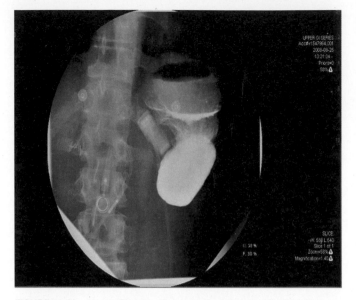

FIGURE 13-20.   **Upper GI series demonstrating slippage of adjustable gastric band.** Note the dilated proximal pouch, failure of contrast passage into the distal stomach, and downward orientation of the band.

Band erosion into the stomach is a relatively rare (about 1%) long-term complication. Patients will present months to years after operation. Some may notice loss of restriction with eating. Others will suddenly develop an infection or fluid collection at their port site. Contrast swallow study usually provides the diagnosis. Confirmation can be made with endoscopy (Figure 13-23). Patients with erosion usually require operative exploration, removal of the adjustable band, and closure of any openings. Occasionally, the eroded band can be retrieved using upper endoscopy. Patients can undergo a second bariatric procedure after healing.

Benefits of Bariatric Operations

Surgical treatment of obesity ameliorates comorbid conditions, reduces mortality, and ultimately decreases health care costs. In a meta-analysis of 22,094 patients, weight

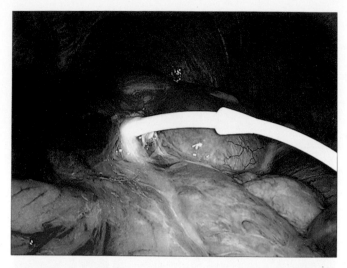

FIGURE 13-22. Intraoperative photo of an acutely dilated proximal gastric pouch secondary to slippage of adjustable band.

loss surgery resolved diabetes in 76% of patients; hypertension was eliminated in 61.7%; obstructive sleep apnea in 85.7%; and high cholesterol levels decreased in more than 70% of patients. Similarly, Christou et al. reported an absolute mortality reduction of 5% when comparing 1,035 patients who underwent weight loss surgery with 5,746 matched controls in a 5-year follow-up. As little as 10% weight loss reduced hypertension, hypercholesterolemia, and type II diabetes, decreased the expected lifetime incidence of heart disease and stroke, and increased life expectancy. Most recently, the Swedish obese subjects (SOS) study found a 28% reduction in the adjusted overall mortality rate in the surgical group compared with conventionally treated controls.

Cost-effectiveness analyses (CEAs) have shown that gastric bypass provides a net savings. In the United States, gastric bypass costs $35,000 per quality-adjusted life year (QALY), and appears to be more cost effective for women than for men, for individuals with a BMI > 40, and for younger individuals. Dialysis, for example, costs more at $50,000 QALY.

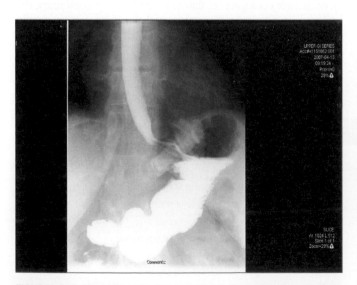

FIGURE 13-21. **Upper GI series demonstrating normal orientation of adjustable gastric band.** Note the difference compared to Figure 13-20.

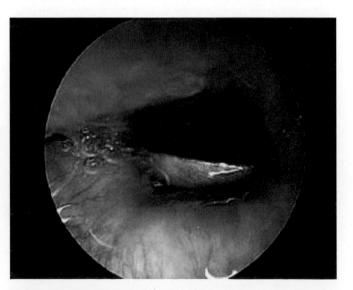

FIGURE 13-23. **Upper endoscopy demonstrating erosion of adjustable gastric band into stomach.**

In the United Kingdom, comparison with nonsurgical management of obesity demonstrates that weight loss operations were indeed more cost effective at £11,000 per QALY. After weight loss surgery, Snow et al. found $240,566.04 dollars per year cost savings on medications alone. Weight loss improves comorbid conditions, and decreases medications of chronic disease, such as diabetes and hypertension. Surgical management is an effective treatment option for severe obesity, improves quality of life, decreases morbidity and mortality, and restores overall health.

NEW FRONTIERS IN BARIATRIC SURGERY

StomaphyX—Gastric Bypass Revision

StomaphyX is an endoscopic incision-free procedure that reduces the stomach volume to help gastric bypass patients get back on track with weight loss. StomaphyX is a new and innovative revisional procedure, approved by the U.S. FDA in 2007 for individuals who have had RNYGB surgery and have regained weight due to pouch or pouch outlet (stoma) enlargement over time. The aim of this procedure is to reduce the volume of the stomach pouch and the stoma to the original gastric bypass size endoscopically without surgery or incisions and with minimal recovery time. It is indicated as a primary procedure for weight loss surgery.

Bariatric Surgery for Adolescents

As in adults, the rates of obesity among youth are on the rise. Experts in pediatric obesity and bariatric surgery recommend that surgical treatment only be considered when adolescents have tried for at least 6 months to lose weight and have not been successful. Candidates should be extremely obese (typically with BMI > 40), have reached their adult height (usually 13 or older for girls and 15 or older for boys), and have serious obesity-related health problems, such as type II diabetes, sleep apnea, heart disease, or significant functional or psychosocial impairment. Psychological evaluation of both patient and parents is important to prepare them for this major surgery and the expectations and long-term follow-up after surgery.

A review of short-term data from the national inpatient sample (the largest inpatient database in the United States) suggests that gastric bypass operations are at least as safe for adolescents as adults. At this time, the adjustable gastric band has not been approved for use in the United States for people younger than age 18, but efforts are currently underway to gain such approval.

Medical Cost and Insurance

Obesity itself is a costly chronic health disease through its association with such major health problems as diabetes, coronary artery disease, and hypertension, which consume a significant amount of money for therapy. However, most of these medical problems improve significantly after surgery, making bariatric procedures, which on average cost from $20,000 to $25,000, a very reasonable and appropriate therapy. Medical insurance coverage varies by state and insurance provider. In 2004, the U.S. Department of Health and Human Services reduced barriers to obtaining Medicare coverage for obesity treatments. Bariatric surgery may be covered if it is medically appropriate and if it is performed to correct an obesity-related illness.

thePoint ✳ Go to http://thePoint.lww.com/activate and use your scratch-off code on the inside cover of this book to access bonus chapters, question bank, videos, and more.

SAMPLE QUESTIONS

Questions

Choose the best answer for each question.

1. A 60-year-old man comes to the emergency room because of hematemesis and bright red blood per rectum. He reports a history of gnawing epigastric pain radiating to the back and improved with eating. His past medical history is significant only for frequent headaches and back pain, for which he takes nonsteroidal anti-inflammatory drugs (NSAIDs) and over-the-counter medications. On physical exam, he is pale, hypotensive, and tachycardic. After resuscitation, initial upper endoscopy reveals evidence of an upper gastrointestinal hemorrhage and an ulcer in the posterior duodenal bulb. Which blood vessel is the most likely source of bleeding?
   A. Left gastric artery
   B. Right gastric artery
   C. Common hepatic artery
   D. Gastroduodenal artery
   E. Superior mesenteric artery

2. A 63-year-old man came to the office because of epigastric pain of 2 months' duration not relieved with antacids. He has a history of an adenomatous gastric polyp removed 3 years ago. At upper endoscopy, he was found to a have another gastric polyp in his antrum that, on endoscopic ultrasound, appeared to be superficial and not associated with any enlarged lymph nodes. Pathological analysis of the polyp reveals evidence of adenocarcinoma invading into the submucosa. On clinical staging, there is no evidence of distant metastasis. The next step in therapy for this patient is
   A. repeat endoscopy in 1 year.
   B. chemotherapy.
   C. chemoradiotherapy.
   D. gastric wedge resection.
   E. subtotal gastrectomy.

3. A 34-year-old woman is being evaluated for epigastric pain and is found to have an ulcer in the anterior duodenal bulb on upper endoscopy. Rapid urease testing of a mucosal biopsy of the antrum of the stomach is positive. In addition to omeprazole, appropriate therapy at this time would include a 2-week course of omeprazole, metronidazole, and
   A. amoxicillin and metronidazole.
   B. tetracycline and cephalexin.
   C. clarithromycin and amoxicillin.
   D. cephalexin and metronidazole.
   E. bismuth and cephalexin.

4. A 53-year-old woman comes to clinic for evaluation for weight loss. She has recently diagnosed diabetes, asthma, sleep apnea, and hypertension. Her BMI is 38 kg/m². Which of the following weight loss options is most appropriate for this patient?
   A. A very low calorie diet
   B. A low-calorie diet
   C. Sibutramine
   D. Orlistat
   E. Gastric bypass

5. A 42-year-old woman comes to the emergency room with epigastric pain radiating to right upper quadrant. She underwent a laparoscopic adjustable gastric band 6 months ago. She has lost approximately 80 lbs over the 6 months. She is afebrile with stable vital signs. A right upper quadrant ultrasound is shown below. Which of the following medications would have been most effective in preventing this complication?
   A. Sucralfate
   B. Ursodeoxycholic acid
   C. Cholestyramine
   D. Calcium citrate
   E. Omeprazole

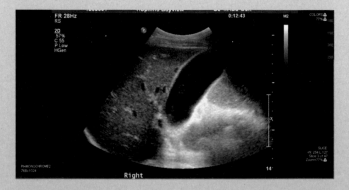

Answers and Explanations

1. Answer: D

The patient presents to the emergency room with evidence of a massive upper gastrointestinal hemorrhage (hematemesis with bright red blood with hypotension and tachycardia). His symptoms of gnawing epigastric pain radiating to the back and improved with eating suggest a posterior bulb duodenal ulcer. Ulcers in this location can erode into the gastroduodenal artery as it passes behind the first portion of the duodenum, causing massive gastrointestinal hemorrhage. The left gastric artery arises from the celiac axis. The common hepatic artery divides into the gastroduodenal and proper hepatic arteries. The right gastric artery arises from the proper hepatic artery. The superior mesenteric artery is a branch off the aorta.

(Anatomy; Benign Duodenal Ulcer/Uncomplicated Duodenal Ulcer/Clinical Presentation and Evaluation; Complicated Duodenal Ulcer/Clinical Presentation and Evaluation)

2. Answer: E

This patient has an early stage gastric cancer (i.e., no evidence of metastasis or perigastric lymph nodes) on clinical staging and is a candidate for potentially curative resection. Patients with minimal evidence of gastric wall invasion (i.e., mucosal or submucosal invasion) do not require any preoperative therapy and should proceed straight to surgical resection. In this patient with an antral lesion, a subtotal gastrectomy is indicated with frozen section analysis of surgical margins to ensure adequate resection. Wedge resection is not recommended. In patients with evidence of greater gastric wall invasion (i.e., invasion to and beyond the lamina propria), perioperative chemotherapy with epirubicin, cisplatin, and 5-fluorouracil has been demonstrated to provide a survival benefit.

(Malignant Gastric Disease/Adenocarcinoma of the Stomach)

3. Answer: C

All patients presenting with duodenal ulceration should undergo testing for the presence of *Helicobacter pylori* infection. The rapid urease test can be performed on antral stomach biopsies and is indicative of infection if positive. If *H. pylori* infection is present, it should be eradicated. First-line therapy includes acid suppression with clarithromycin and amoxicillin or clarithromycin and metronidazole for a minimum of 7 days. Traditional quadruple therapy is a second-line treatment and consists of acid suppression with bismuth, metronidazole, and tetracycline for a minimum of 7 days.

(Benign Duodenal Ulcer/Uncomplicated Duodenal Ulcer Disease)

4. Answer: E

This patient has type II obesity with the life-threatening comorbidity of sleep apnea. As such, she qualifies for surgical intervention according to 1998 NIH guidelines. Weight loss surgery is the only treatment option to demonstrate sustained, substantial weight loss. Gastric bypass, therefore, is indicated. Very low calorie diets are not recommended for weight loss by the NIH guidelines. Although low-calorie diets, sibutramine, and orlistat are all options in treating obese patients, those individuals who qualify for surgery should undergo it if they are deemed appropriate candidates.

(Surgical Treatment of Obesity/Treatment)

5. Answer: B

This patient has developed symptomatic cholelithiasis following rapid weight loss after a bariatric procedure. The ultrasound shows several echogenic stones within the gallbladder. Without pharmacotherapy, the risk of gallstone formation during this period approaches 30%. The prophylactic use of ursodeoxycholic acid decreases the risk of gallstone formation to approximately 2%. Sucralfate is used to promote healing of anastomotic ulcers. Cholestyramine is used in the treatment of alkaline reflux gastritis to bind bile salts. Calcium citrate is given to bariatric patients to prevent calcium deficiency and subsequent osteoporosis. Omeprazole is a proton pump inhibitor used in the treatment of anastomotic ulcers.

(Surgical Treatment of Obesity/Complications of Bariatric Operations/Late Complications)

14
Small Intestine and Appendix

JOHN D. MELLINGER, M.D. • SERGE DUBÉ, M.D. • CHARLES M. FRIEL, M.D. •
ALAN E. HARZMAN, M.D. • DAVID W. MERCER, M.D.

Objectives

1. Describe basic small intestinal and appendiceal anatomy and physiology.

2. Describe the physiology of small intestinal digestion and absorption of carbohydrates, fats, and proteins.

3. Describe the common etiologies, signs, and symptoms of small bowel mechanical obstruction, and contrast them with those of paralytic ileus.

4. Discuss the complications of small bowel obstruction (SBO), including fluid and electrolyte shifts, vascular compromise of the small bowel, and sepsis.

5. Outline the appropriate laboratory tests and radiographs that are used in the diagnostic evaluation of a patient with a suspected SBO.

6. Discuss the clinical appearance of small bowel strangulation and the potential difficulty of making that diagnosis.

7. Compare and contrast mechanical SBO with colon obstruction.

8. Outline a treatment plan for a patient with SBO. Discuss the indications for operative therapy.

9. Describe the various clinical presentations of a patient with Crohn's disease, and explain how they can differ from the presentation of a patient with ulcerative colitis.

10. Outline a diagnostic approach for a patient with Crohn's disease.

11. Discuss the medical and surgical treatment plans for patients with Crohn's disease. Describe the complications associated with the disease process, and explain when surgery is indicated.

12. Discuss the clinical presentation of a patient with acute mesenteric ischemia (AMI).

13. Describe the causes of AMI.

14. Discuss the diagnostic evaluation of patients with mesenteric ischemia.

15. Outline a therapeutic approach to patients diagnosed with mesenteric ischemia.

16. Discuss the relative frequency of the most common benign and malignant small bowel tumors.

17. Discuss the clinical presentation and diagnostic approach to the following types of small bowel tumors: adenocarcinoma, carcinoid, and lymphoma.

18. Describe the carcinoid syndrome, and list the features of a carcinoid tumor that suggest it may be malignant. List the features that must be present for carcinoid syndrome to occur.

19. Discuss the role of surgery in the management of patients with small bowel tumors.

20. Discuss the location, frequency, size, and various clinical presentations of a patient with Meckel's diverticulum.

21. Describe the treatment of Meckel's diverticulum that is incidentally found at surgery and the treatment of one that is symptomatic.

22. Describe intestinal malrotation and its potential complications, as well as their management.

23. Discuss the signs, symptoms, and differential diagnosis of acute appendicitis, and describe how diseases that mimic it may be differentiated.

24. Outline the diagnostic workup of a patient with suspected appendicitis, and describe the laboratory findings that would support the diagnosis.

25. List and discuss the common complications of appendicitis and subsequent appendectomy, and explain how each can be prevented or managed.

26. Describe the presentation and management of appendiceal carcinoid and its significance as an incidental finding.

Diseases of the small intestine and appendix constitute some of the most common surgical emergencies. Acute appendicitis, mechanical small bowel obstruction (SBO), paralytic ileus, and Crohn's disease are particularly frequent problems encountered in the care of the patient with abdominal complaints. In normal settings, the small bowel is an amazingly prolific organ with regard to its physiology, having digestive, nutritional, immunologic, and endocrine functions. Alteration of these functions by disease and iatrogenic intervention can have profound implications for patient management. A thorough understanding of the physiology and pathophysiology of these organs is thus fundamental to the care of the surgical patient.

This chapter focuses on the anatomy, physiology, and pathophysiology of the small intestine and appendix. Diseases including those mentioned above, as well as some of the common vascular, neoplastic, developmental, and diverticular diseases of these organs, are reviewed. Medical and surgical management, including important differential diagnostic considerations, are detailed.

ANATOMY

Small Intestine

The small intestine is composed of three segments: the duodenum, jejunum, and ileum. The duodenum extends from the pylorus to the ligament of Treitz. The jejunum consists of the first 40% of small bowel distal to the duodenum. The ileum consists of the remaining 60%. The duodenum is retroperitoneal, whereas the jejunum and ileum are tethered on a mesentery that extends from the left upper quadrant to the right lower quadrant. The duodenum itself is divided into four segments, including the duodenal bulb (first portion) and descending duodenum (second portion), which harbors the major and minor duodenal papillae. In 90% of cases, the minor papilla allows drainage of the dorsal pancreatic duct (accessory duct of Santorini), and the major papilla drains the common bile duct and the main pancreatic duct (duct of Wirsung). The third and fourth portions are defined by their respective proximal and distal relation to the superior mesenteric vessels, as these structures course anterior to the duodenum. The jejunum has more prominent plica circulares and longer vasa recta than the ileum (Figure 14-1). The blood supply to the small intestine is primarily via the superior mesenteric artery (SMA), with the duodenum also being supplied by the gastroduodenal artery, originating from the celiac axis via the common hepatic artery. Venous drainage parallels the arterial supply, with the majority of the venous effluent coursing through the superior mesenteric vein (SMV), which is joined by the splenic and inferior mesenteric veins to constitute the portal vein. Lymphatic drainage is via lacteals and lymphatic channels paralleling the venous drainage, ultimately joining at the cisterna chyli in the upper abdomen below the aortic hiatus of the diaphragm. The terminal ileum has an abundance of lymphatic tissue known as Peyer's patches and terminates at the ileocecal valve. In addition to these concentrations of lymphatic tissue, the gut also possesses prominent populations of lymphatic cells in the lamina propria and the mucosa. Together these populations comprise what is termed gut associated lymphoid tissue (GALT). Follicular B cells from the periphery of Peyer's patches, and similar lymphoid nodules throughout the gut may migrate to mesenteric nodes and from there to the bloodstream via the thoracic duct. These cells can then return to the mucosa adjacent to their area of origin as B2 memory cells, forming a population of cells known as mucosa-associated lymphoid tissue (MALT). The nerve supply to the small intestine and appendix is mediated through the autonomic nervous system. Parasympathetic fibers originate from the vagus nerve and traverse to the gut via the celiac plexus. Sympathetic fibers travel via the splanchnic nerves from ganglion cells in the superior mesenteric plexus. Pain fibers activated by intestinal distension communicate primarily via sympathetic visceral afferent fibers.

Appendix

The appendix arises from the cecum at the confluence of the taenia coli and is accompanied by an adjacent mesentery, the mesoappendix, in which courses the appendiceal artery as a terminal branch of the ileocolic artery. It is also rich in lymphatic tissue and may be positioned variably in relation to the cecum, including retrocecal and, rarely, truly retroperitoneal locations.

PHYSIOLOGY

The primary function of the small intestine is digestion of food and absorption of the ingested water, electrolytes, and nutrients into the bloodstream. This is accomplished through a complex set of processes that include intestinal motility, the activity of digestive enzymes, the secretion of digestive juices, and absorptive processes predicated on both simple diffusion and active transport. Autonomic and endocrine regulation of all these processes is abundant and critical to their coordination.

Motility

Intestinal motility allows for mixing, propulsion, and storage of enteric contents. The enteric nervous system, which includes intrinsic neural plexuses and autonomic extrinsic neural pathways, governs this motility. Submucosal (Meissner's) and myenteric (Auerbach's) plexuses help perform intrinsic regulatory functions and receive input from local receptors in the mucosa and smooth muscle of the gut. Acetylcholine functions as the primary excitatory neurotransmitter at the myenteric plexus level, and vasoactive intestinal peptide (VIP) and somatostatin are the prominent inhibitory neurotransmitters. Extrinsic control is exerted from the central nervous system

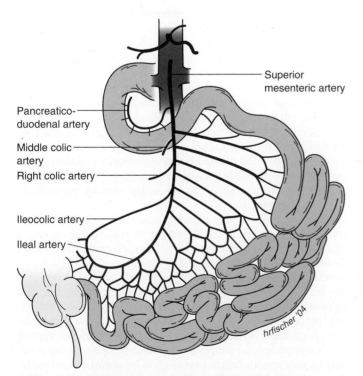

Superior mesenteric artery

Pancreatico-duodenal artery

Middle colic artery

Right colic artery

Ileocolic artery

Ileal artery

hrfischer '04

FIGURE 14-1. Anatomy of the small intestine demonstrating vascular anatomy of the varying segments. Note longer vasa recta in jejunum versus ileum.

through parasympathetic, primarily excitatory, pathways via the vagal and pelvic parasympathetic nerves, and through sympathetic, primarily inhibitory, channels networked via sympathetic ganglia. In general, the enteric nerves determine whether contraction occurs, and intrinsic myogenic control determines the pattern of contraction. Several dozen additional peptides, often referred to generically as gastrointestinal (GI) hormones, provide an additional level of control and coordination through endocrine and paracrine effects on the gut itself, as well as the biliary tract and pancreas (see below). Segmenting contractions allow for mixing function, and peristaltic contractions for propagative function. Tonic contractions are also seen and help to preserve baseline muscle tonicity.

A cyclic pattern of digestive activity is observed during fasting, which involves muscular contractions that migrate from the duodenum to the terminal ileum. This is referred to as the migrating motor complex (MMC), or interdigestive myoelectric complex (IDMEC). The MMC has four distinct phases, which are characterized by differing levels of electrical depolarization activity and corresponding intestinal contraction. Phase 1 is quiescent, with no spikes (larger electrical fluctuations) or contractions. Phase 2 has accelerating and intermittent spike and contractile activity. Phase 3 is characterized by a sequence of high amplitude spiking activity and corresponding strong, rhythmic gut contractions. Phase 4 is a subsequent brief period of intermittent spike activity before the return to quiescence. The duration of the entire cycle is 90 to 120 minutes, and the migration, which begins in the foregut, takes 2 hours to migrate down the small intestine. Eating abolishes the cycle and induces intermittent contractile activity. This fasting cycle may have a role in "housecleaning" the gut during the interdigestive period and preventing stasis and bacterial overgrowth in the distal small bowel. The ileocecal valve itself facilitates normal emptying phases and limits bacterial overgrowth that otherwise could occur secondary to reflux of colonic contents.

Microbiology

Compared with the colon, the small bowel in healthy patients contains few bacteria. Bacterial growth is actively retarded by the small intestinal environment and by peristalsis. Due to the acidic condition of the stomach, the bacterial load in the stomach and duodenum is minimal, measuring only 10^2 to 10^3 colony forming units (cfu)/mL. Progressing distally, the bacterial counts in the small intestine increase gradually, reaching a high of about 10^8 cfu/mL in the terminal ileum. Once in the colon, the bacterial load increases considerably, reaching 10^{12} cfu/mL, a 10,000-fold increase over the ileum and a 1 billion fold increase over the stomach and duodenum. In the proximal small bowel, the composition of the bacteria is mostly facultative gram-positive organisms. Progressing down the small bowel, the composition shifts so that the bacteria within the terminal ileum are similar to the colon, with a majority being gram-negative anaerobes. For these reasons, the infectious complications associated with a perforated small intestine are often less severe than those associated with a perforated colon. However, in certain diseased conditions, bacterial overgrowth can be seen within the small intestine. Stasis is a major risk factor for small bowel overgrowth and can be the result of medical disorders, such as diabetes or scleroderma, but may also result from a small bowel stricture causing a prolonged partial bowel obstruction. Typically the flora associated with small bowel bacterial overgrowth has a similar composition of the colon and therefore may alter infectious complications if surgery is required under these conditions.

Fluid and Nutrient Absorption

The secretion of 5 to 10 L/day of digestive fluid by the salivary glands, stomach, biliary tree, pancreas, and intestine itself is handled primarily by the small intestine, which absorbs 80% of the resulting succus entericus on a daily basis. The small bowel does this isosmotically, without concentrating the enteric contents intraluminally. In the jejunum, fluid is resorbed following the gradient created by Na^+ coupled nutrient absorption, and it is here that the majority of small intestinal fluid is absorbed. Na^+ is the major ion that dictates osmotic gradients favorable for water absorption, and Cl^- is the usual driving force for secretion. Hormones, peptides, drugs, toxins, and immunologic factors may all impact this delicate isosmotic balance and foster increased delivery of succus to the colon, with resulting diarrhea.

The major nutrient substrates absorbed by the small intestine are fats, carbohydrates, and proteins. Each has its own digestive and absorptive requirements. Fat digestion involves a crucial intraluminal phase, which allows the eventual delivery of a water-insoluble nutrient into an aqueous environment. Ingested fat (triglycerides and cholesterol esters) is mechanically broken down into small droplets that are then digested intraluminally by salivary and pancreatic lipase into free fatty acids and monoglycerides complexed with calcium. Bile salts then act as a detergent to allow formation of micelles containing these smaller substrates as well as fat-soluble vitamins. The micelle dissociates at the enterocyte apical membrane, delivering the free fatty acids, cholesterol, and monoglycerides to the cell membrane, where they can permeate the lipid regions of the membrane into the cell without requirement for specific carriers. Inside the enterocyte, triglycerides are reconstituted from the absorbed constituents and packaged into chylomicrons suitable for subsequent lymphatic transport. Only medium chain triglycerides are capable of being absorbed directly into the portal system without going through the chylomicron–lymphatic pathway. The majority of fat absorption occurs in the duodenum and upper jejunum, although the bile salts that facilitate fat digestion are resorbed primarily in the terminal ileum.

Carbohydrate digestion begins with salivary amylase. The process is completed in the jejunum and is accomplished by the intraluminal breakdown of complex starch into oligosaccharides, primarily by pancreatic amylase, and the subsequent breakdown of oligosaccharides by brush border enzymes into glucose, galactose, and fructose. Glucose and galactose are then absorbed via Na^+ coupled carrier transport, and fructose by facilitated diffusion. This system of digestion, which limits the osmotic load of the smaller monosaccharides to a step accomplished at the border of the enterocyte membrane just prior to absorption, serves to minimize osmotic pressure in the intestinal lumen.

Dietary proteins are, like fat, absorbed primarily in the duodenum and jejunum. Digestion begins in the stomach via the action of gastric pepsin, although protein digestion is still efficient in the absence of this step. Cholecystokinin secretion by proximal intestinal endocrine cells is stimulated by the presence of polypeptides in the intestinal lumen, and in turn stimulates pancreatic secretion of peptidases (including precursors of trypsin, chymotrypsin, elastase, and carboxypeptidase), which break the polypeptides down further to oligopeptides and amino acids. These compounds are polar and require specific carrier proteins to be absorbed across the enterocyte membrane. This absorption is coupled to Na^+ transport, which is driven by a favorable electrochemical gradient, thus allowing the amino acids to be accumulated against a concentration gradient.

In addition to the above general mechanisms controlling the absorption of fluid and nutrients from the small intestine, several important substances are absorbed in specific areas of the digestive tract. Vitamin B_{12}, complexed with gastric intrinsic factor, is absorbed in the terminal ileum. The fat-soluble vitamins A, D, E, and K, as well as bile salts, are also absorbed primarily in this area. Calcium and iron are absorbed primarily in the duodenum and proximal small bowel. Knowledge of these specific patterns of specialized absorption can facilitate a comprehension of disease states that can result from segmental intestinal disease or resection.

Endocrine Function

The small intestine is the largest endocrine organ in the body. A variety of hormonal signals act in endocrine, paracrine, autocrine, and neurotransmitting functions. Collectively, these substances help to regulate intestinal secretion and motility, and provide trophic influences on the GI organs, including the gut mucosa, liver, and pancreas. Secretin, cholecystokinin, motilin, gastric inhibitory peptide (GIP), VIP, gastrin releasing peptide, somatostatin, neurotensin, peptide YY (PYY), and glucagon-like peptide 2 (GLP-2) are prominent among the agents elaborated by the small bowel that impact these processes. Secretin is produced by duodenal S cells in response to acid or bile and stimulates pancreatic production of bicarbonate and water. Cholecystokinin is released by proximal small bowel mucosa in response to fatty acids and certain amino acids and facilitates gallbladder emptying and pancreatic enzyme secretion (formerly also called pancreozymin). Motilin is produced in the jejunum and helps coordinate stomach and lower esophageal sphincter function with small intestinal activity during fasting. GIP is produced by jejunal K cells and stimulates insulin release in response to luminal carbohydrate and fat. VIP stimulates pancreatic and intestinal secretion, inhibits gastric secretion, and functions primarily as a neuropeptide. Neurotensin is secreted in response to fat, stimulates pancreatic exocrine secretion, facilitates fat absorption, and has important mucosal trophic effects. Gastrin-releasing peptide stimulates release of all intestinal hormones except secretin, helps regulate gastric acid and gastrin secretion (enterogastrone function), and has important mucosal trophic effects as well. Somatostatin is found in many organs, including the small bowel, and acts as an "off" switch for intestinal hormone, gastric, and pancreatic secretion, as well as intestinal motility. PYY is found in the distal small bowel and proximal colon; it affects gastric and pancreatic secretion and provides trophic influences on the intestinal mucosa. GLP-2 is one of a family of peptides previously termed enteroglucagon and is a potent small intestinal trophic hormone. Our understanding of the various roles of these agents and their interactions with other regulatory systems, including the gut neural system, continues to expand and offers the potential for therapeutic manipulation. Examples of the latter include the use of somatostatin to suppress pancreatic and GI fistula output, or to regulate neuroendocrine tumors of the intestinal tract, and the use of erythromycin as a motilin agonist to stimulate gastric motility.

Immune Function

The immune function of the small intestine is significant in protecting the body against a host of pathogens that gain access via the GI tract. Antigen processing and the development of cellular and humoral immunity, coordinated via the GALT, plays a complementary role to the functions of peristalsis, enzyme and mucus secretion, and competitive influences of the intestinal microflora in protecting against disease. The synthesis and secretion of immunoglobulin A (IgA), in particular by plasma cells in the lamina propria, is a paramount function of the gut immune system. Such IgA is secreted into the intestinal lumen and serves to suppress bacterial growth and adherence to epithelial cells. IgA also can neutralize bacterial toxins and viruses.

DISEASES OF THE SMALL INTESTINE

Small Bowel Obstruction

The most frequent indication for surgery on the small intestine is bowel obstruction. With obstruction, the lumen of the small intestine is blocked causing the small bowel effluent to back up, resulting in abdominal distension, nausea, and vomiting. SBOs are classified as complete, in which no effluent can pass through the point of obstruction, or partial, if there is some passage of small bowel contents. Depending on the mechanism of the obstruction, the mesentery of the small intestine can be compromised causing strangulation of the intestine with resulting ischemia and potentially bowel necrosis. A closed loop obstruction refers to a type of complete obstruction where a portion of small intestine is obstructed both proximally and distally. A closed loop obstruction is at high risk for strangulation and requires immediate surgical attention.

Etiology of Small Bowel Obstruction
Extrinsic Causes

Potential etiologies for SBO are listed in Table 14-1. The most common causes of SBO are in fact extrinsic to the small bowel itself. In industrialized nations postsurgical adhesions, or scar tissue, is the most frequent cause of SBO. Adhesions are present in at least two-thirds of patients who have undergone prior intraperitoneal surgery and in more than 90% of patients who have had two or more prior intra-abdominal operations. These adhesions can cause kinking of the small intestine, resulting in an obstructed bowel. Overall, 5% to 10% of patients who have had prior abdominal surgery will subsequently have symptoms of SBO. Postsurgical, adhesive SBO thus constitutes a significant public health problem in industrialized countries. Adhesions may less frequently be the cause of obstruction during or following acute inflammatory illnesses of the peritoneal organs managed without surgery, such as acute diverticulitis, cholecystitis, appendicitis, pelvic inflammatory disease, or endometriosis.

In areas of the world where abdominal surgery is uncommon, hernia, usually inguinal or umbilical, is the most common cause of SBO. Under these circumstances, a loop of small intestine protrudes through the defect in the abdominal wall and becomes entrapped in the hernia sac. The kinking of the intestine at the neck of the hernia creates the bowel obstruction. If rapidly identified, the bowel can be pushed back into the abdominal cavity, alleviating the bowel obstruction. Such a hernia is considered reducible. However, if the bowel is not rapidly reduced, then swelling and distention will occur. Soon, even with pressure, the bowel cannot be returned into the abdominal cavity. The hernia is now considered irreducible

TABLE 14-1	Classification of Adult Mechanical Intestinal Obstructions

Intraluminal

Foreign bodies

Barium inspissation (colon)

Bezoar

Inspissated feces

Gallstone

Meconium (cystic fibrosis)

Parasites

Other (e.g., swallowed objects, enteroliths)

Intussusception (usually associated with tumor in adults)

Polypoid, exophytic lesions

Intramural

Congenital (rare in adults)

  Atresia, stricture, or stenosis

  Web

  Intestinal duplication

  Meckel's diverticulum

Inflammatory process

  Crohn's disease

  Diverticulitis

  Chronic intestinal ischemia or postischemic stricture

  Radiation enteritis

  Medication induced (nonsteroidal antiinflammatory drugs, potassium chloride tablets)

Neoplasms

  Primary bowel (malignant or benign)

  Secondary (metastases, especially melanoma)

Traumatic (e.g., intramural hematoma of duodenum)

Extrinsic

Adhesions

Congenital

  Ladd or Meckel's bands

  Postoperative

  Postinflammatory (after PID)

Hernias

  External

  Internal

Volvulus

External mass effect

  Abscess

  Annular pancreas

  Carcinomatosis

  Endometriosis

  Pregnancy

  Pancreatic pseudocyst

Used with permission from Saund M, Soybel DL. Ileus and bowel obstruction. In: Mulholland MW, et al. eds. Greenfield's Surgery: Scientific Principles & Practice. 4th ed. Philadelphia, PA: Lippincott Williams & Wilkins, 2006:769.

and the bowel obstruction persists. Frequently, an irreducible hernia has a very narrow neck, which also obstructs the blood flow to the obstructed segment, resulting in strangulation of the affected bowel. Persistent strangulation eventually leads to intestinal necrosis. Therefore, to prevent this dreaded complication, a SBO caused by an irreducible hernia is considered a surgical emergency, requiring immediate operative intervention. A hernia in which only the antimesenteric portion of the small bowel in entrapped, or so-called Richter's hernia, may present as an irreducible mass without bowel obstruction, since the lumen is not completely compromised with persisting patency along the mesenteric aspect. Rarely, SBO can be caused by internal hernias related to mesenteric defects or recesses in an area where the bowel transfers from a retroperitoneal to an intraperitoneal location (e.g., paraduodenal). Since obstructed small bowel within an internal hernia is also at high risk for strangulation, urgent surgical intervention is indicated. A modern clinical example of this is the internal hernias that develop after a laparoscopic gastric bypass. After this procedure, small mesenteric defects can be created through which small bowel can herniate, causing obstruction and potentially strangulation. Obstructions in this scenario therefore require prompt surgical intervention since delays can prove catastrophic.

Metastatic peritoneal cancer, or carcinomatosis, is another common cause of extrinsic SBO. Metastatic peritoneal implants, commonly from ovarian or colon cancer, may compress the small bowel lumen, causing an intestinal obstruction. Unfortunately, this process is often multifocal and therefore may be incurable, but palliative management to relieve the obstruction remains appropriate even in such settings.

Other less common causes of extrinsic SBOs include volvulus and the SMA syndrome. Volvulus, which is the twisting of the small bowel, usually on its mesentery, may occur because of postsurgical adhesive fixation of the bowel, or as a function of congenital malrotation or bands. A closed loop of intestine results, causing the obstruction. Since this twisting often involves the mesentery, a suspected small bowel volvulus is at high risk for strangulation and requires immediate attention (Figure 14-2). Finally, a, duodenal obstruction may be seen in patients with the SMA syndrome. In this setting, typically evolving in a setting of rapid and significant weight loss, the third portion of the duodenum may be compressed by the acute

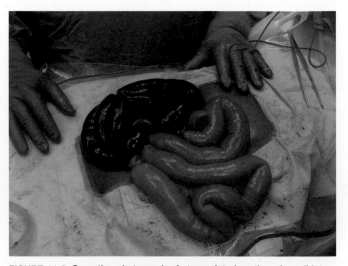

FIGURE 14-2. Operative photograph of strangulated portion of small intestine and adjacent normal small intestine. The strangulation was due to an adhesive band leading to a volvulus of the strangulated segment.

angle between the SMA at its takeoff from the aorta and the aorta itself. Diagnosis often is made with lateral arteriography or other imaging studies, which, in the appropriate clinical setting, document the point of obstruction at this specific location.

Intrinsic Causes

Diseases intrinsic to the small bowel often cause thickening of the bowel wall. If this process continues, the lumen slowly becomes compromised forming a stricture within the small intestine. While liquid may pass, any solid or undigested particles may not be able to pass through the narrowed lumen, causing crampy abdominal pain. Strictures can be classified as benign or malignant. The most common cause for a benign stricture is from Crohn's disease (see below). Other less common causes of a benign stricture include radiation enteritis, ulcers associated with chronic nonsteroidal anti-inflammatory drug (NSAID) use and anastomotic strictures following a previous small bowel resection. Malignant strictures can be caused by any primary small bowel malignancy, such as adenocarcinoma, GI stromal tumors or lymphoma, or by a tumor metastatic to the small intestine, such as malignant melanoma. Bowel obstructions from strictures are often incomplete and more commonly have an insidious onset. Many patients will note weeks of crampy abdominal pain with associated weight loss. Since the mesentery is not compromised, strangulation is not likely. Most malignant strictures will eventually require surgery, but many benign strictures may resolve with nonsurgical options.

Intraluminal Causes

Less commonly, a SBO results from the intraluminal impaction of a foreign body. In general, most foreign bodies that can be swallowed and negotiate the pylorus will pass through the small bowel. However, in some patients the ileocecal valve produces a slight narrowing that may form a barrier for some larger foreign bodies. In these situations, the foreign body becomes impacted at the valve and a bowel obstruction develops. Phytobezoars are concretions of poorly digested fruit and vegetable fiber that can be the cause of an intraluminal obstruction. So-called gallstone ileus, in which a large gallstone erodes through the gallbladder into an adjacent loop of adherent intestine in the setting of cholecystitis, can also be an etiology for SBO, particularly in the elderly population. The stone typically migrates to the distal small bowel and causes obstruction of the intestinal lumen, usually at or near the ileocecal valve.

Intussusception, in which a portion of the intestine telescopes on itself leading to obstruction, can occur spontaneously in small children. Intussusception in adults is uncommon and usually is due to peristalsis acting on a "lead point" such as an intraluminal polyp or tumor. Therefore, even if the intussusception were to resolve, a thorough evaluation of the small intestine, usually with a small bowel follow through, is warranted.

Pathophysiology

Fluid deficits frequently evolve as a function of emesis, decreased absorption, and hormonally stimulated secretion triggered by luminal distension. As the process progresses, "third space" losses due to bowel wall edema and transudation of fluid into the peritoneal cavity may also occur. Electrolyte abnormalities can vary with the location of the obstruction and duration of illness.

The most serious complication of SBO is strangulation of the involved intestine. In this setting, more common with closed loop and high grade or complete obstructions, the bowel becomes ischemic and eventually infarcts as edema and kinking of the mesentery impact mesenteric vascular patency. Local or systemic sepsis, and frank perforation of the affected bowel, may supervene. A number of clinical and laboratory parameters have been used in an attempt to predict progression of obstruction to the point of strangulation. Fever, tachycardia, leukocytosis, and localized abdominal tenderness have most commonly been cited as indicators of a higher risk of strangulation. In some series, the risk of strangulation has increased from 7% when one of these signs is present to 67% when all four are noted. However, it is critical to recognize that bowel infarction may evolve even in the absence of these signs, and all four can be present without infarction having occurred. However, if any one of the four is present, prompt surgical intervention is advised since the risk of strangulation does increase. The risk of infarction also appears to rise in patients with high-grade obstruction who are managed nonoperatively for more than 24 to 48 hours, assuming there are no signs of resolution in that time frame.

Clinical Presentation and Evaluation

History

Common presenting symptoms of SBO are detailed in Table 14-2. A detailed past medical history, including notation of prior abdominal surgeries or illnesses, is of utmost importance. Patients should also be asked about prodromal bulges or focal pain that may herald the presence of a hernia. Individuals with vague and chronic symptomatology prior to the onset of

TABLE 14-2	Symptoms and Signs of Bowel Obstruction			
Symptom or Sign	**Proximal Small Bowel (Open Loop)**	**Distal Small Bowel (Open Loop)**	**Small Bowel (Closed Loop)**	**Colon and Rectum**
Pain	Intermittent, intense, colicky, often relieved by vomiting	Intermittent to constant	Progressive, intermittent to constant, rapidly worsens	Continuous
Vomiting	Large volumes, bilious and frequent	Low volume and frequency; progressively feculent with time	May be prominent (reflex)	Intermittent, not prominent, feculent when present
Tenderness	Epigastric or periumbilical; quite mild unless strangulation is present	Diffuse and progressive	Diffuse, progressive	Diffuse
Distention	Absent	Moderate to marked	Often absent	Marked
Obstipation	May not be present	Present	May not be present	Present

Used with permission from Saund M, Soybel DL. Ileus and bowel obstruction. In: Mulholland MW, et al. eds. *Greenfield's Surgery: Scientific Principles & Practice,* 4th ed. Philadelphia, PA: Lippincott Williams & Wilkins, 2006:770. Adapted from Schuffler MD, Sinanan MN. Intestinal obstruction and pseudo-obstruction. In: Sleisenger MH, Fordtran JS, eds. *Gastrointestinal Disease.* 5th ed. Philadelphia: WB Saunders, 1993:898.

frank obstructive symptoms may have underlying disease states, such as inflammatory disease or neoplasia. The typical onset of acute SBO is marked by colicky abdominal pain in the periumbilical region, given the midgut autonomic innervation pathways of the majority of the small intestine. Pain may become steadier as peristaltic activity lessens and generalized bowel distension progresses with the diathesis. As mentioned above, pain and tenderness that begin to localize in a more somatic pattern should heighten concern for bowel ischemia and peritonitis with attendant parietal peritoneal irritation. Nausea and vomiting are prominent complaints in many patients, although the onset of these symptoms may be delayed in more distal obstructions due to small bowel capacitance. Abdominal distension is also more prominent with distal obstruction for the same reason and may be unimpressive with very proximal obstructions. Constipation, and in particular the lack of any flatus (obstipation), is a particularly ominous sign for higher grade obstruction, but may not be immediate given the potential for passage of air and stool already in the colon at the onset of illness. Conversely, in partial SBO, passage of stool, including even loose stools, and some flatus may persist despite the obstructive process.

Examination

Patients with SBO typically present after a period of pain, often associated with nausea and vomiting, and attendant fluid and electrolyte disturbance. Patients may appear acutely distressed in the early, colicky phases of the illness or may appear lethargic as dehydration and electrolyte disturbances ensue. Tachycardia, dry mucous membranes, decreased skin turgor, and even relative hypotension may be seen in more advanced cases. The abdomen is frequently distended, again depending on the location of the obstruction, and may be tympanitic if the intestine is distended with air or dull to percussion if the bowel loops are fluid filled or ascites has evolved. On auscultation, high-pitched sounds and rushes may be noted early in the illness, and a dearth of bowel activity is characteristic as distension progresses or peritonitis ensues. Surgical scars and areas of potential herniation should be carefully examined. In obese patients, areas of focal contour change, erythema, or tenderness near a surgical scar may be the only clue to bowel incarceration within an otherwise occult hernia. Diffuse mild tenderness is frequent and often will improve after acute decompression via a nasogastric tube, assuming bowel ischemia has not already occurred. Patients with impressive persistent tenderness or more advanced peritoneal signs such as percussion tenderness, rebound tenderness, and fear of movement may have already progressed to advanced disease, and such findings should prompt more urgent surgical intervention.

Radiographic Studies

An abdominal series including supine and upright abdominal films and an upright chest radiograph are the most valuable initial studies. These studies may document other processes, which can mimic the presentation of SBO. Specific inspection should be made for renal or biliary calculi, pneumoperitoneum ("free air"), pneumatosis intestinalis, pneumobilia, and pneumonia. In the absence of confounding illness, typical findings would include bowel distension proximal to the point of obstruction and collapse of the bowel, manifest by nonvisualization on the radiograph, distal to the same point (Figure 14-3). Air fluid levels may be seen on upright films and denote lack of normal propulsive activity in affected loops of

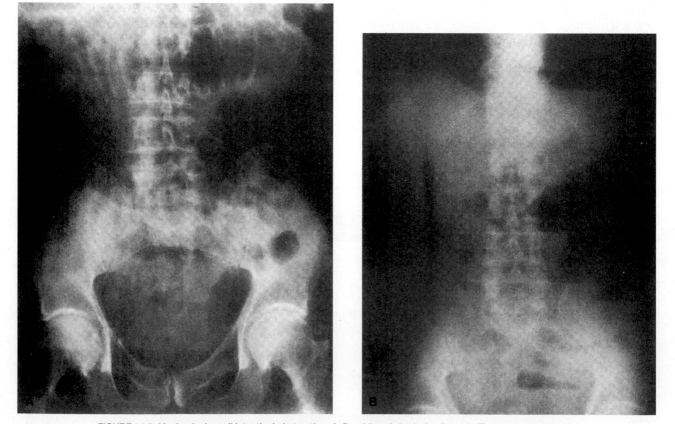

FIGURE 14-3. Mechanical small intestinal obstruction. A, Decubitus abdominal radiograph. There are many centrally located loops of air-filled small intestine and no gas at the periphery of the abdomen. Valvulae conniventes are shown. B, Upright abdominal radiograph. Multiple air-filled levels are seen.

intestine. Focal loops of intestine that are persistently abnormal on serial films may represent closed loop obstruction. It is important to recognize that fluid-filled loops of obstructed bowel may blend with other soft tissue densities on radiography and mislead the clinician who does not see a "typical" obstructive pattern. On the other hand, if the bowel is massively distended with air, it may be difficult to distinguish the small and large bowel. In such settings, water-soluble contrast enema may help to exclude the possibility of a large bowel obstructive mechanism.

Computed tomography (CT) may be very useful in settings of diagnostic confusion, given its ability to delineate confounding illnesses such as nephrolithiasis, diverticulitis, and pancreatitis, or mesenteric vascular disease. It also has the capacity to demonstrate dilated, fluid-filled small intestinal loops, which as noted above can be missed on plain films and may even demonstrate a transition zone between dilated and decompressed small intestine, documenting SBO as the source of illness (Figure 14-4). It can accomplish many of these goals even without administration of oral contrast and is assuming a more prominent role in evaluating the patient with suspected SBO.

Contrast studies of the small intestine are useful in the patient with persistent partial obstructive symptoms, or when it is difficult to distinguish paralytic ileus from mechanical obstruction. It is important before pursuing such studies to be confident one does not need to exclude colonic obstruction or mesenteric occlusive disease, since the contrast enema and angiogram used to evaluate for these entities may be obscured by the contrast used for the small bowel follow through study. Small bowel contrast studies are usually not necessary in the

acute, high grade setting, in which clinical findings, plain film results, and CT are typically adequate to guide management.

Laboratory Data

Laboratory data are not specific in SBO but may be of value in excluding other pathologies and guiding resuscitation. Leukocytosis, particularly if it persists despite nasogastric decompression and fluid resuscitation, may be a sign of progression toward ischemia. Electrolytes should be closely monitored. A hypokalemic, "contraction" alkalosis is common in patients with advanced dehydration. Hyperamylasemia may be seen with SBO, but if it is marked in degree, it may heighten the suspicion for acute pancreatitis as a confounding illness. Urinalysis is important in excluding evidence for urinary infection or stone disease as a source of symptoms. Lactic acidosis, particularly in the setting of adequate volume administration, may signal bowel ischemia, although frank infarction may be seen without acidosis and its absence should not be over interpreted in the patient who is failing to resolve with appropriate nonoperative measures.

Differential Diagnosis

Paralytic ileus is the most frequent differential diagnostic entity considered in the setting of possible SBO. In this process, bowel motility is suppressed as a consequence of systemic or inflammatory illness, and the bowel may become distended and the patient obstipated in a pattern not unlike that of SBO, despite the lack of a mechanical obstruction. Narcotics, bed rest, trauma, hypothyroidism, electrolyte deficiencies (especially potassium, calcium, magnesium, and phosphate), anesthesia, psychotropic medication, and systemic or peritoneal inflammatory illnesses or sepsis are all common causes of ileus. Pain, nausea and emesis, and abdominal distension may all be seen similar to the pattern of SBO, although subtle differences may be noted in the pattern of these symptoms (Table 14-3). Typically, plain films will demonstrate diffuse bowel dilation, including both the small and large intestine, without evidence of a transition zone (Figure 14-5). Contrast enema to exclude colonic obstruction, and, if this condition is excluded, small bowel contrast study may be required in cases where the distinction between ileus and mechanical obstruction remains difficult.

The development of a postoperative ileus (POI) is common following major abdominal surgery. The cause of POI is multifactorial, but is related to the stress of surgery, fluid and electrolyte imbalances, and pain management, especially with narcotics. After major GI surgery, bowel function is slow to return and is the major reason for the longer hospitalizations

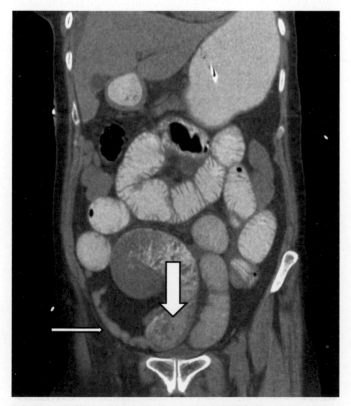

FIGURE 14-4. CT scan demonstrating mechanical SBO. The thick, vertical arrow points to dilated bowel proximal to the point of obstruction. The thin horizontal arrow points to the decompressed distal small bowel, with a clear transition point between these two segments evident on the scan.

TABLE 14-3	Characteristics of Paralytic Ileus and Small Intestinal Obstruction
Paralytic Ileus	**Small Intestinal Obstruction**
Minimal abdominal pain	Crampy abdominal pain
Nausea and vomiting	Nausea and vomiting
Obstipation and failure to pass flatus	Obstipation and failure to pass flatus
Abdominal distension	Abdominal distension
Decreased or absent bowel sounds	Normal or increased bowel sounds
Gas in the small intestine and colon on x-ray	Gas in the small intestine only on x-ray

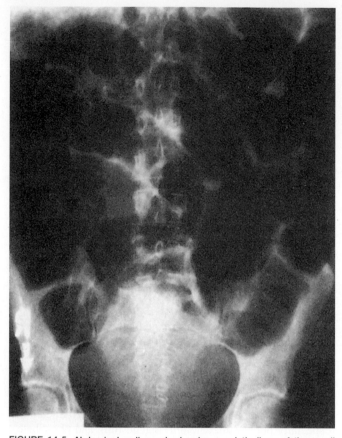

FIGURE 14-5. Abdominal radiograph showing paralytic ileus of the small bowel. This condition is differentiated from mechanical SBO and colonic obstruction by air in the distal sigmoid colon and rectum.

observed following colonic surgery compared with many other abdominal operations. To try and minimize POI, many institutions use a "fast-track" protocol to help limit the duration of the POI. These programs usually include the avoidance of nasogastric tubes, early ambulation, the avoidance of fluid overload and the early introduction of a diet following major GI surgery. Recently, a new medication has also been approved to decrease the length of POI. Alvimopan is an opioid antagonist that specifically targets the mu receptor responsible for the GI side effects of opioids. Alvimopan, which does not cross the blood–brain barrier, therefore selectively blocks the peripheral receptors contributing to POI without significantly altering the central analgesic effects of opioids. In several randomized, placebo-controlled trials, the use of alvimopan seems to have decreased the length of POI and has slightly shortened the hospital stay without a significant impact on pain control. Because of this, the Food and Drug Administration (FDA) has recently approved alvimopan for the treatment of POI and this medication is now available in many hospitals. How this will ultimately affect POI and hospital costs still remains to be seen.

Treatment

Treatment for SBO begins with resuscitation. Correction of fluid and electrolyte deficits should commence even as initial diagnostic studies are being accomplished. Typically, this will include intravenous volume replacement with isotonic solutions, tailored and supplemented as dictated by any specific electrolyte abnormalities encountered. It is important to establish euvolemia before aggressively replacing electrolytes such as potassium, since rapid rises in the serum level may be

encountered if renal perfusion has not been restored. Frequent assessment of urine output via a Foley catheter is the best simple tool for assessing adequacy of volume replacement and may be supplemented in the setting of complicated cardiac disease by invasive central pressure monitoring, if necessary. In adults, an hourly urine output of at least 0.5 mL/kg is usually indicative of adequate volume resuscitation. Nasogastric decompression is commenced via nasogastric tube placement to control emesis, relieve intestinal distension proximal to the obstruction, lower the risk of aspiration, and allow monitoring of ongoing fluid and electrolyte losses. The patient is given nothing per mouth and followed closely for response to initial resuscitation.

If the obstruction is partial or low grade and there is a history of prior abdominal surgery with no palpable hernia, the obstruction is likely adhesive in nature, with an approximately 80% chance of resolution if the above measures are followed. Patients who have incarcerated herniae should have reduction of the same, if possible, and close observation thereafter to ensure that the obstructive process resolves. It is important to be aware that occasionally a "reduction en mass" can occur, in which the hernia sac is reduced with the contents as a unit, and therefore the contents may remain compromised despite being internalized. An unsuccessful reduction may manifest as persistent pain or tenderness, with or without inflammatory examination or laboratory signs. Repair of the hernia following resolution of any obstructive signs should then be accomplished to prevent recurrence. Nonreducible herniae should be urgently repaired following rapid volume resuscitation and correction of any severe electrolyte disturbances. Individuals who have no prior surgery or externally demonstrable herniae on which to blame the obstruction should be prepared for surgery, provided the diagnosis seems clear, since a high percentage of such patients will have conditions such as neoplastic lesions or internal herniae that will require operative management. Similarly, patients with complete or high grade obstructions should generally be prepared for prompt surgical intervention, since in this setting the likelihood of resolution is diminished and the risk of bowel ischemia heightened. Patients in whom nonoperative therapy is initially justified should be taken to surgery if there is not definite clinical and radiologic improvement within 24 to 48 hours, or sooner if there is evidence of deterioration as manifest by exam changes, fluid requirements, radiologic signs, or laboratory parameters. The risk of bowel compromise increases after that time frame provided there is no evidence of improvement. Settings in which a longer period of observation and conservative, nonsurgical management may be appropriate include early postoperative obstructions, the majority of which may resolve within 2 weeks as acute, bulky adhesions and associated postoperative bowel edema begin to mature and resolve, respectively. Patients with known carcinomatosis, with recurrent obstructions in the setting of multiple prior operations and a known hostile abdomen, or with known radiation enteritis may also be candidates for a longer period of nonoperative management.

If surgery is required, preoperative antibiotics are given to cover gram-negative aerobes and anaerobes, which may proliferate in the normally sterile, but now obstructed and stagnant, small bowel. At laparotomy, adhesions are mobilized, herniae reduced and repaired, and the bowel carefully inspected to ensure integrity of its blood supply. If there is question in regard to bowel viability, intraoperative assessment with fluorescein dye or Doppler ultrasound to assess perfusion may augment clinical evaluations of bowel viability such as color, bleeding, and peristalsis. No test is foolproof, and if the surgeon has significant concern, a second-look operation in 24 hours may be appropriate. Care to not be overly aggressive in resection is especially important in patients with underlying Crohn's disease, or when the amount of remaining small intestine is approaching the 100 cm range, after which there would be a high likelihood of dependence on long-term parenteral nutrition. Clearly compromised bowel should be resected. If neoplasia is found, an appropriate resection is accomplished. In general, it is possible to reanastomose the small bowel primarily, although delay of this until a second look operation in the acute and questionably viable setting, or following temporary stoma diversion in complicated situations, is occasionally necessary. If intussusception is found in the adult, resection because of the high likelihood of a lead point lesion should be accomplished. In children, spontaneous intussusception is often able to be managed nonoperatively with pneumatic or contrast enema reduction.

A number of series have now been published evaluating the use of laparoscopy in SBO. While success with this approach in a modest number of cases is well documented, hazards with laparoscopic access and bowel manipulation in the face of distension limit the widespread application of this technique, particularly in the multiply reoperated and surgically hostile abdomen. Interest in this area, and successful use particularly with uncomplicated adhesive obstructions, will likely continue to evolve in the future.

Complications

Wound infection, anastomotic leak, abscess, peritonitis, and fistula formation may all complicate operative intervention for SBO, especially when bowel infarction and/or resection have occurred. Overall, mortality is <1% for laparotomy in the setting of uncomplicated SBO but may exceed 25% when strangulation or perforation has occurred. With extensive resection, short bowel syndrome can eventuate and necessitate long-term parenteral access and nutritional support. Recurrent obstruction may also be seen, as in any postlaparotomy patient. Interest in prevention of recurrent obstruction with chemical or barrier devices intended to limit adhesion formation continues, although to date there is insufficient evidence of efficacy to justify routine use. Currently, a commercially available barrier composed of sodium hyaluronate and carboxymethylcellulose has been shown to be effective in decreasing adhesions after laparotomy. However, it has not been proven to diminish the incidence of recurrent bowel obstruction in prospective studies.

Crohn's Disease of the Small Intestine

Significance and Incidence

Crohn's disease, first described in 1932, has a worldwide prevalence of 10 to 70 cases per 100,000 population. A detailed understanding of its underlying cause remains elusive. It occurs primarily in industrialized nations and appears to be related to underlying genetic as well as environmental factors. First-degree relatives of affected patients have a demonstrably higher risk of the disease than the general population, and disease concordance is significantly higher in monozygotic than dizygotic twins, suggesting a genetic correlation. The *IBD1* locus on chromosome 16 has been identified as a consistent linkage in kindreds with high incidences of Crohn's disease.

It is likely that multiple genomic regions may be involved, and the precise genes and gene products that may predispose to the disease continue to be elucidated. Environmental factors that have been implicated include NSAIDs use and smoking. Current understanding would suggest that, under the influence of predisposing genetic and environmental factors, sustained mucosal immune responses to luminal microflora are responsible for the disease.

The timing of onset of disease has a bimodal distribution, with an early peak in the late teens and early twenties, and a later one in the sixth and seventh decades. The distribution of the disease can be anywhere from the mouth to the anus, although small intestinal and colonic involvement are most common. The ileocecal area is involved in 40% to 50% of patients, the small intestine only in 30% to 40%, and isolated colonic involvement is seen in 20%. The disease may go into prolonged remission but tends to have a recurring course with intermittent flares or exacerbations, and is not curable. As such, it is a significant public health problem.

Pathophysiology

Crohn's disease is a chronic, transmural inflammatory condition of the alimentary tract and may include extraintestinal manifestations affecting the skin, eyes, mouth, joints, and biliary system (see also Clinical Presentation below). Inflammatory bowel disease patients, including those with Crohn's disease, appear to have an increased number of surface adherent and intracellular bacteria in the bowel epithelium, and may have genetically determined abnormal host immune responses that allow for continued immune activation and changes in the epithelial mucosal barrier. The end result of this sustained immune and inflammatory response, mediated by a wide range of cytokines, arachidonic acid metabolites (including prostaglandins), and reactive oxygen metabolites (including nitric oxide), is tissue destruction and clinically manifest disease. As outlined above, it appears likely, based on current understanding, that a combination of genetic, environmental, and microflora-induced events leads to the evolution of disease in a complex, synergistic fashion. No specific genetic alteration, infectious agent, or environmental stimulus single-handedly explains this process.

Crohn's disease can be distinguished from chronic ulcerative colitis (CUC) by a number of its clinical features, although approximately 10% of cases remain "indeterminate" after careful investigation. This may include patients treated for years for CUC, including with total proctocolectomy and pouch reconstruction, who later develop manifestations of Crohn's disease. Common distinguishing features are detailed in Table 15-6, Chapter 15, Colon, Rectum, and Anus. Recognized distinctions include the tendency of Crohn's to involve segments of the GI tract other than the colon, with areas of sparing ("skip areas") between affected areas. Transmural involvement and the associated tendency to develop fistulae, as well as the presence of noncaseating granulomata on histology, are also characteristic of Crohn's. Ulcerative colitis, on the other hand, is a mucosal disease, always involves the rectum, and may spread in confluent fashion proximally in the colon, but without skip areas. It does not affect the small intestine (except as so-called backwash ileitis). Because of its transmural nature and tendency to have periods of remission and exacerbation, Crohn's also may lead to the development of fibrotic strictures and obstructive symptomatology.

On gross inspection, the bowel involved with Crohn's may demonstrate fat wrapping or creeping of the mesenteric fat

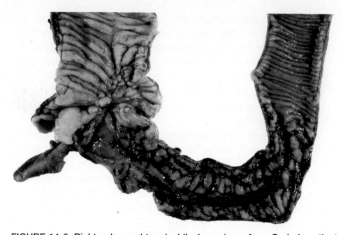

FIGURE 14-6. Right colon and terminal ileal specimen from Crohn's patient demonstrating narrowing of the diseased segment related to chronic transmural inflammation.

up onto the bowel serosa, and the bowel itself may appear thickened (Figure 14-6) and erythematous. The mesentery is often thickened and shortened and harbors lymphadenopathic nodes. Adherence of inflamed loops of bowel to the parietes, bladder, and other loops of intestine, with or without frank fistula formation, may be seen. If fistulization occurs, abscesses may also be noted, including retroperitoneal and intra-abdominal abscesses. With repeated episodes of inflammation, the bowel wall may become increasingly fibrotic, resulting in the formation of fibrostenotic strictures. Perianal fistulae are a particularly vexing manifestation of Crohn's and are more common in patients with colorectal involvement than in patients with isolated small bowel disease.

The bowel mucosa may exhibit aphthoid ulceration, fissures, and crypt abscesses on endoscopic and histologic review. Noncaseating granulomata are characteristic and are seen in 60% of cases histologically, although they may be missed on endoscopic biopsy, which typically samples only the mucosa.

Clinical Presentation

The common presenting triad of Crohn's includes abdominal pain, diarrhea, and weight loss. The symptoms are typically gradual in onset and progressive over time, although a waxing and waning of symptom severity is common. The pain can be related to partial obstruction due to edema and, in more established cases, fibrosis. In such settings, patients may have associated nausea and vomiting, and may notice increased symptoms when higher residue foods are consumed. Right lower quadrant pain is frequent, based on the frequency of ileocecal involvement, although other areas may well be affected depending on disease distribution. Bleeding is uncommon with Crohn's, in contradistinction to ulcerative colitis, in which bloody diarrhea is a relatively frequent presentation. As the disease progresses, constitutional symptoms including malaise, fatigue, fever, weight loss, and anorexia are common.

Perianal involvement, particularly irregular and multiple anal fistulae, should heighten the concern of Crohn's disease. Fissures and abscesses may also occur. Perianal manifestations are most common in patients with colonic involvement, although they can be seen in patients who otherwise appear to have isolated small bowel disease. Occasionally, intervention on what appears to be a simple perianal abscess or fistula will

lead to poor wound healing or incomplete response to treatment, which may be a harbinger of Crohn's.

Extraintestinal manifestations of Crohn's are more common when colonic disease is present, and may include ocular (conjunctivitis, iritis, uveitis, iridocyclitis, episcleritis), skin (pyoderma gangrenosum, erythema nodosum), joint (ankylosing spondylitis, hypertrophic osteoarthropathy, arthritis), and biliary manifestations (sclerosing cholangitis, pericholangitis, granulomatous hepatitis), as well as vasculitis and aphthous stomatitis. Often these manifestations will respond to control of the underlying bowel disease.

Nutritional losses frequently accompany Crohn's disease due to diminished oral intake and impaired absorption, particularly with terminal ileal disease. Hypoalbuminemia, deficiencies of fat-soluble vitamins (A, D, E, and K), and deficiencies of vitamin B_{12} may be seen. Gallstones are frequent in long-standing disease, due to lithogenic bile brought on by loss of terminal ileal bile salt reabsorption. Growth retardation and developmental delays are accordingly common in younger patients. Nutritional support, given parenterally or enterally depending on the patient's presentation, can correct these deficits and is a critical part of early treatment in the patient with more advanced disease.

While some patients present with urgent issues such as acute bowel obstruction or abscess, the majority of patients presents with a more indolent course. There are no laboratory studies specific for the diagnosis, and careful evaluation of the history and presenting findings is important in triggering diagnostic suspicion. In the nonemergent setting, endoscopic and contrast evaluations of the GI tract will often help establish the likely diagnosis. Colonoscopy with visualization of the terminal ileum, or barium enema with inspection of the terminal ileum as well, and small bowel contrast studies (Figure 14-7) are the most useful diagnostic evaluations. Findings may include ulceration, edema, stricture, or fistula formation. In patients with signs or symptoms of abscess or mass effect, or when other diagnostic possibilities are also under consideration, CT may be very helpful and may demonstrate phlegmon, abscess, bowel thickening, partial obstruction, and, occasionally, fistulae. Enteroclysis study of the small intestine may be helpful when standard small bowel follow through is inconclusive. This test involves intubation of the small intestine with injection of air and contrast to allow mucosal detail to be outlined more precisely than can be achieved with standard small bowel contrast examination or CT enterography. Endoscopic biopsies may be helpful, but because they sample primarily mucosa, often fail histologically to prove the diagnosis of Crohn's. Esophagogastroduodenoscopic examination and/or upper GI contrast examination may also be important in the patient suspected of having foregut involvement. Capsule endoscopy, discussed more fully later in this chapter, has been employed increasingly for diagnosis of Crohn's as well as other small intestine pathology in settings where standard endoscopic and radiologic assessments are inconclusive. It is important to rule out a stricture before doing such a study, as the capsule may be retained at the stricture if this is not recognized. Cystography or cystoscopy, and detailed vaginal examination, may also be helpful in the patient with suspected urinary or vaginal fistulae.

Differential Diagnosis

Crohn's disease and ulcerative colitis may be hard to distinguish, particularly when the involvement is primarily colonic

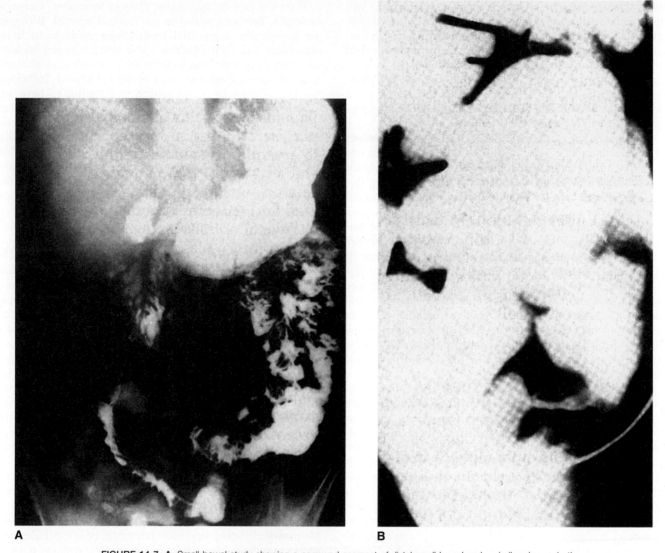

A   B

FIGURE 14-7. A, Small bowel study showing a narrowed segment of distal small bowel and a similar change in the antrum of the stomach. The mucosal pattern of the bowel is altered by pseudopolyps, and the valvulae conniventes are absent. The upper small bowel suggests skip areas of Crohn's involvement, whereas the distal bowel is narrowed and contiguously involved with Crohn's disease. **B,** Small bowel study showing the "string sign of Kantor" in the terminal ileum adjacent to the cecum, with proximal dilation of the ileum.

and diffuse. Other colitides may also be hard to differentiate in the acute setting, although they generally lack the prodromal illness common in the Crohn's patient. Acute appendicitis, acute regional ileitis due to *Yersinia* infection, pelvic inflammatory disease, and tuberculosis of the bowel may also be confounding diagnostic possibilities.

Treatment
Medical Therapy
Medical management of Crohn's disease can include a variety of measures that control symptoms, compensate for side effects of the disease, and impact the underlying inflammatory process. Symptom management can include analgesic therapy and suppression of bowel motility, as well as wound care measures for patients with fistulae. Compensatory therapy typically includes fluid, and often nutritional, management, preferably using enteral approaches, although parenteral administration and complete bowel rest are not uncommonly required for severe disease. Control of the inflammatory diathesis can often be achieved with an expanding array of pharmacologic agents.

Antidiarrheal agents including loperamide, diphenoxylate, codeine, and cholestyramine may help in symptom management. They should be used with care and have their greatest utility in patients with chronic diarrhea related to short bowel from prior resections or chronic diarrhea not associated with obstructive features. They can lead to paralytic ileus, bacterial overgrowth, and even toxic megacolon if used injudiciously. Cholestyramine has its greatest efficacy in patients with bile salt-induced diarrhea due to ileal disease and/or resection. Simple lactose avoidance and/or use of lactase supplementation may also help with diarrheal symptomatology.

Nutritional support is often required in patients with chronic and subacute presentations. Enteral nutrition, with its capacity to preserve mucosal and hepatic cellular structural integrity and function, its lower cost, and its superior safety profile, is preferable. Elemental diets have not been demonstrated to be superior to standard enteral formulae, and while they have the theoretical appeal of minimizing the work of digestion, are generally not palatable and require tube administration. Patients with obstructive features, severe disease, and fistulae (especially proximal small bowel fistulae) will often require parenteral administration. Replacement of vitamins including those absorbed in the terminal ileum as outlined above is frequently necessary. In severely malnourished patients, refeeding syndrome should be anticipated as feedings are commenced. Particular attention to the serum phosphate and potassium levels is necessary in this regard, since chronic depletion becomes taxed by the sudden need to process and store intracellular energy substrates.

A broad array of pharmacologic agents can assist in inducing and maintaining disease remission. Sulfasalazine was one of the first agents recognized to have efficacy, particularly for colonic disease, when it was noted that patients taking this drug for arthritic complaints would often note improvement if they had concomitant colitis. In the distal ileum and colon, intestinal bacteria remove the sulfonamide moiety of sulfasalazine, and the 5-aminosalicylate component is thereby released where it may exert anti-inflammatory effects. It appears this effect may be due to the inhibition of nuclear factor kappa B, which is a potent inflammatory cytokine. It may also limit production of prostaglandins and leukotrienes and assist as a scavenger of reactive oxygen metabolites. Newer preparations of 5-aminosalicylic acid (mesalamine) allow delivery of this agent without the sulfonamide moiety to the more proximal small bowel based on pH-dependent or slow release matrices.

Corticosteroids have significant efficacy in Crohn's disease, particularly when it is unresponsive to 5-aminosalicylate compounds. Topical agents are useful for disease limited to the distal colon, but do not impact small bowel disease. Prednisone in doses up to 60 mg/day can be used orally for more severe disease. A clinical response is seen in the majority of patients within 7 to 10 days of treatment. Intravenous steroids such as hydrocortisone or methylprednisolone can be used for patients unable to tolerate enteral dosing. Budesonide, which is 90% eliminated on first-pass metabolism in the liver, offers the hope of luminal steroid benefit while minimizing systemic toxicities. The latter correlate with the dose and duration of therapy and include hypertension, cataracts, osteoporosis, weight gain, striae, and adrenal suppression. Budesonide has its greatest effect on terminal ileal and right-sided colonic disease and is slightly less efficacious, overall, than conventional corticosteroids.

Immunosuppressive and immune modulating agents including azathioprine, 6-mercaptopurine, methotrexate, cyclosporine, tacrolimus, and mycophenolate mofetil may be useful, particularly in patients unresponsive to steroids, or as part of a strategy to minimize steroid requirements and toxicity in patients remaining dependent on the same. Azathioprine and 6-mercaptopurine, to which azathioprine is metabolized in red blood cells, take 3 to 6 months to achieve effect. They have been shown to be of value in preventing relapse of disease once remission has been medically or surgically induced, a benefit that steroids lack. GI side effects including liver function abnormalities and pancreatitis may be seen with these agents, as may bone marrow toxicity. Methotrexate may also have remission-sustaining benefits. Cyclosporine has been found to be of use in fistulous Crohn's disease unresponsive to other therapies including steroids and antibiotics (especially metronidazole). Particular concern for nephrotoxicity is required with cyclosporine therapy, and prophylaxis for *Pneumocystis carinii* pneumonitis is recommended in patients on continued treatment with this agent.

Over the past decade, a new class of treatment, known as biologics, has been added to the medical arsenal. Biologics are genetically engineered medications made from living organisms and their products. The first approved biologic for Crohn's disease was infliximab, a chimeric monoclonal antibody directed against tumor necrosis factor-α. Infliximab has been shown in recent prospective studies to have significant efficacy in patients with steroid-resistant, moderate to severe Crohn's disease. This agent also has documented effectiveness in the management of enterocutaneous fistulae associated with Crohn's disease (including perianal fistulae) and is effective, although expensive, as maintenance therapy. Its major drawback is infusion reactions, thought to be due to the mouse component of the antibody. Because of these reactions, the intravenous infusions must be done in a monitored setting, resulting in very expensive infusion costs. More recently, adalimumab has been approved for the treatment of moderate to severe Crohn's. Adalimumab is also a monoclonal antibody directed against tumor necrosis factor-α. Since adalimumab is 100% human there are less adverse reactions compared with infliximab. Furthermore, adalimumab is administered via a subcutaneous injection and therefore can be done at home. The latest biologic to be approved is certolizumab. As with adalimumab, there seem to be fewer reactions to certolizumab since there is no mouse component. Certolizumab is also a subcutaneous injection but has the added benefit of longer half-life and therefore less frequent administration. Interestingly, despite the fact all these agents seem to work on a similar mechanism, patients may have different responses to different biologics. Therefore, if one seems to be losing its efficacy it may be reasonable to try a different agent.

While a number of other agents are also being investigated as potential treatments for Crohn's, including growth hormone and thalidomide, one class in particular is worthy of brief mention. Probiotics, living organisms as an oral supplement facilitating intestinal microbial balance, have been shown to reduce relapse rates in conjunction with mesalamine therapy and to reduce pouchitis in patients with inflammatory bowel disease who have undergone colectomy and ileal pouch reconstruction. Given the current understanding of microbial stimuli triggering sustained mucosal inflammatory responses as a pathophysiologic mechanism in Crohn's patients, these nonimmunosuppressive agents may offer hope in future management strategies.

Surgical Therapy

Surgical therapy in Crohn's patients is reserved for complicated disease and disease refractory to medical management (Table 14-4). Complications that may require surgical management can include enteric fistulae, obstruction, and

TABLE 14-4	Indications for Surgery, Crohn's Disease

Perforation
Fibrotic stricture
Acute complete bowel obstruction
Chronic partial bowel obstruction
Fistula (e.g., enterocutaneous, enterovesical, enterovaginal)

perforation. Hemorrhage is rarely an indication for surgical intervention in Crohn's disease. Many fistulae can be managed medically, but enterovesical fistulae usually require medical management to prevent recurring urosepsis and eventual renal dysfunction. Because of the likelihood of recurrence of Crohn's disease after surgery (as high as 40% within 5 years and 75% within 15 years of operation), the basic surgical strategy is one of disease management rather than radical extirpation. Thus, with small intestinal disease, limited bowel resection to grossly normal bowel is typically accomplished. There is no need to achieve microscopically normal margins, and indeed overly aggressive resection may predispose the patient long-term to short bowel syndrome, given the propensity for recurrent disease. When recurrence is seen, it is most commonly proximal to the site of prior disease, although this is not always the case. In the setting of fibrotic, chronic strictures, stricturoplasty may be employed to relieve obstructive symptoms and minimize bowel resection.

Because patients with Crohn's often have bacterial colonization of the small intestine and at least partial obstructive pathology, mechanical bowel preparation (when possible) and antibiotic prophylaxis are advisable. Septic, anastomotic, and wound complications are not uncommon. Primary anastomosis is usually possible, although temporary stomas may be required in the setting of advanced peritonitis or the septically complicated patient on immunosuppressive medical therapy. Removal of the appendix to prevent future diagnostic confusion has traditionally been recommended at the time of management of small intestinal Crohn's disease, provided the base of the appendix at the insertion to the cecum is not itself involved, in which case fecal fistula may complicate the appendectomy.

Patients with fistulae who fail to respond to medical management can be managed with resection of the communicating bowel and simple debridement or limited excision of the communicating cutaneous or nonenteric visceral tract. For patients with established abscesses, percutaneous drainage and optimization of medical management, with delayed surgical intervention if necessary, is appropriate. If perianal fistulae fail to respond to medical management, options can include simple drainage of abscesses and placement of setons to ensure ongoing drainage. More aggressive strategies would include fecal diversion or even proctectomy. As a general rule, surgical intervention is limited and conservative for the patient with minor perianal disease, and aggressive incisions or debridements are avoided because of the potential for non-healing of larger postsurgical wounds. Diversion is reserved for the patient with recurring septic insults or perineal soiling despite medical and limited surgical management, and proctectomy for end stage disease unresponsive to other measures. Nearly all patients coming to surgical therapy will require perioperative nutritional support. At the time of any operative intervention, inspection of the entire bowel for skip lesions should be made, and careful documentation of the length of bowel resected and length of small intestine remaining should be made for future reference. As a general rule, patients who maintain 100 cm of small intestine will be able to sustain themselves on oral intake, although the absorptive health of the remaining intestine and presence of an intact ileocecal valve can impact this significantly.

Complications

The complications of Crohn's disease frequently dictate changes in medical or surgical management strategies, indeed define the clinical behavior of the disease, and are therefore substantially outlined in the preceding section. Malnutrition, obstruction, fistulous disease, and electrolyte disturbances are all in this category. The most frequent complications of medical management include medication side effects, particularly with steroids and immunosuppressive agents, and progression of the disease when resistant to medical therapy. Surgical treatment can be complicated by wound infection, short bowel syndrome (see below), wound healing problems (particularly in patients on preoperative immune suppression), and fistulae, which may result from anastomotic leaks following resection. Anal incontinence can complicate advanced perianal disease or be a consequence of overly aggressive surgical approaches that compromise sphincter integrity. Given the chronicity of the illness and the frequent requirement for repeated surgical intervention and care, the surgeon often forms a close and ongoing relationship with the patient suffering from recurring and complicated Crohn's disease.

Short bowel syndrome is worthy of specific mention at the close of this section, since Crohn's disease of the small intestine can lead to this problem. A fuller discussion of the general management of short bowel syndrome in general follows later in this chapter. Overall, Crohn's disease accounts for approximately one-fourth of short bowel cases, typically due to recurring disease and repeated surgical interventions over a period of years. As mentioned previously, the syndrome is rare if at least 100 cm of adult intestinal length can be maintained.

Mesenteric Ischemia

Mesenteric ischemia is a devastating surgical emergency related to vascular compromise of the midgut, including the small bowel and proximal colon. The major blood vessel supplying this portion of the intestine is the SMA and the venous drainage is through the SMV. In addition to the SMA, there are extensive collaterals that exist from primarily the celiac axis that can help protect the intestine from an acute drop in splanchnic flow. However, with a prolonged period of impaired blood flow, the bowel will become ischemic, which progresses rapidly to bowel death. Unfortunately this is a difficult diagnosis to make and delays often result in significant bowel necrosis and an overall mortality that remains high.

Pathophysiology

There are four major etiologies for acute mesenteric ischemia (AMI) (Table 14-5). SMA embolisms usually originate from the heart and are frequently associated with atrial fibrillation. In this scenario, thrombus forms within the heart, which can become dislodged. If clot passes down the SMA, it will then lodge as the vessel narrows, oftentimes just distal to the take off of the middle colic artery, completely occluding downstream

TABLE 14-5	Causes for Acute Mesenteric Ischemia
Cause	**Frequency (%)**
SMA embolism	50
SMA thrombosis	20
SMV thrombosis	5
Nonocclusive mesenteric ischemia	25

flow. SMA thrombosis is frequently associated with other significant vascular diseases. Patients typically will have evidence of severe atherosclerotic disease in other organ systems (i.e., associated coronary artery disease, peripheral vascular disease, chronic renal insufficiency, etc.). Patients may have a history that includes pain with eating ("intestinal angina"), food fear, and weight loss, indicating a chronic stenosis of the SMA. If the vessel then forms an acute thrombosis, AMI may occur. In contrast to SMA embolism, SMA thrombosis usually begins at the origin of the SMA and is more likely to lead to complete small bowel infarction. SMV thrombosis is often the result of a hypercoagulable state, such as patients with antithrombin III deficiency or a factor V Leiden mutation. Clot forms within the SMV, obstructing venous outflow. This results in venous hypertension, increased bowel wall edema and finally decreased arterial flow. Nonocclusive mesenteric ischemia (NOMI) is generally diagnosed in the intensive care unit (ICU) setting in critically ill patients. As with SMA thrombosis, these patients often have a history of other significant atherosclerotic diseases. When patients are in severe shock, blood may be shunted away from the GI tract. Initially, this process may be beneficial, as the body shunts blood to maintain cerebral blood flow. However, if this process continues, there can be significant vasospasm of the splanchnic circulation, resulting in ischemia to both the small and large intestine. Regardless of the mechanism, prolonged ischemia (e.g., >12 hours) is likely to progress to bowel necrosis. This relatively short window highlights the need for a rapid and immediate diagnosis if we hope to impact on the high mortality of this disease.

Clinical Presentation

Classically, the pain associated with AMI is rapid in onset and severe. Despite this severe pain, the abdominal exam is often unimpressive. This is the classic "pain out of proportion to physical exam," and is often the reason there is a significant delay in diagnosis. The astute physician must recognize this pain pattern, especially if there are associated risk factors for mesenteric ischemia, such as atrial fibrillation or severe atherosclerotic disease in other organ systems. Unfortunately, once a patient develops physical findings of peritonitis, small bowel infarction has usually already occurred and mortality is high.

SMV thrombosis tends to have a more insidious onset. Patients may have pain for several days for even weeks before a diagnosis is made. The pain can be diffuse and nonspecific. Patients with NOMI may have minimal abdominal pain and what pain they may have is frequently overshadowed by the other complex medical problems resulting in the nonocclusive ischemia. The predominant clinical feature of NOMI is hemodynamic instability, which is the primary cause of this entity.

As with the physical findings, laboratory studies are very nonspecific. Currently, there is no lab value that is diagnostic for mesenteric ischemia. Unfortunately, even normal lab values do not rule out the possibility of this disease in the right clinical scenario. While some patients may develop an elevated white blood cell count and a metabolic acidosis, these findings do not have to be present to pursue this diagnosis and may only be late findings suggesting bowel infarction. Waiting for both physical findings and laboratory values to become abnormal only contributes to delays in diagnosis, which negatively impacts overall survival. However, in patients with abdominal pain with a persistent metabolic acidosis, a diagnosis of mesenteric ischemia should be entertained.

Diagnosis

In order to save patients from this devastating problem, a rapid diagnosis must be made and a treatment plan immediately instituted. The diagnosis is ultimately made by direct visualization of the vascular tree. The gold standard is the mesenteric arteriogram. This should allow the physician to determine if the SMA is occluded as well as the status of the other mesenteric vessels. Delayed films should be taken to obtain a venous phase to determine if the SMV is thrombosed. NOMI will show associated spasm and narrowing of the vascular tree. These studies not only make the diagnosis but are critical for therapeutic planning as well. In many institutions, high resolution CT scans have replaced mesenteric arteriogram as the initial study of choice. These studies can provide excellent visualization of the vascular tree, but have the added benefit of imaging the other intra-abdominal organs if the diagnosis of mesenteric ischemia is not confirmed. Furthermore, the CT scan can identify other ominous signs of bowel infarction, such as bowel wall thickening, pneumatosis (air within the bowel wall), or portal venous air.

Treatment

The initial treatment is rapid resuscitation and correction of any metabolic abnormalities. Frequently antibiotics are administered since there is a high likelihood of necrotic intestine. Ultimately the primary goal of treatment is to rapidly restore blood flow to the gut, resect obviously necrotic bowel and minimize any reperfusion injury, which may progress despite restoring blood flow. For patients with an SMA embolism, immediate embolectomy is indicated. This is done via a laparotomy, at which time the viability of the small bowel can be assessed. The SMA is isolated and an arteriotomy is performed. A catheter can then be placed directly into the artery above the clot. A balloon is then inflated and the catheter removed, pulling the clot out of the SMA. For SMA thrombosis, revascularization is often required since the SMA is often chronically narrowed by severe atherosclerotic disease. This can be done by an SMA bypass procedure or, more recently, an SMA endovascular stent. For SMV thrombosis, the primary treatment is supportive as well as prompt anticoagulation with intravenous heparin. If there is any suspicion of bowel necrosis, an exploratory laparotomy or laparoscopy must be done with resection of any infarcted bowel. For NOMI, the treatment is directed at the underlying pathology and aggressive resuscitation efforts. Since vasospasm is a major component of this disease, drugs that induce additional spasm, such as α-adrenergic vasopressors and digoxin, should be avoided. Invasive monitoring is often necessary to optimize cardiac output and therefore mesenteric blood flow. As with SMV thrombosis, if bowel infarction is suspected, then direct visualization via laparotomy or laparoscopy is mandatory.

Once blood flow is restored, obviously necrotic bowel should be resected. Ischemic-appearing bowel can be left in situ, as this bowel may survive once the blood flow is restored. A primary anastomosis is often avoided with the plan for a second look operation in 12 to 24 hours. At the second laparotomy, the surgeon should be able to tell which bowel has survived, resect any additional bowel that has necrosed, and restore continuity. A third look is rarely needed but could be done if clinically indicated. While waiting for the second look procedure, the patient returns to the ICU for supportive care. If there is a mesenteric catheter in place, intra-arterial papaverine can be infused, which can relieve much of the associated vasospasm and improve blood flow to the newly vascularized intestine.

Complications

Unfortunately, patients with AMI are often quite ill. Even under the best of circumstances there are frequent medical and surgical complications, including respiratory failure, renal failure, intra-abdominal infections, and anastomotic breakdown. A prolonged ICU stay may be necessary. These problems are often exacerbated by the many comorbidities these patients tend to have. Furthermore, once there is bowel infarction, these complications are often more severe and devastating. Frequently there is a large amount of necrotic small bowel. When this occurs, the surgeon and the patient's family can be faced with difficult choices as survival may be predicated on complete removal of the small bowel with resulting short gut syndrome. For elderly patients with significant comorbidities, survival under these circumstances is unlikely and the surgeon, after consultation with the patient's family, may choose to close the abdomen and forgo further therapy. Overall mortality from AMI remains high with survival limited to those with a rapid diagnosis and treatment plan.

Small Bowel Tumors

A variety of tumors can arise from the epithelial and mesenchymal components of the small intestine. Tumors are much less common in the small intestine than in the colon and rectum, despite the greater length and absorptive surface area of the small bowel. Small bowel tumors may present with obstructive symptoms, bleeding, or symptoms of metastatic disease. They may also act as lead points for intussusception. Diagnosis is most commonly made by contrast evaluation, enteroclysis, or CT enterography in particular.

Endoscopic evaluation of the duodenum and proximal jejunum, as well as of the terminal ileum, has also been used to diagnose these lesions. Until recently, endoscopic evaluation of the intervening small intestine has been difficult, often requiring specialized instruments, which are tedious to employ, or operative assistance. Capsule endoscopy has recently emerged as a technology that may assist greatly in the diagnosis of small bowel lesions including tumors. With this technique, the patient swallows a capsule-sized device equipped with light emitting diodes, batteries, and a complementary metal–oxide–semiconductor (CMOS) chip that transmits two images per second to a unit worn on the waist, where images are stored for later downloading and interpretation. Early experience with this technology has demonstrated its potential to document small bowel pathology, including the presence of otherwise occult tumors, in a minimally invasive fashion. Double balloon enteroscopy, a technique in which a balloon-fitted endoscope and a balloon-fitted overtube are used to repetitively accordion the small intestine in an antegrade (per os) and/or retrograde (transanal) fashion, has also been useful in visualizing up to two-thirds of the small intestine otherwise inaccessible to more standard endoscopic approaches.

Benign Tumors

Benign small intestinal tumors are much more common than malignant lesions. Most are asymptomatic. Both sexes are equally affected, with a peak incidence in the sixth decade.

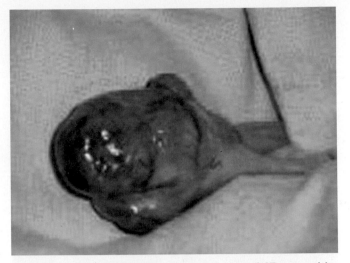

FIGURE 14-8. Operative photograph of a small bowel GIST tumor arising from the antimesenteric border of the intestine.

The most common of these lesions have traditionally been referred to as leiomyomas, which occur most commonly in the jejunum. Many of these lesions, which can occur anywhere in the digestive tract, are on the benign end of a spectrum of mesenchymal tumors of the GI tract and are now referred to as GI stromal tumors (GISTs) (Figure 14-8). These lesions arise from the interstitial cells of Cajal. Lesions in this category can be diagnosed by immunohistochemical determination of their expression of the c-kit proto-oncogene protein, also known as CD117. Benign lesions in this category show fewer mitoses than their malignant counterparts, generally are of smaller size, and lack features such as necrosis, nuclear pleomorphism, and invasive or metastatic behavior. Even benign-appearing lesions may cause overlying mucosal ulceration or obstructive symptoms, particularly if they reach a large size, and may manifest delayed local recurrence. Lipomas may also rarely demonstrate these features, are more common in men, and occur most commonly in the duodenum or ileum.

Other nonepithelial, benign small bowel lesions may include hemangiomas, hamartomas, lymphangiomas, and neurogenic tumors such as schwannomas and neurofibromas. Hemangiomas are an important potential cause of occult bleeding and constitute 5% of benign small bowel lesions. These lesions are often multiple, as can be seen in Osler-Weber-Rendu syndrome. Capsule enteroscopy may offer particular promise in delineating hemangiomas, given their potential for multiplicity and the fact that they do not show up on standard contrast studies. For actively bleeding lesions, angiography may also be useful. Hamartomas are usually isolated and typically asymptomatic. They can be a cause of bleeding or intussusception, particularly in the pediatric population. Multiple hamartomas may be seen in association with Peutz-Jeghers syndrome, an autosomal dominant trait also associated with mucocutaneous hyperpigmentation.

Epithelial benign lesions of the small intestine include tubular, villous, and Brunner's gland adenomas. Brunner's gland adenomas occur primarily in the duodenum and are usually asymptomatic, as are most tubular adenomas. Adenomas with villous histology are more likely to harbor malignancy (overall risk 30%—increasing with lesion size), and should be excised for this reason (Figure 14-9). Duodenal carcinoma of

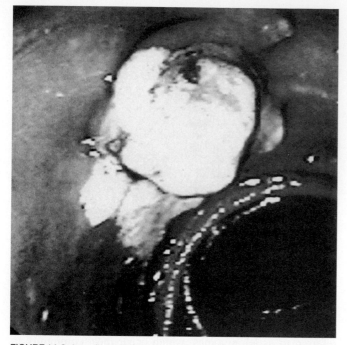

FIGURE 14-9. Ampullary villous adenoma. Reconstruction of the biliary and pancreatic ducts was necessary after local excision of the tumor.

the periampullary region, typically arising from a preexisting benign adenoma, is the most common malignancy affecting individuals with familial polyposis after proctocolectomy, and the duodenum and papilla should be kept under endoscopic surveillance in patients with this diagnosis.

Malignant Tumors

A variety of malignant tumors can affect the small intestine, although these constitute only 2% of all GI tract malignancies. Overall, malignant tumors are slightly more common in males than females, and the average age at presentation is in the sixth decade.

Adenocarcinomas

Adenocarcinomas account for approximately half of all small intestinal malignancies. They are most common in the duodenum, with decreasing incidence as one moves distally in the small bowel. Obstruction, often associated with weight loss, is the most common presentation. Small intestinal obstruction in the absence of hernia or prior abdominal surgery and associated adhesions should heighten one's concern that a small intestinal neoplasm may be present. Occult bleeding and anemia may also be noted. In a younger individual, occult small intestinal bleeding is frequently due to small bowel neoplasia. Massive bleeding is rare. Lesions in the periampullary region may present with painless jaundice and, rarely, otherwise unexplained pancreatitis. Nearly half of small intestinal adenocarcinomas are diagnosed at the time of operation.

Surgical intervention should include wide resection of the involved bowel with margins to facilitate removal of the associated mesenteric lymphatic drainage pathways. Adjuvant therapies have little demonstrated efficacy, and 5-year survival is generally poor, in the 10% to 30% range, reflecting the tendency toward delayed diagnosis predicated on advanced, symptomatic disease. As mentioned above, endoscopic screening of the periampullary region in particular may allow earlier diagnosis in patients with genetic polyposis syndromes and known associated risk.

Carcinoid Tumors

Carcinoid tumors arise from the Kulchitsky cells in the crypts of Lieberkühn. These cells are part of the amine precursor uptake and decarboxylation (APUD) system. They are sometimes called argentaffin cells because of their histologic staining characteristics. Malignant behavior correlates with lesion size; metastasis occurs in only 2% of patients with primary tumors <1 cm in size, but in 90% of those with primary tumors larger than 2 cm. Between 40% and 50% of all GI carcinoids originate in the appendix, with the small intestine being the second most common GI site. Small intestinal carcinoids are most common in the ileum and may be multicentric in as many as 30% of patients.

Obstruction is the most common presenting finding in patients with small intestinal carcinoid. This is usually not due to the size of the primary lesion, but rather an intense desmoplastic reaction that characteristically occurs in the adjacent bowel mesentery. Bleeding and intussusception are less common. Many patients do experience nonspecific symptoms including anorexia, fatigue, and weight loss. The diagnosis is often made at laparotomy. Surgical treatment consists of wide excision of the bowel and adjacent mesentery, which may require right hemicolectomy with terminal ileal lesions. If resectable liver metastases are noted at the time of operation, they should also be removed.

The carcinoid syndrome is a complex of manifestations that metastatic intestinal carcinoids may demonstrate. Episodic cutaneous flushing (especially of the head and trunk), bronchospasm, intestinal cramping and diarrhea, vasomotor instability, pellagra-like skin lesions (due to diversion of tryptophan from niacin synthesis to formation of serotonin and other 5-hydroxyindoles), and right sided valvular heart disease may be seen (Figure 14-10). These attacks may be spontaneous or may be triggered by exertion, excitement, alcohol, anesthesia, or tumor manipulation. These manifestations are related to the elaboration of 5-hydroxytryptamine (serotonin) by the tumor. This substance is degraded on delivery to the liver via the portal vein into 5-hydroxyindole acetic acid (5-HIAA), as well as other vasoactive peptides including 5-hydroxytryptophan, kallikrein, histamine, and adrenocorticotropic hormone (ACTH). It is not entirely clear which combination of these substances is responsible for the syndrome. The liver is highly effective in clearing serotonin and its metabolites from the bloodstream when delivered via the portal vein. Thus, for the syndrome to occur, the bowel lesion must have metastasized to the liver to allow delivery to the venous circulation in a postportal location, or the primary lesion must be in another location not draining via the portal system, such as the lungs, gonads, or rectum. The syndrome is confirmed, when suspected, by urinary measurement of 5-HIAA. Serum measurement of serotonin or chromogranin A may also be confirmatory. Treatment is via resection, when this is possible.

Lymphoma

The small intestine is the most common site of extranodal lymphoma, although only 5% of all lymphomas are found there. Lymphoma accounts for 10% to 15% of all small bowel malignancies. Again, the fifth and sixth decades are the periods of highest incidence. The ileum is the most common site of involvement, given the concentration of lymphoid tissue

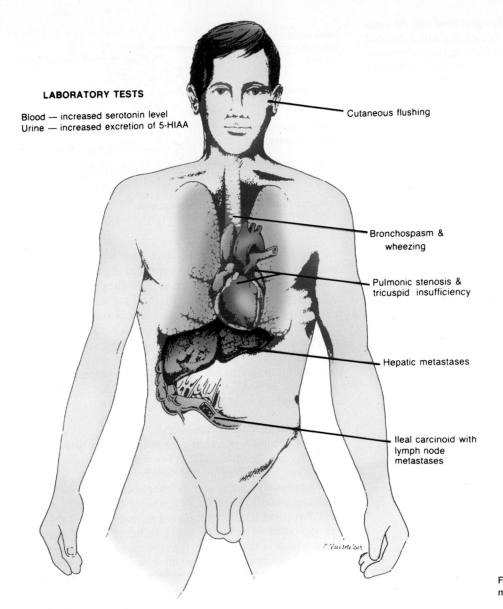

LABORATORY TESTS

Blood — increased serotonin level
Urine — increased excretion of 5-HIAA

Cutaneous flushing

Bronchospasm &
wheezing

Pulmonic stenosis &
tricuspid insufficiency

Hepatic metastases

Ileal carcinoid with
lymph node
metastases

FIGURE 14-10. Clinical manifestations of malignant carcinoid syndrome.

in Peyer's patches in that region. Although more commonly described in the stomach in association with chronic gastritis associated with *Helicobacter pylori* infection, so called MALT lymphomas may occur in the small intestine and are found in a subset of patients with small intestinal lymphoma. While the majority of patients present with nonspecific symptoms such as vague abdominal pain, weight loss, fatigue, and malaise, up to one-fourth may present as abdominal emergencies (perforation, hemorrhage, obstruction, and intussusception). Nodularity and thickening of the bowel wall on contrast studies or CT scan, often with associated mesenteric adenopathy on CT, may allow preoperative suspicion of the diagnosis. Surgical resection is usually accomplished, often with subsequent chemotherapy and/or radiation, depending on the type of lymphoma and stage of disease. Overall 5-year survival is in the 20% to 40% range. Patients diagnosed prior to laparotomy and treated with chemoradiation without surgical resection may experience bowel perforation from tumor lysis, particularly when there is extensive involvement of the bowel wall.

Gastrointestinal Stromal Tumors

As mentioned above, most mesenchymal tumors of the GI tract, formerly referred to as leiomyosarcomas if malignant, are now referred to as GIST lesions. They can have a spectrum of clinical behaviors from benign to malignant, may occur anywhere in the small intestine, have a peak incidence in the sixth decade, and can present with obstruction, bleeding, or perforation. GIST lesions universally exhibit c-kit protein expression, as noted above in the discussion of benign tumors. Malignant mesenchymal lesions that do not exhibit this expression may still be classified as true leiomyosarcomas. Small bowel GISTs appear to have a worse prognosis than similar lesions of the esophagus and stomach. Wide excision with adjacent mesentery is performed, and malignant behavior is predicted from mitoses, evidence of invasive behavior, and tumor necrosis. Overall, approximately 50% of patients will demonstrate recurrence within 2 years. For patients with metastatic GIST lesions, impressive responses may be seen with imatinib, a tyrosine kinase inhibitor used also in patients with chronic myelogenous leukemia. This agent also may be used as neoadjuvant treatment in patients presenting with advanced disease. Several other newer agents in this category of tyrosine or multiple kinase inhibitors are now available for patients who no longer respond to imatinib (e.g., sunitinib, nilotinib, and sorafenib).

Congenital Abnormalities

Meckel's Diverticulum

Significance and Incidence

Meckel's diverticulum is the most common congenital anomaly of the small intestine and represents a remnant of the embryonic vitelline, or omphalomesenteric, duct. It is present in approximately 2% of the population, has a 2:1 male:female predominance, has two types of mucosae, and is typically located within 2 feet of the ileocecal valve ("rule of twos"). Symptoms due to Meckel's diverticula are rare, and are increasingly so as the patient harboring the diverticulum ages. Accordingly, symptoms may develop in 5% of infants harboring the diverticulum, in only 1.5% of individuals at age 40, and extremely rarely in elderly patients, with an overall lifetime risk of symptomatic disease in not more than 4% of the affected population.

Anatomy

Meckel's diverticula evolve when there is incomplete obliteration of the vitelline duct, which arises from the midgut and typically closes between the 8th and 10th week of gestation (Figure 14-11). The diverticulum arises from the antimesenteric border of the ileum, usually within 60 cm (2 feet) of the ileocecal valve (Figure 14-12). Its blood supply is from the vitelline vessels, arising from the ileal blood supply.

Pathophysiology

The cells lining the vitelline duct have pluripotential capabilities. As a result, it is not uncommon to find heterotopic mucosa within the diverticulum. The most common type of such mucosa is gastric (50%). Less frequently, pancreatic and colonic mucosa may be found in the diverticulum. Gastric mucosa in particular, because of its capacity to produce acid in direct proximity to small bowel mucosa, may cause ulceration of the adjacent small intestinal mucosa and hemorrhage. Benign tumors including lipomas, leiomyomas, neurofibromas, and angiomas have been described in diverticula as well. Such tumors may act as a lead point for intussusception and bowel obstruction.

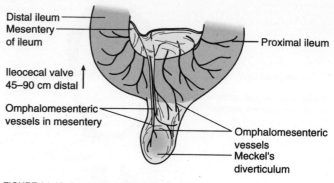

FIGURE 14-12. Anatomy of Meckel's diverticulum.

Persistence of the vitelline duct itself can also cause a variety of problems. If there is complete persistence, a sinus from the umbilicus to the ileum may result, presenting as an enteric fistula at the umbilicus itself. If the umbilical end of the duct only remains patent, an umbilical sinus may result. If the duct obliterates but leaves a fibrous cord remnant, this remnant may act as a point of fixation of the small intestine to the abdominal wall and facilitate bowel obstruction. The diverticulum may also become occluded with fecal material and become inflamed, presenting in a fashion very similar to acute appendicitis.

Clinical Presentation and Evaluation

The most common presenting illnesses related to Meckel's diverticula are listed in Table 14-6 and include obstruction, hemorrhage, inflammation, and umbilical fistula.

Hemorrhage presents with bright red or maroon blood per rectum, is usually painless, and is most common in infants under 2 years of age. Diagnosis can be made 90% of the time with radionuclide scanning using technetium-99m pertechnetate, which is taken up by the ectopic gastric mucosa and delineates the presence of the diverticulum. The positivity of this test may be enhanced by cimetidine or pentagastrin administration, but this is not usually required.

Intestinal obstruction can occur because of volvulus of the small bowel around the diverticulum, or the constrictive effect of a mesodiverticular band (Figure 14-13). Intussusception may also occur, with the diverticulum acting as a lead point. The latter may present with a palpable right-sided mass and the passage of "currant jelly" stool. Air or contrast enema,

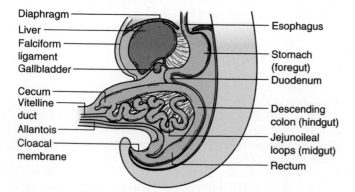

FIGURE 14-11. Embryonic development of Meckel's diverticulum.

TABLE 14-6	Clinical Presentation in Meckel's Diverticula[a]

Clinical Presentation	Frequency (%)
Hemorrhage	23
Ileus	31
Intussusception	14
Diverticulitis	14
Perforation	10
Miscellaneous (e.g., fistula, tumor)	8

[a]Occurrence in 1,044 cases of Meckel's diverticula compiled from previously published reports.
Adapted with permission from Scharli AF. In: Freeman NV, Burge DM, Griffiths DM, Malone PSJ, eds. Surgery of the Newborn. Edinburgh, Scotland: Churchill Livingstone, 1994.

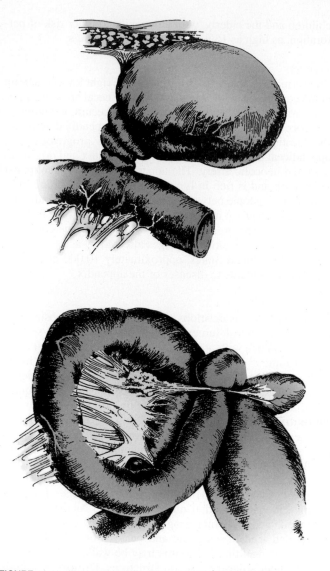

FIGURE 14-13. Obstruction caused by a mesodiverticular band.

particularly in the pediatric population, can facilitate reduction of the intussusception in the acute setting if no bowel compromise has evolved, but subsequent resection of the diverticulum and release of any fibrous attachments should be accomplished.

Diverticulitis closely mimics acute appendicitis, and hence a Meckel's diverticulum should be sought if a patient, especially a younger one, is being explored for suspected appendicitis and is found to have a normal appendix. Less common complications can include iron deficiency anemia, malabsorption, foreign body impaction, perforation, and incarceration in a hernia (Littre's hernia), including inguinal, femoral, and umbilical herniae.

Differential Diagnosis

Acute appendicitis, SBO from other causes, and regional enteritis present similarly to, and are more common than, disease related to Meckel's diverticulum. Lower GI bleeding, except in the very young patient, is much more commonly due to other pathologies including diverticular disease of the colon and angiodysplastic lesions. Meckel's diverticulum is accordingly appropriately considered in small children presenting with lower abdominal pain, obstruction, lower GI bleeding, or umbilical drainage, and should be regarded as a consideration of secondary priority in older patients, in whom other pathologies are far more likely. Studies oriented toward the identification and exclusion of such processes, particularly in the older patient, may help in excluding more common pathologies and may include endoscopic and contrast studies of the GI tract. Patients with acute obstructive and inflammatory presentations dictating surgical intervention will typically have the diagnosis established at surgery. Patients with atypical, subacute presentations and negative workup for other processes may benefit from Meckel's scans, small bowel contrast studies, or even laparoscopy to establish the diagnosis.

Treatment

Resection of the diverticulum is curative and appropriate for the patient presenting with complications related to it. When the diverticulum is broad based, segmental bowel resection may be required to adequately remove all ectopic tissue. Laparoscopic resections are being accomplished and are an option when a Meckel's diverticulum is found to be the source of disease during laparoscopic exploration for suspected appendicitis or obstruction. There is continued controversy regarding the most appropriate management when an asymptomatic diverticulum is found incidentally at the time of surgery for other purposes. In the younger patient, especially, the low morbidity of resection may be justified as a preventive measure. However, this potential benefit is small and clearly diminishes as the patient ages and the likelihood of symptomatic disease decreases. Settings in which resection may be considered in patients outside the pediatric age range include when the diverticulum has a narrow base, when a mesodiverticular band is present, or when heterotopic tissue is evident. Incidental resection may also be appropriate in patients with hostile abdomens who would be difficult to reexplore, for example, in the setting of multiple adhesions and recurring SBO or pending radiation therapy. Ideally, the base of the diverticulum is closed transversely so as to minimize luminal narrowing.

Malrotation

Intestinal malrotation is due to abnormalities of rotation and fixation of the intestinal tract between the 4th and 10th weeks of gestation. The 270° rotation of the proximal midgut places the duodenum in the retroperitoneum, behind the superior mesenteric vessels. The later 270° rotation of the distal mid-gut places the cecum in the right lower quadrant and the transverse colon draped anterior to the superior mesenteric vessels. When these two turns are incomplete or not made at all, a variety of anatomic abnormalities can exist. Although these may be asymptomatic or present at any age, the most common manifestation is midgut volvulus in an infant with an incomplete rotation. The proximal mid-gut fails to rotate beyond the midline, remaining to the right of the superior mesenteric vessels, with the duodenum covered anteriorly by Ladd's bands. The distal mid-gut also only rotates 90° to 180°, and the cecum becomes fixed to the abdominal wall in the right upper quadrant, near the duodenum. While the Ladd's bands themselves may cause a mild degree of obstruction, more serious problems occur because the beginning and end of the small intestine are fixed only in the right upper quadrant by the duodenum, the cecum and their mesentery. This allows the small bowel to twist spontaneously around its mesentery into the surgical emergency known as *small bowel volvulus*.

Like other types of volvulus, this impedes the venous and then arterial blood flow to the small intestine, rapidly leading to ischemia and necrosis. Early symptoms include bilious emesis, with progression to distention, tenderness and shock being late findings due to irreversible necrosis. The most quick, accurate and common method of evaluation for midgut volvulus is a radiographic upper GI series. Once identified, midgut volvulus is treated by emergent laparotomy, with detorsion of the bowel, division of the Ladd's bands, broadening of the mesentery, and placement of the small intestine on the right and colon on the left side of the abdomen. Appendectomy is usually performed, as the appendix would lie in the left upper quadrant with the cecum, making a later case of appendicitis difficult to diagnose. Malrotation that does not present with volvulus can be difficult to diagnose, especially in adults. These cases are approached on an individual basis, with surgical decision making based on the anatomic abnormality and the patient's symptoms.

Short Bowel Syndrome

Short bowel syndrome, sometimes referred to as "short gut," is defined as <200 cm of in-continuity small intestine in an adult. This is usually the result of one or more small bowel resections, for example from Crohn's disease, multiple SBOs or ischemia caused by embolism, necrotizing enterocolitis, midgut volvulus or strangulation in a hernia. The effect of the resection(s) depends on the degree of absorption of nutrients and fluid within the remaining gut. In response to loss of length, the human gut responds with dilation and an increase in villous height. In some cases, increased intake may be all that is required to maintain nutrition. While the ileum may adapt to absorb more nutrients, loss of the terminal ileum results in permanent loss of absorption of vitamin B_{12} and bile salts. Patients with <60 cm of small intestine with an intact colon, or with <100 cm without a colon, will often require total parenteral nutrition (TPN). However, TPN has many risks (e.g., line sepsis, hyperglycemia, hepatic injury, gallstones, venous access complications), and a long-term strategy of dietary modification and supplementation as the gut adapts is preferable. In patients with long-term intestinal failure, small bowel transplantation (discussed in Chapter 23, Transplantation) or an intestinal lengthening procedure may provide relief from TPN. Lengthening may be accomplished by dividing the bowel down its length, leaving one half of the mesentery and terminal vessel branches on each side, and then anastomosing the ends (Bianchi procedure) Alternatively, staggered perpendicular double staple lines can be fired into the bowel from each side, creating an elongated shape out of the cylinder of bowel (serial transverse enteroplasty [STEP] procedure) Overall, short bowel syndrome is a devastating problem with therapy aimed at providing a good quality of life for these unfortunate patients.

DISEASES OF THE APPENDIX

Acute Appendicitis

Significance and Incidence

Acute appendicitis is the most common emergent surgical illness, affecting approximately 5% of the population. The majority of patients are between the ages of 5 and 35 and typically present in the first 24 to 48 hours of illness. Atypical presentation and delayed diagnosis are more common in children and the elderly, with an attendant higher risk of perforation, as high as 15% to 25%, in those settings.

Anatomy

The vermiform appendix is located in the right lower quadrant at the confluence of the taenia coli on the cecal apex. It can be in a variety of positions in relation to the cecum, including in a retrocecal position. The location of the appendix determines the location of tenderness as the disease progresses. The appendiceal artery travels in the mesoappendix and originates from the ileocolic artery. The appendix is lined by columnar epithelium and is rich in lymphatic follicles, which are most numerous in people between 10 and 20 years of age. Individuals in this age group may harbor as many as 200 such follicles in the organ. The presence of this lymphatic tissue correlates closely with the predominant ages affected by acute appendicitis. In the United States, approximately 10,000 deaths per year are attributable to diseases of the appendix.

Pathophysiology

Acute appendicitis develops as a consequence of obstruction of the appendiceal lumen. Lymphoid hyperplasia, seen in 60% of patients with appendicitis, is the most common etiology of luminal obstruction. An accumulation of fecal material, or fecalith, is noted histologically in 35% of patients. Viral illnesses that elicit lymphoid hyperplasia are a frequent prodrome to the onset of appendicitis in the young. As the appendiceal lumen becomes compromised, mucus secretion by the epithelium leads to distension of the appendix distal to the narrowed lumen, with eventual compromise of venous outflow as the organ becomes increasingly turgid, and ultimately, ischemic. Necrosis and bacterial proliferation in the stagnant, ischemic environment may supervene. Bacterial toxins can lead to further mucosal damage. As the swelling, infection, and ischemia progress, they may become transmural and lead to gangrene and perforation. If perforation occurs, the resulting peritonitis may be walled off by omentum or other adjacent visceral structures. Diffuse peritonitis can also develop if the process is not localized, as may more frequently be the case in younger children who lack well developed omentum. If the process is not controlled, spread of infection into the portal system via the venous effluent (pylephlebitis) may result, giving rise to air in the portal system or liver abscesses.

Clinical Presentation and Evaluation

The above pathophysiology correlates closely with the historical pattern of pain classically described by the patient with acute appendicitis. Initial discomfort is due to luminal distension and is perceived as poorly localized, periumbilical pain, consistent with the midgut origin of the appendix and its corresponding pattern of autonomic innervation. As the disease progresses to the point of transmural inflammation, irritation of the adjacent parietal peritoneum occurs, which is innervated somatically rather than autonomically and is perceived in localized fashion at the point of irritation, most commonly in the right lower quadrant. The initial pain may be associated with anorexia, nausea, and, in some cases, vomiting. Repetitive vomiting and diarrhea may be harbingers of a mimicking illness such as gastroenteritis. Low-grade fever and leukocytosis are common, but not universal, and may be more pronounced as the disease progresses.

On examination, the patient will classically exhibit tenderness in the region of McBurney's point, located one third of the distance from the anterior superior iliac spine to the umbilicus. If the appendix lies inferior to the cecum, pain on rectal and/or pelvic examination may also be present. Signs of peritoneal irritation including rebound tenderness, percussion tenderness, and, in advanced cases, involuntary guarding and hyperesthesia may be present. Pain in the right lower quadrant on palpation of the left lower quadrant (Rovsing's sign) is another sign of a focal right lower quadrant process, as is perceived pain in that area with gentle movement such as heel tap or, historically, jostling during transport. Other physical signs that may be present, depending on the position of the appendix, may include pain with right hip extension (psoas sign), which suggests an inflamed retrocecal appendix lying against the iliopsoas muscle, and pain with passive rotation of the flexed right hip (obturator sign), suggesting inflammation adjacent to the obturator internus muscle in the pelvis.

If the appendix perforates, there may be temporary improvement in visceral pain due to decompression of the turgid organ, but increasing peritonitis soon follows. Peritonitis becomes more likely as the duration of symptoms extends beyond 24 hours and may be associated with high fever and leukocytosis with left shift.

In the pregnant patient, the appendix is often displaced into a more cephalad position and may confuse the diagnostician. The leukocytosis of pregnancy may further confuse the picture. A high level of suspicion is warranted in this setting, since progression to perforation and peritonitis is associated with a fetal death rate of 35% or more. When pregnant patients are taken to surgery, the displaced position of the appendix must be taken into consideration when making the incision.

Radiologic studies may aid in the diagnosis of acute appendicitis, particularly in atypical settings. Plain abdominal films are rarely helpful, although a right lower quadrant fecalith may be seen in a minority of cases and supports diagnostic suspicion. Barium enema has been used historically, with nonvisualization of the appendix being interpreted as presumptive evidence of luminal obstruction and possible appendicitis, but there is a 10% to 15% false positive and false negative rate with this study. More recently, ultrasound has been found to be quite sensitive, with the classic finding being the presence of a noncompressible tubular structure with corresponding focal tenderness in the right lower quadrant. As in all ultrasonic examinations, the quality of the exam depends both on the technician and the interpreting physician's experience with interpretation. CT can also provide evidence for the diagnosis and help exclude other confounding pathology. Findings on CT scan may include distension of the appendix, fecalith identification, nonfilling of the appendix with enteral contrast, inflammatory changes in the surrounding fat, abscess formation, and free fluid (Figure 14-14). In the patient with fairly classic symptoms and findings, additional tests such as these are unnecessary and not cost effective. However, in the setting of less typical findings, such studies can be useful in guiding therapy.

Differential Diagnosis

The differential diagnosis of right lower quadrant pain includes a variety of enteric, urologic, musculoskeletal, and gynecologic conditions. Common entities that may mimic acute appendicitis include pelvic inflammatory disease, pyelonephritis, gastroenteritis, inflammatory bowel disease,

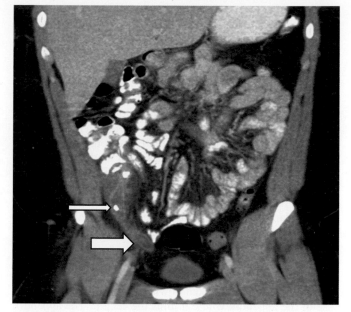

FIGURE 14-14. CT scan showing a distended appendix with thickening of the wall at the tip (*large arrow*) and a fecalith in the appendiceal lumen (*small arrow*).

endometriosis, ovulatory pain (Mittelschmerz), and ruptured or hemorrhagic ovarian cyst. Meckel's diverticulitis, cecal or sigmoid diverticulitis, acute ileitis, cholecystitis, and perforated peptic ulcer disease may also have features similar to appendicitis in some settings. It is particularly important to consider and exclude entities in the differential diagnosis that are managed nonoperatively, which may include urinary tract infections or stones, hepatitis, pelvic inflammatory disease, right lower lobe pneumonia, and ovulatory or menstrual pain. Conversely, in cases of diagnostic uncertainty, close observation and/or operative intervention may be necessary to prevent progression of appendicitis into its more advanced and complicated stages. Accordingly, it has traditionally been deemed appropriate to find a normal appendix in 10% to 20% of explored patients to minimize the chance of missing a progressing appendicitis until it has reached the point of perforation. With increased use of the CT scan in equivocal cases, the incidence of false positive appendicitis should be reduced to 5%. This must be discussed with the patient during the informed consent process.

Given the above differential diagnosis, all patients should have a careful history taken and a physical examination performed to exclude confounding illnesses. A careful urinary and gynecologic evaluation especially should be included. Laboratory studies including a complete blood count (CBC) with differential and a urinalysis should be routinely carried out. Abdominal films, chest radiography, and more advanced studies such as CT or ultrasound should be used selectively when they will impact patient management by excluding other pathology or documenting disease that the clinician suspects but cannot confirm. A CT scan may also be helpful in determining the presence of an abscess or phlegmon that may be better initially treated nonoperatively, especially when symptoms have been present for several days.

Treatment

Appendectomy is the primary treatment for acute appendicitis. Appropriate preoperative preparation should include intravenous fluid resuscitation and antibiotic coverage suitable for colonic flora. A second-generation cephalosporin, broad-spectrum penicillin, or combination of a fluoroquinolone and anaerobic coverage with metronidazole are frequently employed antimicrobial strategies. If the appendix has not ruptured, antibiotics may be discontinued within the first 24 hours postoperatively. If frank peritoneal perforation and contamination or abscess are found, antibiotics are typically continued until the patient is afebrile, has a normal white blood cell count, and has regained GI function.

Once the decision to operate has been made, it should be accomplished expeditiously, since the possibility of perforation increases after the first 24 to 36 hours of illness. Appendectomy may be appropriately accomplished either via an open or laparoscopic approach (see Chapter 25, Surgical Procedures, Techniques, and Skills [online]). The former is commonly done through a muscle splitting incision centered on McBurney's point in the right lower quadrant. If appendicitis is found, the appendix is mobilized into the wound and the mesoappendix taken down, allowing isolation of the base of the appendix where it joins the cecum. The appendix is removed after ligature control of its base. The stump may be left or inverted, with the latter approach being used when there is concern over the viability of the tissue at the appendiceal base. If the patient presents with more advanced peritonitis and/or significant diagnostic uncertainty, a lower midline incision may be more appropriate to allow wider access to the pelvic peritoneal cavity. Laparoscopic appendectomy is also a well-attested option. In most series, it has been associated with slightly less postoperative pain and lower wound infection rates than standard appendectomy. Conversely, some early studies have suggested higher postoperative abscess rates with laparoscopy in perforated appendicitis. Equipment costs, particularly if a stapler is used to control the appendiceal base, make it typically more expensive than standard appendectomy. Laparoscopy may be a particularly attractive option in the setting of diagnostic uncertainty, since it allows inspection of the peritoneal cavity before committing to a given operative exposure. If the appendix is normal with either open or laparoscopic evaluation, possible confounding pathology should be sought for and excluded. Typically this would include inspecting the gynecologic organs, the terminal ileum for Meckel's diverticulum or Crohn's disease, and inspecting or palpating the sigmoid, gallbladder, and right colon for pathology that would explain right-sided abdominal complaints.

Occasionally, the patient presenting with advanced findings may be found to have a palpable mass on examination and corresponding localized abscess on CT or ultrasound. Such patients may be treated nonoperatively with percutaneous radiologic drainage of the abscess and antibiotics. The subject of subsequent interval appendectomy is controversial; historically this has been advised at a 6- to 8-week interval after the acute episode. More recent evaluations of this strategy have documented that most patients do not go on to have recurrent acute appendicitis, and in view of this, so-called interval appendectomy may not be necessary.

Complications

Postoperative wound infection is the most common complication of appendectomy. Pelvic abscess is not uncommon, particularly when there has been frank perforation and peritoneal soilage. Fecal fistula can also be seen and should raise the

concern of Crohn's disease at the cecal base. If, in the setting of advanced inflammation, the surgeon is not careful to clearly delineate the appendiceal base, appendiceal remnants may be left and be a source of recurrent problems in rare instances. In settings of significant contamination, wound infection can be minimized by leaving the skin open to heal by secondary intention or delayed primary closure (see Chapter 7, Wounds and Wound Healing).

Incidental Appendectomy

Appendectomy done at the time of another surgical procedure is known as an *incidental appendectomy*. The rationale for an incidental appendectomy is to prevent future cases of appendicitis. However, incidental appendectomy has been a controversial topic in general surgery for many years. Proponents of this procedure note the technical ease of removing a normal appendix. It can be done quickly, is unlikely to increase the morbidity of the primary procedure, and has the added benefit of preventing future appendicitis and the associated hospital and surgical costs associated with this disease. Opponents of this procedure believe that incidental appendectomy, and incidental surgery in general, is unnecessarily meddlesome. They acknowledge the technical ease of the procedure and agree the additional morbidity should be minimal. However, they would argue, any morbidity from an "unnecessary" procedure is unacceptable and therefore not worth even the small chance of a problem. Furthermore, the true cost savings is minimal since many normal appendices need to be removed to prevent a single case of future appendicitis. The immediate costs of these additional procedures, measured in operating room time and equipment, is likely to minimize any future savings. Finally, the surgeon must remember that appendicitis is a disease of young people, while incidental appendectomies have been most commonly performed in older patients already past the peak incidence of this disease. For all of these reasons, the *routine* incidental appendectomy in *all* patients has fallen out of favor and is not recommended.

If an incidental appendectomy is not routinely advocated, are there select patients who would benefit from this procedure? The answer is yes. Clearly, younger patients, who are at the greatest risk of future appendicitis, will get the most benefit from this procedure. Therefore, patients <20 years old are the best candidates. For this reason, pediatric surgeons are more likely to perform an incidental appendectomy. For patients 20 to 40 years old, the benefits are less clear, so an incidental appendectomy is up to the discretion of the operating surgeon. For patients older than 40 years of age, the benefits drop further and incidental appendectomy should probably be avoided. Regardless of age, incidental appendectomy should certainly be done if an appendiceal lesion is discovered at the time of exploration. Other special circumstances that may justify incidental appendectomy would be the noncommunicative patient or if the position of the appendix is greatly altered by the index operation. Under both of these circumstances, future appendicitis may be very difficult to diagnose and therefore the associated morbidity more significant, justifying an incidental appendectomy.

Regardless of patient age, the operating surgeon must remember that an incidental appendectomy should only be done under optimal conditions. Conditions that should caution the surgeon are emergency surgery associated with hemodynamic instability, an appendix that is difficult to identify (thereby requiring additional dissection or exposure), or if the patient has Crohn's disease affecting the base of the cecum, which may predispose to a postoperative fistula. Under all of these circumstances, the risks increase and therefore do not justify an incidental appendectomy.

Appendiceal Tumors

Appendiceal tumors may include carcinoid, carcinoma, and mucocele. Carcinoid tumors of the appendix account for approximately half of GI carcinoids. The vast majority of appendiceal carcinoids are benign, although they can be a ource of luminal obstruction and appendicitis. Lesions <2 cm in size are usually treated adequately by simple appendectomy. As the size of the carcinoid increases, the possibility of malignancy and lymphatic spread also increases. For lesions larger than 2 cm in diameter, a right hemicolectomy to allow wider removal of the lymphatic drainage pathway is accordingly recommended.

Mucoceles are often a consequence of luminal obstruction and may be related to underlying carcinoma of the appendix, which constitutes <1% of all appendiceal disease. Symptoms of acute appendicitis often are associated with these lesions at presentation. Patients who have unusual or unexpected findings at the time of surgery may have such underlying neoplasia, and an oncologic resection (right hemicolectomy) should be considered if the suspicion warrants. Perforated mucoceles and carcinomas, and some such lesions that have not grossly perforated, may be associated with pseudomyxoma peritonei either at the time of presentation or during subsequent follow up. The overall cure rate for appendiceal adenocarcinoma is in the 50% to 60% range at 5-year follow-up.

thePoint ✳ Go to http://thePoint.lww.com/activate and use your scratch-off code on the inside cover of this book to access bonus chapters, question bank, videos, and more.

SAMPLE QUESTIONS

Questions

Choose the best answer for each question.

1. A 43-year-old woman comes to the emergency department with a 3-day history of abdominal distention, nausea, and vomiting. She also reports decreased urine output over the last 24 hours. She has a history of total abdominal hysterectomy 5 years ago for benign disease. She does not take any medications. Her pulse is 110 beats/minute. Her abdomen is distended and there is mild diffuse tenderness. Bowel sounds are hyperactive. The rest of her exam is normal. Serum electrolytes are sodium—140, chloride—90, bicarbonate—32, and potassium—4.0. Which of the following is the most appropriate initial intravenous fluid to administer to this patient?
   A. D5 ½ normal saline with 40 mEq KCl/L
   B. Lactated Ringer's solution
   C. Normal saline
   D. Colloidal starch solution
   E. 5% albumin in normal saline

2. A 38-year-old man has undergone four operations for Crohn's disease in the last 10 years and recently underwent the last of these for treatment of recurrent disease proximal to a prior ileocolic anastomosis. Which of the following agents is most useful for managing acute exacerbations rather than helping to maintain him in remission from active disease?
   A. Azathioprine
   B. Infliximab
   C. Prednisone
   D. Methotrexate
   E. 6-mercaptopurine

3. A 65-year-old woman comes to clinic with a vague history of diffuse abdominal discomfort over the past 3 weeks. She denies any history of trauma or prior abdominal surgery and has no known stigmata of peripheral vascular disease. She takes vitamin D and calcium supplements. On exam, she has diffuse mild to moderate subjective tenderness without guarding or peritoneal signs. She is in sinus rhythm on EKG. Which of the following is the most likely diagnosis?
   A. Superior mesenteric artery thrombosis
   B. Superior mesenteric artery embolus
   C. Nonocclusive mesenteric ischemia
   D. Mesenteric venous thrombosis
   E. Aortic dissection

4. A 63-year-old woman comes to clinic with symptoms of nonspecific abdominal pain. Her past medical history is unremarkable. She takes vitamins and calcium supplements. A recent CT scan shows a small bowel mass lesion. Laboratory evaluations show an elevated serum level of c-kit protein, with normal chromogranin A. Which of the following intestinal tumors is this consistent with?
   A. Hamartomas
   B. Brunner's gland adenoma
   C. Gastrointestinal stromal tumor
   D. Carcinoid tumor
   E. Osler-Weber-Rendu lesion

5. A 24-year-old female graduate student comes to the emergency department because of abdominal pain for the past 12 hours. Initially she had vague mid-abdominal pain that has localized to the RLQ about 3 hours ago. She is otherwise healthy and takes no medications. Her temperature is 37°C. There is guarding and rebound tenderness in the right lower quadrant and a positive Rovsing's sign. A CT scan shows fat stranding around a dilated appendix. At surgery, there is a 2.5-cm firm, smooth yellowish mass at the base of an inflamed appendix. There is no evidence of perforation and no other abnormalities are found. Frozen section biopsy is consistent with a neuroendocrine tumor. Which of the following is the most appropriate management at this time?
   A. Appendectomy to include the tumor
   B. Cecectomy
   C. Subtotal colectomy
   D. Right hemicolectomy
   E. Appendectomy followed by chemotherapy

Answers and Explanations

1. Answer: C

Potassium should not be added until volume restoration is achieved, lactated Ringer's may worsen metabolic alkalosis because the lactate is converted to bicarbonate in the liver, and colloidal solutions do not correct the hypochloremia and electrolyte imbalances and are not called for in resuscitating the hypovolemic dehydrated patient.

2. Answer: C

All other agents have been successfully used in remission maintenance strategies.

3. Answer: D

Others typically present with more acute or sudden symptomatology.

4. Answer: C

The elevated c-kit level is specific to gastrointestinal stromal tumor (GIST) tumors and is the key information leading to this answer. The other small bowel lesions mentioned could present with similar vague symptoms but are not associated with the c-kit proto-oncogene mutation and associated serum protein marker. Carcinoid tumors may be associated with elevated levels of 5-HIAA (5-hydroxyindole acetic acid) on 24 urine testing. Osler-Weber-Rendu lesions are telangiectasias and may be associated with bleeding and characteristic visible telangiectasias in other mucosal areas including the oral cavity and skin. Hamartomas may be associated with Peutz-Jeghers syndrome. Brunner's gland adenomas are seen in the proximal duodenum, where these glands are part of the mucus and alkaline mucosal protection mechanism of the proximal small intestine.

5. Answer: D

This patient has a carcinoid tumor. A right hemicolectomy is needed because of the heightened risk of lymph node metastases. A simple appendectomy would not be appropriate for a carcinoid at the base of the appendix but would be appropriate for a carcinoid tumor <2 cm at the tip of the appendix. Cecectomy would not adequately sample the regional lymph nodes, and a subtotal colectomy is not necessary. Adjuvant chemotherapy is not indicated for a localized carcinoid tumor.

15
Colon, Rectum, and Anus

MERRIL T. DAYTON, M.D. • GERALD A. ISENBERG, M.D. • JAN RAKINIC, M.D. •
J. SCOTT THOMAS, M.D. • JUDITH L. TRUDEL, M.D.

Objectives

1. List the differential diagnosis, initial management, diagnostic studies, and indications for medical versus surgical treatment in a patient with left lower quadrant pain.

2. Describe the clinical findings of diverticular disease of the colon.

3. Discuss five complications of diverticular disease and their appropriate surgical management.

4. Differentiate ulcerative colitis from Crohn's disease of the colon in terms of history, pathology, x-ray findings, treatment, and risk of cancer.

5. Discuss the role of surgery in the treatment of patients with ulcerative colitis and Crohn's disease.

6. List the signs, symptoms, and diagnostic aids for evaluating presumed large bowel obstruction.

7. Discuss at least four causes of colonic obstruction in adults, including the frequency of each cause.

8. Outline a plan for diagnostic studies, preoperative management, and treatment of volvulus, intussusception, fecal impaction, and obstructing colon cancer.

9. Given a patient with mechanical large or small bowel obstruction, discuss the potential complications if the treatment is inadequate.

10. Identify the common symptoms and signs of carcinoma of the colon, rectum, and anus.

11. Discuss the appropriate laboratory, endoscopic, and x-ray studies for the diagnosis of carcinoma of the colon, rectum, and anus.

12. Using the TNM (tumor, node, metastasis) classification system, discuss the staging and 5-year survival rate of patients with carcinoma of the colon and rectum.

13. Discuss the anatomy of hemorrhoids, including the four grades encountered clinically, and differentiate internal from external hemorrhoids.

14. Describe the symptoms and signs of patients with external and internal hemorrhoids.

15. Outline the principles of management of patients with symptomatic external and internal hemorrhoids, including the roles of nonoperative and operative management.

16. Outline the symptoms and physical findings of patients with perianal infections.

17. Outline the principles of management of patients with perianal infections, including the role of antibiotics, incision and drainage, and primary fistulectomy.

18. Describe the symptoms and physical findings of patients with anal fissures.

19. Outline the principles of management of patients with anal fissures.

20. Name the two most common cancers of the anal canal and describe their clinical presentation.

21. Describe the recent changes in the approach to the treatment of anal canal cancers.

22. Describe the presentation and treatment of anal condyloma.

23. Describe the diagnostic workup and treatment for lymphogranuloma venereum.

24. Name the causative agent in herpetic proctitis.

The colon and rectum are the terminal portion of the alimentary tract. Neither organ is biologically essential; one can live a virtually normal life without one's colon or rectum. Paradoxically, although the colon is much less vital for nutrition, fluid maintenance, and overall homeostasis than the small intestine, disease is far more common in the colon and rectum. Conditions such as diverticulosis coli, colonic polyps,

adenocarcinoma of the colon and rectum, and ulcerative colitis affect a large number of patients in the United States, and the economic, social, and personal costs are enormous.

The anus, anal canal, and anal sphincters play a critical role in continence, a function that is important for comfortable social interaction. Benign conditions (e.g., hemorrhoids, anal fissures) are common and result in frequent visits to the physician as well as a large expenditure for nonprescription medications. These are the reasons why understanding colorectal physiology, anatomy, and pathology are so important.

ANATOMY

The large intestine may be divided into several parts (Figure 15-1). The cecum is the largest part and is the site where the small bowel joins the colon. There is no distinct division between the cecum and the ascending colon, which is partially fixed posteriorly in the right gutter of the posterior abdominal cavity and is therefore a retroperitoneal structure. The hepatic flexure, just inferior to the liver, is the bend in the ascending colon where it becomes the transverse colon, which is suspended freely in the peritoneal cavity by the transverse mesocolon. The transverse colon bends again at the spleen (splenic flexure) and again becomes partially retroperitoneal. The descending colon remains retroperitoneal down to the sigmoid colon, which is a loop of redundant colon in the left lower quadrant. The distal sigmoid colon, which is intraperitoneal, becomes the rectum at the sacrum and becomes partially retroperitoneal. The rectum continues to the anal sphincters that form the short (3 cm) anal canal.

The rectum is 15 cm long. Its origin is marked by anatomic change from the colon. The teniae coli disperse and disappear at approximately the level of the sacral promontory. As a result, the longitudinal muscle layer becomes a continuous, homogeneous layer. In addition, the proximal rectum is covered by peritoneum anteriorly, but not posteriorly, down to approximately 10 cm above the anal verge, where the rectum becomes an extraperitoneal structure. The proximal rectum is attached to the retroperitoneum posteriorly, and is therefore not covered by peritoneum at that level. The clinical importance of knowing what part of the rectum is intraperitoneal is that a full-thickness rectal biopsy taken from higher than 8 to 9 cm above the anal verge carries the potential risk of free perforation into the peritoneal cavity.

The anal canal extends from the anorectal junction (dentate, or pectinate, line) to the anal verge (Figure 15-2). The dentate line marks the junction between the columnar rectal epithelium, which is insensate, and the squamous anal epithelium, which is richly innervated by somatic sensory nerves. For this reason, pathologic conditions that arise below the level of the dentate line cause severe pain. Immediately proximal to the dentate line are longitudinal folds called the columns of Morgagni (rectal columns). Perianal glands normally

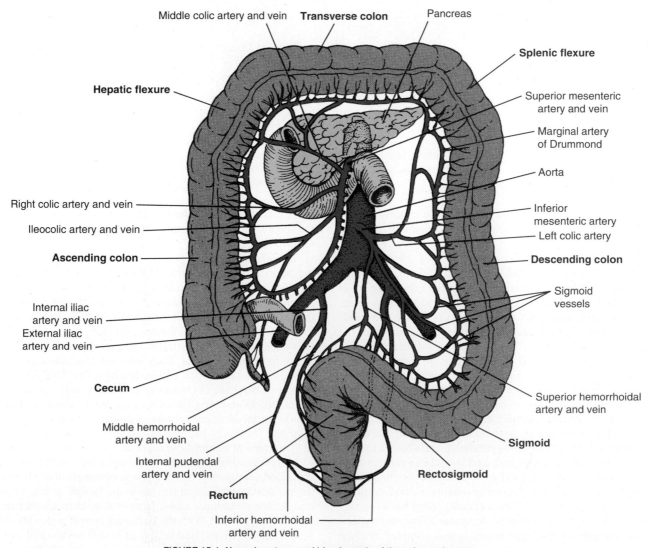

FIGURE 15-1. Normal anatomy and blood supply of the colon and rectum.

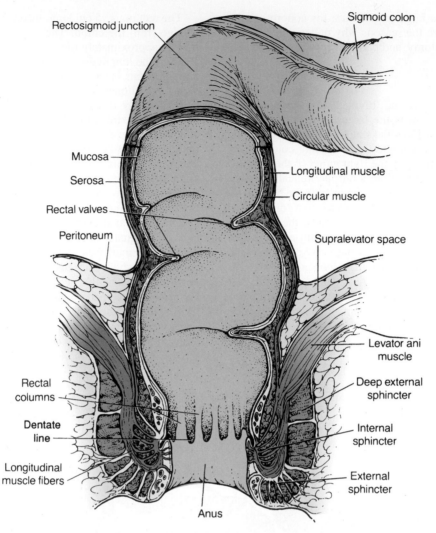

FIGURE 15-2. Normal anatomy of the anorectal canal.

discharge their secretions at the base of these columns, at the level of the anal crypts. Perirectal abscesses usually originate in this area.

The blood supply to the colon (see Figure 15-1) is more complex than that to the small bowel. Like the small intestine, the ascending colon and proximal half of the transverse colon are supplied by branches of the superior mesenteric arteries, whereas the distal half of the transverse colon, descending colon, and sigmoid colon are supplied by branches of the inferior mesenteric artery. The importance of understanding this complex arterial blood supply is that in certain areas of the colon (e.g., splenic flexure) at the junction of two separate blood vessel systems, the blood supply may be relatively poor. For this reason, anastomoses in this region would carry a higher risk of ischemic complications. Another unique aspect of the arterial blood vessels to the colon is the marginal artery of Drummond. This vessel runs parallel to and about 2 to 3 cm from the descending colon wall and is a collateral that connects the middle colic and left colic systems. Its clinical relevance lies in the fact that it provides adequate blood supply to the descending colon even if the left colic artery has to be sacrificed during sigmoid or distal descending colon surgery. The venous drainage of the large bowel is less complex because most branches accompany the arteries and eventually drain

into the portal system. The inferior mesenteric vein drains into the splenic vein, which joins with the superior mesenteric vein to form the portal vein.

The arterial supply to the rectum is derived from a branch of the inferior mesenteric artery (superior hemorrhoidal artery) for the upper rectum, and from branches of the internal iliac arteries (middle hemorrhoidal arteries) and the internal pudendal arteries (inferior hemorrhoidal arteries) for the middle and lower rectum. Veins from the upper rectum drain into the portal system through the inferior mesenteric vein. The middle and inferior rectal veins drain into the systemic circulation through the internal iliac and pudendal veins. This difference in venous drainage is critical to remember when considering rectal tumors and possible sites of metastatic disease. Hemorrhoids are physiologic venous cushions that connect the two systems. They may become distended or thrombose, leading to symptoms of hemorrhoid disease.

Lymphatic drainage of the large intestine parallels the arterial blood supply, with several levels of lymph nodes between the periaortic plexus and the paracolic lymph nodes. In general, tumor metastases move from one level to another in an orderly progression, with the paracolic lymph nodes involved first, followed by the middle tier of lymph nodes, and last by the periaortic lymph nodes. However, lymph node drainage is

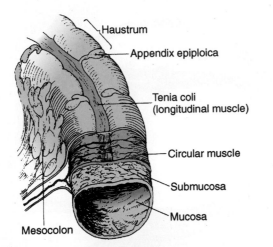

FIGURE 15-3. Oblique cross section showing the layers of the colon wall. (Reprinted from Hardy JD. *Hardy's Textbook of Surgery,* 2nd ed. Philadelphia, PA: Lippincott-Raven, 1983, with permission.)

not as precise as in breast cancer and therefore, sentinel lymph nodes are not as relevant in colon cancer.

The bowel wall of the colon has the same layers as the small intestine: mucosa, submucosa, muscularis, and serosa (Figure 15-3). The major histologic difference is that the colon has no villi (i.e., the mucosal crypts of Lieberkühn form a more uniform surface with less absorptive area). As mentioned earlier, another major difference is that the outer longitudinal smooth muscle layer is separated into three bands (teniae coli) that cause outpouchings of bowel between the teniae (haustra).

The anal sphincter mechanism resembles a tube enclosed in a funnel. The tube is the internal sphincter, which is a continuation of the circular muscular layer of the rectum. This involuntary sphincter is made of smooth muscle. The funnel is the external sphincter, which is a striated voluntary muscle. The external sphincter has three parts: the subcutaneous, superficial, and deep portions. The deep portion is in continuity with the levator ani muscles, which form the base of the pelvic floor. Understanding the anatomy of the sphincters is critical to the diagnosis and treatment of perirectal pathology.

Innervation of the colon is primarily from the autonomic nervous system. Sympathetic nerves pass from the spinal cord through the sympathetic chains and sympathetic ganglia to postganglia that end in Meissner's and Auerbach's plexuses in the bowel wall. Sympathetic stimulation causes inhibition of colonic muscular activity. Parasympathetic innervation comes through the vagus nerve for the colon proximal to the midtransverse colon. The distal transverse colon and beyond is innervated by branches from the second through the fourth sacral cord segments. Parasympathetic activity results in stimulation of colon muscle activity. However, the most important control of colon activity appears to be mediated by regional reflex activity that occurs in the submucosal plexuses (patients with spinal cord transection continue to have relatively normal bowel function).

PHYSIOLOGY

The colon and rectum play some role in maintaining body homeostasis via three main functions: (1) they absorb water and electrolytes from liquid stool, (2) through fermentation, they help digest some starches and protein that are resistant

to digestion and absorption by the small bowel, and (3) they serve as storage for feces. The colon harbors a greater number and variety of bacteria than any other organ in the body. It is host to more than 400 types of bacteria, most of which are anaerobes; *Bacteroides fragilis* is the most common anaerobic colonic organism. The most common aerobes are *Escherichia coli* and enterococci. Colonic bacteria perform a number of important functions for the host including degradation of bile pigments, production of vitamin K, and fermentation of undigested starches and proteins, producing short-chain fatty acids that are absorbed by the colon. As this digestive function represents only a small portion of the digestion and absorption of nutrients that take place in the body, surgical resection of the entire colon and rectum does not impact a person's capacity to maintain normal nutrition. The relatively high number and variety of colonic bacteria do increase the risk of infection during colon surgery. Earlier studies suggested the need to "clean out" the colon ("bowel prep") prior to surgery to lower infection rates. However, more recent studies have cast doubt on the value of the "bowel prep" and a number of surgeons do not do a formal "bowel prep" currently.

The small bowel delivers some 1 to 2 L of chyme to the cecum each day. Up to 90% of the water contained in chyme is absorbed, mostly in the ascending and transverse colon, leaving <200 mL of fluid evacuated daily in solid stool. This amount is a relatively small fraction of the total water absorbed in the intestinal tract. The colon actively absorbs sodium and chloride, and secretes bicarbonate and potassium in exchange. The left portion of the colon and the rectum store solid fecal material permitting defecation at a socially acceptable time and place. The anorectum regulates the final evacuation of solid stool.

Bacterial fermentation also produces approximately 800 to 900 mL/day of colonic gas. The composition of colonic gas varies among individuals and is influenced substantially by diet. Most is passed as flatus, 70% of which is nitrogen (N_2) derived from swallowing air. Other gases include oxygen, carbon dioxide, hydrogen, methane, indole, and skatole. Indole and skatole give colonic gas its characteristic odor.

Colonic motility is unique among organs of the alimentary canal because of the multiple types of contraction patterns, including segmentation and mass contractions. These contractions are characterized by the contraction of long segments of colon, resulting in mass movement of stool. Movement of residue through the colon occurs at a slower rate (18 to 48 hours) than through the small bowel (4 hours). Colonic transit is accelerated by emotional states, diet, disease, infection, and bleeding. Disorders of colonic motility are very prevalent in North America.

The physiology of anal continence is the result of complex interactions between sensory and involuntary and voluntary motor functions. When stool distends the proximal rectum, the internal sphincter relaxes, allowing sensory sampling of the rectal contents. This very sensitive mechanism allows, among other things, the passage of gas without incontinence to stool. Defecation involves a complex interplay among the pelvic floor muscles, rectum, and distal colon, coordinating the relaxation and contraction of several muscle groups. In addition to physiologic weakening of sphincter muscles with advancing age, injury to the sphincter mechanism, either iatrogenic (postsurgical) or postobstetrical contributes to the frequency with which incontinence is seen in adult patients.

The normal frequency of defecation is approximately every 24 hours, but individual variation from 8 to 72 hours is frequent. Any patient who has a significant change in bowel habits should be evaluated for the possibility of serious disease. Severe or new onset constipation (ability to pass flatus, but not stool) and obstipation (inability to pass stool or flatus) are examples of changes that should be evaluated.

COLON AND RECTUM

Diagnostic Evaluation

Patients who have signs or symptoms that are referable to the colon or rectum may be evaluated by several modalities. The digital rectal examination is an important means of detecting many disease processes, including tumors or polyps, abscesses, ulcers, hemorrhoids, and occult colorectal bleeding. There is no downside to performing a rectal examination, but the tendency to defer the digital rectal examination because of patient discomfort or physician inconvenience can result in missing a critical diagnosis.

Although rigid sigmoidoscopy was the standard method of visualizing the distal colon and rectum for many years, it has largely been replaced by fiberoptic flexible sigmoidoscopy. This method provides a higher diagnostic yield and is much more comfortable for the patient. This examination allows visualization of the last 30 to 65 cm of the colorectal complex and results in detection of 60% of colorectal neoplasms. In addition to detecting polyps and neoplasms, it can aid in detecting sites of hemorrhage, ascertaining the etiology of obstruction, evacuating excessive colonic gas, and removing foreign bodies from the rectum. Because of the frequency of colorectal disease, this examination should be an integral part of the routine examination of patients who are older than 50 years of age. In the absence of other symptoms, flexible sigmoidoscopy should be performed every 3 to 5 years, although increasingly many clinicians are shifting to simply doing a full colonoscopy if a study is indicated.

The most accurate diagnostic tool is fiberoptic **colonoscopy**. This instrument allows visualization of the entire colon and rectum and the last few centimeters of terminal ileum. It also provides diagnostic and therapeutic options that were not previously available without surgical intervention (e.g., polyp removal, colonic decompression, stricture dilation, hemorrhage control, biopsy of tumors or inflammatory conditions, foreign body removal). After the patient undergoes thorough bowel preparation and mild sedation, the device is inserted into the anus and advanced to the cecum with a steering mechanism located on the handle (Figure 15-4). Colonoscopy has essentially replaced barium enema for screening, diagnosis, and postoperative follow-up. It is the primary diagnostic modality to evaluate lower gastrointestinal (GI) bleeding of unknown etiology, inflammatory bowel disease, stricture, equivocal barium enema findings, postoperative colonic surveillance, pseudo-obstruction, and polyps (Figure 15-5).

An abdominal series (flat plate and upright radiograph) should be obtained on any patient who has significant abdominal pain. This series is helpful in detecting pneumoperitoneum, large bowel obstruction (e.g., volvulus, tumor), paralytic ileus, appendicolith, and less common diseases. Both the flat plate and the upright x-ray must be obtained, not simply an abdominal flat plate.

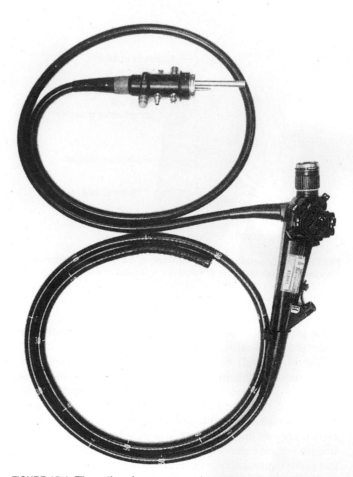

FIGURE 15-4. Fiberoptic colonoscope used for diagnostic and therapeutic maneuvers in the colon.

Barium enema is a radiological diagnostic test during which contrast medium (barium) is introduced under mild pressure to fill the entire colon. As in colonoscopy, a mechanical bowel prep is necessary to empty the bowel prior to the test. A tube is inserted into the rectum, and a contrast medium is introduced under mild pressure to fill the entire colon. When the entire colon and rectum are filled with barium, the study is termed a *single contrast barium enema*. Double-contrast barium enema, using air insufflation while some intraluminal barium

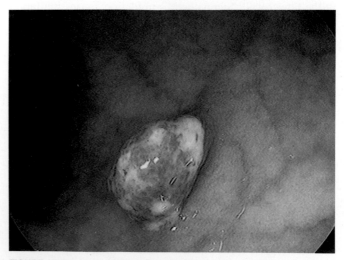

FIGURE 15-5. A polyp detected during colonoscopy.

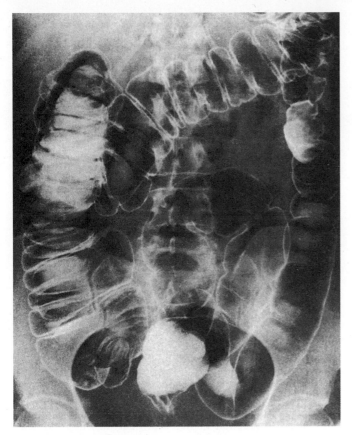

FIGURE 15-6. Normal air-contrast barium enema.

reconstructed images of the colon. Complete cleansing of the colon is required, but sedation is not. The colon is insufflated with air, and the patient is scanned in both the supine and prone positions. The computer software then reconstructs the images for viewing. The ability of CT colography to reliably diagnose colonic polyps and cancers is approaching that of colonoscopy, but remains most sensitive for lesions larger than 1 cm. The American Cancer Society recently included CT colography as an acceptable screening method for colorectal neoplasms; however, many insurance providers do not yet pay for it in this indication.

Technetium-labeled red blood cell scanning is used in the evaluation of lower GI bleeding. This is done when bleeding is less rapid and the patient is reasonably stable. Blood is drawn from the patient and the erythrocytes labeled with radiolabeled technetium; the cells are then retransfused into the patient. A gamma camera is used to detect the activity of the radioisotope, which will collect at the bleeding site. As many lower GI bleeds will have stopped by the time the patient is evaluated, many tagged red blood cell (RBC) scans are nondiagnostic; however, a positive scan is most often followed by mesenteric angiography in an attempt to pinpoint the bleeding site.

Angiography is useful in detecting the source of moderate or rapid colonic bleeding. It is not helpful in patients with slow, chronic blood loss. Nuclear scan (tagged RBC scan) is helpful in identifying bleeding sites in the colon and is more sensitive but less specific than angiography. Capsule endoscopy, a test during which a capsule swallowed by the patient takes video pictures at regular intervals while peristalsis carries it through the bowel, has not yet been perfected for evaluation of the colon.

remains in the colon is particularly sensitive in detecting polyps and small lesions (Figure 15-6). Barium enema may be helpful in diagnosing tumors, diverticulosis, volvulus, and sites of obstruction.

Virtual colonoscopy or CT colography is a promising, relatively new radiological diagnostic test that combines computed tomography (CT) scan capability and computer virtual reality software (Figure 15-7). It uses low-dose, high-resolution helical CT technology to produce three-dimensional

Terminology

Understanding the treatment of colonic diseases requires familiarity with terms that are unique to this organ. **Colostomy** is the surgical procedure in which the colon is divided and the proximal end is brought through a surgically created defect in the abdominal wall (Figure 15-8). The distal end of the bowel is either oversewn and placed in the peritoneal cavity as a blind limb (**Hartmann's procedure**) or brought out inferiorly to the colostomy through the abdominal wall as a **mucous fistula**. Its purpose is nearly always to divert stool

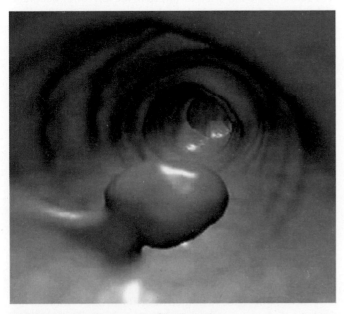

FIGURE 15-7. Image generated by CT colography.

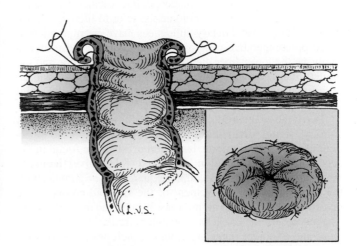

FIGURE 15-8. Lateral and anterior appearance of an end colostomy. (Way L. *Current Surgical Diagnosis*, 7th ed. Stamford, CT: Appleton & Lange, 1985. Reproduced with permission from the McGraw-Hill companies).

from a diseased segment distally in the colon or rectum or to protect a distal anastomosis. A **loop colostomy** is created by bringing a loop of colon through a defect in the abdominal wall, placing a rod underneath, and making a small hole in the loop to allow stool to exit into a colostomy bag. An **ileostomy** is a similar procedure in which ileum is brought through the abdominal wall to divert its contents from distal disease or, in proctocolectomy, to serve as a permanent stoma.

Stomas can be temporary or permanent. Whether for ileostomy or colostomy, stomas are usually performed when stool needs to be diverted for one of the following reasons: (1) to allow healing from a distal anastomosis before bowel continuity is restored; (2) the ends of the bowel are not suitable for an immediate anastomosis after resection (e.g., severely inflamed bowel, questionable vascular supply); (3) when the conditions are not right for proceeding (e.g., severe fecal peritonitis, patient too unstable or too sick to tolerate the procedure); and (4) when there is not enough bowel left for reanastomosis (abdominoperineal resection [APR]).

Other terms that often confuse medical students include **proctocolectomy, abdominoperineal resection (APR),** and **low anterior resection (LAR).** "Procto" is the Greek synonym for the Latin word "rectum." **Proctocolectomy** is operative removal of the entire colon and rectum (e.g., for ulcerative colitis or polyposis syndromes). **Abdominoperineal resection**, which is used in the surgical treatment of very low rectal cancers, is the operative removal of the lower sigmoid colon and the entire rectum and anus, leaving a permanent proximal sigmoid colostomy. **Low anterior resection**, which is used to surgically treat cancers in the middle and upper sections of the rectum, is removal of the distal sigmoid colon and approximately one-half of the rectum, with primary anastomosis of the proximal sigmoid to the distal rectum.

Benign Colonic Disorders

Diverticular Disease

Diverticular disease develops at different rates in different countries with widely varying dietary habits, suggesting the probable influence of diet on the development of this condition. The incidence of diverticular disease is progressive from the fifth to the eighth decade of life, and 70% of elderly patients may have asymptomatic diverticula. Clearly, there is some influence of the aging process on the incidence, but whether it is related to general relaxation of the colonic tissue or to lifelong dietary habits is not clear. Dietary influences have been implicated based on comparative geographic epidemiology; these studies implicate the lower-fiber diet found in Western Europe and the United States. Some postulate that lower stool bulk results in higher generated luminal pressures for propulsion. The resultant increased work causes hypertrophy that leads to diverticulosis.

Two types of diverticula are found in the colon. **Congenital,** solitary, **"true" diverticula** (full wall thickness in the diverticular sac) are uncommon, but when present, are found in the cecum and ascending colon. **Acquired (false) diverticula** are very common in Western countries, and 95% of patients with the condition have involvement of the sigmoid colon. These diverticula are mucosal herniations through the muscular wall. The muscles of the colon have an inner circular smooth muscle layer and a thinner outer layer, which includes three longitudinal bands, the teniae. The most favorable area for herniation occurs where branches of the marginal artery penetrate the wall of the colon (Figure 15-9). The etiology of herniation

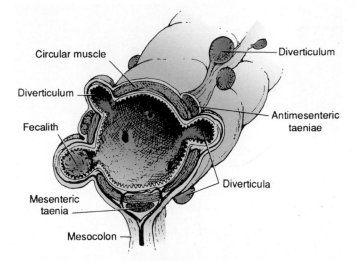

FIGURE 15-9. Mucosal herniation characteristic of diverticulosis. Most herniations occur at a site where the blood vessel penetrates the bowel wall.

is probably related to the colon's exaggerated adaptation for fecal propulsion. One theory suggests that diverticular disease results from higher than normal segmental contractions of the sigmoid colon that lead to high intraluminal pressure. These high intraluminal pressures are confined to the segments that have diverticula. Specifically, the sigmoid colon has localized pressure increases because of segmentation between contraction rings. Contraction of the wall generates high-pressure zones within the segment. As a result, herniation occurs at the weakest point, near the vascular penetration of the bowel wall.

Diverticulosis

General use of the term diverticulosis is reserved for the presence of multiple false diverticula in the colon. This condition is most often an asymptomatic (80%) radiographic finding when a barium enema or colonoscopy is performed for some other diagnostic purpose (Figure 15-10A,B). Nevertheless, certain symptoms are attributed to diverticula in the absence of either inflammation or bleeding.

Clinical Presentation and Evaluation Symptoms include recurrent abdominal pain, often localized to the left lower quadrant, and functional changes in bowel habits, including bleeding, constipation, diarrhea, or alternating constipation and diarrhea. The physical examination is most often unremarkable, or it shows mild tenderness in the left lower quadrant. By definition, fever and leukocytosis are absent. Additional roentgenographic findings may include segmental spasm and luminal narrowing. Endoscopic evaluation of the lumen generally does not show anything except the openings of the diverticula.

Treatment Management of asymptomatic patients with diverticular disease is controversial. Although certain public health organizations recommend a diet with increased fiber content, no specific definition of fiber dietary content has been given for the normal adult. Patients are encouraged to consume fresh fruits and vegetables, whole-grain breads and cereals, and bran products. Pharmacologic preparations of fiber (e.g., psyllium seed products) are more expensive but are more likely to be taken by patients than large amounts of fruits and vegetables with an equivalent amount of fiber.

Diverticulitis

Diverticulitis describes a limited infection of one or more diverticula, including extension into adjacent tissue. The condition

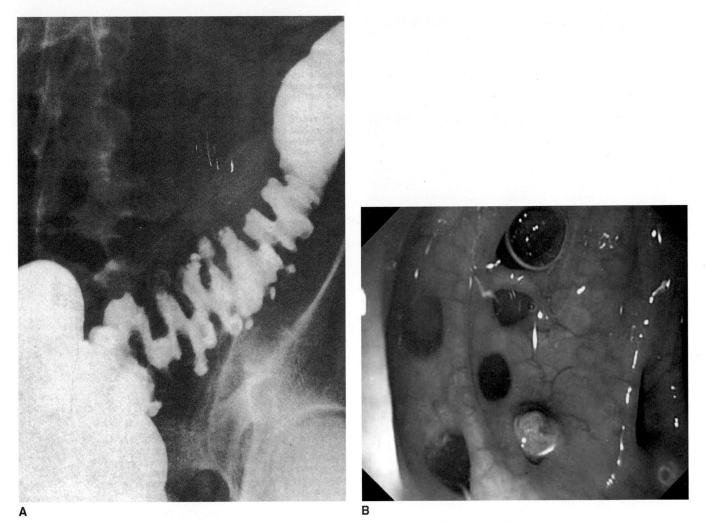

FIGURE 15-10. A, Sigmoid diverticulosis shown on barium enema. **B,** Diverticular openings seen during routine colonoscopy.

is initiated by obstruction of the neck of the diverticulum by a fecalith. The obstruction leads to microperforation that results in swelling in the colon wall or macroperforation that involves the pericolic tissues.

Clinical Presentation and Evaluation The clinical presentation depends on the progression of infection after the perforation. If the perforation is small, it may spontaneously regress. If it is large, it may be confined to pericolic tissues and abate after treatment with antibiotics. The process may enlarge to form an extensive abscess adjacent to the colon or in the mesenteric fat that remains contained, eventually requiring percutaneous or surgical drainage. It may burrow into adjacent hollow organs, resulting in fistula formation. Occasionally, the diverticulum freely ruptures into the peritoneal cavity, causing peritonitis and requiring urgent exploration.

Approximately one-sixth of patients with diverticulosis have signs and symptoms of diverticulitis. The hallmark symptoms of diverticulitis are left lower quadrant abdominal pain (subacute onset), alteration in bowel habits (constipation or diarrhea), occasionally a palpable mass, and fever. Occasionally, free perforation with generalized peritonitis occurs, but the most common picture is one of localized disease. When cicatricial obstruction develops secondary to repeated bouts of inflammation, the patient will have distension, high-pitched bowel sounds, and severe constipation or obstipation. Fistula formation may be associated with diarrhea, stool per vagina

(colovaginal fistula), pneumaturia and recurrent urinary tract infections (colovesical fistula), or skin erythema with a furuncle rupturing and associated stool drainage (colocutaneous fistula). The clinical spectrum is a function of the complications of the diverticular perforation, including abscess formation, fistula development, and partial or total obstruction. Of all life-threatening complications that arise from diverticulitis, 44% involve perforation or abscess, 8% involve fistula, and 4% involve obstruction.

Diagnostic evaluation of diverticulitis or its complications is directed by the clinical presentation. If acute diverticulitis is suspected, abdominal radiographs are obtained to rule out pneumoperitoneum; a barium enema is contraindicated in the acute phase. Barium enema may be obtained 2 to 3 weeks after the episode to confirm the clinical impression. If the patient has obstructive symptoms or evidence of a fistula (e.g., pneumaturia), a contrast enema is indicated. If free perforation has occurred, upright abdominal radiographs show pneumoperitoneum. CT scan is the best diagnostic tool to confirm the diagnosis and determine if an abscess is present (Figure 15-11).

Colovesical fistula is the most common type of fistula encountered in diverticulitis, with a complication occurring in approximately 4% of cases. The differential diagnosis includes carcinoma of the colon, cancer of other organs (e.g., bladder), Crohn's disease, radiation injury, and trauma as a result

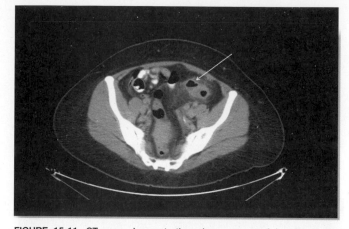

FIGURE 15-11. CT scan demonstrating abscess caused by diverticular perforation.

of foreign bodies. Some patients are symptom-free or mildly symptomatic. However, others have refractory urinary tract infections, fecaluria, and pneumaturia. The most common physical finding is a palpable mass, and leukocytosis secondary to urinary tract infection is frequently found. The diagnostic triad includes barium enema, cystography, and contrast CT scan. However, in a patient with no demonstrable lesion, a dye marker (e.g., methylene blue) can be instilled into the bladder or rectum. Again, CT scan has emerged as the most sensitive test.

Treatment Treatment of the complications of diverticular disease is directed at the specific complication (Table 15-1). Treatment of acute diverticulitis is initially medical in 85% of cases. It consists of admitting the patient to the hospital, instituting intravenous hydration, giving the patient nothing by mouth (NPO), and administering intravenous antibiotics (usually broad coverage of gram-negative coliforms as well as coverage for anaerobes, particularly *B. fragilis*) for 5 to 7 days. Most patients respond to nonoperative treatment and do not require further therapy. However, a subsegment of this group has repeated bouts of acute diverticulitis, requiring hospitalization. Some surgeons believe that any patient who has had two severe bouts of diverticulitis requiring hospitalization should be scheduled for elective sigmoid colectomy (the site of the problem in 95% of cases). However, studies of the natural history of diverticulitis in large groups of patients have shown that while some patients have subsequent episodes of diverticulitis it is the initial episode that is the most severe. Considering the costs and complications associated with resection of the sigmoid colon, this has prompted a shift in how many patients with diverticulitis are approached. At present, most surgeons manage patients with uncomplicated diverticulitis on a case-by-case basis. A person who has one episode of diverticulitis every 3 years is most likely to be managed nonsurgically as described above. However,

TABLE 15-1	Indications for Surgery in Diverticular Disease
Perforation	
Obstruction	
Intractability	
Bleeding	
Fistula	

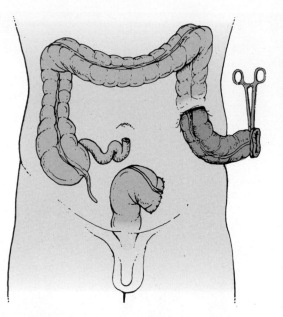

FIGURE 15-12. Operative therapy for diverticular disease usually involves resection of the sigmoid portion of the colon. If the operation is done for acute perforation or obstruction, the segment may be resected, a diverting colostomy brought to the abdominal wall, and the distal rectal stump oversewn (Hartmann procedure). A second stage of the operation involves colostomy takedown and anastomosis to the rectal stump.

a patient who has episodes of uncomplicated diverticulitis requiring hospitalization several times a year is more likely to be advised to consider elective sigmoid colon resection.

Small abscesses adjacent to the colon or within the colonic mesentery may respond to bowel rest and intravenous antibiotics. Larger abscesses are most often treated initially by percutaneous drainage, along with bowel rest and IV antibiotics. Most often, patients in these situations are advised to undergo sigmoid colon resection with reanastomosis after abscess resolution, as it is generally felt that these patients remain at high risk for recurrent abscess formation. In the case of perforation, obstruction, or abscess not amenable to percutaneous drainage, immediate surgical resection of the diseased sigmoid colon is indicated, with a temporary diverting colostomy and a Hartmann procedure (Figure 15-12). In most cases, no attempt at a primary reanastomosis should be made in this setting of unprepared bowel because of the high risk of infection and bowel leak. Intestinal continuity may be reestablished with a colostomy closure after 3 months, when adhesions are felt to be less hostile. In highly selected cases of perforation or obstruction with minimal peritoneal soilage, resection and primary anastomosis may be considered by surgeons experienced in management of these types of situations. If the disease is refractory or a fistula is present, the patient may undergo elective formal sigmoid colectomy with primary anastomosis.

The treatment for colovesical fistula is surgery. Primary closure of the bladder and resection of the sigmoid colon with primary anastomosis is the usual treatment. However, in the presence of severe infection, the colon anastomosis may be delayed and a temporary colostomy performed. Generally, the operation is successful, and recurrence is rare. Similarly, colovaginal fistula is treated with fistula division with sigmoid colon resection and reanastomosis; the opening in the vagina is most often allowed to close by secondary intention. Most colovesical and colovaginal fistula surgery is done electively, as patients are rarely ill from these fistulas.

Diverticular Bleeding

Diverticulosis is occasionally associated with GI hemorrhage. Lower GI bleeding is the primary symptom in 5% to 10% of all patients with diverticular disease. Bleeding from diverticula is occasionally massive (diverticulosis is the most common cause of massive lower GI bleeding) and may be lethal. Massive bleeding is defined as bleeding that is sufficient to warrant transfusion of more than four units of blood in 24 hours to maintain normal hemodynamics. Of all patients with bleeding distal to the ligament of Treitz, approximately 70% have diverticulosis as the source of the bleeding. Approximately 25% of the time, the bleeding is massive.

Clinical Presentation and Evaluation The patient generally has profuse bright or dark red rectal bleeding and hypotension. Unfortunately, the age, sex, and symptoms of patients with bleeding diverticular disease are the same as those with cancer and other lesions. Patients with cancer are unlikely to bleed as severely as patients with diverticulosis, but carcinomas bleed more frequently.

After the history, physical examination, and resuscitation with volume expanders and blood transfusions, the diagnostic approach to the patient with lower GI hemorrhage includes insertion of a nasogastric tube with aspiration until bile is seen (to rule out an upper GI source) and rectal examination including proctoscopy to rule out severe hemorrhoidal bleeding (e.g., portal hypertension) or ulcer. The diagnostic procedure of choice to rule out lower GI sources of bleeding is colonoscopy. Before a colonoscopy can be performed, a mechanical bowel prep using lavage must be completed to clear the colon of stool and old blood. If massive bleeding continues, angiography is the next diagnostic procedure of choice. If the bleeding is intermittent or angiography is indeterminate, colonoscopy after rapid colonic lavage is the preferred modality. Some institutions utilize nuclear scans as their first diagnostic test because it may be more sensitive than colonoscopy and angiography. In addition to diverticulosis, the differential diagnosis includes angiodysplasia, solitary ulcers, varices, cancer, and, rarely, inflammatory bowel disease.

Treatment Most diverticular bleeding will stop without intervention. Mesenteric angiography is useful in detecting the source of moderate or rapid colonic bleeding, defined as a bleeding rate of 0.5 mL/minute or more. Identification of the bleeding site allows surgical resection of the colon, if needed, to be more precise. Mesenteric angiography can also be used in intervention. Vasopressin can be instilled through the angiography catheter just at the bleeding site, successfully stopping bleeding in over 80% of cases. However, since >50% will rebleed, vasopressin instillation is used as a temporizing measure, allowing patients to be resuscitated and then taken for colon resection when more stable, usually within 8 to 12 hours. Similarly, transcatheter embolization with tiny coils can be done to stop bleeding acutely, but is associated with a 6% to 22% risk of ischemia and infarction of the involved bowel segment. For this reason, coil embolization is most often used to temporize as described above, with surgical resection of the involved bowel segment after the patient is resuscitated and stabilized. If the bleeding does not cease spontaneously, surgical resection of the involved segment of colon is indicated.

Ulcerative Colitis and Crohn's Disease of the Colon

Ulcerative colitis is an idiopathic inflammatory bowel disorder that involves the mucosa and submucosa of the large bowel and rectum. It has a bimodal distribution with regard to age. The first, and largest, peak (two-thirds of all cases) includes ages 15 to 30, whereas the second, smaller peak (one-third of all cases) occurs at approximately age 55. The disease is slightly more common in Western countries, and its annual incidence is 10 per 100,000 population. A family history of ulcerative colitis is positive in 20% of patients, suggesting a genetic predisposition.

Crohn's disease is a transmural disease that can involve any portion of the alimentary canal. In a minority of patients, disease is limited to the colorectal region. Like ulcerative colitis, it occurs in a bimodal distribution. Although it more commonly occurs in the region of the terminal ileum, when it occurs exclusively in the colorectum, it is often confused with ulcerative colitis. Gross differences that may be used to distinguish it from ulcerative colitis include rectal sparing, skip lesions (in which diseased segments alternate with normal segments), aphthous sores, and linear ulcers. Crohn's disease is discussed in greater detail elsewhere. This section focuses on ulcerative colitis.

The exact etiology of ulcerative colitis is unknown. Infections, immunologic, genetic, and environmental factors are implicated, but none is proven. The female:male occurrence ratio among patients with ulcerative colitis is 5:4. There is an increased incidence of the disease among Jews, but it is uncommon among blacks and Native Americans.

Pathologic findings include invariable involvement of the rectum (>90%) with variable proximal extension. Occasionally, the rectum alone is involved (ulcerative proctitis). In contrast to Crohn's disease, skip areas of normal bowel between diseased segments are not seen. The mucosa is initially involved, with lymphocyte and leukocyte infiltration that then involves the submucosa with microabscess formation. The crypts of Lieberkühn are commonly affected (crypt abscesses), but muscle layers are rarely involved. The coalescing of these abscesses and erosion of the mucosa lead to pseudopolyp formation, which is identified readily on endoscopic examination. Approximately one-third of the patients affected with ulcerative colitis have pancolitis, in which the entire colon is severely involved.

In addition to the material contained here, the student should refer to Chapter 14, Small Intestine and Appendix, for a discussion of ulcerative colitis and Crohn's disease.

Clinical Presentation and Evaluation

The clinical presentation of ulcerative colitis is variable. The disease may have a sudden onset, with a fulminant, life-threatening course, or it may be mild and insidious. Patients often have watery diarrhea that contains blood, pus, and mucus, accompanied by cramping, abdominal pain, tenesmus, and urgency. To varying degrees, patients have weight loss, dehydration, pain, and fever. Fever is usually indicative of multiple microabscesses or endotoxemia secondary to transmural bacteremia. Approximately 55% of patients have a mild, indolent course; 30% have a moderately severe course that requires large doses of prednisone or sulfasalazine (Azulfidine) or other 5-ASA compounds; and 15% have a fulminant, life-threatening course. The fulminant presentation is often associated with massive colonic dilation secondary to transmural progression of the disease and destruction of the myenteric plexus (toxic megacolon). Patients have severe constitutional symptoms related to sepsis, malnutrition, anemia, acid-base disturbances, and electrolyte abnormalities.

Extraintestinal manifestations occur in a small percentage of patients, including ankylosing spondylitis, peripheral arthritis, uveitis, pyoderma gangrenosum, sclerosing cholangitis, pericholangitis, and pericarditis. The amount of information obtained on physical examination depends on the acuteness and severity of the disease process at the time of examination. If the patient is seen in a quiescent phase, there may be few or no findings; if the patient is seen in an acute phase, there may be a finding of an acute abdomen.

The mainstay of diagnosis is endoscopy with biopsy. Typical endoscopic findings include friable, reddish mucosa with no normal intervening areas, mucosal exudates, and pseudopolyposis (Figure 15-13A,B). A secondary diagnostic study is barium enema, in which mucosal irregularity may be seen. Frequently, shortening of the colon, loss of normal

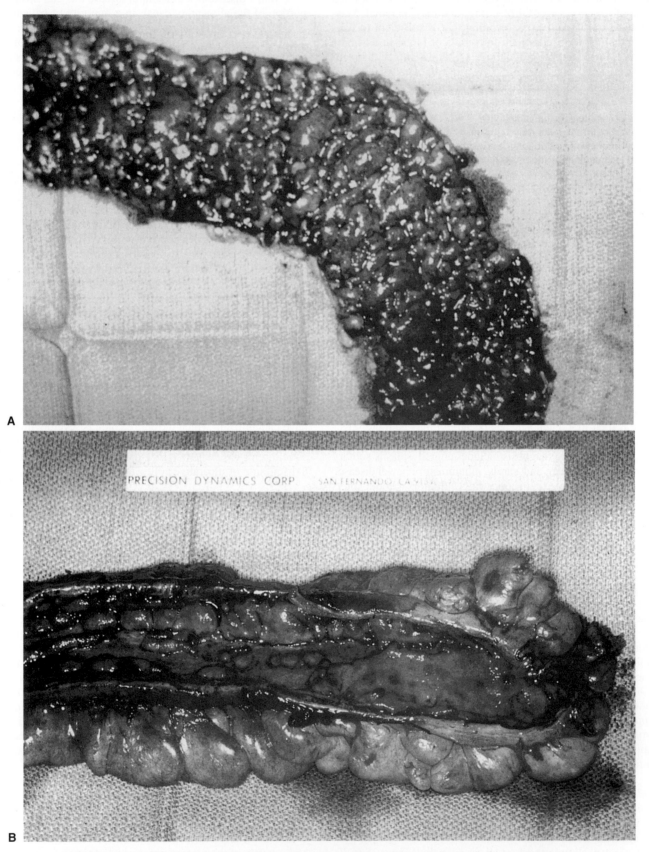

FIGURE 15-13. A, Severe ulcerative colitis showing pseudopolyps, deep ulceration, and friability. **B,** Severe Crohn's colitis showing linear ulcers and "cobblestoning."

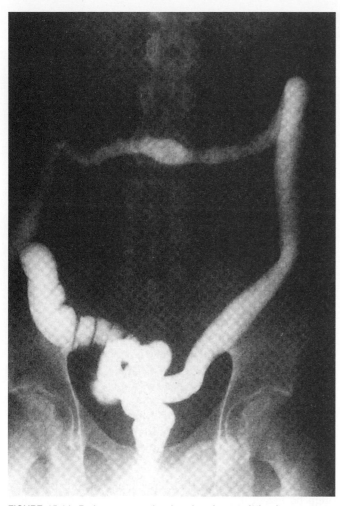

FIGURE 15-14. Barium enema showing the characteristic changes associated with chronic ulcerative colitis. Shown are loss of the haustral pattern, ulcerations, and foreshortening. Because of these changes, the colon is said to resemble a "lead pipe."

haustral markings, and a "lead-pipe" appearance may be seen (Figure 15-14). No specific laboratory tests are diagnostic for ulcerative colitis; however, leukocytosis and anemia may be present. Serologic markers, such as perinuclear antineutrophil cytoplasmic antibodies (pANCA), a group of IgG antibodies commonly elevated in autoimmune disease, may corroborate the diagnosis.

The differential diagnosis includes other inflammatory or infectious disorders, including Crohn's disease, infectious colitis, and pseudomembranous colitis. The disease that is most commonly confused with ulcerative colitis is Crohn's disease of the colon. In approximately 10% of cases, there is an overlap of features; this type of colitis is called indeterminate colitis. Its clinical behavior appears to be more like ulcerative colitis than Crohn's disease, however. Table 15-2 shows distinguishing characteristics of both disease processes.

Treatment

Medical therapy is usually the initial treatment. It is successful in approximately 80% of cases. In mild disease, the treatment is primarily symptomatic, with the use of antidiarrheal agents that slow gut transit (e.g., loperamide) and bulking agents (psyllium seed products) that result in semiformed, less watery stools. In moderate disease, sulfasalazine or mesalamine-based preparations should be tried because they

induce remission in approximately half of all patients initially. In severe disease, most patients respond dramatically to steroid administration. Unfortunately, because of potential severe side effects, the dose is tapered and minimized whenever possible. Recent studies demonstrate efficacy of an anti-tumor necrosis factor (anti-TNF) monoclonal antibody (infliximab [Remicade]) in treating patients with Crohn's disease, especially in the presence of fistulae. While this treatment is more effective in patients with Crohn's disease of the small bowel, patients with primary colonic involvement also have significant response rates. Trials are currently in progress to determine efficacy in ulcerative colitis. Elimination of milk from the diet is occasionally helpful. Supportive therapy, including physical and emotional support, is important. Close interaction between the medical and surgical teams offers these patients the best possible care.

Major complications are toxic megacolon, colonic perforation, massive hemorrhage, serious anorectal complications, and carcinoma development after years of disease. Initial therapy for toxic megacolon is aggressive medical care, including gastric decompression, antibiotics, intravenous administration of fluids, hyperalimentation, and elimination of all other medications, specifically anticholinergics. The goal is to convert these patients to a more stable condition and have a semielective procedure. The majority will have a recurrence of the megacolon without surgery. Emergency surgery can be very difficult because of a paper-thin colon wall.

Surgical therapy is indicated when medical therapy fails or surgically treatable complications ensue (e.g., hemorrhage, perforation, obstruction, dysplasia, or carcinoma). Because of the increased risk of carcinoma, long-standing ulcerative colitis is also an indication for surgical intervention. The risk increases 1% to 2% per year after the initial 10 years of disease. In the past, the definitive operative procedure for ulcerative colitis was total proctocolectomy with permanent ileostomy. In the past, procedures were devised to maintain fecal continence, including an operation that involves constructing a reservoir with a continence-producing nipple valve out of the small intestine (Kock's continent ileostomy). This operation has met with limited success. Subtotal colectomy with ileoproctostomy is attempted in some patients who have less severe rectal involvement and absolutely no perianal problems. Unfortunately, this operation does not cure the disease and subjects the patient to the risks of recurrent disease or the development of a malignancy in the remaining remnant. Total colectomy with proctectomy and ileoanal pull-through (Figure 15-15A–D) is now the operation of choice. The procedure is performed with a surgically constructed ileal reservoir, thereby sparing the patient a permanent abdominal ileostomy. Because patients with toxic megacolon, perforation, or other complications have much higher morbidity and mortality rates, early surgery may be indicated and may require additional stages.

Colonic Obstruction and Volvulus
Obstruction of the Large Intestine

Only 10% to 15% of intestinal obstruction in adults is the result of obstruction of the large bowel. The most common anatomic site of colonic obstruction is the sigmoid colon. The three most common causes are adenocarcinoma (65%), scarring associated with diverticulitis (20%), and volvulus (5%). Inflammatory disorders, benign tumors, foreign bodies, fecal impaction, and other miscellaneous problems

TABLE 15-2	Comparison of Ulcerative Colitis and Crohn's Colitis	
	Ulcerative Colitis	**Crohn's Colitis**
Symptoms and signs		
Diarrhea	Severe, bloody	Less severe, bleeding infrequent
Perianal fistulas	Rare	Common
Strictures or obstruction	Uncommon	Common
Perforation	Free, uncommon	Localized, common
Pattern of development		
Rectum	Virtually always involved	Often normal
Terminal ileum	Normal	Diseased in majority of patients
Distribution	Continuous	Segmented, skip lesions
Megacolon	Frequent	Less common
Appearance		
Gross	Friable, bleeding granular exudates, pseudopolyps, isolated ulcers	Linear ulcers, transverse fissures, cobblestoning, thickening, strictures
Microscopic	Inflamed submucosa and mucosa, crypt abscesses; fibrosis uncommon	Transmural inflammation, granulomas, fibrosis
Radiologic	Lead-pipe, foreshortening, continuous, concentric	String sign in small bowel; segmental, asymmetric internal fistulae
Course		
Natural history	Exacerbations, remissions, dramatic flare-ups	Exacerbations, remissions, chronic, indolent
Medical treatment	Initial response high (>80%)	Response less predictable
Surgical treatment	Curative	Palliative
Recurrence	No	Common

account for the remainder. Obstructive adhesive bands, which are often seen in the small bowel, are extremely uncommon in the colon.

Clinical Presentation and Evaluation Signs and symptoms include abdominal distension; cramping abdominal pain, usually in the hypogastrium; nausea and vomiting; and obstipation. Radiologic and CT findings show distended proximal colon, air-fluid levels, and no distal rectal air (Figure 15-16A, B).

Physical examination usually shows abdominal distension, tympany, high-pitched metallic rushes, and gurgles. On palpation, a localized, tender, palpable mass may indicate a strangulated closed loop or an area of inflamed diverticular disease.

An important element that affects the clinical expression of large bowel obstruction is whether the ileocecal valve is competent. If it is incompetent, the signs and symptoms produced are indistinguishable from those of routine small bowel obstruction. If the ileocecal valve is competent, as is the case in approximately 75% of patients, a "closed loop" obstruction occurs between the ileocecal valve and the obstructing point distally. Massive colonic distension results, and the cecum may reach a diameter of 12 cm, increasing the possibility of perforation, with or without gangrene. It is critically important for the clinician to distinguish between complete large bowel obstruction and partial large bowel obstruction. Patients with complete large bowel obstruction have obstipation that includes a history of no flatus or stool passage for 8 to 12 hours. On the other hand, patients with partial large bowel obstruction describe the passage of some gas or stool. Distinguishing between the two is important because a patient with complete bowel obstruction should undergo emergent operation. Those with partial large bowel obstruction may often be treated by nasogastric decompression and intravenous fluids with resolution of the acute obstruction. This distinction has important surgical ramifications because patients with partial large bowel obstruction can then be prepared for surgery by cleaning out the large intestine, thus avoiding a colostomy.

The appropriate diagnostic techniques include plain films of the abdomen. In patients in whom the cecum measures more than 12 cm and a definitive lesion cannot be delineated, laparotomy is undertaken. The use of water-soluble contrast enema confirms the diagnosis of colonic obstruction and identifies the exact location. If the obstruction is shown on plain abdominal films, barium enema is not necessary. Barium should never be given orally in the presence of suspected colonic obstruction because it may accumulate proximal to the obstruction and cause a barium impaction. Colonoscopic examination plays a major role in Ogilvie's syndrome (localized paralytic ileus of the colon without mechanical obstruction); otherwise, it is reserved for the occasional case of volvulus for decompression or those patients who may need colonic stent placement.

Treatment All patients with large bowel obstruction should be treated with intravenous fluids, nasogastric suction, and continuous observation until the diagnosis is established and definitive therapy is undertaken. Potentially lethal complications of large bowel obstruction are perforation, peritonitis, and sepsis. The major causes of severe colonic obstruction leading to these complications include carcinoma of the colon, with or without perforation; diverticulitis; sigmoid volvulus; and cecal volvulus.

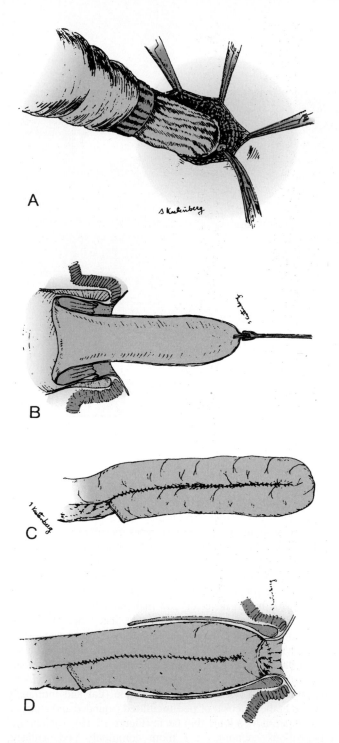

A

B

C

D

FIGURE 15-15. Ileoanal pull-through is the operation of choice for definitive treatment of ulcerative colitis and familial polyposis syndrome. **A,** After removal of the entire colon, the mucosa is stripped away from the muscular layers of the rectum. **B,** This dissection is continued down to the dentate line, and the mucosa is everted out through the anus and resected. **C,** A small reservoir is constructed from the terminal ileum using a J-shaped configuration. **D,** This J-shaped pouch is then pulled through the muscular cuff and anastomosed to the dentate line to create a neorectum.

Emergency laparotomy is undertaken for acute large bowel obstruction with cecal distension beyond 12 cm, severe tenderness, evidence of peritonitis, or generalized sepsis. Perforation caused by volvulus, obstructing cancers, or diverticular strictures usually requires laparotomy with the appropriate surgical procedures, usually resection and diverting colostomy.

Patients with a large bowel obstruction due to cancer and without peritonitis may undergo colonic stent placement that allows decompression without the need for urgent surgery and colostomy.

For the occasional case of Ogilvie's syndrome in which there is idiopathic, enormous dilation of the right side of the colon without mechanical obstruction (pseudo-obstruction), the current therapy is IV neostigmine administration (inhibits breakdown of acetylcholine), which results in contraction of the affected colon. If unsuccessful, fiberoptic colonoscopy, with decompression and placement of a long rectal decompression tube is utilized. Cecostomy may be necessary in cases of recurrence.

The various conditions that lead to large bowel obstruction result in differing prognoses, most of which depend on the patient's age and the comorbidity of existing diseases, particularly cardiovascular disease. Unfortunately, the overall death rate of patients who have a cecal perforation approaches 30%. Thus, prompt surgical intervention is critical.

Volvulus of the Large Intestine
Volvulus is rotation of a segment of the intestine on the axis formed by the mesentery (Figure 15-17). The most common sites of occurrence in the large bowel are the sigmoid (70%) and cecum (30%). Volvulus accounts for 5% to 10% of cases of large bowel obstruction and is the second most common cause of complete colonic obstruction. Stretching and elongation of the sigmoid with age is a predisposing factor. The first occurrence of volvulus in more than 50% of cases is in patients 65 years of age or older. For unknown reasons, patients who are confined to psychiatric institutions or nursing homes have an increased risk for this disease. Volvulus also occurs in patients who have a hypermobile cecum because of incomplete fixation of the ascending colon at the time of intrauterine development. This condition allows the cecum to twist about the mesentery, forming a closed-loop obstruction at the entry and exit points, with major pressure at the sites of the twist. The vessels are partially occluded, and circulatory impairment leads to prompt gangrene and perforation.

Clinical Presentation and Evaluation The patient has abdominal distension, which is often massive; vomiting; abdominal pain; obstipation; and tachypnea. Physical examination shows distension, tympany, high-pitched tinkling sounds, and rushes. Diagnostic studies include abdominal x-ray films and water-soluble contrast enemas. Abdominal radiographs show a massively dilated cecum or sigmoid without haustra that often assumes a kidney bean appearance. Water-soluble contrast enema study shows the exact site of obstruction, with a characteristic funnel-like narrowing that often resembles a bird's beak or an ace of spades. CT scan also has a characteristic appearance (Figure 15-16B).

Treatment Sigmoidoscopy with rectal tube insertion to decompress sigmoid volvulus is the recommended initial treatment for that location. Emergency operation is performed promptly if strangulation or perforation is suspected or if attempts to decompress the bowel are unsuccessful. Surgical therapy involves resection without anastomosis and the construction of a temporary colostomy. Most patients with sigmoid volvulus are easily decompressed and subsequently require elective resection, except for very high-risk elderly patients. Cecal volvulus is always treated surgically, rarely with cecopexy (suturing the cecum to the parietal peritoneum) and most commonly with right hemicolectomy with ileotransverse colostomy.

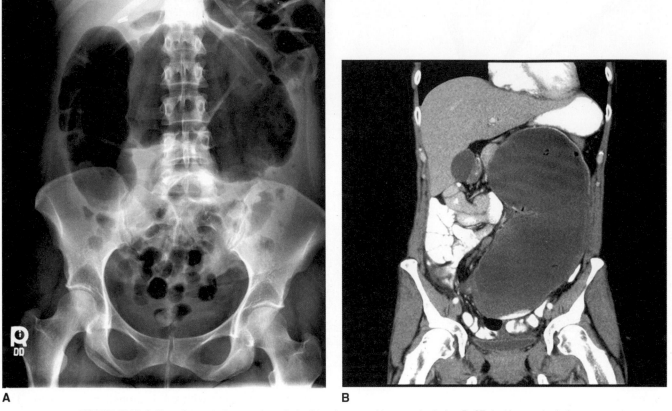

A　　　　　　　　　　　　　　　　　　**B**

FIGURE 15-16. **A,** X-ray demonstrating massive colonic distension caused by a cecal volvulus. **B,** CT showing cecal volvulus.

Polyps and Carcinoma of the Colon and Rectum

Colorectal Polyp

Polyp is a morphologic term that is used to describe small mucosal excrescences that grow into the lumen of the colon and rectum. A variety of polyp types have been described, all with different biologic behaviors (Table 15-3). Approximately

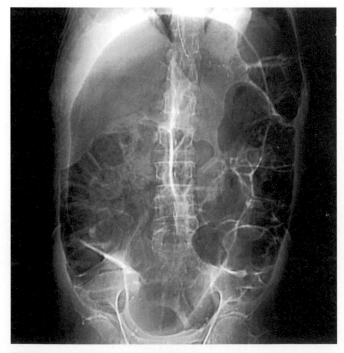

FIGURE 15-17. Volvulus of the sigmoid colon.

5% of all barium enema and 5% to 10% of colonoscopic studies show polyps. Approximately 50% occur in the rectosigmoid region, and 50% are multiple.

Distinguishing among polyp types is important because some types are clearly associated with carcinoma of the colon. Inflammatory polyps (pseudopolyps) are common in inflammatory bowel disease and have no malignant potential. Hamartomas (juvenile polyps and polyps associated with Peutz-Jeghers syndrome) similarly have very low malignant potential and often spontaneously regress or autoamputate. They may be safely observed. However, polyps that fall into the general category of "adenoma" are clearly premalignant, and appropriate vigilance is indicated. Three subdivisions of adenomas are described: (1) tubular (Figure 15-18), (2) tubulovillous, and (3) **villous adenoma.** Most polyps are either **sessile** (flat and intimately attached to the mucosa) or **pedunculated** (rounded and attached to the mucosa by a long, thin neck; (Figure 15-19). Tubular and tubulovillous adenomas are more commonly pedunculated, whereas villous adenomas are more commonly sessile. Evidence for malignant potential includes (1) the high incidence of cancer associated with the polyps in familial polyposis syndrome or Gardner's syndrome, (2) simultaneous occurrence of cancers and polyps in the same specimen, (3) carcinogens that experimentally produce both adenomas and cancers in the same model, and (4) lower cancer risks associated with those who have polyps removed. Approximately 7% of tubular, 20% of tubulovillous, and 33% of villous adenomas become malignant. Villous adenomas >3 cm in diameter have a greater probability of malignancy.

Clinical Presentation and Evaluation

Polyps are usually asymptomatic, but occasionally bleed enough to cause the patient to seek medical evaluation. They are most

TABLE 15-3	Comparison of Colonic Polyps			
Type	**Frequency**	**Location**	**Malignant Potential**	**Treatment**
Tubular	Common: 10% of adults	Rectosigmoid in 20%	7% malignant	Endoscopic excision
Villous	Fairly common, especially in the elderly	Rectosigmoid in 80%	33% malignant	Surgical removal
Hamartoma	Uncommon	Small bowel	Low; uncommon	Excise for bleeding or obstruction
Inflammatory	Uncommon, except in IBD	Colon and rectum	None	Observation
Hyperplastic	Fairly common	Stomach, colon, and rectum	None	Observation

IBD, inflammatory bowel disease.

commonly detected during routine endoscopic surveillance. Occasionally, a family history of polyps causes the patient to seek endoscopic screening.

Treatment

Treatment of adenomatous polyps involves colonoscopic polypectomy. If some cannot be safely removed colonoscopically, biopsy should be performed and a segmental resection of the colon done if the lesion is a villous adenoma or is large, ulcerated, dysplastic, or indurated. For disease conditions that are characterized by extensive polyposis (familial polyposis syndrome or Gardner's syndrome), the operation most commonly performed is total colectomy and **ileoanal pull-through**.

Carcinoma of the Colon and Rectum

Cancer of the colon and rectum is a major cause of death in the United States. The American Cancer Society estimates that over 55,000 people die of this disease annually. Approximately 140,000 to 145,000 new cases are identified each year. Although a large number of factors are associated with the development of this disease, theories about its etiology center on the impact of intraluminal chemical carcinogenesis. There are various theories as to whether these carcinogens are ingested or are the result of biochemical processes that occur intraluminally from existing substances that are found normally in the fecal stream. Geographic epidemiologic studies show that certain populations have a very low incidence of cancer of the colon and rectum, apparently as a result of identifiable dietary factors (e.g., high fiber, low fat), although social customs and a lack of environmental

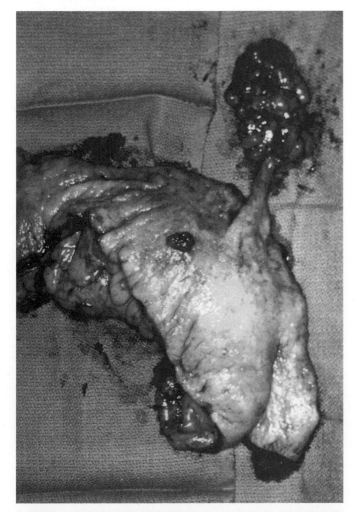

FIGURE 15-18. Large tubular adenoma in a resected segment of the sigmoid colon.

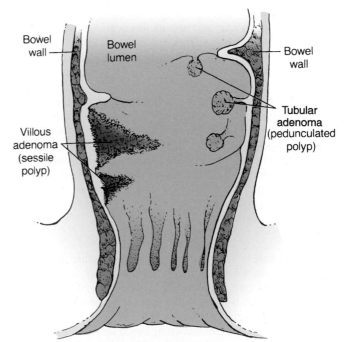

FIGURE 15-19. Characteristic appearance of a villous adenoma (sessile polyp) compared with a tubular adenoma (pedunculated polyp). Sessile polyps tend to be more difficult to manage because they are difficult to remove endoscopically and because their malignant potential is greater.

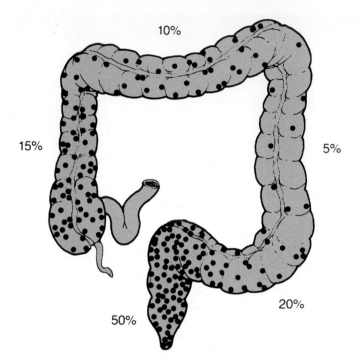

FIGURE 15-20. Frequency distribution of adenocarcinoma of the colon and rectum.

carcinogens cannot be excluded. Certain health agencies promote a low-fat, high-fiber diet as protective against cancer of the colon and rectum. Chemoprevention by ingestion of such agents as carotenoids and other antioxidants has been suggested, but the efficacy of this measure is unproven. There is good evidence that prostaglandin inhibitors such as aspirin and sulindac significantly lower the risk of polyp formation and colon cancer when taken on a regular basis.

Most large bowel cancers occur in the lower left side of the colon, near the rectum (Figure 15-20), although recent studies suggest a slow shifting to right-side lesions. Synchronous (simultaneously occurring) tumors develop in 5% of patients, whereas 3% to 5% of patients have metachronous tumors (a second tumor developing after resection of the first). A family history of colon cancer is an important risk factor for colon cancer in first-degree relatives.

Familial polyposis syndrome, Gardner's syndrome, and the cancer family syndrome (hereditary nonpolyposis colon cancer [HNPCC]) clearly show that certain patient subsets are genetically predisposed to cancer of the colon. Other predisposing diseases include ulcerative colitis, Crohn's colitis, lymphogranuloma venereum, and certain polyps (described previously).

The peak incidence of colon cancers occurs at approximately 70 years of age, but the incidence begins to increase in the fourth decade of life.

Screening

Of all GI cancers, more progress has been made in improving cure rates in colorectal cancer than any other; currently, the 5-year survival rate is 65% (SEER database, NCI). There is little question that this improvement is the direct result of two factors: (1) an effective screening instrument, colonoscopy, and (2) effective strategies for screening based on risk factors. Mild risk factors include age, diet, physical inactivity, obesity, smoking, race, and alcohol. Intermediate risk groups include those with a personal history of colorectal cancer or adenoma, as well as those with a strong family history. Follow-up studies have revealed that individuals with one first-degree relative with colorectal cancer have a twofold increased risk of colorectal cancer, and those with two first-degree relatives have a sixfold increased risk. Patients at high risk for developing colorectal cancer are those with familial colorectal cancer syndromes (familial polyposis, Gardner's, and HNPCC) and patients who have had ulcerative or Crohn's colitis for more than 10 years.

For patients with average risk, the American Cancer Society guidelines recommend that, beginning at age 50, both men and women should follow one of these screening options:

Tests That Find Both Polyps and Cancer
1. Flexible sigmoidoscopy every 5 years*
2. Colonoscopy every 10 years
3. Double-contrast barium enema every 5 years*
4. CT colonography (virtual colonoscopy) every 5 years*

Tests That Mainly Find Cancer
1. Fecal occult blood test (FOBT) every year*
2. Fecal immunochemical test (FIT) every year*
3. Stool DNA test (sDNA), interval uncertain*

Colonoscopy should be done if test results are positive.

It is important to note that CT colonography is a newer test and the final results for its use as a screening method remain unclear. However, it is an important tool when evaluating the obstructed colon or in a patient that can't be evaluated by colonoscopy or barium enema.

If the patient has intermediate risk, the screening should begin at age 40 and be done more frequently than every 10 years (e.g., every 3 to 5 years). In the high-risk group, screening is a function of duration of disease. In inherited polyposis groups, blood tests are now available to rule out the disease in familial polyposis and HNPCC. For patients unable to access the blood tests, screening should begin in the teen years, since full expression of the disease can occur by age 20. Patients who have had ulcerative or Crohn's colitis for 10 years or more should begin annual colonoscopic surveillance with biopsies. Serious consideration should be given to prophylactic total colectomy with ileoanal pull-through in both high-risk groups before an invasive cancer develops.

Clinical Presentation and Evaluation

The clinical signs and symptoms of colorectal cancer are determined largely by the anatomic location. Cancers of the right colon are usually exophytic lesions associated with occult blood loss, resulting in iron deficiency anemia (Table 15-4). At advanced stages of the disease, patients may have a palpable right lower abdominal mass. Recent retrospective studies indicated that the incidence of right colon cancers is increasing at a greater rate than that of left colon cancers. Right-sided lesions may account for as many as one-third of all new cases seen, with most diagnosed at a late stage. Cancers that arise primarily in the left and sigmoid colon are more frequently annular and invasive (Figure 15-21), resulting in obstruction and macroscopic rectal bleeding (see Table 15-4). Cancers of the rectum also cause a symptom complex of rectal bleeding, obstruction, and, occasionally, alternating diarrhea and constipation. Tenesmus occurs with far advanced disease.

Any patient older than 30 with a change in bowel habits, iron deficiency anemia, or rectal bleeding should undergo a complete examination of the colon and rectum by colonoscopy.

TABLE 15-4	Symptoms of Colon and Rectal Cancers		
	Site of Cancer		
Symptom	**Right Colon**	**Left Colon**	**Rectum**
Weight loss	+	+/0	0
Mass	+	0	0
Rectal bleeding	0	+	+
Tympany	0	0	+
Virchow's node	+	0	0
Blumer's shelf	+	+	0
Anemia	+	0	0
Obstruction	0	+	+

If rectal bleeding occurs, workup for a possible malignancy should be initiated, even if the apparent source is a benign lesion (e.g., hemorrhoid) unless the patient is younger and rapidly responds to treatment.

Bright red rectal bleeding should always be evaluated by an examination of the perianal region and digital rectal exam. The value of preoperative total colonoscopy lies in its ability to detect the 3% to 5% of patients with synchronous colon cancers, allowing better planning of surgical therapy. CT of the abdomen is frequently performed before surgery. Preoperative blood tests should evaluate the patient's overall nutritional status and should include liver function tests and a **carcinoembryonic antigen (CEA)** study. Results of the antigen study are elevated in many GI malignancies and, although it is not specific for colorectal cancer, it may be useful in following patients after resection to detect recurrence.

Diagnostic studies showing an obstructing lesion in the sigmoid colon that occurs in the presence of diverticula should raise the suspicion for malignancy. Because both conditions may coexist and it is occasionally impossible to distinguish between the two, the surgeon should proceed with a "cancer operation," which includes a wide lymph node resection, whenever there is any question. Diverticular stricture, polyps, benign tumors, ischemic stricture, and Crohn's colitis are included in the differential diagnosis.

Treatment

The surgical treatment used by most surgeons includes adequate local excision of the tumor, with a length of normal bowel on either side, and resection of the potentially involved lymph node draining basin found in the mesentery that is determined by the vascular supply. Removal of the lymphatics that drain the tumor region should be part of the operation because nodal involvement is present in more than 30% of specimens. Colorectal cancer may also spread hematogenously, intraluminally, or by direct extension or peritoneal seeding (Blumer's shelf on rectal examination). The most common organ involved in distant colorectal metastases is the liver.

Patients whose colon tumors are no longer confined to the bowel and are adherent to extraperitoneal structures in the pelvis, upper abdomen, or other area should have en bloc resections (which include resection of the tumor and any other invaded structure) whenever possible, with the area being subsequently marked with metal clips to identify it as a site of potential recurrence. When the small bowel is involved, it should be included en bloc in the resection. Studies indicate that small bowel involvement does not change the stage-for-stage prognosis. Similarly, a partial cystectomy or total hysterectomy should be performed with the resection if the tumor is adherent to these organs. Bilateral oophorectomy is recommended by some in menopausal or postmenopausal women to remove occult ovarian metastasis and improve staging.

Tumors of the cecum and ascending colon are treated with right hemicolectomy that includes resection of the distal portion of the ileum and the colon to the midtransverse colon with an ileo-midtransverse colon anastomosis (Figure 15-22). Hepatic flexure lesions are best treated by an extended right colectomy that includes resection to or beyond the level of midtransverse colon. Lesions in the transverse colon are resected based on location with respect to the middle colic vessels. Cancers to the right of the middle colic artery have an extended right hemicolectomy; those to the left, a partial left colectomy. Splenic flexure and left-sided lesions are treated with a left hemicolectomy that includes resection from the level of the midtransverse colon to the sigmoid. Sigmoid colon lesions are treated with sigmoid resection. Obstructing or perforating tumors may prevent primary anastomosis and should be treated with resection, diverting colostomy, and Hartmann's pouch or mucous fistula. A more recent approach to obstructing cancers is the use of metallic stents that can be placed endoscopically or with fluoroscopic guidance. When successfully placed, the stents prevent the need for emergency surgery and colostomy by opening the obstructed colon. This can serve as a bridge to elective resection or palliation if the patient has advanced metastatic disease.

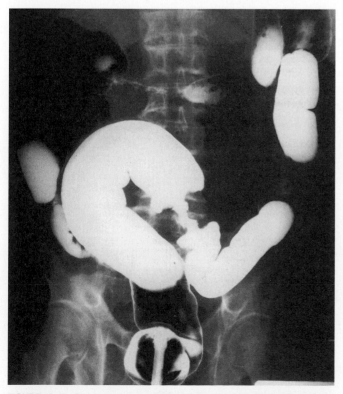

FIGURE 15-21. Carcinoma of the sigmoid colon causing high-grade obstruction and showing a classic "apple core" lesion.

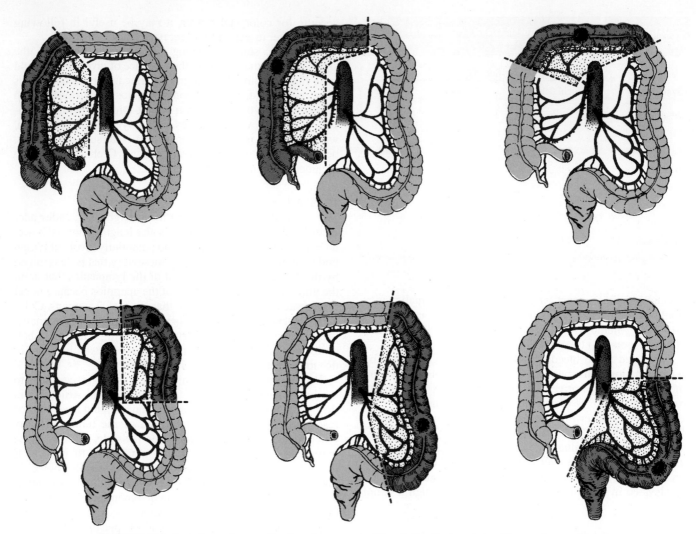

FIGURE 15-22. Indicated operative resection for colon cancer in different sites. The boundaries of the resection are dictated by lymphatic drainage patterns that parallel the blood supply.

Tumors in the upper and middle one-third of the rectum are treated with LAR with primary anastomosis. Total mesorectal excision (TME) is an important part of this technique in which all perirectal fat is removed by compulsively staying in the correct plane laterally. Tumors in the lower one-third of the rectum require specialized procedures (either APR with permanent end sigmoid colostomy or proctectomy and coloanal anastomosis) (Figure 15-23). When the expertise and equipment are available, selected patients with increased comorbidities and rectal lesions that are smaller than 2 cm, exophytic, mobile, superficial, and well differentiated may be treated with transanal full-thickness resection of the lesion, local laser ablation, or electrocoagulation.

Recent developments in minimally invasive surgery involving the use of the laparoscope suggest that laparoscopic resection of colon cancers can be done safely and effectively. A number of studies show that the operation can be done with resection of an acceptable number of lymph nodes. The procedure is usually done with a small abdominal incision to facilitate removal of the bowel containing the tumor and to assist in the anastomosis. Further experience is needed to determine whether laparoscopy can be done safely and with the same oncologic results for resection of rectal tumors.

The use of adjuvant therapies in the treatment of colon and rectal carcinoma generated considerable research in the last several decades. The main outcome from the randomized trials with 5-fluorouracil (5-FU) as a single agent in an adjuvant setting was that no improvement occurred in the disease-free interval, nor was there an increase in cure rate compared

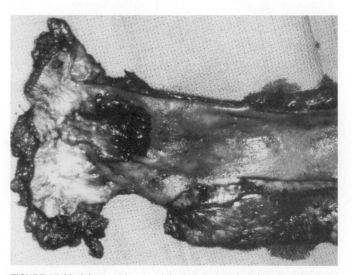

FIGURE 15-23. Adenocarcinoma of the low rectum invading the anal canal and requiring APR.

with surgery alone. However, subsequent studies showed conclusively that 5-FU used in combination with levamisole or leucovorin lowers the mortality rate in patients with Stage III tumors. The recent development of a new chemotherapeutic agent, oxaliplatin, has excited GI oncologists because it appears to be twice as effective as 5-FU alone in reducing cancer recurrence in high-risk patients as well as treating patients with metastatic colorectal cancer. FOLFOX (5-FU, leucovorin and oxaliplatin) is the standard treatment regimen currently. A number of new biologic agents show promise in achieving even better results especially with hepatic metastases (bevacizumab, cetuximab).

Because of their significant rate of recurrence (20%) despite the most radical surgical procedure, rectal tumors that have completely penetrated the rectal wall, with or without lymph node metastases, are treated additionally by radiation combined with 5-FU. Endorectal ultrasound or MRI is used to stage the depth of penetration of the tumor in the rectal wall. Preoperative chemoradiation (neoadjuvant therapy) is generally accepted as the best time to give therapy. This allows shrinkage of the tumor leading to a more complete resection and reduces the complications from postoperative radiation. Occasionally, it also causes enough tumor shrinkage in a very low rectal cancer to allow sphincter preservation.

Prognosis

Dukes first proposed a system of staging large bowel cancer more than 50 years ago. Subsequent modifications have been made, particularly those by Astler and Coller. The American Joint Committee on Cancer developed the TNM system (Table 15-5); this is what is most commonly used today.

TABLE 15-5	TNM Staging System
Primary Tumor (T)	
TX	Primary tumor cannot be assessed
T0	No evidence of primary tumor
Tis	Carcinoma in situ; intraepithelial tumor or invasion of the lamina propria
T1	Tumor invading the submucosa
T2	Tumor invading the muscularis propria
T3	Tumor invading through the muscularis propria into the subserosa, or into nonperitonealized pericolic or perirectal tissues
T4	Tumor directly invading other organs or structures or perforating the visceral peritoneum
Regional Lymph Nodes (N)	
NX	Regional lymph nodes cannot be assessed
N0	No regional lymph node metastasis
N1	Metastasis in 1–3 pericolic or perirectal lymph nodes
N2	Metastasis in ≥4 pericolic or perirectal lymph nodes
N3	Metastasis in any lymph node along the course of a named vascular trunk or metastasis to ≥1 apical node (when marked by the surgeon)
Distant Metastasis (M)	
MX	Presence of distant metastasis cannot be assessed
M0	No distant metastasis
M1	Distant metastasis

Other attempts have been made to look at clusters of prognostic factors (e.g., tumor markers, size of the lesion) and elements that are not included in Dukes' original classification, which was based on the depth of invasion. The most important prognostic variable is lymph node involvement.

For patients who have had curative resection and for whom no adjuvant therapy is appropriate, the question of follow-up surveillance is of maximal importance. The exact interval varies between institutions. A frequently used approach is a visit every 3 months for 2 years, every 6 months for 3 years, and then yearly until 10 years postresection. Visits include physical examination and measurement of carcinoembryonic (CEA) levels. Colonoscopy is usually performed at 1 and 2 years postoperatively and then every 2 to 3 years after. Most recurrences occur in the first 18 to 24 months. The use of carcinoembryonic antigen is well established, with recurrence suggested not only by the absolute level of this antigen, but also by a progressive rise. A progressive rise mandates a complete evaluation of the patient, including CT or MRI of the chest, abdomen, and pelvis. A potentially important new diagnostic modality used to detect widespread metastases in colorectal cancer is the positron emission tomography (PET) scan. This technique relies on administering radioactive positrons, which collide with electrons in diseased tissue that then emit gamma rays sensed by a color monitor. It is currently the most sensitive test to detect recurrent colorectal cancer. Occasionally, a second-look operation is required to detect the source of undiagnosed CEA elevation. The prognosis of colon and rectal carcinoma depends on the classification detailed in Table 15-5. For patients who have recurrences, the effective management of liver metastases, pelvic and anastomotic recurrences, and solitary pulmonary metastases has been demonstrated.

ANUS AND RECTUM

Diagnostic Evaluation

The anus and rectum are the site of many conditions that cause pain, protrusion, bleeding, discharge, or a combination of these. Most people complain generally about their "hemorrhoid problem"; it is up to the physician to distinguish between various pathologies that may present similarly.

Examination of the perianal and rectal area is an integral part of every physical examination. The importance of gentleness and empathy cannot be overemphasized. A complete history must be obtained before the examination; this information alone suggests the diagnosis in more than 80% of the cases. Gentle parting of the buttocks allows inspection that may show fissures, skin tags, hemorrhoids, fistulae, tumors, and dermatologic or infectious conditions. Gentle digital examination may show tumors, polyps, fluctuation, and sphincter weakness.

Anoscopic examination is mandatory because many visible lesions are not palpable. It may be deferred, however, in the presence of acute pain. The anoscope is a beveled instrument devised to examine the anal canal. It allows better detection of more distal lesions than the rigid or flexible proctosigmoidoscope. Flexible sigmoidoscopy and colonoscopy, however, are the instruments of choice for a proper evaluation of the rectum because they best allow exact localization of rectal lesions. Preparation is minimal with use of an enema prior to examination.

Rectal Prolapse (Procidentia)

Rectal prolapse is intussusception of a full-thickness portion of the rectum through the anal opening. This condition occurs most commonly in thin, asthenic women who have weak rectal attachments and may involve from 4 to 20 cm of rectum protruding through the anal opening. The entity must be distinguished from mucosal prolapse, which is eversion of 2 to 3 cm of rectal mucosa through the anal opening but which is not full thickness. They can be distinguished by the concentric, circumferential mucosal folds seen in true prolapse compared to the radial pattern of folds seen in mucosal or hemorrhoidal prolapse (Figure 15-24).

Clinical Presentation and Evaluation

Symptoms of prolapse include rectal pain or pressure, mild bleeding, incontinence, mucous discharge, and a wet anus. On rare occasions, the prolapse cannot be reduced and ischemia results. The prolapse commonly occurs after each bowel movement and must be manually reduced.

Treatment

Management of true rectal prolapse involves an intra-abdominal procedure including sigmoid resection (redundant bowel) with rectopexy (suturing the bowel wall to the presacral fascia to immobilize it). Recurrence rates are <5% if the procedure is correctly performed. For high-risk patients, a procedure can be done in which the entire resection is done through the perineum, but recurrence rates are much higher. Treatment of mucosal or hemorrhoidal prolapse is a three-column hemorrhoidectomy.

Hemorrhoids

Hemorrhoids are vascular cushions located in the anal canal. Hemorrhoidal disease, which most often causes hemorrhoidal protrusion or bleeding, is usually precipitated by constipation and straining at stool. Pregnancy, increased pelvic pressure (ascites, tumors), portal hypertension, and excessive diarrhea may influence the development of hemorrhoidal symptoms.

Hemorrhoids are usually found in three constant positions: left lateral, right anterior, and right posterior. It is preferable to refer to the actual anatomic position of the anorectal processes because with the old "o'clock" system, 12 o'clock is variable depending on the patient's position. In the modern ambulatory setting, most patients are examined either in the left lateral (Simm's) or the knee-chest position, which change the terms of reference by 90° to 180°.

Hemorrhoids are classified as either internal or external. **Internal hemorrhoids** originate above the dentate line; external hemorrhoids are located below the level of the dentate line. Because the rectal mucosa above the dentate line is insensate, bleeding from internal hemorrhoids is usually painless. Conversely, external hemorrhoids are covered by richly innervated anoderm and usually cause pain when thrombosis occurs.

Clinical Presentation and Evaluation

A patient with hemorrhoids has symptoms of hemorrhoidal protrusion or bleeding. In cases of protrusion, the hemorrhoids are graded according to the level of prolapse. First-degree internal hemorrhoids do not prolapse; the anoscope must be used to visualize them. Second-degree internal hemorrhoids prolapse with defecation and return spontaneously to their anatomic position. Third-degree internal hemorrhoids prolapse with defecation and require manual reduction. Fourth-degree hemorrhoids are not reducible (Figure 15-25). There is no classification for external hemorrhoids; they are either present or absent. Mixed hemorrhoids are a combination of internal and external hemorrhoids.

Bleeding may be minimal, appearing only on toilet paper, or it may occasionally be severe enough to cause anemia. It is usually bright red, coats the stool (rather than being mixed with it), and is painless, unless there is thrombosis, ulceration, or gangrene.

Treatment

Treatment is based on the presence of symptoms and the degree of disease (Table 15-6). Asymptomatic hemorrhoids are best left alone; cosmetic treatment is not indicated. Bulk-forming agents (e.g., psyllium derivatives) and avoidance of constipation are recommended. First-degree internal hemorrhoids are treated with topical agents or, if bleeding, with injection

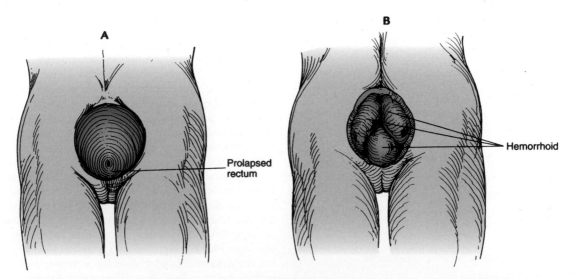

FIGURE 15-24. A, True rectal prolapse is characterized by concentric, circumferential mucosal folds. **B,** Mucosal prolapse is characterized by radial folds separating the mucosa. (Reprinted from Polk HC Jr., et al. *Basic Surgery,* 5th ed. St. Louis, MO: Quality Medical Publishing, 1995, with permission.)

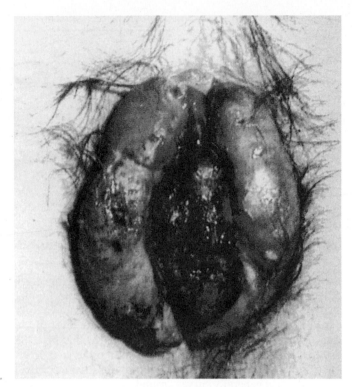

FIGURE 15-25. Fourth-degree hemorrhoids associated with thrombosis.

sclerotherapy or infrared coagulation. Larger first-degree hemorrhoids may be banded as well. Second-degree internal hemorrhoids and some third-degree hemorrhoids are treated with banding. Formal surgical hemorrhoidectomy is used for fourth-degree hemorrhoids, for mixed third-degree hemorrhoids with a large external component, and in some emergency situations (e.g., an acute hemorrhoidal attack with gangrene, severe ulceration). Procedures vary from excision to hemorrhoidopexy (PPH stapler).

External hemorrhoids usually cause few problems. Contrary to popular belief, hemorrhoids do not itch or burn; it is the perianal skin that is the site of pruritus ani. However, large external hemorrhoids may interfere with perianal hygiene and

thus be indirectly associated with pruritus. In these cases, excision may be indicated. It is usually done under local anesthesia.

Some patients may have severe perianal pain and a lump close to the anus after a bout of constipation or prolonged sitting. Examination shows an obvious thrombosed external hemorrhoid. This condition is self-limited and resolves progressively over 7 to 10 days; creams, suppositories, and topical adjuncts are useless. If the patient is seen early in the course of the disease (the first 24 to 48 hours), treatment consists of excision of the thrombosed hemorrhoid under local anesthesia. If the patient is seen later in the course of the disease, spontaneous resolution is usually underway and conservative treatment is indicated. Ulceration of the overlying skin with bleeding is an indication for excision. Sitz baths and a mild nonnarcotic analgesic are recommended.

Perianal Infections: Abscess and Fistula-in-Ano

Abscess

Most anorectal abscesses are believed to start with obstruction of the perianal glands that are located between the internal and external sphincters (intersphincteric space). These glands normally discharge their secretions at the level of the anal crypts that are located at the base of the columns of Morgagni. The term "of cryptoglandular origin" describes the origin of perirectal abscesses. As the early intersphincteric abscess (Figure 15-26, *left*) increases in size, it tends to spread along the planes of lesser resistance and to manifest fully as a perianal abscess (Figure 15-26, *right*). It may also manifest as an ischiorectal abscess in the ischiorectal fossa, located outside the external sphincter mechanism and below the level of the levator ani muscles (Figure 15-27, *left*). If the infection spreads above the levators it becomes a supralevator abscess (Figure 15-27, *right*), which may be very difficult to diagnose clinically. Perianal and ischiorectal abscesses are the most common. They account for as many as 70% of perirectal abscesses.

TABLE 15-6	Internal Hemorrhoids: Classification and Treatment

Degree	Definition	Treatment
First	Bulge in the anal canal lumen; does not protrude outside the lumen	*Asymptomatic*: take bulking agents; avoid constipation; increase water intake
		Symptomatic: same treatment as asymptomatic; rubber-band ligation; infrared coagulation
Second	Protrudes with defecation. Reduces spontaneously	Conservative management (see above) or rubber-band ligation
Third	Protrudes with defecation	*Selected cases*: rubber-band ligation
	Must be reduced manually	*Mixed*: surgical hemorrhoidectomy
Fourth	Protrudes; permanently incarcerated	Surgical hemorrhoidectomy

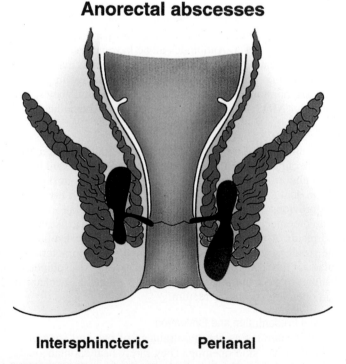

Anorectal abscesses

Intersphincteric   **Perianal**

FIGURE 15-26. Progression of intersphincteric abscess to perianal abscess.

Anorectal abscesses

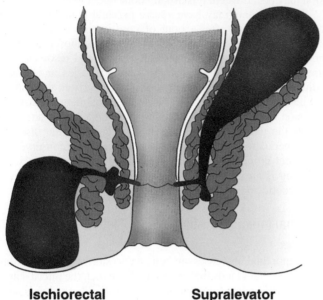

Ischiorectal   Supralevator

FIGURE 15-27. Simple intersphincteric abscesses may progress to more complex ischiorectal and supralevator abscesses.

Clinical Presentation and Evaluation

Except for early intersphincteric abscesses and supralevator abscesses, perianal pain and swelling are readily apparent in perirectal abscesses. Spontaneous drainage of pus may occur. The cardinal signs of infection (pain, fever, redness, swelling, and loss of function) are usually present.

Treatment

Treatment is complete and thorough drainage of the abscess. Failure to adequately drain the abscess results in ongoing pain, sepsis, and overall treatment failure. Sometimes initial drainage can be performed in the outpatient setting with local anesthesia; however, for larger and more complex lesions, the most effective surgical drainage can best be done in the operating room with adequate anesthesia. Antibiotics alone have no role in the primary treatment of an abscess. However, antibiotics may be used in conjunction with surgical incision and drainage in patients who are immunocompromised; those who have diabetes, leukemia, or AIDS; or those who are undergoing chemotherapy.

Fistula-in-Ano

After drainage of a perirectal abscess, the patient has a 50% chance of having a chronic **fistula-in-ano**. An anorectal fistula is an abnormal communication between the anus at the level of the dentate line and the perirectal skin, through the bed of the previous abscess. Fistulae are named in relation to the sphincter mechanism (Table 15-7). Intersphincteric fistulae are the result of perianal abscesses, transsphincteric fistulae are the result of ischiorectal abscesses, and suprasphincteric fistulae are the result of supralevator abscesses. Extrasphincteric fistulae bypass the anal canal and the sphincter mechanism and open high up in the rectum.

Clinical Presentation and Evaluation

Fistulae manifest as chronic drainage of pus and sometimes stool from the skin opening. They rarely heal spontaneously, and surgical correction is indicated to eliminate the symptoms.

TABLE 15-7	Perianal Infections
Abscess: acute phase	
Intersphincteric	
Perianal	
Ischiorectal	
Supralevator	
Fistula: chronic phase	
Intersphincteric	
Transsphincteric	
Suprasphincteric	
Extrasphincteric	

Goodsall's rule helps the examiner to predict the trajectory of the fistulous tract and the probable location of the internal anal opening (Figure 15-28). An imaginary line is drawn from the right lateral to the left lateral position at the level of the anus. For external openings located anterior to this line, the fistula tract usually goes radially straight into the anal crypt. For external openings located posterior to this imaginary line, the fistula tract generally curves around, and the internal opening is in the posterior midline position. However, the greater the distance between the anus and the external opening, the less reliable and helpful Goodsall's rule becomes. The trajectory of complex anal fistulae is unpredictable. Crohn's fistulae do not follow this rule.

Treatment

Fistulotomy consists of unroofing the fistula tract, allowing the fistula to heal slowly by secondary intention. Judgment must be exercised to avoid cutting a large portion of the sphincter muscle, which may precipitate incontinence.

Preliminary identification of the fistula tract by gentle insertion of a probe into the external skin opening, through the tract, until the internal anal opening is found, allows intraoperative evaluation of the structures that need division. Staged fistulotomy with a seton stitch permits immediate division of all nonsphincteric structures and suture encirclement of the sphincter involved. Over the next few weeks, the sphincter muscle is progressively divided by tightening the seton to avoid incontinence.

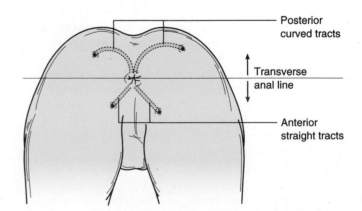

FIGURE 15-28. **Goodsall's rule.** (Schwartz SI, et al. *Principles of Surgery*, 6th ed. New York, NY: McGraw-Hill, 1994. Reproduced with permission of the McGraw-Hill Companies).

Initial reports of a new technique that involved injection of the fistula tract with fibrin glue suggested that a high percentage of cases would result in closing fistulae without surgery. However, subsequent larger series showed disappointing outcomes with this technique. More recently, a technique has been described using a decellularized collagen plug wedged in the fistula tract with suture closure of the internal opening. Initial series appear promising but larger series need to be done to confirm its efficacy.

Anal Fissures

The most common cause of severe localized anorectal pain is **anal fissure.** While hemorrhoids often cause discomfort and mild pressure symptoms, they rarely cause the severe pain associated with fissures. That pain is dramatically increased during bowel movements and is often associated with streaks of blood in the stool. Anal fissures are painful linear tears in the lining of the anal canal, below the level of the dentate line. They are most often located posteriorly in both sexes, but women also have anterior anal fissures. They occur in the posteroanterior plane because pelvic muscular support is weakest along this axis. Ectopic lateral fissures suggest an unusual diagnosis (e.g., Crohn's disease, leukemia, sexually transmitted disease, malignancy).

Clinical Presentation and Evaluation

Fissures are secondary to local trauma, either from constipation or excessive diarrhea. Pain typically starts with defecation and may persist from minutes to hours. It is disproportionate to the size of the lesion. If bleeding is present, it is usually minimal and bright red.

If the history suggests an anal fissure, gentle retraction of the buttocks will reveal the tear at the anal verge. Rectal examination is unnecessary and usually associated with severe pain and significant sphincter spasm. In cases of chronic recurrent anal fissures, the classic triad of an external skin tag, a fissure exposing the internal sphincter fibers, and a hypertrophied anal papilla at the level of the dentate line is pathognomonic.

Treatment

Treatment is based on the duration and severity of the symptoms. Acute anal fissures usually respond to conservative treatment, avoidance of diarrhea or constipation, bulk laxatives to keep bowel movements atraumatic, and a mild nonnarcotic analgesic. Sitz baths are helpful for comfort. Topical agents (procainamide, nitroglycerin) that relax the sphincter may be useful. Botox injection also has had some success. If conservative treatment fails, or if the fissure is chronic, surgery is recommended. Several surgical options are available. In uncomplicated cases, the operation of choice is a partial lateral internal sphincterotomy. A small portion of the internal sphincter is cut, which releases the sphincter spasm, relieves pain, and allows the fissure to heal. The operation carries a small risk of minor incontinence.

Anal Malignancy

Perianal and anal canal malignancies are rare, accounting for only 3% to 4% of all anorectal carcinomas. There are essentially two types of anal cancers: epidermoid carcinoma (a generic type that includes squamous cell, basaloid, cloacogenic, mucoepidermoid, and transitional carcinomas) and malignant melanoma. The anus is the third most common site for malignant melanoma, after the skin and the eyes.

Clinical Presentation and Evaluation

Either type of malignancy may cause pain, bleeding, or a lump. Delay in diagnosis is often a consequence of both patient and physician neglect. In cases of malignant melanoma, lymph node involvement and widespread metastases are common at presentation. The diagnosis is often delayed because of the lack of pigmentation of these lesions (amelanotic melanoma). Examination should include palpation of the inguinal lymph nodes, a site of potential metastasis.

Treatment

In the past, APR and permanent colostomy were the mainstays of treatment for both types of cancer. This approach has been almost completely abandoned in epidermoid cancers in favor of combined modality chemotherapy and radiation therapy, using a protocol of pelvic radiation with infusion of 5-FU and mitomycin C. With this treatment, 5-year survival rates range from 82% to 87%. Surgery is indicated in cases in which residual tumor is present after radiation and chemotherapy. APR is indicated in this setting.

Prophylactic inguinal node dissection is not recommended unless clinically palpable nodes are present because of the high morbidity associated with this procedure. Synchronous inguinal node metastasis is an ominous sign, and survival rates are poor. Conversely, metachronous inguinal node involvement has a better prognosis. Inclusion of the groins in the radiated fields decreases the incidence of metachronous lymph node involvement without adding much morbidity.

For malignant melanoma, the prognosis is dismal, regardless of the treatment. For good-risk patients, APR is a reasonable option to maximize survival and local control.

Anorectal Sexually Transmitted Diseases

More than 20 sexually transmitted diseases can be present in the anorectal area. Therefore, it is important to inquire about a complete sexual history in patients with anorectal symptoms.

Anal Condylomas

Anal condylomas are caused by human papilloma virus. They are the most common anorectal infection affecting homosexual men, but may also be seen in heterosexual men and women and even children. Transmission at birth and by close contact with infected patients has been reported.

Anal condylomas are more common in homosexual men who practice anal-receptive intercourse. The lesions are found perianally, intra-anally, on the penis, and in the urethra. In women, the lesions may be found in the vagina, vulva, cervix, or urethra. Condylomas acuminata are pink or white papillary lesions. They vary in size from <1 mm to large cauliflower-like lesions. They bleed easily, and difficulty in maintaining perianal hygiene leads to pruritus ani. Discomfort and pain are often present.

Various topical caustic agents (bichloracetic acid, podophyllin) and local destructive therapies (electrocoagulation, cryotherapy, laser excision) have been tried with mitigated success. Regardless of the technique, the recurrence rate is high (10% to 50%). Persistent causative sexual behavior obviously increases the recurrence rate. Women with anal condyloma or who are partners of men with condyloma must see their gynecologist; HPV is associated with cervical cancer.

Chlamydia and Lymphogranuloma Venereum

Chlamydial infections are among the most common sexually transmitted diseases. Chlamydial proctitis is increasing in both men and women who practice anal-receptive sex. The disease usually begins as vesicles and progresses to an ulcer. Inguinal adenopathy is a prominent sign. The rectal symptoms are tenesmus and pain. Patients who have lymphogranuloma venereum usually have hematochezia. Sigmoidoscopy may show a friable, ulcerating, erythematous mucosa. Biopsy findings are not definitive. The microimmunofluorescent antibody titer is the test of choice; however, the complement fixation test is still used. Most patients are successfully treated with tetracycline or doxycycline. Erythromycin is reserved for those who are insensitive to tetracyclines.

Gonorrhea

Neisseria gonorrhoeae infections of the rectum account for as many as 50% of the cases of gonorrhea in homosexual men. Evaluation and follow-up of patients with rectal gonorrhea require cultures of the urethra, rectum, and pharynx. Most patients have nonspecific complaints, including pruritus, tenesmus, and hematochezia. Sigmoidoscopy shows a thick, yellow mucopurulent discharge. The rectal mucosa ranges from normal to erythematous and edematous. Culture and Gram stain are used for organism identification. Treatment is ceftriaxone 250 mg given once intramuscularly along with concurrent treatment for Chlamydia infection. Emerging

antibiotic resistance requires the physician to check current CDC guidelines regarding appropriate therapy.

Herpes Simplex Virus

Herpes simplex virus type 2 causes herpetic proctitis. The infection is acquired by direct inoculation. Approximately 15% of homosexual men with rectal symptoms have only this virus identified by rectal culture. The symptoms begin 4 to 28 days after inoculation. The majority of patients have pain and burning worsened by bowel movements. Some patients have a syndrome that is characterized by lumbosacral radiculopathy associated with sacral paresthesias. Symptoms include impotence; lower abdominal, buttock, and thigh pain; and urinary dysfunction. Lesions include vesicles with red areolae, ruptured vesicles, and aphthous ulcers. The usual locations include the perianal skin, anal canal, and lower rectum. Patients who are seen in the relapsing stage may report a history of crusting lesions followed by healing. Scrapings for cytologic examination show intranuclear inclusion bodies and giant cells. Treatment is aimed at relieving symptoms: sitz baths, topical anesthetics, and analgesics. Acyclovir has benefit in the acute and relapse phases. Continuous suppressive therapy is warranted only in the most severe cases.

thePoint ✳ Go to http://thePoint.lww.com/activate and use your scratch-off code on the inside cover of this book to access bonus chapters, question bank, videos, and more.

SAMPLE QUESTIONS

Questions

Choose the best answer for each question.

1. A 57-year-old man comes to clinic with complaints of foul-smelling urine and two urinary tract infections treated with antibiotics by his primary care physician over the past 6 weeks. He has no pain at this time. Two months ago, he was seen in the emergency department with 2 days of left lower quadrant pain and constipation and was treated with oral antibiotics for diverticulitis. His past history is otherwise negative. His only medication is ciprofloxacin. He is afebrile and vital signs are normal. A urine sample is cloudy with sediment. What is the next best step in diagnosis?

   A. Plain radiographs of the abdomen

   B. Ultrasound of the abdomen and pelvis

   C. Barium enema

   D. CT scan of the abdomen and pelvis

   E. Diagnostic cystoscopy

2. A 62-year-old woman is seen in the emergency department with dark red rectal bleeding and hypotension. Initial hemoglobin is 7.2. She is given intravenous fluids and two units of packed red blood cells but continues to have large amounts of bloody stools. Nasogastric tube effluent is clear bilious fluid. The best choice for identification of the bleeding site at this time is

   A. rigid proctoscopy.

   B. bowel prep followed by colonoscopy.

   C. tagged red blood cell nuclear scan.

   D. mesenteric angiography.

   E. diagnostic laparoscopy.

3. An 85-year-old male nursing home resident is brought to the emergency department with 3 days of painless abdominal distention and obstipation. He appears to be in no pain, but his abdomen is massively distended and tympanitic. Plain abdominal films show a kidney-bean-shaped air-filled structure suspicious for cecal volvulus. The best management at this point is

   A. observation if the cecum is <12 cm in diameter.

   B. contrast enema decompression.

   C. colonoscopic detorsion, leaving a rectal tube.

   D. operative detorsion and fixation of the cecum to the abdominal wall.

   E. right colon resection.

4. A 41-year-old man is seen in clinic with bright red rectal bleeding, seen on the toilet tissue intermittently over the last several months. He is an insurance agent, exercises regularly, and eats a well-balanced diet. He denies changes in bowel habits. Family history is unremarkable. His vital signs are normal. His abdomen exam is normal. Digital rectal exam is normal, and blood is identified on the examining finger. Anoscopy shows no other pathology. What is the next best step in diagnosis?

   A. Fecal occult blood test

   B. Complete blood count (CBC): if normal, no further evaluation is indicated

   C. Barium enema

   D. Flexible sigmoidoscopy

   E. Colonoscopy

5. A 24-year-old woman is seen in clinic with anal pain. Examination shows a fissure in the anterior midline of the anal canal. Digital rectal exam cannot be performed due to pain. The next step in management should be

   A. sitz baths, bulking agent, and reassurance.

   B. intramuscular penicillin and oral tetracycline for sexually transmitted disease.

   C. evaluation for Crohn's disease.

   D. evaluation for leukemia.

   E. biopsy to rule out neoplasm.

Answers and Explanations

1. Answer: D

CT scan remains the most sensitive test for diagnosis of enterovesical fistula and location of the portion of the intestinal tract involved. Plain radiographs may show air in the bladder, but not the etiology. Ultrasound has no role. Barium enema identifies the fistula <50% of the time. Cystoscopy usually identifies only bullous edema within the bladder.

2. Answer: D

While rigid proctoscopy may be done, it is unlikely to identify a source of massive bleeding. The patient is unlikely to be sufficiently stable for the colonoscopy prep or the time required for it. Tagged RBC scan is more sensitive than angiography for identifying active bleeding, but much less specific for identifying the source of bleeding and is not as useful in massive bleeds. Diagnostic laparoscopy would not elucidate the bleeding source. Mesenteric angiography is much more specific for identifying the source and offers the potential for therapy (angiographic embolization) to control bleeding as well in selected cases.

3. Answer: E

Observation occurs in Ogilvie's, not volvulus. Contrast enema decompression is not useful in cecal volvulus. Colonoscopic detorsion is useful for sigmoid volvulus, but considered unwise in cecal volvulus due to associated risks. Cecopexy carries a high rate of revolvulus.

4. Answer: E

In the absence of an obvious source in the anus or distal rectum, further evaluation of the colon is needed. Fecal occult blood test (FOBT) is irrelevant with a history of visible rectal bleeding. CBC is unlikely to be helpful. Flexible sigmoidoscopy only examines part of the colon. While barium enema may identify an abnormality anywhere in the colon, it is not as specific as colonoscopy.

5. Answer: A

The presentation is classic for traumatic anal fissure. Fissures off the midline generally prompt evaluation for other etiologies.

16
Biliary Tract

O. JOE HINES, M.D. • JULIANE BINGENER, M.D. •
FREDERICK D. CASON, M.D.• MICHAEL EDWARDS, M.D. • MARY ANN HOPKINS, M.D.

Objectives

1. Outline the factors that contribute to the formation of the three most common types of gallstones.

2. Describe the epidemiology of gallstone disease as it relates to patient evaluation and management.

3. Discuss the most useful laboratory tests and imaging studies to evaluate patients with diseases of the biliary tract.

4. Describe the management of asymptomatic gallstones found incidentally on radiologic studies or at celiotomy.

5. Compare and contrast the (1) clinical presentation, (2) laboratory and radiologic findings, and (3) management of a patient with chronic cholecystitis (biliary colic) and a patient with acute cholecystitis.

6. List the differences in the clinical presentation and evaluation of a jaundiced patient with choledocholithiasis and a jaundiced patient with biliary obstruction secondary to malignancy.

7. Describe the clinical presentation, evaluation, and management of a patient with (1) acute cholangitis and (2) acute suppurative cholangitis. Highlight the differences between the two conditions.

8. Describe the clinical presentation, evaluation, and management of a patient with acute gallstone pancreatitis.

9. Outline the clinical presentation, evaluation, and management of a patient with gallstone ileus. Contrast these with the corresponding features of other types of small bowel obstruction.

10. Outline the epidemiology, clinical presentation, evaluation, and management of carcinoma of the gallbladder.

11. Outline the clinical presentation, evaluation, and management of carcinoma of the extrahepatic biliary ducts.

12. List the common causes of benign strictures of the common bile duct, and describe the clinical features of patients who have such strictures.

13. Outline the various options available to treat stones in the gallbladder and the extrahepatic biliary ducts.

14. Outline the indications for cholecystectomy. Discuss the advantages of the laparoscopic approach over open cholecystectomy.

15. Compare and contrast the complications associated with laparoscopic cholecystectomy with those associated with open cholecystectomy.

16. Outline the postoperative management of a patient after (1) cholecystectomy and (2) common bile duct exploration.

Diseases of the gallbladder and bile ducts are common in the adult population of North America. These conditions can be life threatening and may require a detailed understanding in order to effectively triage patients. Approximately 15% of adults have gallstones, and more than 600,000 cholecystectomies are performed annually in the United States, accounting for more than $5 billion in health care costs. Accurate clinical assessment, including pertinent history and accurate physical examination, yields valuable information about the diagnosis of common diseases of the biliary tract. Laboratory tests are helpful in distinguishing among various causes of jaundice, and imaging studies play a pivotal role in confirming the diagnosis of biliary tract disease. To minimize the risk of iatrogenic injury, the surgeon must possess the skills to recognize common variations in the anatomy of the biliary tract and to perform careful dissection of the vital structures during surgery. This dictum was reemphasized in recent years with the meteoric rise in the popularity of **laparoscopic cholecystectomy,** which has replaced open cholecystectomy as the preferred operation for most patients with gallstone disease.

ANATOMY

The origin of the biliary tree is an outgrowth from the foregut. Three buds from this diverticulum become the liver, ventral pancreas, and gallbladder. Ultimately, the gallbladder is located in the right upper quadrant of the abdomen under the anatomic division of the right and left lobes of the liver. Normally it is a thin-walled, contractile, pear-shaped organ measuring 10 × 5 cm and consists of the fundus, body, and neck, which narrows joining the cystic duct. Synonyms for the gallbladder neck are the *infundibulum* or **Hartmann's pouch**. The gallbladder contains approximately 50 mL of bile when distended and is mostly covered by peritoneum while the remainder is attached to the liver. In some patients, the gallbladder is completely covered by peritoneum and in others embedded in the liver.

The right and left hepatic ducts join to form the common hepatic duct, which is connected to the cystic duct to form the common hepatic duct. The cystic duct is lined by the spiral valves of Heister, which provide some resistance to bile flow from the gallbladder. In the hepatoduodenal ligament, the common bile duct lies to the right side of the patient, the proper hepatic artery to the left side, and the portal vein posterior to both of these. The right hepatic artery gives off the cystic artery before traversing into the right hepatic lobe. The cystic artery lies in the triangle of Calot, which is the anatomic area that is bound by the inferior margin of the liver superiorly, the common hepatic duct medially, and the cystic duct laterally. The common bile duct passes through the head of the pancreas, usually joins the pancreatic duct within 1 cm of the wall of the duodenum to form a common channel, and then empties into the second portion of the duodenum through the ampulla of Vater. Bile flow into the duodenum is regulated in part by the sphincter of Oddi, which encircles this common channel. The most common anatomic configuration of this region is shown in Figure 16-1, which demonstrates the usual relations of the important ductal and arterial structures. However, the anatomy of the extrahepatic biliary system varies considerably from individual to individual, and many anomalies are reported. To prevent inadvertent injury to the extrahepatic bile ducts and related structures during cholecystectomy, anticipation of anomalous anatomy and careful, bloodless dissection are vitally important.

The bile tree receives both parasympathetic and sympathetic innervation. The parasympathetic nerves regulate motor and secretory functions of the biliary tree, and the sympathetic afferent fibers mediate the pain experienced during biliary colic.

PHYSIOLOGY

The liver produces 500 to 1000 mL of bile per day secreted by the hepatocytes and ductal epithelium. Bile contains cholesterol, bile acids, phospholipid (primarily lecithin), conjugated bilirubin, and protein. Primary bile acids are synthesized from cholesterol in the liver and are conjugated with glycine or taurine before they are excreted in the bile. Conjugated bile acids and lecithin form vesicles and micelles, which bring the cholesterol into solution in bile. Cholesterol is most soluble in a mixture that contains at least 50% bile acids and smaller amounts of lecithin. The electrolyte composition of hepatic bile is similar to that of plasma.

Once in the duodenum, bile acids traverse the small intestine, and most are returned to the liver through the portal blood where they are reconjugated and promptly reexcreted. Small amounts of bile acids are reabsorbed passively throughout the small intestine, but most of the reabsorption occurs actively at the level of the terminal ileum. Thus, there is an effective mechanism for enterohepatic circulation of bile acids. Depending on the duration of gastric emptying (e.g., quantity of the meal, fat content), the same bile acid molecules may recirculate two or three times after a meal. Normally, approximately

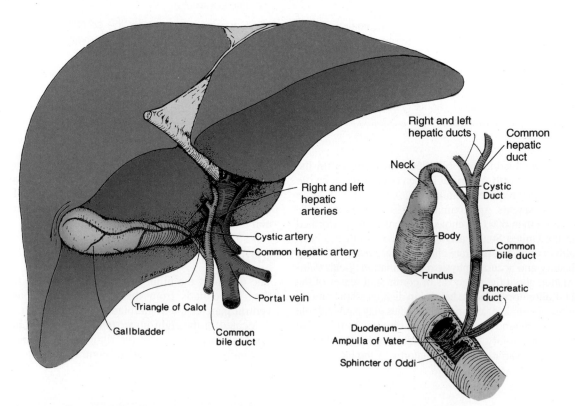

FIGURE 16-1. Anatomy of the gallbladder, porta hepatis, and extrahepatic bile ducts.

5% of bile acids escape reabsorption in the ileum. They are deconjugated or dehydroxylated by intestinal bacteria, rendering them less water soluble, or are adsorbed to intraluminal particulate matter. To keep the bile acid pool relatively constant, the lost bile acids are replaced by hepatic synthesis of new bile acids through a negative feedback mechanism. The liver can compensate for a loss of as much as 20% of the bile acid pool by the synthesis of new bile acids. Greater losses lead to a diminished bile acid pool, hence decreasing bile acid concentration and making the bile more lithogenic (prone to stone formation).

Bilirubin is actively excreted by hepatocytes into bile as a conjugated water-soluble diglucuronide (direct bilirubin). Conjugated bilirubin is responsible for the green-brown color of bile and the brown color of stool. Extrahepatic obstruction to the flow of bile by benign or malignant diseases leads to the accumulation of predominantly conjugated (direct) bilirubin, which is water soluble and is excreted in the urine, making it dark. In contrast, hemolytic diseases, which cause excessive breakdown of heme, and hepatocellular diseases, which preclude adequate conjugation of bilirubin, lead to the accumulation of predominantly unconjugated (indirect) bilirubin, which is fat soluble and is not excreted in the urine.

The volume of bile secreted into the intestine is determined by hepatic secretion, gallbladder contraction, and the resistance provided by the sphincter of Oddi. When the sphincter of Oddi is closed, most hepatic bile is diverted into the gallbladder for storage and concentration. The gallbladder concentrates the bile by absorbing Na^+, Cl^-, and water at rates as high as 20% per hour. The ingestion of a meal causes the gallbladder to contract and the sphincter of Oddi to relax. This mechanism is mediated by cholecystokinin and vagal action (autonomic nervous system) of the gallbladder along with relaxation of the sphincter of Oddi. The result is a slow, sustained emptying of most of the gallbladder bile into the duodenum. Simultaneously, hepatic bile flow is increased because of the addition of (1) water and bicarbonate secretion and (2) the continuous return of bile acids through the enterohepatic circulation—most of which have just been emptied into the duodenum from the gallbladder.

Bile in the duodenum is important for alkalinizing acid gastric chyme, making luminal contents isoosmolar, and digesting and absorbing fats and the fat-soluble vitamins (A, D, E, and K). Hence, obstructive jaundice or external bile diversion may cause problems with fat assimilation (steatorrhea) and blood coagulation (prolonged prothrombin time secondary to vitamin K malabsorption).

GALLSTONE DISEASE

Epidemiology of Gallstones

The incidence of gallstones increases with age, and women are affected approximately three times more often than men. The prevalence of gallstone disease among white women who are younger than 50 years of age is 5% to 15%; in older women, it is approximately 25%. Among white men who are younger than 50 years of age, the prevalence is 4% to 10%; in older men, it is 10% to 15%. Gallstone disease also tends to cluster in families. Native Americans have an extremely high prevalence of gallstones; more than 50% of men and 80% of women have mixed stones by the age of 60 years. Obesity (excessive cholesterol biosynthesis), multiparity (altered steroid metabolism,

lithogenic bile, gallbladder hypomotility), high-dose estrogen oral contraceptives, some cholesterol-lowering agents (alteration of cholesterol and bile acid biosynthesis), rapid weight loss (increased bile saturation index and gallbladder stasis), and prolonged total parenteral nutrition (hyperconcentration of bile and gallbladder stasis) all predispose to the formation of stones. Patients who have had rapid weight loss following bariatric surgery may form gallstones. Diseases that diminish the bile acid pool like Crohn's disease involving the terminal ileum or resection of the terminal ileum increase the incidence of gallstones. Patients with hemolytic disorders and alcoholic cirrhosis tend to form pigment stones.

Patients may be able to prevent gallstone formation by avoiding obesity, following a high-fiber diet to diminish the enterohepatic circulation of dehydroxylated bile acids, eating meals at regular intervals to diminish gallbladder storage time, and eating foods with low levels of saturated fatty acids to diminish the nucleation of lithogenic bile.

Pathogenesis of Gallstones (Cholelithiasis)

The most common type of gallstones in the Western population is mixed containing a high proportion of cholesterol along with bile acids and lecithin. These stones account for approximately 75% of all types of gallstones. The relative concentrations of cholesterol, bile acids, and lecithin must be maintained within a fairly limited range to maintain the cholesterol in solution. A change in the relative concentrations of cholesterol, bile acids, and lecithin favors the formation and precipitation of cholesterol crystals (Figure 16-2). Precipitation of cholesterol as crystals tends to occur if the bile is lithogenic and supersaturated with cholesterol. These crystals, in the presence of enucleating factors, may agglomerate to form gallstones and entrap other components of bile including bilirubin, mucus, and calcium in the process. Most mixed stones do not contain enough calcium rendering them radiolucent. Occasionally, a single large stone forms and is composed almost entirely of cholesterol (cholesterol solitaire). Incomplete emptying of the gallbladder affords ideal conditions for agglomeration; for this reason, most stones form in the gallbladder rather than in the other parts of the

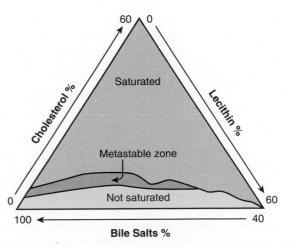

FIGURE 16-2. The molar percentages of cholesterol, lecithin, and bile salts in bile plotted on triangular coordinates. A relative change in the concentrations of these components can lead to supersaturation of the bile with cholesterol, increasing the likelihood of gallstone formation. In the metastable zone, there is supersaturation of cholesterol, but its precipitation occurs extremely slowly.

biliary tree. The source of most stones found in the biliary ducts (**choledocholithiasis**) is the gallbladder. However, bile stasis and infection involving the bile ducts may predispose to the formation of primary bile duct calculi within the ducts, although this is uncommon.

Pigment stones are of two types, black and brown. Black pigment stones account for approximately 20% of all biliary stones and are generally found in the gallbladder. They typically form in sterile gallbladder bile and are commonly associated with hemolytic diseases and cirrhosis. In chronic hemolysis, there is hypersecretion of bilirubin conjugates in the bile and greater secretion of monoglucuronides compared with diglucuronides, which favors the precipitation of pigment stones. In contrast, brown stones are associated with infected bile. They are found primarily in the bile ducts and are soft. Pigment stones often contain enough calcium rendering them radiopaque.

Gallbladder sludge is amorphous material that contains mucoprotein, cholesterol crystals, and calcium bilirubinate. It is often associated with prolonged total parenteral nutrition, starvation, or rapid weight loss. Gallbladder sludge may be a precursor of gallstones.

Diagnostic Evaluation

History and Physical Examination

The identification of biliary tract disease requires a focused history and careful physical examination. Narrowing the differential diagnosis and determining the cause of the biliary tract disease can be accomplished by gathering valuable clues that point to either an acute or a chronic condition. If the patient is jaundiced, the history can suggest either obstructive or hepatocellular disease and may indicate an underlying malignancy. Specific physical findings may also yield useful information that can help with the evaluation.

The hallmark of gallstone disease is pain referred to as **biliary colic.** The pain is usually steady, fairly severe, and located in the right upper quadrant or, less commonly, epigastrium of the abdomen sometimes going through to the back at the same level. The pain is visceral, often described as dull or aching and may last from 1 to 4 hours. The pain is thought to be secondary to increased pressure in the gallbladder that results from contraction against a stone that is impacted in the cystic duct. Typical biliary colic is caused by obstruction and is not associated with acute inflammation or infection. The pain tends to occur postprandial, may be after a large or fatty meal, but it may have no relation to meals and awaken the patient at night. The patient may seek urgent evaluation in an emergency room in order to address the pain. Nausea and vomiting may accompany biliary colic. The pain is seldom relieved by anything but time and potent analgesics. The patient is most commonly well before the onset of pain and then again within minutes to a few hours after the pain subsides.

Acute cholecystitis is the acute inflammation and infection of the gallbladder. These patients experience more localizing tenderness that is steady or crescendo in nature localized in the right upper quadrant of the abdomen or in the epigastrium. The pain lasts longer than 3 to 4 hours and may continue for several days. It is mediated by somatic sensory nerves since the parietal peritoneum is usually irritated. It may be accompanied by nausea, vomiting, and systemic manifestations of an inflammatory process including fever, tachycardia, and, in more severe cases, hemodynamic instability.

In patients with jaundice, the presence of light-colored stools and dark, tea-colored urine suggests extrahepatic biliary obstruction. Patients with malignancies (e.g., carcinoma of the pancreas) generally have dull, vague, or insignificant upper abdominal pain. A history of marked weight loss is often present in patients with malignant conditions. Pruritus is believed to be caused by high tissue concentrations of reabsorbed conjugated bile acids and is often present in patients with obstructive jaundice.

On physical examination, a patient with biliary colic usually appears uncomfortable and restless, whereas a patient who has pain associated with inflammation and acute cholecystitis tends to be still because the pain is aggravated by movement. The pulse rate may be high secondary to pain, inflammation, or infection. Fever often accompanies acute cholecystitis but not biliary colic, and high fever may be present with gangrene of the gallbladder or if the patient has cholangitis. Low blood pressure signifies severe dehydration or septic shock. The abdomen of patients with biliary colic is soft, but some tenderness may be found in the right upper quadrant. Once the pain subsides, the abdomen is nontender between episodes of colic. In acute cholecystitis, examination of the abdomen may show a positive **Murphy's sign**. A Murphy's sign is the cessation of inspiration because of pain on deep palpitation of the right upper quadrant when the visceral peritoneum overlying the gallbladder is inflamed. Once the inflammation spreads to the adjacent parietal peritoneum, abdominal examination shows localized guarding and may demonstrate rebound tenderness. A tender mass representing the inflamed gallbladder may also be palpable in the right upper quadrant of the abdomen in acute cholecystitis. The presence of a nontender, palpable gallbladder with jaundice suggests underlying malignant disease, such as carcinoma of the pancreas and is known as **Courvoisier's sign** (see Chapter 17, Pancreas). In the presence of a malignant obstruction of the common bile duct, the gallbladder is passively distended as a result of back pressure and is palpable in the right upper quadrant. If a stone is the cause of the distal ductal obstruction, the site of origin of the stone is generally a diseased thick-walled gallbladder, which is incapable of passive distension.

Laboratory Tests

A number of laboratory tests aid in the diagnosis and management of biliary tract disease. Liver function tests are helpful in detecting hyperbilirubinemia and providing information about the underlying disease process. The serum level of unconjugated (indirect) bilirubin increases in hemolytic disorders, whereas the conjugated (direct) fraction is elevated with extrahepatic biliary obstruction or cholestasis. Alkaline phosphatase (ALP) is synthesized by the biliary tract epithelium. Serum ALP levels increase as a result of overproduction in conditions that cause extrahepatic biliary obstruction or, less commonly, from cholestasis resulting from a drug reaction or primary biliary cirrhosis. The serum level of this enzyme is moderately elevated in hepatitis, and it may also be elevated as a result of bone disease. ALP of hepatobiliary origin may be differentiated from that originating from bone by confirming its heat stability. The concomitant elevation of gamma-glutamyl transferase (GGT) also indicates that the source of the elevated ALP is the biliary tract. Aspartate aminotransferase (AST) and alanine aminotransferase (ALT) are released from hepatocytes, and serum levels of both enzymes are increased significantly in various types of hepatitis. AST and ALT are also often elevated with biliary obstruction, particularly when it is acute. As a rule, however, the increase in ALP and GGT are greater than the increase in the levels of AST and ALT in biliary obstruction. The converse suggests hepatitis. If the biliary ductal system is partially obstructed (e.g., by a primary or metastatic neoplasm), ALP is released into the serum from the obstructed ducts, but the serum bilirubin may be normal. International normalized ratio (INR) is often elevated (prothrombin time is often prolonged) in patients with obstructive jaundice as a result of the malabsorption of vitamin K. In obstructive jaundice, the water-soluble conjugated (direct) bilirubin is excreted in the urine. On the other hand, urobilinogen is produced in the intestine as a result of bacterial metabolism of bilirubin. Then it is reabsorbed from the intestine and secreted in the urine. Bile duct obstruction leads to the reduction of urobilinogen in the urine because the excretion of bilirubin into the intestine is blocked.

The hemoglobin or hematocrit may be elevated if the patient is dehydrated. Leukocytosis with a shift to the left suggests acute inflammation and infection. Serum amylase and lipase may be slightly elevated in both acute cholecystitis and acute cholangitis, but marked elevations suggest acute pancreatitis.

Imaging Studies

Imaging studies are very helpful in establishing the definitive diagnosis in patients who have clinical features that suggest biliary disease. They are also useful in a variety of therapeutic interventions. Table 16-1 lists commonly used imaging studies and their diagnostic and therapeutic potential.

The initial study of choice for patients with biliary disease is **ultrasonography**. The study is noninvasive, quick, relatively inexpensive, and does not entail the use of radiation. Ultrasonography has replaced the **oral cholecystogram** for routine workup of patients with biliary colic. For stones in the gallbladder, both the sensitivity and the specificity of this study are approximately 95%. Ultrasonography can successfully detect stones as small as 3 mm in diameter, and sometimes smaller stones and debris like gallbladder sludge may be seen (Figure 16-3). Ultrasonography is highly sensitive for detecting dilation of the bile ducts and may provide information on whether the site of biliary obstruction is intrahepatic or extrahepatic. The bile duct is generally considered dilated if it is larger than 7 mm. However, the ultrasound is less helpful for visualizing stones in the bile ducts because of the overlying structures like the duodenum, which can contain air. If the gallbladder is distended and the ducts are dilated, the site of obstruction is likely to be distal to the junction of the cystic duct and the common hepatic duct. The finding of a thickened gallbladder wall or pericholecystic fluid supports the diagnosis of acute cholecystitis. Additionally, ultrasonography provides information about the liver and pancreas.

Rarely, gallstones are visible utilizing plain radiographs (Figure 16-4). Approximately 10% to 15% of gallstones contain sufficient calcium to render them radiopaque. Other findings on a plain x-ray include air in the biliary tree that is present as a result of communication between the biliary and gastrointestinal (GI) tracts secondary to a pathologic fistula or a connection created by a previous procedure. Also, air in the lumen or wall of the gallbladder may be seen in **acute emphysematous cholecystitis.**

Computed tomography (CT) is not the preferred test for the diagnosis of cholelithiasis because of the lower sensitivity in detecting gallstones, the higher cost compared with

TABLE 16-1	Imaging Studies Commonly Used in the Diagnosis and Management of Biliary Disease
Imaging Procedure	**Diagnostic or Therapeutic Potential**
Plain abdominal radiograph	Calcified gallstone
	Air in the biliary tree
	Air in the gallbladder wall or lumen
Ultrasonography	Stones in the gallbladder (possibly in duct)
	Thickened gallbladder wall
	Pericholecystic fluid
	Ultrasonographic Murphy's sign
	Dilation of intrahepatic and extrahepatic ducts
	Liver lesion
	Pancreatic mass
Radionuclide scan (HIDA scan)	Filling of gallbladder
	Filling of bile ducts
	Passage of bile into the duodenum
Computed tomography (CT)	Pancreatic mass
	Dilation of intrahepatic and extrahepatic ducts
	Liver lesion
Magnetic resonance cholangiography (MRC)	Stones in gallbladder or bile ducts
	Dilated or strictured bile ducts
	Masses in liver, pancreas, or ducts
Transhepatic cholangiogram (PTC)	Detecting bile duct obstruction
	Draining obstructed bile duct
	Bypassing bile duct obstruction with stent
	Obtaining cytology specimen
	Detecting bile leak from ducts
	Extracting bile duct calculus
Endoscopic retrograde cholangiopancreatography (ERCP)	Detecting bile duct obstruction
	Draining obstructed bile duct
	Inserting stent to bypass obstruction or control bile leak
	Detecting pancreatic duct obstruction
	Obtaining cytology specimen
	Detecting bile leak from ducts
	Extracting bile duct calculus
	Obtaining biopsy of a neoplasm
	Performing sphincterotomy

ultrasonography, and the risks of radiation. CT scan may be useful to assess patients with severe acute biliary disease, to rule out other causes of biliary obstruction, or identify an alternate diagnosis. Recently, the advent of CT cholangiography has been shown to reliably display anatomic detail of the biliary tree. For some patients CT scan can be used to guide percutaneous needle aspiration for Gram stain, cytology, or core needle biopsy for histology to establish a definitive diagnosis.

Magnetic resonance cholangiography (MRC) refers to selected MR imaging of the biliary and pancreatic ducts, which is helpful in demonstrating common duct stones and other

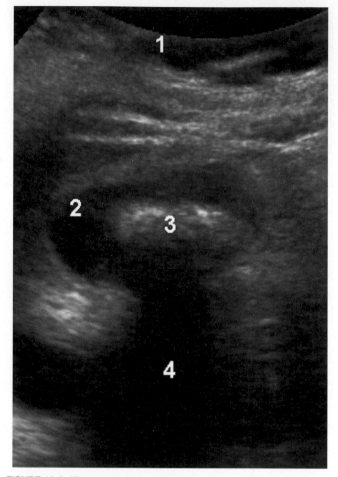

FIGURE 16-3. Ultrasound of the gallbladder showing gallstones. 1. Anterior abdominal wall; 2. Gallbladder; 3. Stones; 4. Acoustic shadow.

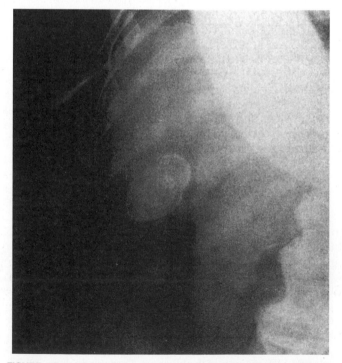

FIGURE 16-4. Plain radiograph of the abdomen showing gallstones (frequency <10%).

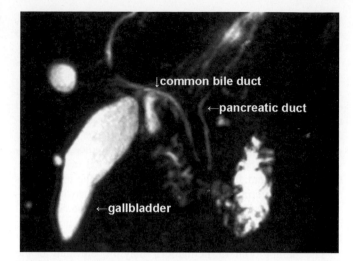

FIGURE 16-5. Magnetic resonance cholangiogram (MRC). MRC demonstrating the gallbladder and common bile duct. The pancreatic duct is also displayed.

biliary tract abnormalities (Figure 16-5). It is commonly utilized as a first test now before **percutaneous transhepatic cholangiogram (PTC)** or an **endoscopic retrograde cholangiopancreatogram (ERCP)**. An MRC may be all that is needed, but usually provides preliminary data before a more invasive imaging test. The obvious advantages of this diagnostic procedure are that it is noninvasive and does not involve the use of radiation.

Radionuclide biliary scanning (HIDA scan) involves the intravenous injection of a ^{99m}technetium-labeled derivative of iminodiacetic acid. The radionuclide is excreted by the liver into the bile in high concentrations. Then it enters the gallbladder (if the cystic duct is patent) and duodenum. The normal gallbladder begins to fill within 30 minutes. Visualization of the common bile duct and duodenum without filling of the gallbladder after 4 hours indicates cystic duct obstruction, which supports the diagnosis of acute cholecystitis (Figure 16-6A, normal; Figure 16-6B, absent gallbladder filling). The sensitivity and specificity of the HIDA scan for diagnosing acute cholecystitis are 95% to 97% and 90% to 97%, respectively. False-positive results may occur in patients who are receiving total parenteral nutrition or those who have hepatitis. The scan is also of value in identifying a suspected bile leak after surgery. However, the HIDA scan is not useful for showing stones in either the gallbladder or the common bile duct.

In patients with obstructive jaundice with evidence of extrahepatic obstruction on ultrasonography, detailed radiographic visualization of the biliary ductal anatomy may be helpful in confirming the diagnosis and planning therapy. Direct injection of contrast agent into the ducts is necessary in these cases. This may be achieved by performing a **PTC** or **ERCP**. PTC involves inserting a thin needle through the skin and body wall, into the liver parenchyma, and injecting contrast medium directly into the intrahepatic bile ducts. Dilated bile ducts facilitate this procedure, yielding a success rate of more than 95%. If the ducts are of normal caliber, the test is successful only 70% to 80% of the time. PTC is particularly valuable for visualizing the proximal ductal system. It can also be used to obtain a cytologic diagnosis, extract stones, and aid in the placement of a biliary drainage catheter into the obstructed bile ducts. ERCP requires a skilled endoscopist, who cannulates the sphincter of Oddi and injects contrast medium to obtain a picture of the biliary and pancreatic ductal anatomy. This study is particularly valuable in patients with

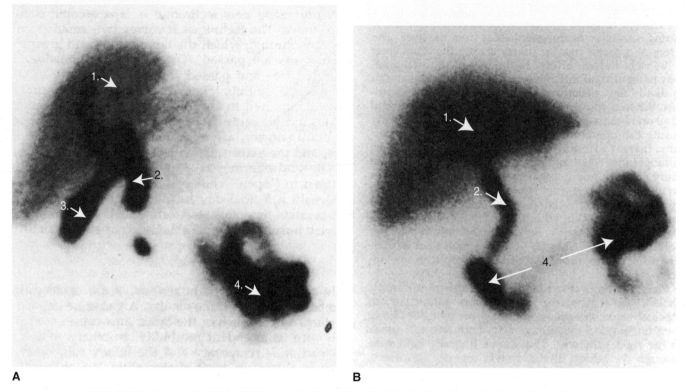

A   B

FIGURE 16-6. Radionuclide biliary (HIDA) scans. A, With and **B,** without visualization of the gallbladder. 1. Liver; 2. Common bile duct; 3. Gallbladder; 4. Activity in intestine.

suspected ampullary lesions because a diagnostic biopsy specimen can be obtained. Further, endoscopic brushing of an obstructed site may provide a cytologic diagnosis. In addition, ERCP can be used to perform a sphincterotomy, which involves cutting the sphincter of Oddi with an electrosurgical current through a wire attached to the ERCP catheter. This facilitates the extraction of biliary calculi and placing a stent through an area of bile duct obstruction. If coagulopathy is present, it must be corrected before either PTC or ERCP.

Figure 16-7 shows an algorithm for the evaluation of a jaundiced patient.

Clinical Presentation and Treatment of Gallstone Disease

Asymptomatic Gallstones

The majority of patients with gallstones will remain asymptomatic. Of these individuals, approximately 1% to 2% per year will develop symptoms or complications of gallstone disease. Thus, two-thirds of individuals remain free of symptoms or complications after 20 years. Although complications secondary to gallstones may occur at any time, most patients experience symptoms for some time before a complication develops. Thus, in adults, prophylactic cholecystectomy is not indicated for asymptomatic gallstones. However, after patients have symptoms of biliary colic, they are at increased risk for complications and should consider elective cholecystectomy. The risk of gallbladder carcinoma in patients with gallstones is too low to justify cholecystectomy for asymptomatic gallstones.

Acute Cholecystitis

The underlying pathology in acute cholecystitis is similar to that of biliary colic, except that there is sustained obstruction of the cystic duct in this condition and it is associated with inflammation and infection. The inflammation extends beyond the visceral peritoneum overlying the gallbladder to involve the parietal peritoneum. Left untreated, complications of empyema, gangrene, or perforation of the gallbladder may result from progression of the disease process. Most patients with acute cholecystitis have a history of biliary colic or dyspepsia. The pain of acute cholecystitis is constant. It is located in the right upper quadrant of the abdomen or the epigastrium and may radiate to the back. Nausea and vomiting are common. The patient is usually febrile, and on examination, the patient has tenderness in the right upper quadrant and a positive Murphy's sign. Once inflammation progresses to involve the parietal peritoneum, the patient has rebound tenderness and guarding. A tender mass is palpable in the right upper quadrant in approximately 20% of cases. Rarely, generalized peritonitis with rebound tenderness may be present if the disease has progressed to free perforation.

The differential diagnosis is long but should include acute hepatitis, acute pancreatitis, perforated peptic ulcer, and acute appendicitis. A careful history, physical, and diagnostic evaluation will lead to an accurate diagnosis in most patients. Laboratory studies demonstrate a leukocytosis and a left shift. Mild increases in the AST, ALT, and ALP are common. Patients may have a mild hyperbilirubinemia, but a significant elevation in the serum bilirubin suggests a common bile duct stone. On occasion, the patient will demonstrate a slight elevation of the serum amylase.

Ultrasonography is very helpful in making a definitive diagnosis. In addition to detecting gallstones with a high degree of accuracy, the study often shows specific characteristic findings of acute cholecystitis, such as a distended gallbladder, thickened gallbladder wall (>3 to 4 mm), pericholecystic fluid collection, and ultrasonographic Murphy's sign. This sign is elicited by demonstrating the presence of the most tender spot directly over

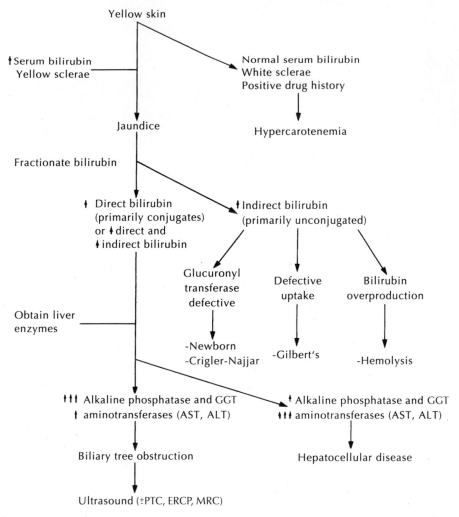

FIGURE 16-7. Algorithm for the evaluation of a jaundiced patient. PTC, percutaneous transhepatic cholangiogram; ERCP, endoscopic retrograde cholangiopancreatogram.

the sonographically localized gallbladder with the ultrasound probe. This sign is present in 98% of patients with acute cholecystitis. Ultrasonography can also provide additional information about the liver, intrahepatic bile ducts, common bile duct, and pancreas.

If there is any suspicion of an intestinal perforation, plain radiographs of the chest and abdomen should be obtained. Upright views are necessary to exclude pneumoperitoneum from another underlying cause of the acute abdomen. Plain x-rays may also show gallstones if they are radiopaque. However, the finding of stones does not in itself establish the diagnosis of acute cholecystitis. Sometimes the patient will undergo evaluation for abdominal complaints by CT scan. The CT can show gallbladder wall thickening and pericholecystic stranding (Figure 16-8), but this imaging test can sometimes miss subtle inflammation of the gallbladder.

HIDA scan is rarely utilized to establish the diagnosis of acute cholecystitis, but may be useful in confirming the diagnosis in cases with a strong clinical suspicion of this diagnosis with ultrasonographic evidence to support the diagnosis. Nonvisualization of the gallbladder after 4 hours of the study indicates cystic duct obstruction and is interpreted as positive for acute cholecystitis. However, certain patients (e.g., individuals receiving total parenteral nutrition, those who have fasted for a long time) may demonstrate

nonvisualization of the gallbladder on HIDA scan, yielding a false-positive result.

The initial management of acute cholecystitis includes withholding oral intake, administering intravenous fluids, and

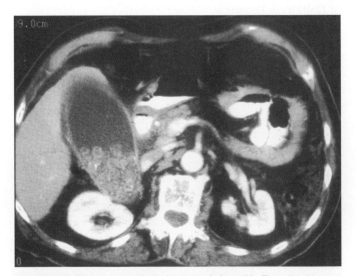

FIGURE 16-8. CT scan of a patient with acute cholecystitis. The gallbladder contains multiple gallstones, has a thick wall, and is surrounding by stranding and edema.

starting antibiotic therapy. The bacteria commonly associated with acute cholecystitis are *Escherichia coli, Klebsiella pneumoniae,* and *Streptococcus faecalis.* Most cases can, therefore, be covered with antibiotics that address gram-negative aerobes and enterococcus. Parenteral analgesics may be administered judiciously after the diagnosis is confirmed and further plans for therapy are made. A nasogastric tube is rarely required, but is recommended when vomiting occurs.

Most patients are best served by early cholecystectomy within a few days of presenting. Once the patient has benefited from some hydration and antibiotic treatment, surgery is indicated. This approach prevents the potential complications of gangrene, perforation, and sepsis, and makes the surgical procedure easier than if it were performed later in the course of the disease, when the inflammatory reaction is more severe. However, the procedure should be delayed if major medical problems must be addressed, and performed earlier if perforation or abscess is suspected. The cholecystectomy may be performed laparoscopically, but may require an open procedure if bleeding or poor definition of the anatomy leads to technical difficulty. As with all urgent or emergent operations, surgery for acute cholecystitis is associated with slightly higher mortality and morbidity rates compared with those for elective cholecystectomy, often as a result of underlying cardiovascular, pulmonary, or metabolic disease.

Patients with acute cholecystitis who are too ill to undergo cholecystectomy may require **cholecystostomy**. This procedure involves the percutaneous placement of a tube under ultrasound guidance through the liver into the gallbladder. This allows for the decompression of the gallbladder by draining the contents of the gallbladder. It is an effective approach for patients who are poor candidates for surgical management.

Acute gangrenous cholecystitis is associated with a morbidity rate of 15% to 25% and a mortality rate of 20% to 25%. Patients with this condition tend to be older and generally have more serious comorbid conditions than patients with simple acute cholecystitis. Often these patients will present with a more serious systematic illness with a higher leukocytosis. Treatment includes stabilization of the medical condition, administration of broad-spectrum antibiotics, and performance of emergency cholecystostomy or cholecystectomy.

Acute emphysematous cholecystitis results from gas-forming bacteria and is associated with a higher risk of gangrene and perforation compared with nonemphysematous cholecystitis. It generally affects older individuals, and diabetes mellitus is present in 20% to 50% of these patients. The classic findings on plain radiographs include air within the wall or lumen of the gallbladder, an air-fluid level within the lumen of the gallbladder, or air in the pericholecystic tissues. Air in the bile ducts may also be seen. Patients with acute emphysematous cholecystitis should receive broad-spectrum antibiotics, including coverage for anaerobes. In addition, they should undergo emergency cholecystectomy.

Although most patients with acute cholecystitis have associated calculi, acute cholecystitis can occur without calculi. **Acute acalculous cholecystitis** may complicate the course of a patient who is being treated for other conditions in a medical or surgical intensive care unit. Many patients are receiving total parenteral nutrition and mechanical ventilatory support and are immunosuppressed. Establishing the diagnosis of acute acalculous cholecystitis can present significant difficulty. The clinical features resemble those of acute calculous cholecystitis; however, the patient often cannot give a coherent history, and the associated conditions result in complex physical findings that are less revealing and more difficult to interpret. Ultrasonography or CT scan is helpful in establishing the diagnosis. Ultrasonography may show gallbladder distension, a thickened gallbladder wall, pericholecystic fluid, and a sonographic Murphy's sign. HIDA scan may help to establish the diagnosis, but it often yields a false-positive result and is associated with a specificity of only 38% in such cases. After the diagnosis is established, the management is similar to that of patients with acute calculous cholecystitis.

Chronic Cholecystitis

Biliary colic is the classic and most common symptom associated with chronic calculous cholecystitis. Characteristic features of biliary colic were described earlier. Nausea and vomiting may accompany this pain. Other associated symptoms include intolerance to fatty foods, flatulence, belching, and indigestion. These symptoms are encompassed by the collective term *dyspepsia.* However, the symptoms of dyspepsia are nonspecific and may be secondary to other diseases. Because the condition is not associated with acute infection, fever and chills are absent. Palpation of the abdomen during the episode of biliary colic may elicit tenderness in the right upper quadrant or the epigastrium, but there are no clinical signs of peritoneal irritation. The abdomen is generally soft, and bowel sounds are active. Between episodes of biliary colic, the abdomen shows no specific abnormality. The differential diagnosis among others includes angina pectoris, peptic ulcer disease, gastroesophageal reflux, ureteral obstruction, and irritable bowel syndrome.

Because biliary colic is not associated with acute inflammation, the total and differential leukocyte counts are within the normal range. In addition, liver function tests may be entirely normal. Typically, biliary colic is distinguished from acute cholecystitis by the presence of the characteristic clinical features described previously and by the absence of leukocytosis. Ultrasonography is the preferred study for evaluation of the biliary tract in these patients. If the results of ultrasonography are negative, it can be repeated again.

Management of the episode of biliary colic includes administration of parenteral analgesics, for severe pain, and observation. After cholelithiasis is confirmed, the optimum treatment is elective cholecystectomy. In most cases, the laparoscopic approach is used. An intraoperative **cholangiogram** may be added to evaluate the biliary ducts for stones and to delineate the biliary anatomy. If the operative cholangiogram performed during the laparoscopic cholecystectomy shows common duct calculi, the duct should be explored, or the patient may be referred subsequently for ERCP and sphincterotomy to extract the stones.

In patients with comorbid conditions that preclude the performance of safe cholecystectomy and in those who refuse surgery, oral dissolution therapy may be considered. Generally, though, this approach is not effective. Ursodeoxycholic acid is the most commonly administered agent. The patients must take the medication for at least 6 months and more likely a year. Patients with small single stones are the best candidates. Oral dissolution therapy yields a dissolution rate of 90% for stones smaller than 5 mm and a dissolution rate of 60% for calculi smaller than 10 mm. However, in approximately 50% of these patients, the gallstones recur within 5 years of discontinuing the therapy. **Extracorporeal shock wave lithotripsy (ESWL)** has been used to manage gallstone disease in selected patients, but support for this procedure has waned as these patients are at increased risk for postprocedural pancreatitis and may form new stones following the procedure.

Choledocholithiasis and Acute Cholangitis

In approximately 15% of patients with gallstones, the stones pass through the cystic duct and enter the common bile duct, resulting in choledocholithiasis. Although the smaller stones that enter the common bile duct can progress further into the duodenum, choledocholithiasis may lead to biliary obstruction, cholangitis, or pancreatitis.

Patients with choledocholithiasis may have a history of previous episodes of biliary colic. If the stone is causing obstruction of the bile duct, the patients will present with jaundice accompanied by light-colored stools and dark, tea-colored urine. The jaundice associated with choledocholithiasis may fluctuate in intensity compared with the progressive jaundice caused by malignant disease. If infection supervenes, **acute cholangitis** will develop. It is characterized by jaundice, right upper quadrant abdominal pain, and fever associated with chills (**Charcot's triad**). Acute cholecystitis is differentiated from acute cholangitis by the lack of biliary obstruction and jaundice. The infection accompanying acute cholangitis can progress to the presence of pus in the biliary ducts, resulting in **acute suppurative cholangitis**. In this condition, the patient may also be hypotensive and demonstrate mental confusion in addition to Charcot's triad. These five features together constitute **Reynold's pentad**. Examination of the abdomen may be unremarkable in a patient with choledocholithiasis or may reveal tenderness in the right upper quadrant if cholangitis is present. Rebound tenderness is not usually found, even in the presence of acute cholangitis. The etiology of obstructive jaundice or cholangitis includes choledocholithiasis, periampullary malignancy, and stricture. **Mirizzi's syndrome**, a condition in which a large stone in the gallbladder compresses the common hepatic duct, can also lead to obstructive jaundice.

The diagnostic evaluation of jaundice associated with probable choledocholithiasis starts with laboratory studies described previously. In patients with cholangitis, the leukocyte count is elevated. Bile duct obstruction leads to elevation in total bilirubin, with a predominance of the direct fraction, marked elevation of serum ALP and GGT, and mild elevations of AST and ALT. Serum amylase and lipase may also be mildly elevated. Ultrasonography is the best initial imaging study in patients with choledocholithiasis and cholangitis. It often shows dilated intrahepatic and extrahepatic ducts along with the presence of gallbladder stones, suggesting that stones are the likely cause of the common duct obstruction. As stated previously, stones in the common bile duct are frequently missed on ultrasonography. MRC, CT cholangiography, ERCP, or PTC are the best suitable studies to define the specific site and determine the source of the bile duct obstruction. Figure 16-9 shows a cholangiogram demonstrating the typical meniscus sign in the distal common bile duct, indicating that the obstruction is secondary to stones. The advantage of ERCP is that not only can the diagnosis be established, but the stones also can be extracted.

The management of patients with choledocholithiasis varies with the clinical situation. A patient with choledocholithiasis without evidence of cholangitis should undergo elective extraction of stones from the common duct. Extraction is most commonly achieved endoscopically but may be performed operatively. Any clotting abnormalities should be corrected

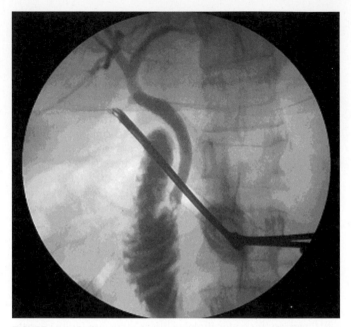

FIGURE 16-9. Cholangiogram demonstrating a stone in the distal common bile duct.

by giving parenteral vitamin K or administering fresh frozen plasma before an invasive procedure. The management of acute cholangitis, especially acute suppurative cholangitis, requires *urgent intervention*. A patient with cholangitis is hydrated with the administration of intravenous fluids, given antibiotics, and placed at bowel rest. The patient will likely need monitoring in an intensive care unit. Blood cultures are obtained, and broad-spectrum antibiotic should be initiated targeting gram-negative rods. Vomiting or abdominal distension resulting from paralytic ileus requires the insertion of a nasogastric tube. More than 70% of patients with cholangitis respond to this treatment algorithm. When the patient has recovered from the acute episode, a cholecystectomy should be performed if gallstones were the etiology for the biliary obstruction. If a patient does not respond to this therapy, urgent decompression of the bile duct through ERCP, PTC, or open surgery can be lifesaving.

When stones are detected in the bile duct by any type of imaging, the calculi can be removed by ERCP and sphincterotomy, and the patient can then undergo elective laparoscopic cholecystectomy. The success rate with ERCP and sphincterotomy in these cases is >90%, with a complication rate of approximately 5% to 10%. If the surgeon is experienced in advanced laparoscopic biliary surgery, laparoscopic cholecystectomy and extraction of the bile duct calculi through the cystic duct or choledochotomy is an option. Open bile duct exploration is still a good option, but endoscopic or laparoscopic stone removal has become the procedure of choice. If the gallbladder was previously removed, the bile duct calculi should be removed endoscopically with ERCP and sphincterotomy. Endoscopic intraluminal lithotripsy can be used to break large stones. The fragments can then pass spontaneously or be removed with ERCP and sphincterotomy or PTC. If the stones cannot be removed by these methods, an open procedure is necessary.

Acute Biliary (Gallstone) Pancreatitis

Gallstones are a very common cause of pancreatitis and may be attributed to transient or persistent obstruction of the ampulla of Vater by a large stone or the passage of small stones and biliary sludge. Management of patients with acute biliary pancreatitis includes initial resuscitation and supportive care, with correction of any existing fluid deficits. If the pancreatitis is mild to moderate in severity, a laparoscopic cholecystectomy can be performed safely, often within the first 48 to 72 hours of admission. By this time, the abdominal pain has largely resolved and the serum amylase level is returning to normal. Without a cholecystectomy, as many as 60% of patients will experience recurrent gallstone pancreatitis within 6 months. Of course, some patients with prohibitive coexisting medical conditions may never be surgical candidates. Then, endoscopic sphincterotomy should be performed, which will decrease the incidence of recurrent pancreatitis to between 2% and 5% over 2 years.

In patients with severe pancreatitis (fluid collections, pancreatic necrosis), cholecystectomy should be delayed until the pancreatitis has resolved, some weeks or even months later. Antibiotics are added for severe pancreatitis and for the management of septic complications. If acute cholecystitis was present, an interval *cholecystostomy* may be required. Emergent endoscopic sphincterotomy with stone extraction may be life saving in some patients with severe biliary pancreatitis. It should be used when a patient with pancreatitis is known to have gallstones, a high suspicion of choledocholithiasis is present, and the clinical course does not improve within 24 to 36 hours with normal resuscitative efforts.

Gallstone Ileus

Gallstone ileus accounts for <1% of all cases of intestinal obstruction. It occurs more commonly in women than in men (3.5:1 ratio). Although the word "ileus" is part of the name, it is a misnomer as this condition is a mechanical obstruction. Gallstone ileus results from the erosion of a large stone through the gallbladder directly into the small intestine, creating an internal fistula between the gallbladder and the intestinal tract, usually at the level of duodenum. Passage of the stone along the length of the small intestine may cause episodes of partial small bowel obstruction until the stone becomes impacted in a narrow portion of the intestine, usually in the distal ileum just proximal to the ileocecal valve. A history of biliary colic or gallstone disease is common. Patients present with the clinical picture of small intestinal obstruction; however, the intermittent nature of the obstruction in the early stages (before impaction of the stone) often results in delay in the diagnosis.

Plain radiographs of the abdomen show findings of small intestinal obstruction and may show air in the biliary tree. Occasionally, a large stone has sufficient calcium to be seen in the intestine. Ultrasonography is useful in documenting gallstones. CT with oral contrast is the preferred diagnostic test, because it can demonstrate air in the biliary tree, a biliary-enteric fistula, the site of obstruction, and the obstructing stone. Historically, a barium study of the small intestine has been used to demonstrate the biliary-enteric fistula and confirm the distal small intestinal obstruction.

The management of gallstone ileus includes placement of a nasogastric tube for decompression of the obstruction and intravenous hydration. Patients should undergo a surgical exploration of the abdomen and an enterolithotomy, an extraction of the stone from the small intestine, to relieve the obstruction. This may be performed with the use of laparoscopy or traditional open surgery. Many of these patients are elderly and will not tolerate prolonged operations, but in a few

select patients who are otherwise healthy, cholecystectomy and definitive correction of the internal fistula may also be performed.

GALLBLADDER CANCER

Gallbladder cancer accounts for <2% of all malignant tumors. Gallbladder cancer rates are the highest among American Indians and among white Hispanic peoples. Within both groups, the incidence of gallbladder cancer is significantly higher in women. Gallbladder cancer arises in the setting of chronic inflammation, and in the vast majority of patients, the source of this chronic inflammation is cholesterol gallstones. The presence of gallstones increases the risk of gallbladder cancer four- to fivefold, but the risk of gallbladder cancer in any one patient with cholelithiasis does not justify cholecystectomy to prevent cancer. Other diseases associated with gallbladder cancer include primary sclerosing cholangitis, ulcerative colitis, liver flukes, chronic *Salmonella typhi*, and *Helicobacter* infection. Porcelain gallbladder, a condition involving calcification of the gallbladder wall, is associated with higher rates of gallbladder cancer (Figure 16-10). Larger gallbladder polyps >1 cm may harbor carcinoma.

Gallbladder cancer may not be suspected preoperatively, since the symptoms overlap substantially with those of calculous disease. Early-stage disease is many times asymptomatic. Most early-stage tumors are found incidentally by the pathologist on histologic review of a gallbladder removed for gallstone disease. Patients with more advanced gallbladder cancer may have vague right upper quadrant pain, weight loss, and malaise. Jaundice is present in approximately 50% of such patients since these cancers tend to spread early through direct extension into the liver and adjacent structures in the porta hepatis causing biliary obstruction, and by metastasizing to the regional lymph nodes and liver. Physical examination may show a mass in the right upper quadrant of the abdomen.

Most gallbladder cancers are adenocarcinomas. Disease localized to the peritonealized surface of the gallbladder is effectively treated with cholecystectomy. Larger tumors

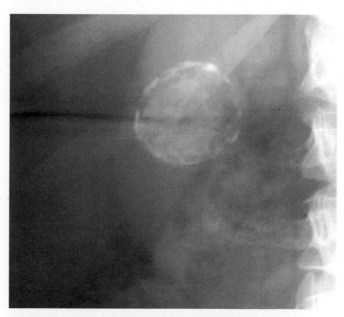

FIGURE 16-10. Plain radiograph of a porcelain gallbladder.

abutting or growing into the liver parenchyma are treated with a liver wedge resection of the gallbladder fossa and a regional lymphadenectomy. Advanced tumors may require a formal liver resection. Porta hepatis lymphadenectomy lacks the standardization associated with other abdominal lymphadenectomies, because of the proximity of vital structures and the organ's lack of a mobile mesentery. Moreover, despite radical approaches, the 5-year survival rate remains poor (<5% at 5 years) unless the cancer is detected incidentally as a small focus within a gallbladder removed for symptomatic stone disease.

EXTRAHEPATIC BILE DUCT MALIGNANCIES

Cancer of the extrahepatic bile ducts is uncommon and referred to as bile duct cancer while cancers of the intrahepatic bile ducts are called cholangiocarcinoma. Bile duct cancer occurs with equal frequency in both sexes, usually affecting individuals between 50 and 70 years of age. As with gallbladder cancer, chronic inflammatory processes often precede the development of overt malignancy. The risk of bile duct malignancy is significantly higher in patients with ulcerative colitis and sclerosing cholangitis. Other risk factors include choledochal cyst and parasitic liver flukes, *Opisthorchis viverrini* or *Clonorchis sinensis*. Approximately one-third of patients with bile duct carcinoma have associated gallstones. Bile duct tumors are usually well circumscribed, and two-thirds of these carcinomas are located above the junction of the cystic duct with the common hepatic duct. Histologically, the lesions are usually mucin-producing adenocarcinomas. In general, bile duct cancers are slow-growing, locally advanced tumors that rarely metastasize to distant sites. However, because of the anatomic relationships of the extrahepatic ducts to the liver, portal vein, and hepatic artery, curative resection of these lesions is the exception rather than the rule.

Common symptoms relate to local growth, impingement on the liver, and obliteration of the bile ductal lumen. Weight loss, abdominal pain, jaundice, and pruritus are common, and if cholangitis is present fever may occur. In contrast to the fluctuating jaundice that is often seen in patients with common duct calculi, the jaundice associated with bile duct cancers is progressive. On physical examination, hepatomegaly may be found. A palpable, nontender gallbladder in a jaundiced patient indicates that the site of the obstructing tumor is distal to the junction of the cystic duct with the common duct and the patients will demonstrate Courvoisier's sign. Distal bile duct malignancies presenting in this manner thus mimic the symptoms of pancreatic tumors.

Laboratory studies show a typical picture of obstructive jaundice, making ultrasound and measurement of fractionated bilirubin good initial studies. Most patients have dilated intrahepatic ducts. However, the absence of intrahepatic ductal dilation does not rule out obstruction, since ducts may be of normal caliber because of incomplete obstruction, tumor ingrowth, or sclerosing cholangitis. Ultrasound, CT scanning, and MRI are helpful in determining the extrahepatic extent of the tumors and providing information about the resectability and invasion of adjacent structures. PTC and ERCP are very helpful in demonstrating lesions, assessing intraductal tumor extent, and obtaining cytologic specimens. PTC is particularly useful for evaluation of the proximal lesions and establishing antegrade access for stenting these lesions.

Tumors in the proximal one-third of the ductal system may involve both the left and right hepatic ducts—a so-called Klatskin tumor. If resection is not possible, the tumor may be traversed with a guide wire and a stent passed through it to relieve the biliary obstruction. Resection of bile duct cancers offers the best chance of survival, although the prognosis after resection of these proximal lesions is poor, with 5-year survival rate of only 5% at best.

Middle-third tumors are best treated by resection and Roux-en-Y hepaticojejunostomy. The 5-year survival rate after resection of middle-third lesions is approximately 10%. Like proximal lesions, the bile duct may be stented with an endoscopic or transhepatic approach. The operation of choice for distal common duct tumors is the Whipple procedure, which involves resecting the distal common duct including the tumor, the pancreatic head, and the duodenum. Three anastomoses, connecting pancreatic remnant, hepatic duct, and proximal GI tract in sequence to a mobilized length of jejunum, must be performed after the resection. The 5-year survival rate after a Whipple procedure for a lesion of the distal third of the common bile duct is approximately 12% to 25%. If resection is not possible, palliation can be achieved through a surgical bypass or biliary stent. If unresectability is determined at operation rather than through preoperative studies, the creation of an operative bypass obviates the need for an indwelling stent and the potential occlusion.

CONGENITAL CHOLEDOCHAL CYSTS

Very uncommonly, cystic enlargements of the bile ducts occur that are thought to be congenital. These are more frequent in females (4:1 female:male) and among the Asian population. Patients may present asymptomatic after an imaging study performed for other reasons, or in the late teens or early 20s with pain and jaundice and rarely an upper abdominal mass. Choledochal cysts are best evaluated by CT scan initially and the specific anatomy determined by MRC or ERCP. Generally, it is recommended that these cysts be resected to address symptoms and the risk of bile duct cancer. Following resection, a Roux-en-Y hepaticojejunostomy is performed to reestablish bile flow. Continued follow-up of these patients is important, since anastomotic structures can occur and patients should be surveyed for malignancy.

BILE DUCT INJURY AND STRICTURE

The majority of bile duct strictures result from iatrogenic injury during an operative procedure. The bile duct is especially susceptible to this because of a limited blood supply and no redundancy. Approximately 75% of injuries occur during simple cholecystectomy and involve division of the bile duct and its vasculature close to the liver. This underscores the importance of recognizing the anatomic variations of the biliary tree correctly and proceeding in a cautious systematic fashion, even during routine cholecystectomy. Injuries can involve the common duct, the hepatic duct, or the left and right hepatic ducts. Although low, the incidence of bile duct injuries associated with laparoscopic cholecystectomy is higher than that associated with open cholecystectomy. This incidence decreases with individual surgeon experience and is higher in operations performed for acute cholecystitis rather than those performed for biliary colic electively. Unfortunately, many iatrogenic injuries that go unrecognized intraoperatively declare themselves as a subhepatic collection, iatrogenic occlusion, or delayed stricture formation.

When bile duct injury or anomaly is suspected intraoperatively, cholangiography should be performed to delineate the anatomy and suspected injury. Injuries to accessory ducts smaller than 3 mm that drain a small amount of liver parenchyma may be ligated. Otherwise the operation should be converted to an open procedure and an operative repair is performed. If the injury involves <50% of the circumference of the duct, and the duct has not sustained significant devascularization, primary repair of this simple injury may be performed. A T tube stent is placed and brought out through another location in the common duct to decompress the duct and stent the repair open. Otherwise, a Roux-en-Y hepaticojejunostomy or choledochojejunostomy should be performed in order to avoid stricturing of a primary repair.

In the early postoperative period, bile duct injury may cause severe abdominal pain, jaundice, drainage of bile from an operatively placed drain or through the wound, signs of acute abdomen, or sepsis. Ultrasonography or CT scan may be obtained to detect or exclude an intra-abdominal bile collection, which is called a *biloma*. Definition of the exact location of the ductal injury requires either ERCP or MRCP. HIDA scan can confirm the presence of bile extravasation, but is less commonly utilized now. A minor leak from an accessory hepatic duct is likely to heal spontaneously and merely requires placement of a percutaneous drainage catheter in the subhepatic space under CT or ultrasound guidance. Leakage from a cystic duct may be treated with ERCP sphincterotomy alone or, more commonly, ERCP sphincterotomy and placement of a stent. If major ductal injury is detected postoperatively, reconstruction will need to be performed but should be delayed while the anatomy is defined, any sepsis resolves, and the local inflammation induced from the bile leak improves.

Late development of stricture leads to obstructive jaundice and recurrent cholangitis. Long-standing strictures may result in biliary cirrhosis and portal hypertension. Diagnosis of strictures is confirmed by MRC, ERCP, or PTC. Cholangitis should be managed with antibiotics and the stricture treated by bypassing the dilated proximal bile duct to a Roux-en-Y loop of jejunum. In the hands of experienced surgeons, excellent outcome of the operative repair is achieved in 70% to 90% of patients. For poor-risk patients, in lieu of dilation, stenting is an option.

Table 16-2 summarizes the common clinical syndromes and complications that can result from cholelithiasis.

BRIEF DESCRIPTION OF SELECTED PROCEDURES

Laparoscopic Cholecystectomy

Laparoscopic cholecystectomy has replaced open cholecystectomy as the preferred approach to the management of gallstone disease in most elective and many emergent situations. When performed electively in an otherwise healthy patient, most procedures can be done as day surgery. If the patient has serious comorbidities, postoperative hospital stay is usually only 24 to 48 hours even after surgery for acute cholecystitis. The main reasons patients can undergo this surgery with such a short hospital stay is the greatly reduced postoperative incisional pain as compared to that with open cholecystectomy.

The advantages of the laparoscopic approach are reduced postoperative pain, wound, and pulmonary complications; the possibility of a short hospitalization; and rapid recovery from the procedure with early return to normal activity. The main risks associated with the laparoscopic approach are related to injury to the bile ducts, intestine, and major vessels usually resulting from blind trocar insertion or the injudicious use of electrocautery. With greater experience of the operating surgeon, the risk of complications diminishes significantly. If anatomy is obscured because of the pathologic process or technical difficulties encountered with the laparoscopic approach, the laparoscopic procedure is converted to an open laparotomy. There is some controversy as to whether cholangiography should be performed routinely or selectively at the time of laparoscopic cholecystectomy. Most surgeons utilize a selective approach. If stones are found in the common bile duct on cholangiography, they may be removed laparoscopically through the cystic duct or an incision in the common bile duct during the same operation or the laparoscopic procedure can be converted to an open common bile duct exploration to extract the stones. Alternatively, ERCP and sphincterotomy and stone extraction may be performed postoperatively

Open Cholecystectomy and Common Bile Duct Exploration

Open cholecystectomy is generally performed through a right subcostal incision. After the abdomen is opened, the gallbladder is exposed and the gallbladder is dissected out of the gallbladder fossa. An intraoperative cholangiogram may be performed through the cystic duct at any time to define the anatomy and confirm or exclude suspected choledocholithiasis. Both the cystic duct and artery are identified and ligated.

A common duct exploration is sometimes performed during a cholecystectomy. Absolute indications for this include a palpable common duct stone and common duct stones visualized on preoperative or intraoperative cholangiograms. Relative indications include jaundice, acute biliary pancreatitis, ductal dilation, and small gallbladder stones. Operative cholangiogram is performed to confirm or exclude stones in the bile duct when only relative indications for bile duct exploration are present.

The procedure for open common bile duct exploration involves mobilizing the duodenum with a Kocher maneuver, identifying the duct and making a small longitudinal incision in the common bile duct. Then the lumen is irrigated with saline using flexible catheters to help flush out stones and debris from the duct. Inflatable balloon catheters are passed both proximally and distally in an attempt to extract stones. A small endoscope (choledochoscope) may be advanced through the opening and the duct thus carefully visualized both proximally and distally to determine whether residual stones are present. A variety of instruments, including stone forceps and collapsible wire baskets are available to remove stones that remain impacted and resist removal by the previous maneuvers. All stones, mucus, and debris are removed from the bile duct, and the duct is irrigated with saline. A T tube is then placed in the lumen of the duct, and the opening in the duct is closed around the T tube. A completion cholangiogram is obtained to ensure that no stones remain in the duct and that contrast flows freely in the duodenum. A closed drainage catheter is often left in the subhepatic space. When there are multiple stones, or the physician believes that there are stones left in the bile duct, it is prudent to perform an anastomosis between

TABLE 16-2	Summary of the Common Clinical Syndromes That Result from Cholelithiasis and the Complications of Cholelithiasis

Syndrome	Etiology	Findings
Biliary colic	Transient cystic duct obstruction	Episodes of upper abdominal pain
		Nonspecific physical findings
		Ultrasound: cholelithiasis
Acute cholecystitis	Sustained cystic duct obstruction	Constant, severe right upper quadrant pain
	Acute inflammation of gallbladder	Elevated temperature
		Murphy's sign
		Rebound tenderness
		Leukocytosis
		Mild hyperbilirubinemia
		Ultrasound: cholelithiasis, with or without other signs of gallbladder inflammation
		HIDA scan: nonvisualization of gallbladder
Choledocholithiasis	Stone in the common bile duct	History of abdominal pain, jaundice, light stool, dark urine
		Laboratory findings: obstructive jaundice picture
		Ultrasound: cholelithiasis with dilated ducts
		CT, MRC, PTC, ERCP—ductal stones
Acute cholangitis	Infected bile; septicemia	History same as choledocholithiasis but acutely ill patient with abdominal pain, jaundice, fever, chills; may also have hypotension and change in mentation (in acute suppurative cholangitis)
		Stone impacted in the common bile duct
		Stricture of the common bile duct (previous biliary surgery)
		Tumor obstructing the common bile duct (especially after an invasive diagnostic procedure that might have seeded the bile with bacteria)
		Laboratory findings: same as choledocholithiasis, plus elevated white blood cell count
		Ultrasound: same as choledocholithiasis, but gallbladder may have been removed previously if the etiology is a stricture
Biliary pancreatitis	Acute pancreatitis	Acutely ill, severe constant epigastric pain, with or without radiation through to the back
		Passage of small stones or sludge through the sphincter of Oddi
		Tenderness, guarding in upper abdomen Markedly elevated serum amylase/lipase
		Ultrasound, CT scan, MRC cholelithiasis, with or without inflammatory mass in pancreas
Gallstone ileus	Cholecystenteric fistula	Elderly debilitated patient
	Very large gallstone(s)	Incomplete bowel obstruction
	Stone obstructing intestine (usually distal ileum)	Radiograph shows bowel obstruction (usually distal small bowel)
		May show air in biliary tree and may see large stone obstructing
		Ultrasound: ± stone in gallbladder and air in biliary tree
		CT: all of the above

CT, computed tomography; ERCP, endoscopic retrograde cholangiopancreatography; HIDA, dimethyl iminodiacetic acid, a radionuclide biliary scan; MRC, magnetic resonance cholangiography; PTC, percutaneous transhepatic cholangiogram.

the bile duct and the GI tract (choledochoduodenostomy or choledochojejunostomy) so that residual stones may pass easily from the duct into the intestine.

The peritoneal drainage catheter is removed within 24 to 48 hours after the T tube has been clamped. Drainage of significant amounts of blood or bile requires further investigation. The typical T tube is left in place for 3 weeks, after which an injection of contrast material in the radiology department is obtained. If the dye flows freely into the duodenum and demonstrates no filling defects, the T tube may be removed. T tubes are typically pulled after an established track is present (3 to 6 weeks). If there is any concern about interpretation of the cholangiogram, the T tube is left in place for a longer period of time and the x-ray study is repeated.

Occasionally, despite thorough common duct exploration, a filling defect is noticed in the postoperative T tube cholangiogram, indicating a missed or retained stone. In approximately 20% of patients, these stones pass spontaneously, especially if they are small. Under such circumstances, the T tube is left in place for 4 to 6 weeks, and the cholangiogram is repeated. If retained stones remain, they may be extracted with the use of ERCP techniques. Alternatively the T tube tract can be utilized to advance a wire basket into the duct under fluoroscopy so that the stones might be retrieved.

In the rare circumstances where none of these methods is successful, operative reexploration of the duct is necessary.

Endoscopic Extraction of Common Bile Duct Stones

Most common bile duct stones are removed by ERCP and sphincterotomy. Sphincterotomy of the sphincter of Oddi is performed by a special cautery wire passed through the duodenoscope into the sphincter. The common duct is then cleared of stones and debris using special balloon catheters or wire baskets also passed through the duodenoscope.

When performed electively, this is usually an outpatient procedure. Any coagulopathy should be corrected before the procedure. If a stone cannot be extracted, jaundice can be relieved by inserting a stent with one end above the stone and the other in the duodenum. This stent is left in place, providing biliary decompression until ERCP extraction can be attempted again or surgical stone removal can be arranged. As well as the risks of ERCP, sphincterotomy and stone manipulation add to the potential complications of postprocedure pancreatitis, GI bleeding (1% to 2%), and duodenal or common duct perforation (0.3%).

thePoint ✳ Go to http://thePoint.lww.com/activate and use your scratch-off code on the inside cover of this book to access bonus chapters, question bank, videos, and more.

SAMPLE QUESTIONS

Questions

Choose the best answer for each question.

1. A 41-year-old woman presents to the emergency department with 18 hours of nausea, right upper quadrant abdominal pain, and fever. She ate a heavy meal the night before and has never experienced similar symptoms. Laboratory evaluation reveals an elevated white blood cell count, normal bilirubin, and slightly elevated aspartate aminotransferase (AST) and alanine aminotransferase (ALT). The most appropriate imaging study to determine the etiology of her symptoms is a(n)
   A. plain abdominal radiograph.
   B. ultrasonography.
   C. endoscopic retrograde cholangiopancreatography (ERCP).
   D. contrast CT scan.
   E. HIDA scan.

2. A 51-year-old woman comes to the emergency department because of fever and abdominal pain. Her temperature is 38.4°C. She is tender with guarding in the right upper quadrant of her abdomen. Her WBC is 17,000/mm³. LFTs and lipase levels are within the normal range. Ultrasound of the right upper quadrant identifies gallstones, a gallbladder wall of 5 mm, and fluid surrounding the gallbladder. The most appropriate antibiotic to treat this condition is
   A. penicillin.
   B. ciprofloxacin.
   C. metronidazole.
   D. cefoxitin.
   E. linezolid.

3. An 83-year-old woman presents to the emergency department with a 2-day history of nausea and vomiting. She has a prior history of a hysterectomy, and on exam, her abdomen is slightly distended and nontender on palpation. Her laboratory evaluation reveals a normal white blood cell count and a metabolic alkalosis. Abdominal x-rays show a small bowel obstruction and air in the biliary tree. Which of the following is the most likely diagnosis?
   A. Colon cancer
   B. Perforated duodenal ulcer
   C. Acute cholangitis
   D. Small bowel obstruction secondary to adhesions
   E. Gallstone ileus

4. A 54-year-old man presents to the clinic with abdominal pain over the past 8 hours. The pain is mid-abdominal and getting worse. Your evaluation has found an elevated white blood cell count, an amylase of 792 U/L, and normal liver function tests. An ultrasound reveals gallstones. Which of the following is the most appropriate management at this time?
   A. Give the patient a prescription for pain medicine and have the patient return to the clinic in 1 week for a checkup.
   B. Admit the patient to the hospital, start antibiotics, monitor the amylase levels, and discharge the patient when the amylase levels have returned to normal.
   C. Admit the patient to the hospital, hold any intake by mouth, and schedule the patient for a cholecystectomy before discharge.
   D. Schedule the patient for emergency exploratory laparotomy.
   E. Call a code, intubate the patient, and admit the patient for treatment in the intensive care unit.

5. A 72-year-old man comes to clinic because his wife noticed that his eyes are yellow. Recently he has found that his urine is dark and the stool light in color. He has recently had a diminished appetite, but otherwise feeling well without other complaints. His past medical history is unremarkable. He smoked cigarettes for 30 years but quit 15 years ago. He is afebrile. Vital signs are normal. He is deeply jaundiced. There is a nontender smooth globular mass consistent with an enlarged gallbladder in the right upper quadrant of his abdomen. The rest of his examination is normal. Which of the following is the most likely diagnosis in this patient?
   A. Pancreatic cancer
   B. Choledocholithiasis
   C. Choledochal cyst
   D. Biliary stricture
   E. Gallstones

Answers and Explanations

1. Answer: B

The patient likely presents with acute cholecystitis. The most sensitive and least invasive imaging study to document the signs of gallbladder wall thickening and pericholecystic fluid is an ultrasound.

2. Answer: D

Most bacteria that infect the biliary tree are Gram-negative rods and include *E. coli* and *Klebsiella*. A second- or third-generation cephalosporin will effectively cover these bacteria. The other choices may target these bacteria as effectively or are reserved for advanced complex infections.

3. Answer: E

By definition, a gallstone ileus results in air in the biliary tree since there is a fistula between the gallbladder and duodenum. If the stone is large enough to obstruct the ileocecal valve, the patient will manifest a bowel obstruction.

4. Answer: C

Most patients with gallstone pancreatitis resolve the episode of pancreatitis with bowel rest and hydration. The incidence of recurrent pancreatitis is high unless the gallbladder is removed. Patients should have a cholecystectomy, therefore, before discharge as long as the patient is a reasonable operative candidate.

5. Answer: A

In order for the patient to present with jaundice and acholic stools, a bile duct obstruction must be present. Gallstones alone do not cause a bile duct obstruction. The other diagnoses may be associated with obstructed jaundice. Given the patient's age and the presentation, it is most likely that this patient has a pancreaticobiliary malignancy.

17
Pancreas

STEVEN B. GOLDIN, M.D., Ph.D. • DIMITRIOS AVGERINOS, M.D. • ALEXANDER A. PARIKH, M.D. •
MOHSEN SHABAHANG, M.D., Ph.D.

Objectives

1. Describe the embryology of the pancreas including ductal development.
2. Describe the anatomic nomenclature used to describe the various segments of the pancreas.
3. Define and classify various types of pancreas divisum.
4. Describe the arterial supply to the pancreas.
5. Describe the venous return from the pancreas.
6. Describe the exocrine functions of the pancreas.
7. Describe the endocrine functions of the pancreas.
8. Define acute pancreatitis.
9. Define chronic pancreatitis.
10. List the common etiologies of pancreatitis.
11. Describe the clinical presentation of a patient with acute pancreatitis.
12. Describe the criteria used for determining the prognosis of an attack of acute pancreatitis.
13. Discuss five potential complications of acute pancreatitis.
14. Discuss the nonoperative management of acute pancreatitis.
15. Describe the indications for surgical intervention in acute pancreatitis.
16. Discuss the mechanism of pseudocyst formation with respect to the role of the pancreatic duct, and list five symptoms and physical signs of pseudocysts.
17. Describe the diagnostic approach to a patient with a suspected pseudocyst, including the indications for and the sequence of tests.
18. Discuss four potential adverse outcomes of chronic pancreatitis as well as the diagnostic approach, treatment options, and management.
19. List four pancreatic neoplasms, and describe the pathology of each with reference to cell type and function.
20. Describe the symptoms, physical signs, laboratory findings, and diagnostic workup of a pancreatic mass on the basis of the location of the tumor.
21. Describe the symptoms, physical signs, laboratory findings, and diagnostic workup of a pancreatic neuroendocrine tumor.
22. Describe Zollinger-Ellison syndrome.
23. Describe the surgical treatment of pancreatic neoplasms, exocrine or endocrine.
24. Discuss the role of adjuvant therapy for pancreatic cancer.
25. Discuss the long-term prognosis for pancreatic cancers on the basis of pathology and cell type.

The pancreas is responsible for a variety of endocrine and exocrine functions. Diseases affecting the pancreas are common and include congenital, inflammatory, infectious, traumatic, and neoplastic processes, which may affect both the endocrine and exocrine functions. The pancreatic exocrine role in digestion was uncovered in the 1800s, and Banting and Best discovered insulin and its role in blood glucose metabolism in Toronto, Canada, in 1921. Frederick Grant Banting and John James Richard Macleod received the Nobel Prize in 1923 for this discovery. Fully understanding the embryology and development, anatomy, and physiology of the pancreas is paramount to understanding the genetic alterations and pathophysiology that may occur in patients with pancreatic disease and the key to understanding, which patients will benefit from surgical intervention.

ANATOMY

The pancreas is a retroperitoneal gland that lies transversely just anterior to the second lumbar vertebra. Normally, the pancreas is 12 to 18 cm in length and weighs between 70 and 110 g. The gland is divided into four distinct parts: head, neck, body, and tail (Figure 17-1).The head of the pancreas is located within the "C-loop" of the duodenum and accounts for approximately 30% of the gland's weight. The superior mesenteric vein defines the junction of the head and neck of the gland. The vascular anatomy is described below. The uncinate process makes up a portion of the head. The neck of the gland is the portion overlying the superior mesenteric vein, and the body extends to the left of the superior mesenteric vein. The tail is the most distal portion of the gland and extends

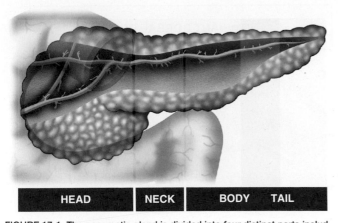

FIGURE 17-1. The pancreatic gland is divided into four distinct parts including the head, neck, body, and tail. The superior mesenteric vein runs under the neck of the gland. Diagram taken from the Internet Encyclopedia of Science. (Drawing by Matthew Campbell.)

toward or abuts the splenic hilum. The anatomic dividing line between the body and the tail is ill defined with lesions of the body or tail usually being managed similarly. The anterior surface of the gland is in contact with the transverse mesocolon and posterior wall of the stomach. Its posterior surface is devoid of peritoneum and abuts the common bile duct, superior mesenteric vessels, inferior vena cava, and aorta.

Embryology and Ductal Anatomy

Understanding the pancreatic embryology and development provides great insight into the pancreatic ductal anatomy. The embryo is 3 to 4 mm in size at 30 days' gestation, when the endoderm lining the duodenum forms the ventral and dorsal pancreatic buds. As the duodenum forms its C-shape, the ventral pancreatic bud rotates clockwise to lie below the dorsal pancreatic bud (Figure 17-2), and by 6 weeks' gestation, the

dorsal and ventral pancreatic buds are contiguous with each other. The parenchyma and ducts of the dorsal and ventral pancreatic buds then fuse during the 8th week. The ventral pancreatic bud forms the inferior portion of the head (the uncinate process), while the dorsal bud forms the remaining portion of the head, body, and tail. The duct of Wirsung (main pancreatic duct) is formed by the fusion of the distal portion of the dorsal pancreatic and the ventral pancreatic ducts. The duct of Wirsung typically forms a common channel with the common bile duct and enters the duodenum at the ampulla of Vater and the sphincter of Oddi (the major papilla). The distal portion of the dorsal pancreatic duct may persist as the duct of Santorini (accessory pancreatic duct) (Figure 17-3A) or be totally obliterated (Figure 17-3B).

When referring to arteries, veins, or ducts, remember that proximal is where the structure begins (e.g., the aorta for arteries, feet for veins, and pancreatic tail for the pancreatic duct) and distal is where they end (e.g., the aorta ends at the common iliac arteries, the veins end at larger proximal veins like the IVC, and the duodenum for the pancreatic duct). Therefore, the proximal pancreatic duct is in the pancreatic tail and the distal pancreatic duct is near the duodenum in the head of the pancreas.

A variety of pancreatic ductal variations occur that are considered variations of normal, since most of the pancreatic secretions empty into the duodenum through the ampulla of Vater (Figure 17-3A, B). Approximately 20% of the population has ventral and dorsal pancreatic ducts that do not fuse completely (Figure 17-3C–E), which results in some variation of the original double duct system with a persistent dominant dorsal duct. The classical description of pancreas divisum has separate dorsal and ventral pancreatic ducts (Figure 17-3C) and occurs in approximately 6% of the population. Other variations include an absent duct of Wirsung (Figure 17-3D), or a filamentous communication between the ventral and dorsal ductal system (Figure 17-3E). These variations, where the majority of the dorsal pancreas empties into the duodenum via the duct of Santorini and a portion of the pancreatic head and uncinate process

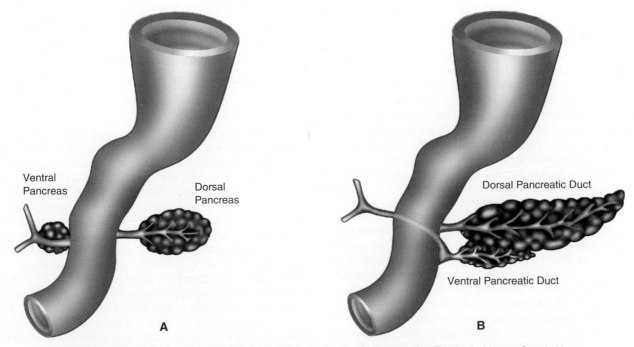

FIGURE 17-2. Dorsal and ventral pancreatic buds. A, Prior to migration. **B,** After migration. (Drawing by Matthew Campbell.)

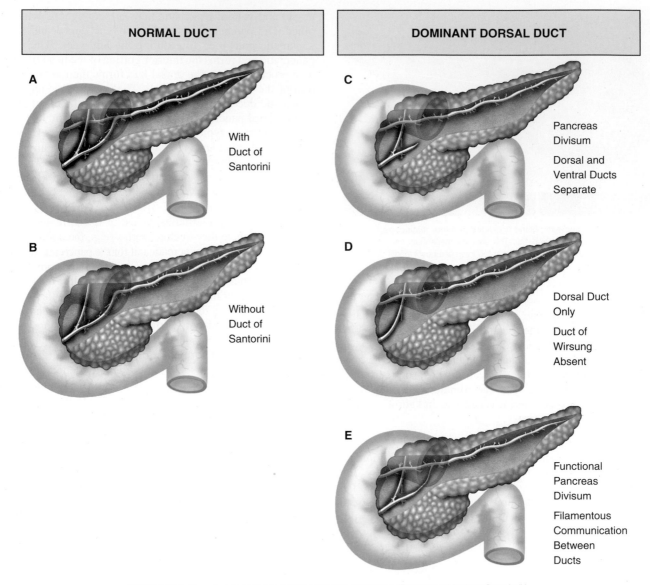

NORMAL DUCT	DOMINANT DORSAL DUCT

A — With Duct of Santorini

B — Without Duct of Santorini

C — Pancreas Divisum / Dorsal and Ventral Ducts Separate

D — Dorsal Duct Only / Duct of Wirsung Absent

E — Functional Pancreas Divisum / Filamentous Communication Between Ducts

FIGURE 17-3. **Common pancreatic ductal anatomic variations.** (Drawing by Matthew Campbell.)

empties via the major papilla, are often grouped together and called "pancreas divisum." The diameter of the major pancreatic duct usually ranges from 1.5 to 2 mm in the tail to 3 to 4 mm in the head. The minor pancreatic duct is usually much smaller and may not allow adequate unobstructed drainage of the body and tail of the gland, which can lead to recurrent bouts of pancreatitis. Figure 17-4 demonstrates an endoscopic retrograde cholangiopancreatography (ERCP) obtained via both major and minor pancreatic ducts. Treatment of pancreatitis will be discussed elsewhere in the chapter.

A second pancreatic developmental anomaly is called annular pancreas. It is less common than pancreas divisum and occurs in 1 out of 12,000 to 15,000 people. Annular pancreas may result from the incomplete rotation of the ventral pancreatic bud, which results in the encirclement of the second portion of the duodenum by a ring of pancreatic tissue. It is one of the causes of duodenal obstruction seen in infants and children. Treatment involves surgical bypass of the pancreatic tissue causing the obstruction (duodenojejunostomy) and specifically avoids division of the pancreatic parenchyma, which would result in a high rate of pancreatic fistula.

PANCREATIC VASCULAR ANATOMY AND INNERVATION

Arterial Blood Supply

Undertaking any surgical procedure requires a thorough understanding of the vascular anatomy. This is particularly true for pancreatic procedures, where a multitude of critically important vascular structures with significant variations are intertwined with the pancreas. In fact, it is the location of these structures that often dictates the type of procedure adopted. For instance, knowledge that the blood supply to the duodenum is interrupted during pancreaticoduodenectomy partially explains why the duodenum is resected during this procedure. Likewise, the splenic artery is closely approximated with the tail of the pancreas and, therefore, distal pancreatectomy also often requires splenectomy to prevent splenic infarction. Patient outcomes often rely upon proper identification of normal or common vascular variations. Lastly, neoplastic invasion of major vascular structures is critically important when determining

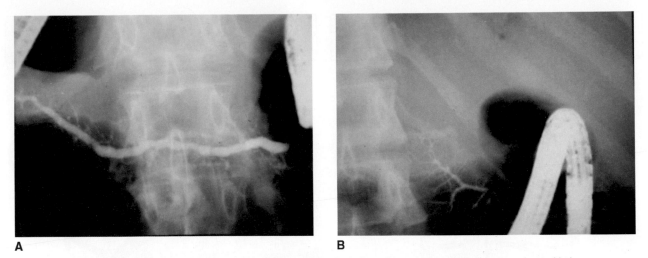

FIGURE 17-4. ERCP study demonstrating pancreas divisum. Both the major and minor ducts have been imaged independently. A, Major pancreatic duct. **B,** Minor pancreatic duct. (Reprinted with permission from Gold SB and Carey LC. Pancreas Divisum. In Cameron JL ed. *Current Surgical Therapy*, 8th ed. Philadelphia, PA: Elsevier Mosby, 2004:473.)

their resectability. Involvement of the celiac axis, superior mesenteric artery (SMA), portal vein, or superior mesenteric vein (SMV) by tumor usually precludes surgical resection.

Celiac Axis

The celiac artery, which is the largest branch of the abdominal aorta, supplies the embryological foregut. It courses from the aorta at a 90° between T12 and L1 just inferior to the diaphragm. Classically, the celiac artery trifurcates into the left gastric, splenic, and common hepatic arteries (Figure 17-5). Multiple common anatomic variations of this classic anatomy exist and involve both the celiac and SMA branches (Figure 17-6). An extensive collateral circulation exists between these vessels due to the importance of maintaining blood flow to the organs they perfuse. Figure 17-6 details the arterial and venous anatomy surrounding the pancreas. The left gastric artery, which lies within the lesser omentum, courses along the lesser curvature of the stomach to anastomose with the right gastric artery, which is a branch of the common hepatic artery. The common hepatic artery supplies a variable number of branches to the pancreas prior to the take off of the right gastric and then gastroduodenal artery (GDA). Following the GDA takeoff, the common hepatic artery becomes the proper hepatic artery, which subsequently divides into the right and left hepatic arteries. The proper hepatic artery usually supplies blood to the duodenum via a retroduodenal artery that courses with the common bile duct. Despite many variations, the right hepatic artery usually passes posterior to the common bile duct. The cystic artery originates from the right hepatic artery in approximately 75% of individuals. The right hepatic artery may be missing or lacking in approximately 20% of individuals, where the blood supply to the right lobe of the liver originates from the SMA. In this case, the artery supplying blood to the right side of the liver is called the "replaced right hepatic artery." If both a right hepatic artery and a supply vessel from the SMA are present, the latter vessel is termed a recurrent or accessory right hepatic artery. The right replaced or accessory vessels usually lie posteriorly, inferiorly, and laterally to the common bile duct and can be injured during pancreaticoduodenectomy or other procedures near the porta hepatis if care is not taken to assess their presence. A replaced left hepatic artery also exists in 20% of the population. A replaced left hepatic artery originates from the left gastric artery and supplies blood to the left side of the liver. This vessel runs with the hepatic branch of the vagus nerve through the lesser omentum. The right gastric artery, as mentioned, courses on the lesser curvature of the stomach to anastomose with the left gastric artery. The gastroduodenal artery courses posterior to the duodenum and anterior to the pancreas. It usually divides into the superior pancreaticoduodenal and right gastroepiploic arteries. The superior pancreaticoduodenal artery runs on the posterior surface of the head of the pancreas and supplies blood to both the duodenum and pancreas via branches that anastomose with vessels from the inferior pancreaticoduodenal artery coming from the SMA. The last branch of the celiac artery is the splenic artery that courses toward the spleen. It lies on the cephalad boarder of the pancreas and its largest branch is called the pancreatic magna (great pancreatic artery). Just before reaching the spleen, the splenic artery provides many short gastric branches to the stomach and the left gastroepiploic artery, which courses along the greater curvature of the stomach to anastomose with the right gastroepiploic artery.

Superior Mesenteric Artery

The SMA is the second largest intra-abdominal aortic branch and supplies blood to the entire embryological midgut. It arises

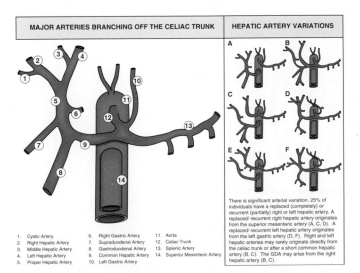

| MAJOR ARTERIES BRANCHING OFF THE CELIAC TRUNK | HEPATIC ARTERY VARIATIONS |

There is significant arterial variation. 25% of individuals have a replaced (completely) or recurrent (partially) right or left hepatic artery. A replaced/ recurrent right hepatic artery originates from the superior mesenteric artery (A, C, D). A replaced/ recurrent left hepatic artery originates from the left gastric artery (D, F). Right and left hepatic arteries may rarely originate directly from the celiac trunk or after a short common hepatic artery (B, C). The GDA may arise from the right hepatic artery (B, C).

1. Cystic Artery	6. Right Gastric Artery	11. Aorta
2. Right Hepatic Artery	7. Supraduodenal Artery	12. Celiac Trunk
3. Middle Hepatic Artery	8. Gastroduodenal Artery	13. Splenic Artery
4. Left Hepatic Artery	9. Common Hepatic Artery	14. Superior Mesenteric Artery
5. Proper Hepatic Artery	10. Left Gastric Artery	

FIGURE 17-5. Celiac artery and its variations. (Drawing by Matthew Campbell.)

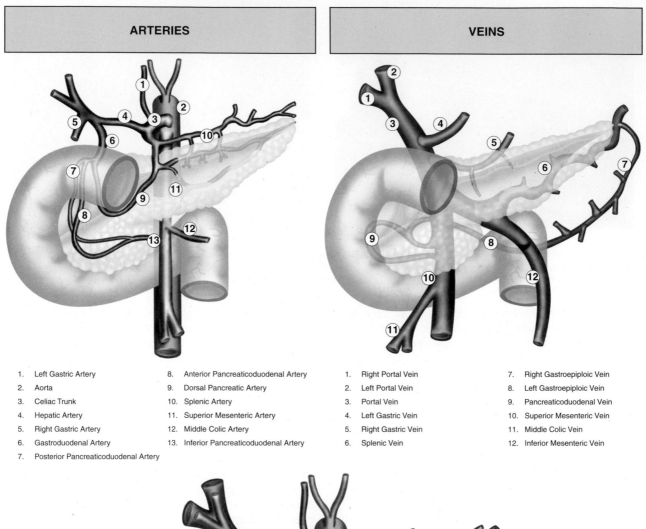

| ARTERIES | VEINS |

1.	Left Gastric Artery	8.	Anterior Pancreaticoduodenal Artery
2.	Aorta	9.	Dorsal Pancreatic Artery
3.	Celiac Trunk	10.	Splenic Artery
4.	Hepatic Artery	11.	Superior Mesenteric Artery
5.	Right Gastric Artery	12.	Middle Colic Artery
6.	Gastroduodenal Artery	13.	Inferior Pancreaticoduodenal Artery
7.	Posterior Pancreaticoduodenal Artery		

1.	Right Portal Vein	7.	Right Gastroepiploic Vein
2.	Left Portal Vein	8.	Left Gastroepiploic Vein
3.	Portal Vein	9.	Pancreaticoduodenal Vein
4.	Left Gastric Vein	10.	Superior Mesenteric Vein
5.	Right Gastric Vein	11.	Middle Colic Vein
6.	Splenic Vein	12.	Inferior Mesenteric Vein

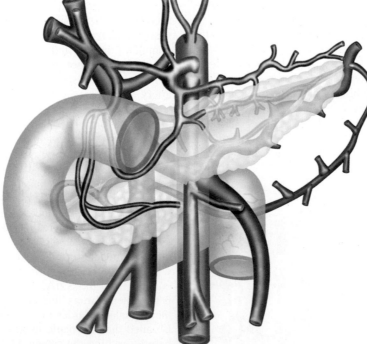

FIGURE 17-6. Arterial vascular arcades supplying the duodenum and pancreas. (Drawing by Matthew Campbell.)

from the aorta 0.5 to 1.5 cm caudal to the celiac artery and is directly posterior to the pancreas. Approximately 1% of individuals have a common SMA and celiac trunk. The SMA leaves the aorta at a 20° to 30° posterior to the body of the pancreas at L1. The artery passes inferiorly, just medial and anteriorly to a portion of the uncinate process where it gives off its first branch, the inferior pancreaticoduodenal artery. This vessel usually takes off from the right side of the SMA due to the relative lack of rotation of this portion of the vessel during development. The artery then passes in front of the third portion of the duodenum where it splits into the anterior and posterior branches that anastomose with pancreaticoduodenal branches of the superior pancreaticoduodenal artery previously described. After passing the duodenum, the SMA enters the root of the mesentery where it supplies the entire small bowel and right colon.

Celiac Axis—Superior Mesenteric Arterial Collaterals

Approximately 21% of individuals have a celiac artery stenosis over 50% at the time of death. Most of these patients are asymptomatic due to the rich collateral vascular supply. The most common collateral pathways involving the celiac artery and SMA surrounding the duodenum and pancreas are shown in Figure 17-6 and involve the pancreaticoduodenal vessels and the dorsal pancreatic artery. The anterior and posterior pancreaticoduodenal arcades are supplied by the gastroduodenal artery superiorly and the SMA inferiorly via its pancreaticoduodenal branches. The dorsal pancreatic artery may arise from a variety of sites including the splenic artery (39%), the right hepatic artery (12%), the SMA (14%), the celiac artery (22%), and elsewhere in 13%. This artery also interconnects celiac artery and SMA at multiple sites prior to dividing into two right and one left branch that also contribute to the pancreaticoduodenal arcades and communicate with caudal pancreatic vessels supplied by the splenic artery. A fourth branch of the dorsal pancreatic artery runs below the pancreas and communicates with the SMA. The collaterals in this region are often extensive and variable due to the large variety of hepatic arterial differences that exist. Not only do the celiac and SMA communicate via collateral circulation, but the inferior mesenteric artery also communicates with the SMA via other collaterals.

Venous Drainage

The venous drainage of the pancreas, duodenum, and spleen corresponds to the arterial supply. Again, recall that when anatomically discussing proximal and distal, the venous portion located closest to the draining organ is proximal, while the segment located more centrally is distal. The veins draining the pancreas lie immediately superficial to the arteries. For instance, the SMV is located anterior and lateral to the SMA. The anterior venous arcade usually drains into the superior mesenteric vein, while the posterior venous arcade usually drains into the portal vein (Figure 17-6). The portal vein is formed where the splenic and superior mesenteric veins fuse, which is posterior to the surgical neck of the pancreas and slightly medial to the common bile duct. The venous drainage of the body and tail of the gland is through branches that enter the splenic and the inferior pancreatic veins. The inferior mesenteric vein may join the portal system anywhere along splenic vein including the splenic–SMV junction. The left gastric vein (coronary vein) drains into the splenic vein or directly into the portal vein. What must be remembered is that all blood flow from the small and large bowel returns via the portal system, and injury to these venous structures may result in bowel infarction.

Innervation

The pancreas receives both sympathetic (greater splanchnic) and parasympathetic (vagus) innervation, which are important in the gland's endocrine functions. Pancreatic pain is also of significant importance and travels by afferent sensory nerve fibers. All innervation passes through the celiac or superior mesenteric ganglion. Pancreatic pain may result from neoplastic or inflammatory processes that may be due to obstruction of the pancreatic duct, a desmoplastic reaction that encompasses a tumor, or pancreatitis. Two major theories are thought to explain pain experienced by patients with pancreatitis, including increased intraductal or intraparenchymal pressures, and a neurogenic theory where immunologically activated cells or noxious substances irritate exposed nerve cells resulting in excruciating pain. Treatment of severe pain may involve blocking the afferent nerves by celiac plexus neurolysis, which may be done by alcohol or neurolytic injection. Neurolysis may be done percutaneously using CT, intraoperatively, or endoscopically using ultrasound.

PHYSIOLOGY

Exocrine

The pancreas plays a major role in digestion and secretes 500 to 800 mL/day of isotonic, alkaline fluid containing electrolytes and digestive enzymes. The sodium and potassium concentrations equal those in plasma. Chloride concentrations vary inversely with bicarbonate secretion, which is very important in digestion. An alkaline environment carries inactive digestive enzymes to the duodenum and neutralizes the acidic duodenal contents. The high bicarbonate concentration results in a fluid with a pH between 7.9 and 9.0 depending upon the stimulatory state of the gland. The major stimulus for bicarbonate production is a duodenal pH of <3, which results in the release of secretin from the duodenal mucosa. Cholecystokinin (CCK) also weakly stimulates bicarbonate production. The intraluminal digestion products including peptides, amino acids, and free fatty acids stimulate the release of CCK. CCK also plays a major role in digestion by stimulating contraction of the gallbladder so that bile mixes with pancreatic secretions and chyme to facilitate digestion and absorption. The nervous system also plays a permissive role in pancreatic secretion with truncal vagotomy and atropine both inhibiting bicarbonate secretion by decreasing cholinergic activity. Truncal vagotomy is commonly done in patients undergoing antiulcer procedures and esophagectomy, and it may also complicate antireflux procedures done at the gastroesophageal junction.

The pancreas also secretes three types of digestive enzymes including amylases, lipases, and proteases. Secretion is stimulated via neural and hormonal factors. CCK, acetylcholine, vasoactive intestinal polypeptide (VIP), and secretin stimulate enzyme secretion. Approximately 20 different digestive enzymes are secreted as inactive precursors (e.g., trypsin and chymotrypsin are secreted as trypsinogen and chymotrypsinogen) that are activated upon contact with the duodenal contents. Amylase is the *only* enzyme secreted in its active form, but it functions best at a pH of 7.0. The exocrine function of the pancreas can be tested in a variety of ways including the secretin test, fecal fat measurement, dimethadione test, Lundh test, triolein breath test, para-aminobenzoic acid test, and the test-meal pancreatic polypeptide tests.

Endocrine

The islets of Langerhans produce a variety of peptide hormones including insulin, glucagon, somatostatin, pancreatic polypeptide, VIP, galanin, serotonin, amylin, pancreastatin, and chromogranin A. Islets are 75 to 150 μm in diameter, make up 1.5% of the pancreas by weight, and are more abundant in the tail of the pancreas. The main endocrine role of islet cells is to control glucose homeostasis with a feedback mechanism that is based upon glucose levels. Alpha cells secrete glucagon in response to low glucose levels, which results in glycogenolysis and rising blood glucose levels. Beta cells constitute 60% of the islets and secrete insulin in response to increased serum glucose levels. Delta cells constitute a small proportion of the islet cells (5% to 10%) and secrete somatostatin, which is a strong inhibitor of pancreatic exocrine secretion. Endocrine function can be assessed using an oral or IV glucose tolerance tests, an intravenous arginine test, and the tolbutamide response test depending upon the specific disorder being evaluated.

PATHOPHYSIOLOGY

Acute Pancreatitis

Acute pancreatitis is a common disease that results from a malfunction in exocrine secretion. The disease ranges in severity from mild and self-limited to severe and life threatening. The Atlanta Classification defines acute pancreatitis as an acute inflammatory process of the pancreas with variable involvement of other regional tissues or remote organ systems. It is associated with elevated pancreatic enzyme levels in the blood and/or urine. The Atlanta Classification system introduces uniformity into the terminology and definition of various terms used to describe acute pancreatitis and its complications. The recommended nomenclature for describing pathologic processes is listed in Table 17-1 while Table 17-2 lists frequently used, but abandoned terms.

Acute pancreatitis is due to acinar cell injury, which allows activation of pancreatic enzymes outside of the pancreatic ducts and digestive tract. This results in the destruction of pancreatic and peripancreatic tissue. Grossly, the gland may be swollen, edematous, hemorrhagic, or even necrotic. Histologic changes range from interstitial edema and inflammation to hemorrhage and necrosis. Even when imaging fails to demonstrate necrosis, glandular destruction does occur on a microscopic level.

Etiology

Alcohol ingestion and biliary calculi account for 85% of cases with the more frequent cause being dictated by the social environment. Other etiologies of pancreatitis include metabolic,

TABLE 17-1	Summary of the 1992 Atlanta Classification
Term	**Definition**
Acute pancreatitis	An acute inflammatory process of the pancreas with variable involvement of other regional tissues or remote organ systems
	Associated with raised pancreatic enzyme levels in blood and/or urine
Severity	
Mild acute pancreatitis	Associated with minimal organ dysfunction and an uneventful recovery; lacks the features of severe acute pancreatitis. Usually, normal enhancement of the pancreatic parenchyma on contrast-enhanced computed tomography
Severe acute pancreatitis	Associated with organ failure and/or local complications such as necrosis, abscess, or pseudocyst
Predicted severity	Ranson score ≥3 or APACHE II score ≥8
Organ failure and systemic complications	
Shock	Systolic blood pressure <90 mm Hg
Pulmonary insufficiency	PaO$_2$ ≤60 mm Hg
Renal failure	Creatinine ≥177 μmol/L or ≤2 mg/dL after rehydration
Gastrointestinal bleeding	500 mL in 24 hr
Disseminated intravascular coagulation	Platelets ≤100,000/mm³, fibrinogen <1.0 g/L and fibrin-split products >80 μg/L
Severe metabolic disturbances	Calcium ≤ 1.87 mmol/l or ≤ 7.5 mg/dL
Local complications	
Acute fluid collections	Occur early in the course of acute pancreatitis, are located in or near the pancreas and always lack a wall of granulation of fibrous tissue. In about half of patients, spontaneous regression occurs. In the other half, an acute fluid collection develops into a pancreatic abscess or pseudocyst
Pancreatic necrosis	Diffuse or focal area(s) of nonviable pancreatic parenchyma typically associated with peripancreatic fat necrosis
	Nonenhanced pancreatic parenchyma >3 cm or involving more than 30% of the area of the pancreas
Acute pseudocyst	Collection of pancreatic juice enclosed by a wall of fibrous or granulation tissue, which arises as a result of acute pancreatitis, pancreatic trauma or chronic pancreatitis, occurring at least 4 weeks after the onset of symptoms, is round or ovoid and most often sterile; when pus is present, the lesion is termed a "pancreatic abscess"
Pancreatic abscess	Circumscribed, intra-abdominal collection of pus, usually in proximity to the pancreas, containing little or no pancreatic necrosis, which arises as a consequence of acute pancreatitis or pancreatic trauma
	Often 4 weeks or more after onset
	Pancreatic abscess and infected pancreatic necrosis differ in clinical expression and extent of associated necrosis

TABLE 17-2	Abandoned Terms
Phlegmon	
Infected pseudocyst	
Hemorrhagic pancreatitis	
Persistent acute pancreatitis	

mechanical, postoperative, traumatic, vascular, infectious, genetic, and autoimmune (Table 17-3). In patients with pancreatitis related to alcohol consumption, the first episode is usually preceded by 6 to 8 years of heavy alcohol ingestion. These patients often experience recurring acute attacks, which are frequently related to continued alcohol consumption. After multiple attacks of acute pancreatitis, the pancreatic ductal system becomes permanently damaged and leads to the development of **chronic pancreatitis**. Alcohol may contribute by causing secretions with a high protein content that precipitate and block small pancreatic ductules. The mechanism by which hyperlipidemia, hypercalcemia, and medications such as corticosteroids, thiazide diuretics, furosemide, estrogens, azathioprine, and dideoxyinosine promote the disease is unknown.

Mechanical causes of pancreatitis include anything that may obstruct the pancreatic duct. This includes gallstones, tumors, trauma, and parasitic diseases among others. Gallstones are the most common mechanical cause of pancreatitis and it is estimated that 60% of nonalcoholic patients with

TABLE 17-3	Etiologic Factors of Acute Pancreatitis
Metabolic	Alcohol, hyperlipidemia, hypertriglyceridemia, hypercalcemia (hyperparathyroidism), uremia, pregnancy, scorpion venom
Mechanical	Cholelithiasis, pancreas divisum, duct obstruction (ascaris, tumor, etc.), ERCP, ductal bleeding, duodenal obstruction, duct obstruction from scar secondary to prior episodes of pancreatitis, sphincter of Oddi dysfunction
Postoperative and traumatic	0.8%–17% gastric procedures, 0.7%–9.3% biliary procedures, direct pancreatic injury or trauma, injury to pancreatic blood supply, obstruction of the pancreatic duct at the duodenum, cardiopulmonary bypass (ischemia)
Vascular	Periarteritis nodosa, lupus erythematosus, atheroembolism
Infectious	Mumps, Coxsackie B virus, cytomegalovirus, *Cryptococcus*, *Enterovirus*, hepatitis A, B, or C, Epstein-Barr virus, herpes simplex virus, echovirus, *Ascaris* infestation
Hereditary— genetic	Hereditary form of autosomal dominant, cystic fibrosis, pancreas divisum, familial pancreatitis, tropical pancreatitis
Autoimmune	Autoimmune pancreatitis
Medications	Many medications may cause pancreatitis
Idiopathic	Unknown

pancreatitis have gallstones. How choledocholithiasis cause pancreatitis is not fully understood and may not be entirely due to reflux of bile into the pancreatic duct. Experimentally, at physiologic pressures, bile does not cause pancreatitis when introduced into the pancreatic duct. It may be that the mixing of bile and pancreatic juice leads to the formation of a highly toxic substance to the pancreas.

Ischemic injuries to the pancreas, secondary to hypotension (e.g., during open heart procedures performed on pump) or devascularization during upper abdominal surgery, may also initiate pancreatitis or play a role in the progression of pancreatic edema to pancreatic necrosis. Postoperative pancreatitis is seen after gastric surgery in as many as 15% of cases and after biliary tract surgery in 10% of cases. Pancreatitis following biliary tract procedures may result from trauma, especially in cases where the common duct has been instrumented. Acute pancreatitis is a complication in 1% of patients who undergo ERCP and may be due to an acute increase in intraductal pressure. Approximately 8% to 10% of cases of pancreatitis have no recognizable etiology (idiopathic pancreatitis), but the majority of these cases may be related to biliary tract sludge or microlithiasis. Therefore, cholecystectomy is recommended in this group.

Clinical Presentation and Evaluation
Patients with acute pancreatitis have noncrampy, epigastric abdominal pain. The character of the pain is variable, and it frequently radiates to the left or right upper quadrant or the back. The pain may be alleviated by sitting or standing. It is associated with nausea and vomiting. Physical examination is characterized by fever, tachycardia, and upper abdominal tenderness with guarding. Patients may develop an adynamic ileus with abdominal distention. Generalized abdominal and rebound tenderness may also occur in severe pancreatitis. In severe acute pancreatitis, blood may dissect into the posterior retroperitoneal soft tissue causing a flank hematoma known as Grey Turner's sign or up the falciform ligament resulting in a periumbilical ecchymosis called Cullen's sign.

Laboratory evaluation usually demonstrates a leukocytosis with an elevated serum amylase and lipase. An elevation of the serum amylase level 1.5 times the normal limit with a lipase value of 5 times the normal limit have a 95% sensitivity in confirming this diagnosis. Used individually, a serum amylase level three times normal has a 95% specificity, but a lowered sensitivity of 61%. The serum amylase rises quickly within the first 12 hours after admission and usually returns to normal after 3 to 5 days. The sensitivity and accuracy of the amylase and lipase levels for diagnostic purposes falls precipitously after several days, and in some patients, including those with end stage chronic pancreatitis, may not be elevated even on admission. Severe cases of pancreatitis can initiate a systemic inflammatory response syndrome (SIRS) with activation of inflammatory mediators (cytokines, lymphocytes, the complement cascade). This SIRS response may look like severe sepsis and cause injury to remote sites and other organs distinct from the pancreas. In severe cases of pancreatitis, there may be abnormal liver chemistries, hyperglycemia, hypocalcemia, elevated blood urea nitrogen (BUN) and creatinine levels, and hypoxemia as a result of injury to the liver, lungs, and kidneys.

The differential diagnosis of acute pancreatitis includes acute cholecystitis, perforated peptic ulcer, mesenteric ischemia, esophageal perforation, and myocardial infarction. Table 17-4 contains a list of possible etiologies of

TABLE 17-4	List of Disease Processes That May Result in Hyperamylasemia

Perforated ulcer	Ovarian tumor or cyst
Ischemic bowel	Lung cancer
Small bowel obstruction	Prostate cancer
Renal failure	Diabetic ketoacidosis
Salivary gland infection	Macroamylasemia
Ectopic pregnancy	

TABLE 17-5	Ranson's Criteria—Prognostic Factors for Major Complications or Death

	Nonbiliary	Biliary
On Admission		
Age	>55	>70
WBC count	>16	>18
Glucose	>200 mg/100 mL	>220 mg/100 mL
LDH	>350	>400
SGOT (AST)	>250	>250
During the Initial 48 Hours		
Hematocrit decrease	>10%	>10%
BUN increase	>5 mg/dL	>2 mg/dL
Calcium	<8 mg/dL	<8 mg/dL
Arterial pO$_2$	<60 mm Hg	—
Base deficit	>4 mEq/L	>5 mEq/L
Fluid sequestration	>6 L	>4 L

hyperamylasemia, which should be considered in the differential of any patient with an elevated amylase level. Patients with suspected acute pancreatitis should be evaluated radiographically with (1) a chest x-ray to look for sympathetic pleural effusions, atelectasis, or hemidiaphragm elevation (suggestive of fluid sequestration), and to exclude free air (pneumoperitoneum); (2) plain and upright abdominal x-rays to evaluate for possible calcifications (indicating chronic pancreatitis), gallstones (though only about 15% of gallstones are radioopaque), local adynamic ileus (or signs of bowel obstruction), or a "cutoff sign" where gas in the transverse colon appears to end abruptly; and (3) ultrasonography to look for gallstones, common duct dilatation, pancreatic enlargement, and peripancreatic fluid collections. Ultrasonography may be of limited value in obese patients or in patients with significant amounts of bowel gas overlying the pancreas.

In most cases, a computed tomography (CT) scan is useful to detect peripancreatic fluid, pancreatic edema, and pancreatic necrosis. Necrosis of the gland and the peripancreatic tissues is a common finding in patients with severe pancreatitis. Pancreatic tissue that does not enhance with IV contrast is interpreted to be devoid of blood flow and thus necrotic. Pancreatic necrosis, however, is not an indication for surgical intervention and most patients with necrosis without infection recover without surgery. Other methods for predicting the presence of pancreatic necrosis include utilization of Ranson's criteria, which are discussed in the next section. Thus, it is possible to predict on admission which patients will develop pancreatic necrosis without subjecting patients to the undesirable consequences of IV contrast including renal dysfunction. Therefore, initial evaluation by CT scans with oral and without IV contrast is recommended when the diagnosis of pancreatitis is certain. When the diagnosis is unclear, a CT scan takes on a larger role in diagnosis and IV contrast may be recommended depending upon the clinical situation. Other imaging modalities including magnetic resonance cholangiopancreatography (MRCP) may benefit selected cases by noninvasively visualizing the bile duct and pancreas.

Prognosis

The patient outcome following an episode of acute pancreatitis is directly related to the severity of the attack. Eighty percent of patients recover from the attack without sequelae, while twenty percent experience complications. The Atlanta Classification discussed previously has introduced uniformity to the description, nomenclature, and definitions regarding acute pancreatitis and its complications. Grading systems for the severity of pancreatitis are used to predict the risk for complications. Ranson developed one of the first grading systems for

pancreatitis, which relies upon readily measured laboratory and clinical variables (**Ranson's criteria**) (Table 17-5). Five variables are measured on admission, and six additional variables are measured over the ensuing 48 hours. The presence of three or more criteria indicates severe pancreatitis and is associated with an increased incidence of local and systemic complications. Clinically, this is very useful, since it predicts which patients may become extremely ill or develop pancreatic necrosis or complications. It should also be emphasized that neither the serum amylase or lipase are included in Ranson's criteria, and hence neither is reflective of the severity of the attack or the likelihood of developing complications, but they are markers of acinar cell damage.

Another prognostic index is the Acute Physiology and Chronic Health Evaluation II (APACHE II) score (Table 17-6). Although this was first used to stratify intensive care unit patients, the scoring system is useful in assessing patients with acute pancreatitis. The APACHE II scoring system is not as simple and straightforward to use as is Ranson's criteria, but also relies upon readily obtainable variables. Numeric scores are assigned to physiologic measurements, age, and preexisting organ insufficiencies to provide a score that reflects the severity of the disease. Patients with APACHE II scores of 8 or greater are considered to have severe acute pancreatitis. The main advantage of the APACHE II system is that a score can be derived at any time during the patient's hospital course, while Ranson's criteria are only prognostic during the initial 48 hours.

Finally, CT scans also yield prognostic information. Emil J. Balthazar et al. developed a grading system based upon CT findings seen in Table 17-7. The severity of the attack was directly related to the development of pancreatic fluid collections. This grading system is easy and fast to use, does not require IV contrast, and helps predict which patients (Group D or E) are at risk for developing significant morbidity. Its main drawback is that pancreatic necrosis is not evaluated, but this does not have significant clinical treatment implications on admission.

TABLE 17-6	Acute Physiological Assessment and Chronic Health Evaluation (APACHE) II Scoring System[a]								

					Point Score				
Physiologic Variable[b]	+4	+3	+2	+1	0	+1	+2	+3	+4
1. Temperature, core (°C)	≥41°	39°–40.9°	—	38.5°–38.9°	36°–38.4°	34°–35.9°	32°–33.9°	30°–31.9°	≤29.9°
2. Mean arterial pressure (mm Hg)	≥160	130–159	110–129	—	70–109	—	50–69	—	≤49
3. Heart rate	≥180	140–179	110–139	—	70–109	—	55–69	40–54	≤39
4. Respiratory rate (nonventilated or ventilated)	≥50	35–49	—	25–34	12–24	10–11	6–9	—	≤5
5. Oxygenation									
(a) FIO$_2$ ≥ 0.5: use A-a DO$_2$	≥500	350–499	200–349	—	<200	—	—	—	—
(b) FIO$_2$ < 0.5: use PaO$_2$ (mm Hg)	—	—	—	—	>70	61–70	—	55–60	<55
6. Arterial pH	≥7.7	7.6–7.69	—	7.5–7.59	7.33–7.49	—	7.25–7.32	7.15–7.24	<7.15
7. Serum Na (mmol/L)	≥180	160–179	155–159	150–154	130–149	—	120–129	111–119	≤110
8. Serum I (mmol/L)	≥7	6–6.9	—	5.5–5.9	3.5–5.4	3–3.4	2.5–2.9	—	<2.5
9. Serum creatinine (mg/dL); double point score for **acute** renal failure	≥3.5	2–3.4	1.5–1.9	—	0.6–1.4	—	<0.6	—	—
10. Hct (%)	≥60	—	50–59.9	46–49.9	30–45.9	—	20–29.9	—	<20
11. WBC (in 1,000s)	≥40	—	20–39.9	15–19.9	3–14.9	—	1–2.9	—	<1
12. Glasgow coma score	Score = 15 – actual GCS								

Acute physiology score is the sum of the 12 individual variable points.

Add 0 points for age <44; 2 points for 45–54 yr; 3 points, 55–64 yr; 5 points, 65–74 yr; 6 points ≥75 yr.

Add chronic health status points: 2 points if elective postoperative patient with immunocompromise or history of severe organ insufficiency; 5 points for nonoperative patient or emergency postoperative patient with immunocompromise or severe organ insufficiency.[c]

13.[d] Serum HCO$_3$ (venous-mmol/L)	≥52	41–51.9	—	32–40.9	22–31.9	—	18–21.9	15–17.9	<15

[a]APACHE II score = acute physiology score + age points + chronic health points. Minimum score = 0; maximum score = 71. Increasing score is associated with increasing risk of hospital death.
[b]Choose worst value in past 24 h.
[c]Chronic health status: Organ insufficiency (e.g., hepatic, cardiovascular, renal, pulmonary) or immunocompromised state must have preceded current admission.
[d]Optional variable; use only if no ABGs.
A-a DO$_2$ = Alveolar-arterial oxygen gradient; FIO$_2$ = fractional inspired O$_2$.
Table printed with permission from Wolters Kluwer Health. Adapted from Knaus WA, Draper EA, Wagner DP, Zimmerman JE: APACHE II: A severity of disease classification system. Crit Care Med. 1985;13:818–829.

Treatment

Medical

Medical therapy for acute pancreatitis can be divided into general supportive therapy including preventing complications such as deep vein thrombosis or peptic ulceration, and the specific treatment of pancreatic inflammation or its complications. In patients with mild bouts of pancreatitis, it is appropriate to withhold food until pain and tenderness resolve and the serum amylase and WBC return to normal. This approach is sensible, since pancreatitis damages the pancreatic parenchyma and/or pancreatic ductal system with the resultant spillage of pancreatic enzymes into areas of the pancreatic gland or abdominal cavity. An elevated amylase level is an indication of continuing leakage of cellular or ductal contents. Stimulation of pancreatic secretion may increase leakage of pancreatic enzymes from the disrupted glandular tissue or ducts resulting in progressive tissue destruction. Thus, efforts to slow pancreatic secretion should be made which include withholding oral feeding.

Following more severe episodes of pancreatitis, it is important to maintain adequate tissue perfusion by monitoring cardiovascular parameters and maintaining adequate intravascular volume. Massive fluid sequestrations can occur in the retroperitoneum due to the inflammatory process, and in severe cases, resuscitation with several liters of isotonic solution may be required. Fluid management is aided by use of a urinary catheter, central venous line, or possibly a pulmonary artery catheter. Electrolytes and blood glucose are carefully managed.

TABLE 17-7	CT Grading System for Acute Pancreatitis

Grade	CT Finding
A	Normal Pancreas
B	Pancreatic enlargement
C	Pancreatic inflammation and/or peripancreatic fat
D	Single peripancreatic fluid collection
E	Two or more fluid collections and/or retroperitoneal air

Respiratory function is monitored carefully, as sympathetic pleural effusions, atelectasis, adult respiratory distress syndrome due to SIRS, hemidiaphragm elevation, and fluid overload may impair oxygenation. Oxygenation is monitored with pulse oximetry or arterial blood gas measurements if necessary. Intubation and aggressive ventilatory support are sometimes required.

Specific inhibition of pancreatic secretion has been attempted with a variety of pharmacologic and mechanical methods. Nasogastric suction has been theorized to decrease secretin release. Practically, however, no obvious clinical benefit is seen in patients without significant nausea, vomiting, or abdominal distention where its use might decrease the risk of aspiration. All pharmacologic attempts at decreasing pancreatic secretion including anticholinergics, somatostatin analogues, inhibitors of the inflammatory cascade, specific enzyme inhibitors (e.g., aprotinin—a proteolytic enzyme inhibitor), and antacids have not demonstrated any significant benefit. Antibiotics have also been used prophylactically in patients with pancreatitis to prevent infection of necrotic material, which is the number one predictor of survival. Prophylactic antibiotics do not have a role in mild or moderate disease since necrosis does not occur. Unfortunately, however, prophylactic antibiotic use in severe disease (more than three of Ranson's criteria) does not alter mortality, but does prolong the time from presentation to infection and alters the resistance spectrum of the infecting pathogens. Antibiotics are important once infection is identified.

Nutritional support must also be provided to malnourished patients and to patients with severe disease who may not eat for a prolonged period. A nasal jejunal feeding tube should be placed and the gastrointestinal tract utilized as the primary mode of nutrition. Tube feeds given distal to the ligament of Treitz do not stimulate pancreatic secretion and should not exacerbate the attack. Total parenteral nutrition may be required in patients without a functional gastrointestinal tract.

Surgical

Surgical indications for acute pancreatitis fall into several categories. The first includes those patients with diagnostic uncertainty. The second indication for surgery includes procedures to prevent further episodes of pancreatitis. Lastly, surgical intervention is frequently undertaken for a variety of complications that may occur. These categories will be discussed below.

First, diagnostic uncertainty may mandate celiotomy (laparotomy) to establish the correct diagnosis and rule out other pathology. As mentioned, other acute surgical conditions can raise serum amylase levels and include a perforated ulcer, gangrenous cholecystitis, or ischemic or infarcted bowel. These conditions often require surgical intervention, but early operative intervention in patients with pancreatic necrosis is directly related to the chance of developing infected pancreatic necrosis and should be avoided if possible.

Second, surgery may be undertaken to prevent further attacks of acute pancreatitis. Patients with mild or moderate pancreatitis due to cholelithiasis should undergo cholecystectomy during the current admission. If imaging or laboratory values are suggestive of choledocholithiasis, an ERCP with sphincterotomy and stone extraction should be done preoperatively to clear the common bile duct. Cholecystectomy, where cholelithiasis is responsible for pancreatitis, reduces the risk of developing another bout of pancreatitis from approximately 50% to around 5%, but does not affect, alter, or augment the attack of pancreatitis, which must run its course.

In patients with severe gallstone pancreatitis, early cholecystectomy should not be done due to the significant morbidity of this procedure in this population. In patients with severe pancreatitis and a gallstone impacted at the ampulla of Vater, ERCP with sphincterotomy and stone extraction is advisable. These patients should then be allowed to recover prior to cholecystectomy. Lastly, the surgical indications for complications will be discussed below.

Complications

Acute pancreatitis may be associated with a variety of complications including those previously discussed such as electrolyte abnormalities, hyperglycemia, hypocalcemia, and a SIRS response, which may affect the renal, gastrointestinal, and respiratory systems. Long-term complications may also effect exocrine function and require pancreatic enzyme replacement. Other complications include coagulopathy and hemorrhage, which are treated by clotting factor replacement, endoscopic procedures, or angiographic embolization. Surgery should be avoided, if possible, due to the inaccessibility of the bleeding vessels and the risk of infecting sterile necrotic collections. Another complication includes common bile duct obstruction due to compression by a fluid collection or intrinsic fibrosis within the head of the pancreas due to pancreatitis. Treatment involves surgical drainage of the fluid collection and a possible biliary bypass via either Roux-en-Y hepaticojejunostomy or choledochoduodenostomy. Gastric outlet obstruction may also occur due to duodenal edema or a mass effect from a fluid collection pushing on the duodenum. Gastric outlet obstruction is treated by nasogastric decompression, fluid and electrolyte repletion, and possible surgical intervention to drain a compressing fluid collection. Another common complication of severe pancreatitis is splenic and/or portal vein thrombosis due to inflammation and edema in the pancreatic head, body, or tail. This may result in sinistral portal hypertension (left-sided portal hypertension) with the formation of large gastric varices that may hemorrhage. Treatment for bleeding gastric varices resulting from sinistral portal hypertension is splenectomy. The most common complications including peripancreatic fluid collections, pseudocysts, and infected pancreatic necrosis are discussed below.

Infected Pancreatic Necrosis

Infected pancreatic necrosis is the number one determinant of mortality, which may be over 40%. The risk of infection is directly related to the extent of necrosis. Infection is almost never present upon presentation and usually occurs after 2 to 3 weeks. When infection occurs, worsening organ dysfunction is usually seen. A CT scan demonstrating edema surrounding the pancreas is shown in Figure 17-7A. Approximately 1 month later, a repeat CT scan demonstrating retroperitoneal air or air within the lesser sac is seen in Figure 17-7B. This retroperitoneal air is diagnostic of infected pancreatic necrosis. Infection by some organisms, however, does not produce air in the retroperitoneum. If the suspicion for infection is high and the patient is deteriorating, a CT-guided needle aspiration of the fluid collection may be appropriate. Fluid obtained should be sent for Gram stain and culture with specific cultures also being sent for yeast. Prior prophylactic use of antibiotics may have substantially affected the organism resistance spectrum. If infection is identified, operative debridement, large-scale drainage, antibiotics, and supportive care are required. Multiple operative procedures may be needed to remove the infected

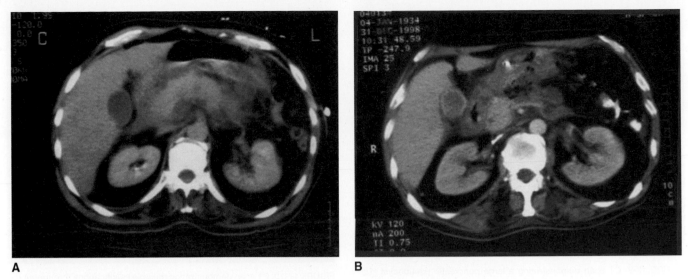

FIGURE 17-7. A, CT scan demonstrating edema and inflammation surrounding the majority of the pancreas. **B,** CT scan after 30 days in the same patient shown above. Air is present within the lesser sac signifying infected pancreatic necrosis.

debris without damaging adjacent structures. Over time, adherent infected necrotic tissue can be removed and large drainage catheters placed to control the expected pancreatic leak. Percutaneous drainage of these infected regions usually fails due to the volume of material that needs to be evacuated as well as the thick rubbery consistency of the material that will not exit through small drains. Examples of tissue removed during pancreatic necrosectomies are shown in Figure 17-8A, B. A pancreatic abscess is different than infected pancreatic necrosis with an abscess being a discrete collection of pus adjacent to the pancreas without underlying necrosis. It is much less common than infected pancreatic necrosis. Treatment is similar to other intra-abdominal abscess and includes external drainage, which can be accomplished by operation or occasionally percutaneously.

Peripancreatic Fluid Collections and Pseudocysts

The most common complication of pancreatitis is the development of a fluid collection in the peripancreatic area or, in more severe cases, at distant locations in the retroperitoneum.

This complication is caused by disruption of the pancreatic duct. Enzymatic fluid collects around the pancreas and is walled-off by surrounding viscera. Patients with peripancreatic fluid collections are at risk of developing complications specific to the collection, therefore these patients should be followed closely with serial imaging studies. Most acute fluid collections resolve spontaneously, but those that persist become **pseudocysts.** A pseudocyst is a collection of peripancreatic fluid contained in a cyst-like structure without an epithelial lining. Pseudocysts may be communicating or noncommunicating, based upon whether the cyst is connected to the pancreatic duct. The wall of the nonresolving fluid collections thickens or matures over 4 to 6 weeks and forms a pseudocyst. This maturation process is required for surgical intervention if external drains are to be avoided. Pseudocysts may grow to large sizes and commonly cause symptoms of epigastric pain, nausea, vomiting, and early satiety. Many of the symptoms are related to compression of adjacent structures including mechanical obstruction of the stomach, duodenum, or common bile duct.

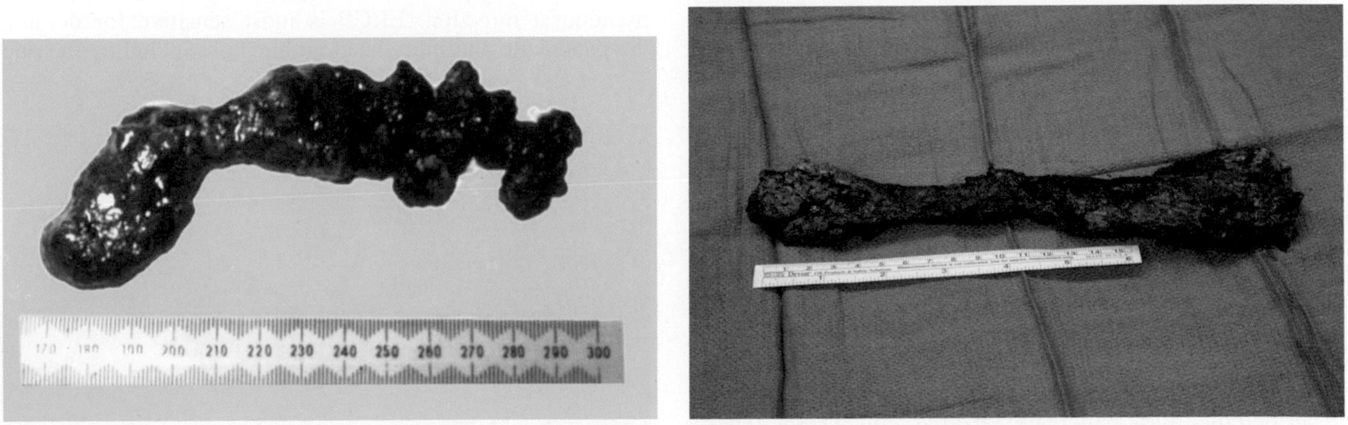

FIGURE 17-8. A, Necrosectomy specimen obtained from the patient with the CT scans shown in Figure 17-7A. The specimen is semisolid with a consistency of cookie dough. Calcified regions are visible from saponification. **B,** Necrosectomy specimen obtained from the pseudocyst shown in Figure 17-9. Pathology demonstrated hemorrhagic necrosis. The specimen is solid with a consistency of material removed from a clogged bathroom drain.

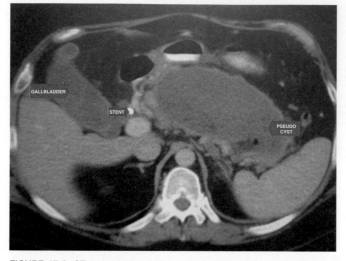

FIGURE 17-9. CT scan demonstrating a large pancreatic pseudocyst. The wall of the pseudocyst is enhancing and thickened. An endostent is also present within the common bile duct due to a stricture that formed in the bile duct due to the episode of pancreatitis.

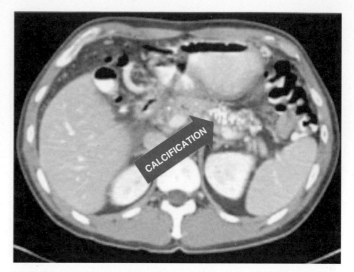

FIGURE 17-10. CT scan demonstrating multiple calcifications throughout the body and tail consistent with chronic pancreatitis.

CT scans are the best imaging studies for pseudocyst evaluation (Figure 17-9). CT scans allow delineation of the cyst walls and their relation to the surrounding structures. This is critically important when planning surgery to address the pseudocyst. Mature pseudocysts may be treated in a variety of manners. Noncommunicating pseudocysts may be aspirated or drained percutaneously. Communicating pseudocysts require internal drainage into the stomach, duodenum, or Roux limb to prevent formation of a pancreatic fistula, since they communicate directly with the pancreatic duct. Internal drainage is accomplished by sewing the cyst wall directly to the stomach or other recipient drainage organ. During the procedure, a portion of cyst wall should be sent to pathology for frozen section evaluation to ensure that the cyst is not a neoplasm. Internal drainage is successful in over 90% of cases.

Chronic Pancreatitis

Etiology

Alcohol consumption is related to approximately 70% of cases of chronic pancreatitis. The incidence of chronic pancreatitis ranges between 5 and 10 new cases per 100,000 population, with a prevalence of 25 cases per 100,000 people. It differs from acute pancreatitis in that the glandular damage is no longer reversible and, in fact, is usually progressive. Each recurring episode of pancreatitis contributes to the formation of a scarred, fibrotic gland with an abnormal ductal system that drains poorly and is easily clogged with debris, which may be related to abnormalities in protein and calcium secretion. When 90% of the gland has been damaged or replaced with scar, endocrine and exocrine insufficiencies occur and are manifested by diabetes and steatorrhea. Steatorrhea may be ascertained by a careful history of foul-smelling light-colored stool that floats with an oily layer seen on the surface of the toilet bowl water. Steatorrhea may be quantified by measuring fecal fat after a prescribed diet. Oral pancreatic enzyme replacement generally aids in treating steatorrhea. Diabetes is best treated with insulin, and for an unknown reason, these patients do not seem as vulnerable to small vessel disease in other organs as other diabetic patients.

Clinical Presentation and Evaluation

The most common symptom of chronic pancreatitis is pain. The pain is usually dull, epigastric in location, and radiates to the back. The pain is initially intermittent, but with progression of disease, becomes constant and unrelenting. In some, pain may be improved by leaning forward and aggravated by the supine position. Food often makes pain worse. Self-medication of pain by increased alcohol ingestion and/or narcotic use with drug dependency is common. Malnutrition and fat-soluble vitamin deficiencies due to malabsorption secondary to exocrine insufficiency and steatorrhea are frequently seen.

Patients with chronic pancreatitis should undergo a variety of imaging studies, depending upon the clinical situation. If the etiology of the disease is not understood, CT, MRCP, and ERCP may play a role in determining other non–alcohol-related causes. CT may show glandular enlargement or atrophy, inflammation, tumors, fluid collections or pseudocysts, pancreatic ductal dilation, or calcifications (Figure 17-10). The liver, gallbladder, and bile ducts are also visualized. MRCP and ERCP may identify pancreas divisum (Figure 17-11), obstructing pancreatic duct stones, or pancreatic ductal strictures. ERCP is an invasive test and carries a small risk of exacerbating pancreatitis, biliary or pancreatic sepsis, or pseudocyst infection. ERCP is most sensitive for defining the pancreatic and bile ductal architecture including the duct

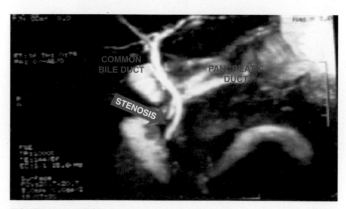

FIGURE 17-11. MRCP demonstrating stenosis of the minor duct and a dilated main pancreatic duct.

size and whether there are strictures, fistulas, or obstruction. Ultrasound is significantly less sensitive in evaluating the pancreas than these other modalities. When the etiology of the chronic disease is understood, imaging is useful for following the progression of the disease and identifies those that would benefit from surgical intervention or those that develop new complications of the disease.

Treatment

Medical treatment for chronic pancreatitis includes treatment of alcoholism, narcotic dependence, and a low-fat diabetic diet with pancreatic enzyme replacement to minimize steatorrhea and hyperglycemia. Medical treatment is the mainstay for patients with chronic pancreatitis, but rarely resolves the pain. Surgery is indicated in various scenarios and includes treatment of some with chronic pain as well as other complications of the disease that have discrete anatomic abnormalities that are potentially related to the pain or to recurrent bouts of acute pancreatitis. Preoperative imaging with CT, ERCP, or MRCP is useful for identifying pancreatic ductal obstructions, strictures, calculi, masses, duct ectasia, pseudocysts, and the surrounding vascular anatomy. CT and MRCP are noninvasive tests, but usually do not show sufficient detail to plan operative intervention. ERCP, although invasive and of some risk, is frequently required when planning surgical intervention and may be therapeutic if ductal stones causing obstruction are identified and removed.

Surgical options for treating chronic pancreatitis fall into two main categories, which include drainage or resectional procedures. Drainage procedures work best on those with a dilated pancreatic duct while resectional procedures are used in patients with nondilated ducts and disease that can be localized to a specific location within the gland. The benefit of drainage procedures includes maximizing the remaining pancreatic tissue and delaying the onset of both exocrine and endocrine insufficiency. Patients with dilated ducts including those with segmental ductal obstructions or dilated ducts that alternate with areas of stricture ("chain of lakes") can undergo ductal decompression into a loop of jejunum, which is called a lateral pancreaticojejunostomy, modified Puestow or Partington-Rochelle procedure. This drainage procedure results in approximately 70% of patients achieving lasting pain relief. Resectional procedures include pancreaticoduodenectomy, distal pancreatectomy, and duodenal-preserving pancreatic head resections (Beger or Frey procedures). When the ductal system is not dilated and no focal disease is identified, total pancreatectomy has been utilized, but is not recommended due to the severe exocrine and endocrine dysfunction that follows and the failure to reliably relieve pain. Pain relief in this group may be attempted via splanchnicectomy (neurolysis), which can be done percutaneously, endoscopically, or surgically, but results have been disappointing without good long-term durability. Other surgical interventions for chronic pancreatitis include those required to treat various complications including biliary strictures and pseudocysts 5 cm or larger that fail to resolve spontaneously.

Pancreatic Neoplasms (Excluding Neuroendocrine Tumors)

General Considerations

Pancreatic neoplasms may be malignant, premalignant, or benign. Malignant neoplasms include pancreatic adenocarcinoma, cystadenocarcinoma, most neuroendocrine

TABLE 17-8	Pancreatic Neoplasms Excluding Neuroendocrine Tumors of the Pancreas
Malignant	
Adenocarcinoma	
Adenosquamous carcinoma	
Mucinous cystadenocarcinoma	
Mucinous noncystic carcinoma	
Acinar cell carcinoma	
Signet ring carcinoma	
Osteoclast-like giant cell tumor	
Pancreaticoblastoma	
Undifferentiated carcinoma	
Lymphoma	
Metastatic disease	
Premalignant	
Mucinous adenoma	
Mucinous cystic neoplasm	
Mixed seromucinous adenoma	
Intraductal papillary mucinous neoplasm (IPMN)	
Solid pseudopapillary neoplasm (Hamoudi tumor)	
Benign Neoplasms	
Serous cystadenoma (microcystic adenoma)	
Pseudocyst	
Simple cyst	
Dermoid cyst	
Teratoma (mature)	

(islet cell) tumors, lymphomas, and other rare neoplasms shown in Tables 17-8 and 17-9. Premalignant lesions include intraductal papillary mucinous neoplasms, mucinous neoplasms, papillary-cystic neoplasms, and most nonmalignant lesions. Benign neoplasms include pancreatic pseudocysts, simple cysts, serous (microcystic) neoplasms, and most insulinomas. Pseudocysts are often recognizable by careful history taking and imaging features. When pseudocysts are removed from the group, benign neoplasms become significantly less

TABLE 17-9	Pancreatic Neuroendocrine Tumors
Benign (majority)	
Insulinoma	
Malignant (majority)	
Gastrinoma	
Glucagonoma	
Somatostatinoma	
VIPoma	
PPoma (pancreatic polypeptide)	
Nonfunctional islet cell	

common than malignant or premalignant tumors and diagnostic uncertainty often results in surgical treatment.

Pancreatic adenocarcinoma is responsible for approximately 6% of all cancer deaths making it the fourth most common cause of cancer death in the United States. In 2009, it is estimated that over 42,470 new cases will be diagnosed and 35,240 deaths will be attributable to this disease in the United States. Approximately 98% of patients diagnosed with pancreatic adenocarcinoma die from their disease despite multimodality treatment. The male:female ratio is between 1.1 and 2.0, but no clear link between female hormones and a protective effect on pancreatic adenocarcinoma has been demonstrated. The lifetime risk of developing pancreatic cancer is approximately 1 in 76 (1.31%), with the principal risk factors being increasing age and cigarette smoking that doubles the risk of developing pancreatic cancer. The etiologic roles of diabetes, pancreatitis, and alcohol in pancreatic carcinoma are controversial. Two thirds of the cases of pancreatic carcinoma occur in the head of the gland but they may also be multicentric. Over 90% of pancreatic cancers are adenocarcinomas that originate from the ductal epithelium, with the remainder being islet cell tumors, lymphomas, and metastatic lesions. Treatment includes resection for all neoplasms except lymphomas and serous cysts irrespective of size.

Genetic Mutations Associated with Pancreatic Cancer

Pancreatic cancer has been associated with three main genetic abnormalities: (1) oncogene activation, (2) tumor suppressor gene inactivation, and (3) overexpression of growth factors or their receptors (Table 17-10).

The most commonly expressed genetic mutation in malignant pancreatic neoplasms occurs in the **K-ras** (Kirsten rat sarcoma) oncogene and at least 75% of pancreatic carcinomas harbor this mutation. The *ras* gene encodes a GTP-binding protein that is involved in growth signal transduction and when mutated, aids in transforming cells. Tumor suppressor genes are also involved in pancreatic cancer and are listed in Table 17-10.

It is now generally believed that pancreatic cancer evolves in a progressive, stepwise fashion, much like that observed for colon cancer. Precursor ductal lesions have been identified, and the stepwise progression toward invasive cancer and metastasis has been related to the accumulated presence of multiple genetic abnormalities. K-*ras* mutations and

HER2/neu overexpression are the earliest changes to occur. Alterations in p16 are found primarily in Pancreatic Intraepithelial Neoplasia-2 (PanIN-2) and PanIN-3. DPC4, BRCA2, and p53 are inactivated during the later stages of cancer progression and are found almost exclusively in invasive lesions.

Pancreatic cancer has been observed to be increased in families with hereditary nonpolyposis colon cancer (HNPCC), familial breast cancer (associated with the BRCA2 mutation), Peutz-Jeghers syndrome, ataxia-telangiectasia, and those with the familial atypical multiple mole melanoma (FAMMM) syndromes. The most important gene in hereditary pancreatic cancer is BRCA2, which accounts for approximately 10% of such cases in Ashkenazi Jews. Patients with hereditary pancreatitis are also at increased risk for developing pancreatic cancer. This is particularly true in those people with a paternal pattern of inheritance who have up to a 75% risk for developing pancreatic cancer. Even in the absence of a familial cancer syndrome or hereditary pancreatitis, individuals with a family history of pancreatic cancer, especially those with two or more pancreatic cancer–affected first-degree relatives, have an increased risk for developing pancreatic cancer.

Clinical Presentation and Evaluation

The signs and symptoms of pancreatic carcinoma relate to the location of the tumor and the tumors effects on local structures. Periampullary tumors often present early with painless jaundice. Most patients have a combination of weight loss, jaundice, and pain as a result of infiltration of the tumor into the peripancreatic region including retroperitoneal nerves carried through the celiac plexus. Invasion of these nerves by tumor often results in pain that is constant, posterior, and epigastric in distribution with radiation to the back as opposed to the intermittent colicky pain that is usually associated with biliary tract disease. A palpable nontender gallbladder associated with painless jaundice is more commonly associated with malignancy (**Courvoisier's sign**), while cholecystitis or obstructive jaundice due to choledocholithiasis is typically painful and associated with tenderness on examination.

The evaluation of jaundiced patients includes serum chemistries. Markedly elevated transaminases (AST, ALT near 1000) are suggestive of hepatitis. Elevation of the total and direct bilirubin, alkaline phosphatase and γ-GGT are suggestive of obstructive jaundice. Transaminases may be mildly elevated into the low hundreds. Liver function studies suggesting obstructive jaundice demand further imaging studies that should begin with ultrasonography. Ultrasound is useful in diagnosing a dilated or obstructed biliary ductal system, liver lesions, cholelithiasis, choledocholithiasis, cholecystitis, and in some cases pancreatic neoplasms. In patients with a history and physical findings suggestive of a pancreatic neoplasm, CT may be a more informative initial diagnostic test. CT provides information about the level of the biliary tract obstruction, delineates the mass and its relation to vital structures, and identifies liver metastases. A high-quality, contrast-enhanced CT scan is required to preoperatively stage the lesion and to determine tumor resectability as defined by the absence of distant spread of disease, ascites, and lack of involvement of the SMV, portal vein (PV), SMA, hepatic artery, vena cava, or aorta. Figure 17-12A shows a normal CT scan of the SMV and SMA, vena cava and aorta. Figure 17-12B shows a CT scan demonstrating an unresectable pancreatic mass involving the SMV–PV junction as seen by contrast ending abruptly in the splenic vein at the pancreatic mass. Endoscopic

TABLE 17-10	Genetic Mutations Associated with Pancreatic Cancer
Type of Mutation	**Name of Gene or Growth Factor**
Oncogenes	K-*ras* (Kirsten rat sarcoma)
Tumor suppressor genes	p53
	p16
	SMAD4/DPC
	DCC (Deleted in Colorectal Carcinoma)
	APC (Adenomatous Polyposis Coli)
	DNA mismatch repair
	Retinoblastoma gene (RB)
Growth factors	EGF receptor
	HER2, HER3, and HER4 receptors

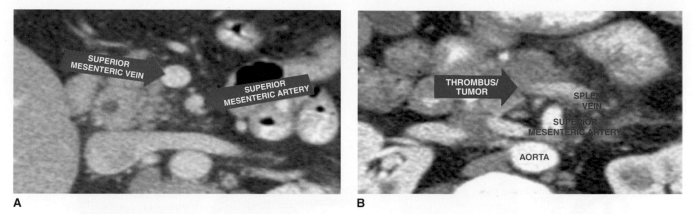

FIGURE 17-12. A, CT scan demonstrating a patent portal and SMV. Neither the SMA nor vein is encroached upon by tumor. **B,** CT scan of an unresectable pancreatic mass secondary to portal-SMV replacement by tumor. An endostent is present in the common bile duct.

ultrasound (EUS) is the newest modality for evaluating pancreatic lesions. Its sensitivity and specificity are similar to that of CT in evaluating the mass and adjacent vasculature. It is not useful for evaluating liver metastases. EUS, unlike CT, however, is invasive and highly operator dependent. MRCP, ERCP, and percutaneous transhepatic cholangiography (PTC) can also delineate biliary and pancreatic ductal anatomy. Palliative drainage of the biliary tract to address symptoms due to hyperbilirubinemia can also be achieved endoscopically or transhepatically in unresectable cases, but preoperative drainage of the biliary system is not routinely indicated when imaging studies suggest a resectable pancreatic tumor. Likewise, biopsy of a pancreatic mass in resectable cases is not indicated due to a high false negative rate and difficulty in establishing the diagnosis. Biopsy and tissue diagnosis are important if neoadjuvant or palliative chemotherapy or radiation therapy is to be undertaken and may be obtained by percutaneous CT- or EUS-guided methods. The diagnostic algorithm for evaluation of a pancreatic neoplasm is shown in Figure 17-13.

Treatment

Obstructive jaundice may result in vitamin K–related coagulopathy due to interruption of the enterohepatic circulation and

malnutrition, which should be corrected. Baseline laboratory studies to evaluate hepatic function and nutritional status include albumin, transferrin, prealbumin, and the prothrombin time. Patients with preoperative studies suggesting resectability should undergo exploration with curative intent if comorbidities permit. Pancreatic head or periampullary lesions are best approached with **pancreaticoduodenectomy (Whipple procedure)**, while body and tail lesions are treated with a distal pancreatectomy that usually includes a splenectomy. Laparoscopy is sometimes done prior to celiotomy to search for metastatic disease not visualized by preoperative imaging studies. Palliation can usually be achieved by endoscopically stenting the biliary tract. Gastric outlet obstruction develops in approximately 10% of patients and requires a palliative gastrojejunostomy. Back pain can be improved with a celiac axis neurolysis.

Pancreaticoduodenectomy involves resection of the distal common bile duct, duodenum, and head of the pancreas as seen in Figure 17-14. The duodenum may be divided just distal to the pylorus or a hemigastrectomy may be required based upon tumor extent. Reconstruction includes a choledochojejunostomy, pancreaticojejunostomy, and gastrojejunostomy. Although mortality for the procedure is <5%, complications are common, but can usually be managed without reoperation. Complications include leakage from any of the anastomoses with the highest rate occurring at the pancreaticojejunostomy. Amylase-rich fluid may leak from the anastomoses with abscess formation and possible sepsis. Pancreatic fistulas may also occur. Anastomotic leakage or disruption is usually managed by drainage and provision of nutrition. Other risks of the procedure include delayed gastric emptying, leak from the other anastomoses, and diabetes.

Prognosis

Most pancreatic cancer patients present with unresectable disease and have a median survival of approximately 6 months even with chemotherapy. Surgical resection extends life to approximately 19 months if negative margins are obtained and adjuvant chemoradiation is tolerated. These patients, however, usually still die from this disease with perhaps 20% surviving 5 years. Poor prognostic indicators include lymph node metastasis, tumor size >3 cm, and perineural invasion.

Adjuvant and Neoadjuvant Treatment for Pancreatic Cancer

Pancreatic cancer has a high rate of recurrence after surgical resection. This is presumably due to the presence of

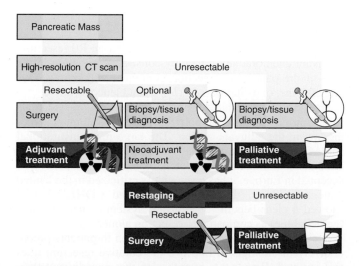

FIGURE 17-13. Algorithm for the evaluation of a pancreatic mass. (Drawing by Matthew Campbell.)

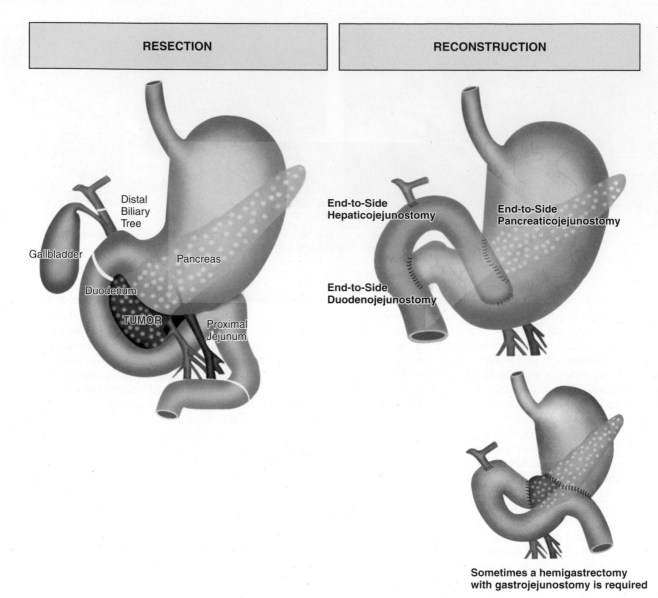

FIGURE 17-14. Pancreaticoduodenectomy. The resection is shown on the left and the right demonstrates the reconstruction with a pancreaticojejunostomy, choledochojejunostomy, and a duodenojejunostomy above or gastrojejunostomy below. The first upper reconstruction is used for pylorus-preserving pancreaticoduodenectomies and the bottom is used when a hemigastrectomy is required. (Drawing by Matthew Campbell.)

micrometastatic disease after surgical resection or tumor stem cells. Due to high recurrence rates, effort has been directed toward developing adjuvant and neoadjuvant therapies to improve survival.

Adjuvant strategies include both the use of systemic chemotherapy as well as the use of chemoradiation. The basis for the use of chemoradiation stems from a small randomized trial published over 20 years ago that suggested that chemoradiation and chemotherapy were better than surgery alone. Since that time, several other trials have been less conclusive. A large multi-institutional study suggested that patients who receive adjuvant chemoradiation therapy for pancreatic adenocarcinoma treated by resection achieve a significant overall survival benefit when compared to patients treated only with surgery. Subset analysis, however, suggests that this benefit is seen only in patients with positive lymph node disease. A recent Mayo Clinic study has also showed a survival benefit with

the addition of chemoradiation therapy after an R0 resection. Adjuvant chemoradiation therapy consists of radiation to the area of the pancreatic resection combined with intravenous gemcitabine, or 5-fluorouracil (5-FU) and leucovorin.

In contrast, there have been two recent randomized trials from Europe that have supported the use of systemic chemotherapy in the adjuvant setting. The large multi-institutional ESPAC-1 trial suggested that chemotherapy was beneficial but that chemoradiation was not. Although this study was well accepted in Europe, it has been widely criticized in the United States. Similarly, the recently published CONKO-1 trial showed a clear benefit for adjuvant systemic chemotherapy (gemcitabine) as compared to resection alone.

Neoadjuvant therapy is treatment given to patients preoperatively in attempts to improve the curative resection rates and survival. Proponents hypothesize that neoadjuvant therapy decreases the chance of leaving behind microscopic or gross disease at the time of resection. Neoadjuvant regimens also allow delivery of radiation to well-oxygenated cancer cells and avoid delays in chemotherapy administration due to complications after resection. Neoadjuvant therapy, however, can delay surgical treatment of pancreatic cancer and carries its own morbidity with some patients never becoming operative candidates after the treatment.

The M.D. Anderson and Fox Chase Cancer Centers have reported neoadjuvant therapy trial results. Most studies involved limited numbers of patients, and most reported on combinations of 5-FU, gemcitabine, or cisplatin with external-beam radiation therapy (EBRT). Patients who underwent neoadjuvant chemoradiation experienced a lower rate of local recurrences and had an excellent median survival. Unfortunately, however, specific treatment regimens have varied between studies, and none of these trials were randomized. Due to variability in study design, size, and treatment algorithms, analysis of the available studies is therefore difficult and confusing. Until large randomized trials comparing neoadjuvant therapy to adjuvant therapy or to resection alone are done, the utility of neoadjuvant therapy in pancreatic cancer is still unclear.

Pancreatic Endocrine Tumors

Pancreatic endocrine tumors (PETs) are known by a variety of synonyms including pancreatic islet cell tumors and pancreatic neuroendocrine neoplasms. PETs are classified as APUDomas (amine precursor uptake and decarboxylation) because it was initially thought they arose from the islets of Langerhans, but it is now believed that they originate from pluripotent stem cells in the ductal epithelium. Approximately 2,500 PETs are diagnosed annually with an incidence of one to five cases per million population. There is no gender predilection and PETs may occur at any age with the peak incidence occurring between the ages of 30 and 60. PETs are much less common than pancreatic adenocarcinoma and comprise approximately 7% of all pancreatic malignancies.

PETs are categorized as functional or nonfunctional depending upon whether they are associated with a clinical syndrome secondary to peptide secretion. Approximately 50% of PETs are nonfunctional. Both functional and nonfunctional PETs secrete peptides that are not associated with a clinically recognizable syndrome including pancreatic polypeptide (PP), chromogranin A (CgA), neurotensin, or ghrelin. Functional PETs also secrete peptides that cause a clinical syndrome. The incidence of functional PETs is 1 per million population for insulinomas, 0.2 to 2 per million for gastrinomas, 0.5 to 1 per 10 million for VIPomas, 1 per 20 million for glucagonomas, and 1 per 40 million for somatostatinomas.

Most PETs occur sporadically, but genetic alterations in PETs have been identified in patients with multiple endocrine neoplasia syndrome type I (MEN 1), von Hippel-Lindau disease, von Recklinghausen's disease, and tuberous sclerosis.

Insulinoma

Insulinomas compromise 20% to 30% of all PETs and are the most common functional PET. The majority (85–% to 90%) are benign, whereas the majority (60%) of all other PETs are malignant. Most insulinomas are solitary, <2 cm in diameter, and distributed equally throughout the gland.

Insulin hypersecretion causes hypoglycemia that is manifested by sweating, hunger, weakness, anxiety, irritability, headaches, blurry vision, incoherence, confusion, personality changes, amnesia, psychosis, peripheral distal neuropathy,

palpitations, diaphoresis, tremors, seizure, and coma. Patients eat frequent meals with high sugar contents and often gain weight attempting to prevent hypoglycemic symptoms. These patients are also frequently diagnosed with psychiatric conditions or epilepsy prior to the correct diagnosis due to the vagueness of their symptoms and erratic behavior often observed.

Diagnosis is confirmed during a monitored 72-hour fast. Health care professionals must monitor the patients for signs and symptoms of hypoglycemia. When these occur, blood sugar levels are measured. Whipple's triad ([1] symptoms and hypoglycemia, [2] a low blood glucose level [40 to 50 mg/dL], and [3] relief of symptoms following the intravenous administration of glucose) is suggestive of insulinoma. There are, however, six diagnostic criteria of insulinoma, which include a documented blood glucose ≤45 mg/dL, concomitant serum insulin levels ≥36 μU/L (≥36 pmol/L; ≥3 μU/L by ICMA), plasma/serum C-peptide levels ≥200 pmol/L, serum proinsulin levels ≥5 pmol/L, serum β-hydroxybutyrate levels ≤2.7 mmol/L, and the absence of sulfonylurea in the plasma and/or urine. When results are indeterminate, a secretin injection test may help make the diagnosis. Normally, secretin stimulates release of insulin from β-cells, but insulinomas do not release insulin in response to secretin and also inhibit the normal response of β-cells to secretin. Thus, patients with insulinomas do not increase insulin production in response to secretin.

Gastrinoma

Gastrinomas were initially identified by Zollinger and Ellison. Gastrinomas account for approximately 20% of the functional PETs. Three-quarters occur sporadically and one-fourth occur as part of the MEN I syndrome. Many gastrinomas are not found in the pancreas with over 50% being located within the duodenal wall. Between 60% and 90% are found within the gastrinoma triangle (Figure 17-15) defined by the junction of the common bile and cystic ducts, the neck and body of the pancreas, and the second and third portion of the duodenum. Gastrinomas, however, can arise almost anywhere in the body

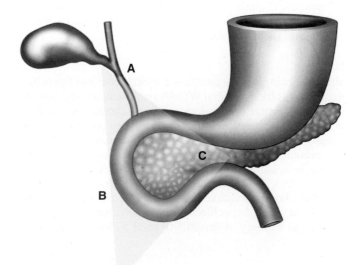

FIGURE 17-15. The gastrinoma triangle. Approximately 90% of gastrinomas are located within the region bounded by the confluence of the cystic and common bile duct (**A**), the junction of the second and third portions of the duodenum (**B**), and the junction of the neck and body of the pancreas (**C**). (Drawing by Matthew Campbell.)

including the liver, ovary, and lymph nodes, are multicentric in half of cases, and tend to metastasize to lymph nodes and the liver (50%). Gastric acid hypersecretion is responsible for the majority of symptoms including intractable abdominal pain, severe esophagitis, and persistent diarrhea, which occur as a result of small bowel mucosal injury, inactivation of lipase, and precipitation of bile salts. Thus, when gastric acid secretion is controlled, symptoms resolve regardless of the gastrin level.

The diagnosis should be considered in all patients with peptic ulcers and diarrhea, familial peptic ulcers, when peptic ulcers are identified in unusual locations, and in patients who develop recurrent peptic ulcers that are resistant to treatment. A fasting serum gastrin level should also be measured in patients requiring gastric surgery for peptic ulcer disease. Gastrin levels >1000 pg/mL in a patient with a gastric pH of <2 is diagnostic. Two-thirds of gastrinoma patients, however, have gastrin levels <1,000 pg/mL and require additional information. In this group, an elevated fasting gastrin level >200 pg/mL, a basal acid output ≥15 mEq/hour, and a positive secretin stimulation test as defined by a >200 pg/mL increase in gastrin after injection of secretin is diagnostic. Calcium infusion may also be used diagnostically when the secretin test is negative to help confirm the diagnosis.

Gastrin levels may also be elevated for a variety of reasons besides a gastrinoma, and prior to making the diagnosis of gastrinoma, these conditions should be considered in the differential diagnosis for any patient with an elevated gastrin level. Hypergastrinemic states includes patients with pernicious anemia or atrophic gastritis, chronic renal failure, use of proton-pump inhibitors, *Helicobacter pylori* infection, and postvagotomy syndromes, G-cell hyperplasia, retained antrum, short bowel syndrome, chronic renal failure, and gastric outlet obstruction.

Glucagonoma

Glucagonomas arise from pancreatic alpha cells. They are more commonly located in the body or tail of the gland. Patients usually present with large lesions and metastatic disease. Symptoms include mild glucose intolerance and in over half of the cases necrolytic migratory erythema, which is a characteristic skin rash. Patients develop frequent deep vein thromboses, thrombophlebitis, weight loss, anemia, cachexia, and psychiatric disorders. A serum glucagon level of 500 to 1000 pg/mL is diagnostic.

VIPoma

VIPomas cause watery diarrhea, hypokalemia, and hypochlorhydria. This triad is called WDHA syndrome, watery diarrhea syndrome, pancreatic cholera syndrome, endocrine cholera, or Verner-Morrison syndrome. The diarrhea is chronic, unresponsive to medical management, large volume (6 to 8 L/day), and present despite fasting. Patients experience dehydration, weight loss, and metabolic acidosis due to excretion of Na^+, K^+, Cl^-, HCO_3^-, and water. VIP also inhibits gastric acid output, stimulates bone resorption, glycogenolysis, and vasodilatation, which can cause hypochlorhydria, hypercalcemia, hyperglycemia, and flushing. A serum VIP level >75 to 150 pg/mL is diagnostic.

Somatostatinoma

Somatostatinomas may arise in the pancreas, ampulla, duodenum, jejunum, cystic duct, or rectum. Somatostatin inhibits production of a variety of hormones including growth hormone, gastrin, insulin, and glucagon. Somatostatin also inhibits intestinal absorption, gastrointestinal motility, and gallbladder contraction. Patients can present in a variety of manners and may develop diabetes, gallstones, and diarrhea with steatorrhea that results in hypochlorhydria. Most patients' symptoms are nonspecific and include pain, weight loss, and a change in bowel habits. Somatostatinomas are usually located in the pancreatic head (60%), are large solitary lesions at the time of diagnosis (>5 cm, range 0.5 to 10 cm), and cause symptoms from local growth or metastases in 70% of cases. A fasting somatostatin level >160 pg/mL and a pancreatic or duodenal mass are diagnostic.

Evaluation

All patients with PETs should undergo a CT or MRI for localization, determination of resectability, and evaluation for metastatic disease. Functional tumors often present at smaller sizes due to the syndrome they produce and can be difficult to image. Radiographically, most PETs look like solid hypervascular lesions. Malignancy is suggested by imaging findings of calcifications, necrosis, and invasion of retroperitoneal structures. EUS may help identify small pancreatic lesions.

When an insulinoma is suspected and CT, MRI, and EUS are unable to localize the lesion, selective arterial calcium stimulation and hepatic venous sampling (ASVS) can be utilized. ASVS also helps to differentiate the 5% of patients with islet cell hyperplasia (nesidioblastosis or noninsulinoma pancreatogenic hypoglycemia syndrome) from those with insulinoma. Insulinoma cells increase secretion of insulin in response to calcium. Calcium gluconate is injected into the gastroduodenal, mid and proximal splenic, and superior mesenteric arteries while insulin levels are obtained from the right hepatic vein. This allows for the area of the pancreas containing the insulinoma to be identified. It does not actually demonstrate the insulinoma, but allows for surgery to be targeted to a specific area of the pancreas. Intraoperative ultrasound can also be helpful in combination with ASVS in identifying the lesion.

Somatostatin scintigraphy (Octreoscan) should also be done for all PETs except insulinoma because it is not readily detected with a sensitivity of <50%. Octreoscan is also very useful for evaluating metastatic disease for PETs. Positron emission tomography using fluorine-18 (F-18) fluorodeoxyglucose (FDG) may also be complementary to Octreoscan and occasionally identifies lesions missed by Octreoscan.

If these localizing studies fail to identify the location of a gastrinoma, the selective arterial secretagogue injection test (SASI) with the arterial injection of calcium or secretin can be used similarly to the ASVS test with measurement of gastrin levels in venous tributaries to localize the gastrinoma to a specific area in the patient.

Treatment

Curative treatment of PETs requires complete surgical extirpation of the primary and all metastatic disease. Resection should not be undertaken if extra-abdominal or bony metastases are identified. Overall survival is significantly better than with adenocarcinoma and long-term survival with metastatic disease is possible. Surgical debulking procedures for liver metastases are also appropriate if at least 90% of the disease can be extirpated.

Benign insulinomas can be treated by enucleation or resection. Laparoscopic techniques might be possible especially with good preoperative localization studies. More aggressive surgery is typically required for malignant PETs. Symptoms of PETs should be controlled preoperatively using somatostatin

TABLE 17-11	Classification of Neuroendocrine Tumors of the Pancreas (WHO Classification 2004)

1. Well-differentiated neuroendocrine tumor

- Benign: confined to pancreas, <2 cm in size, nonangioinvasive, ≤2 mitoses/HPF and ≤2% Ki-67–positive cells
  - ○ Functioning insulinoma
  - ○ Nonfunctioning

- Benign or low grade malignant (uncertain malignant potential): confined to pancreas, ≥2 cm in size, >2 mitoses/HPF, >2% Ki-67–positive cells, or angioinvasive
  - ○ Functioning: gastrinoma, insulinoma, VIPoma, glucagonoma, somatostatinoma, or ectopic hormonal syndrome
  - ○ Nonfunctioning

2. Well-differentiated neuroendocrine carcinoma

- Low grade malignant: invasion of adjacent organs and/or metastases
  - ○ Functioning: gastrinoma, insulinoma, glucagonoma, VIPoma, somatostatinoma or ectopic hormonal syndrome
  - ○ Nonfunctioning

3. Poorly differentiated neuroendocrine carcinoma

- High grade malignant

Table 71 in Tumors of the Pancreas chapter in DeLellis L, Heitz PU, Eng C eds. Pathology and Genetics: Tumours of the endocrine organs, WHO Classification of Tumors. Lyon, France: IARC Press, 2004:175–208. Used with permission.

TABLE 17-12	Proposal for a TNM Classification and Disease Staging for Endocrine Tumors of the Pancreas

T-primary Tumor

TX	Primary tumor cannot be assessed
T0	No evidence of primary tumor
T1	Tumor limited to the pancreas and size <2 cm
T2	Tumor limited to the pancreas and size 2–4 cm
T3	Tumor limited to the pancreas and size >4 cm or invading duodenum or bile duct
T4	Tumor invading adjacent organs (stomach, spleen, colon, adrenal gland) or the wall of large vessels (celiac axis or superior mesenteric artery)
	For any T, add (m) for multiple tumors

N-regional Lymph Nodes

NX	Regional lymph node cannot be assessed
N0	No regional lymph node metastasis
N1	Regional lymph node metastasis

M-distant Metastases

MX	Distant metastasis cannot be assessed
M0	No distant metastases
M1[a]	Distant metastasis

Stage

Disease Stages

Stage I	T1	N0	M0
Stage IIa	T2	N0	M0
IIb	T3	N0	M0
Stage IIIa	T4	N0	M0
IIIb	Any T	N1	M0
Stage IV	Any T	Any N	M1

[a]M1 specific sites defined according to Sobin LH, Wittekind, C, eds. TNM classification of malignant tumours. New York: Wiley-Liss, 2002.
Table taken from Rindi G, Kloppel G, Alhman H, et al. TNM staging of foregut (neuro)endocrine tumors: a consensus proposal including a grading system. Virchows Arch. 2006;449:395–401.

analogues and proton pump inhibitors. Surgery for small gastrinomas can be aided by intraoperative duodenoscopy with transillumination. Pancreatic head lesions are best treated by pancreaticoduodenectomy, while body or tail lesions are best treated with distal pancreatectomy. Metastases should be resected if possible.

Nonoperative palliative treatment includes symptom control and ablative modalities including radiofrequency ablation, cryotherapy, hepatic artery embolization and chemoembolization using cisplatin and doxorubicin, or combinations of these with systemic chemotherapeutic agents.

Somatostatin analogues can control symptoms in almost 100% of patients. These analogues are well tolerated and may briefly stabilize disease progression, but do not prolong survival. Chemotherapy with streptozocin, 5-FU, and doxorubicin can be used as salvage therapy for malignant insulinomas, but has poor efficacy and significant toxicity.

Staging and Prognosis

It was previously believed that histological grading system could not predict the behavior of well-differentiated PETs, but there are now standardized staging systems for PETs. The tumors cytologic and histologic features including mitotic index, nuclear pleomorphism, capsular invasion, or focal vascular invasion cannot determine malignancy which is based upon the findings of metastatic disease or tumor invasion into adjacent organs. In 2004, the World Health Organization (WHO) developed a classification system placing for PETs and

TABLE 17-13	Grading Proposal for Foregut (Neuro)Endocrine Tumors	
Grade	**Mitotic Count (10 HPF)**[a]	**Ki-67 Index (%)**[b]
G1	<2	≤2
G2	2–20	3–20
G3	>20	>20

[a] 10 HPF: high power field = 2 mm², at least 40 fields (at 40× magnification) evaluated in areas of highest mitotic density
[b] MIB1 antibody; % of 2,000 tumor cells in areas of highest nuclear labeling.

placed them into three risk groups (Table 17-11) based upon histologic criteria. This staging system is useful for determining prognosis. Prognostic criteria include the degree of tumor differentiation, size, angioinvasion, and the proliferation index.

The European Neuroendocrine Tumor Society (ENETS) has also established guidelines for the treatment of patients with PETs, and developed a TNM classification system (Table 17-12). The TNM staging system is based upon the WHO classification. The ENETS also proposed a foregut neuroendocrine tumor grading system (Table 17-13). Grades G1 and G2 correspond to well-differentiated PETs while grade G3 is reserved for poorly differentiated tumors. These grading and classification systems still require further validation, but may prove clinically useful.

the Point ✳ Go to http://thePoint.lww.com/activate and use your scratch-off code on the inside cover of this book to access bonus chapters, question bank, videos, and more.

SAMPLE QUESTIONS

Questions

Choose the best answer for each question.

1. A 20-year-old man comes to the emergency department with severe epigastric pain. He has a history of pancreatitis 8 months ago, but no cause was identified. He has otherwise been healthy. He does not smoke or drink alcohol. He takes no medications. His vital signs are temperature—38°C, blood pressure (BP)—130/80 mm Hg, pulse—110/minute, and respirations—18/minute. He has severe epigastric tenderness with guarding. There is no scleral icterus. An ultrasound does not show gallstones. The bile ducts are not dilated. Laboratory studies show:

    Lipase—20,000 units
    Total bilirubin—0.9 mg/dL
    Calcium—9/0 mg/dL

    Which of the following additional findings is most likely to support the diagnosis of pancreas divisum?

    A. An absent duct of Santorini

    B. Separate dorsal and ventral ducts

    C. The majority of pancreatic secretions enter the duodenum via the duct of Wirsung.

    D. Separate common bile duct and pancreatic duct

    E. Dilatation of the pancreatic duct

2. A 50-year-old woman has severe gallstone pancreatitis. She is receiving IV fluid and is receiving nothing by mouth in an effort to slow pancreatic secretion to decrease the amount of active pancreatic enzyme leaking into the disrupted glandular tissue. Which of the following enzymes is produced by the pancreas and secreted in its active form?

    A. Amylase

    B. Trypsin

    C. Chymotrypsin

    D. Cholecystokinin

    E. Gastrin

3. A 42-year-old man comes to the emergency department with severe abdominal pain. He takes no medications. He drinks a quart of vodka daily and smokes one to two packs of cigarettes daily. Temperature is 38°C, BP is 110/90, pulse is 20/minute, and respirations are 24/minute. He has severe epigastric tenderness. Which of the following variables is included in Ranson's criteria *on admission* to predict the severity of this patient's illness?

    A. Calcium

    B. Arterial PO_2

    C. WBC

    D. Base deficit

    E. Total bilirubin

4. A 70-year-old woman is brought to the clinic by her family because of jaundice. She has also had a 20-pound weight loss over the past few months and has recently noticed very dark urine and light-colored stools. She does not have any pain. She is thin. There is a nontender, globular mass in the right upper quadrant. An ultrasound shows dilated intrahepatic and extrahepatic bile ducts with a dilated pancreatic duct and a mass in the head of the pancreas. Mutations in which of the following is most likely associated with this patient's diagnosis?

    A. p53

    B. p16

    C. K-*ras*

    D. DNA mismatch repair

    E. Retinoblastoma (RB) gene

5. A 66-year-old man presented to the clinic with painless jaundice. Further evaluation with CT imaging and endoscopic ultrasonography (EUS) showed a small resectable tumor in the head of the pancreas and no evidence of metastatic disease. EUS-guided biopsy confirmed the diagnosis of pancreatic adenocarcinoma. Pancreaticoduodenectomy is planned. Which of the following statements regarding the role of adjuvant or neoadjuvant therapy for this patient is true?

    A. Adjuvant and neoadjuvant strategies can include radiation and/or chemotherapy.

    B. There is no role for chemotherapy in the adjuvant or neoadjuvant setting.

    C. Neoadjuvant strategies are the standard of care for patients with pancreatic cancer.

    D. The use of neoadjuvant and adjuvant strategies is usually not indicated due to the low recurrence rates in patients with resected disease.

    E. Neoadjuvant therapy is given postoperatively.

Answers and Explanations

1. Answer: B

Pancreatic divisum generally encompasses a variety of anatomic abnormalities whereby the majority of the dorsal pancreas empties into the duodenum via the duct of Santorini and a portion of the pancreatic head and uncinate empty via the major papilla. The abnormalities can include an absent duct of Wirsung and separate dorsal and ventral ducts that do not fuse as well as a filamentous connection between the dorsal and ventral ducts. In the absence of divisum, that is, in the normal state, the dorsal and ventral ducts join and the majority of secretions enter the duodenum via the duct of Wirsung through the major papilla. The common bile duct is separate from the pancreatic duct until they merge at near the ampulla. (Taken from Embryology and Ductal Anatomy).

2. Answer: A

The pancreas secretes a variety of digestive enzymes including amylases, lipases, and proteases. The majority of enzymes including trypsin and chymotrypsin are secreted in their inactive form (trypsinogen and chymotrypsinogen). Amylase is secreted in its active form. Cholecystokinin (CCK) is secreted by the duodenum and leads to the secretion of several pancreatic enzymes, while gastrin is a hormone primarily produced in the antrum. (Taken from Exocrine).

3. Answer: C

Ranson's criteria is one of the grading systems for the severity of pancreatitis that relies on clinical and laboratory values on admission and during the initial 48 hours. On admission, the criteria include age, WBC, serum glucose, serum LDH, and SGOT. Arterial PO_2, calcium, and base deficit are three of six criteria measured during the initial 48 hours. Total bilirubin, although often measured, is not part of the criteria. (Taken from Acute Pancreatitis, Prognosis).

4. Answer: C

The most commonly expressed genetic mutation in pancreatic cancer occurs in the K-*ras* oncogene. It is present in at least 75% of pancreatic carcinomas. Mutations in the p53 tumor suppressor gene are the second most common mutation in pancreatic cancer and the most common genetic event in all human cancers. Mutations in other genes including p16, the retinoblastoma gene, and in the DNA mismatch repair genes also occur but are less common. (Taken from Pancreatic Neoplasms, Genetic Mutations Associated with Pancreatic Cancer).

5. Answer: A

Unfortunately, even after successful surgical resection, the majority of patients with pancreatic cancer will develop recurrence of their disease—both locally and systemically. Due to the high recurrence rates, efforts aimed at developing adjuvant and neoadjuvant strategies have been pursued. Treatment can consist of either chemotherapy alone or with radiation. Treatment can be given preoperatively (neoadjuvant) or postoperatively (adjuvant). Although there are several theoretical advantages of neoadjuvant strategies with promising results, no randomized comparisons have been done versus adjuvant therapy. (Taken from Pancreatic Neoplasms, Adjuvant and Neoadjuvant Treatment for Pancreatic Cancer).

WILLIAM C. CHAPMAN, M.D. • ADNAN A. ALSEIDI, M.D. • JONATHAN R. HIATT, M.D. •
RUSSELL J. NAUTA, M.D. • MICHAEL D. STONE, M.D.

Objectives

1. Understand the natural history of benign tumors of the liver, and describe their appropriate treatment.
2. List four factors that favorably influence the prognosis after resection of hepatic metastasis from colorectal cancer.
3. List the two most common primary hepatobiliary malignancies and their relative frequency.
4. List the steps involved in diagnosing a hepatic mass.
5. Compare and contrast the clinical and pathologic features and the treatment of hepatic adenoma and focal nodular hyperplasia.

6. Identify three major complications of portal hypertension.
7. List four forms of specific therapy for acute variceal hemorrhage in the order in which they are typically applied.
8. List at least three sites of portosystemic collateral channel formation in patients with portal hypertension.
9. List at least four causes of portal hypertension in addition to cirrhosis.
10. List three complications associated with ascites formation in the patient with portal hypertension.

In the liver, mass lesions (tumors, cysts, and abscesses), complications of **portal hypertension,** organ failure, and trauma constitute the vast majority of hepatic diseases for which surgical intervention is warranted.

ANATOMY

While anatomy remains pivotal in treatment of almost any surgical disease, nowhere does this relationship become as paramount as when approaching the liver and surgical hepatic disease. The liver is the largest single gland in the body. In the average adult, it weighs approximately 1200 to 1600 g. It is located below the diaphragm, with its greatest mass to the right of the midline but does extend, to a variable degree, into the left upper quadrant. In the cranial–caudal axis, the liver extends from about the fourth to fifth intercostal space on both sides to just below the costal margin on the right. It is covered by the tough, fibrous Glisson's capsule, which extends into its parenchyma along penetrating vessels, for example, porta hepatis. Except for the bare area, located over its posterior surface near the vena cava, and the gallbladder bed, the liver is invested in peritoneum. Folds or reflections of this peritoneum are named ligaments. Such ligaments, for example, falciform, coronary, and triangular ligaments, attach the liver to the diaphragm and the anterior abdominal wall. Another reflection of the peritoneum is the gastrohepatic ligament (lesser omentum), which extends from the liver to the lesser curvature of the stomach and the first part of the duodenum.

The liver enjoys a dual blood supply, the hepatic arterial and portal venous systems. Twenty-five percent of blood flow to the liver is usually from the hepatic arterial system, while the rest is from the portal veins. Unlike the portal system, the hepatic arterial system can be variable; up to 40% of cases have some variation from the "traditional" branching of the arterial system (Figure 18-1). These variations can be either accessory vessels (an aberrant vessel in addition to the normal branching vessel) or replaced vessels (an aberrant vessel that is present in the absence of the normal branching vessel), or both. Thus, for example, while the hepatic artery commonly arises from the celiac axis, it occasionally is a replaced artery arising from the superior mesenteric artery. The portal vein represents the confluence of drainage from the bowel (superior mesenteric vein) and the spleen (splenic vein). The liver is drained by the right, middle, and left hepatic veins. These drain directly into the inferior vena cava.

Until recently, two separate methods have been used to classify liver anatomy. The first, based on the work of James Cantlie, uses surface anatomy as its bases. The other uses internal vascular and biliary anatomy as the foundation for the classification. The latter method was pioneered by anatomists

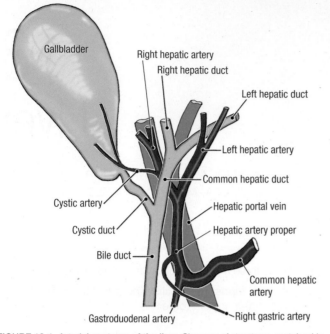

FIGURE 18-1. Arterial anatomy of the liver. Close-up of structures contained in the hepatoduodenal ligament. Tributaries of bile duct and branches of common hepatic artery. (Reprinted with permission from Sauerland EK, ed., *Grant's Dissector*, 12th ed. Baltimore, MD: Lippincott Williams & Wilkins, 1999:66.)

such as Couinaud and Healey. The survival of both methods, for many years, resulted in a confusion that strained medical communication internationally. In an effort to clarify this confusion, the terminology committee of the International Hepato-Pancreato-Biliary Association (IHPBA), at its biannual meeting in Brisbane in 2000, adopted coherent and universal terminology. Based on this adopted nomenclature, the surface-anatomy method will no longer be used. The term "lobe" was dropped from the nomenclature due to multiple definitions. Further, due to the slight difference between Couinaud's and Healey's terminologies, especially in the left liver, neither was completely adopted; a combined nomenclature that is based on the ramification of the arterial and biliary anatomy was introduced. The portal anatomy follows the arterial and biliary anatomy in the right liver; however, due to its role in fetal circulation, it has a different course in the left liver. Thus, the portal anatomy was not used as a basis of classification in the Brisbane 2000–adopted nomenclature.

As a result, while Couinaud's segments were retained in this nomenclature (Figure 18-2), they are used to describe third-order ramification of the arterial and biliary system (Figure 18-3). The first-order ramification will result in liver/hemiliver terminology (Figure 18-4), while the second-order ramification results in the description of "sections" (Figure 18-5).

PHYSIOLOGY

The functional unit of the liver is the lobule. On the periphery of each lobule lie hepatic arterial and portal venous branches. Centrally lies a draining hepatic vein. Blood from the terminal portal venules and hepatic arterioles will converge in the hepatic sinusoids, with which each hepatocyte has intimate contact, and drain centrally into the hepatic venule (Figure 18-6).

The liver performs more than 2000 metabolic functions. Major hepatic functions include protein synthesis, energy metabolism, detoxification, bile production, and the liver's immune reticuloendothelial function. However, many other functions, some not very well understood, exist. The hepatocyte, which is the principal cell of the liver, accounts for most metabolic activity. These cells continually divide and can potentially reproduce the entire cell mass of the liver every 50 days. The cells are aligned in a single layer along the hepatic sinusoids, and they transport essential substrates and hormones intracellularly. The hepatocytes then transport metabolic products either back into the plasma or into the bile canaliculus, which is positioned on the opposite side of this single layer of cells. In this way, the hepatocyte monitors and regulates plasma levels of proteins and ensures that metabolic requirements are met.

The liver also performs many important immunologic functions. **Kupffer cells** line the vascular endothelium and are in close proximity to hepatocytes. These macrophages represent 80% to 90% of the fixed macrophages of the body and are subject to frequent turnover. Their unique position within the liver allows them to interface directly with damaging agents (e.g., endotoxins) from the portal circulation. These cells secrete a variety of effectors on hepatocytes and other cells within the body, including tumor necrosis factor alpha (TNF-α), interleukin 1 (IL-1), interleukin 6 (IL-6), and other important cytokines.

LIVER INJURIES

Despite the substantial protection afforded by the ribs and abdominal musculature, the liver can be injured by penetrating trauma or blunt force injury. Blunt injury can produce a shearing effect of the parenchyma, resulting in a so-called bear claw deformity as parallel capsular lacerations develop and extend into the hepatic tissue.

A focused assessment with sonography in trauma (FAST), ultrasound study, or computed tomography (CT) scan are the usual modalities utilized to detect liver injury, whereas hemodynamic instability is the major reason for operative intervention. Small hematomas or lacerations expected to be self-limiting are often managed nonoperatively. Expanding hematomas and deep lacerations require surgical intervention, as do lacerations involving several Couinaud segments or those in proximity to large blood vessels.

The American Academy for the Surgery of Trauma (AAST) has developed a classification for physical hepatic injury (Table 18-1), reflecting that parenchymal and perivascular injuries in classes III, IV, V, and VI are likely to produce significant bleeding and require surgical intervention.

Hemoperitoneum is an expected finding at laparotomy for liver injury and is approached with four-quadrant abdominal packing. As multiple other organs are often injured, a "damage control" approach to such major abdominal trauma (see Chapter 9, Trauma) is often utilized to avoid shock, coagulopathy, and hypothermia.

While knowledge of the anatomic segmentation of the liver is essential, in the setting of physical hepatic injury, hepatic resection is seldom necessary and is reserved for extensive, near-avulsing parenchymal injury. Suture ligation is more common and is utilized for readily visualized bleeding vessels not amenable to packing.

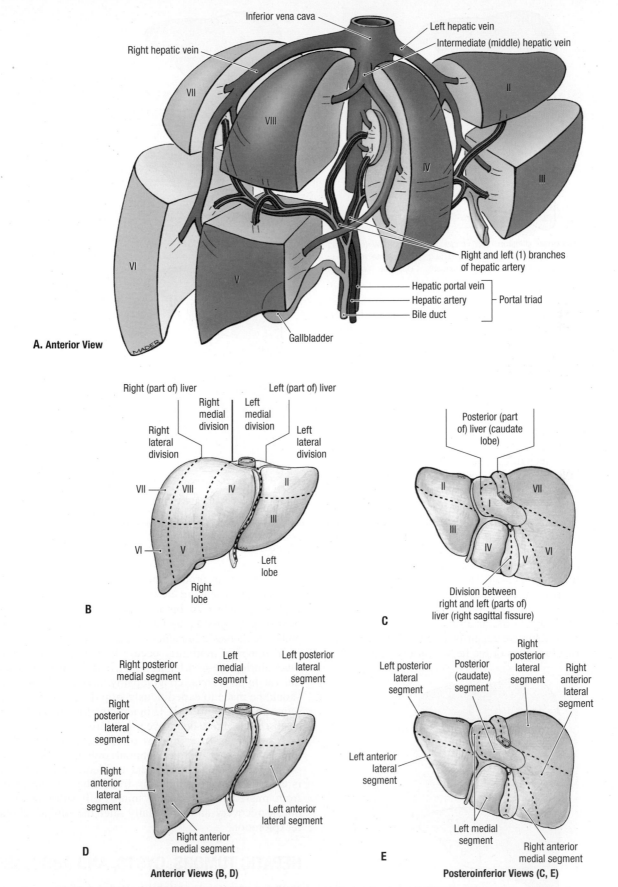

FIGURE 18-2. Couinaud segmental anatomy. A, Anterior view. **B, D,** Anterior views. **C, E,** Posteroinferior views. (Reprinted with permission from Agur AMR, Dalley AF, eds. *Grant's Atlas of Anatomy*, 12th ed. Baltimore, MD: Lippincott Williams & Wilkins, 2009:150.)

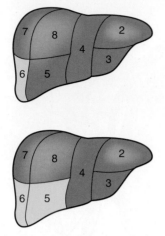

FIGURE 18-3. Third-order division. Top image: Segmentectomy (e.g., segmentectomy 6). Lower image: Bisegmentectomy (e.g., bisegmentectomy 5,6). (Reprinted with permission of Dr. Steven Strasberg. Copyright: Washington University, St. Louis, MO.)

The bleeding comes from injury to branches of the hepatic artery, portal vein, or hepatic veins. Temporary occlusion of the hepatic inflow by application of a vascular clamp to the portal vein and hepatic artery in the porta hepatis (the so-called Pringle maneuver) (Figure 18-7) should stop bleeding from branches of those structures. Ongoing bleeding despite this maneuver can thus be attributed to injury of branches of the hepatic veins. Confirmation of such injury can be achieved by the observation of a reduction in bleeding due to falling central venous pressure when the patient is removed temporarily from mechanical ventilation. Rarely, in injury of the retrohepatic vena cava or hepatic veins, operative shunts to exclude defects in these structures may be placed to facilitate repair (Figure 18-8). Such injuries, however, more often than not, are fatal, as are operations, which require major resection of hepatic parenchyma to control bleeding.

Deep lacerations of the liver may be controlled with omental packing, gauze packing, or inflatable pneumatic devices made with catheters and Penrose drains. The latter are particularly useful in applying pressure to tracts created by bullets or other missiles.

Deep parenchymal lacerations also produce injuries to the bile ducts. Closed suction drains allow evacuation of the bilious effluent until definitive repair can be effected. Injury to intraparenchymal branches of the hepatic artery in proximity

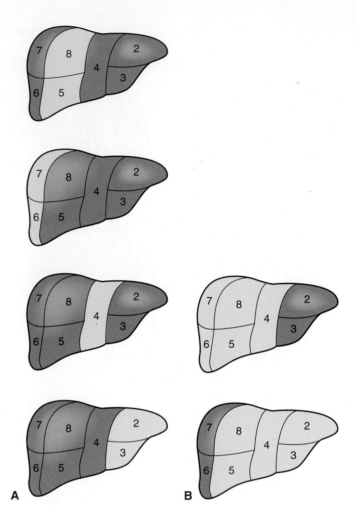

FIGURE 18-5. Second-order division. A, From top to bottom: right anterior sectionectomy, right posterior sectionectomy, left medial sectionectomy (also segmentectomy 4), left lateral sectionectomy. **B**, From top to bottom: right trisectionectomy, left trisectionectomy. (Reprinted with permission of Dr. Steven Strasberg. Copyright: Washington University, St. Louis, MO.)

to bile ducts can produce hemobilia, which may complicate recovery by producing elevated liver function tests and cholangitis secondary to biliary obstruction. Control of hemobilia is often possible by interventional radiologists, who can embolize damaged branches of the hepatic artery.

Incremental morbidity occurs from attempting to do too much during the first laparotomy; in deference to the potential for hypothermia, coagulopathy, and shock, all attempts should be made to expeditiously stop the bleeding, pack, and return the patient to an ICU in anticipation and acceptance of a subsequent, more definitive procedure.

However, as liver injuries often occur with concomitant injuries to other intra-abdominal organs, expeditious, yet complete, operative assessment to identify all such injuries is essential. Ongoing bleeding from other organs or soilage from missed hollow viscus injury will substantially complicate recovery and potentially alter the timing of planned reexploration.

HEPATIC TUMORS, CYSTS, AND ABSCESSES

With the increased availability and use of abdominal imaging techniques, including CT scanning, asymptomatic and incidental liver abnormalities are discovered with greater frequency. An important role of the physician who is treating

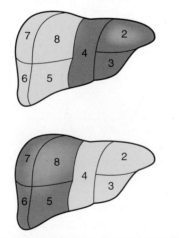

FIGURE 18-4. First-order division. Top: Left hepatectomy or left hemihepatectomy. Bottom: Right hepatectomy or right hemihepatectomy. (Reprinted with permission of Dr. Steven Strasberg. Copyright: Washington University, St. Louis, MO.)

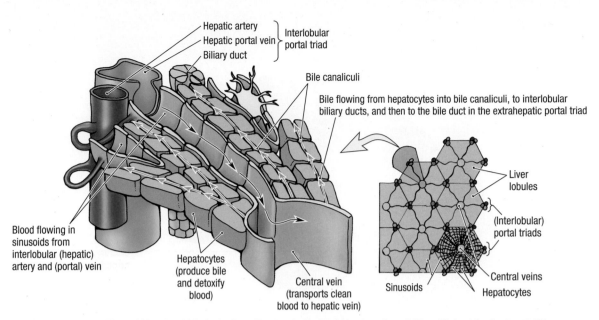

FIGURE 18-6. **Flow of blood and bile in the liver.** (Reprinted with permission from Agur AMR and Dalley AF, eds. *Grant's Atlas of Anatomy*, 12th ed. Baltimore, MD: Lippincott Williams & Wilkins, 2009:151.)

a patient with a newly discovered hepatic abnormality is to determine both the likely etiology of the abnormality and whether further diagnostic or therapeutic measures are needed. Careful patient assessment is needed because incidental benign liver tumors and cysts are common and usually require no specific therapy. On the other hand, some benign liver tumors are resected, if feasible, even in the asymptomatic patient. An important principle is to avoid liver biopsy early in the workup of a newly discovered liver mass in an otherwise asymptomatic patient. Needle biopsy is usually not necessary to determine the most likely diagnosis. It is subject to sampling error and may introduce additional risks of bleeding or tumor seeding in a patient who might undergo tumor resection regardless of the biopsy result. Needle biopsy may be appropriate when the nature of an unresectable tumor remains unknown despite imaging and laboratory tests.

Benign Tumors

Hemangioma

Cavernous hemangioma of the liver is the most common benign liver tumor and occurs in as many as 1% to 20% of the general population. These are probably congenital lesions and are embryologic hamartomas (benign tumors with two distinct cell types). Microscopic evaluation shows endothelial vascular spaces separated by fibrous septa. These lesions may enlarge over the lifetime of an individual. They are five times more common in women and some findings suggest hormonal responsiveness, including enlargement during pregnancy. Cavernous hemangiomas that are larger than 10 cm are defined as giant hemangiomas. Hemangiomas are often incidental findings and require no specific therapy. Liver function tests are usually normal. Ultrasonography may be diagnostic, showing focal hyperechoic abnormalities that are characteristic. Contrast-enhanced CT imaging usually shows a progressive peripheral-to-central prominent enhancement and a central hypodense region.

Most patients are asymptomatic at presentation and remain so in follow-up. Longitudinal studies assessing long-term (>10 years) follow-up in patients with giant cavernous hemangiomas confirm the absence of spontaneous hemorrhage and or rupture. Occasionally, patients with very large hemangiomas have pain, and surgical resection may be considered. Many of these patients have another cause of their pain. Nonresectional strategies used in the past (e.g., radiation, high-dose steroid administration, hepatic artery ligation, embolization) may result in shrinkage but not resolution of these lesions. These lesions may undergo spontaneous thrombosis, which causes transient pain, elevation in hepatic transaminases, and involution on imaging studies.

TABLE 18-1		The American Association for the Surgery of Trauma (AAST) Liver Injury Scale
I	Hematoma	Subcapsular, <10% surface
	Laceration	Capsular tear, <1 cm parenchymal depth
II	Hematoma	Subcapsular, 10%–50% surface area; intraparenchymal, <10 cm in diameter
	Laceration	1–3 cm parenchymal depth, <10 cm in length
III	Hematoma	Subcapsular, >50% surface area or expanding; ruptured subcapsular or parenchymal hematoma; intraparenchymal hematoma >10 cm or expanding
	Laceration	>3 cm parenchymal depth
IV	Laceration	Parenchymal disruption involving 25%–75% of hepatic lobe or one to three Couinaud's segments within a single lobe
V	Laceration	Parenchymal disruption involving >75% of hepatic lobe or >3 Couinaud's segments within a single lobe
	Vascular	Juxtavenous hepatic injuries; i.e., retrohepatic vena cava/central major hepatic veins
VI	Vascular	Hepatic avulsion

Reprinted with permission from Moore EE, et al. Organ injury scaling: spleen and liver (1994 revision). J Trauma 1995;38(3):323–324.

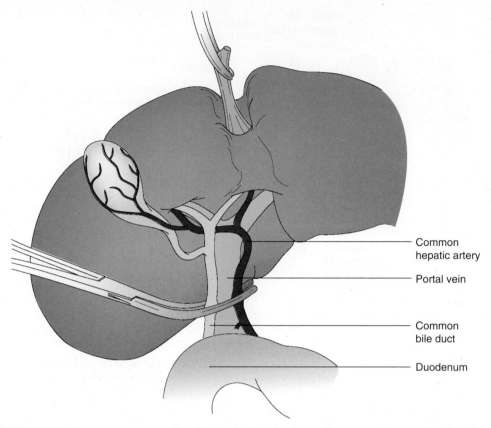

FIGURE 18-7. Pringle maneuver: compression of the portal triad structures with a noncrushing vascular clamp for hepatic inflow control. If possible, clamp times should be limited to 15- to 20-minute intervals. (Reprinted with permission from Mulholland MW et al., eds. *Greenfield's Surgery*, 4th ed. Philadelphia, PA: Lippincott Williams & Wilkins, 2006:430.)

Common hepatic artery

Portal vein

Common bile duct

Duodenum

Focal Nodular Hyperplasia

Focal nodular hyperplasia (FNH) is a well-circumscribed benign lesion, usually found incidentally when ultrasound or CT scanning is performed for some other cause. FNH arises from an arterial malformation. Classic findings are a central scar with fibrous septae and nodular hyperplasia. Unlike hepatic adenoma, bile ducts are scattered throughout. Pain, when present, with these lesions is likely caused by some other process. Liver function tests are usually normal. These tumors do not have malignant potential, and are rarely associated with rupture or hemorrhage.

The major issue in managing FNH lies in differentiating it from hepatic adenoma and hepatocellular carcinoma. CT scanning may demonstrate a classic central stellate scar in larger lesions. Ultrasonography with Doppler may show a characteristic spoke-wheel vascular pattern. MRI scans are most helpful when characteristic patterns of enhancement are seen on arterial, venous, and equilibrium phases. Core-needle biopsy may distinguish this tumor from hepatic adenoma in some but not all cases.

FNH is a benign, regenerative process and should be treated conservatively when the diagnosis is established by imaging. Its growth is not altered by hormonal or oral contraceptive use. When symptoms are present, evaluation should be carried out to exclude other causes. When the diagnosis is in doubt, usually with smaller lesions, resection may be appropriate.

Hepatic Adenoma

A **hepatic adenoma** is a benign tumor that usually occurs in young women between 30 and 50 years of age. Most patients have a history of estrogen exposure, usually in the form of long-standing use of oral contraceptives and occasionally from estrogen replacement therapy. These tumors grossly appear as solitary, unencapsulated masses. Their cut surfaces have a smooth, soft appearance. Microscopically, they appear as sheets of hepatocytes without portal triads or bile ducts.

The clinical presentation is often highly suggestive of hepatic adenoma, but definite preoperative diagnosis may not be possible. CT scanning usually shows a solid hypodense lesion, sometimes with evidence of adjacent hemorrhage (Figure 18-9). ^{99m}Tc sulfur colloid scanning usually shows a corresponding filling defect because these tumors do not contain Kupffer cells and do not take up this tracer. MRI is excellent for characterizing hepatic adenomas, and heterogeneity is the hallmark feature. Needle biopsy may help to establish the diagnosis. Sampling error can make it difficult to distinguish hepatic adenoma from focal nodular hyperplasia or hepatocellular carcinoma on the basis of needle biopsy alone.

Hepatic adenomas can expand and bleed in 20% to 40% of cases, with higher rates seen in women with long-term contraceptive use, pregnancy, and tumors larger than 5 cm. The treatment of hepatic adenoma is consideration of surgical resection for tumors larger than 4 cm. Discontinuation of oral contraceptives may result in shrinkage of these tumors. Bleeding with shock may require emergency operation in some patients while others can be resuscitated, embolized, and undergo delayed, elective surgery. The risk of malignancy in these tumors appears to be about 10% and is increased with large adenomas.

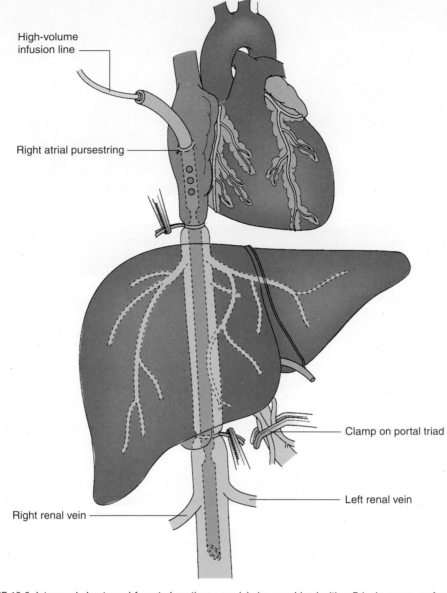

FIGURE 18-8. Intracaval shunt used for retrohepatic venous injuries, combined with a Pringle maneuver for isolation of the retrohepatic vena cava for operative repair. (Reprinted with permission from Mulholland MW et al., eds. *Greenfield's Surgery*, 4th ed. Philadelphia, PA: Lippincott Williams & Wilkins, 2006:431.)

The treatment of choice for these tumors is hepatic resection. Occasionally, patients note tumor regression on withdrawal of hormonal therapy, but this approach should not be used as primary therapy for an otherwise resectable tumor in a healthy patient. Intraoperative ultrasonography is performed in these patients, as in any patient with a hepatic neoplasm, to search for unsuspected additional tumors and to define the relation of the tumor to adjacent portal venous and hepatic arterial structures. Women with a history of hepatic adenoma should use alternative methods of contraception and avoid subsequent use of oral contraceptives. Avoidance of subsequent pregnancy is optimal, but if a patient becomes pregnant, she should undergo periodic assessment with ultrasound surveillance of the liver.

Malignant Tumors

Hepatocellular Carcinoma

Hepatocellular carcinoma (HCC), or hepatoma, accounts for more than 90% of all primary liver malignancies. This tumor usually occurs in patients with underlying liver disease (70% to 80%). It occurs at high rates in areas where hepatitis B is endemic. Although cirrhosis from any cause appears to be associated with the development of HCC, it is also found at increased rates in noncirrhotic chronic carriers of hepatitis B and hepatitis C. Alcohol intake and obesity-related nonalcoholic steatohepatitis (NASH) are other risk factors.

HCC is suspected in any patient with known cirrhosis and sudden clinical decompensation, including worsening jaundice, encephalopathy, or increasing ascites. HCC should be included in the differential diagnosis for any solid liver tumor. Alpha-fetoprotein (AFP) is an α_1-globulin serum marker that is elevated in 60% to 80% of patients with HCC. This tumor marker may also be elevated to 200 to 400 mg/dL in patients with cirrhosis who do not have a hepatoma. Elevations >500 to 1000 mg/dL are almost always associated with HCC.

Any mass larger than 1 cm in a patient with cirrhosis must be investigated for possible HCC. When HCC is suspected, ultrasound, CT, or magnetic resonance scanning may show the

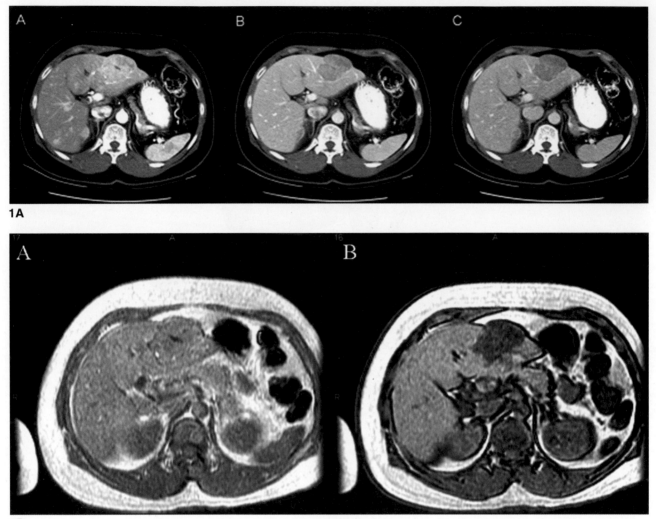

FIGURE 18-9. 1A, Three-phase CT scan of a hepatic adenoma. **Left**: arterial phase; **center**: portal phase; **right**: venous phase. **1B**, In-phase (**left**) and out-of-phase (**right**) MRI of the same hepatic adenoma. As a result of the high fat content of the lesion, the signal cancels out on the out-of-phase image. The lesion, therefore, appears to be nonenhancing. (Reprinted with permission from Mulholland MW et al. eds. *Greenfield's Surgery*, 4th ed. Philadelphia, PA: Lippincott Williams & Wilkins, 2006:962.)

tumor mass. A typical vascular pattern of enhancement on MR arterial phase images followed by washout with residual ring enhancement on delayed imaging is diagnostic (Figure 18-10). If the typical pattern is not seen, biopsy should be considered.

HCC has a propensity for vascular invasion, particularly into portal venous tributaries, and the likelihood of vascular invasion increases with increasing tumor size. Number of nodules, size, and the presence of vascular invasion are important determinants of stage and prognosticators of outcome in these patients.

Treatment for HCC depends on the size of the tumor and the extent of underlying liver disease (Table 18-2). For patients without cirrhosis, liver resection with clear margins is the standard. Unfortunately, surgical resection is often impossible because of the underlying cirrhosis that is common in patients with HCC. Although it is possible to remove as much as 70% of the normal hepatic parenchyma at liver resection, the presence of cirrhosis limits the regenerative capacity of the liver. No specific studies conclusively determine the extent of hepatic parenchyma that can be safely resected in a cirrhotic patient and most surgeons attempt only small peripheral wedge or segmental resections in this setting.

Liver transplantation is appropriate for some patients with HCC because it removes the malignant tumor, eliminates possible sites of recurrence in the remaining diseased liver, and provides hepatic replacement in patients who usually have severely limited hepatic reserve in addition to their tumor. Limitations to the use of liver transplantation in the treatment of patients with HCC include the limited number of donor livers for transplantation and the high cost of this treatment modality. Strict criteria (Milan Criteria: single tumor <5 cm or up to three tumors all ≤3 cms; no vascular invasion) have been developed to guide the use of transplantation for HCC.

Other strategies for local treatment of HCC attempt to destroy tumor cells by heating tumors above 100°C (radiofrequency ablation [RFA], laser ablation, microwave ablation) or by freezing (cryoablation). Both approaches are limited by the "heat sink" from normothermic blood passing by in proximity to the front of thermal change.

Chemoembolization involves the infusion of chemotherapy (usually doxorubicin [Adriamycin]) combined with embolic particles, either gelatin foam or glass microspheres. This process induces tumor ischemia while prolonging chemotherapy dwell times at the site of hepatic tumors. This approach takes

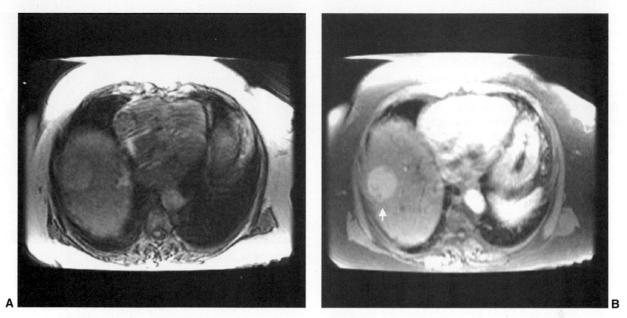

FIGURE 18-10. Hepatocellular carcinoma. A 4-cm lesion in hepatic segment VIII seen before **(A)** and after **(B)** administration of gadolinium contrast on T1-weighted magnetic resonance images. (Reprinted with permission from Maddrey WC et al. eds. *Schiff's Diseases of the Liver*, 10th ed. Ch. 4. Philadelphia, PA: Lippincott Williams & Wilkins, 2007.)

advantage of the preferential arterial blood supply of HCC, while normal hepatocytes receive 70% of their blood and 50% of their oxygen delivery from the portal venous system.

In many centers, combined treatments including transarterial chemoembolization (TACE) with RFA, RFA followed by transplantation, and TACE followed by liver transplantation are used for patients with advanced cirrhosis and small (<5 cm), but unresectable HCC. Recent strategies have used preoperative chemoembolization followed by posttransplant adjuvant chemotherapy in carefully selected patients. Such patients now receive accelerated listing priority by the United Network for Organ Sharing (UNOS).

The fibrolamellar variant of HCC occurs more often in younger patients and often is not associated with underlying cirrhosis. Patients with this tumor usually do not have elevated AFP levels and have a better long-term prognosis after resection than patients with standard HCC. It is unclear whether this improved prognosis is related to the less aggressive nature of the tumor or to the absence of underlying liver disease and a greater resectability rate.

When patients with HCC and cirrhosis undergo successful tumor resection, the remaining liver is the most common site of future recurrence (≥50% of patients), probably because similar etiologic factors are present in the remaining liver (e.g., hepatitis with the formation of second primary lesions) and also from satellite lesions that were not detected at initial resection. Other sites of tumor metastasis include lung and bone. Brain and intraperitoneal metastases are less common.

Cholangiocarcinoma

Cholangiocarcinoma arises from the mucosa of the biliary tree (see Chapter 16, Biliary Tract) and may present in the periphery of the liver, centrally within the liver, or involving the extrahepatic bile ducts. The location determines the nature of the symptoms experienced by the patient. Peripheral tumors may be asymptomatic while central or hilar tumors (Klatskin Tumor) may cause obstructive jaundice and a bile duct stricture on endoscopic retrograde cholangiopancreatography (ERCP). There is often no visible tumor mass on CT scan, while MRCP may show missing segments of the central biliary tree. Jaundice with dilated intrahepatic ducts and a small gallbladder is strongly suggestive of a hilar or central cholangiocarcinoma. These cancers are treated with liver resection. Other rare primary tumors of the liver include angiosarcoma and epithelioid hemangioendothelioma (EHE).

Metastatic Tumors

The most common malignant tumors found in the liver are metastatic, most commonly from a gastrointestinal source. In all patients who die of cancer, 30% to 40% have hepatic metastases at autopsy. Although hepatic metastases usually are associated with extrahepatic disease, in some cases hepatic metastases may be the only site of metastatic disease, indicating the possibility of survival benefit from hepatic-directed therapy. This approach is clearly established for colorectal carcinoma, where successful resection of metastatic

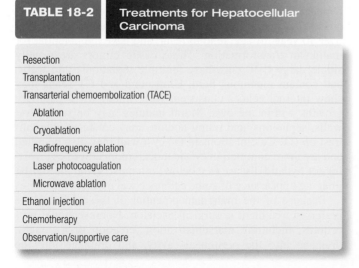

TABLE 18-2	Treatments for Hepatocellular Carcinoma
Resection	
Transplantation	
Transarterial chemoembolization (TACE)	
Ablation	
Cryoablation	
Radiofrequency ablation	
Laser photocoagulation	
Microwave ablation	
Ethanol injection	
Chemotherapy	
Observation/supportive care	

foci can result in 5-year survival rates of 30% to 40% in properly selected patients. Other cancers that may exhibit liver-only metastatic pattern are neuroendocrine tumors, and gastrointestinal stromal tumors (GIST). On rare occasions, hepatic metastases from other sites (breast, melanoma) may be resected for cure in highly selected patients.

With colorectal cancer metastases, patients with fewer and smaller tumors, low CEA levels, a longer (>1 year) disease-free interval, no extrahepatic disease, and node-negative primaries have the best outcomes from liver resection. Surgeons are now more aggressive in treating colorectal metastases because hepatic resection for colorectal cancer now carries a very low mortality rate, and, with the advent of several new and effective chemotherapy drugs, long-term survival is reported with multiple tumors in both lobes and even extrahepatic disease.

Although resection of hepatic metastases may afford long-term survival, most patients (60% to 70%) have recurrence of colorectal carcinoma, and the residual liver is the most common site of recurrence. For this reason, resected patients require careful selection and close follow-up. Ablative therapy techniques (cryoablation and RFA) have been used for metastatic tumors. This therapy is usually reserved for patients with unresectable liver-only tumors. RFA is performed by passing a needle guide into the tumor and radiofrequency energy is used to heat the tumor and a surrounding rim of nontumor parenchyma. Because RFA can be performed through a much smaller probe and can be performed laparoscopically, it is more frequently utilized than cryoablation. The precise role of ablative therapy in the management of hepatic tumors remains to be fully defined.

Hepatic Cysts

Simple Cysts and Polycystic Liver Disease

Cysts of the liver are common, and are identified more frequently with the increased use of CT to investigate many abdominal conditions. Liver cysts may be congenital, or acquired, and the latter may be neoplastic, or infectious. Simple cysts occur in as many as 10% of patients. Most are small, asymptomatic, contain clear serous fluid, and do not communicate with the biliary tree. When multiple, they usually number up to three or four and are scattered throughout the liver.

Simple cysts (Figure 18-11) occasionally may become quite large and be associated with pain, early satiety because of the mass effect, or segmental biliary obstruction from

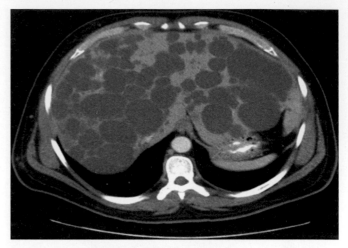

FIGURE 18-12. Polycystic disease.

pressure effects. Intracystic bleeding may occur with larger cysts resulting in symptoms and difficulty differentiating this entity from neoplastic or infectious cysts. Needle aspiration may provide temporary relief of symptoms from simple cysts, but the cyst almost always recurs. For this reason, standard treatment includes unroofing or fenestrating the cyst wall and allowing the cyst fluid to drain into, and be resorbed by, the peritoneal cavity. Surgical resection of simple cysts is not usually required and may be dangerous because large portal and hepatic venous branches may be compressed in the cyst–parenchyma interface and because there is usually no clear plane for resection of the cyst wall.

Polycystic liver disease (Figure 18-12) is an autosomal dominant disorder that causes multiple cysts that are microscopically similar to simple cysts. Unlike simple cysts, however, these cysts are numerous, and progressive enlargement is the norm. Additionally, patients with polycystic liver disease often have polycystic kidney disease that may progress to end-stage renal disease. The hepatic cysts in this condition may be treated with resection of the dominant area of cystic involvement. Simple cyst unroofing alone is rarely effective because of extensive involvement. Some patients have extensive involvement of the entire liver, but even in this situation, it is rare for hepatic synthetic function to be significantly altered.

Cystic Neoplasms

Neoplastic cysts of the liver (cystadenoma or cystadenocarcinoma) are rare. Cystadenomas occur mainly in women over 40 years of age, tend to recur, and have the potential for malignant transformation. These cystic tumors are usually single, large (>10 cm), have multiple septations, thin walls, and contain mucinous fluid. Ultrasound and CT scans may show internal echoes consistent with septations or papillary growths within the cyst. Mural nodules may be seen. Cyst walls, septations, and mural nodules may enhance with contrast on CT. Calcifications in the cyst wall may also be noted and are more common in cystadenocarcinoma. Serologic testing for hydatid disease (see below) is a must, given the similar imaging appearance of some echinococcal cysts.

Because of the malignant potential of these lesions, the preferred treatment is surgical excision. Nonresectional procedures, including marsupialization (creation of a pouch), drainage into the peritoneal cavity, and drainage into the

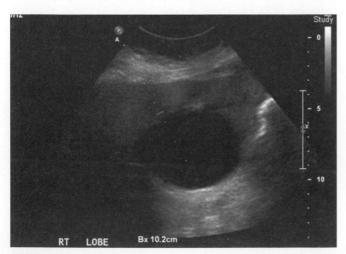

FIGURE 18-11. Simple liver cyst.

gastrointestinal tract, are contraindicated because of a high rate of cyst recurrence and infection.

Hydatid Cysts

Hydatid cystic disease occurs when humans become infected with a parasite, either *Echinococcus granulosus* or *Echinococcus multilocularis,* and become an accidental, intermediate host. The normal life cycle of this parasite involves sheep and carnivores (wolves or dogs). Humans are infected by contact with dog feces. The most common infecting organism is *E. granulosus,* which forms unilocular cysts within the hepatic parenchyma that may grow as large as 10 to 20 cm. Within the larger cysts are multiple daughter cysts that contain innumerable protoscoleces. This disease is commonly manifested by complex liver cysts, which may result in compression of normal liver tissue, secondary pyogenic infection, or biliary fistula with extension into the chest, bronchial tree, or peritoneal cavity.

The diagnosis should be suspected in any patient with a liver cyst (Figure 18-13) who has lived in an endemic region (Mediterranean countries, the Middle and Far East, East Africa, South America, and Australia). Calcifications may be seen on imaging and may be indicative of long-standing indolent infection. Eosinophilia may be seen in one-third to one-half of patients. The diagnosis of Echinococcal infection is confirmed by serologic testing.

If the diagnosis is suspected, *diagnostic* needle aspiration or biopsy should be avoided as these approaches may result in seeding of protoscoleces throughout the abdominal cavity and, possibly, anaphylaxis and shock. After the diagnosis is established, antiparasitic therapy with albendazole is initiated. In some cases of small, unilocular cysts, this therapy alone may be successful in controlling further growth and spread of the disease.

Surgery remains the most effective treatment. The goals of surgery are to remove the parasites and to treat the biliary complications of the disease (fistula). Conservative surgery may be performed to remove the cyst contents and inactivate protoscoleces through the use of scolicidal agents. Prevention of intraoperative spillage, which can lead to intraperitoneal recurrence of hydatid cyst disease, is the critical component of the procedure. The area of cystic involvement is walled off with a scolicidal agent (e.g., hypertonic saline in laparotomy pads). The cyst contents are then carefully evacuated using a closed suction system. This is followed by instillation and reevacuation of a scolicidal agent if the cyst contents are not bile stained or infected. Anatomic or nonanatomic liver resection may be necessary, or elected, to ensure complete cyst removal. In all cases, attention should be paid to connections to the biliary tree, which may leak postoperatively if not recognized and managed appropriately.

Treatment by percutaneous aspiration was discouraged in the past but has now been shown to be successful for selected patients with unilocular cysts in the hands of experienced operators. Using real time imaging, cysts are percutaneously punctured, aspirated, injected with a scolicidal agent, and then reaspirated (with or without a drainage catheter).

Hepatic Abscesses

Pyogenic Abscess

Patients with bacterial liver abscess usually have right upper quadrant pain, fever, and leukocytosis. The alkaline phosphatase level is elevated in most patients. Ultrasound imaging usually shows a hypoechoic mass, often associated with a hyperechoic wall. CT usually shows a fluid density lesion, which may have a hypervascular wall. Although hepatic abscess may develop as a consequence of hematogenous seeding from any site, most result from a gastrointestinal (i.e., diverticulitis or appendicitis) or biliary tract source of infection.

Percutaneous aspiration and drain placement aid in the diagnosis and resolution of the infectious process. Antimicrobial therapy is directed by the results of blood and abscess cultures. Biliary stenting may be required if biliary obstruction contributed to the abscess formation. The source of the bacteria should be identified and treated.

Amebic Abscess

Although rare in the United States, amebic liver abscess is relatively common in regions endemic for amebiasis, including Central and South America. For this reason, it should be considered in immigrants from, or travelers to, these regions. Liver abscess occurs in as many as 10% of patients with amebiasis and the liver is one of the most common sites of extraintestinal infection. Antiamebic antibodies can be found in almost all patients with infection, and is a useful test in patients who are not from endemic areas (many patients from endemic areas, without active amebiasis, will test positive). Percutaneous aspiration shows a sterile fluid that has a characteristic "anchovy paste" appearance. These abscesses respond dramatically to metronidazole. Unlike pyogenic abscesses, they do not require percutaneous drainage.

EVALUATION AND MANAGEMENT OF PORTAL HYPERTENSION

Portal hypertension is defined as an abnormally high pressure in the portal vein or its tributaries. The portal circulation is shown in Figure 18-14. Normal portal venous pressure is 5 to 10 mm Hg; by definition, portal hypertension is present with portal venous pressure above 12 to 15 mm Hg or wedged hepatic venous pressure more than 5 mm Hg above pressure in the inferior vena cava. Wedged hepatic venous pressure is obtained by cannulation of a hepatic vein via a transjugular route.

Most cases of portal hypertension are generalized, with elevated pressure in the portal vein and all of its tributaries. Sinistral, or left-sided, portal hypertension is a relatively uncommon form of portal hypertension where thrombosis of the splenic vein, usually caused by pancreatitis or pancreatic tumor, produces increased pressure in the spleen with splenomegaly and secondary hypersplenism. Another consequence of this disorder is the development of isolated gastric varices with splenic venous return to the portal vein through the short gastric veins, the submucosal veins of the stomach, and the coronary vein. Splenectomy cures this compartmentalized form of portal hypertension.

Cirrhosis causes approximately 90% of all portal hypertension in the United States. Most cases of cirrhosis are caused by hepatitis C and/or chronic ethanol ingestion. Portal vein thrombosis accounts for 50% of cases of portal hypertension in children, often the consequence of umbilical venous catheterization in infancy. Portal hypertension occasionally results from excessive inflow, such as with a large arteriovenous fistula to a portal vein tributary. Obstruction of hepatic venous outflow can transmit high pressure to the portal vein.

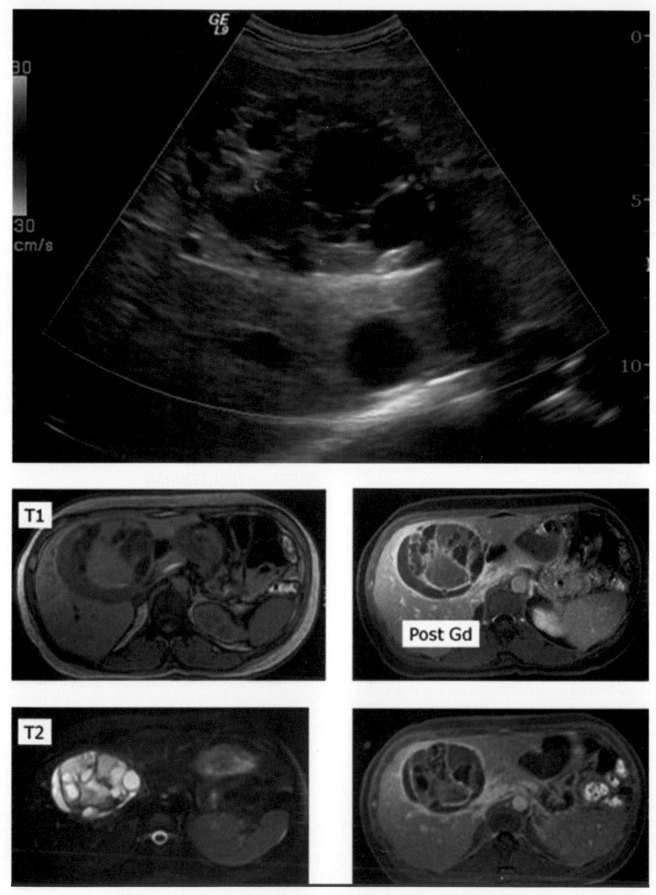

FIGURE 18-13. Hydatid liver disease. Hydatid cyst ultrasound (upper row) and MRI (lower two rows).

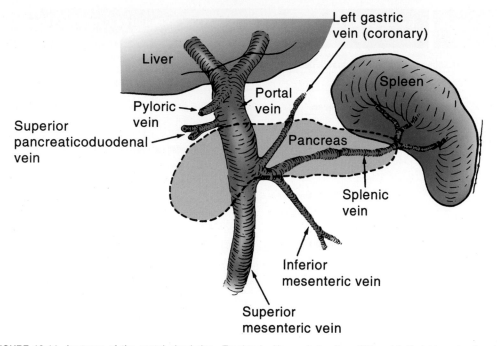

FIGURE 18-14. Anatomy of the portal circulation. (Reprinted with permission from Rikkers LF. Portal hypertension. In: Goldsmith HS, ed. *Practice of Surgery: General Surgery.* Vol. 3, Ch. 4. Philadelphia, PA: Harper & Row, 1981.)

The best-known example of outflow obstruction is the Budd-Chiari syndrome of hepatic venous occlusion, which can result from various thrombotic states or from vascular webs in the vena cava. Congestive heart failure, constrictive pericarditis, and severe tricuspid regurgitation are rare causes of portal hypertension in adults. Schistosomiasis is the most common worldwide cause of presinusoidal portal hypertension but is not found in the United States.

Compensation for elevated portal venous pressure occurs in part by dilation of the portal venous tributaries and in part by the development of collateral channels to the systemic venous system. Collateral portosystemic channels form at sites where portal and systemic veins normally meet (Figure 18-15). These sites include the submucosal veins of the esophagus, which communicate with the azygous system and produce esophagogastric varices; the hemorrhoidal veins, which communicate with the iliac system and produce anorectal hemorrhoids; the umbilical vein, which communicates with veins of the anterior abdominal wall that form the caput Medusae; and retroperitoneal veins, which communicate with the vena cava. Adhesions to the abdominal wall also may carry large portosystemic collateral veins.

Liver transplantation for appropriate and eligible candidates represents definitive treatment for all of the complications of portal hypertension, and some complications are also treated with nontransplant operations. At times, the surgeon is asked to consider operative treatment of other problems such as abdominal wall hernias, which may be exacerbated by portal hypertension. Surgery in patients with portal hypertension represents a formidable challenge and only should be undertaken for well-considered indications. Specific problems include bleeding from collateral vessels when entering and working within the abdomen, hemodynamic abnormalities related to drainage of large volumes of ascites, and postoperative hepatic decompensation related to general anesthesia. A number of scoring systems have been used to predict mortality from complications of portal hypertension, with or without operative therapy; these include the Modified Child-Pugh Classification and Model for End-Stage Liver Disease (MELD) score (Table 18-3) and are discussed further in subsequent sections of this chapter.

Complications of portal hypertension include ascites, hepatic encephalopathy, gastrointestinal variceal bleeding, hepatorenal syndrome, hydrothorax, spontaneous bacterial

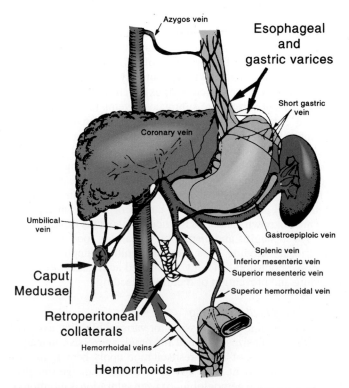

FIGURE 18-15. Sites of portal systemic collateralization. (Reprinted with permission from Rikkers LF. Portal hypertension. In: Goldsmith HS, ed. *Practice of Surgery: General Surgery.* Vol. 3, Ch. 4. Philadelphia, PA: Harper & Row, 1981.)

TABLE 18-3	Two Models Used for Predicting Survival in Patients with Liver Disease (Child-Pugh Score [CPS] and Model of End-Stage Liver Disease [MELD])

Models for Predicting Survival in Patients with Decompensated Cirrhosis

Child-Pugh Score				Model of End-Stage Liver Disease (MELD) Score

	Points Given			MELD = 3.8 Log^{e}TB + 11.2 Log^{e}INR + 9.6 Log^{e}Cr + 6.4
	1	**2**	**3**	
Bilirubin (mg/dL)	<2	2–3	>3	**Variables**
Albumin (g/dL)	>3.5	2.8–3.5	<2.8	TB = Serum total bilirubin (mg/dL)
Prothrombin time(s)	1–3	4–6	>6	INR = International normalized ratio
Ascites	None	Mild	Mod	Cr = Serum creatinine (mg/dL)
Encephalopathy	None	Grade I–II	Grade III–IV	**Rules**
	Classification			Any lab value <1 is rounded to 1
	A	**B**	**C**	Serum creatinine >4 or hemodialysis is rounded to 4
Total points	5–6	7–9	>9	Scores range from 6 (least ill) to 40 (most ill)
				All scores >40 are given a score of 40
				For age ≤12 use the PELD score instead
				A modification for cancer patients exists

Adapted with permission from Pugh RN, Murray-Lyon IM, Dawson JL, Pietroni MC, Williams R., Transection of the oesophagus for bleeding oesophageal varices. Br J Surg. 1973;60:646.

Adapted with permission from Kamath PS, Wiesner RH, Malinchoc M, Kremers W, Therneau TM, Kosberg CL, et al. A model to predict survival in patients with endstage liver disease. Hepatology. 2001;33:464–470.

peritonitis, hepatopulmonary syndrome, and portopulmonary hypertension. Evaluation and management of variceal bleeding, ascites, and encephalopathy will be considered in detail.

Variceal Bleeding

Although ascites and encephalopathy cause substantial morbidity in patients with portal hypertension, bleeding from esophageal varices is the complication associated with the greatest mortality. The fraction of cirrhotic patients with esophageal varices is not known, but only approximately 30% of patients who have varices will experience bleeding.

Esophageal varices are submucosal veins in the short gastric and coronary to azygous collateral venous routes that become dilated and fragile in the presence of portal hypertension. Gastric varices also may be present and are somewhat more difficult to treat. While variceal bleeding is known to occur when the portal systemic pressure gradient exceeds 12 mm Hg, and the risk of variceal rupture varies directly with intraluminal pressure, the exact causes of rupture at a given time are unknown. Theories include spontaneous rupture, erosion by esophagitis and disruption by passing food.

Variceal bleeding is a life-threatening complication of portal hypertension. Therapy is directed at cessation of acute bleeding and prevention of recurrent bleeding.

Cessation of Acute Bleeding

The mortality rate per admission for variceal bleeding exceeds 20% and emphasizes the need for rapid, aggressive management. The ABCs of acute resuscitation apply here as in any ill or injured patient. The airway is secured, oxygen is also administered, and hemoglobin–oxygen saturation is monitored closely. The initial goal of treatment is volume resuscitation with large-bore intravenous lines to maintain tissue perfusion.

Lost blood is replaced with blood and components with the goal of restoring adequate circulatory volume while avoiding excessive volume replacement with crystalloid solutions that may promote ascites formation and also rebleeding, since variceal pressure varies directly with central venous pressure. Urinary output is the best clinical measure of adequate circulatory resuscitation and perfusion. For this reason, a urinary catheter is placed early in the resuscitation, and hemoglobin and coagulation factors are monitored frequently to determine the adequacy of blood component therapy. Short-term antibiotic prophylaxis also is utilized because of the infection risk in these critically ill patients.

It is critical to establish the diagnosis of variceal bleeding and exclude other causes of gastrointestinal hemorrhage early in the course of management so that therapy can be directed properly and specifically. While the diagnoses of cirrhosis and portal hypertension can often be made from the history and physical examination (showing stigmata of portal hypertension such as temporal muscle wasting, parotid enlargement, spider angiomata, gynecomastia, testicular atrophy, ascites, and splenomegaly), numerous studies show that as many as half of acute upper gastrointestinal bleeding episodes in cirrhotic patients originate from nonvariceal sources such as peptic ulcer disease and Mallory-Weiss mucosal tears at the gastroesophageal junction. For this reason, upper gastrointestinal endoscopy is essential to determine the source of bleeding and is performed as early as possible after onset of bleeding. Gastric lavage before endoscopy is beneficial both in achieving a thorough examination and in purging blood from the gut, thereby diminishing risk of subsequent encephalopathy from the added protein load. Lavage is not performed with iced solutions because these cause rapid loss of body temperature, which can hinder the coagulation process. During endoscopy, the diagnosis is made by visualizing the bleeding varix or by documenting the presence of varices and the absence of other bleeding sources.

Pharmacologic Therapy

As pharmacologic therapy for variceal hemorrhage is usually well tolerated with limited adverse effects, even if there is a nonvariceal cause of bleeding, treatment with vasoactive agents is initiated before the diagnosis of variceal bleeding is confirmed. Various agents are utilized.

Intravenous **somatostatin** acts promptly to decrease variceal bleeding by splanchnic vasoconstriction and decrease of portal venous flow. Somatostatin diminishes or halts variceal bleeding in more than 50% of patients and has few clinically significant side effects. Intravenous vasopressin also acts by splanchnic vasoconstriction, but in prospective randomized trials were not as effective as somatostatin in controlling variceal hemorrhage. Also, the vasoconstrictive effect of vasopressin is not limited to the splanchnic circulation and may cause serious ischemic complications such as myocardial infarction and limb ischemia in patients with atherosclerotic disease. As the simultaneous infusion of nitroglycerin with vasopressin ameliorates these complications and may help to stop variceal bleeding, the two drugs usually are used in combination.

Endoscopic Therapy

Endoscopic therapy is effective in approximately 80% of patients with acute variceal hemorrhage. Endoscopic sclerotherapy and band ligation are the two principal procedures that are utilized.

In endoscopic sclerotherapy, small volumes of caustic solutions are injected either into or adjacent to varices to induce edema and scarring and obliterate the variceal lumen. A number of complications can occur, including additional bleeding from torn varices, ulceration of the epithelium over the varix, esophageal perforation, and dissemination of the sclerosing agent to the pulmonary or systemic circulation.

To accomplish luminal obliteration of the varix without many of the complications of sclerotherapy, band ligation of varices is now generally used. This treatment is similar to the banding of internal hemorrhoids. A hollow extension of the endoscope is placed in contact with the epithelium surrounding a varix, and suction is applied to elevate both the epithelium and the underlying varix. A very small rubber band is then used to encircle and tightly gather the varix, thereby obliterating its lumen. Banding is at least as effective as sclerotherapy in the cessation of acute variceal hemorrhage, without the potential morbidity, and has become the preferred form of endoscopic therapy in acute bleeding.

One limitation to both forms of endoscopic therapy is that the varices must be seen clearly for accurate and safe treatment. Massive active bleeding that fills the lumen of the esophagus may preclude endoscopic therapy. Another limitation of endoscopic therapy is that it is much more difficult to apply safely to gastric varices than to esophageal varices.

Luminal Tamponade

When both pharmacologic and endoscopic treatments fail to control variceal hemorrhage, luminal tamponade can be used. The **Sengstaken-Blakemore tube** (Figure 18-16) is one specific device available for luminal tamponade, but a number of other tubes with various modifications are available. All of these devices have a distal port to evacuate the luminal

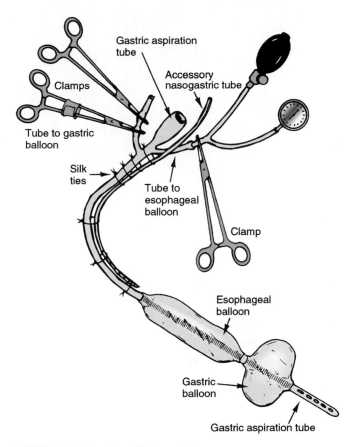

FIGURE 18-16. Sengstaken-Blakemore tube.

contents of the stomach, a large round balloon that places traction on the gastric fundus and occludes the submucosal veins that approach the esophagus, and a more proximal cylindrical balloon to provide direct tamponade to the esophageal varices. If the available device does not have a port proximal to the esophageal balloon to remove swallowed saliva, a second tube is placed for this purpose.

When properly applied, luminal tamponade effectively controls variceal bleeding in approximately 90% of cases. A number of serious complications may occur, including aspiration, airway obstruction, and esophageal injury (ulceration, necrosis, and rupture). Placement and maintenance of these tubes requires experience and a very strict protocol. As rebleeding occurs in half of patients when tamponade is released, and as tamponade can be applied only for a relatively short period of 24 to 36 hours because of the risk of tissue necrosis, subsequent measures are needed for further treatment following use of tamponade.

Transjugular Intrahepatic Portacaval Shunt

A **transjugular intrahepatic portacaval shunt** (TIPS) is an interventional radiologic procedure used to treat various complications of portal hypertension by decreasing portal pressure. A semirigid wire is passed from the internal jugular vein into a large hepatic vein with subsequent puncture of the hepatic vein wall, the intervening hepatic parenchyma, and the wall of a large portal vein branch in the vicinity. An expandable metallic stent covered with polytetrafluoroethylene (PTFE) is then used to dilate and maintain a channel between the portal and hepatic venous branches, effectively creating a portacaval shunt within the liver. The diameter of the channel is adjusted until the reduction in portal pressure is

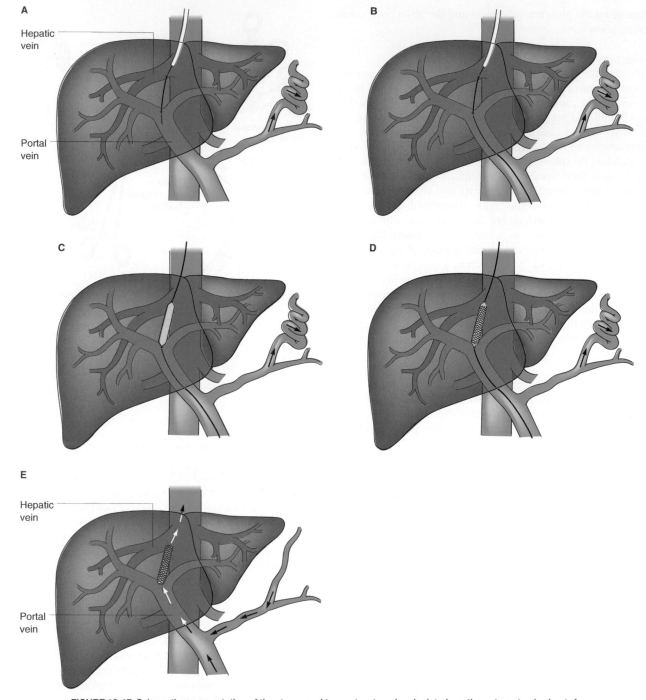

FIGURE 18-17. Schematic representation of the steps used to create a transjugular intrahepatic portosystemic shunt. **A, B,** Via the jugular-hepatic vein route, the portal vein is accessed through the liver parenchyma. **C,** The track is diluted. **D, E,** The stent is then placed over a balloon. (From Zemel G, Katzen BT, Becker GJ, et al. Percutaneous transjugular portosystemic shunt. *JAMA* 1991;266:390, with permission. In Mulholland MW et al., eds. *Greenfield's Surgery.* 4th ed. Philadelphia, PA: Lippincott Williams & Wilkins, 2006:941.)

sufficient to halt the variceal bleeding (Figure 18-17). TIPS is accomplished successfully in approximately 95% of patients and, except in profoundly coagulopathic patients, is highly effective in controlling acute variceal hemorrhage. TIPS complications are discussed below.

After the acute variceal hemorrhage is controlled, attention is turned to correcting ascites, encephalopathy, and other problems including infection and malnutrition. As the risk of repeated bleeding approaches 70% once variceal bleeding has occurred, therapies to prevent recurrent variceal hemorrhage should be initiated following the index bleeding episode.

Prevention of Recurrent Variceal Hemorrhage

A number of options are available to prevent recurrent bleeding. The choice of therapy for an individual patient depends on several factors, including the etiology of liver disease and an estimation of the functional reserve of the liver. The Modified Child-Pugh classification (Table 18-3) uses readily available clinical information to make this estimation. CT angiography (Figure 18-18) may be utilized to show the portal venous anatomy, the presence of portal or splenic vein thrombosis, and the left renal vein and inferior vena cava that are of interest as outflow tracts when surgical shunts are considered.

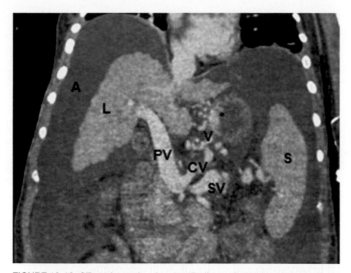

FIGURE 18-18. CT angiography showing findings of portal hypertension and portal venous anatomy including a shrunken, cirrhotic liver (*L*), splenomegaly (*S*), ascites (*A*), esophageal varices (*V*), portal vein (*PV*), splenic vein (*SV*), and coronary vein (*CV*).

Wedged hepatic venous pressure may be obtained to measure the portal systemic pressure gradient.

Options for prevention of recurrent variceal bleeding include medical, endoscopic, radiologic, and surgical therapy. Medical therapy centers on the use of β-blockade to decrease portal venous flow and commonly is used as an adjunct to other treatments. The choice among the more invasive options should consider the functional hepatic reserve, the reliability of the patient to return for additional studies and treatment, and the patient's ongoing access to prompt medical care.

Endoscopic therapy (Figure 18-19) is often used as primary treatment, regardless of the status of hepatic reserve, and TIPS is used increasingly as definitive therapy, either primarily or after failure of endoscopic therapy. The incidence of rebleeding is higher with endoscopic therapy than with

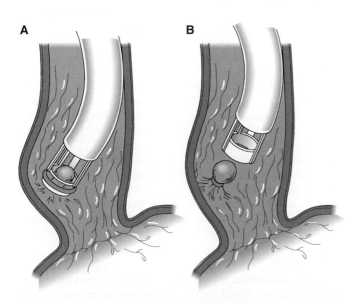

FIGURE 18-19. Endoscopic ligation of esophageal varices. The device used for ligation is based on the standard Barron-type ligator for the treatment of anal hemorrhoids. The esophageal varix is drawn up into the ligating device with suction (**A**), and the base of the varix is ligated with an O-ring (**B**). Up to six varices can be treated at a single session. (Reprinted with permission from Mulholland MW et al. eds. *Greenfield's Surgery.* 4th ed. Philadelphia, PA: Lippincott Williams & Wilkins, 2006:940.)

TIPS, while the incidence of encephalopathy is greater with TIPS than endoscopic therapy. The long-term survival is comparable for the two. Both of these modalities require careful ongoing surveillance. Surgical shunts, although more invasive and associated with greater initial procedural risk, have excellent long-term patency with a low risk of recurrent bleeding. Surgical shunts, now utilized far less frequently than in prior eras, are best suited for Child's A and B patients; the operative mortality in Child's C patients precludes shunting when less invasive options are available. While liver transplantation is performed for liver failure and not for variceal bleeding, all Child's C patients should undergo transplant evaluation.

Endoscopic Therapy

Sclerotherapy and banding, described above for use in acute bleeding, also are used to prevent recurrent bleeding. The aim is to eradicate all visible esophageal varices during a series of endoscopic sessions over the first few weeks and then to identify and treat new varices through continuing surveillance. One problem with endoscopic therapy is that eradication of esophageal varices often leads to the development of gastric varices, for which endoscopic treatment is far less successful. Rebleeding rates approach 60% with endoscopic therapy, but the episodes are generally less severe than the primary episode. Overall failure rate with long-term endoscopic therapy is approximately 30%.

Transjugular Intrahepatic Portacaval Shunt

TIPS is used for acute and chronic variceal bleeding but has two major problems. The first is a rate of encephalopathy that approaches 30%, a problem with any type of portosystemic shunt. The second is a high rate of thrombosis due to intimal hyperplasia along the intrahepatic course of the metallic shunt. Stenosis or occlusion occurs in more than half of patients by 1 year after TIPS placement, with an 18% to 30% incidence of recurrent variceal hemorrhage. TIPS patients are monitored with Doppler ultrasonography every 3 months; if shunt stenosis or occlusion is found, dilation or restenting is needed to prevent recurrent bleeding.

Surgical Therapy

With the advent of endoscopic therapy, TIPS, and liver transplantation, surgical shunting to prevent recurrent variceal hemorrhage is now uncommon. Three forms of surgical shunts have been used.

In **portosystemic** (total) **shunts**, large caliber connections are made between the portal and systemic circulations, either by direct anastomosis or use of an interposition graft. The many options (Figure 18-20) are hemodynamically equivalent. While portosystemic shunts very effectively prevent bleeding and control ascites, they divert portal flow to such a degree that hepatic functional deterioration and encephalopathy occur frequently. Both TIPS and surgically constructed nonselective central shunts allow portal blood to bypass the metabolic actions of the liver. As a result, amino acid imbalances may occur and are believed to play an important role in development of hepatic encephalopathy.

Selective shunts, including the distal splenorenal and coronary–caval shunt, decompress varices and prevent variceal bleeding while preserving portal flow to the liver. They do so by decompressing only the gastrosplenic compartment into the systemic circulation and are as effective as portosystemic shunts at preventing variceal hemorrhage, with much lower rates of encephalopathy. Selective shunts have excellent

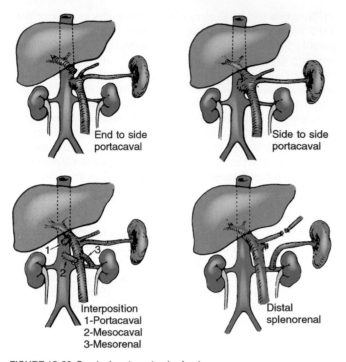

FIGURE 18-20. Surgical portosystemic shunts.

long-term patency. The small bore or partial portacaval shunt, designed to achieve the same goals as selective shunts, is simpler to perform and has excellent long-term patency with much lower rates of encephalopathy than with total shunts.

Nonshunt operations control bleeding by interrupting blood flow to the varices. One option is division and reanastomosis of the esophagus, which is usually done with an end-to-end stapling device. Another is devascularization of the stomach and lower esophagus, usually with splenectomy, to halt flow through the varices. Although nonshunt operations are successful in other parts of the world for certain diseases, they are rarely performed in the United States.

Prognosis
Regardless of the choice of therapy for patients with bleeding varices, the most important predictor of long-term survival is the functional reserve of the liver. Because cirrhosis tends to progress relentlessly, only 50% of patients who have had variceal bleeding survive for 5 years without liver transplantation.

Ascites
Ascites is the accumulation of serous fluid in the peritoneal cavity. In portal hypertension, ascites forms as a result of increased hydrostatic pressure and decreased colloid oncotic pressure caused by deficient protein production. This situation favors transudation of fluid out of the vascular space, into the hepatic parenchyma, and ultimately into the peritoneal cavity. The renin–angiotensin–aldosterone system is involved, as are mediators including nitric oxide, atrial natriuretic peptide, and prostaglandins. Ascitic volumes of 1500 mL or more are detected with physical findings including dependent dullness to percussion and presence of a fluid wave. Ultrasonography or CT can detect volumes as low as 100 mL.

While portal hypertension due to chronic liver disease is by far the most common cause of ascites, ascites may occur with a number of other conditions, including hypoproteinemic states (nephrotic syndrome, protein-losing enteropathy, malnutrition); heart failure; carcinomatosis; tuberculosis; pancreatic, chyle, or bile leakage; and collagen-vascular diseases. The differential diagnosis emphasizes the need for diagnostic paracentesis in the patient with newly diagnosed ascites. Studies on the fluid should include cytology, cell count and differential, amylase, triglyceride and protein levels, pH, and cultures.

In patients with portal hypertension related to cirrhosis and without complicating features, the cell count and differential of ascitic fluid usually shows a predominance of monocytes with a total neutrophil cell count below 250 cells/mL. Cytology shows nonneoplastic cells, amylase level and triglyceride levels are less than or equal to serum levels, and bacterial and fungal cultures are negative. The pH is usually 7.3 or greater in noninfected ascites, and the protein content is usually <2.5 g. Serum-ascites albumin gradient is ≥1.1 g/dL with portal hypertension and <1.1 g/dL with other causes.

Morbidity from ascites due to portal hypertension may be substantial. Umbilical, groin, and other abdominal wall hernias can enlarge dramatically with the added pressure of ascites. The skin overlying hernias can become thinned and ulcerated; rupture of the skin may occur and has been associated with a high mortality rate.

Spontaneous bacterial peritonitis (SBP) occurs in approximately 10% of cirrhotic patients with ascites. It is usually associated with an ascitic fluid white blood cell count of more than 250 cells/mL and a predominance of neutrophils. Most infections are monomicrobial with enteric organisms. The mechanism of inoculation is debated, with theories including gut bacterial translocation, seeding of ascites from other sources, and impaired reticuloendothelial clearance of portal bacteremia. Mortality rate is 50% within 1 year. SBP is treated with aggressive antibiotic therapy, and secondary peritonitis due to perforation of an abdominal viscus or other etiology must be excluded.

Acute renal failure in patients with ascites rarely occurs spontaneously but may be precipitated by overzealous use of diuretics. The more typical scenario is development of hepatorenal syndrome (HRS). The decreased circulating plasma volume in patients with significant ascites leads to decreased renal blood flow, increased circulating levels of aldosterone, and redistribution of renal blood flow. While HRS is classically characterized by oliguria and low urinary sodium concentration in the presence of progressively raising plasma creatinine, it remains a diagnosis of exclusion. Thus, acute tubular necrosis (ATN) and other causes of prerenal disease must remain within the differential diagnosis. There is no clear evidence to show that HRS represents anything other than profound prerenal azotemia secondary to intravascular volume depletion. Renal histology shows no pathognomonic changes. Liver transplantation is the best treatment; vasodilators, octreotide, and alpha-adrenergic agonists (midodrine) have been used with limited success.

Treatment
Medical management effectively controls ascites in more than 90% of patients. Fluid intake is moderately restricted, and sodium intake is limited to <40 mEq/day. Diuresis begins with spironolactone, an aldosterone antagonist, to promote sodium excretion. The dose is gradually increased until urinary excretion of sodium exceeds that of potassium. If further diuresis is necessary, loop or thiazide diuretics are added.

When the ascitic volume severely limits respiration or mobility and rapid decompression is needed, therapeutic paracentesis is performed. Large volumes of ascites (8 to 10 L) can safely be removed in one session. During paracentesis, albumin is administered intravenously (8 g/L removed) to replace protein and avoid hypovolemia.

Rarely, when medical measures and paracentesis fail, more invasive treatment is required. Two types of surgical shunt procedures have been utilized for control of ascites.

Peritoneal venous shunts were popular in the 1970s but are used less frequently today. The shunt tubing, approximately the diameter of intravenous tubing, originates in the peritoneal cavity and runs subcutaneously to insertion in the internal jugular vein. The peritoneal end has multiple side-hole perforations, and the tubing contains a one-way valve that prevents reflux of blood. When functioning properly, these devices restore circulating volume and enhance urinary output. Placement is technically simple, but peritoneal venous shunts have with a number of complications including infection, occlusion of the tubing by proteinaceous debris, congestive heart failure, and disseminated intravascular coagulation. Variceal bleeding may occur as a result of the increased venous pressure associated with increased circulating volume. No survival advantages to the use of these shunts over medical measures have been shown.

TIPS and surgical shunts provide control of ascites by reducing portal pressure. TIPS has now replaced surgical shunting but is not always successful in controlling ascites and, as noted above, may precipitate development of encephalopathy.

Hepatic Encephalopathy

Hepatic encephalopathy is a neuropsychiatric disorder that occurs commonly in patients with severe hepatic insufficiency. Clinical features include confusion, obtundation, tremor, asterixis, and fetor hepaticus, a sweet, slightly feculent smell of the breath noted in advanced liver disease. Four stages of encephalopathy are recognized: Stage I, mild confusion or lack of awareness; Stage II, lethargy; Stage III, somnolent but arousable; Stage IV, coma. Even with normal consciousness, patients with advanced liver disease show impaired psychomotor testing.

The pathogenesis of encephalopathy is not understood. A number of theories have been advanced, including increased circulating levels of nitrogenous toxins, particularly ammonia; the presence of false neurotransmitters such as aromatic amino acids; and the concerted effect of two or more metabolic abnormalities such as alkalosis, hypoxia, infection, and electrolyte imbalances. Ammonia is believed to have a key role. Ammonia in the gut normally enters the portal circulation and is converted to urea by the liver; with hepatocellular dysfunction and portosystemic collaterals (or shunts), ammonia enters the systemic circulation, crosses the blood-brain barrier, and induces neuronal edema.

Certain factors are known to precipitate encephalopathy, including infection, gastrointestinal bleeding, constipation, dehydration, sedatives and opioids, metabolic disorders, and portosystemic shunts. In some cases, the ingestion of even modest amounts of dietary protein will induce encephalopathy.

The diagnosis of hepatic encephalopathy is made clinically. The serum ammonia level is often elevated in encephalopathic patients, but this test lacks sufficient specificity to be diagnostic. Certain electroencephalographic patterns are seen in encephalopathy but also are not diagnostic. Other causes of mental status alterations must be excluded, including acute intoxication, organic brain syndrome and infection, head injury, or central nervous system tumor.

Treatment

Encephalopathy is usually reversible with medical measures. Much of the treatment is empiric and not consistently supported by controlled trials. Any precipitating causes of encephalopathy such as infection should be sought and corrected. The airway is protected, sedation is avoided, and nutrition is supported with moderate restriction of protein intake. In patients who have gastrointestinal bleeding or constipation, the gut is purged.

A number of pharmacologic agents are used. Lactulose, a nonabsorbable disaccharide, is administered by mouth, nasogastric tube, or enema. Lactulose acts as a cathartic and also alters colonic pH, which traps ammonia in the lumen. Intraluminal antibiotics including neomycin, metronidazole, and rifaximin decrease ammonia production by decreasing urease-producing bacterial flora. Zinc supplementation, benzodiazepine receptor antagonists, and probiotics have shown benefit for treatment of encephalopathy in some trials.

END-STAGE LIVER DISEASE AND LIVER TRANSPLANTATION

End-stage liver disease has many recognized complications, some of which are life threatening. Liver transplantation is now considered standard treatment for many causes of acute and chronic liver failure. However, significant risks are associated with the transplant procedure, and it is costly. Additionally, there is limited organ availability, and the procedure commits the transplant recipient to lifelong immunosuppressive therapy, with its inherent risks. Thus, physicians must exercise careful judgment to determine which patients can be treated with medical measures or less complicated surgical procedures and which ones are likely to require transplantation because of disease progression. Please also see Chapter 23, Transplantation, for further discussion regarding liver transplantation.

Indications for Transplantation

Patients who are under consideration for liver transplantation usually have irreversible hepatic failure for which there is no suitable alternative therapy. Thus, for most patients, medical measures are tried initially to treat specific complications associated with cirrhosis and liver failure. Transplantation is considered only when these measures are not effective. Three common severe complications seen in association with end-stage liver disease are hepatic encephalopathy, intractable ascites (which may be associated with spontaneous bacterial peritonitis), and variceal hemorrhage. When these occur as isolated complicating factors in patients with otherwise well-preserved hepatic synthetic function, then attention can be directed toward correcting the isolated problem (e.g., placement of a TIPS). However, when complications occur in the patient with advanced liver disease, they serve as markers of declining hepatic functional reserve, and consideration is usually given to liver transplantation.

Liver transplantation in adults is generally performed for two major indications: chronic, progressive advanced liver disease and **fulminant hepatic failure,** the latter being present for about 5% or less of all liver transplants. Other indications

TABLE 18-4	Absolute Contraindications to Liver Transplantation
Uncontrolled sepsis	
Extrahepatic malignancy	
Active alcohol or substance abuse	
Advanced cardiac or pulmonary disease	

include unresectable malignancies, usually in patients with some underlying liver disease and inborn errors of metabolism in patients who may not have underlying cirrhosis. Table 18-4 lists contraindications to liver transplantation.

Chronic liver disease usually results from either hepatocellular injury (e.g., viral hepatitis, alcohol-induced injury) or cholestatic liver disease (e.g., primary biliary cirrhosis, sclerosing cholangitis) (discussed later). Because of the risks and expense associated with transplantation, patients are usually considered for this procedure when their 1- to 2-year survival rate is estimated at 50% or less. Although it is sometimes difficult to predict expected survival in patients with advanced liver disease, certain markers assist in this prediction. For example, in patients with chronic liver disease, clinical factors that indicate advanced liver disease include nutritional impairment and muscle wasting, hepatic encephalopathy, difficult-to-control ascites, variceal hemorrhage, and renal insufficiency.

Laboratory parameters may be altered depending on the etiology of liver failure. When cirrhosis has a hepatocellular cause, the prothrombin time is prolonged beyond 18 to 20 seconds (international normalized ratio [INR] $\geq$ 2.0). A serum albumin level of <2.5 to 3.0 g/L is associated with diminished hepatic synthetic reserve. Patients whose cirrhosis has a cholestatic etiology may have near-normal prothrombin times and serum albumin values of 3 g/L or greater. However, elevation of the serum bilirubin above 10 mg/dL suggests advanced liver disease in this group. Laboratory parameters are only guides to hepatic functional reserve and must be considered in the context of the clinical condition of the individual patient. When patients have complications of liver disease (e.g., difficult-to-manage ascites, variceal hemorrhage, marginally controlled encephalopathy), the decision to proceed with transplantation rather than to continue observation of the patient is likely to be made.

In an effort to predict the mortality risk (without transplant or other intervention) for patients with chronic end-stage liver disease, MELD was developed (Table 18-3). This scoring system utilizes only three objective parameters, the serum bilirubin, INR, and creatinine. Using these variables, a MELD score is determined, ranging from 7 to 40, and this has been found to correlate with 3-month mortality without transplantation. Currently, patients are generally not considered for liver transplantation based on chronic liver disease until their MELD score reaches 15.

Chronic and Progressive Advanced Liver Disease
Chronic Hepatitis C
Chronic hepatitis C infection is one of the most common indications for liver transplantation today. Hepatitis C was previously categorized under the heading non-A, non-B hepatitis, but molecular techniques allowed identification of this single-stranded RNA virus in 1989. Although it was a common cause of transfusion-associated hepatitis in the past, this risk is now

<0.05% per unit of blood product transfused with current testing of banked blood. Many patients with chronic hepatitis C have such identifiable risk factors as previous drug use, previous transfusions, and multiple sexual partners, but up to 50% have no definable risk factors. Its course is usually slowly progressive, and most patients have chronic infection for 10 to 20 years before complications of liver disease occur or a liver transplant is needed. Only approximately 20% of patients clear the hepatitis C virus in response to acute infection.

After liver transplantation for chronic hepatitis C, reinfection of the transplanted liver is nearly universal, but fortunately, the course of hepatocellular injury is indolent in most patients. New strategies, including antiviral therapies, are under investigation, but no effective measures to prevent allograft infection have been established. Although the short-term results of liver transplantation for hepatitis C are satisfactory in most cases, there can be development of cirrhosis in the allograft leading to graft failure.

Chronic Hepatitis B
Chronic hepatitis B infection, unlike hepatitis C infection, shows a marked propensity to cause significant hepatocellular injury in the transplanted allograft if untreated, with a high incidence of early graft loss and death of the transplant recipient. Although at one time hepatitis B infection was a contraindication to liver transplantation, the use of hepatitis B immunoglobulin (HBIG) to suppress viral expression along with antiviral therapy (e.g., adefovir) has been very effective in preventing recurrence of HBV in the posttransplant period in the majority of patients. Fortunately, the universal use of HBV vaccination in the United States has markedly reduced this as an indication for transplantation. Chronic hepatitis B infection is still endemic in many regions of the world and can be seen in immigrants to the United States.

Alcoholic Liver Disease
Transplantation for alcoholic liver disease is one of the most controversial indications for liver transplantation. With intensive pretransplant screening, including completion of an alcohol rehabilitation program and a period of supervised abstinence (usually $\geq$6 months), the risk of recidivism is <10% to 15%. Of those who consume alcohol after transplantation, continued alcohol use to the point of causing liver disease in the allograft is extremely rare. For reasons that are not well understood, as many as one-third of patients with a history of alcohol abuse also have serologic markers for hepatitis C infection without other known risk factors.

Autoimmune Hepatitis
Autoimmune hepatitis can usually be distinguished from other causes of chronic liver disease on the basis of immunologic and serologic testing. These patients usually have positive antinuclear or other self-directed antibodies. Initial treatment is usually with immunosuppressive medication, including corticosteroids and azathioprine. Patients in whom this treatment fails are usually good candidates for liver transplantation. Recurrent disease does not usually occur in the transplanted liver.

Hemochromatosis
Hemochromatosis is an autosomal recessive disease that causes iron overload as a result of excessive absorption from the intestinal tract. Multiple organs are affected by iron deposition, including the liver, heart, pancreas, spleen, adrenal glands, pituitary, and joints. The peak incidence of liver disease is between 40 and 60 years of age. Men show clinical manifestations and cirrhosis earlier than women, who may

be protected by iron loss during menstruation and childbirth. Treatment in recognized patients is with serial phlebotomy. Withdrawal of 500 mL blood/week is often required until the excessive iron stores are depleted. Effective treatment may reverse many of the damaging effects of iron deposition. Hemochromatosis is associated with a significant risk of hepatocellular carcinoma, up to 200 times that of other patients with cirrhosis. This risk is not fully diminished by phlebotomy. Liver transplantation is effective for patients with hemochromatosis and end-stage cirrhosis, but may be complicated by the preexisting cardiomyopathy and diabetes often found in these patients. The increased absorption of iron continues after liver transplantation, necessitating careful surveillance, even in patients who undergo successful transplantation.

Wilson's Disease

Wilson's disease is a rare autosomal recessive disorder of copper metabolism. Patients have increased deposition of copper in the liver, corneas (Kayser-Fleischer rings), kidneys, brain, and other locations. Patients with Wilson's disease have decreased circulating levels of ceruloplasmin and increased urinary excretion of copper. In normal individuals, excess copper is excreted into bile, but patients with Wilson's disease appear to have diminished biliary excretion. Some patients with Wilson's disease may have acute hepatitis and fulminant hepatic failure, whereas others have chronic progressive liver disease. Patients who have chronic liver disease are initially treated with D-penicillamine, which chelates copper and increases urinary excretion. Liver transplantation is effective in patients with fulminant failure and those in whom initial medical therapy fails. After transplantation, the metabolic defect is corrected, and no further damage from excessive copper occurs.

Alpha₁-Antitrypsin Deficiency

Alpha₁-antitrypsin deficiency is an autosomal dominant disorder that causes varying degrees of lung and liver damage over a patient's lifetime. The diagnosis is established by the determination of low levels of serum alpha₁-antitrypsin levels and confirmed with phenotypic studies. Most patients with liver disease have relatively mild pulmonary involvement, but more advanced pulmonary disease can complicate attempts at liver transplantation. There is no effective medical treatment, except for supportive measures. After liver transplantation, alpha₁-antitrypsin levels return to normal as the recipient takes on the phenotype of the transplanted liver.

Primary Biliary Cirrhosis

Primary biliary cirrhosis (PBC), which primarily affects middle-aged women, causes progressive bile duct destruction, probably from cytotoxic T cells. Patients often have pruritus without jaundice and usually have a positive antimitochondrial antibody finding (AMA ≥ 1/40). The course of the disease may be indolent, with patients living 10 years or longer from presentation. Elevation of the serum bilirubin level is associated with disease progression and usually prompts consideration of liver transplantation.

Primary Sclerosing Cholangitis

Primary sclerosing cholangitis (PSC) is an idiopathic disease that causes chronic fibrotic strictures that can involve any portion of the intrahepatic or extrahepatic biliary tree. One-half to two-thirds of patients also have inflammatory bowel disease, usually ulcerative colitis (UC). The risk of cholangiocarcinoma is increased in patients with primary sclerosing cholangitis, and rapid progression of disease should prompt a search for malignant strictures within the biliary tree. Disease progression in patients with primary sclerosing cholangitis is more variable than in patients with primary biliary cirrhosis. When patients become jaundiced and do not have a correctable biliary stricture (usually with stenting, but occasionally with surgical bypass), transplantation is considered. After transplantation, patients who have primary sclerosing cholangitis and ulcerative colitis require close colonic surveillance because of the increased risk of colon carcinoma.

Fulminant Hepatic Failure

Fulminant hepatic failure occurs when massive hepatocyte necrosis or severe impairment of liver function occurs. These patients do not have evidence of chronic liver disease. Liver dysfunction occurs within 8 to 12 weeks of the onset of symptoms. In these patients, hepatic encephalopathy develops and can progress to coma, brain stem herniation, and death without liver replacement. The INR is usually significantly prolonged, and reversible renal insufficiency (hepatorenal syndrome) may develop. Because these patients do not have chronic liver disease, muscle wasting and portal hypertension usually are not present. For this reason, liver transplantation is technically easier to perform than in the setting of chronic liver disease. However, because of the rapidly advancing nature of liver dysfunction in this setting, most patients die within 1 to 2 weeks of presentation without liver transplantation.

At most centers, fulminant hepatic failure is the indication for approximately 5% to 10% of liver transplantations, at most. Common causes of fulminant hepatic failure include viral infection and hepatotoxic drugs (e.g., anesthetic drugs, acetaminophen, isoniazid). Mushroom poisoning occurs in certain areas of the United States (Pacific Northwest) and Europe, where wild mushrooms are gathered and eaten by unsuspecting individuals.

Because of the rapid progression of fulminant hepatic failure, patients require an aggressive and accelerated workup in addition to aggressive supportive measures. Patients in hepatic coma usually undergo placement of an intracerebral pressure monitor so that adequate cerebral perfusion pressures can be maintained and increases in cerebral pressures minimized. To be successful, liver transplantation must be performed before irreversible brain injury occurs. Some patients with milder forms recover without liver transplantation, but the period of observation cannot extend for too long, or it may not be possible to obtain a suitable donor liver in time to perform a successful transplant. Thus, the decision to proceed with liver transplantation requires careful judgment by the treating physicians, who must weigh the risks of death without a transplant against the potential commitment to lifelong immunosuppression in a patient who might otherwise recover without this procedure. Clinical trials with extracorporeal liver support systems are underway. These systems may prevent cerebral injury while the injured liver recovers or until a suitable donor liver is located. In the future, these systems may successfully assist patients during this critical period.

SAMPLE QUESTIONS

Questions

Choose the best answer for each question.

1. A 52-year-old man with sigmoid colon adenocarcinoma is being evaluated for surgery. Preoperative workup reveals two liver mets. One met encases the right hepatic vein, and the other is in segment 4. There is no evidence of intrinsic liver disease and he is fit for surgery. From an anatomical prospective, which of the following surgical recommendations is most appropriate regarding his liver findings?

A. No appropriate surgical option due to burden of disease

B. Right trisectionectomy

C. Right posterior sectionectomy and resection of segment 4

D. Right anterior sectionectomy and resection of segment 4

E. Right hepatectomy and adjunct treatments for segment 4

2. A 60-year-old woman with chronic hepatitis C is brought to an acute care clinic by her family because of increasing confusion. Physical examination identifies jaundice, spider angiomata, and splenomegaly. Neurologic examination shows the patient to be lethargic; asterixis is present. Which of the following pharmacologic agents is most appropriate for treatment of this condition?

A. Spironolactone

B. Lactulose

C. Somatostatin

D. Ammonia

E. Midodrine

3. A 46-year-old man presents to the emergency department with hematemesis. There have been no prior episodes. He admits to drinking a pint of hard liquor daily for more than 10 years. Upper gastrointestinal endoscopy is performed and shows bleeding esophageal varices. Which of the following is the best management for this patient's bleeding?

A. Emergency surgical portosystemic shunt

B. Luminal tamponade

C. Endoscopic rubber band ligation

D. Transjugular intrahepatic portacaval shunt (TIPS)

E. Peritoneovenous shunt

Questions 4 and 5 are linked (same patient)

4. A 55-year-old man with known cirrhosis presents to the emergency department with severe abdominal pain. He appears ill. Blood pressure (BP) is 90/50 mm Hg, pulse is 110 beats/minute, respirations are 24/minute, and temperature is 38.8°C. The abdomen is distended and tender; a fluid wave is present. Blood test results are Hgb—13 g/dL, WBC—16,500/μL, normal electrolytes, urea nitrogen—10 mg/dL, and creatinine—1.1 mg/dL. A CT scan shows a small shrunken liver, an enlarged spleen, and a large volume of ascites. The ascites is sampled by paracentesis and the results of this analysis are WBC—750 cells/mL with 90% neutrophils; cultures are positive for a single Gram-negative aerobic organism. Which of the following is the most likely diagnosis?

A. Perforated viscus

B. Carcinomatosis

C. Mallory-Weiss tear

D. Spontaneous bacterial peritonitis

E. Hepatorenal syndrome

5. A 55-year-old man with known cirrhosis presents to the emergency department with severe abdominal pain. He appears ill. BP is 90/50 mm Hg, pulse is 110 beats/minute, respirations are 24/minute, and temperature is 38.8°C. The abdomen is distended and tender; a fluid wave is present. Blood test results are Hgb—13 g/dL, WBC—16,500/μL, normal electrolytes, urea nitrogen—10 mg/dL, and creatinine—1.1 mg/dL. A CT scan shows a small shrunken liver, an enlarged spleen, and a large volume of ascites. The ascites is sampled by paracentesis and the results of this analysis are WBC—750 cells/mL with 90% neutrophils; cultures are positive for a single Gram-negative aerobic organism. Which of the following is the most appropriate immediate therapy?

A. Exploratory laparotomy

B. Intraluminal antibiotics

C. Protein restriction

D. Intravenous antibiotics

E. Albumin

Answers and Explanations

1. Answer: B

A. Incorrect. Resection of all disease is achievable via a right trisectionectomy. If further concern regarding the function of the remnant liver exists, the surgeon may choose to employ techniques that hypertrophy the remnant liver (portal vein embolization or two-stage surgery).

B. Correct. It will result in complete surgical removal of liver disease (see answer for "A").

C. Incorrect. The right hepatic vein is encased, thus making a right posterior sectionectomy oncologically unsound.

D. Incorrect. The right hepatic vein is encased, thus making a right anterior sectionectomy oncologically unsound.

E. Incorrect. Inappropriate treatment since segment 4 met is resectable.

2. Answer: B

A. Incorrect. Spironolactone is a potassium-sparing diuretic used in patients with chronic liver disease and fluid retention (peripheral edema and ascites).

B. Correct. Lactulose is a nonabsorbable disaccharide that acts to increase stool transit and convert ammonia to a nonabsorbable ammonium ($NH4^+$). The goal of administration is for patients to have three to five soft stools per day.

C. Incorrect. Somatostatin is a GI peptide that regulates endocrine function. It can be used to decrease mesenteric blood flow in patients with portal hypertensive bleeding.

D. Incorrect. Increased levels of ammonia are associated with the development of hepatic encephalopathy, although it is unclear whether ammonia or an associated middle molecule is responsible for the alterations observed in mental status.

E. Incorrect. Midodrine is a vasoactive antihypotensive oral peptide used in patients with symptomatic orthostatic hypotension.

3. Answer: C

A. Incorrect. Emergency surgical portosystemic shunt procedures are associated with a very high morbidity and mortality rate, especially liver failure. In addition, other measures are usually able to control bleeding so that invasive procedures can be performed on a semielective basis under optimized conditions.

B. Incorrect. Luminal tamponade with a Sengstaken-Blakemore (or similar device) tube is usually employed as a last ditch effort in patients who have failed medical management and endoscopic therapy.

C. Correct. Endoscopic therapy with rubber band ligation has become the procedure of choice in patients with bleeding esophageal varices and should be performed as soon as the diagnosis is made and the patient initially stabilized.

D. Incorrect. Transjugular intrahepatic portacaval shunt (TIPS) is associated with a high rate of liver failure when performed as an emergency procedure in unstable patients. For this reason, TIPS should be performed on an elective basis in patients with well-compensated liver disease.

E. Incorrect. Peritoneovenous shunt placement is occasionally used for patients with intractable ascites but will have no effect on portal hypertension or variceal bleeding.

4. Answer: D

A. Incorrect. A perforated viscus is usually associated with free air on CT and plain films and will almost always show a polymicrobial infection on wound culture. In addition, the WBC count of the ascites in this setting is much greater, typically higher than 10,000.

B. Incorrect. Carcinomatosis can present with ascites, but this is usually gradual in onset and unassociated with severe pain. In addition, the liver size should be normal in size and contour and tumor nodules are usually visible throughout the abdomen.

C. Incorrect. A Mallory-Weiss tear occurs following forceful vomiting and results in significant upper GI hemorrhage. Ascites should not occur in this setting.

D. Correct. Spontaneous bacterial peritonitis (SBP) is thought to occur in the setting of ascites with immunosuppression (cirrhosis) and is a marker of advanced, end-stage liver disease. Bacterial translocation across the gut is thought to be the leading cause in most cases.

E. Incorrect. Hepatorenal syndrome (HRS) may occur in patients with advanced liver failure (cirrhosis) or fulminant liver failure. This condition is usually fatal unless the patient receives a liver transplant. In HRS, the kidneys are grossly and microscopically normal and usually have return of normal renal function, once a normal liver is in place.

5. Answer: D

A. Incorrect. Exploratory laparotomy is never required for SBP, since the cause is bacterial contamination of the ascitic fluid, and this almost always resolves with appropriate antibiotic therapy. In addition, exploratory laparotomy will place the patient at great risk to wound breakdown and ascitic fluid leak, which can be associated with disastrous consequences.

B Incorrect. Intraluminal antibiotics (e.g., neomycin) are sometimes used for treatment of hepatic encephalopathy, but because they are not absorbed from the GI tract, they are ineffective for treatment of systemic infection.

C. Incorrect. Protein restriction is sometimes required for treatment of hepatic encephalopathy but will have no effect on SBP.

D. Correct. In cases of SBP, culture of the ascitic fluid often shows a single organism but may not result in positive growth and clinical treatment decisions are made on an empiric basis, with antibiotic selection usually targeted toward enteric organisms.

E. Incorrect. Intravenous albumin has been shown to be beneficial for the treatment of associated renal insufficiency in patients with cirrhosis and SBP. However, this therapy would be considered an adjunct in their management and not primary treatment of the SBP per se.

19
Breast

GARY L. DUNNINGTON, M.D. • LECIA APANTAKU, M.D. • TED A. JAMES, M.D. •
SUSAN KAISER, M.D., PH.D. • ELIZABETH PERALTA, M.D.

Objectives

1. Categorize the risk factors for breast cancer into major and minor factors.

2. Provide the guidelines for routine screening mammography.

3. Describe the diagnostic workup and management for common benign breast conditions, including breast pain, cysts, fibroadenoma, nipple discharge, and breast abscess.

4. List the diagnostic modalities and describe their sequence in the workup of a patient with a breast mass or nipple discharge.

5. Describe the preoperative evaluation for a patient with breast cancer.

6. Provide the differential diagnosis of a breast lump in a woman in her twenties and in a woman in her sixties.

7. Describe how ductal cancer in situ differs from invasive breast cancer. Describe its role as a risk factor for invasive cancer.

8. Explain the rationale for breast conservation treatment as the preferred therapeutic option for most stage I and stage II breast cancers.

9. Describe the rationale for adjuvant therapy, radiation therapy, and hormonal therapy in the treatment of breast cancer.

10. Describe the expected survival and local recurrence rates after treatment for early breast cancer.

Familiarity with evaluation of the breast and an understanding of breast disease are critically important for primary care physicians and surgeons. This chapter focuses on the evaluation of the patient who is undergoing routine screening as well as the patient who has a breast complaint. Breast surveillance and the appropriate treatment of breast problems have become prominent aspects of health care for women, because breast cancer is common, often curable, and almost always at least treatable. It was estimated that 256,000 people in the United States (237,000 women and 1,900 men) would be diagnosed with breast cancer in 2003, or 32% of all new cancers diagnosed in women. Also in 2009, approximately 40,000 women died of breast cancer, or 15% of all women who die of cancer. The rate of breast cancer in women has shown a slow but steady rise over the past 25 years; presently, it is estimated that one in eight women will develop breast cancer during their lifetime. The death rate has remained relatively stable over the past 70 years, with a recent trend toward decline thought to be related to earlier diagnosis and possibly to improvements in treatment.

ANATOMY

The breast is a heterogeneous structure consisting of skin, subcutaneous tissue, parenchyma, and stroma. Contained within this architecture are glandular, ductal, and connective tissues, as well as blood vessels, nerves, and a rich lymphatic system. The breast parenchyma is divided into 15 to 20 segments that converge at the nipple in a radial pattern. Collecting ducts drain each segment into terminal lactiferous sinuses in the subareolar space. Each segment or lobe is further subdivided into 20 to 40 lobules, which are further divided into 10 to 100 alveoli or tubulosaccular secretory units. The upper outer quadrant of the breast contains a greater amount of glandular tissue.

The breast may extend from the clavicle superiorly to the sixth rib inferiorly and from the midsternal line medially into the axilla laterally (Figure 19-1). Breast tissue often extends into the anterior axillary fold known as the tail of Spence. The breast is located within the superficial fascia of the anterior thoracic wall continuous with the superficial abdominal fascia (Camper's). It rests on the deep posterior fascia overlying the muscles of the pectoralis major, serratus anterior, external oblique, and the rectus sheath. Cooper's ligaments are fibrous bands connecting the deep to superficial layers and provide a suspensory function to the breast. Skin dimpling, produced by retraction of Cooper's ligaments, may be associated with underlying malignancy.

The nipple contains numerous sensory nerves as well as sebaceous and apocrine sweat glands. The areola is a pigmented dermal region surrounding the nipple containing sebaceous glands (montgomery glands).

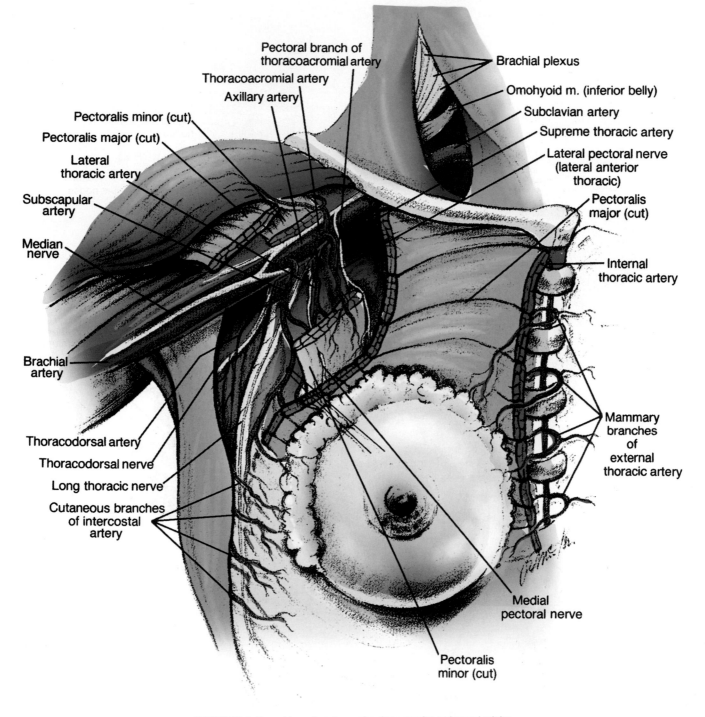

FIGURE 19-1. Normal breast anatomy showing vascular and neural origins.

The breast is a well-vascularized organ and derives its main blood supply from perforating branches of the internal mammary and lateral thoracic arteries. Additional supply is provided from pectoral branches of the thoracoacromial artery and branches of the intercostal, subscapular, and thoracodorsal arteries. The axillary, subclavian, and intercostal veins receive venous drainage from the breast. Lymphatics of the breast are confluent with subepithelial lymphatics over the surface of the body and ultimately communicate with the subdermal lymphatic vessels and subareolar lymphatic plexus of Sappey (Figure 19-2). Lymph flows from the superficial lymphatics into the deep subcutaneous and perilobular lymphatics. The vast majority of lymphatic flow goes to the axilla, with only a minor portion directed to the internal mammary chain.

The concept of lymphatic flow from the breast to axilla forms the basis for sentinel node biopsy. Following injection into the breast of a radioactive tracer and/or blue dye, lymphatic drainage of the breast is thought to follow an orderly pattern, so that drainage is first to the sentinel lymph node and subsequently to the nonsentinel lymph nodes. Consequently, if the sentinel lymph node is negative for malignant cells, involvement of any other node is rare and axillary dissection can be avoided.

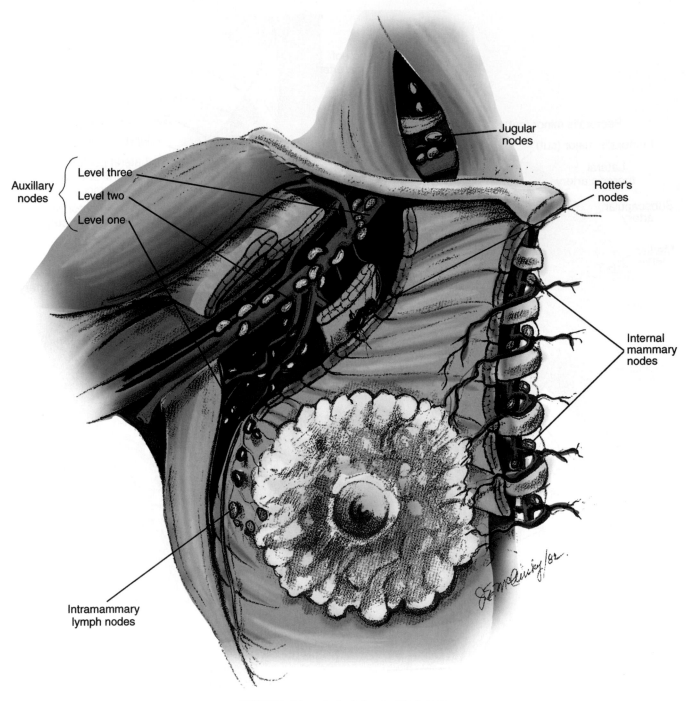

FIGURE 19-2. Lymphatic drainage of the breast.

The axilla is a pyramidal-shaped region located between the upper extremity and thorax. It contains a rich complex of neurovascular and lymphatic structures within a layer of dense connective tissue known as the axillary sheath. Contained within the axilla are two motor branches of the brachial plexus, the long thoracic and thoracodorsal nerves. The long thoracic, thoracodorsal, and intercostobrachial nerves are intimately associated anatomically with the breast and the axillary space. The long thoracic nerve courses vertically along the superficial surface of the serratus anterior muscle in the axilla. It provides motor innervation to the serratus anterior muscle, which abducts and laterally rotates the scapula and holds it against the chest wall. Injury to this nerve, which can occur during mastectomy or axillary dissection, results in a winged

scapula. The loss of the serratus anterior muscle holding the scapula against the posterior chest wall results in a limiting of overhead elevation of the arm above the shoulder. The thoracodorsal nerve, which is located posteriorly in the axillary space, innervates the latissimus dorsi muscle, which adducts, extends, and medially rotates the arm. This nerve is also potentially at risk during axillary surgery. The medial pectoral nerve, named for its origin from the medial cord of the brachial plexus, most commonly pierces the pectoralis minor en route to the pectoralis major while innervating both. The nerve may pass *lateral* to the pectoralis minor muscle, and for this reason, it is vulnerable to injury during axillary dissection. The intercostobrachial nerves, which are the lateral cutaneous branches of the first and second intercostal nerves, course across the axillary space to provide cutaneous innervation to the inner aspect of the upper arm and the axilla. Attempts should be made to identify and preserve the intercostobrachial nerves during an axillary dissection; however, it is acceptable to sacrifice these sensory nerves if they are in the direct path of the specimen. Patients will have a resultant loss of sensation or paresthesia at the medial portion of the upper arm, which resolves over time.

PHYSIOLOGY

The female breast is a modified apocrine gland that undergoes considerable structural and physiologic changes during a woman's lifetime. The mammary glands have evolved as a milk-producing organ, and play a significant role in breast-feeding children. The paired glands develop along the milk lines. A wide range of congenital abnormalities in breast development exists. Polythelia (accessory nipple) can occur anywhere along the milk line from the axilla to the inguinal region. A more rare condition, polymastia (accessory breast tissue), mostly occurs in the axilla. Congenital absence of the breast is called amastia, while a lack of breast tissue development with perseverance of the nipple is termed amazia.

The development of the breast from childhood to adulthood has been categorized into the five Tanner phases. Increased hormonal production by the ovary at puberty causes ductal budding and the initial formation of acini, which are proliferations of the terminal ducts lined with secretory cells for milk production. Periductal connective tissue increases in volume elasticity, vascularity, and in the amount of adipose deposition. The synergistic physiologic effect of both estrogen and progesterone result in full maturation of the ductal and lobular components of the breast. With each menstrual cycle, preovulatory estrogen production stimulates proliferation of the breast ductal system. After ovulation, decreased estrogen and progesterone levels cause a decrease in ductal proliferation. In pregnancy, when estrogen and progesterone levels remain relatively high, there is continued hypertrophy and budding of the ductal system, with associated acinar development. The sudden decrease in hormone levels in the postpartum period, associated with prolactin secretion from the pituitary gland, precipitates the onset of lactation. Postmenopausally, in the absence of the hormonal stimulus for cyclic proliferation of the breast ductal system, breast parenchyma is progressively lost and replaced by adipose tissue. The male breast is anatomically composed of the same heterogeneous tissue as the female breast, but it does not undergo cyclic hormonally related changes.

Physiologic gynecomastia occurs in over one-half of adolescent males. For these young patients the enlarged breasts may be asymmetric and tender secondary to a physiologic excess of plasma estradiol relative to plasma testosterone. This adolescent gynecomastia usually resolves by age 20. In young girls, adolescent or juvenile hypertrophy is a postpubertal persistence of epithelial and stromal growth that can result in very large breasts. Often this occurs in the absence of any systemic hormonal imbalances. Physiologic gynecomastia is also prevalent in a significant percentage of aging men. This is manifested by either bilateral or unilateral breast enlargement often associated with breast tenderness. This gynecomastia is secondary to a relative hyperestrinism with falling plasma testosterone levels and increasing conversion of androgens to estrogens in peripheral tissues. In the absence of a palpable mass or significant symptoms, this condition does not require clinical evaluation. A thorough history and careful physical exam will often be all that is required for most asymptomatic patients without features suggestive of possible malignancy. Less frequently, gynecomastia may be associated with certain drugs or result from pathological conditions such as hepatic, renal, or endocrine disorders. Treatment of gynecomastia is tailored to etiology and symptoms.

CLINICAL PRESENTATION AND EVALUATION: ASSESSMENT OF BREAST CANCER RISK

A complete medical history, risk assessment, and focused physical examination should be obtained from any woman with breast complaints. Table 19-1 summarizes essential elements of the history. Risk assessment is useful primarily in women without complaints, since diagnostic and therapeutic approaches in women who do have complaints are determined by the nature of the problem rather than by the level of risk. In other words, complaints should not be disregarded because the risk is low. Many women who develop breast cancer *do not* have significant risk factors.

Abnormalities occurring in young women, those under the age of 30, are likely to be related to benign pathologies such as fibrocystic changes, cysts, and fibroadenomas. Abnormalities in postmenopausal women, such as pain, nipple discharge, and new masses, are much more likely to be related to malignancies. A solid mass in a postmenopausal woman should be considered suspicious for cancer until proven otherwise. Diagnostic problems most often arise in the intermediate group: women aged 30 to 50, who may have either benign or malignant pathology.

Breast cancer risk factors are statistical associations and do not define causality. A greater number of risk factors (Table 19-2) suggest greater risk, but the nature of these interactions is not well understood and awaits further study.

Hormone replacement therapy (HRT) has long been known to be associated with an increased risk of breast cancer. Recent large, randomized studies have demonstrated an increased risk of breast cancer with estrogen-plus-progestin replacement. The risk of estrogen alone replacement remains somewhat uncertain. These studies have also shown that the only significant benefit of HRT is in treatment of menopausal symptoms, and that it does not decrease the risk of fracture or heart disease.

TABLE 19-1	Key Elements in the History of a Patient with a Breast Complaint

History of current problem (duration, timing, intensity)

Previous breast problems including biopsies

Results of recent mammography

Family history of breast cancer, ovarian cancer

Age at onset of menses and natural or surgical menopause

Age at first full-term pregnancy, number of pregnancies

Use of birth control pills, HRT

Current medications

Past medical and surgical history

TABLE 19-2 | Breast Cancer Risk Factors

Relative Risk	Factor
>4.0	Female
	Age (65+ vs. <65 yr, although risk increases across all ages until age 80)
	Certain inherited genetic mutations for breast cancer (BRCA1 and/or BRCA2)
	Two or more first-degree relatives with breast cancer diagnosed at an early age
	Personal history of breast cancer
	High breast tissue density
	Biopsy-confirmed atypical hyperplasia
2.1–4.0	One first-degree relative with breast cancer
	High-dose radiation to chest
	High bone density (postmenopausal)
1.1–2.0	
Factors that affect circulating hormones	Late age at first full-term pregnancy (>30 yr)
	Early menarche (<12 yr)
	Late menopause (>55 yr)
	No full-term pregnancies
	Never breast-fed a child
	Recent oral contraceptive use
	Recent and long-term use of HRT
Other factors	Obesity (postmenopausal)
	Personal history of endometrium, ovary, or colon cancer
	Alcohol consumption
	Height (tall)
	High socioeconomic status
	Jewish heritage

Adapted with permission from Hulka BS, Moorman PG. Breast cancer: hormones and other risk factors. Maturitas. 2001;38(1):103–113; discussion 113–106.

TABLE 19-3 | Age-Specific Probability of Breast Cancer

If Current Age Is:	The Probability of Developing Breast Cancer in the Next 10 Years Is:	Or 1 in:
20	0.05%	1,837
30	0.43%	234
40	1.43%	70
50	2.51%	40
60	3.51%	28
70	3.88%	26
Lifetime risk	12.28%	8

American Cancer Society, Surveillance Research, 2007.

is 36% to 85% for breast cancer and 16% to 60% for ovarian cancer. In order to best provide options for high-risk screening and prevention, patients suspected to have a hereditary mutation predisposing for breast cancer should be offered further assessment with a genetic counselor and possible genetic testing (Table 19-4). Both maternal and paternal sides of the family history should be considered.

Management of high-risk patients, with or without confirmation of a genetic mutation, often requires the coordination of a multidisciplinary team. High-risk screening with clinical breast exam every 6 months, annual mammography and annual magnetic resonance imaging (MRI) can begin at age 25 or be individualized based on earliest age of breast cancer onset in the family. Although controversial for normal risk patients, high-risk patients may also benefit from regular breast self-exam (BSE). Randomized controlled trials have demonstrated the benefit of chemoprevention with agents Tamoxifen and Raloxifene. The use of these drugs in high-risk individuals results in an approximately 50%

TABLE 19-4 | Guidelines: Referral for Genetic Counseling

Individuals from a family with a known BRCA1 or BRCA2 mutation
Personal history of breast cancer with one of the following:
• Diagnosed at or before age 45
• Diagnosed at or before age 50 with one or more close family relatives diagnosed with breast cancer or ovarian cancer at or before 50[a]
• Diagnosed at or before age 50 with two or more synchronous primary breast cancers
• Diagnosed at any age and two or more close family relatives with breast or ovarian cancer[a]
• Two or more close family relatives with breast or ovarian cancer[a]
• Personal history of ovarian cancer
• Close male relative with breast cancer
• High-risk ethnic background (i.e., Ashkenazi Jewish)
Personal history of male breast cancer
Close family member with one or more of the above criteria

[a]Both maternal and paternal sides of family should be considered. Close family relative includes first, second and third degree blood relatives (risk is greater with first degree).

Major risk factors for breast cancer include female sex, increasing age, family history, and proliferative pathology with atypia on biopsy (i.e., atypical ductal or lobular hyperplasia). The older women get, the more likely they are to be diagnosed with breast cancer, but at the same time, they become less likely to die from it (Table 19-3). Breast cancer in families featuring early age of onset (premenopausal), multiple close relatives, bilateral disease, male breast cancer, and in combination with ovarian cancer are more suggestive of a hereditary predisposition.

It is estimated that approximately 5% to 10% of breast cancers are related to specific genetic mutations inherited from family members. Certain familial cancer syndromes, such as Li-Fraumeni and Cowden's, have been associated with a greater risk of breast cancer. Other genes linked to an increased susceptibility of breast cancer have been identified, including most notably the BRCA genetic mutations. BRCA1 has been mapped to the long arm of chromosome 17 and BRCA2 to the long arm of chromosome 13. The lifetime risk of penetrance (disease expression) in BRCA mutation carriers reduced incidence of breast cancer. The potential risks and side effects of these drugs need to be taken into consideration and discussed with the patient prior to initiating chemoprevention. Patients should also have a careful discussion about risk-reducing bilateral mastectomy as well as risk-reducing bilateral salpingo-oophorectomy. Prophylactic mastectomy is associated with approximately 90% risk reduction of breast cancer. The addition of prophylactic oophorectomy in premenopausal women yields approximately 95% risk reduction of breast cancer, while prophylactic oophorectomy alone is associated with approximately 50% risk reduction of breast cancer and 90% risk reduction of ovarian cancer. Patients electing to undergo prophylactic bilateral mastectomy should be offered the opportunity to explore breast reconstruction options. Patient education is an essential component of risk management, and it is important that all risks, benefits, and alternative approaches are thoroughly discussed with the patient.

Physical Examination of the Breasts

A systematic approach to the physical examination of the breasts includes both inspection and palpation. Important elements in the breast exam are to be thorough while maintaining patient comfort. The examination begins with the patient in the seated position. Both breasts should be exposed to allow for full inspection and assessment for any breast asymmetry, skin changes (e.g., retraction or erythema), or nipple-areolar abnormalities (e.g., scaling of the nipple or nipple inversion). The breasts are inspected first with the arms at the patient's side, and then pressed firmly at her waist in order to contract the pectoralis muscle. This maneuver may accentuate skin retraction associated with a mass. Other maneuvers such as elevating the arms above the head and leaning forward are not routinely necessary; however, they can be utilized as needed (i.e., large pendulous breasts). With the patient still in the seated position, both axillae are examined, with the patient's arm resting over the forearm of the examiner to relax the shoulder musculature, allowing for full assessment of axillary contents. Lymph nodes are best detected as the examiner pushes superiorly in the axilla, and then moves the fingertips inferiorly against the chest wall, trapping lymph nodes between the finger and the chest wall. A careful lymph node examination also involves palpation in the supraclavicular fossae. Palpation of the breasts in the sitting position is discouraged because it often yields false-positive findings for the examiner (as well as for the patient during self-examination). The breasts should be palpated with the patient supine and the arm resting comfortably above the head. This position evenly distributes the breast tissue out over the chest wall, allowing more accurate detection of abnormalities.

There are several different methods of palpating the breast; however, the vertical strip technique is a reliable, evidenced-based method shown to have the lowest incidence of missed abnormalities. Palpation of the breast should encompass all breast tissue and cover the perimeter bordered by the clavicle, sternum, axilla, and inframammary crease. The exam should be performed with a vertical strip pattern covering the entire breast using overlapping dime-sized circular motions of the increasing pressure (light, medium, deep). The pads (not the tips) of the index, middle, and ring fingers are used for palpation. Irregularities are palpated between the skin and the chest wall, not between the two hands of the examiner. The size of any palpable abnormality should be described with the use of a measuring instrument. The examiner should note additional features including mobility, texture, and whether or not there is associated tenderness. The precise location of any abnormality should be described. When annotating location, using the clock-face position and distance from the nipple is helpful (i.e., right breast mass as 12:00, 4 cm from the nipple). It is not necessary to squeeze the nipples during a breast examination, since typically only spontaneous nipple discharge (especially bloody or serous) requires further evaluation. Unilateral nonspontaneous discharge is frequently benign, particularly in younger women. With a history of **spontaneous nipple discharge**, the source of the discharge should be localized with systematic palpation from the outer breast to the nipple circumferentially around the areola. If discharge is identified, the color should be noted, as well as whether it is bloody, whether more than one duct orifice is involved, and whether it is bilateral. Unilateral bloody single-duct spontaneous discharge is more likely to result from an underlying malignancy, especially if it is associated with a mass in the breast. However, the most common cause of unilateral spontaneous bloody nipple discharge is a benign papilloma.

Diagnostic Evaluation

The foundation of breast cancer screening is the annual mammogram. Large prospective studies evaluating the impact of screening mammogram on breast cancer mortality demonstrate a 40% to 45% decrease in breast cancer deaths in a screened population compared to the years prior to screening. Monthly BSE in addition to mammography does not yield additional improvement in breast cancer survival, yet the fact remains that among patients not engaged in screening, such as those under age 40, the majority of breast cancers are diagnosed after a patient reports a self-detected lump. Therefore, women should be encouraged to seek medical attention if a new breast mass or other abnormality is found. The current recommendations for breast cancer screening from the American Cancer Society are shown in Table 19-5).

Mammography

Screening mammography is an x-ray image with two views of each breast: Craniocaudal (CC) and median lateral oblique (MLO), with identifiable markers placed on the nipple and any visible or palpable lesions. Film labels are by convention located on the lateral aspect of a CC view and the superior

TABLE 19-5	American Cancer Society Guidelines for Breast Cancer Screening

Yearly mammograms are recommended starting at age 40 and continuing for as long as a woman is in good health.

Women should know how their breasts normally feel and report any breast change promptly to their health care providers. BSE is an option for women starting in their twenties.

Women at high risk (>20% lifetime risk) should get an MRI and a mammogram every year. Women at moderately increased risk (15%–20% lifetime risk) should talk with their doctors about the benefits and limitations of adding MRI screening to their yearly mammogram. Yearly MRI screening is not recommended for women whose lifetime risk of breast cancer is <15%.

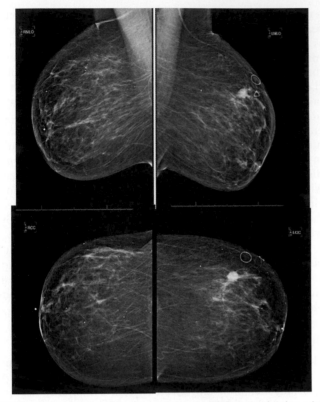

FIGURE 19-3. MLO and CC views of right and left breasts showing a left spiculated lesion.

aspect of an MLO view, allowing the reader to determine the quadrant wherein an abnormality is located (Figure 19-3). The x-ray modality can demonstrate differences in density of breast tissue, architectural distortion of the tissue planes, asymmetry such as unilateral nipple retraction, and calcifications ranging from those associated with benign involutional changes to suspicious microcalcifications that can be described as pleomorphic, clustered, linear, or branching. The findings are scored for level of suspicion according to the Breast Imaging Reporting and Data System (BIRADS) classification (Table 19-6), which corresponds to the need for additional studies or interval follow-up. The assigned score is inherently subjective to the radiologist and includes a comparison to mammograms from previous years.

Additional diagnostic views involve tissue compression and magnification, which can resolve summation artifact, eliminating a perceived density, or enhancing the spiculated contours of an actual mass lesion or cluster of microcalcifications.

TABLE 19-6	BIRADS Classification for Mammogram Findings
Category 0	Needs additional imaging evaluation
Category 1	Negative
Category 2	Benign finding
Category 3	Probably benign finding—short interval follow-up suggested
Category 4	Suspicious abnormality—biopsy should be considered
Category 5	Highly suggestive of malignancy—appropriate action should be taken

Although mammography is an effective tool for screening, it is not a definitive diagnostic study. The false negative rate of mammography is 10% to 20%. Any physical finding or mammographic abnormality must be further evaluated on clinical grounds as well as with additional diagnostic studies usually combined with a biopsy.

Technological advances in mammography include computer-assisted detection (CAD) software that highlights potentially suspicious patterns on a digital image, as well as digital mammography, which is a technique that eliminates photographic film and creates digital images that can be processed to enhance contrast in dense soft tissue. Both of these techniques increase sensitivity and the breast cancer detection rate, at the cost of an increased rate of patient recall for additional diagnostic views.

Ultrasound

Ultrasonography of the breast is a diagnostic adjunct to mammography. It is particularly valuable in characterizing a mammographic density or palpable mass as cystic or solid, and in guiding core needle biopsy. Benign sonographic features of masses include well-demarcated borders, posterior enhancement, and absence of internal echoes (characteristic of cysts). Features suspicious for malignancy include poorly demarcated borders, posterior shadowing, heterogeneous internal echoes, and a "taller than wide" orientation that invades across tissue planes.

Magnetic Resonance Imaging

MRI uses the physical characteristics of fat, water, and intravenous gadolinium contrast in magnetic fields to produce breast images with improved resolution of soft tissues. Dense breast tissue, scar, and implants, which may make mammography less sensitive, do not interfere with MRI diagnosis. In addition to such "problem-solving" applications, MRI has been shown to be a more sensitive screening test than mammography, and is appropriate in women who carry a deleterious BRCA1 or BRCA2 mutation, or who by family history and other risk factors, carry at least a 20% lifetime risk of breast cancer. The development of biopsy equipment compatible with magnetic fields allows MRI-directed breast biopsy when a suspicious lesion is detected by MRI alone.

Tissue Sampling Techniques

The definitive diagnosis of breast lesions depends on microscopic examination of tissue by either cytology (individual cells obtained by fine needle aspiration) or histology (samples of tissue obtained by core needle or surgical biopsy.) Cytology specimens can be air-dried and stained in minutes, providing rapid diagnosis of a suspected malignancy. Histologic specimens provide pieces of tissue that can be processed for special staining techniques to demonstrate invasive versus in situ carcinoma, type of cancer, and the expression of estrogen, progesterone, and human epidermal growth factor 2 receptor (HER-2/neu).

Palpable lesions can be needle biopsied directly, but the majority of lesions are detected radiologically and must be biopsied under radiological guidance. Mass lesions are efficiently biopsied by ultrasound guidance, but microcalcifications and subtle abnormalities require stereotactic localization in the mammography suite (Figure 19-4).

Any needle biopsy must be regarded as only a sampling, and verification that a lesion is benign requires the so-called triple test: concordance between clinical exam, radiographic appear-

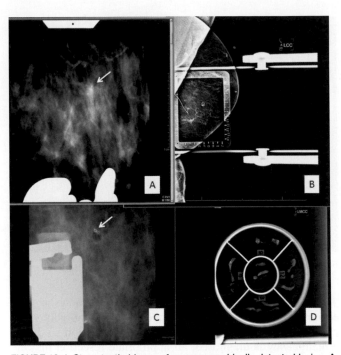

FIGURE 19-4. Stereotactic biopsy of mammographically detected lesion. A, Suspicious microcalcifications (*arrow*). **B,** With patient positioned on a stereotactic biopsy table, the lesion is localized for a core-needle biopsy. **C,** A clip (*arrow*) is deployed at site of biopsy for future reference. **D,** The specimen cores are radiographed to demonstrate targeted microcalcifications.

ance, and pathology. If the needle biopsy results are discordant, an excisional biopsy guided by a localizing wire placed under radiological guidance is necessary. Open excisional biopsy without a prior needle biopsy can lead to less than optimal management of a malignancy due to possible positive margins, cosmetically unfavorable incision placement, and the need to go back to the operating room for lymph node staging.

Evaluation of the Patient with a Breast Mass

The evaluation of a patient presenting with a complaint of breast mass depends on patient age and physical findings. If physical and radiographic examinations show typical areas of fibroglandular tissue without a discrete mass, the patient should be reevaluated in 6 to 12 weeks. If there is a question as to whether the physical findings reveal a specific area of thickening or discrete mass, a workup should be initiated along the lines of the presented algorithm (Figure 19-5). All patients felt to have a discrete, persistent mass require tissue diagnosis.

BENIGN CONDITIONS OF THE BREAST

Breast Pain

Mild, cyclic bilateral breast tenderness and swelling is a common experience a few days preceding the menses and rarely prompts medical consultation. Although it is distinctly

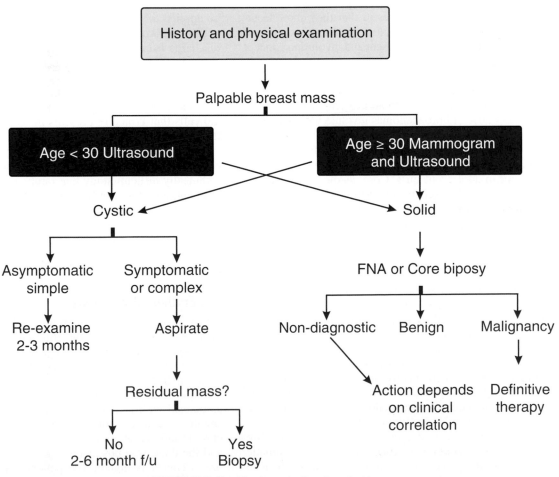

FIGURE 19-5. Algorithm for evaluation of a palpable mass.

unusual for the presence of breast cancer to be signaled by pain, persistent or unilateral pain and tenderness can be a cause of alarm. A thorough clinical evaluation and appropriate diagnostic workup should be performed. Musculoskeletal causes and angina should be considered, and breast imaging such as mammogram and ultrasound should be used to rule out a malignancy. In the absence of any physical or radiological abnormality, reassurance and a follow-up examination in a few months often provide adequate relief.

Hormonal stimulation of glandular breast tissue is thought to be the underlying cause of mastalgia. Discontinuing HRT in postmenopausal women with breast pain is recommended. Other therapeutic measures include use of a compressive elastic style of bra (sport or minimizer bra), decreasing caffeine consumption, nonsteroidal anti-inflammatory analgesics, and evening primrose oil capsules. Danazol, an androgen analogue, is effective in relieving breast pain and tenderness, but it should only be used after failure of the previous measures because of its adverse effects, including deepening of the voice and hirsutism.

Fibroadenoma

Fibroadenoma is a very common benign tumor of the breast. It usually occurs in young women (late teens to early thirties), although it may develop at any age. Typically, the fibroadenoma is 1 to 3 cm in size and is palpated as a freely movable, discrete, firm, rounded mass in the breast. Histologically, fibroadenomas are composed of fibrous stromal tissue and tissue clefts lined with normal epithelium. Fine needle aspiration or core biopsy can establish the diagnosis. Fibroadenomas resemble normal mammary lobules in that they show lactation in pregnancy and involution in menopause, an example of the aberrancies of normal development and involution concept (ANDI) that supports observation rather than excision.

For young women with a typical clinical presentation and cytological diagnosis of fibroadenoma, excision is not required if the fibroadenoma is small (<3 cm). In this group, approximately 50% of fibroadenomas involute within 5 years. Stable fibroadenomas may be followed. Hormonal stimulation during pregnancy may cause rapid growth of a fibroadenoma and require its excision. Giant fibroadenoma is an uncommon benign tumor in adolescent girls. Core needle biopsy should be performed prior to excision to distinguish the relatively rare **phyllodes tumor**, a usually benign (90%) tumor of the stromal elements requiring wide margins of resection to prevent local recurrence.

Breast Cyst

A cyst is the most common cause of breast mass in women in their fourth and fifth decades of life. Cysts may be solitary or multiple, and present as firm, mobile, slightly tender masses, often with less well-defined borders compared to fibroadenomas. Unlike fibroadenomas, the size and degree of tenderness of a cyst typically fluctuates with the menstrual cycle. Screening mammography will frequently detect nonpalpable cysts. Ultrasonography is very useful in demonstrating a simple cyst as a well-demarcated, hypoechoic mass with posterior enhancement of transmission (Figure 19-6).

Such an appearance is diagnostic and does not require biopsy. Aspiration may be performed on large, symptomatic cysts. The resulting fluid may be straw-colored or greenish and cytological analysis is unnecessary.

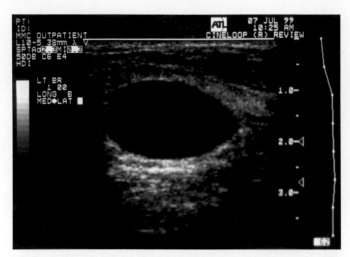

FIGURE 19-6. Sonogram of a simple breast cyst.

The ultrasound appearance of complex cysts shows internal echoes or an associated solid component. Mammography and core needle biopsy are warranted prior to excision so that if a malignancy is diagnosed, an appropriate resection may be planned.

Nipple Discharge

The most common cause of nipple discharge is duct ectasia, a nonneoplastic condition characterized by multiple dilated ducts in the subareolar space. The nipple discharge may be clear, milky, or green-brown. The discharge should be applied to occult blood test paper and further evaluation performed when blood is present. Persistent, spontaneous discharge from a single duct and bloody discharge are considered pathological. The incidence of malignancy is 10% to 15% in unilateral, bloody nipple discharge. An intraductal papilloma is the usual cause in the remaining instances. An intraductal papilloma is a local proliferation of ductal epithelial cells that typically presents in women in their fourth or fifth decade of life.

Systematic palpation around the nipple-areolar complex can frequently identify the discharging duct. A ductogram is a technically difficult study that rarely alters the surgical management, and thus can be avoided. Mammography is important to evaluate for malignancy. In the absence of clinical or radiological evidence of malignancy, duct excision through a circumareolar incision allows definitive histological diagnosis and eliminates the discharge with a cosmetically acceptable result.

The Erythematous Breast

When a woman presents with a breast that is warm, edematous, and erythematous, the differential diagnosis revolves around an infectious process such as mastitis or breast abscess versus malignancy presenting as inflammatory breast cancer. A careful history must be taken to assess risk factors and onset and time course of symptoms. Mastitis is most commonly associated with lactation. In nonlactating women, especially smokers, recurrent retroareolar abscesses may occur with chronic inflammation and fistula formation between the skin and the duct. In a postmenopausal woman, the likelihood of breast cancer is higher. The patient may admit to a known breast lump that was asymptomatic for months or years and is only now brought to attention because of the redness, but inflammatory breast cancer can occur with diffuse breast swelling and no discrete mass.

Physical findings include erythema spreading in a lymphangitic pattern from areola toward the axilla, skin thickening with accentuation of the pores (*peau d'orange*), lymphadenopathy, overall breast enlargement and heaviness, and a mass that may be fluctuant. Pain is not usual in malignancy, while abscesses are exquisitely tender. The nipple can be deformed in either cancer or recurrent retroareolar abscess. Diagnostic imaging includes mammography and ultrasound. In cases where no mass is demonstrated by these modalities, breast MRI is useful. Fine-needle aspiration of a mass can establish the presence of malignancy in minutes, but core-needle biopsies should also be obtained for immunohistochemical studies to plan primary systemic therapy. Punch biopsy of skin may show dilated lymphatic channels carrying malignant cells, but it is not necessary to demonstrate these in order to make a clinical diagnosis of inflammatory breast cancer.

Ultrasound demonstrates drainable fluid collections. Repeated aspiration of a breast abscess combined with antibiotics may allow resolution of the abscess without open drainage. Chronic retroareolar inflammation and mammary duct fistula require antibiotics with coverage of anaerobic organisms followed by excision of the subareolar ducts including the fistula tract. Mastitis in lactating women is usually caused by staphylococci or streptococci. Appropriate antibiotics such as dicloxacillin or clindamycin should bring prompt relief. Breastfeeding may continue on the unaffected breast, while the use of a breast pump is helpful to reduce congestion of the infected breast.

BREAST CANCER

Approximately one of every eight women will have breast cancer in her lifetime. It is the most frequently diagnosed non-skin cancer, and the second leading cause of cancer death in women. Although incidence rates have been increasing, the rate of increase has slowed in the past decade. Approximately 25% of new cancers are in situ. The rise in the detection of ductal carcinoma in situ (DCIS) is a result of the increased use of screening mammography, which detects breast cancers before they are palpable.

The earliest sign of a breast cancer is usually an abnormality on a mammogram. As breast cancers grow, they can produce a palpable mass that is often hard and irregular. Other signs may include thickening, swelling, skin irritation, or dimpling. Nipple changes due to breast cancer can include scaliness and dryness, ulceration, retraction, or discharge.

In most cases of breast cancer, the cause is unknown, but many risk factors such as hormonal and dietary factors have been identified. About 10% of cancers are related to genetic factors. Approximately 1% of breast cancers occur in men.

Histologic Types of Breast Cancer

Ductal cancer in situ (DCIS), also known as intraductal carcinoma, is a preinvasive form of ductal cancer. If not treated adequately, invasive cancer may develop in 30% to 50% of patients over 10 years (Figure 19-7). The typical appearance of DCIS on mammography is microcalcifications; there is rarely a mass on physical examination or mammography. The histologic types of DCIS include solid, cribriform, micropapillary, and comedo-type. DCIS can be classified on the basis of nuclear grades 1, 2, and 3, with grade 1 being the most favorable. Patients with comedo-type necrosis and/or high-grade lesions have an increased risk of recurrence and of the lesion developing into invasive cancer.

Infiltrating ductal carcinoma constitutes approximately 80% of invasive breast cancers. It produces the characteristic firm, irregular mass on physical examination. These masses are characteristically better defined mammographically and histologically than infiltrating lobular cancers.

Infiltrating lobular carcinoma makes up approximately 10% of breast cancers and is often difficult to detect mammographically and on physical examination because of its indistinct borders. It is characterized by a higher incidence of multicentricity in the same breast and by its presence in the contralateral breast.

Tubular carcinoma, a very well-differentiated form of ductal carcinoma, constitutes approximately 1% to 2% of breast cancers. It is so named because it forms small tubules, randomly arranged, each lined by a single uniform row of cells. This subtype tends to occur in women who are slightly younger than the average patient with breast cancer. The prognosis is better than with other infiltrating ductal carcinomas.

Medullary carcinoma, another variant of infiltrating ductal cancer, is characterized by extensive tumor invasion by small lymphocytes and is slightly less well differentiated than tubular carcinoma. It constitutes approximately 5% of breast carcinomas. At diagnosis, it tends to be rapidly growing and large, and it is often associated with DCIS. It less commonly metastasizes to regional lymph nodes and has a better prognosis than the typical infiltrating ductal carcinoma.

Colloid or mucinous carcinoma is also a variant of infiltrating ductal cancer and accounts for approximately 2% to 3% of breast carcinomas. It is characterized histologically by clumps and strands of epithelial cells in pools of mucoid material. It

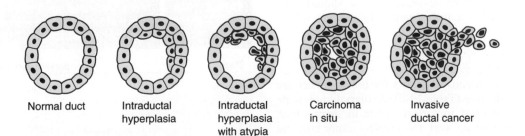

Normal duct   Intraductal hyperplasia   Intraductal hyperplasia with atypia   Carcinoma in situ   Invasive ductal cancer

FIGURE 19-7. The evolution from normal duct to invasive cancer. (Adapted with permission from Love SM. *Dr. Susan Love's Breast Book.* Reading, MA: Addison-Wesley Longman, 1990;192. Copyright 1990, 1991 by Susan M. Love, MD. Reprinted by permission of Addison-Wesley Longman, Inc.)

grows slowly and occurs more often in older women. The pure type has a relatively good prognosis.

True papillary carcinoma accounts for approximately 1% of breast carcinomas. These tumors can be difficult to distinguish histologically from intraductal papilloma, a benign lesion. They tend to be quite small, and even when they metastasize to regional nodes, they have a better prognosis than ductal carcinomas because of their slower rate of growth.

Inflammatory carcinoma accounts for 3% of all breast cancers and presents with skin edema (peau d'orange) and erythema. The skin edema is secondary to dermal lymphatics congested with malignant cells that are generally ductal in origin. Inflammatory carcinoma of the breast has a poor prognosis, with approximately 25% of patients alive 5 years later. Malignancies that rarely occur in the breast include sarcomas, lymphomas, and leukemia.

Paget's disease of the nipple is a cutaneous nipple abnormality, which may be moist and exudative, dry and scaly, erosive, or just a thickened area. The patient may note itching, burning, or sticking pain in the nipple. As time passes, the lesion spreads out from the duct orifice. Histologically, the dermis is infiltrated by Paget's cells, which are of ductal origin, large and pale, with large nuclei, prominent nucleoli, and abundant cytoplasm. Paget's disease of the nipple is seen in approximately 3% of breast cancers and is usually, but not always, associated with an underlying malignancy, which is palpable in half of cases. It may originate in DCIS or in an invasive cancer.

Paget's disease of the nipple is often misdiagnosed as a simple dermatologic eruption and treated with ointments and creams for prolonged periods, during which time the cancer progresses. If a lesion is clinically suspicious for Paget's disease, a nipple biopsy should be done.

Staging

The treatment for breast cancer depends on the likelihood of local recurrence and distant spread. The most common areas of breast cancer metastasis are bone, lung, liver, and brain. The risk for distant spread is related to tumor size and lymph node involvement with cancer. The tumor, node, metastasis (TNM) status defines the patient's stage of disease (Table 19-7).

Besides TNM status, other factors are taken into account when planning therapy for breast cancer. These include the estrogen receptor status, the histopathologic grade of the tumor, and the mitotic index. HER-2/*neu*, an oncogene produced by some tumors, predicts a poorer prognosis as well as the likelihood of a response to Herceptin, a monoclonal antibody.

When the patient's risk for metastatic disease is low (tumor size <5 cm and no palpable lymphadenopathy), only chest radiograph and complete blood count are necessary prior to surgery. Patients with more advanced disease should have chest and abdominal CT scans as well as bone scans before surgical treatment.

Prognosis

The most important prognostic factors for breast cancer are related to stage of disease (Table 19-8). Axillary lymph node status is the single most important factor in determining disease-free and overall survival, followed by tumor size and estrogen receptor (ER) status. Other possible prognostic factors such as growth factors and proteases are being investigated. The risk of developing a second primary breast cancer

TABLE 19-7	TNM Staging System for Breast Cancer

Primary Tumor (T)

Tis	Carcinoma in situ
T1	Tumor ≤2 cm
T2	Tumor >2 cm, ≤5 cm
T3	Tumor >5 cm
T4	Tumor any size with extension to chest wall or skin

Regional Lymph Nodes (N)

N0	No lymph node metastasis
N1	Metastasis in one to three axillary lymph nodes
N2	Metastasis in four to nine axillary lymph nodes
N3	Metastasis in 10 or more axillary lymph nodes

Distant Metastasis (M)

M0	No distant metastasis
M1	Distant metastasis

Stage Grouping

0	Tis	N0	M0
I	T1	N0	M0
IIA	T0	N1	M0
	T1	N1	M0
	T2	N0	M0
IIB	T2	N1	M0
	T3	N0	M0
IIIA	T0	N2	M0
	T1	N2	M0
	T2	N2	M0
	T3	N1	M0
	T3	N2	M0
IIIB	T4	N0	M0
	T4	N1	M0
	T4	N2	M0
IIIC	Any T	N3	M0
IV	Any T	Any N	M1

is approximately 1% per year for the first 15 years. The risk of recurrence, while never reaching 0%, decreases over time.

TABLE 19-8	Five-Year Relative Survival Rates for Patients with Treated Breast Cancer by Stage

Stage	Survival Rate (%)
I	96
II	82
III	53
IV	18

Rates adjusted for deaths from other causes.

Follow-Up

Follow-up for breast cancer patients should include bilateral mammogram 6 months after completion of radiation therapy following lumpectomy and yearly thereafter. After mastectomy, contralateral breast mammogram should be performed annually. Physical examination should be done every 3 to 6 months for 3 years and then annually. Other studies to detect metastasis are not cost-effective and should be performed only when indicated by symptoms or physical findings.

Treatment of Breast Cancer

Breast cancer treatment is a multidisciplinary effort involving radiologists, breast and plastic surgeons, medical and radiation oncologists, pathologists, gynecologists, oncology nurses, social workers, and psychiatrists. It includes local, adjuvant, and neoadjuvant treatment designed to cure, to decrease systemic recurrence, and to increase survival and quality of life.

Cancer is a disorder of individual cells, and treatment, whether local or systemic, is directed at eliminating these abnormal cells. Early stage breast cancer, stage 0, I, or II, is regarded as potentially curable, meaning that once the cancer is treated it may never recur. Later stage breast cancer, stage III or IV, is treatable. In either case, however, surveillance continues for the rest of the patient's life.

Treatment of breast cancer is both local and systemic. Local treatments include surgery and radiation. Systemic treatments are intravenous and oral medicines.

Local Treatments
Surgery
The choice of surgical option should balance the extent of disease with the morbidity of treatment. Noninvasive disease (DCIS) does not require axillary staging unless it is extensive. Lumpectomy is usually feasible in tumors under 4 cm, depending on the size of the breast. Lumpectomy usually mandates postoperative radiation.

There is no statistically significant difference in 5-year survival between lumpectomy with radiation and mastectomy. The two options are essentially equivalent with regard to local recurrence. The type of breast cancer such as ductal versus lobular cancer is not a major factor in choice of surgical treatment. Prophylactic (bilateral simple) mastectomy is an option for patients whose risk is very high.

Lumpectomy, wide excision, segmental, and partial mastectomy all refer to the excision of malignancy with a circumferential margin of microscopically normal tissue. Lumpectomy may be used in the treatment of DCIS and invasive carcinoma, if postoperative radiation will be performed.

Simple, or total, mastectomy removes the entire breast with the pectoralis major fascia. Modified radical mastectomy is simple mastectomy with axillary dissection. Dermal lymphatic involvement, diffuse or multiple tumors, unwillingness or inability to undergo radiation therapy, and the expectation of a cosmetically unacceptable result are indications for mastectomy.

Breast reconstruction, using prosthetic implants or autologous tissue, should be discussed with all mastectomy patients; it can be performed under the same anesthesia as mastectomy or delayed. The breast may be reconstructed using a saline or silicone prosthesis or the patient's own tissue from the abdomen or back. The federal Women's Health and Cancer Rights Act requires health insurers that cover mastectomies to cover some form of breast reconstruction as well.

The Axilla Assessment of the axilla is essential in staging and treating breast cancer. Since the first report of a pilot study in 1993, sentinel node biopsy has become the standard of care for early breast cancer. In a clinically negative axilla, periareolar intradermal injection of a radioactive colloid and/or blue dye in the quadrant of the tumor enables the surgeon to identify the first lymph node that receives drainage from the breast. Typically, only a few nodes will pick up the marker. These nodes may be identified and removed with a much smaller incision, less dissection, and less risk of disrupting the lymphatic drainage of the arm. Staging of the regional nodes is then based upon histopathologic analysis of the sentinel node(s). Axillary dissection, indicated in the presence of a positive sentinel node or a clinically positive axilla, removes the level I (in the axillary fat pad, lateral to the pectoralis major muscle), level II (beneath the pectoralis major muscle), and sometimes level III (superomedial to the pectoralis minor muscle) lymph nodes. Some patients undergoing partial mastectomy and radiation may be treated without axillary dissection with only one or two positive sentinel nodes.

Radiation Treatment
Following lumpectomy, radiation reduces the recurrence rate from about 30% to about 10%. Pregnancy and previous radiation to the same field are absolute contraindications to radiation therapy. Relative contraindications include previous radiation to the same general area, underlying pulmonary disease or cardiomyopathy, significant vasculitis, and inability to lie flat. Omitting radiation may be considered if the patient is at least 70 years old, has a single cancer less than 2 cm. completely excised, and has negative lymph nodes, especially if the tumor is hormone receptor positive.

Whole breast external beam radiation treatments each take only a few minutes and are given 5 days a week for a period of at least 4 to 6 weeks, usually with a "boost" to the tumor bed. Tangential fields (giving the treatments from multiple angles across the chest) spare underlying organs such as the heart and lungs.

Partial breast irradiation, in which the local area of the lumpectomy is radiated more intensively with external beams, radioactive material in a balloon, or radioactive seeds, is briefer and may have superior cosmetic results. Studies are ongoing, and whole breast radiation is still the standard of care.

Systemic Treatments
The development of an increasingly effective array of adjuvant systemic treatments is thought to be largely responsible for the recently seen gradual improvement in breast cancer survival. This remains an area of rapid innovation and frequent change, and it is likely that any particular regimen specified here would be outdated by the time you read this.

Hormonal
Hormonal therapy is generally used after surgery, chemotherapy, and radiation have been completed, although in some situations it may be used as a sole therapy. Selective estrogen receptor modulators (SERMs), particularly tamoxifen, act as estrogen receptor antagonists in breast tissue and as estrogen agonists in bone. They are used to treat estrogen receptor–positive (ER+) tumors, decreasing the incidence of contralateral breast cancer by approximately 40% and decreasing recurrence. There is no benefit beyond 5 years. Tamoxifen is also used for prophylaxis in high-risk women.

Aromatase inhibitors (AIs), such as letrozole, anastrozole, and exemestane, are being used with increasing frequency as an alternative or supplement to tamoxifen. As a class of drugs, they have been shown to decrease circulating estrogen levels by approximately 90% in postmenopausal women, and they may be superior to tamoxifen in prolonging disease-free survival. Multiple regimens are currently in use and in trial.

Chemotherapy

Indications for chemotherapy include node-positive disease or tumors greater than 1 cm in greatest diameter. Increasingly, multiple-gene assays that predict recurrence and response to treatment can be used to decide which patients with early-stage, ER+, node-negative cancers are likely to benefit from chemotherapy and which are not. The most commonly used regimen includes an anthracycline, a taxane, and possibly an alkylating agent. Many regimens are currently under study; the optimal chemotherapy regimen has not been determined. Chemotherapy may be given as the first treatment (called neoadjuvant when given prior to surgery), to reduce or downstage tumors and axillary involvement or to make surgery easier or more cosmetically acceptable.

Cytotoxic chemotherapy refers to chemical agents that kill cells. It is never given as a single agent in the treatment of breast cancer. The best-studied regimen includes cyclophosphamide, methotrexate, and 5-fluorouracil (CMF), which was the standard for many years. It has been superseded by the development of taxanes and inclusion of anthracyclines (which produce a small but significant improvement in survival). The inclusion of a taxane (such as paclitaxel and docetaxel) produces a 20% improvement in 5-year survival.

Biologic therapies for breast cancer are based on physiologic mechanisms, supporting activities of the immune system in targeting specific antigens. Trastuzumab improves survival in patients with HER-2–positive tumors. Other agents in this class are presently being developed.

Treatment of Male Breast Cancer

Mastectomy is the standard surgical treatment of operable breast cancer in men, because the breast is usually small. Most of these cancers are hormone-receptor positive. Evidence-based treatment regimens are difficult to develop because of the rarity of the disease. In general, all modalities of treatment are similar to those for women, including the use of radiation, taxanes, and trastuzumab.

Treatment of Recurrence and Metastasis

Local tumor recurrence in the breast after lumpectomy is treated with mastectomy. If radiation was never given, a small recurrence may be treated with lumpectomy and radiation. Local recurrence after mastectomy is treated with surgical excision, if possible, and radiation to the area, if not contraindicated. Early recurrences are treated with systemic chemotherapy. Local recurrence has a good prognosis in the absence of concomitant systemic recurrence.

Metastatic disease is treated with chemotherapy, including taxanes and biologic treatments. Brain metastases, which are often multiple, are treated with radiation. Bony metastases are treated with radiation and surgical fixation if there is a high risk of fracture. Radioactive strontium (^{89}Sr) is used for widespread and painful bony metastases. Bisphosphonates support bone strength, lessen the risk of fracture, and may reduce bone pain. Second-generation AIs may also be used for both recurrent and metastatic breast cancer.

Complications of Treatment
Surgery

Adverse effects of breast surgery include bleeding, infection, development of seroma, inflammation, pain and tenderness, swelling, and deformity. Some cosmetic problems can be corrected at least in part by plastic surgery. In addition, mastectomy can be complicated by flap necrosis.

Axillary lymph node dissection causes some degree of lymphedema, usually not severe, in up to 25% of patients. Decreased range of motion in the shoulder is almost always overcome by postoperative exercises. Damage to an intercostobrachial nerve may result in loss of sensation to the skin of the inner upper arm; other nerve injury is uncommon. The incidence of these complications is less with sentinel node biopsy, because of the less extensive dissection.

Breast reconstruction may produce an undesirable cosmetic result. Other adverse effects depend on the method of reconstruction. Reconstruction with implants has a somewhat higher risk of infection and in the long term may develop contracture of the capsule. All methods may result in chronic pain. Silicone breast implants have never been shown to cause significant systemic illness, although rupture and leakage can cause local problems and require further surgery. All implants eventually fail. Musculocutaneous flaps from the abdomen or back may cause weakness or deformity in the donor area. Free flaps are particularly vulnerable, but any flap may develop ischemic necrosis.

Radiation Treatment

A common side effect early after radiation treatment is breast edema with altered sensation. Fat necrosis may also occur. Bilateral discrepancy in the size and shape of the breasts is exacerbated by radiation. Chronic changes may progress to fibrosis and hyperpigmentation. Pneumonitis and bone necrosis are rare. There is a low risk of secondary cancers.

Whole breast radiation treatments gradually produce short-term symptoms similar to those of severe sunburn, including weakness and fatigue, skin irritation and redness, pain and tenderness. Long-term adverse effects may include fat necrosis, fibrosis, poor wound healing, deformity, and hyperpigmentation. Pericardial and pulmonary fibroses are rare.

Partial breast irradiation is given over a shorter period of time and a smaller area than whole breast radiation, but the effects are otherwise much the same.

Systemic Treatments

The adverse effects listed here are only the most common or dramatic.

Common side effects of tamoxifen are fatigue, night sweats, hot flashes, fluid retention, vaginitis, and thrombocytopenia. Serious side effects are much less common and include deep vein thrombosis, pulmonary embolism, stroke, hepatotoxicity, and endometrial cancer. AIs cause fewer blood clots than tamoxifen and do not cause endometrial cancer. Adverse reactions include osteoporosis, fractures, muscle and joint pains, and hot flashes.

Chemotherapies in general act on cell reproduction. Normal, necessary cells are affected, and those in bone marrow and the lining of the gut are particularly vulnerable. Common adverse effects of chemotherapy include nausea, vomiting, bone marrow suppression, stomatitis, and alopecia. Resulting problems include infection and bleeding. Recombinant erythropoietin and granulocyte colony-stimulating factor have made it possible to keep hematocrit and neutrophil counts at acceptable levels. Anthracyclines cause dose-dependent cardiotoxicity.

Serious adverse effects of taxanes include anaphylactic reactions, bone marrow suppression, and marked fluid retention. Common adverse effects include gastrointestinal bleeding, nausea, vomiting, diarrhea, fever, chills, rashes, peripheral neuropathies, dyspnea, and tachycardia.

In patients with no preexisting conditions, adverse effects of trastuzumab are usually mild but may include significant cardiac or pulmonary toxicity as well as fever, nausea, vomiting, diarrhea, weakness, headache, anemia, neutropenia, tumor pain, cough, dyspnea, and infusion reactions. Combining trastuzumab with chemotherapy increases cardiac risk.

The common adverse effect of nausea can be treated effectively.

Summary of Treatment

The treatment of breast cancer is a daunting task. It takes a long time and often has many complications and setbacks. It is frightening for the patient; in addition to the fear of death, which lessens over time for most patients, it involves many complex choices with unpredictable outcomes. In addition, it is never over. Unlike early colon cancer, which, if it does not recur within 5 years, can be regarded as cured, and unlike pancreatic cancer, which usually shows rapid progression, most breast cancer has a relatively indolent course and can recur after decades. As mentioned in the beginning, treatment is a team effort, and the most important member of the team is the patient, who must undergo pain, disfigurement, and constant conscientious effort through surgeries, chemotherapy and radiation treatments, follow-up tests, and many visits to doctors.

thePoint ☀ Go to http://thePoint.lww.com/activate and use your scratch-off code on the inside cover of this book to access bonus chapters, question bank, videos, and more.

Primary Hyperparathyroidism

In **primary hyperparathyroidism**, the inverse relationship between PTH and serum calcium is disturbed. Although calcium may remain within normal limits, PTH is elevated relative to the serum calcium level. Serum phosphate is often low and renal function is normal. Primary hyperparathyroidism may be caused by **parathyroid adenoma** (85%), **parathyroid hyperplasia** (15%), or parathyroid carcinoma (<1%). PTH secretion is increased and the homeostatic set point for calcium is reset at a higher value in all three conditions. Excess PTH secretion leads to increased GI calcium absorption, increased urinary calcium excretion, and net bone loss. Adenoma (uniglandular disease) refers to a single enlarged gland and is a benign process. The abnormal gland is rarely palpable preoperatively. Typical adenomas measure about 1 cm in size and weigh 500 to 1,000 mg. Hyperplasia (multiglandular disease) is diagnosed when multiple glands are all grossly abnormal. Hyperplasia is a benign process affecting all glands, but gland enlargement may be asymmetric. Primary hyperplasia most often is sporadic but may be inherited, either alone or as part of a MEN syndrome.

Secondary and Tertiary Hyperparathyroidism

Secondary hyperparathyroidism most often occurs in renal failure patients. Impaired glomerular filtration causes phosphate retention and decreased serum calcium levels. Reduced functional renal mass is available to hydroxylate 25-OH-vitamin D. The resultant lower 1,25-dihydroxy-vitamin D levels lead to less GI absorption of calcium and further hypocalcemia. PTH secretion by all glands is stimulated to restore calcium and phosphorous homeostasis. Continued nephron loss produces chronic overstimulation of PTH secretion, elevated PTH levels, and parathyroid hyperplasia, plus hyperphosphatemia (Figure 20-10). The multiple abnormalities in calcium, phosphate, and vitamin D metabolism have extremely deleterious effects on bone mineralization and may also lead to soft tissue calcium deposition and damage (e.g., tendon rupture, skin necrosis). Secondary hyperparathyroidism can also occur because of low vitamin D levels related to nutritional deficiencies or lack of sun exposure.

An important role for vitamin D is emerging in cardiovascular health, yielding upward revisions of existing normal ranges and dietary recommendations.

In **tertiary hyperparathyroidism**, one or more of the hyperplastic glands of a patient with secondary hyperparathyroidism becomes an autonomous producer of PTH. Most patients with tertiary disease are identified when their PTH levels remain high despite successful renal transplantation. The remaining patients are those who remain on dialysis and spontaneously progress from secondary to tertiary hyperparathyroidism, usually marked by the onset of hypercalcemia. Tertiary disease behaves in most ways like primary hyperparathyroidism, although multiglandular disease is more common than in primary hyperparathyroidism.

Clinical Presentation and Evaluation

Patients with primary hyperparathyroidism have classically presented with the complaints suggested in the mnemonic, "stones, bones, groans, moans, and psych overtones," most often urolithiasis ("stones") or bone diseases including bone resorption with cyst (osteitis cystica) and brown tumor formation ("bones"). Less commonly seen were abdominal pain from peptic ulcers or pancreatitis ("moans"), diffuse joint and muscle pains, fatigue and lethargy ("groans"), and neuropsychiatric abnormalities including depression or worsening psychosis ("psych overtones").

Currently most patients with primary hyperparathyroidism are found when unrelated laboratory testing reveals hypercalcemia. The most common cause of outpatient hypercalcemia is primary hyperparathyroidism, and the most frequent source of inpatient hypercalcemia is malignancy, either via paraneoplastic syndrome or bony metastases. Additional causes include some common medications (e.g., hydrochlorothiazide, lithium, calcium supplements), the inherited hypercalcemia syndromes, and sarcoidosis (Table 20-3).

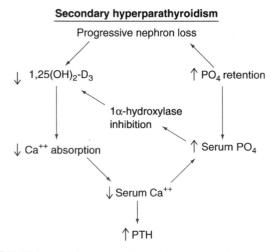

FIGURE 20-10. In secondary hyperparathyroidism, progressive nephron loss leads to phosphate retention, decreased calcium absorption, inhibition of 1α-hydroxylase, and decreased activation of vitamin D. These factors lead to decreased serum calcium and increased secretion of PTH. PTH, parathyroid hormone.

TABLE 20-3	Differential Diagnosis of Hypercalcemia		
Diagnosis		**PTH**	**PTHrP**
Primary hyperparathyroidism		High	Low
Tertiary hyperparathyroidism		High	Low
Familial hypercalcemic hypocalciuria		High, normal, or low	Low
Lithium therapy		High or normal	Low
Paraneoplastic syndrome (humoral hypercalcemia of malignancy)		Low	High
Osteolytic metastases		Low	Low
Multiple myeloma		Low	Low
Drug-induced hypercalcemia[a]		Low	Low
Granulomatous disease		Low	Low
Hypervitaminosis D		Low	Low
Milk-alkali syndrome		Low	Low
Nonparathyroid endocrine disease		Low	Low
Immobilization		Low	Low
Idiopathic		Low	Low

[a]Except lithium induced; see text.

PTH, parathyroid hormone; PTHrP, parathyroid hormone–related peptide.

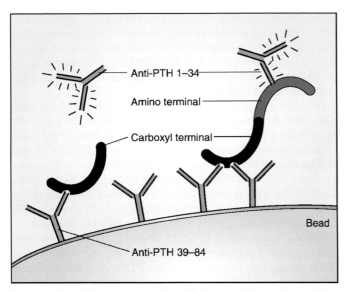

FIGURE 20-11. Intact PTH assay. An antibody recognizing PTH 39-84 binds carboxyl fragments in the midpoint and C-terminus of the molecule. A second antibody recognizes the amino terminal region of PTH (1-34).

History taking should target the classic complaints of primary hyperparathyroidism, but also the now more common, poorly defined constitutional or neuropsychiatric symptoms such as a decreased sense of well-being or behavioral changes. Negative drug and family histories, plus negative system reviews focused on the most common occult malignancies, support a working diagnosis of sporadic primary hyperparathyroidism. Further workup begins with simultaneous serum calcium and PTH levels. Standard PTH assays measure the whole PTH peptide by double antibody techniques and are known as "intact" or "biointact" assays (Figure 20-11). Table 20-3 lists diseases associated with hypercalcemia arranged into those associated with or without elevated PTH. Elevated intact PTH plus hypercalcemia occurs only with primary and tertiary hyperparathyroidism, familial hypercalcemic hypocalciuria (FHH, also called familial benign hypercalcemia), vitamin D deficiency, or lithium-induced hypercalcemia. Urinary calcium and serum vitamin D levels can help differentiate among the causes of increased PTH. A calcium:creatinine clearance ratio of <0.05 indicates FHH. The family history may be confirmatory as can genetic analysis for FHH mutations in the calcium-sensing receptor.

Obtaining a serum parathyroid hormone–related peptide (PTHrP) level might be useful when occult malignancy is a concern (Table 20-3). PTHrP, encoded on chromosome 12 and expressed by almost all cells, may represent a primitive precursor to PTH, which is encoded on chromosome 11 and expressed only by parathyroid cells. The role of PTHrP in normal calcium metabolism is unknown. PTHrP may help maintain calcium homeostasis during pregnancy, since PTHrP, unlike PTH, crosses the placenta. PTHrP shares the same initial 34 N-terminal amino acids with PTH but is a longer peptide and does not cross-react with intact PTH assays. Epithelial tumors may secrete PTHrP and cause hypercalcemia as a paraneoplastic syndrome; the most common is bronchial squamous cell carcinoma. Other PTHrP sources include breast, renal, and ovarian cancers. Bone destruction by primary cancers (e.g., multiple myeloma) or lytic bony metastases causes hypercalcemia without PTHrP elevation. vitamin D analogues are secreted by some tumors

(e.g., lymphoma) and can produce hypercalcemia without PTH or PTHrP elevations.

Increased activation of 25-OH-vitamin D by macrophages in granulomatous lesions (e.g., sarcoidosis) can lead to hypercalcemia without increased PTH or PTHrP. A normal chest radiograph makes sarcoidosis unlikely. Lithium appears to interfere with the calcium-PTH feedback loop; a history of bipolar disorder or a therapeutic lithium level should point to this possibility.

Secondary hyperparathyroidism is present to some degree in most end-stage renal disease patients. Intact PTH levels are often elevated but serum calcium is usually normal. An elevated serum calcium level raises concern for tertiary disease. Serum phosphorus and creatinine are increased, while vitamin D levels are often low. PTH fragments, especially C-terminal ones, have prolonged half-lives and are increased in chronic renal failure. Typical manifestations of disease are bone pain, soft tissue calcifications (calcinosis), and pruritus.

Treatment
Medical
Acute, severe hypercalcemia is managed by large-volume saline infusion to restore intravascular volume and to initiate a saline diuresis, which in turn triggers calciuresis. Loop diuretics (e.g., furosemide) are used adjunctively. Drugs may be added to decrease bone turnover (e.g., bisphosphonates, calcitonin). Acute dialysis is rarely required. Treatment directed at any underlying malignancy or other precipitating condition is added where appropriate (e.g., glucocorticoids for sarcoidosis).

Currently, there is no definitive medical treatment for primary or tertiary hyperparathyroidism. Bisphosphonates (e.g., alendronate [Fosamax]) and selective estrogen receptor modulators (e.g., raloxifene [Evista]) can help to slow and sometimes prevent bone loss. Since these drugs are relatively ineffective in primary and tertiary hyperparathyroidism, they are generally reserved for patients who are prohibitive operative risks. For end-stage renal disease patients, improved techniques of dialysis, better vitamin D supplements, and effective oral phosphate binders have markedly enhanced the medical control of secondary hyperparathyroidism and decreased the incidence of significant bony disease. Cinacalcet (Sensipar), which lowers calcium by activating the calcium-sensing receptor, also is available for use in secondary disease.

Surgical
For patients with overt symptoms or signs of primary hyperparathyroidism (e.g., urolithiasis), operation is clearly indicated. In the absence of major, life-limiting comorbidities, patients with metabolic derangements due to primary hyperparathyroidism (e.g., hypercalciuria, decreased bone density) are also best served by surgery. Operative indications for patients with no or minimal symptoms are somewhat less clear. Outcome data are confounded by the overlap between the constitutional symptoms of primary hyperparathyroidism and the aches and pains of aging. However, today's less invasive parathyroid operations offer a low-risk, lower-cost procedure with rapid convalescence. When compared to the inconvenience and cost of observation with serial metabolic evaluations and the inherent risks of prolonged hyperparathyroidism, surgery is being recommended increasingly for minimally symptomatic patients. Patient selection criteria for parathyroidectomy as developed by the National Institutes of Health include asymptomatic patients <50 years of age (Table 20-4).

TABLE 20-4	NIH Criteria for Parathyroidectomy

Age < 50 OR Any age with any of the following:

Nephrolithiasis
Osteitis fibrosa cystica
Serum calcium >1.0 mg/dL above reference range (typically >11.2)
Hypercalciuria (>400 mg/day)
Bone mineral density T score reduced by >2.5 SD measured at one or more sites
Creatinine clearance reduced by 30% compared to age-matched normal range
History of an episode of life-threatening hypercalcemia
Neuromuscular symptoms: documented proximal weakness, atrophy, hyperreflexia, and gait disturbance

Observation rather than operation is not safe for noncompliant patients. Observation requires active surveillance including biannual serum calcium levels, annual serum creatinine measurement, and annual bone mineral density determination.

For end-stage renal disease patients, renal transplantation remains the most effective long-term treatment for both renal disease and secondary hyperparathyroidism. Parathyroidectomy is sometimes indicated for ongoing bone loss, soft tissue calcifications, or severe pruritus, particularly for patients who are not transplant candidates. Parathyroidectomy is occasionally indicated for patients on lithium who develop hypercalcemia and who cannot be managed with alternative medications (e.g., divalproex sodium [Depakote]).

Operative Strategies *Classic open exploration* for sporadic primary hyperparathyroidism includes visualization of all cervical glands, characterization of the disease by the surgeon based upon operative observations (uniglandular [adenoma] or multiglandular [hyperplasia]), and resection of sufficient parathyroid tissue to restore long-term eucalcemia while not creating hypoparathyroidism. Exploration is typically performed under general anesthesia. Single-gland resection is performed for adenoma; hyperplasia is most often treated by subtotal (three and one-half gland) resection. Familial syndromes (see MEN) introduce other considerations and alternatives such as total parathyroidectomy with forearm autotransplantation and cryopreservation of excised tissue are often performed.

Two *directed* operative strategies, also known as *minimally invasive* or *targeted*, are often applicable to sporadic primary hyperparathyroidism: intraoperative PTH (ioPTH) assay monitoring and radioguidance. Both approaches require that an abnormal parathyroid gland be identified preoperatively to guide the surgeon to the appropriate side of the neck. Such preoperative localization is usually done by sestamibi radionuclide scanning. A nonlocalizing scan precludes radioguided operation. Other imaging modalities (e.g., cervical ultrasonography) may lateralize an abnormal parathyroid gland and still allow an ioPTH-based approach. Both of the directed operations can be performed under cervical block anesthesia combined with conscious sedation or under general anesthesia.

With the *radioguided strategy*, the patient is injected with sestamibi about 2 hours prior to the start of operation. The incision is placed over the point of maximal radioactivity as detected by a handheld gamma probe. Dissection follows the radioactivity signal to expose abnormal parathyroid tissue, which is excised. Radioactivity should equalize throughout the neck after adenoma removal, and the adenoma should have a radioactivity count at least 20% above the neck background count. Failure to meet these radioactivity criteria mandates continued neck exploration.

For the *ioPTH-directed strategy*, a peripheral blood sampling device is inserted before neck exploration and a baseline sample drawn for ioPTH assay, which is an intact PTH assay modified to shorten the turnaround time to 20 minutes. A limited incision is made sufficient to expose and excise the preoperatively localized abnormal parathyroid gland. Serial blood samples for ioPTH are drawn after excision for comparison with a baseline drawn after anesthetic induction. An ioPTH level at 10 minutes postexcision that has fallen into the normal range and has declined by >50% from baseline indicates sufficient parathyroid resection to restore long-term eucalcemia. Time criteria may be modified when PTH degradation kinetics are impaired (e.g., renal disease). Failure of the ioPTH level to drop appropriately leads to continued neck exploration.

Directed parathyroidectomy by either method normally allows patients to be discharged in 24 hours or less. Minimal analgesics are required and convalescence is typically brief. Patients are sometimes discharged on calcium supplements to be weaned as outpatients, depending upon surgeon preference and the patient's access to urgent health care.

Endoscopic parathyroidectomy is a relatively new approach that utilizes very small incisions, which can be placed in locations distant from the neck. General or regional anesthesia is feasible depending upon port placement sites. The abnormal parathyroid gland must be localized by preoperative imaging, and ioPTH monitoring is used to confirm uniglandular disease. Optimal patient selection criteria for endoscopic parathyroidectomy are still evolving. Multiglandular disease and prior neck operations are relative contraindications to an endoscopic approach.

Parathyroid cancer is quite rare and may be recognized intraoperatively by adjacent tissue invasion. Operation includes resection of the primary tumor and the ipsilateral thyroid lobe plus adherent soft tissue and regional lymph nodes. For parathyroid cancer diagnosed postoperatively based upon final histopathology only, reoperation is generally not indicated. Serum calcium and PTH levels are followed in parathyroid cancer patients to detect recurrences. There is no effective adjuvant radiotherapy or chemotherapy. Recurrences are treated by medical control of hypercalcemia plus cinacalcet and by resection of tumor whenever feasible.

Since secondary hyperparathyroidism is always multiglandular, at least subtotal parathyroidectomy (three and one-half gland) should be performed. Total parathyroidectomy with forearm autotransplantation is preferred by some surgeons. Published results are similar for both procedures. More recently, some surgeons have employed total parathyroidectomy without autotransplantation, as patients often have residual rests of cervical parathyroid tissue that suffice for calcium homeostasis. Cervical thymectomy is typically performed with operations for secondary disease, since the inferior glands and many parathyroid rests are near to or within the thymus.

Operations for tertiary hyperparathyroidism are guided by the intraoperative findings, most often multiglandular disease leading to either total parathyroidectomy with forearm autotransplant or subtotal parathyroidectomy. There is limited experience with directed operative approaches to tertiary disease.

Complications The most serious complication of parathyroidectomy, recurrent laryngeal nerve injury, should be extremely rare. Persistent hypercalcemia because of failure to identify the adenoma or all hyperplastic glands occurs in 1% to 5% of patients in most large series. Transient, early postoperative hypoparathyroidism sometimes occurs because of chronic preoperative suppression of the remaining normal parathyroid tissue by the hyperfunctioning gland(s). Patients with established bone disease appear to be at increased risk for early hypoparathyroidism. Permanent hypoparathyroidism should be rare (<1%). Phosphorus as well as calcium should be measured postoperatively, as successful operation typically corrects hypophosphatemia. In the "hungry bone" syndrome, phosphorus is taken up by the bone with calcium and serum phosphorus will remain low. Such patients require supplemental calcium postoperatively until the syndrome resolves.

Reoperative Surgery In the event of persistent or recurrent hypercalcemia, repeat laboratory testing is done first to confirm the diagnosis of hyperparathyroidism. Radionuclide and anatomic imaging studies are then repeated. When conventional imaging is negative, transfemoral selective venous sampling for PTH in the neck and mediastinum may localize the disease source. Most persistent abnormal tissue is found in the neck. Cervical reoperation carries substantially greater risks of recurrent nerve injury and permanent hypoparathyroidism. Mediastinal abnormal parathyroid glands can sometimes be ablated by angioembolization or removed thoracoscopically.

■ ADRENAL GLANDS

ANATOMY

The adrenal glands are small (3 to 5 g each), yellow, triangular-shaped glands located behind the peritoneum of the posterior abdominal wall, closely associated with the upper poles of the kidneys (Figure 20-12). The right adrenal gland lies posterior to the liver, and posterior and lateral to the

inferior vena cava. The left adrenal is lateral to the aorta and just behind the superior border of the pancreatic tail.

The arterial blood supply to the adrenal glands is from three main arteries: the superior adrenal artery branches from the inferior phrenic artery, the middle adrenal artery arises from the aorta, and the inferior adrenal artery is a branch from the renal artery. The adrenal veins are remarkably consistent in their location and drainage, but different by side. The right adrenal vein is 2 to 5 mm long, takes off from the anterior aspect of the adrenal gland, and drains into the posterolateral aspect of the vena cava. The left adrenal vein arises from the lower portion of the gland and travels inferiorly to drain into the left renal vein.

The adrenal gland is divided into two primary areas based on embryological development of the tissue types: the cortex, which is derived from the mesoderm; and the medulla, which arises from neural crest cells. The medulla is the only endocrine organ whose activity is controlled entirely by nervous impulses. The innervation of the adrenal medulla is unusual in that there are no postganglionic cells. Preganglionic fibers from the sympathetic nervous system end directly on the medullary cells.

PHYSIOLOGY: ADRENAL CORTEX

The adrenal cortex has three layers, the outer zona glomerulosa, the middle zona fasciculata, and the inner zona reticularis. Each zone produces its own distinct hormones derived from cholesterol, which is converted to Δ-pregnenolone. The latter serves as the precursor for the glucocorticoids, mineralocorticoids, and androgenic steroids produced by the cortical cells (Table 20-5).

The *zona glomerulosa* produces and secretes mineralocorticoids, of which the most predominant is aldosterone. Aldosterone has a half-life of 15 minutes and is metabolized in the liver. Secretion of aldosterone is primarily regulated by the renin–angiotensin system in a negative feedback fashion, and is also influenced by plasma potassium concentration. In response to a decrease in renal blood flow, the juxtaglomerular cells within the kidney produce renin, which cleaves angiotensinogen into angiotensin I, which is then converted

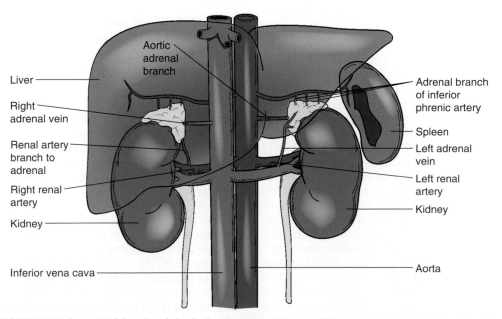

FIGURE 20-12. Anatomy of the adrenal glands showing their relations to adjacent structures and their blood supply.

TABLE 20-5 | Correlation of Adrenal Zones with Disease Syndromes and Abnormal Adrenal Function

Adrenal Zone	Hormone Produced	Normal Function	Hypersecretory Syndrome	Symptoms	Pearls
Zona glomerulosa	Aldosterone	Electrolyte metabolism	Conn's syndrome	Hypokalemia	Insuppressible hyperaldosteronism and suppressed plasma renin
				Hypertension	
				Muscle weakness	
Zona fasciculata	Cortisone	Protein and carbohydrate metabolism	Cushing's syndrome or disease	Buffalo hump	Exclude exogenous intake of glucocorticoids
	Hydrocortisone			Violaceous striae	
				Moon facies	
				Truncal obesity	
				Hypertension	
Zona reticularis	Progesterone	Sexual differentiation	Adrenogenital syndrome	Virilism/feminization	Presents in early childhood
	Androgen			Hyponatremia	
	Estrogen			Hypertension	
Medulla	Epinephrine	Sympathetic response	Pheochromocytoma	Episodic hypertension	10% are:
					Malignant
					Bilateral
					Familial
					Extra-adrenal
	Norepinephrine			Headache	
				Sweating	
				Palpitations	

by angiotensin-converting enzyme (ACE) in the lung to angiotensin II. Angiotensin II directly stimulates aldosterone release from the zona glomerulosa, which increases the exchange of sodium for potassium and hydrogen ions in the distal nephron. Aldosterone results in renal sodium reabsorption while promoting potassium wasting to modulate the body's electrolyte composition, fluid volume, and blood pressure.

The cells within the *zona fasciculata* secrete the glucocorticoid cortisol, stimulated by circulating adrenocorticotropic hormone (ACTH) from the anterior pituitary and suppressed by cortisol feedback inhibition. Cortisol is involved in the intermediate metabolism of carbohydrates, proteins, and lipids. It increases blood glucose levels by decreasing insulin uptake and stimulating hepatic gluconeogenesis. Cortisol also slows amino acid uptake and peripheral protein synthesis while increasing peripheral lipolysis.

Normal individuals produce 10 to 30 mg of cortisol daily in a diurnal rhythm. Cortisol has a half-life of approximately 90 minutes and is metabolized primarily by the liver. The natural by-products of cortisol metabolism can be measured in the urine as *17-hydroxycorticosteroids*. Prolonged effects of high levels of cortisol include induction of a catabolic state, proximal muscle wasting, truncal obesity, insulin-resistant diabetes, impaired wound healing, and immunosuppression.

The cells of the *zona reticularis* respond to ACTH by converting pregnenolone to 17-hydroxypregnenolone, which is then converted to dehydroepiandrosterone (DHEA), the major sex steroid produced by the adrenal glands. DHEA is converted by local tissues into testosterone. Adrenal wproduction of sex hormones is responsible, in part, for the development of male secondary sexual features. Abnormal production can cause virilization in women.

DISEASE STATES

Hyperadrenocorticism (Cushing's Syndrome and Cushing's Disease)

Harvey Cushing, M.D., first described hypercortisolism in 1932. Cushing's syndrome (CS) refers to the signs and symptoms of hypercortisolism, whereas Cushing's disease is hypercortisolism due to an ACTH-producing pituitary adenoma. CS is classified as either ACTH dependent or ACTH independent. ACTH-independent hypercortisolism most commonly results from exogenous corticosteroid administration but can also be caused by adrenocortical tumors including adenomas (10% to 25% of patients with CS), adrenal cortical carcinomas (ACCs) (8%), and bilateral adrenal hyperplasia (1%). ACTH-dependent CS can be caused by excessive ACTH production secondary to the hypothalamus releasing excessive amounts of corticotrophin-releasing hormone (CRH), pituitary adenomas (Cushing's disease), which produce excessive amounts of ACTH, or extrapituitary ACTH-producing tumors such as bronchial carcinoids and small cell lung cancer (5% to 10% of cases). Cushing's disease produces bilateral adrenal cortical hyperplasia and is responsible for approximately 70% of cases of endogenous CS.

Clinical Presentation of Cushing's Syndrome

CS usually presents in the third and the fourth decades, and it has a 4:1 female-to-male preponderance. The classic clinical features include truncal obesity (90%), hypertension (80%), diabetes (80%), weakness (80%), purple striae (70%), hirsutism (70%), moon facies (60%), and a buffalo hump (posterior thorax). A number of other symptoms can be seen including depression, mental changes, osteoporosis, kidney stones, polyuria, fungal skin infections, poor wound healing, menstrual disturbances, and acne. In patients with CS, the diurnal variation in glucocorticoid secretion (high levels in the morning, declining during the day, with lowest levels in the evening) and the ability of the adrenal gland to increase cortisol secretion in response to ACTH stimulation are either lost or blunted. Mild hyperglycemia, glycosuria, hypokalemia, and elevated carbon dioxide content are occasional findings in CS. When CS is due to ectopic ACTH and pituitary tumors, melanotropins are also secreted, leading to increased skin pigmentation.

Diagnosis of Cushing's Syndrome

In patients with suspected CS, a complete history and physical examination looking for the above-mentioned symptoms is critical. It is particularly important to rule out sources of exogenous glucocorticoid exposure and to be aware of medications that might interfere with some screening tests. Initial screening tests measure glucocorticoid hormones or their breakdown products. There are three main screening tests: urinary free cortisol (UFC; at least 2 measurements), late-night salivary cortisol (2 measurements) and 1-mg overnight dexamethasone suppression test (DST). One of these tests should be performed and if there is any abnormal result, with serial testing, one or two of the other tests should also be performed. A 24-hour urinary excretion of free cortisol >300 μg is diagnostic for CS, 45 to 300 μg is indeterminate, and <45 μg is normal although 10% to 15% of patients with CS will have a normal test on serial sampling.

If CS is confirmed by one of the above tests, a workup is performed to determine the subtype of CS affecting the patient. Plasma ACTH measurement segregates patients into ACTH-dependent or ACTH-independent subtypes. In patients with a suppressed ACTH level (<5 pg/mL), the CS etiology is due to a primary adrenal tumor. CT scan, or occasionally MRI, of the abdomen should be performed to localize the mass. Unilateral masses are either adenomas or ACCs and they are usually radiographically distinct because ACCs are rarely <5 cm and because they have different radiographic appearances. Bilateral adrenal tumors can be due to primary pigmented nodular adrenocortical disease (PPNAD), ACTH-independent macronodular adrenal hyperplasia (AIMAH), or bilateral cortisol-secreting adenomas.

If the ACTH level is normal or increased, the patient should have a pituitary MRI. If this shows a pituitary tumor (hypodense, nonenhancing, ≥5 mm) and the clinical picture is consistent with this finding, patients should be treated by transsphenoidal surgery. If the MRI is normal or equivocal, inferior petrosal sinus sampling (IPSS) should be performed. If IPSS does not reveal a pituitary tumor, further workup for ectopic sources of ACTH is required including CT, MRI, neck ultrasound, scintigraphy, and tumor markers.

Treatment: Cushing's Disease
Medical Therapy

Cushing's disease can temporarily be controlled with the use of agents that inhibit steroid biosynthesis such as metyrapone, ketoconazole, or aminoglutethimide. Nearly all patients will eventually develop a tolerance to these medications. This approach is generally reserved for patients who are very poor surgical candidates. A DDT derivative, mitotane, is toxic to the adrenal cortex and has been used in some cases of hyperadrenocorticism with modest success, although its side effects are serious and quite common. Radiation of pituitary adenomas can also be effective; however, resolution of symptoms may take up to a year and recurrence is very common.

Surgical Therapy

The treatment of choice in patients with Cushing's disease caused by a pituitary adenoma is transsphenoidal microadenomectomy, which has an initial cure rate approaching 95%. Recurrent disease necessitating a second exploration produces a cure rate of approximately 50%. If TSS fails, patients may require bilateral laparoscopic adrenalectomy, radiotherapy and/or total hypophysectomy. After bilateral adrenalectomy, Nelson's syndrome, with hyperpigmentation, headaches, exophthalmos, and visual field loss, is seen in about 20% of patients. This results from progression of an ACTH-secreting pituitary adenoma.

Primary Adrenal Cushing's Syndrome
Adrenal Adenoma

Solitary adenomas are the cause of primary adrenal hypercortisolism in 80% to 90% of patients. As a result of the hypersecretion of cortisol and inhibition of ACTH, the remaining adrenal tissue on the ipsilateral side and the contralateral adrenal tissue atrophy and function poorly until the adenoma is removed. The treatment of choice is laparoscopic unilateral adrenalectomy. All of these patients should receive perioperative doses of steroids, and because the remaining adrenal tissue does not function normally for many months, patients should be maintained on maintenance doses of prednisone (5 mg q AM and 2.5 mg q PM) or hydrocortisone until normal adrenal function has returned as determined by normalization of the ACTH stimulation test. This may take as long as 12 to 18 months.

Adrenal Cortical Carcinoma

The standard of care is open unilateral adrenalectomy for ACC (see later section on Adrenal Cortical Carcinoma).

Primary Adrenal Hyperplasia

Primary adrenal hyperplasia, either PPNAD or AIMAH, affects bilateral adrenals and treatment usually requires bilateral adrenalectomy. This is usually performed laparoscopically.

Bilateral Adenomas

Patients with bilateral cortisol-secreting adenomas are ideally treated with bilateral cortical-sparing laparoscopic adrenalectomy.

Primary Aldosteronism

Primary aldosteronism (PA) (Conn's syndrome) was first described by Jerome Conn, MD, at the University of Michigan in 1955. The syndrome is twice as common in women as in men, and most commonly occurs between the fourth and the sixth decades of life. Patients with PA produce excess aldosterone that is not responsive to the rennin–angiotensin axis and that is not suppressed by salt loading. PA has recently been reported in more than 10% of hypertensive patients, and 17% to 23% of patients with resistant hypertension. Although the classic presentation of PA is hypertension and hypokalemia, only a minority of patients (9% to 37%) has hypokalemia. The importance of diagnosing PA is that it is curable, and these patients have higher cardiovascular morbidity and mortality than matched patients with hypertension of other etiologies. PA is usually due to an adrenal adenoma, diffuse hyperplasia, or nodular (adenomatous) hyperplasia of the adrenal cortex. ACC is the cause in <1%.

Clinical Presentation

Excess aldosterone increases total body sodium, decreases potassium levels, and increases extracellular volume resulting in metabolic alkalosis and hypertension. Hypomagnesemia, tetany, and periodic paralysis may also be seen. The classic biochemical findings include persistently elevated plasma and urinary aldosterone levels and decreased plasma renin activity unresponsive to stimulation. Aldosterone is normally secreted in response to a reduced effective blood volume and renal blood flow, sodium depletion or restriction, and potassium loading. It stimulates absorption of sodium at the distal convoluted and cortical collecting tubules. Sodium is reabsorbed at the expense of hydrogen and potassium ions.

Diagnosis

Primary hyperaldosteronism is defined as inappropriate hypersecretion of aldosterone in the absence of activation of the renin–angiotensin system. The diagnosis is suspected in patients with moderate or severe hypertension or drug-resistant hypertension, hypertension and hypokalemia, hypertension and an adrenal lesion or hypertension in a patient with a family history of PA, early-onset hypertension, or the sequelae of hypertension. Fifty-five to sixty percent of these patients have an adrenal adenoma, while 35% to 45% have bilateral hyperplasia. Rarely an adrenal cortical adenoma can be a part of multiple endocrine neoplasia type 1 (MEN-1) syndrome or familial Conn's syndrome. Bilateral adenomas have also been described as having nonfunctional adenomas (incidentalomas) in the presence of bilateral hyperplasia. Secondary hyperaldosteronism is a normal homeostatic response to volume or salt depletion. It is associated with elevated plasma renin activity and elevated or high normal aldosterone levels. It can be seen in association with cirrhosis, nephrotic syndrome, and congestive heart failure.

In these patients, an aldosterone-to-renin ratio (ARR) is the initial screening test. Prior to testing hypokalemia should be corrected, sodium intake should not be restricted; certain medications, like spironolactone, potassium-wasting diuretics, and chewing tobacco should be stopped 4 weeks prior to testing. If a patient has a positive ARR (generally >20 but the number is variable due to different laboratory standard normals), confirmation with oral sodium loading, saline infusion, fludrocortisone suppression, or captopril challenge tests can be used. Once PA has been confirmed, all patients should have a CT scan of the abdomen. Small lesions may be missed, so if the patient is a surgical candidate, adrenal venous sampling can localize the lesion.

Treatment

Patients with unilateral aldosteronomas should have their hypertension and hypokalemia normalized prior to surgical intervention, often with a mineralocorticoid receptor antagonist (like spironolactone). Laparoscopic unilateral adrenalectomy is the treatment of choice in these patients. When adenomas are removed, the blood pressure becomes normal in 70% of cases;

the remainder will require modest antihypertensive therapy. Patients with hyperaldosteronism that cannot be localized to one adrenal gland are managed with spironolactone and symptomatic treatment. In most of these patients, bilateral adrenal hyperplasia (diffuse disease) is the cause of the hyperaldosteronism, and bilateral adrenalectomy is not recommended.

Adrenal Cortical Carcinoma

ACCs are rare tumors with a worldwide incidence of 2 per million people annually. These tumors can occur at any age, but demonstrate a peak incidence in the fourth and fifth decades. They also show a slight left-sided and a female preponderance, are usually unilateral, and symptoms are most often related to hormone hypersecretion (found in 40% to 60%). The prognosis is generally poor with 50% to 70% of patients presenting with extra-adrenal disease (liver, lung) and after resection recurrence occurs in 70% to 80% of patients. Poor prognosis is related with advanced stage and incomplete surgical resection and there is debate about the prognostic significance of tumor grade, hormonal hypersecretion, age, gender, and tumor size.

Most ACCs are large (>6 cm), encapsulated, friable, and have extensive central necrosis and hemorrhage. It is often difficult to differentiate large benign adrenal neoplasms from malignant lesions purely on the basis of cellular characteristics. Venous or capsular invasion and distant metastases are the most reliable signs of malignancy. However, tumor necrosis, intratumoral hemorrhage, marked nuclear and cellular pleomorphism, and the presence of many mitotic figures per high-power field all strongly support the diagnosis of ACC.

Clinical Presentation

Over 50% of patients with ACCs present with CS; 15% present with virilizing, feminizing, and purely aldosterone-secreting carcinomas; and 10% of tumors are found to be hormonally active only by biochemical studies. An abdominal mass is a common finding. Symptoms from metastases including weight loss, weakness, fever, and bone pain are also seen. Children are more likely to have tumors that produce excess androgen. Women with virilizing tumors will have hirsutism, temporal balding, increased muscle mass, and amenorrhea. Boys will present with precocious puberty. Men with virilizing tumors will typically present with gynecomastia, testicular atrophy, impotence, or decreased libido.

Diagnosis

CT scan is the imaging modality of choice for adrenal lesions. Features on abdominal CT that suggest that an adrenal mass is a carcinoma include larger size (8 to 15 cm), irregular borders, heterogeneity, evidence of central necrosis, stippled calcifications (15% to 30% of cases), regional adenopathy, invasion of adjacent structures, and the presence of metastases. ACCs have a predilection for extension through the adrenal vein into either the renal vein (left-sided neoplasms) or the inferior vena cava (right-sided neoplasms). MRI can be helpful in delineating vascular extension.

Treatment

The treatment of choice is surgical excision with total gross tumor removal. Resection is possible in 80% of cases. If patients present with early disease, adrenalectomy and excision of involved regional lymph nodes may be all that is necessary. If there is presence of local invasion or visceral metastases, ipsilateral nephrectomy and resection of contiguous structures or hepatic metastases is indicated. Postoperatively, corticosteroid replacement is usually necessary because of atrophy of the contralateral gland secondary to tumor hypersecretion of cortisol.

Patients with resected localized adrenal carcinoma that is low grade only require follow-up imaging every 3 to 6 months; if biomarkers were elevated, these should be followed. If a resected localized ACC is high grade, NCCN Guidelines recommend considering external-beam radiation to the tumor bed and adjuvant mitotane chemotherapy in addition to the follow-up described for low-grade tumors. If the lesion is metastatic or unresectable and low grade, NCCN guidelines recommend considering resection of the lesion if it is functional and if >90% of the tumor can be resected. In addition, systemic therapy consists of some combination of mitotane with a combination of cisplatin, etoposide, doxorubicin, or streptozocin, optimally as part of a clinical trial. If a metastatic or unresectable tumor is high grade, systemic chemotherapy as described above is considered. For these patients, there is no role for partial resection of the lesion; however, the guidelines do recommend considering external-beam radiation to metastatic sites or to the primary tumor. Recurrence rates are high (70% to 80%) and some studies have shown a survival advantage with resection of disease recurrence in addition to palliation of hormonal symptoms in functional tumors.

The overall prognosis of ACC is poor. Unadjusted 5-year observed survival ranges from 24% to 44% with worse survival in older patients. Patients with negative resection margins have a median survival of 51 months compared with 7 months in patients who had positive resection margins. Survival has been relatively unchanged for the past 20 years.

Incidentally Discovered Adrenal Mass

With increasing use of CT, MRI, and ultrasound, incidentally discovered adrenal masses are becoming more common. Adrenal tumors are usually diagnosed on the basis of clinical symptoms; the incidentally discovered mass is typically asymptomatic and therefore presents a unique challenge for the managing physician. The prevalence of adrenal incidentaloma has been estimated at 0.6% to 5% when upper abdominal CT scans are evaluated. Incidental adrenal lesions are noted on 8.7% of patients on autopsy. The diagnostic approach to the adrenal incidentaloma should consist of clinical, laboratory, and imaging evaluation to rule out hypercortisolism, aldosteronism (if hypertensive), pheochromocytoma, or a malignant adrenal lesion.

Approximately 80% of incidentally discovered adrenal masses are nonfunctioning adenomas, 5% are subclinical CS, 5% are pheochromocytomas, 1% are aldosteronoma, <5% are adrenocortical carcinomas, and 2.5% are metastases to the adrenal gland.

Diagnosis

The initial step is to establish whether a mass is hormonally active. A 1-mg overnight DST is a good initial screening test to evaluate for excess cortisol (subclinical CS). If clinical suspicion is high due to hypertension, obesity, diabetes or osteoporosis, guidelines recommend combining salivary cortisol, dexamethasone suppression, and urine-free cortisol tests.

The next step is to determine if the lesion has radiographic findings concerning for malignancy. If the lesion is <4 cm with heterogeneous, regular borders, the patient should be tested for a hormonally active tumor. If there is no evidence of

an aberrant hormonal milieu, the patient should be followed. If there is evidence of a hormonally active tumor, the patient will likely progress to adrenalectomy. If the CT scan shows a lesion that is ≥4 cm and has features that are indeterminate or consistent with malignancy, a hormonal workup should be completed and the tumor surgically removed as is appropriate based on the suspected etiology.

Finally, the clinician must evaluate if the patient is at risk for metastatic disease, hypercortisolism, aldosteronism, or pheochromocytoma. A patient at risk for pheochromocytoma should have plasma-fractionated metanephrines and normetanephrines, or a 24-hour total urinary metanephrines and fractionated catecholamines checked (see Pheochromocytoma section below). If the lesion does not meet any of the above criteria and occurs in a patient with a history of cancer, a metastatic lesion should be considered. It is very rare that the diagnostic workup necessitates an adrenal biopsy; however, if a biopsy is indicated, the practitioner must be sure that the lesion is not a pheochromocytoma.

Treatment

If there is no evidence of an adrenal tumor requiring surgical excision, patients should have a follow-up radiographic test 3 to 6 months after the initial diagnosis and then annually for 1 to 2 years with evaluation for hormonal disturbances at the time of diagnosis and then each year for 5 years. Patients with subclinical CS, as evidenced by cortisol excess on one of the 4 tests above, should not have elective adrenalectomy unless symptoms of hypertension, diabetes, dyslipidemia, or osteoporosis develop and/or worsen.

All pheochromocytomas should be resected after appropriate preoperative treatment (see Pheochromocytoma section below). In patients with PA with venous sampling showing a unilateral source of aldosterone, laparoscopic total adrenalectomy is indicated. Patients with hyperaldosteronism that is bilateral, or in patients who are not surgical candidates, can be managed with mineralocorticoid receptor blockers. Any tumor with concerning findings on CT, and most lesions >4 cm, should be resected because of the risk for adrenal cancer. If ACC is suspected, open resection of the adrenal is recommended. It is rare that an adrenal metastasis requires resection.

Medulla: Pheochromocytoma

Pheochromocytomas are defined by the World Health Organization (WHO) as tumors arising from catecholamine-producing chromaffin cells in the adrenal medulla. Most are hormonally active with most producing norepinephrine (NE) and epinephrine (EPI) and few producing epi only (mostly MEN-2). Vasoconstriction from alpha-adrenergic stimulation, increased cardiac output from beta-adrenergic stimulation, and hypertension occur as a result. The incidence among hypertensive patients is 0.1% to 2%. They are found in 0.1% of autopsies and constitute about 5% of adrenal tumors found incidentally on CT scans. Similar lesions that arise from extra-adrenal sites are classified by the WHO as extra-adrenal paragangliomas, although many people group these tumors with pheochromocytomas. These extra-adrenal sites may be anywhere from the base of the skull to the pelvis, but are most often para-aortic. Approximately 10% of these tumors are malignant, 10% are bilateral, 10% are found in children, 10% are familial, and 10% are extra-adrenal (rule of 10s).

Ninety-eight percent of pheochromocytomas are located in the abdominal cavity. Other locations include the bladder and the Organ of Zuckerkandl; an area of chromaffin tissue inferior to the take-off of the inferior mesenteric artery and anterior to the aorta. [Repeats second sentence above paragraph]In order to convert NE to EPI, phenylethanolamine-*N*-methyltransferase (PNMT) must be induced. Extra-adrenal tumors do not have a high enough cortisol level around them to induce this enzyme and thus usually only secrete NE. Plasma normetanephrine levels are elevated in 97% of patients with adrenal pheochromocytoma and 100% of patients with extra-adrenal pheochromocytomas. A plasma metanephrine/normetanephrine ratio of <0.2 is indicative of an extra-adrenal tumor.

Clinical Presentation

Although pheochromocytomas may have extremely variable presentations, most have hypertension associated with palpitations, headache, and sweating. These symptoms are a direct result of sustained or paroxysmal secretion of NE and/or EPI. Patients may also experience a sense of impending doom, significant anxiety, weight loss, and constipation. Physical signs of an attack may include pallor, flushing, and sweating. Most attacks are short-lived, lasting 15 minutes or less, and can be precipitated by trauma (including invasive medical procedures), physical activity, exertion, changes in position, alcohol intake, micturition, smoking, or labor. Hypertension can be episodic, sustained or widely fluctuating, and superimposed on sustained hypertension. Fifty percent of these patients have sustained hypertension; however, some patients exhibit only mild clinical symptoms, making the diagnosis difficult. Pheochromocytoma typically presents as a sporadic tumor, but may also be found as a part of the MEN complexes 1 and 2. Pheochromocytomas are also associated with many familial disorders, including von Recklinghausen's disease, von Hippel-Lindau, and Sturge-Weber syndrome.

Diagnosis

Evaluating patients for pheochromocytoma or functional paraganglionoma includes plasma-free metanephrine and normetanephrine or urine metanephrine, chest and abdominal CT or MRI, and genetic counseling. If patients are having bone symptoms a bone scan is indicated, and if there is a suspicion of multiple tumors or if CT is negative, MIBG (metaiodobenzylguanidine) scan/Octreoscan is indicated. Fifteen to twenty percent of patients with pheochromocytomas will have normal plasma or urine catecholamines. Catecholamine levels do not correlate with tumor size.

Treatment

Once the diagnosis of pheochromocytoma is confirmed, patients should be started on alpha-blockade (phenoxybenzamine). Alpha-methyltyrosine can be added if needed. Doses of phenoxybenzamine should be increased until adequate alpha blockade is achieved. During this period, the patient must be kept adequately hydrated to maintain adequate intravascular volume. After the patient is alpha blocked, beta-blockade is used 10 days prior to surgery or if the patient is tachycardic. It is critical to initiate beta-blocker therapy only after adequate alpha blockade has been achieved. Patients with pheochromocytoma have severe peripheral vasoconstriction, increased systemic vascular resistance, and increased cardiac afterload. In order to maintain perfusion, patients compensate by increasing heart rate and stroke volume. Therefore, if a beta-blocker is initially given, the mechanisms by which the patient has compensated for the severe vasoconstriction are removed, and cardiovascular collapse can occur.

If the pheochromocytoma is resectable, laparoscopic adrenalectomy is the procedure of choice. Postoperatively, patients should have physical exam including blood pressure and catecholamines checked initially every 3 months and then every 6 months for three years and then annually after four years with imaging studies as indicated. Patients must have long-term follow-up after resection because 10% to 15% of patients with pheochromocytoma will recur.

Patients with locally unresectable pheochromocytoma should have a cytoreductive resection if possible, alpha-blockade and possible radiation therapy without alpha-methyltyrosine and/or beta-blockade following the principles noted above. If patients have distant metastases, they can have the same therapy as that for locally unresectable tumors. Other alternatives include systemic chemotherapy (dacarbazine, cyclophosphamide, vincristine), or 131I MIBG treatment. Both locally unresectable and patients with distant metastases should have physical exam including blood pressure and catecholamines checked every 3 to 4 months with imaging studies as indicated clinically.

Treatment of Complications

The morbidity and complications associated with adrenalectomy are typically a consequence of the underlying adrenal pathology. For example, among patients who are undergoing adrenalectomy for CS, the increased susceptibility to infection, deep venous thrombosis, poor wound healing, and mild glucose intolerance are primarily consequences of hypercortisolism.

Intraoperative complications include hypertension and hemorrhage secondary to inadvertent injury to the adrenal vein, especially during right adrenalectomy. Hemorrhage can be avoided by using meticulous surgical technique. The surgeon should secure control of the venous drainage of the adrenal gland and divide the adrenal vein before manipulating any tumors. The risk of significant changes in blood pressure during adrenalectomy for pheochromocytoma is minimized with adequate preoperative preparation that includes volume replacement and adrenergic blockade. Intraoperative hypertension, usually associated with manipulation of the pheochromocytoma, is managed with nitroprusside.

Perhaps the most important postoperative complication of adrenalectomy is the onset of occult **adrenal insufficiency** or Addisonian crisis as a result of inadequate glucocorticoid (cortisol) replacement. Patients who undergo unilateral adrenalectomy for an adrenal cause of CS are treated with hydrocortisone perioperatively because the contralateral adrenal gland is assumed to be suppressed until proven otherwise. Patients who undergo bilateral adrenalectomy for Cushing's disease (adrenal hyperplasia) or bilateral pheochromocytomas require lifelong glucocorticoid replacement. Patients who undergo unilateral adrenalectomy for PA, pheochromocytoma, or a nonfunctional adrenal tumor (e.g., adrenal cyst, myelolipoma) do not need cortisol replacement.

Another important cause of adrenal insufficiency is long-term corticosteroid therapy and the ACTH and adrenal suppression that are a result of such treatment, when it has been longer than a week. These patients cannot respond normally to the stress of surgery by increasing their secretion of cortisol and become relatively adrenal insufficient in the perioperative period, unless adequate replacement is given.

Postural hypotension or dizziness, nausea, vomiting, abdominal pain, weakness, fatigability, hyperkalemia, and hyponatremia are common symptoms and signs of adrenal insufficiency. The patient may not have all of these findings, but the presence of any one of them in a patient in the correct clinical setting raises the index of suspicion. When adrenal insufficiency is suspected in an unstable patient, it is appropriate to draw blood to measure cortisol and then immediately to give the patient parenteral steroids (100 to 200 mg hydrocortisone IV). Treating a patient with a dose of hydrocortisone that is not needed has no significant consequence; however, missing the diagnosis of adrenal insufficiency could lead to death.

After the surgical resection of any adrenal gland, it is the responsibility of the managing physician to document the presence of an intact or recovered hypothalamic–pituitary–adrenal (HPA) axis before weaning postoperative cortisol replacement. The standard method is to establish that the patient has adequate adrenal reserve (i.e., demonstrate the ability of the remaining adrenal gland to respond appropriately to ACTH). This can be done with an ACTH stimulation test, which involves administering 250 mg synthetic ACTH by IV bolus or IM injection after a baseline plasma cortisol level is drawn. Plasma cortisol is then measured at 30 and 60 minutes. The test should be performed before 9:00 AM, and only if there are no known contraindications. If the baseline cortisol level is 20 mg/dL or greater and increases more than 7 mg/dL, then the HPA axis is normal. If the cortisol level is <20 mg/dL and increases <7 mg/dL, then the HPA axis is abnormal. Until the HPA axis is normal, the patient needs maintenance hydrocortisone.

■ MULTIPLE ENDOCRINE NEOPLASIA SYNDROMES

Familial endocrine tumor syndromes, inherited as autosomal dominant conditions, are divided into three types: **MEN-1, MEN-2A,** and **MEN-2B.** Another autosomal dominant condition, **familial medullary thyroid carcinoma (FMTC),** is also inherited, but it is associated only with **medullary thyroid carcinoma** and no other endocrine abnormalities.

MULTIPLE ENDOCRINE NEOPLASIA TYPE 1

MEN-1 is an inherited endocrine disorder that combines parathyroid hyperplasia with other endocrine neoplasms, usually pancreatic islet cell and anterior pituitary tumors. Many other endocrine and nonendocrine tumors occur, but less commonly. Carcinoid tumors and lipomas are the most frequent (Table 20-6).

Multiple Endocrine Neoplasia Type 1 Genetics and Screening

MEN-1 is an autosomal dominant disorder with a high degree of penetrance but variable expression (i.e., 50% of the offspring will have the syndrome, but each child may not express all component diseases). The causative gene in MEN-1 is a tumor suppressor gene located on the long arm of chromosome 11 that encodes the protein **menin.** Inactivating germline mutations can occur across a wide region of the gene. The heterogeneity of mutations complicates genetic screening for MEN-1. Specific mutations as detected by the MEN-1 germline mutation test have been localized for 80% of MEN-1 kindreds. More complex testing may allow carrier identification when the MEN-1 germline mutation test is negative. Genetic test results are useful for MEN-1 patient counseling

TABLE 20-6	Multiple Endocrine Neoplasia Type I: Gland Involvement	
Glands and Sites Involved	Type of Disease	Estimated Penetrance by Age 40 (%)
Parathyroid	Hyperplasia	90
Pancreas	Islet cell tumors	70
Pituitary	Adenoma	35
Adrenal	Adenoma or carcinoma	25
Enterochromaffin system	Carcinoid tumor	15
Soft tissue	Lipoma	30
	Facial angiofibroma	85
	Collagenoma	70

but, unlike MEN-2, do not mandate therapeutic interventions. Periodic biochemical screening is required for MEN-1 carriers and for patients in whom DNA-based tests are not possible.

Biochemical screening should begin during the second or third decade of life. Concomitant history and physical examination should seek evidence for MEN-1 component diseases. Screening of MEN-1 carriers is performed annually. When DNA tests are not feasible or informative, individuals at 50% risk (i.e., first-degree relatives of known MEN-1 patients) should be screened every 3 years. Screening includes tests for the common lesions of MEN-1 (calcium, prolactin, fasting glucose and insulin, gastrin). Other tests are added based upon individual patient evaluation and family history. Patients from MEN-1 kindreds with known mutations who have negative genetic testing do not require further genetic or biochemical screening.

Calcium and PTH levels should be measured in all patients newly presenting with pancreatic islet cell tumors, since the absence of hyperparathyroidism virtually excludes MEN-1.

Multiple Endocrine Neoplasia Type 1 Parathyroid Disease

Primary hyperparathyroidism is the most common endocrine disorder in MEN-1, occurring in over 90% of cases, but represents only about 3% of all cases of primary hyperparathyroidism. The mean age of onset is 25 years, much younger than for sporadic primary hyperparathyroidism. The clinical manifestations are similar for MEN-1 and for sporadic disease, including asymptomatic hypercalcemia, constitutional and neuropsychiatric complaints (weakness, fatigue, irritability, depression), urinary tract findings (urolithiasis, hypercalciuria), abdominal pain (peptic ulcer disease, pancreatitis), and bone disease (decreased bone density, bone pain, fractures). As for sporadic disease, MEN-1 hyperparathyroidism is diagnosed by serum calcium and PTH levels. Assessment of metabolic disease (e.g., hypercalciuria, osteoporosis) may guide therapeutic recommendations for minimally symptomatic patients.

Hyperparathyroidism in MEN-1 affects all parathyroid glands, although the hyperplasia may be asymmetric. The neoplastic genetic stimulus is not eliminated by

of disease, despite total thyroidectomy and extensive lymph node dissections. Distant metastases are to lung, liver, and bone. Survival rates after thyroidectomy in MEN-2A currently are intermediate between FMTC and MEN-2B, but could approach 100% using genetic screening. Management of persistent or recurrent postoperative hypercalcitonemia is controversial.

Nearly 50% of MEN-2A patients will develop pheochromocytomas. The tumors are almost always in the adrenal glands and are very rarely malignant. Symptoms, if present, are similar to those for sporadic pheochromocytoma. The biochemical diagnosis is made by measuring plasma or urinary catecholamines. Tumors detected only by screening often produce lesser amounts of catecholamines. Tumor localization is primarily by CT scan. MIBG radionuclide scan or MRI is sometimes helpful. Bilateral adrenalectomy is performed when bilateral adrenal imaging abnormalities are present. When the disease appears unilateral, treatment is controversial, ranging from unilateral adrenalectomy with close follow-up to bilateral resection. The 50% risk of contralateral tumor development must be balanced against the lifelong risk of Addisonian crisis. Unilateral adrenalectomy is currently preferred for most patients, and laparoscopic adrenalectomy is often feasible. Screening for pheochromocytoma should precede all operations for MTC, and, when screening is positive, adrenalectomy should precede thyroidectomy.

Nearly 25% of MEN-2A patients will develop primary hyperparathyroidism; the disease is less severe and presents at a later age than in MEN-1. The disease always affects all four glands, although hyperplasia may be asymmetric. Symptoms are similar to those in patients with sporadic disease. Diagnosis is made using blood calcium and PTH levels. Either total parathyroidectomy (four glands) with forearm autotransplantation or subtotal resection (three and one-half glands) is appropriate. Resected parathyroid tissue can be cryopreserved for later reimplantation if permanent hypoparathyroidism develops. If abnormal parathyroid glands are encountered during thyroidectomy for MTC, at least subtotal parathyroidectomy is appropriate, even for normocalcemic patients. Screening for pheochromocytoma should precede parathyroid operations, and, when screening is positive, adrenalectomy should precede parathyroidectomy.

Multiple Endocrine Neoplasia Type 2B

Patients with MEN-2B have a characteristic phenotype with features evident soon after birth. They include marfanoid habitus, prognathism, puffy lips, bumpy tongue, and hyperflexible joints. Corneal nerve hypertrophy is seen on slit-lamp examination. RET testing is confirmatory. Among the MEN/FMTC syndromes, MTC is most aggressive in MEN-2B, with distant metastases reported as early as the first year of life. RET-positive patients should undergo thyroidectomy and central neck lymphadenectomy before age 6 months.

The presentation, diagnosis, and management of pheochromocytoma in MEN-2B patients are identical to those of MEN-2A. Hyperparathyroidism is absent in MEN-2B. Ganglioneuromas occur at multiple sites in MEN-2B patients, and in the colon can lead to severe constipation and megacolon.

Familial Medullary Thyroid Carcinoma

MTC is least virulent in FMTC, and patient survival exceeds that for MEN-2A, MEN-2B, and sporadic MTC. The age of onset of MTC is later in FMTC kindreds than in MEN-2A or MEN-2B kindreds. In small kindreds, distinguishing MEN-2A from FMTC may be difficult, since MTC is the first manifestation of both syndromes. FMTC patients should therefore undergo thyroidectomy in early childhood, similar to MEN-2A patients. Definitive diagnosis of FMTC is made using RET testing plus rigorous kindred criteria that include longitudinal observation of multiple kindred members. Equivocal cases should be classified as MEN-2A so that potentially curative thyroidectomy is not delayed and so that pheochromocytoma is not missed. By definition, FMTC has no other associated familial endocrinopathies.

 ☀ Go to http://thePoint.lww.com/activate and use your scratch-off code on the inside cover of this book to access bonus chapters, question bank, videos, and more.

SAMPLE QUESTIONS

Questions

Choose the best answer for each question.

1. A 20-year-old woman is seen in clinic because of a thyroid nodule. She is asymptomatic and her past medical history is unremarkable. She takes no medications. There is a 1-cm firm, solitary, nodule in the lateral aspect of the left lobe of the thyroid. A radionuclide scan showed no uptake of tracer in the nodule. Ultrasonography shows a solid, homogenous 1-cm mass. Fine-needle aspiration cytology shows a follicular neoplasm. What is the next best step in management?
   A. Irradiation (radioactive iodine)
   B. Thyroid suppression with thyroxine
   C. Incisional biopsy and enucleation if benign
   D. Total thyroidectomy
   E. Left thyroid lobectomy

2. A 50-year-old woman is seen in clinic because of weight loss, restlessness, and palpitations. She also has noted leg swelling and excessive hair loss. Her past medical history is unremarkable. She takes no medications. She is afebrile. On exam, she is tachycardic and has a fine tremor. She has mild exophthalmos. Her thyroid is smooth and uniformly enlarged. TSH levels are low and T3 and T4 levels are elevated. What is the next best step in management?
   A. Radioactive iodine
   B. Early operation
   C. Propranolol
   D. Antithyroid medication
   E. Thyroxine suppression

3. A 25-year-old otherwise healthy woman is found to have a serum calcium of 10.9 mg/dL (normal 8.2 to 10.2 mg/dL) during a well-woman preventive medicine visit. A parathyroid hormone (PTH) level returns 75 pg/mL (normal 13 to 65 pg/mL). She is asymptomatic. She takes no chronic medications. Family history discloses that her mother has hypercalcemia that has never required medication or operation. Physical examination is normal. The patient is most likely to have which of the following laboratory findings?
   A. Low calcium:creatinine clearance ratio
   B. Decreased serum vitamin D level
   C. Elevated serum PTHrP level
   D. Hypomagnesemia
   E. Hyperphosphatemia

4. A 40-year-old healthy woman is found to have a serum calcium level of 11 mg/dL during a preventive medicine visit. She is otherwise healthy and takes no medications. There is no family history of endocrine disease. Serum phosphorus is 2.4 mg/dL and PTH level is 90 pg/mL. Sestamibi scan is without focal uptake. Cervical ultrasonography demonstrates a 15-mm ovoid hypoechoic solid soft tissue mass immediately adjacent and lateral to the inferior pole of the right thyroid lobe. Which one of the following is the most appropriate treatment recommendation for this patient?
   A. Observation and repeat laboratory studies in 6 months
   B. Begin daily oral furosemide
   C. Begin saline and bisphosphonates intravenously
   D. Radioguided parathyroidectomy
   E. Targeted parathyroidectomy with intraoperative PTH monitoring

5. A 35-year-old woman is seen in clinic because of weight gain and abnormal hair growth. She has gained 15 kg in 6 months, most notably in her torso. She denies increased appetite and has not changed her daily activity patterns. She has been emotionally labile and her previously regular menses have become irregular (periods are shorter or missed altogether). On examination, she has truncal obesity and hirsutism. The most likely primary cause of her symptoms is due to hyperfunction of which one of the following?
   A. Pituitary basophils
   B. Pulmonary enterochromaffin (Kulchitsky) cells
   C. Adrenal medullary cells
   D. Adrenal cortical cells
   E. Ovarian epithelial cells

Answers and Explanations

1. Answer: E

This patient should undergo a thyroid lobectomy. Even though an FNA showing follicular cells is only 5% likely to be a malignancy, most endocrine surgeons would recommend excision because of that concern. Radioactive iodine is inappropriate because it would destroy normal thyroid and leave the nodule. Suppression with levothyroxine to suppress thyroid-stimulating hormone (TSH) to below normal limits is associated with accelerated osteoporosis and cardiac irregularities. Suppression to within normal range could be a temporizing maneuver. Incisional biopsy and enucleation are inappropriate because neither will allow examination of the interface between the nodule and normal thyroid and potentially not allow the diagnosis of a follicular variant of papillary thyroid carcinoma. Total thyroidectomy is unnecessarily aggressive. (Thyroid Nodule)

2. Answer: D

The patient has Graves' disease. Initial treatment should be with antithyroid medication to suppress thyroxine production. Radioactive iodine as the first line of treatment is inappropriate because as many as 75% of patients have been reported to have sustained remission after 3 to 6 months of treatment with antithyroid drugs. Early operation is too aggressive when nonoperative methods of treatment are available. Propranolol may be used as an adjunct to antithyroid medications but used alone does not help suppress the thyrotropin receptor antibodies (TRAbs) that are responsible for Graves' disease. The highest rates of remission are associated with elimination of these antibodies. Thyroxine suppression will be ineffective since the patient already has high levels of T4. (Hyperthyroidism/Graves' Disease/Treatment)

3. Answer: A

This asymptomatic patient with mild elevations of calcium and intact PTH levels and a family history of benign hypercalcemia most likely has FHH, familial hypercalcemic hypocalciuria. The diagnosis can be confirmed by a 24-hour urine collection for calcium and creatinine, which should show calcium <100 mg/24 hours and a calcium:creatinine ratio <0.05. FHH does not affect vitamin D, magnesium, or phosphorus levels in the serum. FHH is not associated with production of parathyroid hormone–related protein. (Parathyroid/Secondary and Tertiary Hyperparathyroidism/Clinical Presentation and Evaluation)

4. Answer: E

This patient has early sporadic primary hyperparathyroidism. While she is asymptomatic, she meets the NIH consensus criterion for parathyroid operation of age <50 years. The absence of focal sestamibi uptake precludes radioguided parathyroidectomy since the gamma probe cannot be used to guide the surgeon to the lesion. The sonogram shows a mass consistent with an enlarged right inferior parathyroid gland, so that a targeted approach to parathyroidectomy using ioPTH monitoring is possible. (Primary Hyperparathyroidism/Treatment Surgical)

5. Answer: A

This patient has symptoms and signs of hypercortisolism (Cushing's syndrome). The most common cause of Cushing's syndrome in adults is an adrenocorticotropic hormone (ACTH)-secreting tumor of the pituitary basophils (Cushing's disease). Women in the third and fourth decades of life are the typical patients. Cushing's disease accounts for 70% of cases of Cushing's syndrome. Bronchial carcinoid tumors (arising from Kulchitsky cells) are a source of ectopic ACTH production. Ectopic ACTH syndrome causes about 15% of Cushing's syndrome in adults. The adrenal medulla does not produce glucocorticoids; tumors of the medulla are pheochromocytomas and produce excess catecholamines. A tumor of ovarian epithelial cells could lead to menstrual irregularities through excess sex steroid production but would not produce hypercortisolism. (Adrenal Glands/Disease States/Hyperadrenocorticism/Clinical Presentation/Diagnosis)

21

Spleen and Lymph Nodes

JAMES C. HEBERT, M.D. • GINA L. ANDRALES, M.D. • PATRICK FORGIONE, M.D. •
KENNITH H. SARTORELLI, M.D. • WARREN D. WIDMANN, M.D.

Objectives

1. Describe the anatomy and physiology of the spleen and lymph nodes.

2. Discuss the workup and management of a patient with splenic injury.

3. Discuss the role of splenectomy in patients with hematologic abnormalities.

4. Distinguish between splenomegaly and hypersplenism, and discuss their causes.

5. Discuss the associated risks and long-term consequences of splenectomy.

6. Discuss the means available to lessen the harmful consequences of splenectomy.

7. Describe the workup of a patient with lymphadenopathy.

8. Describe the evaluation of a patient suspected to have lymphoma.

9. Describe the role of the surgeon in the staging and treatment of Hodgkin's lymphoma and non-Hodgkin's lymphoma.

To the ancients, the function of the spleen was an enigma. In times past, mirth and fleet-footedness were attributed to the spleen. We now realize that the spleen, the largest mass of lymphoid tissue in the body, along with the lymph nodes, thymus, Waldeyer's ring (tonsils and adenoids), and the gut-associated lymph tissue, plays a key role in maintaining the integrity of an individual's immune status. The spleen and lymph nodes often undergo changes in structure and function as a result of a variety of pathologic conditions, and the role of the surgeon in treating diseases involving the spleen and lymph tissue has evolved as our understanding has of the physiology of the lymph organs in both health and disease.

SPLEEN ANATOMY AND PHYSIOLOGY

The spleen develops from the dorsal mesogastrium by the sixth week of gestation. The spleen resides in the left upper quadrant of the abdomen, bounded by the diaphragm superiorly and the lower thoracic cage anterolaterally and posteriorly (Figure 21-1). The spleen is intimately associated with the tail of the pancreas, stomach, left kidney, colon, and diaphragm by a series of suspensory ligaments that are also derived from the dorsal mesogastrium. The splenorenal, gastrosplenic, splenocolic, and splenophrenic ligaments provide direct fixation of the spleen to the left upper quadrant. The short gastric vessels run through the gastrosplenic ligament. The splenic vessels and the tail of the pancreas traverse the splenorenal ligament. Laxity of the splenic ligaments leads to excessive mobility of the spleen, which may be associated with symptoms from

torsion in any of the other quadrants of the abdomen (wandering spleen). This condition is treated with splenopexy and returning the spleen to the left upper abdomen. The spleen is encased in a capsule that becomes thin and fibrotic by adulthood. Traction on the spleen or its supporting ligaments by blunt or operative trauma may cause bleeding from capsular avulsion. The normal spleen weighs between 75 and 150 g.

The spleen is an extremely vascular organ that receives approximately 5% of the cardiac output. The organ has a potential dual arterial blood supply. The splenic artery provides the primary inflow, but when the splenic artery is occluded, the short gastric arteries provide collateral flow from the left gastric artery (Figure 21-2A). The splenic artery is a branch of the celiac artery and courses along the superior border of the pancreas, cranially to the splenic vein. The splenic artery then branches into two distinct patterns, the distributive or magistral patterns. With the distributive pattern, the splenic artery branches into 6 to 13 branches starting approximately 3 to 13 cm from the splenic hilum; these branches then enter the spleen over three-fourths of its hilar surface. With the magistral pattern, the splenic artery branches into three or four large branches as it enters the splenic hilum, and these branches insert over one-fourth of the hilar surface of the spleen. The distributive pattern of splenic artery branching is seen in 70% of people. There are usually four to six short gastric arterial branches from the left gastroepiploic artery. Vexing bleeding from the short gastric vessels can be encountered during splenectomy or operations on the stomach (e.g., fundoplication).

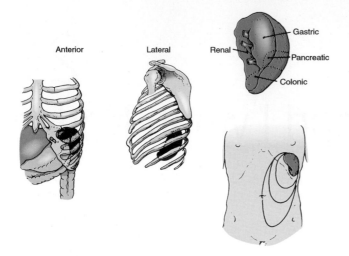

FIGURE 21-1. Normal external relations of the spleen. (Used with permission from Moore KL and Dailey AF, eds., *Clinically Oriented Anatomy*. 5th ed. Baltimore, MD: Lippincott Williams & Wilkins, 2005.)

Venous drainage of the spleen occurs through the splenic and short gastric veins. The course of the splenic vein is caudal to and parallels the splenic artery. The splenic vein joins the superior mesenteric vein to form the portal vein (Figure 21-2B).

A variety of developmental disorders affect the spleen. The most common developmental anomaly is the presence of **accessory spleens** in addition to a normal spleen. Accessory spleens are found in 10% to 30% of the population and are believed to result from failure of separate splenic masses in the dorsal mesogastrium to fuse. These splenic buds are then carried to various locations by the migration of the splenic ligaments. The most common sites for accessory spleens, in order of decreasing frequency, are the splenic hilum, splenocolic ligament, gastrocolic ligament, splenorenal ligament, and omentum (Figure 21-3). Failure to identify and remove accessory spleens may lead to relapse of various hematologic disorders after splenectomy.

Polysplenia is the presence of multiple small spleens, with no normal spleen. Polysplenia is associated with multiple anomalies, including severe cardiac defects, and biliary atresia. Bilateral left-sidedness is a condition characterized by normally unpaired organs having mirror image organs, usually two spleens, one on each side, and often associated with cardiac anomalies. Absence of the spleen (asplenia), a life-threatening condition, is also associated with severe cardiac anomalies and bilateral right-sidedness (Ivemark syndrome). Splenogonadal fusion is a rare disorder of development, in which splenic tissue is found in the left scrotum, often attached to the testicle.

The spleen has several distinct functions, including hematopoiesis, blood filtering, and immune modulation. The function of the spleen is intimately related to its microstructure. Central to its microstructure is its microcirculation (Figure 21-4). A trabecular meshwork of fibrous tissue joins the fibroelastic capsule to the hilum of the spleen and surrounds the entering blood vessels. Blood enters the splenic parenchyma through central arteries that branch off the trabecular arteries. These central arteries course through the **white pulp,** where they are surrounded by periarterial lymphatic sheaths that consist primarily of T lymphocytes and macrophages that can process soluble antigens. Some blood flows into surrounding lymphatic follicles where

B lymphocytes can proliferate in germinal centers. Mature antibody-producing cells (plasma cells) are found here. Blood that leaves the white pulp flows into a marginal zone, where it is directed either back to the white pulp or through terminal arterioles into the **splenic cords of Billroth** in the **red pulp** (open circulation). In the reticular network of the cords, which have no endothelial cells, blood percolates slowly and comes into contact with numerous macrophages before they enter the endothelial-lined sinuses that connect with the splenic vein branches. The red pulp is the site of removal of antibody-sensitized cells and particulate material. In some pathologic conditions, blood is shunted from the marginal zone directly into the sinuses (closed circulation) (depicted in the lower portion of Figure 21-4), bypassing much of the critical filtering function.

The spleen is a site of fetal extramedullary hematopoiesis, but this activity usually ceases by birth in normal humans.

In its capacity as a blood filter, the spleen culls abnormal and aged erythrocytes, granulocytes, and platelets from the nearly 350 L/day of blood that passes through it. As red blood cells near the end of their lives, (normal RBC lifespan 110 to 120 days) they lose membrane integrity as a result of declining adenosine triphosphate levels. As a result, they are marked for destruction. Abnormal and senescent red blood cells cannot deform appropriately to enter the splenic sinuses through the fenestrations in the endothelium. Therefore, they are removed in the red pulp. In addition, as red blood cells deform to enter the splenic sinuses as they leave the red pulp, cellular inclusions are pinched off from the cells. This "pitting" function removes nuclear remnants, such as **Howell-Jolly bodies,** from red blood cells. It also removes other red blood cell inclusions, such as **Heinz bodies** (denatured hemoglobin) and **Pappenheimer bodies** (iron inclusions). Therefore, when a patient has undergone splenectomy, these nuclear remnants should be present, and their presence can be assessed by viewing a peripheral blood smear. If they are not present after splenectomy, this should raise the suspicion of an accessory spleen.

The role of the spleen in the sequestration and destruction of granulocytes and platelets under normal circumstances is not well understood. Normally, one-third of the body's platelets are stored in the spleen. Abnormal splenic processing of platelets occurs in several diseases and causes marked thrombocytopenia. Splenectomy is usually followed by transient thrombocytosis.

The spleen is part of the reticuloendothelial system and plays an important role in the immune system. It provides both nonspecific and specific immune responses. A nonspecific response has two arms: (1) clearance of opsonized particles and bacteria by fixed splenic macrophages and (2) opsonin production. **Opsonins** that are produced by the spleen include properdin, tuftsin, and fibronectin. Properdin activates the alternative pathway of the complement system. Tuftsin facilitates macrophage phagocytosis. The specific immune response of the spleen includes antigen processing and antibody production by splenic lymphocytes present in the white pulp. The spleen is the body's largest source of immunoglobulin M (IgM), and splenectomy causes a marked decrease in IgM and opsonin production. Because of its mass and its position in the circulation, the spleen probably plays a major role in modulating the systemic cytokine response to infection. However, little is understood about this role.

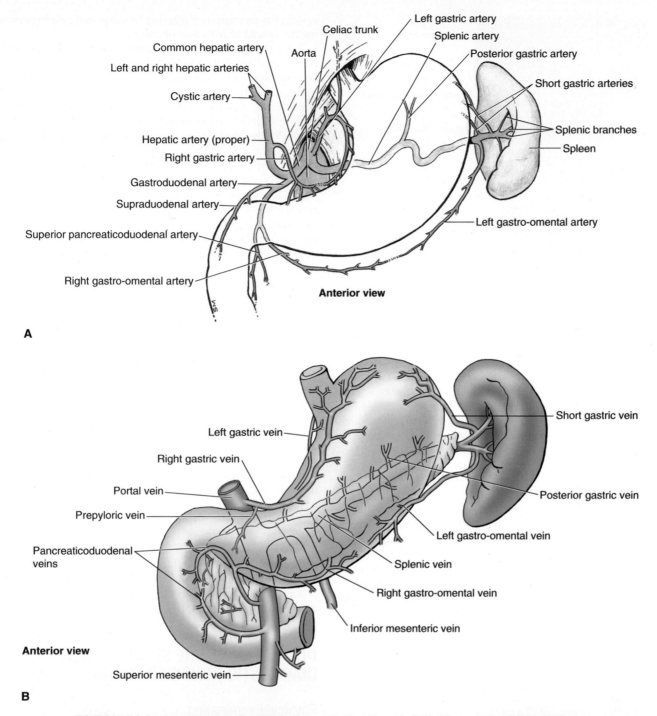

FIGURE 21-2. **A**, Arterial supply to the spleen. (Used with permission from Moore KL, Dailey AF, eds., *Clinically Oriented Anatomy*. 5th ed. Baltimore, MD: Lippincott Williams & Wilkins, 2005.) **B**, Venous supply to the spleen. (Used with permission from Moore KL and Dailey AF, eds., *Clinically Oriented Anatomy*. 5th ed. Baltimore, MD: Lippincott Williams & Wilkins, 2005.)

LYMPH NODES AND LYMPHATICS ANATOMY AND PHYSIOLOGY

The lymphatic system includes a series of lymphatic capillaries and vessels that collect fluid from the interstitial space and transport the fluid through one or a series of filters (lymph nodes) back to the bloodstream (Figure 21-5). While much of the excess fluid reaching the extracellular space is reabsorbed by the blood capillaries due to the osmotic gradient created by the proteins within the capillaries (Starling hypothesis), as much as 3 L of fluid may fail to be absorbed each day. Unlike blood capillaries, the lymphatic capillaries are composed of highly fenestrated endothelium that lacks a basement membrane. A plexus of these capillaries originates in the extracellular spaces of most tissues where, because of their highly fenestrated structure, excess fluid as well as proteins, intestinal fat, bacteria, some whole cells, and other debris can enter them. The lymphatic capillaries coalesce into larger lymphatic vessels that anastomose frequently.

Afferent lymphatic vessels enter lymph nodes that are situated throughout the course of the lymphatic vessels. Like the spleen, the nodes function as filters facilitated by their

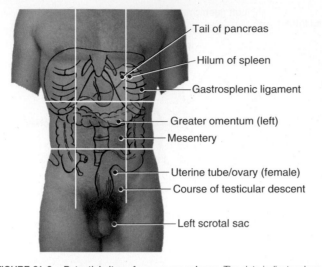

FIGURE 21-3. Potential sites of accessory spleens. The dots indicate where potential accessory spleens may be located. (Used with permission from Moore KL and Dailey AF, eds., *Clinically Oriented Anatomy*. 5th ed. Baltimore, MD: Lippincott Williams & Wilkins, 2005.)

anatomy and large populations of reticuloendothelial cells and lymphocytes, which are important in regulating local immune responses. The lymph exits the nodes via efferent vessels as it courses to other nodes or directly into the bloodstream. Like veins, lymphatic valves determine the direction of flow, and muscle contraction facilitates the movement of lymph, the fluid collected by the lymphatic capillaries. Lymph collected from the right side of the head, neck, and chest as well as the right upper limb drains to the right lymphatic duct that enters into the junction of the right subclavian and right jugular veins (right venous angle). Lymph from the rest of the body drains via the thoracic duct to enter the junction of the left internal jugular and the left subclavian veins (left venous angle). Lymph is similar to plasma fluid. When the system is functioning properly, the amount of extracellular fluid remains constant and debris does not accumulate in the extracellular space. Edema, increased interstitial fluid, results when the system is overwhelmed.

In addition to transporting fluid and macromolecules from the interstitial space back to the bloodstream, the lymphatic

system has an important filtering function that aids in preventing the spread of infection or cancer.

Like the spleen, the microanatomy of the lymph nodes is arranged to facilitate this filtering process (Figure 21-6). Lymph nodes are surrounded by a capsule with fibrous trabeculae radiating to the hilum. Within a lymph node are four main zones: (1) the cortex, containing lymphoid follicles (rich in B cells) and germinal centers (sites of B-cell activation); (2) the paracortex, populated mainly with T lymphocytes; (3) the medullary cords; (4) sinuses. Lymph enters through the capsule via afferent lymph vessels into the subcapsular sinuses then through the cortical sinuses followed by the medullary sinuses and ultimately exits via the efferent vessels. Blood, which carries circulating lymphocytes, enters the node through a small artery at the hilum. This divides into an arcade of arterioles that supply blood-to-blood capillary beds within the medulla and cortex. Throughout each zone, an interstitial space is separated by endothelium from an intravascular space and an intralymphatic space. Within the sinuses, this is simple flat endothelium with fenestrations to allow passage of material. Free cells consisting of lymphocytes and macrophages populate the sinuses and are free to enter or leave the capillaries through these fenestrations. Within the deep cortical zone, or paracortex, is a specialized region populated mainly by T lymphocytes, the thymus-dependent zone, so called because its cells are depleted following neonatal thymectomy. Postcapillary venules, high endothelial venules, course through the paracortex and the thymus-dependent zone before forming collecting veins that ultimately leave from the hilum. Recirculating lymphocytes recognize and adhere to this specialized endothelium in these high endothelial venules and squeeze through from the blood to the lymph. T cells that are activated within the lymph node can leave to recirculate via the efferent lymphatic vessels that leave the hilum. B cells that enter the node make their way to the lymphoid nodules or follicles and their extensions along the medullary cords. Activated B cells proliferate within the germinal centers of secondary lymphoid follicles, which also contain regulatory macrophages and T lymphocytes. B cells differentiate into plasma cells within the cords and produce antibodies that are primarily of the IgG class.

DISORDERS OF THE SPLEEN—GENERAL DIAGNOSTIC CONSIDERATIONS

Physical Examination

It is difficult to palpate a normal spleen because of its size and position. The long axis of the spleen is located deep to behind and perpendicular to the 10th rib in the midaxillary line. The normal adult spleen is approximately 12 cm long and 7 cm wide. Palpation and percussion are used to determine estimate the size of the spleen. The edge of an enlarged spleen may be palpated at the costal margin and may extend into the left iliac fossa. Rarely, it crosses the midline into the right iliac fossa (see Figure 21-1). A spleen that is enlarged secondary to a hematologic condition usually is not tender. Therefore, discomfort on palpation alerts the clinician to the possibility of splenic infection, splenic infarction, or splenic rupture. Palpation of the spleen is performed bimanually with the patient lying flat (Figure 21-7) or with Middleton's method (Figure 21-8).

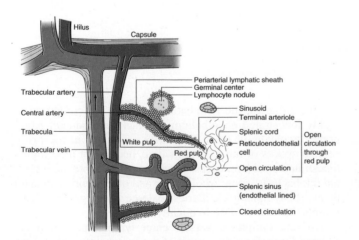

FIGURE 21-4. Microanatomy of the spleen, with its functional components, showing both open and closed circulations.

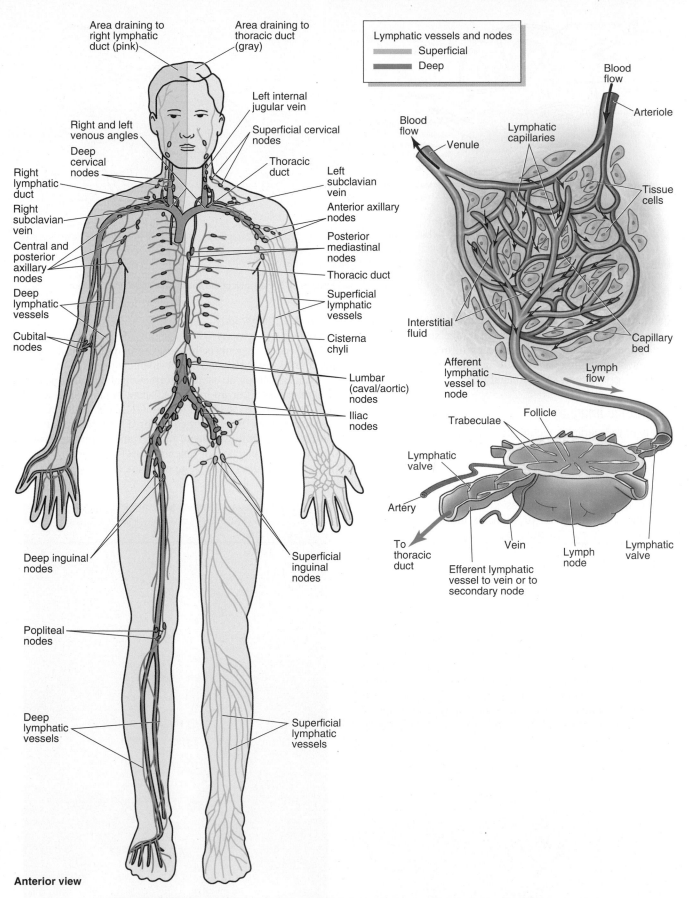

Anterior view

FIGURE 21-5. Lymphatic system. The lymphatic system includes lymphatic vessels, lymphatic ducts, lymphatic trunks, lymph nodes, lymphoid tissue, and lymph organs, such as the spleen. *Black arrows* indicate the flow (leaking) of interstitial fluid out of blood vessels and (absorption) into the lymphatic capillaries. (Used with permission from Moore KL and Dailey AF, eds., *Clinically Oriented Anatomy*. 5th ed. Baltimore, MD: Lippincott Williams & Wilkins, 2005.)

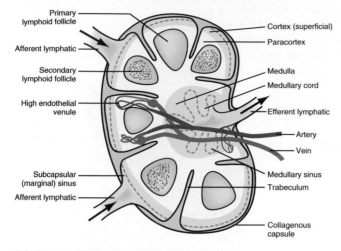

FIGURE 21-6. Microanatomy of a lymph node.

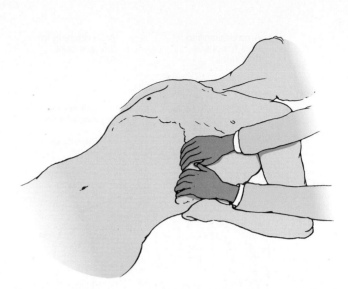

FIGURE 21-8. Palpation of the spleen with Middleton's method.

Estimation of splenic size by percussion relies on the dullness of the percussion note caused by the solid spleen in the left upper quadrant. However, feces in the colon and/or fluid in the stomach may also result in a dull percussion note and may falsely suggest splenomegaly.

Radiographic Imaging

A variety of radiographic techniques are available to aid in the diagnosis and treatment of disorders of the spleen.

Plain Abdominal Roentgenogram

Plain films of the abdomen rarely show the normal spleen. However, splenomegaly is suggested when there is displacement of the colon inferiorly or stomach, medially, or the left diaphragm is elevated. At times an enlarged splenic shadow is seen (Figure 21-9). Fractures of the lower left ribs suggest concomitant splenic rupture.

Ultrasound

Ultrasound is a useful tool for evaluation of splenic size. Sonography may show splenomegaly, splenic cysts, or splenic abscesses (Figure 21-10). Abdominal ultrasound is one of the best ways to rapidly evaluate trauma patients for the presence of blood within the abdomen (see discussion in the abdominal trauma section of Chapter 9, Trauma). However, gas within the intestines may interfere with visualization of the spleen and other abdominal structures. Sonography and Doppler imaging can be used to obtain information about the patency of splenic vessels.

Computed Tomography

Computed tomography (CT) scanning done with intravenous and oral contrast agents is the most useful imaging technique to determine splenic size and detect splenic injury (Figure 21-11). CT scans also provide useful information about other potential disease processes or injuries in adjacent organs. Splenic cysts and abscesses are clearly shown by CT scans, and percutaneous drainage can be performed under CT guidance. CT scans can be used to follow splenic injuries and to obtain information about the patency of splenic vessels, but sonography is preferred, as it does not require radiation of the patient.

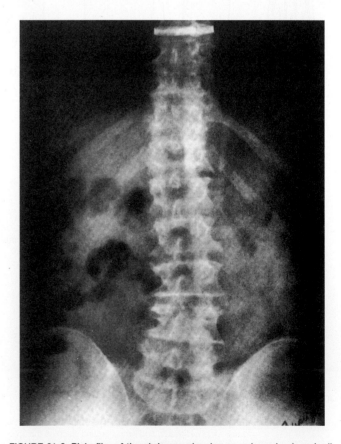

FIGURE 21-9. Plain film of the abdomen showing an enlarged spleen (radiopaque shadow in the left upper quadrant).

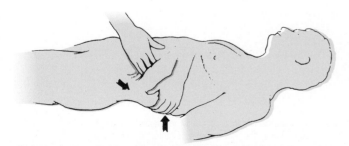

FIGURE 21-7. Bimanual palpation of the spleen.

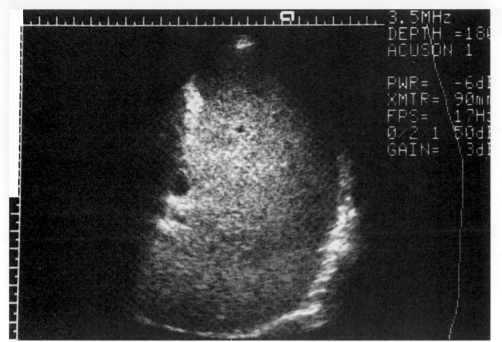

FIGURE 21-10. Ultrasound of the left upper quadrant showing an enlarged spleen. In this case, splenomegaly is secondary to myelofibrosis.

Radionuclide Scans

Colloid suspensions of technetium are taken up by the reticuloendothelial system and subsequent imaging gives information about splenic size and function. Radionuclide scans are helpful in searching for missed accessory spleens in cases in which splenectomy failed to control the underlying hematologic disorder, or in cases with later return of the hematologic disorder after a period of improvement. Radionuclide scans can also help differentiate an accessory spleen from a tumor in the tail of the pancreas. Splenosis results in uptake in aberrant positions.

Angiography

Thin slice rapid CT angiography has replaced splenic artery catheterization for evaluation of the spleen in stable patients after sonography shows intra-abdominal fluid in cases of trauma. CT angiography is also useful in showing splenic vein thrombosis and aids in planning portal venous decompressive procedures. Angiography is also helpful in the evaluation of splenic tumors. Splenic artery embolization may be a useful adjunct to lessen bleeding in cases undergoing elective laparoscopic or open splenectomy. Partial splenic embolization is used to control hypersplenism in children with portal hypertension and to control bleeding in patients with splenic injuries.

Surgical Disorders of the Spleen

The spleen is subject to a variety of disorders that may require surgical intervention (see Table 21-1). Trauma is the most common reason for splenectomy. Alternatives to total splenectomy (e.g., partial splenectomy, embolization to control bleeding, and, image-guided percutaneous drainage procedures) are often used successfully.

Splenic Trauma

The spleen is the most commonly injured organ following blunt abdominal trauma and the second most commonly injured organ after penetrating abdominal trauma. Traditionally, injuries to the spleen were treated with prompt splenectomy. However, recognition of **overwhelming postsplenectomy infection (OPSI)** coupled with a better understanding of the immunologic function of the spleen, led to attempts at splenic preservation in the hemodynamically stable patient when feasible. In unstable patients with ruptured spleens, expeditious splenectomy remains the standard of care. The deliberate induction of splenosis following stabilization of the patient by splenectomy remains controversial.

Clinical Presentation and Evaluation

Three general mechanisms that cause splenic injury are penetrating wounds, blunt compressive forces, and blunt deceleration injuries. The damage produced by penetrating injuries depends on the device used to create the injury (firearm vs. knife). Penetrating trauma, particularly with firearms, often involves the spleen parenchyma and splenic vasculature as

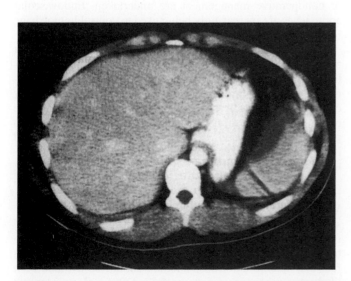

FIGURE 21-11. CT scan of the abdomen showing a subcapsular hematoma of the spleen.

TABLE 21-1	Indications for Splenectomy

Splenic rupture (repair of the spleen is preferred in certain patients)

  Trauma

  Spontaneous

  Iatrogenic injury

Hematologic disorders

  Hemolytic anemias

  Hereditary spherocytosis

  Hereditary elliptocytosis

  Thalassemia minor and major (rarely)

  Autoimmune hemolytic anemia not responsive to steroid therapy

  Idiopathic thrombocytopenic purpura

  Immunologic thrombocytopenia associated with chronic lymphocytic leukemia or systemic lupus erythematosis

  Thrombotic thrombocytopenic purpura (rarely)

Hypersplenism associated with other diseases

  Inflammation

  Infiltrative diseases

Congestion

Leukemia and lymphoma (rarely)

Other diseases

  Splenic abscess (often associated with drug abuse or AIDS)

  Primary and metastatic tumors

  Splenic cysts

  Splenic artery aneurysm

  Bleeding gastric varices secondary to splenic vein thrombosis

AIDS, Acquired immune deficiency syndrome.

TABLE 21-2	Grades of Splenic Trauma

Grade	Description
I	Hematoma: Subcapsular <10% surface area
	Laceration: <1 cm deep
II	Hematoma: Subcapsular 10%–50% surface area
	Parenchymal <5 cm diameter
	Laceration: 1–3 cm deep, not involving trabecular vessels
III	Hematoma: Subcapsular >50% surface area
	Parenchymal >5 cm diameter
	Any expanding or ruptured
	Laceration: >3 cm deep or involving trabecular vessels
IV	Laceration: Segmental vessels involved with devascularization <50%
V	Completely shattered spleen or hilar vascular injury with devascularization

well as adjacent organs. Because of the fixation of the spleen by the splenic ligaments, the spleen is prone to blunt compressive injuries as well as capsular avulsion from rapid decelerations. Compressive forces more easily injure the spleen in children as the compliant thoracic cage of children provides little protection to the spleen from blunt forces. In children, ribs are flexible and rarely fracture. However, in adults, while the ribs may provide some protection to the spleen, rib fractures are present in 20% of spleen injuries. In the absence of external penetrating trauma, penetrating wounds of the spleen may be caused by fractured ribs. A scale of severity for splenic injuries was devised by the American Association for the Surgery of Trauma (Table 21-2). Such scales are useful for predicting which patients will stabilize initially; once the patient is stabilized, the scale no longer predicts which patients will become unstable and require splenectomy. All patients should be resuscitated according to the guidelines of the Advanced Trauma Life Support Course of the American College of Surgeons.

In evaluating patients for splenic injury, the physician should look for signs and symptoms of local peritoneal irritation and acute hemorrhage. Signs of peritoneal irritation include left upper quadrant tenderness to palpation and pain medial to at the top of the left shoulder joint (**Kehr's sign/ omalgia**). Percussion dullness of the left flank (**Ballance's sign**) suggests intraperitoneal bleeding. When evaluating

patients with penetrating trauma, it must be remembered that the diaphragm and underlying spleen may ascend as high as the fourth intercostal space during inspiration. Any penetrating injury from the level of the nipples down may traverse the peritoneal cavity, and patients with signs of intraperitoneal hemorrhage who are unstable and do not respond to the standard resuscitation fluids should undergo prompt laparotomy.

The evaluation of patients with blunt abdominal trauma is complicated by the high incidence of concomitant neurologic and orthopedic injuries. Isolated splenic injury occurs in only 30% of patients. Hemodynamically unstable patients who have signs of blunt abdominal trauma require prompt laparotomy. Stable patients who have signs of abdominal injury and those whose neurologic status is impaired require evaluation with ultrasound, CT scan, and only rarely with diagnostic peritoneal lavage. If splenic injury is present, several treatment options exist.

Treatment

Splenectomy is performed if the spleen is extensively injured (grade V) or if the patient is profoundly unstable. In stable patients, attempts at splenic preservation with splenorrhaphy or nonoperative management are undertaken. Endovascular approaches are increasingly being used to control hemorrhage in splenic trauma.

Splenorrhaphy is operative repair of the spleen. If at least 50% of the splenic volume is preserved, the immune function of the spleen should remain intact. Techniques of splenorrhaphy include debridement of devitalized tissue followed by compression with microcrystalline collagen, pledgeted suture repair, and the creation of polyglycolic acid mesh slings to provide hemostatic compression. Splenorrhaphy is abandoned if the patient has persistent hypotension or extensive additional intra-abdominal injuries.

Splenic autotransplantation by placing splenic fragments in the omentum or peritoneal cavity remains controversial. While cases of spontaneous splenosis have been shown to preserve some degree of splenic function, especially the pitting function, with a resultant normal blood smear, the preservation of immune function remains in doubt, and most surgeons feel that splenic autotransplantation should be avoided as it likely does not protect patients from OPSI and may lead to a high risk of bowel obstruction requiring further surgery that is associated with troublesome bloody adhesions. A few surgeons favor splenosis and argue that risk of late sepsis is suggestively lessened in trauma patients who have developed extensive splenosis spontaneously. By carefully placing splenic fragments into omental pockets and then studying patients 6 months or more following the autotransplantation, significant uptake on splenic isotope scans is demonstrated. Furthermore, they argue that the reported cases of problems of late bowel obstructions from adhesions associated with splenosis relate to cases of spontaneous splenosis and not to those with deliberate and careful induction of splenosis.

Nonoperative management of splenic injuries is the treatment of choice in hemodynamically stable children, or in children in whom hemodynamic stability is achieved with rapid resuscitation. Nonoperative management has also gained acceptance in adults. For nonoperative therapy to be successful, the patient must be hemodynamically stable, or become stable rapidly with resuscitation, and generally, such patients have an isolated splenic injury, usually grades I to III injuries by CT scan. Protocols must be followed including treatment. Treatment is undertaken in a very controlled environment by a surgical team experienced in the management of splenic trauma. While protocols vary from institution to institution, usually, the patient is observed at bed rest initially in an intensive care unit. The combination of serial vital signs, examinations, sonographic studies, and checking of the hematocrit/hemoglobin demonstrate which patients are stable and can be transferred to floor care. If the patient shows any signs of shock or has evidence of continued bleeding, then prompt laparotomy is undertaken. Patients who remain hemodynamically stable are followed closely. Duration of hospitalization and recommendations for activity restriction vary. Without clear evidence-based guidelines, the course of management is dictated by clinical judgment. The American Pediatric Surgical Association has published evidence-based guidelines for the nonoperative management of pediatric injuries. CT or ultrasound may be used to check for splenic healing before the patient is allowed to return to full activity. However, the utility of repeat imaging is not well established. Nonoperative therapy is successful in more than 90% of children and 70% of adults. The success rate has been improved by advances in CT imaging that denote arterial bleeding by a contrast blush and the application of angiographic embolization to control splenic arterial bleeding. Concerns about nonoperative therapy include delayed splenic rupture, risk of transfusions, and missed associated injuries. Although these concerns are real, they are not borne out by experience to outweigh the benefit of splenic preservation or morbidity of splenectomy.

Disorders of Splenic Function

Disorders of the spleen are classified as either functional or anatomic. Functional disorders are considered in terms of too little function (**hyposplenism** and **asplenia**) or excess function (**hypersplenism**). Congenital asplenia or hyposplenism is extremely rare. Splenectomy is the most common reason for the asplenic state, although other conditions (e.g., sickle cell anemia) may lead to a functional asplenic state. The size of the spleen is not related to its hematologic function. Splenomegaly (anatomic enlargement of the spleen) is caused by a variety of conditions (Table 21-3) and should not be confused with hypersplenism (excessive function of the spleen).

Hypersplenism is characterized by **cytopenia** (anemia, leukopenia, and thrombocytopenia, alone or in combination) and

TABLE 21-3	Classification of Splenomegaly (Based on Degree of Enlargement)	
Slight	**Moderate**	**Great**
Chronic passive congestion	Rickets	Chronic myelocytic leukemia
Acute malaria	Hepatitis	Myelofibrosis
Typhoid fever	Hepatic cirrhosis	Gaucher's disease
Subacute bacterial endocarditis	Lymphoma (leukemia)	Niemann-Pick disease
Acute and subacute infection	Infectious mononucleosis	Thalassemia major
Systemic lupus erythematosus	Pernicious anemia	Chronic malaria
Thalassemia minor	Abscesses, infarcts	Leishmaniasis
	Amyloidosis	Splenic vein thrombosis
		Reticuloendotheliosis (hairy-cell leukemia)

normal or hyperplastic cellular precursors in the bone marrow. Cytopenia results from increased sequestration of the cells in the spleen, increased destruction of cells by the spleen, or production of antibody in the spleen leading to increased sequestration and destruction of cells. Hyposplenism also occurs with normal or enlarged spleens (multiple myeloma, sickle cell anemia).

There are three hematologic disorders of splenic function for which splenectomy may be helpful: **hemolytic anemia, immune thrombocytopenic purpura** (ITP), and cytopenia associated with splenomegaly from other diseases (secondary hypersplenism).

Hemolytic Anemia

Splenectomy may aid in the management of hereditary hemolytic anemias and some cases of acquired immune hemolytic anemias. Hereditary hemolytic anemias are classified into three broad areas: membrane structural abnormalities, metabolic abnormalities, and **hemoglobinopathies** (Table 21-4).

Hereditary spherocytosis, an autosomal dominant trait, is characterized by abnormally shaped, rigid red cells as a result of a deficiency in membrane proteins essential for deformability, such as spectrin, ankyrin, or band 3. These rigid erythrocytes cannot pass through the splenic sinuses and become sequestered in the red pulp. Splenectomy is usually indicated because it allows red cells to survive and hematocrit to reach near-normal values postoperatively. An intraoperative search for an accessory spleen is also performed. Patients may present with symptomatic cholelithiasis (black pigment stones—see Chapter 16, Biliary Tract), hemolytic episodes, or aplastic crisis. Splenectomy is considered curative. However, the decision to proceed with splenectomy should be guided by careful consideration of the risks and benefits. Additionally, following splenectomy, there is no risk of postviral hemolytic crises that can be fatal. An intraoperative search for accessory spleens is integral to the procedure as remaining accessory spleens can hypertrophy and reproduce the symptoms. Because of the careful removal of the intact spleen and all accessory splenic tissue, these patients are at risk for OPSI Since the risk of

TABLE 21-4	Hereditary Hemolytic Anemias		

Type	Inheritance	Defect	Usefulness of Splenectomy
Abnormal Membrane Structure			
Spherocytosis	Autosomal dominant	Deficiency in spectrin (membrane component essential for deformability)	Usually
		Rigid erythrocytes cannot pass through splenic vasculature and are sequestered, leading to progressive splenomegaly	Usually
Elliptocytosis	Autosomal dominant	Decreased levels of spectrin; relatively mild in most cases	Rarely
Pyropoikilocytosis	Autosomal recessive	Rare variant of spherocytosis	Usually
Xerocytosis	Autosomal dominant	Water loss leading to increased concentration of hemoglobin	Rarely
Hydrocytosis	Autosomal dominant	Abnormality in erythrocyte Na^+/K^+ transport	Often
Metabolic Abnormalities			
Pyruvate kinase deficiency	Autosomal recessive	Decreased ATP generation leads to membrane destruction	Rarely
G6PD deficiency	Sex-linked recessive	Pentose phosphate shunt is blocked and membrane is injured by oxidation injury from certain drugs (e.g., sulfamethoxazole, ASA, phenacetin, nitrofurantoin)	Never
Hemoglobinopathies			
Sickle cell	Autosomal recessive (homozygous more severe)	Valine substitute for glutamic acid at position 6 of β-chain of HbA; rigid, sickle-shaped cells at low O_2	Rarely
Thalassemias	Many varieties	Deficits in the synthesis of one or more subunits of Hb	Rarely

ATP, adenosine triphosphate; ASA, aminopsalicylic acid; Hb, hemoglobin.

OPSI is much greater in young children, operation should be delayed until after 4 to 5 years of age.

Other types of membrane structural abnormalities are less common, but may require splenectomy. Cholecystectomy is often performed concomitantly with splenectomy as many patients with spherocytosis and other membrane structural abnormalities have gallstones at the time splenectomy is contemplated, and all of these patients should have gallbladder ultrasonography to look for gallstones. Because the ongoing hemolysis will be terminated by splenectomy, there is no indication to remove a normal gall bladder that does not contain any stones or sludge.

Hemolytic anemias caused by metabolic abnormalities (e.g., pyruvate kinase deficiency, glucose-6-phosphate dehydrogenase [G6PD] deficiency) are not responsive to splenectomy. In G6PD deficiency, the erythrocyte membrane is injured by certain oxidizing drugs, such as chloramphenicol, chloroquine, certain vitamin K preparations, Dapsone, primaquine, and probenecid, which should be avoided.

Hemoglobinopathies, which are abnormalities in hemoglobin structure, can lead to red cell deformity and subsequent hemolytic anemia. Sickle cell disease is an autosomal recessive disease. The disease is manifest in a mild form in the heterozygous state and is more severe in the homozygous state. In sickle hemoglobin, valine is substituted for glutamic acid at position six of the β-chain of hemoglobin A. This substitution causes a conformational change in structure that leads to the formation of a rigid sickle-shaped red cell at low oxygen saturations. In addition to hemolytic anemia, sickle cells cause an increase in blood viscosity that leads to stasis and subsequent thrombocytosis. Ischemia occurs as a result and leads to fibrosis in a variety of organs. Most patients with homozygous sickle cell anemia become functionally asplenic because of repeated splenic infarcts and fibrosis. Rarely, splenectomy is

indicated in sickle cell patients with splenomegaly in hemolytic crisis. This treatment is usually confined to those treated early in the disease but is rarely required. Recently, partial splenectomy has shown some efficacy in children in ameliorating the frequency and severity of hemolytic crises while preserving some of the spleen's immunological function.

Thalassemias are characterized by deficits in the synthesis of one or more subunits of hemoglobin. There are many varied types. In thalassemia major (homozygous β-thalassemia), splenectomy is beneficial in reducing the requirements for transfusion, the physical discomfort from massive splenomegaly, and the potential for rupture. In thalassemia minor (heterozygous β-thalassemia), splenectomy can decrease the need for transfusion and the problems associated with iron overload. In general, patients who have thalassemia and undergo splenectomy are at the highest risk for OPSI. For this reason, alternatives to total splenectomy (e.g., splenic embolization, partial splenectomy) are preferred in these patients.

Acquired autoimmune hemolytic anemias are caused by exposure to chemicals, drugs, infectious agents, inflammatory processes, or malignancies. In many cases, a cause is not readily identified. Red blood cells from patients with autoimmune hemolytic anemias are coated with immunoglobulin, complement, or both, which results in a positive direct Coombs' test. Coombs'-negative hemolytic anemia is usually secondary to drugs, toxins, or infectious agents, and is best treated by removing the responsible agent. Patients with Coombs'-positive hemolytic anemia should receive corticosteroid therapy and treatment for any underlying disorders. Splenectomy is indicated when steroids are ineffective, when high doses are required, and when toxic side effects develop during steroid treatment. Splenic sequestration studies and red cell survival studies may help to select patients who will respond to splenectomy. Further, anemias associated with warm reactive antibodies (usually IgG) do not include complement activation. They are associated with splenic sequestration and usually respond to splenectomy. Hemolytic anemias associated with cold reactive antibodies (usually IgM) are characterized by complement binding and agglutination. Hemolysis occurs in peripheral locations in response to cool environmental temperatures. Thus, splenectomy is not indicated for hemolytic anemia associated with cold reactive antibodies.

Thrombocytopenia

Thrombocytopenia has a variety of causes (Table 21-5). Splenectomy is appropriate only in idiopathic, immune-mediated thrombocytopenias (those in which a cause cannot be found). These platelet disorders are usually characterized by the coexistence of a low platelet count, a normal or increased number of megakaryocytes in the bone marrow, and the absence of other hematologic disorders or splenomegaly. The medication history is important, particularly the history of the use of drugs that interfere with platelet function (e.g., aspirin) or other therapeutic agents that are known to cause thrombocytopenia.

Patients with thrombocytopenia often have multiple petechiae (pinpoint lesions that result from breakage of small capillaries or increased permeability of the arterioles, capillaries, or venules). Petechiae occur in areas of the body that encounter pressure and are characteristic of thrombocytopenia. A confluence of petechiae results in purpura. Ecchymoses are extensive purpuric lesions and sometimes such hemorrhages spread along fascial planes. Ecchymoses are more suggestive of a coagulation disorder than of thrombocytopenia.

If the platelet count is low and coagulation disorders were ruled out by appropriate laboratory tests, then all medications should be discontinued. Antiplatelet antibodies are found in 85% of patients with ITP. The bone marrow is evaluated to determine whether the thrombocytopenia is the result of decreased production of platelets by assessing the number of megakaryocytes. In disorders of platelet destruction (e.g., ITP), the bone marrow shows either normal or increased numbers of megakaryocytes.

Immune Thrombocytopenic Purpura Acute ITP usually occurs after an acute viral infection. It has an excellent prognosis in children younger than 16 years of age. Approximately 80% of these patients have a complete, permanent, spontaneous recovery without therapy. Chronic ITP is primarily a disease of young adults. It affects women more often than men. Patients are best treated initially with a course of corticosteroid therapy. If patients do not respond with an elevated platelet count and are refractory to advanced medical therapy such as gamma globulin or monoclonal antibody, splenectomy is performed (ITP is the number one hematologic abnormality requiring splenectomy). In patients who respond to steroid therapy, splenectomy is recommended if thrombocytopenia recurs after steroids are tapered. Patients who initially respond to steroid therapy may fare better after splenectomy than those who do not respond to steroids; however, this remains questionable. Patients who have any sign of intracranial bleeding during steroid therapy require emergent splenectomy. Of patients who undergo splenectomy, 75% to 85% respond permanently and require no further therapy. If platelet counts are <20,000, platelets should be available for transfusion. Transfusion of platelets should not be performed before the splenic artery is clamped because transfused platelets are rapidly destroyed in the spleen. For patients who do not respond or who relapse after splenectomy and who do not improve with corticosteroids, treatment with vincristine and γ-globulin shows some success. Increasingly, gamma globulin is being used in preparation for splenectomy in patients who do not respond well to steroids. Recurrence of ITP may be related to persistent splenic tissue after splenectomy, either as overlooked accessory spleens or as splenosis in cases in which the splenic capsule was ruptured and parenchyma remained in the abdominal cavity.

Thrombotic Thrombocytopenic Purpura Thrombotic thrombocytopenic purpura is a disease of the arteries or capillaries. It is characterized by thrombotic episodes and low platelet counts. The constellation of clinical features in virtually all cases consists of fever, purpura, hemolytic anemia, neurologic manifestations, and signs of renal disease. Plasma pheresis, a therapy aimed at removing plasma-derived factors that cause platelet aggregation, is usually successful, either alone or in combination with antiplatelet therapy, whole-blood exchange transfusions, and steroids. Splenectomy is arguably indicated if these measures fail.

HIV-Associated Thrombocytopenia Infection with HIV may lead to HIV-associated thrombocytopenia. HIV-positive patients and those with AIDS and symptomatic HIV-associated thrombocytopenia that is resistant to medical therapy appear to benefit from splenectomy. Sustained resolution of thrombocytopenia is seen in 60% to 80% of these patients. Splenectomy is performed without an undue increase in morbidity and mortality rates. Splenectomy does not appear to accelerate the conversion rate to AIDS in HIV-positive patients.

Hypersplenism Associated with Other Diseases

A number of clinical syndromes are characterized by destruction of various formed elements of the blood. The cardinal features include splenomegaly; some reduction in the number of circulating blood cells affecting granulocytes, erythrocytes, or platelets in any combination; a compensatory proliferative response in the bone marrow; and the potential for correction of these hematologic abnormalities by splenectomy. Both infiltrative and congestive forms of splenomegaly are associated with hypersplenism (Table 21-6). In patients with splenomegaly, sequestration of both red cells and platelets occurs. Red cell transit time through the spleen increases proportionately

TABLE 21-5	Classification of Thrombocytopenia

Decreased production

Hypoproliferation (toxic agents, sepsis, radiation, myelofibrosis, tumor involvement of marrow)

Ineffective platelet production (megaloblastic anemia, Guglielmo's syndrome)

Splenic sequestration (congestive splenomegaly, myeloid metaplasia, lymphoma, Gaucher's disease)

Dilutional loss (after massive transfusion)

Abnormal destruction

Consumption (disseminated intravascular coagulation)

Immune mechanisms

Splenectomy sometimes indicated (idiopathic thrombocytopenic purpura, chronic lymphocytic leukemia, systemic lupus erythematosus)

Splenectomy not indicated (drug-induced thrombocytopenia, neonatal thrombocytopenia, posttransfusion purpura)

TABLE 21-6	Diseases Associated with Hypersplenism

Congestive diseases of the spleen

Portal hypertension

Splenic vein thrombosis

Infiltrative diseases of the spleen

Benign conditions (Gaucher's disease, Niemann-Pick disease, amyloidosis, extramedullary hematopoiesis)

Neoplastic conditions (leukemias, lymphoma, Hodgkin's disease, primary tumors, metastatic tumors, myeloid metaplasia)

Miscellaneous diseases

Felty's syndrome (rheumatoid arthritis, splenomegaly, neutropenia)

Porphyria erythropoietica

Sarcoidosis

with splenomegaly. Platelet survival is not usually affected; however, platelet sequestration by the enlarged spleen is increased. For this reason, thrombocytopenia usually develops before anemia in patients with hypersplenism associated with splenomegaly.

Hypersplenism is suggested by splenomegaly. Peripheral blood smears may show pancytopenia, isolated thrombocytopenia, anemia, or leukopenia. Most cases of hypersplenism, however, show pancytopenia. The bone marrow is usually hyperplastic. In myelofibrosis, bone marrow examination shows an increased deposition of collagen. The diagnostic approach is dictated by the accompanying features (e.g., hematologic findings, lymphadenopathy, portal hypertension, liver dysfunction, systemic infection). For a variety of reasons, splenectomy is indicated for patients with splenomegaly and hypersplenism. Splenectomy is indicated for hypersplenism if the platelet count is <50,000, with evidence of bleeding; if the neutrophil count is <2000, with or without frequent intercurrent infections; or if the patient has anemia requiring blood transfusion. In myelofibrosis with myeloid metaplasia as well as other cases of extramedullary hematopoiesis, splenectomy is indicated only when the clinical evidence suggests that the compensatory hematopoietic function of the enlarged spleen is outweighed by accelerated sequestration and destruction of red cells.

In most cases of secondary hypersplenism, splenectomy does not completely alleviate the cytopenia. Postoperatively, however, a dramatic increase in the number of platelets may occur and may be associated with thrombosis and thromboembolism, particularly in patients with myelofibrosis. Splenic and portal vein thromboses as well as the more common deep vein thromboses in the lower extremity veins may develop, especially if there is postoperative thrombocytosis. Close postoperative monitoring of platelets is essential with initiation of antiplatelet therapy if needed. Hydroxyurea is the treatment of choice when there is significant postsplenectomy thrombocytosis.

Congestive Splenomegaly Hypersplenism associated with **congestive splenomegaly** as a result of liver failure and the vascular consequences of portal hypertension requires treatment of the hypertension rather than splenectomy. Splenectomy is contraindicated as the primary treatment in this setting.

Splenectomy, with ligation of the splenic vein, eliminates the possibility of performing a selective splenorenal shunt procedure, which is a more appropriate treatment for congestive splenomegaly caused by portal hypertension. In this setting, splenectomy may also lead to splenic and portal vein thrombosis and complicate potential liver transplantation.

Infiltrative Splenomegaly In benign cases of **infiltrative splenomegaly** (e.g., Gaucher's disease, an autosomal recessive disorder that causes abnormal accumulation of glucocerebrosides in the reticuloendothelial cells), partial splenectomy and splenic embolization are used instead of splenectomy to treat hypersplenism and abdominal discomfort caused by massive splenomegaly.

Felty's Syndrome Some patients with rheumatoid arthritis have leg ulcers or other chronic infections, with associated splenomegaly and neutropenia. In these patients, circulating antibodies against neutrophils are found. Splenectomy is controversial because the response is unpredictable. Splenectomy is usually performed for **Felty's syndrome** when severe recurrent infections or intractable leg ulcers occur.

Hematologic Malignancies

Splenectomy is not indicated for acute leukemia. For patients with chronic leukemia, splenectomy is indicated for some cases of hypersplenism and for symptoms associated with massive splenomegaly.

Leukemic reticuloendotheliosis (hairy cell leukemia) is an indolent, progressive form of chronic leukemia. Ongoing hepatomegaly and splenomegaly occur as the disease progresses and the leukemic cells infiltrate the spleen and liver. In the recent past, splenectomy was believed to be an important therapeutic intervention early in the treatment of hairy cell leukemia. Recently, α-interferon and 21-deoxycoformycin were introduced as first-line treatments. Splenectomy is now reserved primarily for palliating cytopenias and symptoms of splenomegaly.

Splenectomy as part of a staging laparotomy to match treatment with extent of disease is now rarely performed for Hodgkin's disease because of improvements in imaging technologies and changes to more systemic forms of therapy. Splenectomy for non-Hodgkin's lymphoma is rarely indicated except in patients with massive splenic enlargement that causes local pressure on the abdominal viscera, or symptomatic hypersplenism.

Further Technical Aspects of Considerations for Splenic Surgery

Splenectomy may be accomplished by traditional open means or by minimally invasive techniques. Open splenectomy is performed with either a midline incision or a left subcostal incision. The keys to safe splenectomy are early mobilization of the spleen and control of the splenic vasculature. Complete mobilization of the spleen is mandatory for partial splenectomy and to evaluate and repair splenic injuries. It is important not to take the short gastric vessels too close to the stomach to avoid injury of the gastric wall. Care is also taken to avoid injuring the tail of the pancreas at the splenic hilum. Splenectomy for hematologic disease is not complete until a thorough search for accessory spleens is made. Drains are not routinely left after splenectomy.

Increasingly, laparoscopic splenectomy has supplanted open splenectomy as the preferred approach for all indications except for trauma. The principles for laparoscopic splenectomy are the same as those for open splenectomy. However, it is necessary to morselize the spleen in special bags that are removed through the small incisions. Occasionally, surgeons make a larger lower abdominal incision to remove very large spleens in fragments.

Consequences and Complications of Splenectomy

Hematologic Changes

In a normal patient, after the spleen is removed, the white blood cell count increases by an average of 50% over baseline. In some cases, the number of neutrophils increases to 15,000 to 20,000 mm³ in the initial postoperative period. The white blood cell count usually returns to normal within 5 to 7 days. Elevation beyond this period suggests infection. In some patients, the elevation of the white count is permanent. In such cases, there is a normal differential count.

The peripheral smear of a patient who underwent splenectomy routinely shows Howell-Jolly bodies (nuclear remnants), nucleated red cells, Heinz Bodies (hemoglobin precipitates), Pappenheimer bodies, and pitted red cells on phase microscopy. Some red blood cells may show abnormal morphology. The absence of these findings after splenectomy for hematologic disease suggests that an accessory spleen was missed. A radionuclide spleen scan may be useful for identifying retained splenic elements.

The platelet count increases by 30% between 2 and 10 days after splenectomy and usually returns to normal within 2 weeks. **Thrombocytosis** (platelet count > 400,000/mm³) occurs in as many as 50% of patients. Theoretically, this increase predisposes the patient to thrombotic complications (e.g., deep vein thromboses in the lower extremities, thrombosis of the mesenteric veins, and possible pulmonary embolism). However, little evidence supports a correlation between absolute platelet count and thrombosis. Most thromboses and pulmonary emboli occur in patients who have myeloproliferative disorders. Postoperative therapy with platelet inhibitors (e.g., aspirin, dipyridamole) has been used in patients who have myeloproliferative disease and platelet counts >400,000/mm³ and in all other patients after splenectomy if the platelet count is >750,000/mm³. Treatment continues until the platelet count returns to normal. Anticoagulation with heparin or warfarin therapy is not beneficial and should be avoided. For more extreme elevations of the platelet count, treatment with hydroxyurea is indicated.

Immune Consequences

The risk of OPSI varies with the age of the patient at the time of splenectomy and the reason for splenectomy. In otherwise normal children, the potential risk of OPSI is approximately 2% to 4%. In adults, it is approximately 1% to 2%. Patients who undergo splenectomy for hematologic disorders are at the highest risk. The overall incidence of OPSI in postsplenectomy patients is 40 times that of the general population, and these patients remain at risk for the rest of their lives. OPSI usually does not occur in the immediate postoperative period. Residual functioning splenic tissue may lessen the risk as evidenced by the lower incidence of postsplenectomy sepsis in trauma patients in whom retained accessory spleens and the development of splenosis are likely to account for some residual immune protection.

Overwhelming infections are usually caused by encapsulated organisms. *Streptococcus pneumoniae* (pneumococcus) is the most common agent (75%), followed in decreasing frequency by *Haemophilus influenzae, Neisseria meningitidis,* β-hemolytic streptococcus, *Staphylococcus aureus, Escherichia coli,* and *Pseudomonas.* Viral infections, most commonly herpes zoster, may be severe in splenectomized patients. Some parasitic infections (babesiosis, malaria) also overwhelm the splenectomized host.

Overwhelming infections with encapsulated bacteria (e.g., pneumococcus) are insidious in onset, often mimicking a cold or flu. However, within a few hours, patients may become septic, and death may ensue rapidly (24 to 48 hours) despite vigorous antibiotic therapy. Adrenal infarction causing adrenal insufficiency is often associated with these infections (Waterhouse-Friderichsen syndrome).

Polyvalent pneumococcal polysaccharide vaccines are given after total splenectomy or conservative splenic operation for trauma. Patients with splenic trauma who are managed nonoperatively are also vaccinated. Neither the surgeon nor the patient should consider this vaccine full protection against overwhelming postsplenectomy sepsis. Both clinical and experimental evidence suggests that splenectomized patients may not respond well to pneumococcal polysaccharide antigens. Children who are younger than 2 years of age also do not become effectively immunized. In addition, pneumococcal types that are not contained in the vaccine (or other bacteria) may cause overwhelming sepsis. Patients who undergo elective splenectomy should be immunized well in advance of surgery. The exact timing for immunization is unknown, but longer than 1 week before surgery is probably sufficient. However, many of the patients who undergo splenectomy are being treated with steroids and this may lessen the immune response. In such patients, delayed immunization after steroids have been discontinued may be preferred. After splenectomy, it is wise to wait until the patient is nutritionally intact and recovers from other injuries before administering the vaccination. Vaccinations against *H. influenzae* type B and *N. meningitidis* are available and should be considered for asplenic patients. Pneumococcal conjugate vaccines are now available and recommended for children; however, their efficacy after splenectomy is not clearly defined. When dealing with trauma patients, there is concern that some may not return for their postoperative visits and thus if not immunized before discharge, they may not be immunized at all.

Long-term antibiotic prophylaxis with oral penicillin is a reasonable approach in immunologically compromised patients (e.g., renal transplant recipients), those receiving chemotherapy, and children younger than 6 years of age who undergo splenectomy. This approach does not provide definite prophylaxis for a number of reasons, including lack of compliance, inconvenience, and the development of bacterial resistance.

People who undergo splenectomy should carry identification that explains their medical condition. They should also be instructed to contact their physician at the first sign of any minor infection (e.g., cold, sore throat). Antibiotics should be prescribed and the patient followed closely. While these general principles are frequently put forth, there is no evidence that they result in measurable changes in outcome.

Other Complications After Splenectomy

Morbidity and mortality rates after splenectomy are relatively low. Older patients and those with severe underlying conditions have the highest morbidity and mortality rates.

Atelectasis is the most common complication after splenectomy. It is usually caused by ineffective coughing with reduced respiratory excursions secondary to pain due to high abdominal incisions and irritation of the diaphragm. Atelectasis usually resolves within 2 to 3 days if it is properly treated. Improperly treated, atelectasis can progress to pneumonia. Small left-sided pleural effusions are common and may be associated with atelectasis and/or diaphragmatic irritation. When the effusion is large and the patient has a persistent fever, it is more likely that the patient has developed a subphrenic abscess. Subphrenic fluid may collect in the residual space postsplenectomy. Such fluid may be bland and this situation occurs secondary to bleeding, inflammation, or leakage of pancreatic fluid as a result of injury to the tail of the pancreas. Abscesses are more likely to develop if the gastrointestinal (GI) tract has been is opened. The placement of prophylactic drains increases the risk of subphrenic abscess. These drains are rarely used unless a pancreatic injury is identified. Subphrenic abscesses are usually apparent within 5 to 10 days after surgery. Signs include fever, left upper quadrant pain, omalgia, left pleural effusion, prolonged atelectasis, pneumonia, and prolonged leukocytosis. Ultrasonography and CT scanning are useful for identifying abscesses. Once identified, they should be drained promptly either percutaneously with image guidance or operatively.

Injury to the pancreas occurs in 1% to 5% of patients who undergo splenectomy. It may be clinically unrecognized and cause mild hyperamylasemia or may cause clinical pancreatitis, pancreatic fistula, or pancreatic pseudocysts. Serum amylase or lipase determination on the second to fourth day after surgery may help to identify those patients with the pancreatic injury. Symptoms and signs (nausea and vomiting, abdominal distension, abdominal pain, and pulmonary complications, such as those seen with a subphrenic abscess) usually develop within 4 to 5 days after splenectomy.

Likewise, injury to the stomach may occur when a portion of the stomach is included in the ligation of the short gastric vessels with resultant necrosis and fistulization from the stomach into the left upper quadrant. This injury may lead to the development of a subphrenic abscess or gastrocutaneous fistula. Some surgeons advocate nasogastric decompression for 2 to 3 days after splenectomy to avoid gastric distension with "slipping off" of the sutures on the short gastric vessels and prevent complications; however, data to support this is lacking. Care is taken to avoid thermal or direct injury to the gastric wall, and oversewing any area of question may be advisable to prevent problems.

Brisk bleeding may occur in the course of splenectomy, especially when the spleen is massively enlarged and traction on the splenic ligaments is applied. Additionally, dilated veins are typically fragile. Preparatory splenic artery occlusion by endovascular techniques may lessen this risk of hemorrhage, but this has not been subjected to rigorous evaluation. Such splenic artery occlusion may result in splenic infarction. It also does produce an elevation in the platelet count, which may be beneficial in some cases.

Persistent hemorrhage after splenectomy occurs in <1% of cases. It most commonly occurs in patients who undergo splenectomy for thrombocytopenia, especially those in whom the platelet count does not respond to splenectomy. Reoperation is necessary if bleeding continues after any coagulation abnormalities are corrected or if hemodynamic instability occurs.

The spleen and its functions were an enigma to the ancients. The same remains true today, perhaps to a lesser degree, with many problems as yet unsolved including the circulation of the spleen, the role of splenosis, the optimal time for immunizations in patients who will undergo splenectomy or have had splenectomy performed as an emergency procedure, and the treatment of postsplenectomy thrombocytosis. Today's students may give us the answers. History tells us that it was a medical student who first suggested that splenectomy might aid in the treatment of ITP!

DISORDERS OF LYMPH NODES

Lymphadenopathy

Normal lymph nodes are usually small (<1 cm), and tend to be larger in adolescents than in adults. Lymph nodes usually are not palpable, except in the inguinal regions of healthy individuals, arguably because of chronic low-level trauma and low-grade infection in the lower extremities. Lymphadenopathy, enlarged lymph nodes, can be caused by a number of diseases and drugs. Localized lymphadenopathy involves only one region such as an axilla, while generalized lymphadenopathy involves more than one region. Diagnosing the cause for lymphadenopathy relies on a careful history and physical examination, and distinguishing between localized and generalized lymphadenopathy can be useful in diagnosis.

Careful history should be taken to focus on symptoms and/or signs of infection or malignancy; dermatological disease; exposures such as to cats and other animals, raw meat, insect bites, high risk sexual behaviors, intravenous drug use, and travel. A history of fever, night sweats, and weight loss suggests chronic infections such as tuberculosis, lymphoma, or other malignancy. A careful drug history should be obtained as some drugs can cause lymphadenopathy. Tables 21-7 and 21-8 list common causes of regional and generalized lymphadenopathy.

A complete physical examination should be performed. The presence of an enlarged spleen in association with lymphadenopathy suggests diseases such as infectious mononucleosis, lymphoma, or leukemia. All lymph node regions should be palpated. Abnormal nodes are >1 cm in diameter. Tender nodes imply a more rapid enlargement as often seen with acute infections of the skin and soft tissues. Hard nodes are often found with cancers and rubbery nodes with lymphomas. Nodes are usually freely mobile, but may become fixed to surrounding tissues by inflammation or invasive malignancy. Matted nodes are nodes fixed to each other by inflammation of tumor.

Some infections with certain strains of streptococci and staphylococci involve and spread via the lymphatics. Red streaks (lymphangitis) can be seen running from the site of infections to locally draining lymph nodes that become enlarged, tender, and can occasionally suppurate (lymphadenitis). Patients with lymphedema (see also Chapter 22, Diseases of the Vascular System) are at risk for developing lymphangitis often without an obvious source.

Anterior cervical lymphadenopathy often is due to infections of the head or neck, while posterior cervical lymphadenopathy should make one suspicious of lymphoma in the absence of other signs and symptoms. Hard cervical nodes, particularly in older patients with a history of smoking, suggest metastatic squamous cell carcinoma.

Supraclavicular lymphadenopathy usually suggests malignancy. Cancers of the right lung or esophagus are associated with right supraclavicular adenopathy, while GI and other abdominal malignancies are associated with left supraclavicular adenopathy (Virchow's node) where the thoracic duct

TABLE 21-7	Causes of Regional Lymphadenopathy
Regional Lymph Nodes	**Common Causes**
Occipital	Scalp infections, rarely lymphoma or metastatic cancer
Posterior auricular	Rubella
Anterior auricular	Conjunctival and eyelid infections
Posterior cervical	Chronic infections (e.g., toxoplasmosis), metastatic cancer, lymphoma, tuberculosis
Submental	Dental infections
Anterior cervical	Oral cavity and pharyngeal infections, metastatic squamous cell cancer, lymphoma, tuberculosis
Supraclavicular	Metastases from intrathoracic and intraabdominal (left side) cancers, lymphoma, rarely infections
Axillary	Upper extremity infections, cat-scratch disease, metastatic breast cancer, lymphoma
Epitrochlear	Hand infections, viral disease (children), sarcoidosis, tularemia
Inguinal	Lower extremity infections, lymphogranuloma venereum, gonorrhea, herpes, lymphoma, metastatic rectal cancer
Pulmonary hilar	Metastatic lung cancer, sarcoidosis, tuberculosis, histoplasmosis, coccidioidomycosis
Mediastinal	Hodgkin's lymphoma, sarcoidosis, metastatic cancer
Intra-abdominal/retroperitoneal	Lymphoma, metastatic cancer

empties into the left venous angle of the left subclavian and left internal jugular vein.

Axillary lymphadenopathy can be associated with infections such as cat scratch disease, where the nodes become quite large and tender and often suppurate. In the absence of upper extremity infections or lesions, malignancy, particularly cancer of the breast, must be ruled out.

Epitrochlear lymphadenopathy is always abnormal, often related to infections, metastatic cancers, or lymphoma.

Generalized lymphadenopathy suggests systemic disease. Patients with HIV infection develop nontender lymphadenopathy involving the cervical, occipital, and axillary nodes. This is presumed to be related to the development of an

TABLE 21-8	Causes of Generalized Lymphadenopathy
Infections	Influenza, infectious mononucleosis, rubella, cytomegalovirus, tuberculosis
Systemic disease	HIV infection, sarcoidosis, Addison's disease, hyperthyroidism, hypopituitarism, leukemia, lymphoma
Drugs	Allopurinol, atenolol, captopril, carbamazepine, cephalosporins, gold, hydralazine, penicillin, phenytoin, primidone, pyrimethamine, quinidine, sulfonamides, sulindac

immune response to the virus. Tuberculosis can present with lymphadenopathy, and can mimic malignancies. Infectious mononucleosis classically presents with fever, pharyngitis, and lymphadenopathy with symmetrical involvement of the posterior cervical nodes more than the anterior cervical nodes. Generalized lymphadenopathy may be associated with leukemias. Lymphadenopathy is often seen with metabolic diseases such as Addison's disease, hyperthyroidism, and hypopituitarism.

General Diagnostic Considerations

In addition to a complete blood count and differential, additional laboratory studies should be obtained as needed to rule out specific suspected causes. Imaging studies may be useful. Chest radiographs can show enlarged mediastinal nodes and associated pulmonary infections or tumors. Computed tomography (CT) and magnetic resonance imaging (MRI) have replaced lymphangiography for assessing lymphadenopathy.

Lymph node biopsy should be performed if the cause of nodal enlargement is not obvious. Fine-needle aspiration (FNA) biopsies for cytology are useful when metastatic carcinoma is suspected or in areas where open biopsies are not easily obtained without an extensive operation. False negative FNA biopsy is not uncommon, and repeat FNA or open biopsy should be considered if the initial FNA biopsy is negative and suspicion remains.

Open biopsy allows examination for abnormal cells and abnormal architecture, which is important for the diagnosis of lymphomas. In cases of generalized lymphadenopathy, the order of preference for biopsy is cervical, supraclavicular, axillary, and inguinal. Inguinal nodes are often enlarged and often show chronic reactivity secondary to chronic minor trauma. Node biopsy specimens should be transferred quickly to the lab in a fresh, sterile state. Tissue from the specimen can be submitted for culture. If lymphoma is suspected, a frozen section should be performed. If lymphoma is diagnosed by frozen section, tissue should be processed for immunologic markers by specialized staining and flow cytometry. By using specific monoclonal antibodies, the specific cell type of origin of the lymphoma can be determined.

Hodgkin's Lymphoma and Non-Hodgkin's Lymphoma

Lymphomas are malignancies that arise in the lymphoid tissues of the body. Collections of lymphoid cells occur in the lymph nodes, the white pulp of the spleen, Waldeyer's ring, the thymus gland, and lymphoid aggregates in the submucosa of the respiratory and GI tracts (**Peyer's patches**). The two major subgroups of malignant lymphoma are **Hodgkin's lymphoma** (13%) and **non-Hodgkin's lymphoma** (87%). Lymphomas are classified based on immunohistopathologic standards (Table 21-9). Lymphomas originate from **B cells, T cells,** histiocytes, or other lymphoid cells.

Hodgkin's Lymphoma
Incidence and Etiology

The incidence of Hodgkin's lymphoma follows a bimodal curve, with peaks in young adulthood (late 20s) and in older adults (mid 70s). The average age of a patient with Hodgkin's lymphoma is 32 years. The incidence in the United States has declined significantly since the 1980s, and the National Cancer Institute estimates there will be approximately 8510 new cases in 2009.

TABLE 21-9	Lymphoid Neoplasms Recognized by the International Lymphoma Study Group

B-cell Neoplasms

I. Precursor B-cell neoplasm: precursor B-lymphoblastic leukemia/lymphoma

II. Peripheral B-cell neoplasms

    1. B-cell chronic lymphocytic leukemia, prolymphocytic leukemia or small lymphocytic lymphoma

    2. Lymphoplasmacytoid lymphoma or immunocytoma

    3. Mantle cell lymphoma

    4. Follicle center lymphoma, follicular

        Provisional cytologic grades: I (small cell), II (mixed small and large cell), III (large cell)

        Provisional subtype: diffuse, predominantly small cell type

    5. Marginal zone B-cell lymphoma

        Extranodal (MALT-type with or without monocytoid B cells)

        Provisional subtype: nodal (with or without monocytoid B cells)

    6. Provisional entity: splenic marginal zone lymphoma (with or without villous lymphocytes)

    7. Hairy cell leukemia

    8. Plasmacytoma or plasma cell myeloma

    9. *Diffuse large B-cell lymphoma*[a]

        Subtype: primary mediastinal (thymic) B-cell lymphoma

    10. Burkitt's lymphoma

    11. *Provisional entity: high-grade B-cell lymphoma, Burkitt-like*[a]

T-cell and Putative NK-cell Neoplasms

I. Precursor T-cell neoplasm: precursor T-lymphoblastic lymphoma or leukemia

II. Peripheral T-cell and NK-cell neoplasms

    1. T-cell chronic lymphocytic leukemia or prolymphocytic leukemia

    2. Large granular lymphocyte leukemia

        T-cell type

        NK-cell type

    3. Mycosis fungoides or Sezary syndrome

    4. *Peripheral T-cell lymphomas, unspecified*[a]

        Provisional cytologic categories: medium cell, mixed medium and large cell, large cell, or lymphoepithelioid cell

        Provisional subtype: hepatosplenic $\gamma\delta$ T-cell lymphoma

        Provisional subtype: subcutaneous panniculitic T-cell lymphoma

    5. Angioimmunoblastic T-cell lymphoma

    6. Angiocentric lymphoma

    7. Intestinal T-cell lymphoma (with or without associated enteropathy)

    8. Adult T-cell lymphoma or leukemia

    9. Anaplastic large cell lymphoma, CD30+, T- and null-cell types

    10. Provisional entity: anaplastic large-cell lymphoma, Hodgkin's-like

Hodgkin's Lymphoma

I. Lymphocyte predominance

II. Nodular sclerosis

III. Mixed cellularity

IV. Lymphocyte depletion

V. Provisional entity: lymphocyte-rich classical Hodgkin's lymphoma

[a]*These categories probably include more than one disease entity.*

The etiology of Hodgkin's lymphoma is unknown. Various theories are postulated, including infectious causes (e.g., Epstein-Barr virus). The cellular origin of Hodgkin's lymphoma is also uncertain, although it may involve the monocyte–macrophage cell line.

Clinical Presentation and Evaluation

Hodgkin's lymphoma usually causes asymptomatic cervical lymphadenopathy (60% to 80%). Supradiaphragmatic disease occurs initially in 90% of young adults who have Hodgkin's lymphoma. In older adults, however, the likelihood of subdiaphragmatic disease is 25%. Systemic symptoms (fever, night sweats, and loss of more than 10% of body weight) indicate a worse prognosis. Hodgkin's lymphoma may be localized or disseminated. Patients also may have signs and symptoms because of the mass effect of mediastinal or retroperitoneal disease.

All patients must undergo a thorough evaluation, including a complete physical examination. Particular attention is paid to the peripheral lymph node regions. A chest radiograph is also needed. The next step is excisional biopsy of an enlarged, abnormal lymph node. If multiple sites are enlarged, biopsy is performed on cervical rather than axillary or inguinal nodes, since these sites are more likely to show reactive changes and therefore be nondiagnostic. After the histologic diagnosis is made, a bone marrow biopsy is obtained. Finally, the liver, spleen, and retroperitoneal nodes are evaluated with CT scan.

In the past, staging laparotomy was an important part of the pretreatment evaluation of a patient with Hodgkin's disease. Staging laparotomy includes splenectomy and biopsy of the splenic hilar, celiac, porta hepatis, mesenteric, paraaortic, and iliac nodes. Bilateral wedge and needle biopsies of the liver are also performed. In an attempt to maintain fertility after radiation treatment in premenopausal women, the ovaries are positioned in a retrouterine site and sutured to presacral fascia (oophoropexy). Now, staging laparotomy rarely plays a role in the evaluation of patients with Hodgkin's disease. Its use is limited to patients with minimal stage disease. The issue for the physician is differentiating patients who may have limited disease treatable by radiation from those who have more extensive disease and need chemotherapy. Over the last few decades, the need for staging laparotomy has decreased as imaging studies have permitted greater accuracy in staging, and treatment patterns have changed with greater use of chemotherapy. For example, staging laparotomy is not necessary in patients who have a large mediastinal mass and in older patients who have mixed- or lymphocyte-depleted histology. These patients require systemic therapy, and laparotomy does not alter the course of treatment.

Staging

The Revised European-American Classification of Lymphoid Neoplasms/World Health Organization (REAL/WHO) classification system groups Hodgkin's lymphoma histologically into five categories: nodular lymphocyte predominate, lymphocyte rich, nodular sclerosis, mixed cellularity, and lymphocyte depleted. Nodular sclerosis is the most common histologic type (relative frequency of 70%). Histologically, Hodgkin's lymphoma appears as a tumor with a large reactive background of lymphocytes, eosinophils, and plasma cells, with a few malignant mononuclear cells and multinuclear giant cells (Reed-Sternberg cells). The Reed-Sternberg cell has a classic "owl eye" appearance (Figure 21-12). This cell must

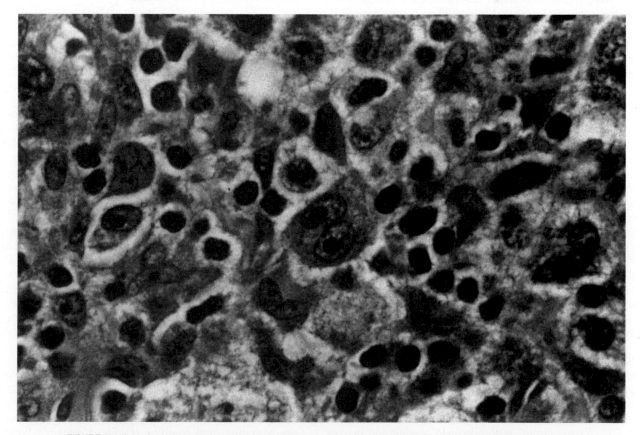

FIGURE 21-12. Hodgkin's lymphoma, mixed cellularity subtype. A classic, diagnostic bilobulated Reed-Steinberg cell is surrounded by a variety of cell types, including malignant Hodgkin's cells and benign small lymphocytes and histiocytes (hematoxylin and eosin 1000×). (Courtesy of Dr. Rogers Griffith, Department of Pathology, Rhode Island Hospital, Providence, Rhode Island.)

TABLE 21-10	Cotswolds Staging for Hodgkin's Lymphoma

Stage	Findings
I	Involvement of a single lymph node region or lymphoid structure (e.g., spleen, thymus, Waldeyer's ring) or a single extralymphatic organ or site
II	Involvement of two or more lymph node regions on the same side of the diaphragm (hilar nodes, when involved on both sides, constitute stage II disease); localized contiguous involvement of only one extralymphatic organ or site and lymph node region on the same side of the diaphragm (IIE). The number of anatomic regions involved should be indicated by a subscript (e.g., II_3)
III	Involvement of lymph node regions on both sides of the diaphragm (III), which may be accompanied by involvement of the spleen (III_S), of or by localized contiguous involvement of only one extralymphatic organ site (III_E), or both (III_{SE})
III_1	With or without involvement of splenic, hilar, celiac, or portal nodes
III_2	With involvement of para-aortic, iliac, and mesenteric nodes
IV	Diffuse or disseminated involvement of one or more extralymphatic organs or tissues, with or without associated lymph node involvement (involved organs should be identified by a symbol)
Designations Applicable to any Disease Stage	
A	No symptoms
B	Fever (temperature >38°C, drenching night sweats, unexplained weight loss >10% of body weight within past 6 months
X	Bulky disease (a widening of the mediastinum by more than one-third of the presence of a nodal mass with a maximal dimension >10 cm)
E	Involvement of a single extranodal site that is contiguous or proximal to the known nodal site
CS	Clinical Stage
PS	Pathologic stage (as determined by laparotomy)

Used with permission of the American Society of Clinical Oncology. The original source for this material is: Lister T, Crowther D, Sutcliff S, et al. Report of a committee convened to discuss the evaluation and staging of patients with Hodgkin's disease: Cotswolds meeting. J Clin Oncol. 1989;7:1630.

be present for the diagnosis of Hodgkin's lymphoma to be made. Reed-Sternberg cells are also present in other disorders, including mononucleosis and other inflammatory conditions, and with phenytoin (Dilantin) therapy.

The Cotswolds classification is used to stage Hodgkin's lymphoma (Table 21-10). This classification identifies patients as stage A (asymptomatic) or stage B (fevers, night sweats, and weight loss). Stage classification is based on the involvement of single, multiple, or disseminated sites of one or more extralymphatic organs.

Treatment

The treatment of Hodgkin's lymphoma is determined by staging. Radiation therapy plays a role in the treatment of early-stage disease (stages I and II). When used, radiation is administered in doses of 30 to 40 Gy to areas of known involvement and to neighboring nodal basins that are likely to represent the next area of spread. Chemotherapy, with or without radiation therapy, is recommended for advanced disease.

Chemotherapy significantly alters the prognosis of patients with Hodgkin's lymphoma, with cure achieved in 80% of cases. Two common regimens are nitrogen mustard, vincristine, procarbazine, and prednisone (MOPP); and doxorubicin (adriamycin), bleomycin, vinblastine, and dacarbazine (ABVD).

Prognosis

The prognosis for patients with Hodgkin's lymphoma is excellent. Risk factors include the stage of disease at the time of treatment and the histology. The lymphocyte-predominant group appears to have the best prognosis, followed by the nodular-sclerosis group. With adequate staging and therapy, 80% of patients are cured. The risk of a second tumor after treatment (thought to be secondary to the treatment) continues to increase with time. The risk of leukemia reaches a plateau of approximately 3% at 10 years.

Non-Hodgkin's Lymphoma

Non-Hodgkin's lymphomas consist of a diverse group, representing a large spectrum of malignancies. Their histology, immunology, and clinical characteristics are heterogeneous.

Incidence and Etiology

Since 1970, the incidence of non-Hodgkin's lymphoma has nearly doubled. According to the National Cancer Institute, 65,980 new cases of non-Hodgkin's lymphoma will be diagnosed in 2009. It is the seventh most common cancer, representing 4% of all cancers in the United States. Non-Hodgkin's lymphoma appears to be associated with HIV, although the increased incidence is not entirely explained by the rise in the number of cases of AIDS.

As with Hodgkin's lymphoma, the etiology of most types of non-Hodgkin's lymphoma is unclear. The incidence appears to increase in association with immunosuppression. Patients with AIDS and those who undergo organ transplantation are at increased risk for this disorder. Viruses can cause specific lymphomas. Epstein-Barr virus infection is associated with Burkitt's lymphoma, and human T-cell lymphoma virus-1 is associated with a T-cell lymphoma that is found in the Caribbean Islands.

Clinical Presentation and Evaluation

Most patients with non-Hodgkin's lymphoma are asymptomatic at presentation, although 20% have systemic symptoms (fever, night sweats, or weight loss). Patients may have enlarged lymph nodes, with GI symptoms that include nausea, vomiting, and bleeding. Unlike Hodgkin's lymphoma, non-Hodgkin's lymphoma tends to be disseminated. Patients may have symptoms secondary to the extent of spread. Some

TABLE 21-11	International Non-Hodgkin's Lymphoma Prognostic Factors Project			
Category	Risk Factors[a] (*n*)	Complete Response Rate (%)	2-yr Survival (%)	5-yr Survival (%)
Low risk	≤1	87	84	73
Low-intermediate risk	2	67	66	50
High-intermediate risk	3	55	54	43

[a]Risk factors include age (≥60 yr), Stage (I/II vs. III/IV), extranodal sites (≤1 or >1), performance status (Eastern Cooperative Oncology Group ≤1 vs. 2), and lactic dehydrogenase level (normal vs. abnormal).
Adapted with permission from The International Non-Hodgkin's Lymphoma Prognostic Factors Project. A predictive model for aggressive non-Hodgkin's lymphoma. N Engl J Med. 1993;329:987–994. Copyright 1993 Massachusetts Medical Society. All rights reserved.

dramatic presentations include superior vena cava syndrome, acute spinal cord compression, MALT lymphomas, and meningeal involvement. MALT represents lymphomas that occur outside the lymph nodes (GI tract, thyroid, breast, or skin).

The evaluation of patients with non-Hodgkin's lymphoma begins with a complete history and physical examination. Next, diagnostic studies are performed, including complete blood count, liver function tests, chest radiograph, and CT scan of the chest, abdomen, and pelvis. Bone marrow biopsy is then performed. Patients with intermediate-grade non-Hodgkin's lymphoma with bone marrow involvement and those with high-grade non-Hodgkin's lymphoma may require lumbar puncture because central nervous system involvement is increased in these groups. Staging laparotomy is usually not indicated because these patients tend to have disseminated disease, in contrast to those with Hodgkin's lymphoma, who tend to have localized disease that progresses by involvement of contiguous node basins.

Classification and Staging
Many histologic classification systems are used for non-Hodgkin's lymphoma. These include the Rappaport and the Working Formulation systems as well as the REAL/WHO (Table 21-9). The latter system incorporates morphology, immunophenotype, and genetic characteristics to give a comprehensive list of diseases with distinct clinical characteristics. The stage is determined with the Ann Arbor system, although this system is somewhat limited because non-Hodgkin's lymphoma tends to occur in disseminated form. In 1993, the International Non-Hodgkin's Lymphoma Prognostic Factors Project devised a new classification system (Table 21-11) that groups patients based on risk of relapse. This system is used in conjunction with staging information to determine the optimal patient treatment plan.

Treatment
The treatment of non-Hodgkin's lymphoma is variable, depending on the histologic subtype, the stage, and the risk of relapse. Surgery, radiation therapy, and chemotherapy are the treatment options. The primary role of surgery is for diagnosis, although it is sometimes an important aspect of treatment. Localized gastric and small-bowel non-Hodgkin's lymphoma may be effectively treated with resection (see Chapter 13, Stomach and Duodenum, and Chapter 14, Small Intestine and Appendix). Surgery may also be indicated to treat complications (perforation, obstruction) of the disease or those associated with treatment (perforation). Radiation therapy is useful in localized non-Hodgkin's lymphoma, although this presentation is unusual. Radiation therapy is also used for complications related to mass effect (e.g., superior vena cava obstruction, spinal cord compression).

Non-Hodgkin's lymphoma tumors are primarily treated with chemotherapy. A variety of agents and treatment protocols are used. The response to chemotherapy and the duration of remission are related to tumor grade and stage.

Prognosis
To determine the prognosis, tumor grade and stage are considered. Low-grade tumors tend to follow an indolent course, and if left untreated, patients often survive 5 years or longer. On the other hand, high-grade tumors may progress rapidly if they are not treated and may result in death. These high-grade tumors respond well to chemotherapy. Factors that affect responsiveness in patients with high- and intermediate-grade tumors have been defined. The prognosis is poor in patients who are older than 60 years of age, have systemic symptoms (fever, night sweats, weight loss), and have bulky disease, and in those who have extranodal disease and bone marrow or GI involvement.

SAMPLE QUESTIONS

Questions

Choose the best answer for each question.

1. A 27-year-old woman is brought to the emergency department by her husband 16 hours after the onset of fever, malaise, sweats, vague abdominal pain, and increasing confusion. She has no chronic illnesses and takes no medications. Ten years ago, she underwent splenectomy for a ruptured spleen sustained when she was kicked by a horse. She recalls receiving vaccinations at that time when she was discharged from the hospital. Now her temperature is 39°C. Vital signs are pulse—125/minute, blood pressure (BP)—85/40 mm Hg, and respirations—30/minute. She is confused. There are diffuse petechiae over her trunk. Her abdomen is soft and nontender with a long, well-healed midline incisional scar. Laboratory values are WBC—26,000 mm³, sodium—125 mEq/dL, potassium of 6.0 mEq/dL, and glucose of 60 mg/dL.

   After the patient is stabilized, a CT scan is performed, which shows bilateral adrenal infarcts with adrenal hemorrhage. Infection with which of the following microorganisms is the most likely cause for her current infection?

   A. *Escherichia coli*

   B. *Pseudomonas aeruginosa*

   C. *Clostridium perfringens*

   D. *Streptococcus pneumoniae*

   E. *Bacteroides fragilis*

2. A 45-year-old woman comes to clinic because of bleeding gums when she brushes her teeth and heavy menstrual bleeding. She has a history of immune thrombocytopenic purpura that was unresponsive to corticosteroids at that time and underwent splenectomy 15 months ago. Her platelet count 2 months after splenectomy was 175,000/mm³. Her physical exam today reveals scattered petechiae and a few purpuric lesions on her forearms. Platelet count today is 30,000/mm³. A peripheral smear shows normal red cell morphology and no red cell inclusions. What is the next best step in management?

   A. Platelet pheresis

   B. Bone marrow aspiration for analysis

   C. Radionuclide spleen scan

   D. Corticosteroid therapy

   E. Platelet transfusion

3. A 23-year-old man is brought to the emergency department 30 minutes after a motorcycle crash. He is awake and complaining of severe abdominal and left chest pain. Oxygen therapy and IV fluids were started at the scene. Blood pressure on admission was 90/60 with a pulse of 110/minute and respirations were 18/minute. A chest tube was placed on the left that yielded only a small amount of bloody fluid. Breath sounds are only slightly diminished at the left base and there is no tracheal deviation. After 2 L of normal saline, his BP is 80/50. A FAST exam shows a large amount of fluid in the abdomen and what appears to be a fractured spleen. In addition to blood transfusion, the most appropriate management is

   A. admission to the surgical intensive care unit for further resuscitation.

   B. arteriography and attempt embolization of the splenic artery.

   C. abdominal CT scan with IV and oral contrast.

   D. exploratory laparotomy.

   E. dopamine infusion at 10 μg/kg/min.

4. A 29-year-old woman is seen in clinic with fatigue and weakness. She recently had a urinary tract infection treated for 7 days with trimethoprim/sulfamethoxazole and stopped taking this 2 days ago. She takes no other medications. She has a history of glucose-6-phophate dehydrogenase deficiency. Her pulse is 100. She appears pale. Otherwise her physical exam is normal. Hematocrit is 22%. What is the most likely mechanism for her anemia?

   A. Spectrin deficiency

   B. Sensitization of red blood cells by membrane-bound antibody

   C. Conformational change in hemoglobin

   D. Decreased ATP

   E. Oxidation injury of the cell membrane

5. A 19-year-old man comes to clinic because of a left neck mass. He first noticed a firm nontender mass just above his clavicle about a month ago. He has not had any recent infections. He has a cat that has been a pet for 4 years. He has also had nighttime sweats, but he has not taken his temperature. He does not use tobacco products and does not drink alcohol. He is now afebrile. On physical exam, there is a 3-cm, firm, nontender mass in the supraclavicular fossa. The rest of the physical exam is normal. What is the most likely diagnosis?

   A. Cat scratch disease

   B. Reactive lymphadenopathy

   C. Hodgkin's lymphoma

   D. Addison's disease

   E. Metastatic esophageal cancer

Answers and Explanations

1. Answer: D

Overwhelming postsplenectomy infection (OPSI) is most often caused by encapsulated organisms such as the *Pneumococcus.* She received vaccination after splenectomy, and therefore she is still at higher risk for developing OPSI with pneumococcus than someone who was vaccinated prior to splenectomy. Pneumococcal sepsis can lead to adrenal infarction (Waterhouse-Friderichsen syndrome). While the other organisms can cause severe infections, her clinical presentation is most likely due to pneumococcal sepsis.

2. Answer: C

The correct answer is to obtain a radionuclide spleen scan to look for a missed accessory spleen. Accessory spleens can hypertrophy and sequester platelets just like a normal spleen. For this reason, it is important to look for and remove all accessory splenic tissue at the time of splenectomy. Platelet pheresis has no role at this time. If no accessory splenic tissue is identified on a radionuclide scan, further evaluation with a bone marrow aspirate may be necessary but not at this time. She did not respond initially to steroids so it is unlikely she will respond at this time. Platelet transfusion is not indicated at this time as she is not actively bleeding.

3. Answer: D

The correct answer is to perform an exploratory laparotomy. This patient is in shock and appears to have a severe splenic injury with continued hemorrhage. This is not amenable to no operative treatment. Admission to the intensive care unit is necessary to monitor patients for nonoperative management; however, this patient is too unstable. It takes time to organize an angiography team, and this patient is too unstable. A CT scan is needed before an attempt at angiographic control of splenic hemorrhage in order to rule out other injuries. This patient remains hypotensive because of continued rapid intra-abdominal hemorrhage and needs control of the bleeding, which is best accomplished at the time of laparotomy. Dopamine will not stop the bleeding.

4. Answer: E

Glucose-6-phosphate dehydrogenase deficiency is a sex-linked recessive trait. The pentose phosphate shunt is blocked and red cell membranes are injured by oxidation injury from certain drugs such as sulfamethoxazole, aspirin, phenacetin, or nitrofurantoin. Spectrin deficiency, a membrane component essential for deformability, is seen in spherocytosis. Sensitization of red cell membranes by membrane-bound antibody is the result of acquired hemolytic anemia. Conformational change in hemoglobin is seen in sickle cell anemia. Decreased production of ATP leading to membrane destruction is the mechanism by which pyruvate kinase deficiency causes hemolysis.

5. Answer: C

The correct answer is Hodgkin's disease. The presence of night sweats and the identification of a large, nontender firm node suggest Hodgkin's disease as opposed to a benign reactive adenopathy. Cat scratch disease usually presents with painful, suppurative adenopathy. There is usually generalized mild lymphadenopathy associated with Addison's disease. He has no risk factors for esophageal cancer, and the node is firm rather than hard, which would be more characteristic of metastatic cancer.

22

Diseases of the Vascular System

JAMES F. MCKINSEY, M.D. • JAMES ALEXANDER, M.D. • ARNOLD BYER, M.D. • GREGORY S. CHERR, M.D. • BRUCE L. GEWERTZ, M.D. • PETER F. LAWRENCE, M.D. • PETER R. NELSON, M.D.

Objectives

Arterial Disease: Atherosclerosis, Aneurysms, Peripheral Arterial Occlusive Disease, and Cerebrovascular Insufficiency

1. Describe five risk factors for the development of atherosclerosis.

2. List three specific sites that have a predilection for atherosclerotic plaque, and explain why this predilection exists.

3. List three ways to retard the atherosclerotic process.

4. List at least two clinical sequelae of atherosclerosis.

5. Describe the pathophysiology of intermittent claudication, and differentiate this symptom from leg pain from other causes.

6. List the common sites and relative incidence of arterial aneurysms.

7. Discuss the risk factors for development of aneurysms.

8. Discuss the indications and contraindications for repair in patients with nonruptured abdominal aortic aneurysms (AAAs).

9. List the symptoms, signs, differential diagnosis, and diagnostic and management plans for a patient with a rupturing AAA.

10. Compare the presentation, complications (i.e., frequency of dissection, rupture, thrombosis, and embolization), and treatment of thoracic, abdominal, femoral, and popliteal aneurysms.

11. Discuss alternative management options for aneurysms at different sites.

12. Define and discuss the common complications of aneurysm procedures.

13. List the criteria to help differentiate among venous, arterial, diabetic, and infectious leg ulcers.

14. Describe the medical management of arterial occlusive disease of the lower extremities.

15. Describe the endovascular and surgical treatment options available for chronic occlusive disease of the distal aorta, iliac, superficial femoral, popliteal, tibial, and peroneal arteries.

16. List four indications for amputation, and discuss the methods used to select the amputation site.

17. Describe the clinical manifestations, diagnostic workup, and indications for procedures for chronic renal artery stenosis.

18. Describe the natural history and causes of acute arterial occlusion, and differentiate between embolic and thrombotic occlusion.

19. List six signs and symptoms of acute arterial occlusion, and outline its management (e.g., indications for medical, endovascular, and surgical treatment).

20. Define and differentiate among the following:
    A. Amaurosis fugax
    B. Transient ischemic attacks (TIAs)
    C. Cerebrovascular accident (stroke)

21. Outline the diagnostic methods to evaluate carotid stenosis.

22. Discuss the management of a patient with asymptomatic carotid artery disease.

23. Outline a management and treatment plan for patients with TIAs and stroke due to carotid disease.

24. Differentiate between hemispheric and vertebrobasilar symptoms.

Venous Disease: Superficial Vein Thrombosis, Deep Vein Thrombosis, Pulmonary Embolus, Chronic Venous Insufficiency, Venous Ulcers, and Varicose Veins

1. Identify several anatomic locations where deep vein thrombosis originates.

2. Discuss the clinical factors that lead to an increased incidence of deep vein thrombosis.

3. Describe three common operations associated with a high risk of developing deep vein thrombophlebitis.

4. Describe four methods of preventing the development of deep venous thrombosis in surgical patients.

5. Identify the noninvasive testing procedures used to diagnose superficial and deep vein thrombosis.

6. Outline the differential diagnosis of acute unilateral leg pain or unilateral swelling.

7. Discuss the treatment of a patient with septic superficial thrombophlebitis

8. Describe the methods used to administer anticoagulant and thrombolytic agents for treatment of venous thrombosis, and describe the contraindications to therapy.

9. Describe the clinical syndrome of pulmonary embolus, and identify current methods of preventing pulmonary embolism.

10. Discuss a procedure used in patients with deep venous thrombosis to prevent pulmonary embolism.

11. Describe the management of a patient with varicose veins.

12. Outline the diagnostic evaluation and management of patients with venous ulcers.

Vasospastic Diseases, Thoracic Outlet Syndrome, and Lymphatic Disorders

1. Describe the anatomic mechanisms that cause each of the three variants of thoracic outlet syndrome (TOS).

2. Discuss the management of neurogenic TOS.

3. Discuss the management of arterial aneurysms due to TOS.

4. Discuss the diagnosis and management of Paget-Schroetter syndrome due to TOS.

Vascular Trauma

1. List the indications for arterial imaging in a patient with a possible arterial injury to the extremities.

2. In a patient with recent trauma, outline the diagnostic options and alternative treatment options for suspected arterial injury.

Vasospastic and Lymphatic Disorders

1. List five underlying diseases or disorders associated with vasospastic changes in the extremities, and discuss their diagnosis and treatment.

2. Define lymphedema praecox, lymphedema tarda, primary lymphedema, and secondary lymphedema.

3. Explain the pathophysiology of lymphedema.

4. Discuss the treatment of lymphedema.

■ ARTERIAL DISEASE

ANATOMY

The vascular system consists of a network of branching, interconnected blood vessels that conduct the blood flow to and from the heart and throughout the body. The components of the vascular system are divided into arteries, veins, and lymphatics. These are not passive conduits but dynamic and responsive tissues that continuously interact with the blood elements and are under endocrine and neural influences. The three layers of the arterial wall are the intima, media, and adventitia (Figure 22-1). The internal elastic lamina separates the intima from the media, and the external elastic lamina separates the media from the adventitia.

The endothelium, which is derived from hemangioblasts, lines the inner aspect of the intima. Given the large number of blood vessels, the collective mass of endothelial cells is greater than that of the liver. The endothelial layer is responsive both to cellular and soluble blood components and to the dynamics of blood flow. The endothelium functions as an antithrombotic surface that expresses proteins C and S, antithrombin 3, prostacyclin, thrombomodulin, heparin, and tissue plasminogen activator (TPA). Conversely, it also modulates hemostasis by

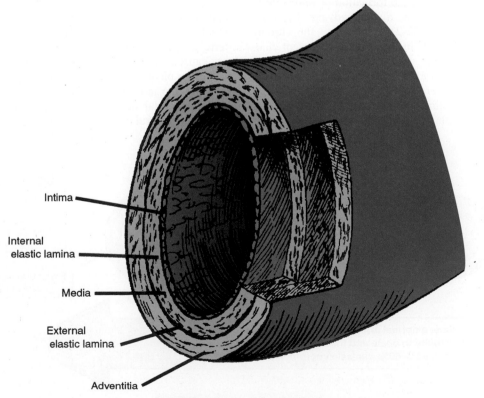

FIGURE 22-1. Layers of the arterial wall.

contributing von Willebrand factor, thromboxane, coagulation factor V, and platelet-activating factor (PAF). Endothelial cells generate vasoactive agents such as nitric oxide, which results in vasodilation and angiotensin-converting enzyme, which facilitates vasoconstriction. They have LDL receptors on their surface and produce lipoprotein lipase. In addition, they are an important source of growth factors such as platelet-derived growth factor (PDGF), which modulates their interactions with the cellular elements of the blood.

The media is the thickest layer of the arterial wall. It is composed chiefly of smooth muscle cells, along with a connective tissue matrix that includes elastin, collagen, and proteoglycans. The smooth muscle cells are predominantly aligned circumferentially around the lumen such that contraction will produce vasoconstriction and relaxation will yield dilation. The smooth muscle cells and surrounding matrix are organized into discrete bundles or lamellae. Larger vessels, which have more lamellar units stacked in cross section, have their own blood supply, the vasovasorum, which penetrates from the adventitia. Arteries with fewer lamellar units are oxygenated directly by diffusion of blood-borne oxygen from within the lumen.

The adventitia is the outermost layer. It extends beyond the external elastic lamina and is composed of connective tissue, fibroblasts, capillaries, and neural fibers. The adventitia is rich in collagen. It is the site of vessel nutrition and neural innervation and is important in containing hemorrhage after trauma or aneurysmal rupture.

ATHEROSCLEROSIS

The most common cause of arterial stenosis and occlusion is atherosclerosis, a degenerative disease that is characterized by endothelial cell dysfunction, inflammatory cell adhesion and infiltration, and the accumulation of cellular and matrix elements. These processes lead to the formation of fibrocellular plaques. In the end stages of the disease, advanced plaques impede blood flow (Figure 22-2) and lead to the chronic syndromes of angina pectoris in the heart, intermittent claudication in the legs, and organ-specific syndromes such as renovascular hypertension. More sudden events (e.g., myocardial infarction [MI], stroke, atheroembolism) are caused by unstable plaques that may rupture into the arterial lumen causing acute thrombosis at the plaque, or distal emboli.

Risk factors for the development of atherosclerosis include cigarette smoking, hypertension, abnormalities in cholesterol metabolism (elevated levels of low-density lipoprotein and depressed levels of high-density lipoprotein), diabetes mellitus, obesity, coagulation disorders, and regions of turbulence within the arterial circulation. It appears that smoking is a greater risk factor for peripheral atherosclerosis than for coronary atherosclerosis. The common thread is that all these factors cause injuries to the arterial wall. The Framingham Study has shown that the presence of multiple risk factors compounds the risk (Figure 22-3).

The first signs of atherosclerosis may appear early in adolescence as lipid- and macrophage-laden fatty streaks on the endothelial surface. These lesions progress to fibrous plaques consisting of macrophages encapsulated by collagen and elastin. As the fibrous plaque matures, regions within the plaque become necrotic and eventually rupture, leading to plaque ulceration. Within these complex plaques, regions of microcalcification develop and can progress to significant calcium deposits.

Although atherosclerosis is usually considered a systemic disease, plaques tend to localize in specific regions. The most common sites of atherosclerotic plaques are within the coronary arteries, the carotid bifurcation, the proximal iliac arteries, and the adductor canal region of the distal superficial femoral arteries. Regions of arterial bifurcation are also predisposed to the development of atherosclerotic plaques because of turbulence at the flow divider that results in regions of low shear stress and flow stagnation (Figure 22-4). This stasis allows greater contact time between the vessel wall and lipids and other atherogenic factors in the blood.

Common sequelae of atherosclerosis are (1) MI or angina pectoris as a result of coronary atherosclerosis; (2) **transient ischemic attack (TIA)** or stroke as a result of carotid bifurcation atherosclerosis; and (3) lower extremity ischemia that can cause difficulty in walking, rest pain, or gangrene. Less common clinical presentations are renal hypoperfusion due to renal artery stenosis and small bowel ischemia due to mesenteric stenosis or occlusion. The symptoms of arterial stenosis are caused by either gradual, progressive occlusion from an enlarging plaque that limits distal flow, or by sudden thrombosis of the artery superimposed on an underlying plaque. Sudden arterial occlusion does not allow for the development of collateral arterial channels, but gradual stenosis of the

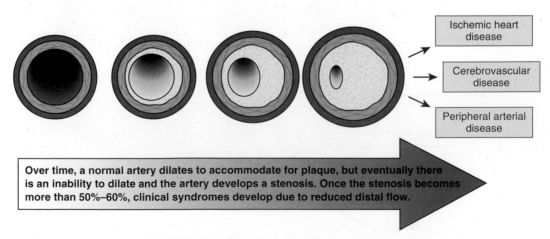

Ischemic heart disease

Cerebrovascular disease

Peripheral arterial disease

Over time, a normal artery dilates to accommodate for plaque, but eventually there is an inability to dilate and the artery develops a stenosis. Once the stenosis becomes more than 50%–60%, clinical syndromes develop due to reduced distal flow.

FIGURE 22-2. Time course of human atherosclerosis.

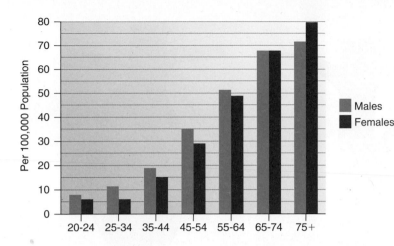

FIGURE 22-3. Risk factors and age. Risk factors are both modifiable and nonmodifiable. Smoking, hypertension, diabetes, lipid disorders, obesity, and sedentary lifestyle are cumulative risk factors that increase with age.

artery may allow for the development of arterial collaterals to maintain distal perfusion. Plaque ulcerations often become a nidus for platelet deposition and thrombus formation. Distal embolization of this material may produce an acute occlusive event and sudden onset of symptoms.

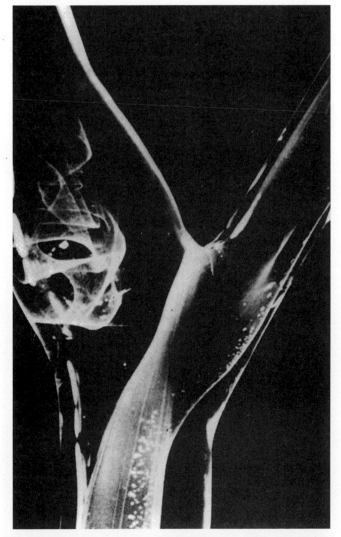

FIGURE 22-4. Glass model of the carotid bifurcation. Hydrogen gas bubbles show the streamlining of flow fields at the carotid flow divider and the complex counterrotating helical pattern at the arterial wall opposite the flow divider. (Reprinted with permission from Zarins CK, Glagov S. Arterial wall pathology in atherosclerosis. In: Rutherford RB, ed. *Vascular Surgery*. 4th ed. Vol. 1. Philadelphia, PA: WB Saunders, 1996:214.)

Atherosclerosis is a progressive disease manifested by the development of symptomatic ischemic syndromes. The best way to retard its progression is to modify atherosclerotic risk factors. Programs that use a combination of risk factor modification and specific pharmacologic agents that retard the progression of atherosclerosis, such as antiplatelet agents, β-blockers, statins, antihypertensives, and nutritional supplementation have been shown to dramatically reduce the incidence of cardiovascular events. Exercise has a protective effect by increasing the level of high-density lipoproteins, which enhance the transport and metabolism of other lipids.

ANEURYSMS

An aneurysm is a focal dilation of an artery to more than one-and-a-half times its normal diameter. Aneurysms may be either "true" aneurysms, which include all three layers of the arterial wall, or "false" aneurysms (**pseudoaneurysms**), which do not include all three layers of the arterial wall and occur secondary to trauma, infection, or disruption of an arterial bypass anastomosis. Many times the outer wall or the capsule of a pseudoaneurysm is only a thickened fibrous membrane. Aneurysms are also classified by their shape. A fusiform aneurysm is diffusely dilated whereas a saccular aneurysm is an eccentric outpouching of an otherwise normal-appearing artery (Figure 22-5).

Aneurysms may occur in any location within the arterial tree, but are most common in the infrarenal aorta, iliac arteries, and popliteal arteries (Table 22-1). Aneurysms also have a predilection to form at arterial branch points. It is estimated that 3% of all men older than 70 years of age have an aortic aneurysm, but patients with high-risk factors may have an incidence of up to 10%. Aneurysmal formation is a systemic and familial disease. A patient with one popliteal aneurysm has more than a 50% chance of having an aneurysm in the contralateral popliteal artery and a 50% chance of harboring an AAA. Approximately 20% of patients with AAAs have a first-degree relative with the same disease.

The majority of aneurysms are associated with atherosclerosis. While the precise etiology is not known, atherosclerosis likely impairs the diffusion of nutrients and predisposes to metalloproteinase-mediated arterial wall degeneration. Recent studies have demonstrated increased levels of matrix-metalloproteinase-2 (MMP-2) and MMP-9 in early AAA, and an abundance of MMP-9 levels in patients with larger AAA. The poorly developed vasovasorum of the

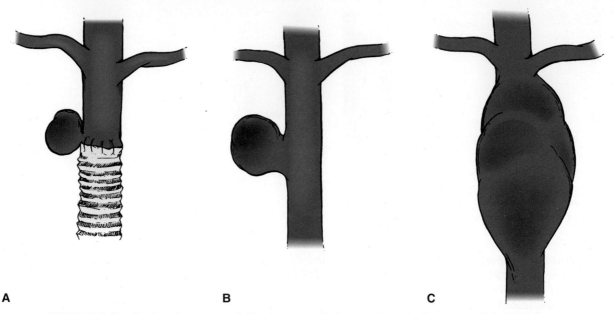

A B C

FIGURE 22-5. Classification of aneurysms. **A**, Pseudoaneurysm. **B**, Saccular atherosclerotic aneurysm. **C**, Fusiform atherosclerotic aneurysm.

infrarenal aorta likely contributes to this effect, explaining the predilection of aneurysm formation in this location. Less common causes of aneurysm formation include connective tissue disease (Marfan's syndrome, Ehlers-Danlos syndrome), infection (mycotic aneurysm), cystic medial degeneration, disruption of anastomotic connections (anastomotic pseudoaneurysm), and trauma (traumatic pseudoaneurysm) (Table 22-2).

The most serious complication of aneurysms is their propensity for enlargement and rupture. The growth rate of aneurysms is variable; although most AAAs enlarge at an average rate of approximately 0.3 cm/year, the range of expansion rates is wide; some aneurysms double in size over a few months. The size of an aneurysm is important because the risk of rupture is diameter dependent. According to a modification of the law of Laplace, the larger and thinner an aneurysm grows, the higher its tangential wall stress (J):

$$J = P \times r/t,$$

where P, intraluminal pressure; r, aneurysm radius; and t, wall thickness.

As the diameter increases at the aneurysmal portion of the artery, the velocity of the blood flow decreases, which also can

TABLE 22-1	Localization and Incidence of Abdominal Aneurysms
Location of Aneurysm	**Incidence**
Abdominal aorta	1.5%–3.0%
Common iliac artery	20%–40% present with AAA
	0.03% isolated, without AAA
Splenic artery	0.8%
	60% of all splanchnic artery aneurysms
Renal artery	0.1%
Hepatic artery	0.1%
Superior mesenteric artery	0.07%
Celiac axis	0.05%

AAA, abdominal aortic artery.

TABLE 22-2	Etiology of Aneurysmal Disease
Congenital
Idiopathic
Tuberous sclerosis
Turner's syndrome
Poststenotic dilation (e.g., aortic coarctation)
Inherited abnormalities of connective tissue
Marfan's syndrome
Ehlers-Danlos syndrome
Cystic medial necrosis
Dissection
Infection
Mycotic
Posttraumatic
Infection of existing aneurysm
Inflammatory
Aneurysms that enlarge/rupture during pregnancy
Splenic artery
Mesenteric vessels
Renal artery
Aneurysms associated with arteritis
Takayasu's disease
Giant cell arteritis
Polyarteritis nodosa
Systemic lupus erythematosus
Pseudoaneurysm
Nonspecific aortic aneurysms: "atherosclerotic"

result in thrombus formation along the wall. Such thrombi can embolize to the more distant arterial circulation, especially when they occur in peripheral aneurysms.

Clinical Presentation of Aneurysms

Aneurysms are often discovered as asymptomatic pulsatile masses on routine physical examination or during diagnostic tests, such as ultrasound, computed tomography (CT) scan, or MRI performed for other conditions. Approximately 20% of aneurysms cause symptoms, including pain, thrombosis, distal embolization, or rupture, which is the most life-threatening occurrence (Figure 22-6). The clinical presentation reflects the location of the aneurysm. Abdominal and thoracoabdominal aortic aneurysms tend to be discovered during routine examination; when such aneurysms rupture, they present as a clinical catastrophe with acute back pain and hemodynamic collapse. Popliteal and femoral aneurysms rarely rupture but laminated thrombus along the wall can dislodge and embolize into the arteries of the calf and foot, causing acute arterial ischemia. Extracranial carotid artery aneurysms, which are relatively rare, may cause cerebrovascular ischemia, including TIA or stroke, when they embolize.

As noted above, the diagnosis of aortic and peripheral artery aneurysms is often made during a routine physical examination. If an aneurysm is suspected, the patient should undergo a diagnostic evaluation. The best and most cost effective screening test for most aneurysms is ultrasonography. A well-performed ultrasound assesses the size and general location of the aneurysm with more than 95% accuracy. If the diagnosis of AAA of significant size is established, the patient should undergo CT scanning to evaluate the full extent of the aneurysm, its precise location (infrarenal or suprarenal), and better assess the need for

intervention. In the past, most AAAs were further evaluated with invasive contrast angiography, but because of improvements in the performance and interpretation of CT scans, most patients proceed to operation without angiography. CT angiography is also advised for peripheral artery aneurysms to plan the arterial reconstruction.

Treatment of Aortic Aneurysms

The natural history of AAA is to enlarge and rupture; as a consequence, patients with large AAA have a greatly decreased life expectancy compared with age-matched controls. The risk of rupture is directly related to the diameter of the aneurysm; most clinical studies show that a 4-cm AAA has an annual risk of rupture of <1% (5-year risk of rupture is 5% to 6%), but the annual rate increases to more than 10% when the AAA reaches 6 cm (Figure 22-7).

The treatment of smaller aneurysms is being carefully studied. Two recent projects, the United Kingdom Small Aneurysm Trial and the VA Cooperative Small Aneurysm study, demonstrated equivalent "all cause" mortality in patients with asymptomatic AAA between 4 and 5.5 cm, whether they were treated medically or surgically. Another study evaluated the role of endovascular treatment of small <5 cm AAAs and found that there was no advantage to the treatment of these small aneurysms compared to observation. This would indicate that men may be followed if their AAAs are asymptomatic and <5.0 to 5.5 cm. In contrast to this recommendation, women have a fourfold increased risk of rupture in aneurysms >5 cm. A >5 cm aneurysm represents a proportionately greater enlargement due to the smaller initial size of the female aorta. It is generally recommended that "good risk" women with AAA >4.5 cm be considered for repair.

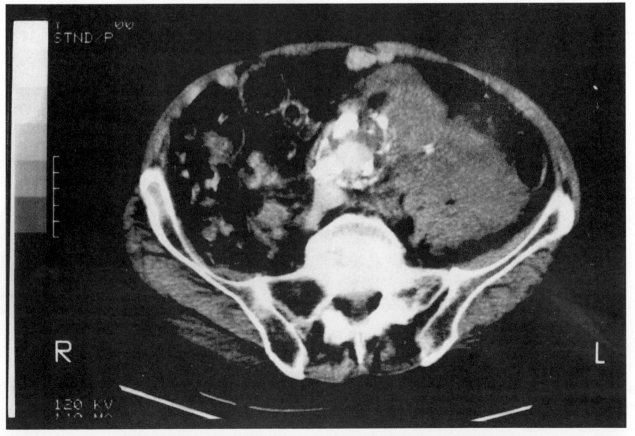

FIGURE 22-6. CT scan of a calcific AAA with a contained rupture into the left retroperitoneum.

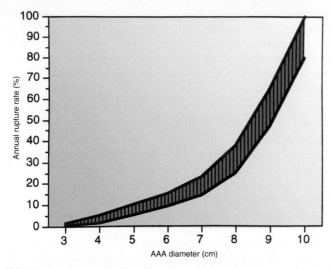

FIGURE 22-7. The annual risk of aneurysm rupture according to size. AAA, abdominal aortic artery. (Reprinted with permission from Sampson LN, Cronenwett JL. Abdominal aortic aneurysm. *Probl Gen Surg*. 1995;2:385–417.)

The elective open surgical treatment of AAAs is usually accomplished with a midline abdominal or left flank retroperitoneal incision. Advantages of the retroperitoneal incision are ease of access to the perirenal and suprarenal aorta and decreased postoperative pulmonary dysfunction. It is a particularly useful alternative approach for those patients that have a "hostile abdomen" secondary to previous intraperitoneal operations or inflammatory aneurysms. Disadvantages of the retroperitoneal approach include slightly more difficult access to the right iliac system and inability to evaluate the intraperitoneal contents.

During the operative approach, the normal infrarenal aorta and distal arteries are dissected and isolated. After heparinization, the aorta is clamped and the aneurysm incised. A prosthetic graft is sewn in place and covered with the residual aneurysm sac (Figure 22-8). Aneurysms that involve the more proximal (suprarenal) portions of the abdominal or thoracic aorta are technically more challenging, requiring suprarenal or supraceliac clamping and risk renal and intestinal ischemia, but good results are consistently reported in modern series. The operative mortality for elective repair of an infrarenal AAA is <3% to 5% in good-risk patients, but a thoracoabdominal aneurysm repair has a higher operative mortality.

The evolution of sophisticated catheter techniques and devices has led to the development of the endovascular graft as an alternative to traditional operative AAA repair. Endografts have now become the standard of care for many aneurysms. The procedure involves placing a bifurcated prosthetic graft with wire supports that attach to the uninvolved aorta

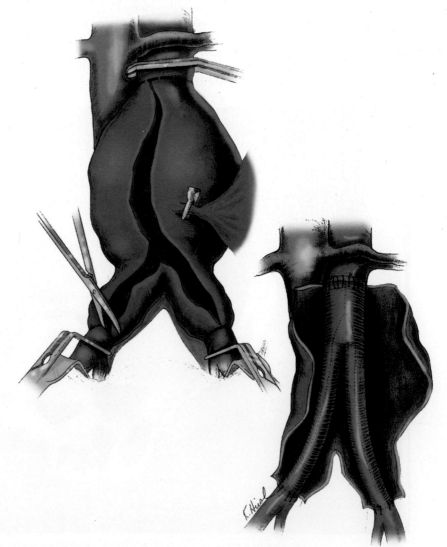

FIGURE 22-8. Repair of an AAA and a bilateral iliac artery aneurysm with an aortoiliac bypass graft. (Reprinted with permission from Zarins CK, Gewertz BL. Aneurysms. In: *Atlas of Vascular Surgery*. New York, NY: Churchill Livingstone, 1989:51.)

above the aneurysm and to the iliac vessels distal to the aneurysm. The graft is initially loaded into a delivery catheter and introduced from a remote access site in the femoral artery into the infrarenal aorta and iliac arteries (Figure 22-9). The attachment to the aorta and the iliac vessels is accomplished through outward radial force of self-expanding stents or hooks that embed in the aortic wall. Endovascular repair of AAAs has been shown to be associated with decreased perioperative mortality, decreased blood loss, a shortened hospital stay, and a more rapid return to normal activity. Recent studies have also shown decreased short-term mortality with endovascular repair (~ 1.5%) compared to conventional open aortic repair (~ 3%). Endografts with branches to the renal and mesenteric arteries are increasingly being used and have significantly reduced the procedural mortality.

The disadvantages of endovascular repair include the need for regular follow-up requiring annual abdominal ultrasound or CT scans, an increased rate of secondary interventions to correct problems with the fixation of the aortic graft, leakage of blood into the aortic aneurysm sac, and the risk of renal dysfunction secondary to the contrast agents used for visualization of the graft.

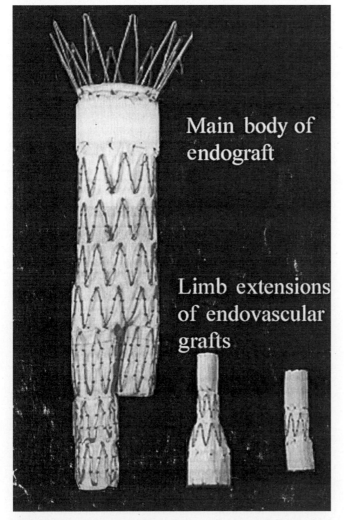

FIGURE 22-9. Example of an endovascular aortic stent graft (Zenith; Cook, Inc., Bloomingdale, Indiana.) There is a main body of the graft that is implanted in the aorta just below the renal arteries and then limb extensions that are intussuscepted into the gates for extension into the iliac arteries. The diameter of the distal aspect of the extension limbs comes in multiple sizes to allow for treatment of different-sized iliac arteries.

Patients who have rupture of an aneurysm will succumb unless they are immediately treated. Those patients with the classic triad of back pain, hypotension, and a pulsatile abdominal mass should be taken to the operating room immediately for repair. These patients should be judiciously resuscitated with fluid and blood products while being prepared for operation. Current practice is a technique of "permissive hypotension" with a restriction of volume resuscitation such that the blood pressure is titrated to maintain a systolic blood pressure between 70 and 80 mm Hg with monitoring of mental status and organ perfusion. This technique strives to minimize ongoing blood loss through the aortic defect. Despite advances in surgical critical care, the 30-day mortality of open ruptured aneurysm repair remains as high as 40% to 70%. Many survivors have major complications, including renal dysfunction, MI, and cerebrovascular accident. Endografts are being increasingly used to repair ruptured AAAs with improved results (reduction in mortality to 20% to 30%), especially in those centers that perform a large number of elective AAA endografts.

Complications of Aortic Aneurysm Repair

Immediate complications after elective repair of aortic aneurysms include MI, renal failure, colonic ischemia, distal emboli, and hemorrhage. Long-term complications include aortic graft infection, **aortoenteric fistula**, and graft thrombosis. Gradual disruption of the proximal or distal anastomotic suture lines, unassociated with infection, may cause anastomotic pseudoaneurysms to form.

After aortic repair, colonic ischemia can result from the disruption of pelvic arterial collateral flow, ligation of the inferior mesenteric artery, or perioperative hypotension. The patient with postoperative colonic ischemia usually presents with colonic emptying, occult blood diarrhea, or abdominal pain. Patients who experience diarrhea immediately postoperatively, with or without blood, should undergo sigmoidoscopy to further evaluate the sigmoid colon and rectum. If the colon is frankly infarcted, the affected colonic portion should be resected and a colostomy performed. If the colon inner lumen appears ischemic but without frank necrosis, the patient is treated with blood pressure support and broad-spectrum antibiotics. Frequent repeat sigmoidoscopy is used to assure that the ischemia has not progressed to frank necrosis. As with all complications, prevention is far more desirable than treatment after the fact. Colonic ischemia can be prevented by reimplanting a patent inferior mesenteric artery into the prosthetic graft in patients anatomically predisposed to poor colonic blood flow.

Graft infection following open repair and prosthetic graft replacement is a devastating complication with a mortality exceeding 50%. Any patient with a history of aortic graft implantation presenting with sepsis should be urgently evaluated by blood cultures, indium-111–labeled WBC scanning, and most definitively by CT scanning to search for perigraft fluid. Treatment consists of graft removal and extra-anatomic bypass in clean fields to restore pelvic and lower extremity perfusion. Other treatment options include systemic antibiotics, in situ prosthetic graft replacement, or autogenous replacement.

Aortoenteric fistula is another serious late complication of AAA replacement with prosthetic grafts. This complication most commonly presents with sudden upper gastrointestinal

(GI) bleeding ("herald bleed"), which may be limited in quantity initially. CT scans or bleeding scans are often inconclusive. The best diagnostic procedure is direct evaluation with upper endoscopy, using an orally placed colonoscope. Since communication generally occurs between the third portion of the duodenum and the proximal aortograft anastomosis, it is important that the endoscopist fully evaluate the entire duodenum. Endoscopic findings can vary from an irregular erythematous region in the third portion of the duodenum to the observation of the aortic graft through the duodenal wall.

Prompt surgery is the procedure of choice. Because there continues to be a controversy among vascular surgeons as to the precise etiology of this complication, the specific findings at surgery and the surgeon's experience strongly influence treatment. Treatment generally entails duodenal repair, graft removal, and extra-anatomic bypass or, in select patients, simple repair of the duodenum and in situ aortic graft replacement with a nonprosthetic graft such as cryopreserved aorta.

Endoleak is a complication associated with the endovascular repair of aortic and iliac aneurysms. An endoleak represents leakage of blood into the aneurysm sac. Endoleaks are classified as types I to IV. A type I endoleak represents a leak at either the proximal or distal attachment site. This is associated with a high rate of expansion and rupture, and should be repaired with either placement of an additional stent graft or replacement of the endovascular graft with an open repair. A type II endoleak represents persistent flow into and out of the aneurysm sac from lumbar or inferior mesenteric arteries. Generally, type II endoleaks are not treated unless there is expansion of the aneurysm sac or symptoms. Type III endoleaks occur from a modular disconnection between components of the stent graft or a tear in the fabric of the graft. They should be repaired when identified. A type IV endoleak is due to diffusion of blood and serum through the graft and generally will resolve once anticoagulation is reversed at the conclusion of the surgical procedure.

Peripheral Aneurysms

Popliteal artery aneurysms classically cause either distal emboli or thrombosis. Such distal emboli may cause "blue toe syndrome," in which a mural thrombus embolizes to the digital vessels of the foot, resulting in localized thrombosis and gangrene. Complete thrombosis of a popliteal artery aneurysm has a poor prognosis and a 50% amputation rate. The morbidity rate is high because a popliteal artery aneurysm generally thromboses only after it has showered multiple emboli to the lower extremity, thrombosing the outflow vessels. This sequence has prompted the initial use of thrombolytic therapy to lyse the obstructed outflow vessels before arterial reconstruction. Popliteal aneurysms should be considered for repair if they exceed 2 cm in diameter or if there is evidence of thrombus formation in the aneurysm or distal embolization. Preoperative angiography (computed tomographic angiography (CTA) or magnetic resonance arteriography [MRA]) is essential for planning the reconstruction and/or delivery of thrombolytic (clot dissolving) therapy to recanalize thrombosed distal vessels.

Popliteal aneurysm repair can be accomplished with either open surgery or a covered stent graft. The preferred surgical conduit is saphenous vein graft, because of its superior patency record for below-the-knee (BKA) revascularization. Popliteal aneurysms that have recently been treated with covered stent grafts, especially in high-risk patients or in patients whose popliteal aneurysm only involves the region of the popliteal artery proximal to the knee joint, have demonstrated comparable results to open repair.

Femoral artery aneurysms are less morbid than popliteal aneurysms as they embolize and thrombose less frequently. Treatment is by interposition bypass grafting.

AORTIC DISSECTION

Aortic dissection is one of the most common aortic diseases; it results from a tear in the intima into the media of the aortic wall. This tear is a result of weakening in the wall due to trauma from hypertension, structural changes from atherosclerosis, or other diseases such as Marfan's and Ehler-Danlos syndromes that predispose to medial degeneration and disruption. Once the tear in the aortic wall is created, the dissection can extend (or "propagate") proximally or distally as a pulsatile blood column traveling through the media of the thoracic and abdominal aorta in the "false" lumen. This creates a "double-barreled" aorta with the false lumen often occupying 50% or more of the aortic circumference. In some cases, the origins of critical arterial branches can be compromised with ischemia of the spinal cord, intestines, or kidneys. This occurrence complicates repair in that preservation of flow must be maintained to these critical branches while the flow to the false lumen is corrected. Dissections classically begin in the thoracic aorta and are classified as A or B by their site of origin. Stanford Type A dissections involve the ascending thoracic aorta and may or may not extend into the descending thoracic aorta, while Stanford Type B begin in the descending aorta distal to the left subclavian artery and often extend into the abdominal aorta.

Most dissections present with severe acute chest pain described as "tearing." The pain is differentiated from other cardiac problems by pain location, radiation, severity of pain, and timing. Complications from an ascending aortic dissection relate to retrograde or antegrade propagation of the dissection. With retrograde dissection toward the aortic valve, the origins of the coronary arteries can be obstructed, resulting in acute myocardial ischemia. The dissection can also extend into the aortic valve leaflets and result in acute aortic valve insufficiency. The most devastating complication is proximal extension of the dissection into the aortic root and free rupture into the pericardial sac causing cardiac tamponade. Dissection can also extend into the brachiocephalic vessels and cause stroke. The diagnosis of an aortic dissection is confirmed by transesophageal echocardiography, CT scan, or angiography.

Type A dissections are usually managed by emergent surgery. In contrast, many Type B dissections are treated successfully by lowering blood pressure and heart rate and decreasing the velocity of left ventricular contraction (dp/dt) to reduce the stress on the arterial wall. Surgery or aortic stent grafting for Type B dissection is indicated for those dissections that compromise flow in the mesenteric, renal, or iliac arteries producing ischemia of the respective organs. Surgery is also indicated for Type B lesions that form large enough aneurysms that threaten to rupture. Indeed, enlargement of a chronic dissection with aneurysm formation is the main indication for elective repair.

PERIPHERAL ARTERIAL OCCLUSIVE DISEASE

Peripheral arterial disease (PAD) is characterized by occlusions or stenoses (partial occlusions) of the arteries of the lower extremities. Specific symptoms are dictated by the number and severity of occlusions, the degree of collateralization, and the patient's tolerance to limitations in walking distance.

Stenosis or occlusion of the aorta and iliac arteries (aortoiliac occlusive disease) is more common in adults between 45 and 65 years of age. The predilection to aortoiliac disease is increased by cigarette smoking, hypertension, and hyperlipidemia. Disease confined below the inguinal ligament is known as femoropopliteal occlusive disease. The most common site of disease is the distal superficial femoral artery (SFA) within the adductor (Hunter's) canal. Femoropopliteal occlusive disease may be asymptomatic unless a patient participates in extensive exercise, since collateral blood flow from the profunda femoris artery can usually provide sufficient foot and calf blood flow at rest. Involvement of the arteries below the popliteal trifurcation is called tibial occlusive disease. Tibial occlusive disease is common in patients with diabetes, end-stage renal failure, and advanced age.

Physiology

Large atherosclerotic plaques occlude the arterial lumen, impede blood flow, and diminish blood pressure distal to the stenosis. The loss of pressure due to reduction in a vessel's diameter is described by Poiseuille's law. While it was originally formulated for a cell-free "Newtonian" liquid and not a cellular fluid like blood in a pulsatile system, it does provide a reasonable description of the flow dynamics:

$$\Delta P = 8QL\eta/\pi r^4$$

where ΔP, change in pressure; Q, volume of blood flow; L, arterial length; η, density; and r, arterial radius.

The loss in pressure is directly proportional to the volume of blood flow and the arterial length but inversely proportional to the fourth power of the radius. Hence, a decrease in radius has the most profound effect on ΔP. In general, ΔP is small until the reduction in diameter or "stenosis" is reduced by 50% in diameter or 75% in cross-sectional area (Figure 22-10); at that point, pressure and flow past the point of narrowing decrease exponentially with greater narrowing.

Enlargement of an atherosclerotic plaque is the leading cause of development of symptoms of peripheral vascular arterial occlusive disease. Studies have shown that as a plaque grows, the vessel initially adapts and enlarges its overall diameter. Once maximal enlargement is attained, this compensation is exhausted, and the luminal area is progressively decreased by the atherosclerotic process (Figure 22-11). Other less common causes of arterial occlusive disease include Buerger's disease (thromboarteritis obliterans), cystic adventitial disease, and compression of arteries by aberrant muscular bands (e.g., popliteal artery entrapment syndrome and cervical rib).

Clinical Presentation

Ischemia of the lower extremity can progressively cause intermittent claudication, ischemic rest pain, skin ulceration, and gangrene. The degree of ischemia determines the presentation. Claudication, from the Latin *claudatio* (to limp), is characterized by reproducible pain in a major muscle group that is precipitated by exercise and relieved by rest. The joints

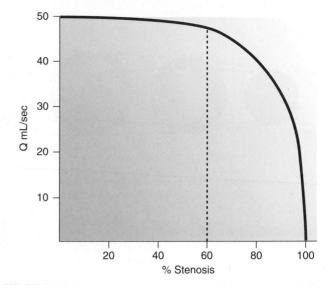

FIGURE 22-10. Relationship between degree of stenosis and flow. Focal accumulation of plaque occurs at sites of turbulence and reduced shear stress. When plaque forms, reduction in flow only occurs when 60% to 70% of the artery diameter is narrowed.

and foot are spared because they have little muscle mass. The mechanism is straightforward; these patients maintain adequate arterial perfusion at rest but their arterial occlusions prevent the augmentation of blood flow necessary to meet the metabolic demands of active muscles during exercise. The result is conversion to anaerobic metabolism and painful local metabolic acidosis. The muscle groups that are affected by claudication are always one level "downstream" from the level of arterial obstruction. Hence, aortoiliac occlusion classically causes Leriche syndrome, defined by impotence, lower extremity claudication, and muscle wasting of the buttocks. Occlusion of the SFA causes calf, but not thigh, claudication since the thigh blood supply comes from the profunda femoris artery.

The natural history of untreated claudication is generally benign. In one landmark population study (Framingham), the risk of major amputation was only 5% within 5 years if claudication was treated conservatively. With cessation of cigarette smoking and an organized exercise program, as many as 50% of patients with claudication improved or completely resolved their symptoms. The most common cause of death in patients with claudication is the systemic manifestation of atherosclerosis, such as cardiac or cerebral events.

Ischemic rest pain indicates more advanced peripheral ischemia. Most commonly, patients have pain in the toes and metatarsal heads while lying down at night. Temporary relief is achieved by dangling the legs over the side of the bed or walking. By making the feet more dependent, gravitational hydrostatic pressure increases arterial pressure and temporarily enhances oxygen delivery. Rest pain is caused by nerve ischemia of tissues that are most sensitive to hypoxia. Nocturnal cramps in the calf muscle are unassociated with impairment of blood flow and can be distinguished from true rest pain by the location of the pain (calf vs. distal foot) and the absence of advanced ischemic changes in the skin.

Ulceration of the skin of the toes, heel, or dorsum of the foot can occur as a result of arterial insufficiency. Even minor trauma such as friction from an ill-fitting shoe, poor nail care, or a small break in the skin can lead to progressive ulceration in the setting of insufficient arterial flow. Ulcers due to

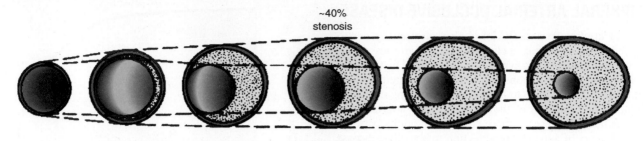

~40%
stenosis

FIGURE 22-11. Proposed arterial adaptation to enlarging atherosclerotic plaques. Initially, the artery enlarges to maintain the luminal diameter despite the enlarging plaque. After the plaques create a stenosis of more than 40%, the artery can no longer adapt, and a luminal stenosis develops. (Reprinted with permission from Glagov S, Weisenberg E, Zarins CK, et al. Compensatory enlargement of human atherosclerotic coronary arteries. *N Engl J Med*. 1987;316:1371.)

arterial insufficiency are usually painful, except in patients with diabetes who often have associated peripheral neuropathy. Ischemic ulcers may have a punched-out appearance and a pale or necrotic base. By comparison, ulcerations due to venous insufficiency usually occur at the level of the medial or lateral malleolus ("gaiter zone").

Diabetic ulcerations are painless and are located on the plantar or lateral aspect of the foot, in areas of pressure. They are a direct result of the neuropathy of diabetes. Because of the injury to the autonomic, motor, and sensory nerves, the skin becomes dry and the foot can become deformed (Charcot's foot) and insensate. The changes associated with diabetes are worsened by the arterial occlusive process that often accompanies diabetes.

The outlook for patients with rest pain or ulceration is far worse than that for patients with claudication. If untreated, nearly 50% of patients with rest pain come to amputation for intractable pain or gangrene within a short period. Dry and wet gangrene are differentiated clinically. Dry gangrene is mummification of the digits of the foot without associated purulent drainage or cellulitis. Wet gangrene is associated with ongoing infection. The severely ischemic foot is a nidus for the colonization and growth of bacteria, and is generally malodorous with copious purulent drainage. The outlook is ominous with likely sepsis and immediate limb loss unless the necrotic tissue is removed and the limb is revascularized. The most common cause of a major limb amputation is diabetes, and a diabetic with a limb amputation has a 2-year survival rate of 50%.

Evaluation

Routine evaluation of patients with peripheral arterial disease includes a thorough physical examination and noninvasive vascular testing. A search for coexisting cardiovascular disease is mandatory. Inspection of the legs and feet may show loss of hair on the distal aspect of the leg, muscle atrophy, color changes in the leg, and ulcers or gangrene. Patients with severe PAD often have Buerger's sign (dependent rubor). When the foot is dangled, pooling of oxygenated blood in the maximally dilated arteriolar bed distal to an arterial occlusion causes the foot to appear ruborous (red). When the extremity is elevated, hydrostatic pressure decreases, pooled blood drains, and the foot becomes white (pallor).

Intermittent claudication can be differentiated from musculoskeletal or neurogenic pain by a careful history, physical examination, and noninvasive vascular evaluation. Neurogenic lower extremity pain is usually not located in major muscle groups and is rarely precipitated by exercise. Straightleg raised

lifts and findings of sensory examinations may be abnormal. Musculoskeletal pain is often present at rest. Pain secondary to spinal stenosis is relieved by bending forward while walking. It often radiates down the limb and is not relieved immediately by resting.

Physical examination should include investigation of the presence and character of the arterial pulse in the groin (femoral artery), in the popliteal fossa (popliteal artery), in the dorsum of the foot (dorsalis pedis artery), and posterior to the medial malleolus (posterior tibial artery). All pulses should be confirmed by Doppler ultrasound.

Patients with extremity ischemia should be examined with continuous-wave Doppler ultrasound (Figure 22-12). The Doppler probe emits 2- to 10-MHz ultrasonic waves that are reflected by flowing red blood cells and detected by a receiving crystal. The frequency shift between the transmitting and the receiving crystals is proportional to the velocity of the moving particles and provides a qualitative assessment of the degree of stenosis. Normally, a triphasic waveform is seen, representing the forward flow of systole, reversal of the arterial velocity waveform against the relatively high-resistance vascular bed, and resumption of forward flow during diastole. If proximal stenosis is present, the pulse volume from cardiac contraction loses kinetic energy crossing the area of stenosis and does not have enough energy to recoil against the vascular outflow bed. As a result, the Doppler signal becomes biphasic. With further progression of proximal arterial stenosis, the

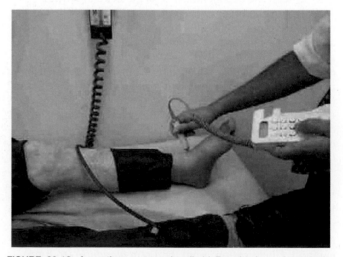

FIGURE 22-12. A continuous wave handheld Doppler is an inexpensive instrument that can be used at the bedside to both grade the quality of arterial signals and measure ankle or arm arterial pressures.

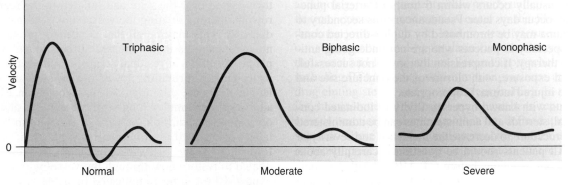

FIGURE 22-13. A Doppler ultrasound instrument provides an analog display of blood flow velocity (waveform). With progressive occlusion, the waveform changes from triphasic to biphasic to monophasic.

waveform becomes widened and it eventually becomes monophasic (Figure 22-13).

In addition to this qualitative assessment of disease, the systolic pressure within the arteries of the foot can be determined. A blood pressure cuff is inflated in the calf and then slowly deflated while the Doppler signal is monitored. The pressure at which a signal "reappears" is the systolic pressure within the artery. The pressure is normalized for all patients by dividing the ankle pressure by the systolic blood pressure in the arm and calculating the **ankle-brachial index** (ABI). In general, an ABI > 0.9 is normal, an ABI <0.8 is consistent with claudication, whereas an ABI <0.4 is usually associated with rest pain or tissue loss. If the clinical assessment is confusing, patients should be observed while walking on a treadmill. Claudicators will drop their ABI when symptoms occur while patients with other causes of leg pain will not show any change in pressure measurements.

Advances in ultrasound technology have led to anatomic correlation using arterial duplex scanning. Duplex scanners provide visualization of blood flow within the artery in two dimensions and can also calculate the velocity of flowing blood. In regions of significant stenosis, high-velocity jets are seen as blood travels through the narrow lumen.

Diagnostic Imaging in Vascular Disorders

Patients with severe lifestyle-limiting claudication, rest pain, or gangrene should undergo diagnostic MRA or CTA. Contrast arteriography, performed with a percutaneous femoral artery puncture, is used when diagnosis is combined with a planned therapeutic procedure.

MR angiography and CTA do not require puncture of an artery and therefore do not have puncture site complications. In these studies, the dye is injected into a central vein, and timing of the images is critical to obtain quality studies. The risk of contrast complications still exists, though small. Gadolinium (MRA contrast agent) may rarely cause subcutaneous fibrosis in patients with renal failure, and most CTA contrast agents may exacerbate renal insufficiency. Lower doses of all agents are reducing the risk of these complications.

Angiography involves puncture of a peripheral artery, with passage of an intravascular catheter for selective injection of arteries (Seldinger technique) (Figure 22-14). A needle and then a guide wire are percutaneously inserted into the femoral artery and advanced into the aorta under x-ray guidance. A catheter is then inserted over the wire into the aorta. After removal of the wire, a liquid contrast agent is injected into the catheter. This contrast mixes with the blood and is radiopaque. Wherever blood travels, so does the contrast, and regions of enlargement (aneurysms) or narrowing (stenosis) are visualized. When the catheter is removed the puncture site is either compressed manually or closed with a permanent or absorbable mechanical device.

The principal complications of angiography include bleeding or thrombosis at the puncture site caused by the insertion of the catheter, formation of a pseudoaneurysm at the puncture site, hypersensitivity reaction to the iodinated dye, and contrast-related renal toxicity. The latter complication is most common in diabetic patients. Bleeding may be immediate or delayed and may lead to a pseudoaneurysm later. The initial presentation of local bleeding often includes paresthesias in the involved limb because of compression of adjacent nerves.

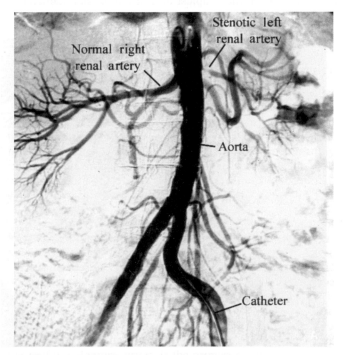

FIGURE 22-14. Example of an angiogram of the abdominal aorta. A proximal left renal artery stenosis is visualized.

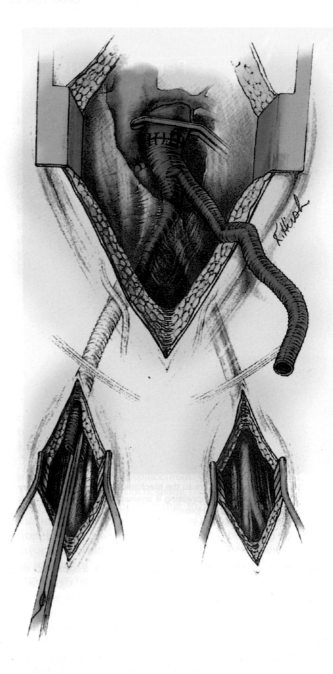

FIGURE 22-17. Aortobifemoral bypass graft showing the creation of the retroperitoneal tunnels to the groins. (Reprinted with permission from Zarins CK, Gewertz BL. Aneurysms. In: *Atlas of Vascular Surgery*. New York, NY: Churchill Livingstone, 1989:125.)

patency rate of >90%. When aortofemoral bypass graft limb occlusion occurs, it is usually caused by the progression of distal outflow disease, which limits blood flow through the graft.

If the patient has an occluded aorta and is a prohibitive surgical risk for an intra-abdominal procedure or has had multiple intra-abdominal procedures or infections ("hostile" abdomen), extra-anatomic bypasses are considered. Extra-anatomic bypasses include axillary artery-to-femoral artery bypass grafts and femoral artery to femoral artery bypass grafts. These grafts typically use prosthetic conduits tunneled from one artery to the other in the subcutaneous tissue. In critically ill patients, this procedure actually may be performed with local anesthesia and intravenous sedation. The patency rates for extra-anatomic bypasses are lower than those for aortofemoral bypass grafts, but still acceptable. Occlusions typically occur due to neointimal hyperplasia at the anastomoses or due to progression of distal disease, but can also occur secondary to the longer length of the bypass graft and/or

graft compression or kinking within the subcutaneous tunnels. Systemic anticoagulation is often used to improve patency.

In patients with ischemic rest pain and occluded superficial femoral arteries with proximal profunda femoral artery stenoses, opening the stenoses by profundaplasty combined with femoral endarterectomy can increase lower leg perfusion through collaterals and relieve most symptoms. However, if the ischemia has progressed to tissue loss or gangrene, it is unlikely that profundaplasty alone can adequately increase arterial inflow into the leg to heal the ulcerative lesions. In this case, arterial bypass must be performed.

Patients who have infrainguinal occlusive disease can often be treated with bypass of the occluded segment. Bypass to the popliteal artery above the knee is performed with either the patient's own (autologous) vein or a prosthetic graft; both have comparable initial results. In contrast, prosthetic bypasses to arteries below the knee function more poorly. These distal bypass procedures are best accomplished with autologous vein (Table 22-3). Saphenous vein bypass grafts are harvested

TABLE 22-3	Outcomes of Infrainguinal Arterial Bypasses	
Graft Type	2-yr Patency (%) Primary/Secondary	4-yr Patency (%) Primary/Secondary
Above-knee femoropopliteal, PTFE	75	60
Above-knee femoropopliteal, vein	80	70
Below-knee femoropopliteal, PTFE	60	40
Below-knee femoropopliteal, vein	75–80/90	70–75/80
Femoral-tibial bypass, PTFE	30	20
Femoral-tibial bypass, vein	70–75/80–90	60–70/75–80

PTFE, polytetrafluoroethylene.

and either reversed so that the venous valves are in the same direction as arterial flow, or alternatively, in situ bypasses can be performed in which the saphenous vein is left in its normal anatomic position and the vein valves are disrupted with a valvulotome. This approach allows a better size match between the artery and the vein and can often be performed with minimal incisions. Disadvantages of in situ bypass include endothelial injury during passage of the valvulotome and the possibility of missing a valve cusp (retained valve).

In situations where ipsilateral saphenous vein is not available, alternative conduit must be used. Contralateral saphenous may be used if available but caution must be taken to consider the circulation in the other leg and the potential need for its own bypass. Upper extremity veins can also be a valuable source of conduit. Cephalic and basilic veins can often be harvested and combined to create a composite graft long enough to accomplish a leg bypass. If no adequate venous conduit is available, prosthetic bypass to the tibial level can still be used. Outcomes can be improved with the use of a vein patch or cuff at the distal anastomosis in an effort to improve the hemodynamics of this critical connection. Bypass grafts to the vessels in the foot are now routinely used for limb salvage.

Postoperative duplex ultrasound surveillance of vein bypass grafts is useful in identifying anastomotic and midgraft stenoses that, if uncorrected, could lead to graft failure. The combination of duplex graft surveillance and either balloon angioplasty or surgical repair of stenotic lesions results in higher long-term patency of the saphenous vein bypass graft. The "assisted" patency rates of these vein grafts approach 90% at 2 years post-bypass. In contrast, if a stenosis of a saphenous vein graft is allowed to progress to occlusion before it is revised, the patency rate at 2 years is only 30%.

Immediate complications of arterial bypass graft procedures include postoperative bleeding from the anastomotic sites, graft thrombosis, wound infection, and lymphatic leakage that results in a lymphocele (lymphatic fluid collection). Because many patients with peripheral arterial occlusive disease have concomitant coronary artery disease, renal insufficiency, or pulmonary obstructive disease, other serious postoperative cardiopulmonary complications are always a concern in the postoperative period.

In summary, lower extremity revascularization must be individualized to each patient. Claudication can be adequately treated by risk factor modification, especially smoking cessation and structured exercise. Interventions in this setting should be justified by advanced, debilitating symptoms that

restrict daily activities or threaten an individual's livelihood. A percutaneous approach for intervention using any of the techniques described may be the most appropriate first line of treatment in this setting, reserving more invasive approaches for more advanced disease. For limb-threatening disease such as rest pain, tissue loss, or gangrene, a bypass is often the best option. Interventional techniques in this setting should be used for high surgical risk patients. In either case, the best long-term results require the appropriate use of antiplatelet or anticoagulant therapy, ideal medical management of other risk factors, and vigilant surveillance with reintervention if needed.

Amputation may be the only option in some patients with severe rest pain or gangrene who are not candidates for revascularization. In general, the more distal the amputation is, the better the rehabilitation potential. Distal amputations include toe, transmetatarsal, and Syme's (ankle) amputations. If arterial inflow is inadequate and an arterial bypass cannot be performed, then a BKA or above-the-knee (AKA) amputation may be required.

It is important to choose the appropriate site for amputation to ensure adequate wound healing. A BKA is often the lowest level that will heal; it is important to attempt to preserve the knee joint, because significantly more energy is required to ambulate with an AKA prosthesis.

AKA is required when profound ischemia and gangrene extend to the knee. At this higher amputation level, healing is likely, even in advanced ischemia. AKA amputation is also indicated in patients who are bedridden or represent a high surgical risk because of other medical conditions.

CHRONIC INTESTINAL ISCHEMIA

The visceral arterial supply includes the celiac axis, superior mesenteric artery (SMA), and inferior mesenteric artery. If one of these visceral vessels becomes stenotic or occluded, the other two vessels, through the gastroduodenal artery and marginal artery can supply significant collateral flow (Figure 22-18). If the gastroduodenal artery is not well developed or there is occlusion of two of the three major arterial pathways to the visceral organs, patients may experience visceral ischemic symptoms. Once two vessels are occluded, symptoms become very common.

The clinical manifestations of chronic intestinal ischemia include postprandial abdominal pain and weight loss.

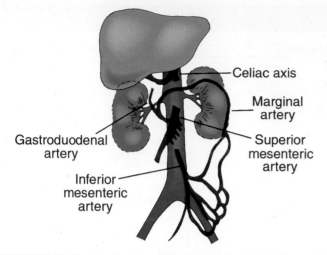

FIGURE 22-18. The intestinal circulation is characterized by three main vessels: the celiac axis, SMA, and inferior mesenteric artery. Collaterals connect these vessels so that chronic occlusion of one vessel is well compensated.

Postprandial pain usually occurs within an hour after meals and ranges from a persistent epigastric ache to severe, disabling, cramping pain. Many patients have a fear of food because of the intimidation of postprandial pain and limit their oral intake. This factor accounts for the significant weight loss seen in many patients. The malnutrition associated with chronic visceral ischemia can be severe and frequently is mistaken for carcinomatosis or primary visceral malignancies. Associated symptoms of systemic atherosclerotic disease are often present (e.g., coronary artery disease, claudication, cerebrovascular accident).

The diagnosis is based on an accurate history and physical examination as well as duplex ultrasound studies, CTA, and mesenteric angiography of the visceral vessels. Noninvasive duplex scans assess the flow within the visceral vessels as well as the presence of a proximal arterial stenosis. The limitation of the duplex scan is its inability to evaluate the visceral vessels if a significant amount of bowel gas is present or if there is significant calcification in the visceral vessels. Therefore, CT or MR angiograms are the best diagnostic study. They are used to show hemodynamically significant lesions of at least two of the three major visceral vessels and evidence of collateral flow circumventing the stenotic mesenteric vessel. Catheter angiograms are only used for interventions.

Treatment

Mesenteric revascularization usually provides symptomatic improvement and prevents catastrophic mesenteric infarction. Mesenteric revascularization should be considered in patients who have symptoms consistent with mesenteric ischemia as well as angiographic evidence of significant visceral occlusive disease.

Proximal mesenteric artery balloon angioplasty and stenting is being used much more frequently in treatment of chronic mesenteric ischemia, for both thrombotic occlusions and preocclusive stenoses. While the long-term durability of angioplasty/stenting is not quite as good as surgical bypass (approximately 70% PTA vs. 90% surgical over 3 years), the immediate morbidity is much less, favoring the use of these techniques in older and nutritionally depleted patients.

Surgical revascularization options include endarterectomy of the proximal visceral vessels or bypass with synthetic

grafts. Autogenous vein is only used when infection is a significant risk. Many experienced surgeons routinely revascularize at least two of the visceral vessels to maximize the durability of the repair. Bypass routes are either retrograde or antegrade bypass to the SMA and celiac axis. The antegrade bypass from the supraceliac aorta is preferable due to the direct course of the bypass graft and a decreased risk of kinking, but this procedure is more stressful due to the need to temporarily occlude the aorta above the celiac artery. Retrograde bypasses can originate from either the infrarenal aorta or an iliac artery but are more prone to kink when the mesentery is returned to its normal position.

RENOVASCULAR HYPERTENSION

Renovascular hypertension accounts for approximately 5% of the cause of hypertension, but this disease is responsible for a disproportionately high proportion of curable hypertension, especially in children and young adults. Atherosclerosis is the most common cause of renal artery stenosis, but occurs in older patients. **Fibromuscular dysplasia** and posttraumatic dissections are less common causes but are, in fact, more amenable to treatment. Although most patients with renal artery stenoses are asymptomatic, these obstructive lesions may be associated with poorly controlled blood pressure (renovascular hypertension) or renal insufficiency (ischemic nephropathy). Other causes of surgically correctable hypertension include pheochromocytoma, aldosterone-secreting tumors, and descending thoracic aortic coarctation.

Atherosclerotic renal artery lesions usually occur in the proximal portion of the renal artery and often represent an extension of an aortic plaque into the renal artery ostium. In contrast, fibromuscular dysplasia most commonly involves the middle to distal portion of the renal artery, with sparing of the proximal aspect of the renal artery (Figure 22-19). Fibromuscular dysplasia is a hyperplastic, fibrosing process of the intima, media, or adventitia. It occurs in children (equal sex

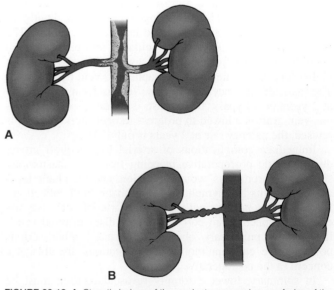

FIGURE 22-19. A, Stenotic lesions of the renal artery cause hypoperfusion of the kidney and activation of the renin–angiotensin system. As a result, significant hypertension occurs. Atherosclerotic lesions usually involve the origin to the middle portion of the renal artery. B, Fibromuscular hyperplasia involves the middle to distal portion of the renal artery.

distribution) or in the second to fourth decade (more common in women). Bilateral involvement is seen in as many as 50% of cases.

Critical stenosis of the renal artery causes decreased blood pressure and flow to the kidney as well as decreased glomerular filtration. This change stimulates the renal juxtaglomerular apparatus to produce renin, which catalyzes the conversion of angiotensinogen to angiotensin I. Angiotensin-converting enzyme then converts angiotensin I to angiotensin II, a potent vasoconstrictor. Angiotensin II also stimulates the production of aldosterone, causing sodium retention and increased plasma volume. This combination of vasoconstriction and sodium retention causes a hypertensive state. With progression of bilateral renal artery stenoses, patients may have inadequate blood flow to support renal function and may develop ischemic nephropathy.

Most untreated patients have profound diastolic hypertension with diastolic pressures occasionally exceeding 120 mm Hg. An epigastric or flank bruit may be noted on auscultation of the abdomen and suggests turbulent flow within the renal artery.

Renal artery stenosis should be suspected with the onset of hypertension in patients younger than 35, worsening of previously well-controlled blood pressure, uncontrolled hypertension despite three or more antihypertensive medications, flash pulmonary edema, or severe hypertension with a rapid decline in renal function. For patients with suspected renal artery stenosis, screening studies include renal duplex scan, renal function studies, and CT or MR angiography.

Renal duplex ultrasonography can assess the flow velocity profile in both renal arteries as well as the juxtarenal aorta. A significant difference in renal artery velocities (renal artery:aorta ratio > 3.5) suggests the presence of a hemodynamically significant renal artery stenosis. The duplex scan can also determine renal parenchymal size and assess whether one of the kidneys is atrophying as a result of ischemia. With an experienced technologist, the sensitivity and specificity of renal artery duplex ultrasonography for detecting significant renal artery stenosis is >90%.

A functional test for renovascular hypertension is the captopril challenge test. Captopril, an angiotensin II–converting enzyme inhibitor, prevents the conversion of angiotensin I to angiotensin II. Because of the blockage of synthesis of angiotensin II, more renin is produced and plasma renin levels are elevated after captopril administration. A positive captopril test also leads to a decrease in the glomerular filtration rate because of the blockage of the effect of angiotensin II on the efferent arteriole of the renal glomeruli. Without the vasoconstriction of the efferent renal arteriolar bed, there is decreased outflow resistance and less of a pressure gradient to allow for renal filtration.

CT or MR angiography can reliably detect renal artery stenosis. Unfortunately, CT scan is associated with the use of potentially nephrotoxic intravenous contrast agents that can worsen renal function, and MR angiography does not identify calcium and may overestimate the severity of stenosis. Also, these studies are expensive for use as screening tools. Catheter renal arteriography not only detects renal artery stenoses but also assists in determining kidney size by evaluating the postinjection nephrogram. At the time of renal angiography, a pressure gradient can be measured using a pressure sensing wire or a small catheter that is attached to a pressure monitor and withdrawn across the region of suspected stenosis.

A greater than 10 mm Hg pressure gradient is consistent with a significant renal artery stenosis.

Treatment

In young patients with fibromuscular dysplasia, antihypertensive medications are often ineffective in controlling severe renovascular hypertension. For example, angiotensin II–converting enzyme inhibitors, usually very effective drugs for hypertension, should be avoided in cases of bilateral renal artery stenoses because these drugs decrease glomerular filtration by altering postglomerular capillary tone. In the worst circumstances, they may cause acute renal failure.

In patients with severe hypertension and hemodynamically significant renal artery stenoses, renal revascularization should be considered. Fibromuscular dysplasia responds exceptionally well to percutaneous transluminal balloon angioplasty without stenting in all age groups. Current experience with fibromuscular disease in pediatric patients and young adults suggests that more than 95% of patients are cured or significantly improved with renal artery angioplasty. Atherosclerotic lesions of the proximal renal artery are most frequently treated with both angioplasty and stenting, as angioplasty alone is associated with a high rate of restenosis. Unfortunately, few patients are cured of their hypertension after angioplasty/stenting for atherosclerotic renal artery stenosis, although a significant portion may have improved blood pressure control. The procedure may be complicated by worsening renal function from contrast nephrotoxicity or atheroembolism. Since the risk of surgical intervention for failure of endovascular treatment of renal artery stenosis is the same as for primary surgical procedures, many vascular specialists recommend angioplasty/stenting as the initial method of treatment for renal artery stenosis. Open surgical bypass is reserved for those patients that fail endovascular intervention. A recent study comparing revascularization to medical therapy suggested limiting revascularization to a very selective group of patients.

Surgical treatment for renal vascular hypertension is performed in patients who have recurrent stenosis after angioplasty. It is also performed when lesions are not correctable with angioplasty. Surgical interventions include endarterectomy of the atherosclerotic lesions and bypass to the renal artery from the aorta, iliac, hepatic, or splenic arteries.

ACUTE ARTERIAL OCCLUSION

Acute occlusion of an extremity or visceral vessel can cause limb, intestinal, or life-threatening ischemia. Etiologies of acute arterial occlusion include in situ thrombosis of preexisting atherosclerotic occlusive disease, arterial emboli from another site, penetrating and blunt trauma, and thrombosis of a preexisting arterial aneurysm. Patients with preexisting arterial occlusive disease may have a history of claudication or intestinal angina before arterial thrombosis occurs. These patients may already have a well-developed collateral bed and may therefore develop less acute symptoms. In contrast, patients with arterial emboli, vascular trauma, or thrombosis of a preexisting aneurysm are usually asymptomatic before the arterial occlusion occurs and may have more profound ischemic symptoms.

The classic presentation of limb-threatening acute arterial occlusion includes the "six Ps": *p*allor, *p*ain, *p*aresthesia, *p*aralysis, *p*ulselessness, and *p*oikilothermia (change in temperature). These changes are limited to the area distal to the region of acute arterial occlusion. For example, with femoral artery occlusion, the ischemic changes occur in the distal thigh, calf, or foot.

The great majority (80%) of arterial emboli originate in the left side of the heart. Thrombi form in the left atrium in patients with atrial fibrillation and in hypokinetic regions of previous MI. These thrombi can dislodge and embolize to the peripheral circulation. Nonthrombotic emboli can also occur from detached fragments of atherosclerotic lesions of the aorta and aortic valve. Mural thrombi within thoracic, abdominal aortic, and popliteal aneurysms can also cause distal embolization. The most common site of embolic occlusion is the femoral artery. Other common sites are the axillary, popliteal, and iliac arteries, the aortic bifurcation, and the mesenteric vessels.

Acute mesenteric ischemia results from arterial occlusion (embolus or thrombosis), mesenteric venous occlusion, or nonocclusive mesenteric ischemia (especially vasospasm). Embolization to the SMA accounts for approximately 50% of all cases of acute mesenteric ischemia; 25% of cases occur secondary to thrombosis of a preexisting atherosclerotic lesion. Most emboli to the SMA lodge just distal to the origin of the middle colic artery, approximately 5 to 10 cm from the origin of the SMA (Figure 22-20). Nonocclusive mesenteric ischemia accounts for an additional 25% of cases of acute mesenteric ischemia. The etiology of nonocclusive mesenteric ischemia is multifactorial, but usually involves moderate to severe mesenteric atherosclerotic lesions in association with a low cardiac output state or the administration of vasoconstricting medications, such as digitalis.

Acute mesenteric venous occlusion usually involves the superior mesenteric vein and its branches. It is an infrequent but life-threatening condition generally in patients with portal hypertension or hypercoagulability, and in elderly patients with a history of poor oral intake and dehydration. It presents as acute abdominal pain with early lab values pointing toward intestinal ischemia. Diagnosis is aided by CT scan with IV contrast, which shows the thrombus within the mesenteric veins, as well as thickened bowel wall.

Treatment

Treatment of acute mesenteric venous thrombosis is anticoagulation; prompt surgery with venous thrombectomy is only performed for an acute abdomen; if the bowel is viable, continued systemic anticoagulation with heparin and second look surgery within 24 hours to assess bowel viability is recommended.

Irrespective of the arterial bed involved, patients with acute arterial occlusion require rapid evaluation and diagnosis to prevent limb-, bowel-, or life-threatening ischemia. Anticoagulation with intravenous heparin is administered to prevent further propagation of the thrombus, but heparin does not lyse existing clot. Contraindications to anticoagulation include a history of GI bleeding, a new neurologic deficit, head injury, ongoing sites of active bleeding, and antibodies to heparin. Aggressive fluid resuscitation and correction of ongoing systemic acidosis should be performed. Patients who are in critical condition may require inotropic cardiac support. Interventions should not be significantly delayed to allow for correction of the acidosis because the ongoing ischemia is usually the primary contributor to the acid–base disturbance.

In cases of limb-threatening ischemia, immediate surgical thrombectomy or embolectomy is performed. Preoperative arteriography may be of benefit in patients who have a history of arterial occlusive disease to determine the sites of potential bypass. In contrast, in previously normal patients with sudden acute ischemia, arteriograms should be avoided and immediate surgical revascularization performed with the exploration based on the level at which pulses are absent.

The surgical approach is directed toward rapidly reperfusing the threatened extremity or organ. Reperfusion can be accomplished by embolectomy, endarterectomy, or surgical bypass. The results of revascularization are variable and depend on the extent of the occlusive disease and the duration of ischemia. In embolic occlusion, embolectomy is performed through peripheral vessels with specialized balloon-tipped catheters. Complete thrombectomy is performed both proximally and distally. Distal thrombectomy is essential because nearly one-third of patients with arterial occlusions have additional thrombus past the point of occlusion. Pathologic evaluation should be performed of all emboli, especially in the absence of atrial fibrillation, to ensure that the embolus is not of malignant origin.

After extremity or organ revascularization, the reperfused organ is examined to determine the extent of tissue damage and the potential for edema. If there is lengthy extremity ischemia (>4 hours), fasciotomy is often required to decompress the muscular compartments and prevent compression of the arteries, nerves, and veins (i.e., compartment syndrome).

Unfortunately, the mortality rate from acute arterial occlusion is relatively high. This high rate is related to the advanced age of the patient population as well as to comorbid factors such as severe myocardial disease. In the case of embolic arterial occlusion, postoperative long-term anticoagulation must be considered because one-third of patients have recurrent emboli within 30 days if not anticoagulated.

In patients who have acute arterial occlusion but present prior to profound ischemia, thrombolytic therapy should be

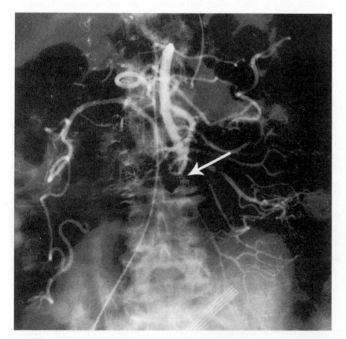

FIGURE 22-20. Acute embolus of the proximal SMA (*arrow*).

considered. The goal of thrombolysis is to reperfuse the limb or organ gradually, causing fewer systemic effects. It also spares the patient a surgical procedure with the attendant complications. This approach requires arterial cannulation of the area proximal to the area of occlusion and administration of a thrombolytic agent such as tPA. If therapy is unsuccessful or if there are signs of progressive critical ischemia, thrombolytic therapy is aborted and surgical revascularization is performed.

In any acute arterial occlusion involving the extremities, systemic ischemia-reperfusion syndrome may be expected. It is characterized by compartment syndrome, hyperkalemia, metabolic acidosis, myoglobinuria, and renal and pulmonary insufficiency. Vigorous hydration, alkalinization of the urine by IV route, and fascial decompression are all-important treatments in this setting.

CEREBROVASCULAR INSUFFICIENCY

Arterial cerebrovascular insufficiency can result from occlusive, ulcerative, or aneurysmal disease of the carotid or vertebral arteries. The most devastating complication of cerebrovascular insufficiency is stroke. Stroke is the third leading cause of death in North America and the leading cause of long-term disability. Each year, more than 500,000 new strokes and 200,000 stroke-related deaths occur. The medical cost of managing patients after stroke is estimated at $40 billion per year.

Strokes are caused by infarction or hemorrhage within the cerebral hemispheres. Approximately one-third of strokes are caused by **embolism** from atherosclerotic plaques in the carotid arteries of the neck. Although medical management, including antihypertensive, hypocholesterolemic, and antiplatelet agents, may help to prevent carotid atheroembolism, the most effective strategy is either removal of the plaque through carotid endarterectomy (CEA) or carotid stenting.

Blood reaches the brain through the paired carotid and vertebral arteries (Figure 22-21). The right and left carotid arteries originate from the innominate artery and the aortic arch, respectively. The vertebral arteries arise from the proximal portions of the subclavian arteries. The common carotid arteries in the neck bifurcate into the external carotid arteries (which supply the muscles of the face) and the internal carotid arteries. The internal carotid arteries have no branches in the neck, but they enter the petrous portion of the skull and give rise to the ophthalmic artery of the eye and the anterior and middle cerebral arteries that serve the cerebral cortex. The paired vertebral arteries form a single blood vessel within the brainstem (basilar artery) and then give rise to the posterior cerebral arteries and the arteries of the cerebellum. The arteries of the anterior and posterior circulation are part of a rich collateral network of vessels (circle of Willis) that is composed of the P1 segments of the posterior cerebral arteries, the posterior communicating arteries, the A1 segments of the anterior cerebral arteries, and the anterior communicating artery. Theoretically, an intact circle of Willis allows cerebral perfusion to be maintained in the face of occlusion or stenosis of one or more of the main branches. Unfortunately, this collateral network is complete in <25% of people.

Approximately 15% of the cardiac output is directed to maintain cerebral perfusion. The resting total cerebral blood flow is 100 mL/minute/100 g brain matter, with as much as 50 to 60 mL/minute/100 g directed to the more cellular gray matter and 20 mL/minute/100 g to the less cellular white matter. Cerebral ischemia can result once the total perfusion is <18 mL/minute/100 g brain matter. Cerebral infarction can occur after the cerebral perfusion decreases to <8 mL/minute/100 g.

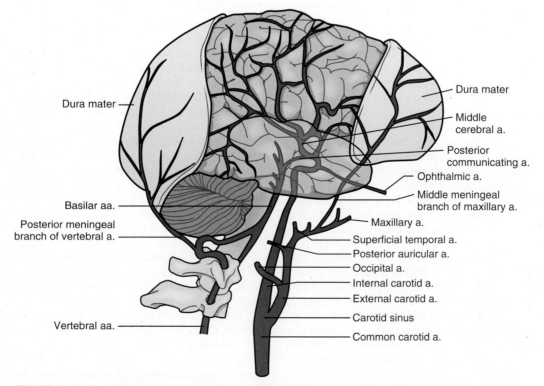

FIGURE 22-21. **The cerebrovascular anatomy has multiple interconnecting arteries, although the Circle of Willis is complete in only 25% of patients.** Occlusion of one vessel may not lead to cerebral ischemia if the other vessels are patent.

A number of mechanisms maintain cerebral blood flow in the face of systemic hypotension or fixed lesions in the carotid and vertebral arteries and intracerebral branches. Baroreceptors located at the carotid sinus sample and regulate blood pressure and heart rate. Further, cerebral vessels dilate in response to decreased perfusion pressure (autoregulation). This change is probably mediated by local receptors in the vascular smooth muscle and by autoregulatory autocoids (e.g., nitric oxide).

Although cerebral ischemia occasionally results from systemically induced decreased blood flow, atheroembolism is by far the most common cause of cerebral infarction. Cerebral embolism may originate from any source between the left atrium and cerebral arteries, including the atrial appendage, left ventricle, aortic valve, aortic arch, carotid bifurcation, carotid siphon, or small vessel intracranial disease. The most common source of emboli is an atherosclerotic lesion at the carotid bifurcation. Experimental models show that the carotid bifurcation contains areas of low and oscillatory shear stress. This finding may account for the transfer of circulating lipids to predisposed segments of the carotid bifurcation and the development of occlusive plaques. Like any lesion in the body, most plaques are eventually covered with a fibrous cap, or scar, and separated from the circulation. Occasionally, however, the fibrous cap is disrupted, allowing embolism of exposed plaque elements or laminated thrombus. Less common causes of carotid arterial occlusive disease include fibromuscular dysplasia, Takayasu arteritis, arterial dissection, and trauma.

Hypoperfusion can cause neurologic deficits in the watershed areas between the perfused territories of the main cerebral arteries, where collateral flow is marginal. Sudden thrombosis of the carotid artery can cause massive cerebral infarction or may be asymptomatic if there is adequate collateral circulation from the contralateral carotid artery and the basilar artery (silent occlusion).

Clinical Presentation

Symptoms of cerebral vascular insufficiency are classified according to the location of the deficit, its duration, and the presence of cerebral infarction. These symptoms can be either transient or permanent. **Amaurosis fugax** (fleeting blindness) is a transient monocular blindness that is caused by emboli to the ophthalmic artery. Classically, amaurosis fugax is described as a curtain of blindness being pulled down from superior to inferior and involving the eye ipsilateral to the carotid lesion. TIAs are short-lived, with often repetitive changes in mentation, vision, or sensorimotor function that are completely reversed within 24 hours. Most TIAs last only a few minutes before they resolve completely. Because TIAs often involve the middle cerebral artery distribution, patients often have contralateral arm, leg, and facial weakness. A stroke-in-evolution is a rapid progressive worsening of a neurologic deficit. A cerebral infarction, or **cerebrovascular accident**, is a permanent neurologic deficit, or stroke. Cerebral CT scan or MRI of a patient who had a stroke shows a region of nonviable cerebral tissue. MRI diffuse weighted imaging generally is the most sensitive in detecting cerebral infarction. Atherosclerotic carotid artery disease is not the only etiology of these clinical presentations. TIAs are also caused by migraines, seizure disorders, brain tumors, intracranial aneurysms, and arteriovenous malformations (AVMs).

The severity of the neurologic deficit is determined by the volume and location of the ischemic area of the brain. The most commonly involved area is the perfused territory of the middle cerebral artery (parietal lobe), which is the main outflow vessel of the carotid artery. Hypoperfusion of the middle cerebral artery causes contralateral hemiparesis or hemiplegia and, occasionally, paralysis of the contralateral lower part of the face (central seventh nerve paralysis). Difficulty with speech (aphasia) is noted if the dominant hemisphere is involved. The left hemisphere is dominant in nearly all right-handed people and most left-handed people.

Patients with ischemia of the brain tissue that is supplied by the anterior cerebral artery have contralateral monoplegia that is usually more severe in the lower extremity. Posterior cerebral artery ischemia is usually related to obstruction of both vertebral arteries or the basilar artery. Dizziness or syncope may be accompanied by visual field defects, palsy of the ipsilateral third cranial nerve, and contralateral sensory losses.

As with most syndromes of vascular insufficiency, the diagnosis is usually suggested by the history alone. A carefully elicited history may also localize the neuroanatomic deficit and the offending arterial lesion. Physical examination should include a thorough neurologic examination as well as a search for evidence of arterial occlusive disease in other vascular beds. The classic finding in a patient with carotid stenosis is a cervical bruit (high-frequency systolic murmur) heard during auscultation with a stethoscope placed at the angle of the jaw. Unfortunately, there is little correlation between the degree of stenosis and the pitch, duration, or intensity of the bruit. A minimal stenosis can produce a loud bruit, but a near-total occlusion may not produce a bruit at all. A bruit can also be produced from other cervical blood vessels or transmitted from the aortic valve. Because of the close proximity of the carotid artery to the ear, some patients actually note a buzzing or heartbeat in their ear referred from the carotid stenosis. During ophthalmologic examination, small, yellow refractile particles (Hollenhorst plaques) may be seen at the branch point of the retinal vessels. These plaques are cholesterol emboli from a carotid artery, aortic arch, or aortic valve plaque. Fisher plugs are due to platelet emboli and are not refractile.

Noninvasive tests can determine the extent of carotid artery stenosis without the use of arteriography. Candidates for noninvasive testing include patients with cerebrovascular symptoms, those with cervical bruits, and, in some cases, those who are undergoing major vascular procedures (e.g., coronary artery bypass grafting). Noninvasive, yet direct, evaluation of the extracranial carotid arterial vessels is obtained with Doppler ultrasound. The nature of the plaque (soft, calcific, or ulcerated) and its precise location (common versus external versus internal carotid artery) can be determined with duplex ultrasound. The accuracy of imaging is enhanced by combining B-mode ultrasound with Doppler-derived assessments of blood flow velocity (duplex scan). In more than 90% of patients with carotid bifurcation plaque, no further diagnostic test is needed to institute therapy. A limitation of duplex scanning is the inability to assess the intracranial circulation and the origins of the common carotid arteries from the aortic arch. Occasionally, visualization of the carotid bifurcation is impaired by calcification of the vessels.

The definitive study of the extracranial carotid arterial system is arteriography. Arterial injections offer the clearest definition of carotid plaques and potential ulcerations (Figure 22-22). Arteriography is indicated in patients who have a potential aortic arch or intracranial lesion, those with uncertain symptoms, and those in whom the carotid stenosis cannot be clearly visualized on duplex ultrasonography.

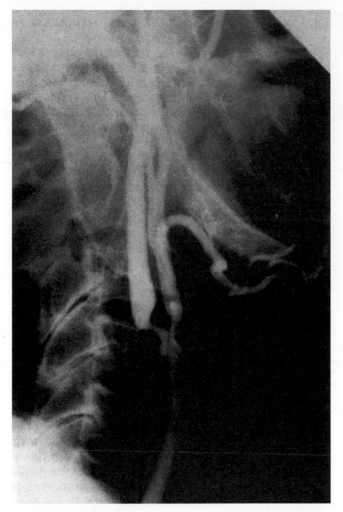

FIGURE 22-22. Angiogram of an internal carotid stenosis showing an ulcerative and stenotic atherosclerotic lesion at the carotid bifurcation in a patient who has TIAs.

Complications are rare, but can be devastating. They include cerebrovascular accident (approximately 0.5% of cases). As a consequence, most diagnostic angiograms today employ CT technology, which does not require arterial catheterization. These CT angiograms nearly match catheter-based studies in detail and diagnostic quality.

Recent improvements in CTA, cerebral MRI, and MRA have led to increased application in patients with carotid occlusive disease. CTA with 3-D reconstruction is as accurate as catheter angiography for carotid and intracerebral vascular evaluation. MRI is useful for evaluation of the brain tissue for infarction, tumor, AVM, and hemorrhage. MRA also provides detailed visualization of the carotid arterial system without requiring arterial puncture and injection (Figure 22-23).

Treatment

Medical therapy for cerebrovascular disease is directed at the control of risk factors (hypertension, smoking, diabetes, and hyperlipoproteinemia) and anticoagulation (warfarin) or administration of antiplatelet drugs (aspirin, clopidogrel). Anticoagulation and antiplatelet therapies are most commonly used in patients with ulcerative nonstenotic lesions or severe intracerebral disease because surgical therapy would not change the natural history of the disease process. A prospective rand-

omized study (North American Symptomatic Carotid Endarterectomy Trial [NASCET]) evaluated the treatment of patients with internal carotid artery stenosis and cerebrovascular symptoms. After 2 years of follow-up, researchers found that in symptomatic patients who had more than 70% ipsilateral stenosis and were managed with antiplatelet therapy alone, the risk of cerebrovascular accident or death was approximately 26% compared with 9% in patients who were treated with operative repair of the carotid through CEA. The risk in symptomatic patients with 50% to 69% stenosis was also reduced with CEA.

Asymptomatic patients with documented 60% or greater carotid stenosis were studied in the Asymptomatic Carotid Atherosclerosis Study (ACAS). The risk of stroke in the medically managed group was calculated at 11% in 5 years. CEA reduced the risk to 5%. While not as a dramatic as the reduction in symptomatic patients, these findings firmly established the role of CEA in the prevention of stroke in properly selected patients with significant carotid stenosis. However, aggressive risk factor management, which was not used during ACAS, makes surgical and medical treatment of asymptomatic carotid stenosis comparable.

In experienced hands, the morbidity and mortality rates for CEA are <2%. Recurrent lesions may occur in as many as 10% of endarterectomized arteries, so long-term follow-up with serial ultrasonography is advised. Restenosis within 2 years usually represents intimal hyperplasia, whereas late recurrence is usually a manifestation of recurrent atherosclerosis.

Carotid angioplasty with placement of a metallic stent (carotid stenting) has been evaluated and is being used with increasing frequency to treat symptomatic carotid stenosis. The recent CREST trial showed comparable overall results: patients with carotid angioplasty had more postprocedure strokes but fewer MIs, and patients who underwent endarterectomy had fewer strokes but more MIs. More recent studies have shown that there is a significant learning curve associated with carotid artery stenting and only experienced interventionalists should be performing these procedures.

All patients with carotid stenosis, whether asymptomatic or symptomatic, must be on antiplatelet (aspirin or clopidogrel) therapy, statins, and β-blocker therapy, unless one is contraindicated.

VERTEBRAL BASILAR DISEASE

The classic syndrome of vertebral basilar insufficiency is subclavian steal syndrome, which is associated with subclavian or innominate artery occlusive disease. Symptoms occur when an occlusive lesion that is located proximal to the origin of the vertebral vessel decreases perfusion pressure in the subclavian artery. The vertebral artery then functions as a collateral pathway to the arm circulation. During arm exercise, vascular resistance in the arm decreases, and flow is reversed in the vertebral artery. As a result, basilar arterial blood flow and perfusion pressure are decreased (Figure 22-24). Symptoms of posterior cerebral and cerebellar ischemia are common and include light-headedness and syncope correlated with arm exercise. Supraclavicular bruits are often detected, and blood pressure in the ipsilateral brachial artery is usually reduced by at least 15 mm Hg. Because of the increased length of the left subclavian artery relative to the right, there is a three-to-four times increased incidence of left subclavian stenosis and subclavian steal syndrome.

In patients with associated carotid artery stenosis, CEA alone may relieve the symptoms of vertebral basilar

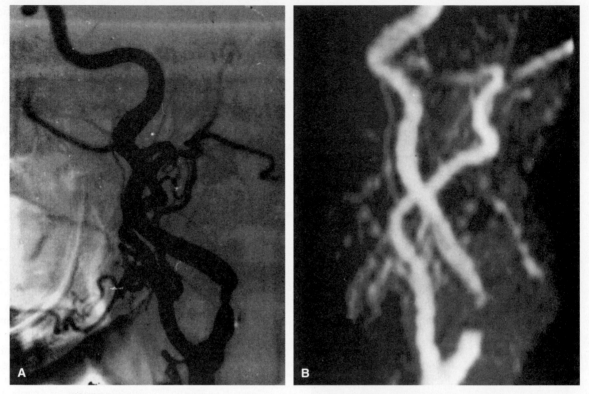

FIGURE 22-23. **A,** A conventional cerebral angiogram. **B,** A magnetic resonance angiogram in the same patient.

insufficiency by increasing collateral flow to the posterior cerebral artery and cerebellum. However, in most symptomatic patients with subclavian steal syndrome, the most effective procedures are either carotid–subclavian bypass, reimplantation of the subclavian artery into the proximal common carotid artery, or subclavian angioplasty. These procedures restore normal blood flow to the subclavian artery and allow antegrade perfusion of the vertebral artery.

■ VENOUS DISEASE

Venous disease is one of the most common medical conditions affecting adults. Approximately 40% of adults have some form of venous disease including varicose veins, **postthrombotic syndrome**, venous ulcers, and telangiectasias (spider veins). An adult has a 6% probability of having a venous ulcer within his or her lifetime. The incidence of venous diseases increases with age, so that 70% of adults over the age of 70 have some form of chronic venous disease.

Acute venous disease, primarily deep vein thrombophlebitis (DVT), is responsible for many unexpected deaths in hospitalized patients, particularly postsurgery. The Surgeon General has recently issued a "call to action" for physicians to reduce preventable deaths from DVT by using more aggressive prevention measures. Currently, all surgical patients must have consideration given to some form of prophylaxis when they undergo a procedure that has a significant risk of DVT.

ANATOMY

The venous system is divided into central and peripheral systems. The central venous system includes the inferior and superior vena cava, iliac veins, and subclavian veins.

The peripheral venous system includes the upper and lower extremity venous systems as well as the venous drainage of the head and neck region. The extremity veins are further classified as either superficial or deep (Figure 22-25). The superficial system of the lower extremity is composed of the great and small saphenous veins and their tributaries. The deep venous system is composed of the large veins that travel with the major arteries of the extremity. The common femoral, femoral, and profunda femoral veins parallel the arteries of the same names. Recently, the "superficial femoral" vein

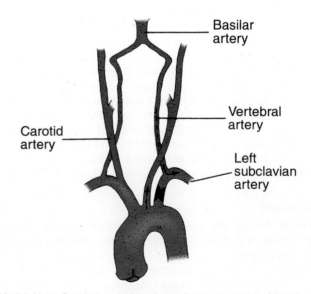

FIGURE 22-24. **Subclavian steal syndrome.** Proximal occlusion of the left subclavian artery causes retrograde flow of blood through the left vertebral artery, "stealing" blood from the basilar circulation and causing transient dizziness and syncope with arm exercise.

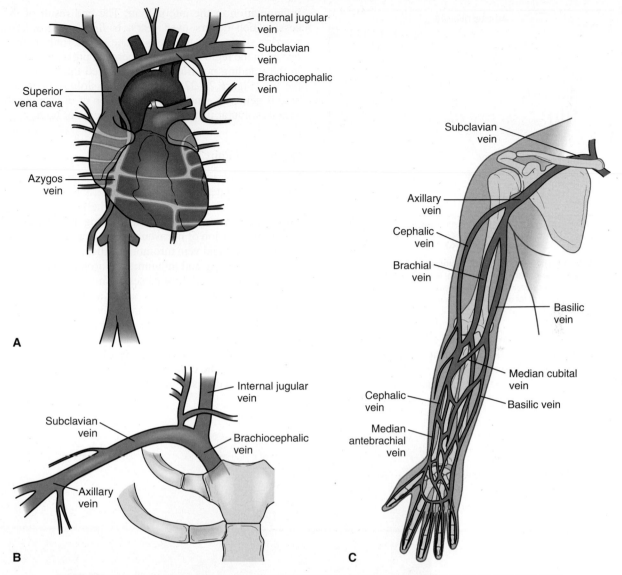

FIGURE 22-25. A, The chest wall, upper limb, and head drain into the superior vena cava. **B,** Blood from the upper limb, neck, and face drain into the axillary and external jugular veins, respectively. **C,** The arm veins drain from both superficial and deep veins into the axillary and subclavian veins.

was renamed the "femoral" to avoid confusion and assure appropriate concern for the risk of pulmonary embolism if this deep vein develops phlebitis. The anterior tibial, posterior tibial, and peroneal veins are almost always paired; therefore, the calf has six primary deep veins, in contrast to three primary arteries.

Unidirectional flow back to the heart is maintained by a series of bicuspid vein valves. These vein valves prevent reflux of blood back toward the lower extremity during standing. The superficial and deep venous systems are connected by perforating veins that direct blood from the superficial system to the deep system. Incompetence of the valves in the deep or perforating veins, as a result of congenital defects, scarring, or distension, allows retrograde flow from the deep system into the superficial system. If severe and long-standing enough, such reflux will cause varicosities, chronic venous insufficiency, and eventually venous ulcerations. Venous ulcers are an important health care problem, resulting in disability, lost workdays, huge costs, and serious lifestyle changes.

PHYSIOLOGY

The muscular compartments of the calf are critically important in the venous circulation. Muscular contraction increases pressure within the compartments, forcing blood back to the heart. Unlike the deep veins, the superficial veins are not surrounded by muscular compartments and therefore are not emptied by muscular contraction. The venous pressures in the standing and supine position reflect the critical role of the valves, muscular contraction, and the position of the patient (Figure 22-26).

PATHOLOGY

In 1856, Virchow identified a triad of risk factors for DVT. It included stasis, venous endothelial injury, and hypercoagulable states. Although many other risk factors, including pregnancy, the use of oral contraceptives, a history of DVT, surgical procedures, sepsis, and obesity appear independent, they can all be placed into one of these categories. Bony and soft tissue trauma to the legs is one of the most common causes of endothelial injury and DVT.

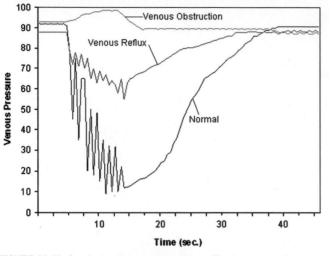

FIGURE 22-26. Graph showing venous pressure. The lower extremity venous pressure starts high, but with walking, the pressure is significantly reduced. When walking is completed, the pressure rises gradually. When there is venous insufficiency, the pressure does not fall as rapidly and then returns to a higher pressure.

Once the valves are damaged from DVT, the ambulatory venous pressure becomes much higher and results in stasis and venous distension, which may injure the venous endothelium and allow protein to leak into the subcutaneous tissue, causing inflammation in the interstitium. The end result of this process, which occurs over years, is *lipodermatosclerosis*, or scarring of the subcutaneous tissue in the limb. It invariably occurs in the region of the leg where the pressure is the highest in the standing position, which is called the "gaiter zone" of the leg (Figure 22-27). The pathophysiology of venous disease is generally caused by obstruction of the venous system, venous valvular insufficiency, or elements of both.

Superficial Vein Thrombosis

Thrombosis of a superficial vein (SVT) causes swelling, erythema, and tenderness along its course. Patients with varicose veins are at risk for thrombosis of the superficial veins and SVT. In addition, there are many iatrogenic causes of SVT, including insertion of intravenous catheters and sclerotherapy. When a superficial vein thromboses, there is often pain associated with swelling and inflammation around the vein. Patients who have superficial thromboses are managed with nonsteroidal anti-inflammatory agents and warm compresses. Occasionally, the vein is so tender that the best treatment is excision of the involved vein. After the thrombosed vein is transected, the thrombus can be extracted and there is immediate pain relief. In addition, thrombectomy of superficial thrombosed veins improves the cosmetic appearance of the skin overlying the vein and reduces pigmentation of the skin.

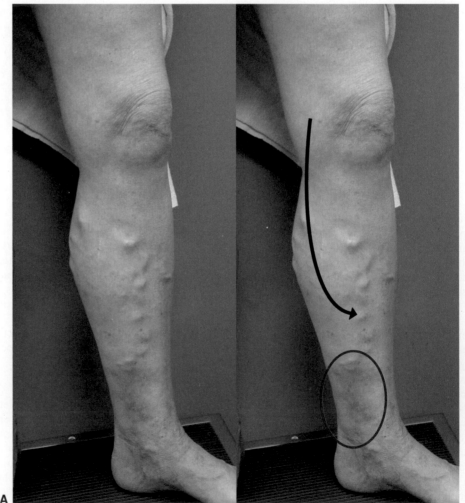

FIGURE 22-27. A, Varicose veins often occur when the proximal saphenous vein becomes incompetent and there is reflux down the saphenous vein and into the tributaries. **B,** This reflux causes visible varicosities and even pigmentation in the "gaiter" zone at the level of the ankle, which is circled in purple.

A   B

Deep Vein Thrombosis

Approximately 500,000 patients per year have DVT. If pulmonary thromboembolism occurs, in-hospital mortality rates are 10%.

Clinical Presentation

As many as 50% of episodes of hospital-acquired DVT are asymptomatic. The remaining patients have local pain secondary to inflammation and edema. DVT of the left iliac venous system is more common than that of the right iliac venous system because of the potential for compression of the left iliac vein by the aortic bifurcation and crossing of the right iliac artery (May-Thurner syndrome; Figure 22-28). Unfortunately, in a small percentage of patients, the first symptom of DVT is pulmonary embolism.

Diagnosis

Physical examination of a patient with a lower-extremity DVT may show unilateral extremity swelling or pain. Calf pain precipitated by dorsal flexion of the foot (Homan's sign) is present in fewer than 50% of cases. Because the accuracy of diagnosis based on clinical and physical examination alone is only 50%, more objective diagnostic studies are needed to confirm the presence of DVT before treatment. In addition to DVT, the differential diagnosis of acute edema and leg pain includes trauma, ruptured plantaris tendon, infection, lymphangitis, muscle hematoma, and ruptured Baker's cyst.

The accuracy of duplex ultrasound (duplex scan) is >95% in diagnosing DVT because it can characterize venous blood flow and visualize the venous thrombus (Figure 22-29). A Doppler ultrasound can document the loss of the normal augmentation of venous flow with distal compression and the variation of venous flow with respiration. Normally, lower extremity venous flow decreases with inspiration as a result of increased intra-abdominal pressure. The accuracy of duplex scanning is decreased in the tibial veins because of the difficulty in visualizing these small veins within the muscular compartments. In unusual cases, CT scans of the abdomen and pelvis, with intravenous contrast material, may aid in the diagnosis of pelvic and vena caval thrombosis. Use of blood tests that measure the degradation of thrombus (D-dimer) can also be used as a screening test for DVT, particularly in the outpatient and ER setting where it is costly to bring in a technician to test each patient with duplex ultrasound who has leg pain. D-dimer is a sensitive, but not specific screening test for DVT and should be followed by duplex ultrasound if it is positive. Venography is rarely performed for diagnosis of DVT but is frequently used prior to thrombolysis of DVT.

Evaluation for hypercoagulability with measures of protein C, protein S, antithrombin 3, factor V Leiden, prothrombin mutation, and anticardiolipin antibodies should be performed in patients with spontaneous (unprovoked) DVT.

Prophylaxis

DVT and pulmonary embolus are significant risks for patients undergoing major surgery. Preoperative prophylaxis has an impact in reducing DVT and should be used routinely for patients who undergo major surgical procedures. Prophylactic measures include mechanical therapy (intermittent segmental compression device [SCD]), early ambulation, and pharmacologic therapy (with subcutaneous heparin or warfarin). Patients can be stratified for risk of DVT; advanced age, long procedures, patients with cancer, and patients with prior DVT are particularly vulnerable.

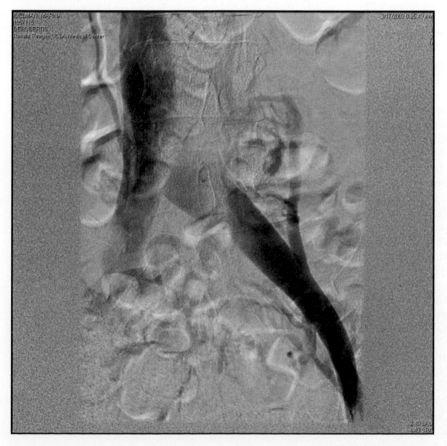

FIGURE 22-28. This venogram of the iliac veins and vena cava shows compression of the left iliac vein by the right iliac artery. The area of compression, when severe, leads to May-Thurner syndrome, in which a patient develops left leg swelling with exercise and venous thrombosis distal to the site of compression.

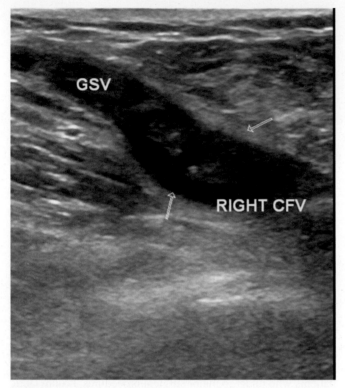

FIGURE 22-29. Duplex scan. GSV, great saphenous vein; CFV, central femoral vein.

Treatment

The goals of treatment of DVT include decreasing the risk of pulmonary embolus, preventing further propagation of the venous thrombus, and reducing the damage to the deep venous valves, so that long-term chronic venous insufficiency does not occur. Primary therapy includes anticoagulation with heparin; this can be administered in both inpatients and outpatients. After the patient is adequately anticoagulated with heparin, long-term anticoagulation is begun with warfarin (Coumadin). Warfarin therapy is monitored to maintain a therapeutic international normalized ratio (INR) of 2 to 3. Sodium warfarin inhibits the vitamin K–dependent factors for both the procoagulant factors (II, VII, IX, X) and the anticoagulant factors (protein C and protein S). Because the half-lives of protein C and protein S are less than those of the procoagulant factors, for a short time after the initiation of warfarin therapy, even appropriately treated patients may become hypercoagulable. Warfarin skin necrosis is a rare but catastrophic complication of this rare hypercoagulable state that can cause significant loss of skin. For this reason, heparin anticoagulation is maintained during the beginning of warfarin therapy. Contraindications to anticoagulation therapy include bleeding diathesis, GI ulceration, recent stroke, cerebral AVMs, recent surgery, hematologic disorders (e.g., hemophilia), and bone marrow suppression as a result of chemotherapy.

Anticoagulation therapy prevents further propagation of the thrombus but does not actually dissolve or lyse the existing thrombus. Fibrinolysis occurs gradually through the endogenous plasminogen system or may be stimulated by the administration of an exogenous thrombolytic agent such as tPA. Definite indications for thrombolytic therapy include subclavian vein thrombosis, acute renal vein thrombosis, and acute superior vena cava occlusion by the thrombus. Recently, the recommendation of the International Society for Chest Physicians lists thrombolysis in patients with DVT as level 2b and should

be considered in all healthy patients with iliofemoral DVT. In addition, mechanical thrombectomy devices are increasingly being used, since they allow concentration of the agent in the vein that is occluded, and limit the dissemination of the agent into the systemic circulation. Mechanical devices also reduce the time needed to recanalize the occluded deep vein and therefore reduce complications from thrombolysis. It is still uncertain whether venous valvular function can be preserved with successful thrombolytic therapy, but evidence is supporting a more aggressive approach for most patients with DVT who are otherwise healthy. Contraindications to thrombolysis include recent surgery or trauma and recent bleeding. Mechanical thrombectomy has fewer contraindications due to the isolation of the thrombolytic agent in the thrombosed vein. Surgical thrombectomy is rarely indicated and is usually reserved for cases of limb-threatening ischemia. Even in complete iliofemoral thrombosis with massive edema (phlegmasia cerulea dolens or phlegmasia alba dolens), mechanical thrombectomy devices or thrombolysis are the primary treatment modalities.

PULMONARY EMBOLISM

Pulmonary embolism results from the migration of venous clots to the pulmonary arteries. Clots may originate in any large vein, especially those that arise from the iliac, femoral, and large pelvic veins. Patients with hypercoagulable conditions are predisposed to DVT and pulmonary embolism.

Clinical Presentation

Patients with pulmonary embolism may have no specific clinical findings or may have massive cardiovascular collapse. The classic clinical presentation (Table 22-4) includes pleuritic chest pain, dyspnea, tachypnea, tachycardia, cough, and hemoptysis. Right-sided heart strain is seen on EKG.

Prevention

The use of support hose and prophylactic anticoagulation is indicated in patients who have a high risk of pulmonary embolism, with the indications being similar to those who have a high risk of DVT and were mentioned above.

Diagnosis

The definitive diagnosis of pulmonary embolism is made by CT scan of the chest, ventilation–perfusion lung scan, or pulmonary angiogram. A wedge-shaped or lobar defect seen on perfusion scan without a ventilation deficit indicates a high probability of pulmonary embolism. Chest CT scan often

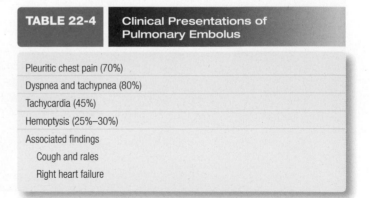

TABLE 22-4	Clinical Presentations of Pulmonary Embolus
Pleuritic chest pain (70%)	
Dyspnea and tachypnea (80%)	
Tachycardia (45%)	
Hemoptysis (25%–30%)	
Associated findings	
Cough and rales	
Right heart failure	

shows both the thrombus in the pulmonary artery and the infarcted lung parenchyma. Pulmonary angiogram has specificity and a sensitivity of >98%, but it is an invasive procedure.

Chest radiography is rarely diagnostic for pulmonary embolus. A pleural effusion is present in as many as one-third of patients with pulmonary embolus. The classic wedge-shaped region of atelectasis from a pulmonary embolus is rarely noted. Chest radiography is most useful for ruling out other potential pulmonary pathology.

Treatment

The primary therapy for pulmonary embolism is anticoagulation to prevent further emboli and clot propagation. If the patient is hemodynamically unstable, inotropic support may be required. If the patient remains stable but is compromised as a result of the pulmonary embolus, thrombolytic therapy is considered. There is no direct correlation between clot size, cardiopulmonary dynamics, and other risk factors and survival in patients with acute embolism. Multiple small emboli cause cardiovascular collapse as often as massive emboli.

If a patient with lower-extremity or pelvic venous thrombus has a contraindication to anticoagulation or has had a pulmonary embolism while anticoagulated (failure of anticoagulation), a mechanical filter device can be placed in the inferior vena cava. This device traps emboli before they reach the pulmonary artery. Vena caval filters are permanent or removable and can be placed with a percutaneous catheter from either the internal jugular vein or the femoral vein.

VARICOSE VEINS

Incidence

Venous disease, including varicose veins, spider veins, and postthrombotic limbs with edema and ulcers, is among the most common diseases in the United States. It is estimated that more than 40% of the adult population has varicose veins and that 6% of adults will develop a venous ulcer during their lifetime. In addition, the recurrence of the end-stage manifestation, venous ulcers, is high, and most patients live for long periods with open ulcers, punctuated with periods of healing. Consequently, venous problems are not only extremely common but also important to the entire health care system.

Anatomy

Knowledge of venous anatomy is critical to understanding venous disease. The superficial, perforating, and deep systems interconnect (Figure 22-30), with blood flowing from the superficial to the deep system, and with valves preventing reflux from proximal to distal and from the deep to the superficial systems. Since 85% to 90% of the venous return is in the deep system, establishing its presence and patency is a key to treatment, and removal of the superficial veins has little consequence on blood flow physiology as long as the deep system is patent.

Primary Varicose Veins

Superficial veins often are not associated with other perforating or deep venous involvement and therefore are considered "primary." The most common cause of primary varicose veins is the development of incompetence of the venous valve at the junction of the saphenous vein with the femoral vein in the inguinal region. Incompetence of this valve results in proximal vein dilation and progressive incompetence of distal valves and veins. Eventually, the dilated vein results in incompetence of the entire saphenous vein as well as tributary (branch) veins. The visible portion of the incompetent veins is usually in the calf, where they are closer to the skin. In spite of proximal incompetence, many patients request treatment only when the calf veins become visible.

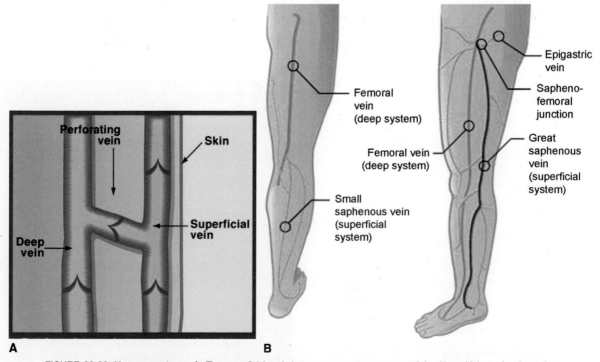

FIGURE 22-30. Venous anatomy. A, The superficial and deep venous systems are parallel, with multiple perforating veins connecting them. **B,** The superficial and deep venous systems are illustrated in two drawings of the leg.

Symptoms

Superficial varicose veins cause symptoms of heaviness and fatigue after prolonged standing, night cramps, and occasionally ankle edema, superficial thrombophlebitis, or hemorrhage from superficial veins.

Diagnosis

Although physical examination is helpful in establishing the presence of varicose veins, the critical determinant of the approach to treatment is the competence of the saphenofemoral junction valve, which cannot be determined by physical examination. Duplex ultrasound is the best diagnostic test for valve incompetence and should be used in all patients with symptoms. If the saphenous vein is not assessed for competency, then an incompetent saphenous vein may be left in place, leading to recurrence. Venography is now rarely used and may cause phlebitis. Plethysmography assesses reflux in the superficial and deep system, but has little role in primary varicose vein evaluation.

Treatment

The treatment of primary varicose veins has changed dramatically in the past 10 years, and, like many areas of surgery, has become less invasive.

1. "Stripping" of the saphenous vein. The saphenous vein may be removed by a technique of stripping, where the vein is exposed at each end and then removed by passing a disposable or metal catheter up the vein from the ankle or knee. A suture is tied around the vein at the saphenofemoral junction and the vein is then removed or "stripped." This technique is being used less frequently, since it is associated with a slightly longer patient recovery with more postoperative pain than minimally invasive approaches.

2. Saphenous ligation. Ligating the saphenous vein flush with the femoral vein in the fossa ovalis can eliminate the saphenous reflux. Although this technique eliminates reflux, there is a higher recurrence with ligation than with stripping. Ligation is particularly indicated in patients with very large proximal saphenous veins that measure >1.5 cm.

3. Endovenous closure with radiofrequency ablation (RFA) (Figure 22-31) or endovenous laser therapy of the saphenous vein. This technique is the least invasive and is performed by accessing the saphenous vein below the knee with a needle, using ultrasound guidance. A wire is then passed into the vein, followed by a sheath and then a radiofrequency or laser catheter. After the catheter has been

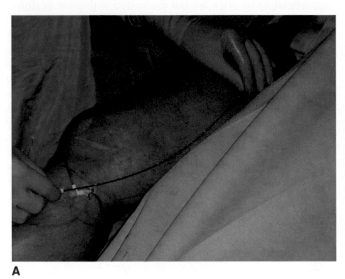

A

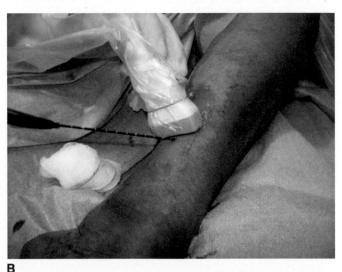

B

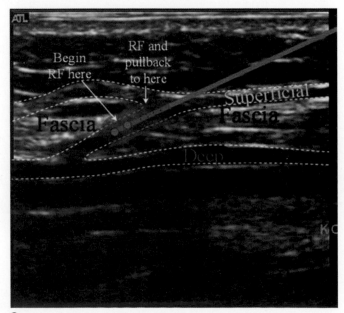

C

FIGURE 22-31. Endovenous closure with RFA. Endovenous ablation of the great saphenous and perforator veins is performed by placing a catheter into the vein and then heating the tip of the catheter until the vein contracts, closing the incompetent vein.

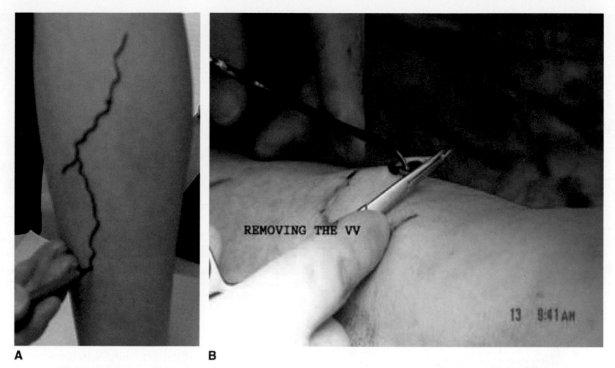

FIGURE 22-32. Microphlebectomy or "stab" phlebectomy is a technique for removing tributary or branch veins by making a small incision adjacent to the vein, which is marked in the standing position (A), and then removing it with a crochet-hook-like instrument (B). The ends of the avulsed veins are not tied and bleeding is controlled with compression.

passed up to the saphenofemoral junction, the catheter is used to heat the vein. The heat contracts collagen and thromboses the vein, leading to closure.

4. Branch vein excision by micro incision (stab phlebectomy) (Figure 22-32). The tributary branches of the saphenous vein can be removed with small incisions that allow the vein to be visualized and removed with small crochet hooks, instruments, or clamps. The resulting scars are very small and nearly invisible.

CHRONIC VENOUS INSUFFICIENCY

Chronic venous insufficiency is a direct result of local venous hypertension. Causes of venous hypertension include deep venous valvular incompetence, venous obstruction as a result of intrinsic or extrinsic compression, and reflux from perforating veins.

The clinical manifestations of chronic venous insufficiency are chronically swollen legs, hyper-pigmentation, and venous ulceration. The leg is typically swollen and pigmented in the "gaiter" zone of the ankle. The pigmentation is a reflection of inflammation and chronic venous hypertension, which is worsened in the standing position. The term "lipodermatosclerosis" refers to the end stage of venous hypertension, when the chronic venous hypertension leads to pigmentation and fibrosis of the tissue around the ankle.

Diagnosis

Physical examination shows an orange-brown skin discoloration at the level of the ankle (Figure 22-33) with hemosiderin deposition, lower extremity edema, superficial varicosities, and/or ulceration. Venous stasis ulceration usually occurs at the medial and lateral malleoli of the ankle. These chronic changes in the lower extremity occur as a result of venous hypertension

and are usually postthrombotic, but may also be caused by congenital deep valvular incompetence and severe obesity.

Noninvasive vascular laboratory evaluation includes venous duplex ultrasonography, which allows visualization of venous flow as well as reflux through incompetent deep and perforator venous valves. Likewise, a duplex scan can directly visualize a deep vein chronic occlusion or note the inability of the vein to be compressed secondary to venous thrombus. If the noninvasive duplex scan is not diagnostic, MRI/MRV or CT venogram may be necessary.

Treatment

The initial management of chronic venous insufficiency with lower extremity lipodermatosclerosis is the use of gradient compression stockings. Unfortunately, compliance is poor in many patients, since they do not see the immediate benefit of the support hose and dislike the cost of the hose and the discomfort associated with wearing the hose. In patients with venous ulceration, wound care is required to promote healing. A medicated, tightly applied dressing of three or four layers (Figure 22-34) should be used for compression. Stripping/removal or closure with RFA or laser of the refluxing superficial veins, as well as interruption of perforating veins, may be necessary to heal venous ulcers. If the wound does not heal, but the refluxing veins and edema are controlled, split-thickness skin grafting may accomplish wound healing.

■ VASCULAR TRAUMA

Blood vessels are injured directly by penetrating trauma (e.g., stab and gunshot wounds), blunt trauma (especially fractures of the long bones), and during surgical exposure other structures adjacent to blood vessels. In high-speed collisions and

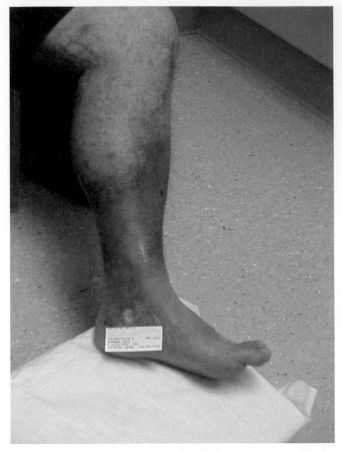

FIGURE 22-33. Lipodermatosclerosis occurs in the "gaiter zone" of the calf and ankle and is a combination of pigmentation and subcutaneous fibrosis.

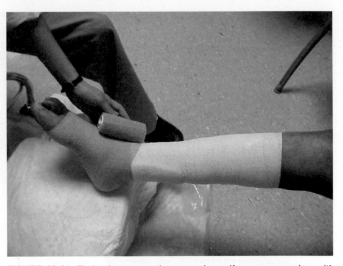

FIGURE 22-34. To heal, venous ulcers require uniform compression with pressures of 30 to 40 mm Hg, which reduces the leg edema and collapses the superficial and perforating veins.

falls, vessels may be torn by the shear stress of sudden acceleration or deceleration. While patients with arterial injuries may have obvious signs such as hemorrhage and absence of distal pulses, the signs of vascular injury are often subtle. Hemorrhage may be occult and confined to soft tissue or body cavities. Other findings associated with vascular injury include arteriovenous fistulae (associated with "to-and-fro" murmurs or palpable **thrills**), neurologic deficits and paresthesias (as a result of nerve compression by adjacent hematomas), or organ-specific deficits that reflect obstruction of the main arterial supply (e.g., cerebral infarction with carotid artery injuries). A common misconception is that a patient who has an arterial injury must have a reduced or absent distal pulse; however, diminished pulses only occur if the injury restricts blood flow. Further, the presentation is commonly delayed; intimal flaps from deformation or stretching of the endothelial layer may not cause thrombosis for hours or days.

Immediate diagnosis and treatment of arterial injuries is indicated to avoid excessive blood loss and to restore extremity or organ blood flow. If the diagnosis is missed on initial evaluation, late complications may be much more difficult to treat. These late complications include pseudoaneurysms, high-volume arteriovenous fistulae with high-output cardiac failure, and delayed thrombosis from untreated intimal dissections.

The poor reliability of physical diagnosis in accurately assessing the location and extent of vascular injury mandates diagnostic studies whenever arterial injury is suspected. If the patient has a viable extremity with an ABI of 1.0, then limb-threatening arterial injury is unlikely and the vessels that are near the region of trauma can be further evaluated by duplex ultrasound studies. If the extremity is ischemic, angiography is indicated unless the delay puts the limb or organ at risk. Because of the tremendous concussive energy of high-velocity missiles, extensive damage can result even if the vessels are not in the direct line of the penetrating bullet. Certain types of blunt trauma (especially dislocation of the knees and elbows) are so often associated with arterial injury that duplex ultrasonography or arteriography is prudent even if no symptoms are present.

Although the consequences of venous injury are not as severe as those of arterial trauma, venous laceration must be considered in any patient who has evidence of excessive blood loss and no arterial lesion on angiography. Magnetic resonance venography may be able to confirm and localize the injury, although operative exploration to control bleeding may be more expedient. Venous injury also predisposes the patient to the development of deep venous thrombosis.

Repair of vascular injuries may be as simple as ligation of noncritical vessel or lateral suture (suture repair of the side of the vessel). In some cases, bypass grafts are needed, with resection of the vessel. In these cases, it is preferable to use an autologous vein from an uninjured extremity, because this type of conduit has higher patency and low infection rate, even in the face of contamination. When both arteries and veins of an extremity are injured, repair of both results in a higher limb salvage rate.

■ OTHER VASCULAR DISORDERS

ARTERIOVENOUS MALFORMATIONS AND ARTERIOVENOUS FISTULAE

Arteriovenous malformations (AVMs) result from abnormal embryologic development of the maturing vascular spaces, producing pathologic arteriovenous connections that involve small and medium-sized vessels. There is an equal male:female ratio, and the lower extremities are involved two to three times as often as the upper extremities. Although lesions are present at birth, most become clinically significant only in the second and third decade as they gradually enlarge. On palpation, a vibration or "thrill" is often noted over the level of the arteriovenous connection and an accompanying bruit can usually be auscultated. A mass may also be present and cutaneous extension may result in a discolored or pigmented area marking the lesion. Intra-abdominal and retroperitoneal AVMs are less common but can pose more complex diagnostic and management challenges. Diagnosis generally starts with physical examination, but is confirmed with duplex ultrasound and MRI/MRA. CT angiography/ venography may also be useful for delineation of feeding vasculature and conventional angiography/venography may be required for definitive diagnostic purposes as well as therapeutic intervention.

The management of symptomatic, localized congenital AVMs is surgical excision. Symptoms usually consist of pain and swelling associated with the lesion. Significant musculoskeletal disability may result depending on the size and location of the AVM. In larger AVMs, skin ulceration and bleeding are troublesome complications. Rarely, congenital arteriovenous fistulae produce cardiac enlargement and heart failure as a result of increased blood flow. Finally, the location and potentially disfiguring appearance of some AVMs may warrant treatment even in the absence of symptoms.

The treatment of large or diffuse lesions can be extremely difficult and is associated with a high recurrence rate. An alternative or adjunct to surgery is percutaneous intra-arterial embolization of the main feeding artery and/or intravenous sclerosis of the outflow veins to decrease the amount of blood that is shunted from the arterioles to the venules. Treatment approaches can sometimes be directed by flow findings on duplex. High-flow lesions generally have a significant arterial component and require embolization prior to either surgery or sclerotherapy. Low-flow, primarily venous lesions can either be managed conservatively, or can be sclerosed primarily. In either case, significant soft tissue necrosis and even marked skin ulceration and complex wounds can result. Therefore, these are best treated in a multidisciplinary fashion with a team including vascular, radiologic, plastic, and pediatric surgeons, along with other wound care specialists.

Acquired arteriovenous fistulae are abnormal communications between the arteries and veins, but they usually result from iatrogenic injuries (arterial catheterizations) or penetrating trauma (gunshot or knife wounds). These fistulae are often associated with a false aneurysm and involve large vessels (common femoral artery–common femoral vein fistula). A palpable thrill or audible bruit may be present. Diagnosis is confirmed by duplex ultrasound examination. Venous hypertension, extremity swelling, and venous stasis changes may occur with long-standing arteriovenous fistulae.

All large acquired traumatic arteriovenous fistulae should be repaired to prevent the development of complications (e.g., cardiac failure, local pain, aneurysmal formation, limb length discrepancy in children, chronic venous hypertension). Direct ultrasound-guided compression of postcatheterization arteriovenous fistulae can be effective, especially if the patient is not anticoagulated. Operative intervention requires complete dissection and separation of the involved vessels and appropriate vascular repair. Depending on their location, some arteriovenous communications can be excluded interventionally using covered stent grafts.

VASOSPASTIC DISORDERS

Episodic digital vasospasm involving the hands and feet was first described by Maurice Raynaud in 1862. Raynaud's syndrome is cold or emotionally induced episodic digital ischemia. As many as 90% of patients are female, and 50% have an associated autoimmune disease (e.g., scleroderma, lupus erythematosus, rheumatoid arthritis, Sjögren's syndrome). Some develop Raynaud's syndrome from work-related overuse of vibratory machinery. Unilateral Raynaud's syndrome is more common in men and is often associated with proximal arterial disease of the large vessels such as subclavian stenoses or occlusions.

The classic Raynaud's attack has three distinct phases, which occur in sequence (white, blue, red). Exposure to cold initially causes profound vasospasm and blanching of the digits (white). After approximately 15 minutes, cyanosis is evident, caused by venous filling with delayed venous emptying (blue). Later, the digits and hands become hyperemic as vasospasm lessens and flow to the digits is restored (red).

The diagnosis of Raynaud's syndrome is made from the history and physical examination. Coexistent symptoms of connective tissue disorders are often elicited. Laboratory tests (sedimentation rate, complement assay, antinuclear antibody assay) often confirm the immunologic disorders associated with the syndrome. It is important to document all pulses palpated. Doppler evaluation may be helpful if pulses are difficult to feel.

Treatment consists of discontinuing any medications that cause reduced cardiac output or promote vasospasm and that are associated with Raynaud's syndrome (ergotamines and β-blockers). Other pharmacologic agents, especially α- and calcium channel–blocking agents, may be used to decrease the tendency toward vasospasm. Sympathetic blocks with xylocaine are occasionally used for temporary relief, although surgical sympathectomy is not a particularly effective treatment since sympathetic fibers regenerate over time. Revascularization of an ischemic extremity may markedly improve the symptoms in patients with arterial occlusive disease.

THORACIC OUTLET SYNDROME

TOS is a constellation of clinical problems related to compression of the brachial plexus (neurogenic), arteries (aneurysm and emboli), and veins (Paget-Schroetter syndrome). The neurogenic syndrome is often seen in young and middle-aged women. Symptoms are caused by compression or irritation of the brachial plexus as nerves pass through the thoracic outlet and the costoclavicular space.

Anatomic causes of the syndrome include an elongated transverse process of the seventh cervical vertebra; a fully developed cervical rib; congenital bands in the outlet related to the cervical rib, middle scalene muscle, or anterior scalene muscle; and a narrowed costoclavicular space, often because of a previously fractured rib or clavicle, with callus formation (Figure 22-35).

Paresthesias of the arm and hand reflect neurologic compression and are much more common than arterial symptoms. When arterial symptoms occur, they include coldness of the hand and arm, pallor, and muscle fatigue. In rare cases, stenosis of the subclavian artery causes an aneurysm (Figure 22-36)

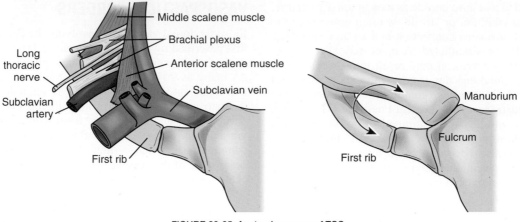

FIGURE 22-35. Anatomic causes of TOS.

and/or emboli to the hand. Subclavian vein thrombosis (Paget-Schroetter syndrome) may also occur (Figure 22-37).

Evaluation of these patients involves a detailed history and a thorough physical examination to document localized scalene muscle tenderness and radicular phenomena. Adson's test (disappearance of the radial pulse on arm abduction and external rotation of the shoulder), said to be indicative of TOS in the early literature, is now considered relatively nonspecific. Cervical spine radiographs are obtained to identify cervical ribs. Nerve conduction velocity across the outlet and local anesthetic injection of the anterior scalene muscle are used to determine the etiology of symptoms. Angiography is recommended only if arterial occlusion or embolization is suspected. Venography is used in patients with duplex scan confirmation of thrombosis of the subclavian vein.

After the diagnosis is confirmed, nonsurgical treatments, including physical therapy and Botox injection of the anterior scalene muscle, are attempted in patients with neurogenic TOS. If symptoms persist, surgical decompression of the outlet may be warranted. The most commonly used procedure is resection of the first thoracic rib, removal of any cervical ribs, and division of the anterior scalene muscle. Patients with TOS without a cervical rib can have either a transaxillary approach with first rib resection or supraclavicular anterior scalenectomy for decompression of the thoracic outlet. Patients with vasculogenic TOS (artery or vein) require thrombolysis of clot, followed by decompression

of the thoracic inlet and occasionally surgical repair of the affected artery or vein.

LYMPHATIC DISORDERS

The lymphatic system serves a number of functions, including the return of proteins and extracellular fluid that are lost from the capillary circulation, and the removal of bacteria and foreign materials from the extracellular space. Lymphedema occurs when transcapillary fluid flux into the extracellular space exceeds the capacity of lymph transport to return that fluid to the circulation. In these situations, protein-rich fluid accumulates in the limb and relative stasis of the fluid ensues.

Primary lymphedema is classified as either congenital lymphedema (present at birth), lymphedema praecox (usually starting at 10 to 15 years of age), or lymphedema tarda (starting after 35 years of age). The lymphangiographic appearance further divides primary lymphedema into hyperplasia, in which numerous dilated lymphatic vessels are present, and hypoplasia, in which lymphatics are few in number and small in caliber. Secondary or acquired lymphedema occurs after recurrent infection, radiation, surgical excision, or neoplastic invasion of regional lymph nodes.

Patients with lymphedema usually have diffuse painless enlargement of the extremities. Elevation of the extremity is often of little help, as elevated venous pressures are not usually a major factor in the accumulation of fluid. Similarly, diuretics often are of little benefit. With time, the soft "pitting" edema becomes "woody" as progressive fibrosis of the connective tissue occurs. Superimposed infection (cellulitis) of the extremity will accelerate the fibrotic process and exacerbate lymphedema.

Treatment includes both medical and surgical management, neither of which can cure the process. The use of high-pressure support hosiery, avoidance of prolonged standing, lymphatic massage, sequential compression devices, and meticulous foot care to minimize infection are the primary medical therapies. If infection develops, erythema and lymphangitis may ensue. This should be treated aggressively with antibiotics, elevation, and bed rest. Patients with long-standing acquired lymphedema are at an increased risk of lymphangiosarcoma and should be followed closely with biopsy of any suspicious changes.

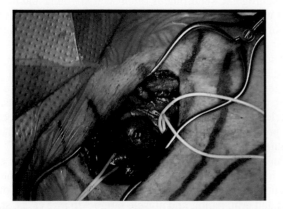

FIGURE 22-36. Aneurysm of subclavian artery. This photograph shows a subclavian artery aneurysm, which formed distal to compression from TOS.

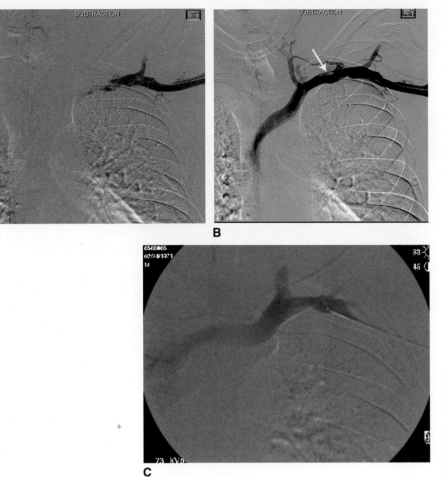

FIGURE 22-37. Subclavian vein thrombosis. Venograms demonstrating lysis of an axillo-subclavian vein secondary to PS. **A,** The occluded vein before crossing of the lesion with a wire. **B,** The vein after it has been recanalized, although there is still some residual clot within the vein (*arrow*). **C,** The vein after complete resolution of the thrombus and removal of the first rib. This follow-up venogram was performed 4 months after the initial presentation and lysis.

Surgical intervention is considered only if medical management fails to adequately control symptoms. Surgical approaches fall into two categories: reconstruction of the lymphatic drainage (lymphangioplasty) and excision of varying amounts of subcutaneous tissue and skin. Unfortunately, the results of surgery are often disappointing and should be reserved for patients with extensive edema who have failed medical therapy and are in such distress from the lymphedema that amputation is a viable consideration.

thePoint ✳ Go to http://thePoint.lww.com/activate and use your scratch-off code on the inside cover of this book to access bonus chapters, question bank, videos, and more.

SAMPLE QUESTIONS

Questions

Choose the best answer for each question.

1. A 68-year-old man comes to the office because he noted a pulsatile bulge in his abdomen for the past 2 years, and it is becoming more prominent. He has a remote history of MI, and his only risk factors are one pack per day of smoking and hypertension, controlled with a diuretic. His physical exam is normal except for a pulsatile, nontender mass above his umbilicus, which measures 7 cm. What is the best initial test for this patient?

A. CT scan with contrast of the abdomen and pelvis

B. MRI/MRA of the abdomen and pelvis

C. Duplex ultrasound of the abdomen

D. Arteriogram

E. Plain film of the abdomen

2. A 70-year-old woman responds to an advertisement for cardiovascular screening, which includes an ABI, an EKG, an ultrasound for AAA, and a carotid duplex ultrasound. She is told that she has a stenosis in her left carotid artery of 50% to 70%, and no significant stenosis in the right carotid bulb. What should your recommendation to her be?

A. Carotid endarterectomy

B. Carotid angiogram

C. Carotid stent

D. High-dose aspirin

E. Repeat carotid duplex ultrasound

3. A 50-year-old type 1 diabetic woman has developed an ulcer that penetrates into the fat on the plantar aspect of the left foot, under the ball of her big toe. She has foot swelling so pulses are not palpable, but she has good capillary refill in the toes. The ulcer is not painful and is not clinically infected. What is the next best step for this problem?

A. Big toe amputation

B. IV antibiotics

C. Measure ankle brachial index and toe pressures

D. Angiography

E. Non–weight bearing and continued observation

4. A 55-year-old man has degenerative hip disease and must undergo a total hip replacement. His BMI is 36.3. He is otherwise healthy and has never had an episode of deep venous thrombosis. The most appropriate DVT prophylaxis for him is:

A. support hose intra- and post-op

B. sequential compression intra- and post-op

C. venacaval filter

D. aspirin pre- and post-op

E. low molecular weight heparin pre- and post-op

5. A 35-year-old woman comes to the office because of an ulcer on the skin of her left ankle. She developed pigmentation in her left medial ankle several years ago and then developed a superficial, painless ulcer in the center of the pigmented area 2 months ago. She had been in excellent health prior to that. She works as a schoolteacher and is on her feet most of the day. She has been unable to heal it with local wound care and comes to see you for treatment. Which of the following diagnostic tests would be most useful?

A. Ankle brachial index

B. Wound culture

C. Labs tests for autoimmune disease

D. Venous duplex ultrasound

E. Ulcer biopsy

6. A 25-year-old man comes to the office because of right arm weakness. He is an elite swimmer, who is otherwise healthy, but is now unable to compete due to arm weakness. On exam his left arm is stronger than his right and he has a reduced right radial pulse with shoulder elevation. The best approach to his problem is:

A. physical therapy

B. change in type of physical activity

C. angiogram and arterial repair

D. MRI followed by first rib resection

E. MR venogram, followed by thrombolysis

Answers and Explanations

1. Answer: A

All of the tests offered above will diagnose an aneurysm; an astute clinician needs to determine the most cost effective of available tests. The diagnosis of aneurysm, based on a large AAA by physical exam, is not in doubt, so the key to management is selecting the one test that can size the aneurysm, determine the anatomy, determine whether he is a candidate for an endovascular graft, and allow for pre-op planning. Only a CTA provides all of this information. An ultrasound is the best and most cost-effective test for screening, which is not necessary in this situation since his aneurysm has already been diagnosed. MRI/MRA can show most aspects for planning, except for assessing the aortic wall for calcium, which can help determine whether he is a candidate for an endograft. Arteriography has been replaced by CTA, since an arteriogram does not show the aortic wall or thrombus in the aneurysm sac, which is important for procedural planning. A plain film can assess for the presence and size of an aneurysm, but does not allow for procedural planning.

2. Answer: E

Carotid stenosis is often found by screening studies but must be confirmed by another diagnostic test before treatment. Of the options available, only repeat duplex ultrasound is a low risk diagnostic test. When a screening study is abnormal, confirmation of the findings with a repeat full-length study is often the best approach to confirm the findings. An angiogram carries a risk of stroke and has little additional information that cannot be obtained with an MR angiogram or CTA. The decision for treatment in an asymptomatic patient should be preceded by risk factor modification with low dose antiplatelet therapy, statins, and β-blockers. Carotid stent is not approved in asymptomatic patients and CEA should not be performed in asymptomatic women until their stenosis becomes >80%.

3. Answer: C

This patient has a mal perforans ulcer, which is a neuropathic ulcer on the ball of the foot due to changes in the motor, sensory, and autonomic nerves in the extremity. The absence of ulcer pain, in itself, tells you that she has a severe peripheral neuropathy. She is at risk for a major amputation unless she has adequate blood supply to heal, good local wound care with offloading of the ulcer, and then good footwear once the ulcer is healed. The presence of blood supply is critical to preventing amputation, and physical exam is not accurate for assessing perfusion, so she needs noninvasive testing, including an ABI, toe pressures, and assessment of tissue perfusion around the ulcer. If she has a significant pressure deficit in the foot, then an angioplasty or bypass is needed to provide enough blood supply to heal the ulcer. Amputation and IV antibiotics will not be effective if there is inadequate blood supply.

4. Answer: E

This patient represents a high risk for DVT post-op due to his risk factor of obesity and the procedure that he is undergoing, total hip arthroplasty. Orthopedic procedures carry one of the highest risks of DVT due to the relationship between the procedure and the deep veins and the post-op immobilization often required. Of the options presented, only low molecular weight heparin (LMWH) has been demonstrated to prevent DVT in high-risk patients. Support hose are used primarily in low risk patients. Sequential compression is useful for all patients pre- and post-op, but is not as successful in preventing DVT in high-risk procedures. A venacaval filter does not prevent DVT—it merely protects the patient from DVT progressing to pulmonary embolism. Aspirin is more effective for prevention of arterial thrombosis and has minimal effect on preventing DVT.

5. Answer: D

Based on the location and description, as well as the age of the patient and absence of significant other medical problems, this patient has chronic venous insufficiency, the pigmentation represents lipodermatosclerosis, and the venous ulcer is likely due to reflux in the superficial, perforator, and deep venous systems. An ABI is unlikely to be helpful in a woman at her age, with the ulcer in its current location. Wound cultures are helpful occasionally in management of venous ulcers, but not to diagnose them, and the location and age make both serum autoimmune disease tests and biopsies unlikely to make the diagnosis.

6. Answer: D

This patient has signs and symptoms of neurogenic TOS, which is commonly associated with physical activity and repetitive sports. Since he already exercises regularly, physical therapy (PT) is unlikely to help. He is an elite swimmer and is unlikely to give up his lifestyle unless there are no other options. Even though his pulse is diminished, this is a common finding in many patients and the primary problem is thoracic outlet compression, not intrinsic arterial disease. MRI can help determine the location of compression and other pathology, such as cervical rib. Following MRI, a first rib resection, with cervical rib removal if present, is a treatment that is likely to return him to normal function. His symptoms are primarily neurogenic, and not venous, which would be arm swelling, arm pain, and prominent veins. Therefore, venography and thrombolysis are unlikely to be needed.

23
Transplantation

HILARY SANFEY, M.D., B.CH. • MITCHELL H. GOLDMAN, M.D. •
OSCAR H. GRANDAS, M.D. • SUSAN LERNER, M.D.

Objectives

1. List the organs and tissues that are commonly transplanted, and give the statistics for graft survival for organs from living related and deceased donors for each organ.

2. List the criteria used to establish death for the purpose of organ and tissue donation.

3. Given a potential donor, list the acceptable and exclusionary criteria for the donation of each organ and tissue.

4. Define autograft, isograft, allograft, xenograft, orthotopic graft, and heterotopic graft.

5. List the current forms of immunosuppression for transplantation, and describe their mechanisms of action and specific side effects.

6. Distinguish among hyperacute, accelerated acute, acute, and chronic rejection in terms of pathophysiology, interval from transplant, histology, and prognosis.

Until the middle of the 20th century, the failure of any organ essential to life was uniformly fatal. However, technologies to sustain life despite transient organ failure were slowly developed. Two examples are early dialysis for acute renal failure and the refinement of respirators for respiratory insufficiency. The experimental techniques of organ and tissue transfer were attempted in humans, mostly in the form of kidney transplantation and skin grafting. Early attempts at kidney transplantation failed because the understanding of immunology did not evolve as rapidly as the surgical techniques for organ replacement. Now, because of improved understanding of immunology and the evolution of modern day organ and tissue preservation, end-stage failure of many organs essential to life no longer dooms the patient. In addition, tissues that are not vital to life (e.g., cornea, bone, skin, dura) can be transplanted, improving the quality of many lives.

ORGAN AND TISSUE DONATION

Organ transplantation can be a lifesaving therapy for many patients with organ failure. Organs and tissues for transplantation come from either deceased donors or living donors. Although grafts from living related donors have the advantages of increased graft survival, ready availability, and immediate graft function, deceased donors are the major sources of graft tissues. The organ donation and transplantation community in the United States continues to undergo dramatic and sustainable change for better performance and quality. The rate of growth in the yearly number of deceased donors has shown an increase since 2002 (Figure 23-1). However, the number of living donors declined during the same time period (Figure 23-1 and Table 23-1).

Between 1998 and 2002, deceased donors (at least one organ recovered) had increased at an average rate of 99 donors per year. Since 2002, the number of deceased donors increased by an average of 380 donors per year. This trend appears to have reached a plateau and the number of donors in 2007 increased by only 67 from 2006. The average increase in deceased donors contrasts with a faster increase, followed by a slower increase and then a decline in the number of living donors in the 1998 to 2007 time periods. The number of deceased donors has continued to exceed the number of living donors over the past several years. There continue to be increases in the use of organs from donors after cardiac death (DCD) and expanded criteria donors (ECD). Finally, the national transplant environment has changed in response to the increased regulatory oversight and new requirements for donation and transplant provider organizations.

The total number of organ donors has increased by 39% over the past decade (Table 23-1). This rise is most notable for an almost tenfold increase in the number of donations after cardiac death (DCD) and a threefold increase in living liver donors. Both of these factors are reflective of the need to expand the donor pool to meet the demands of an increasing recipient waiting list. Recently, there has been an acceptance of the concept of "emotionally" related or voluntary unrelated living donation of kidneys. Spouses, distant relatives, friends, and even strangers who have expressed an interest in donation without remuneration are being accepted as donors in an attempt to alleviate the shortage of donors for the growing waiting list.

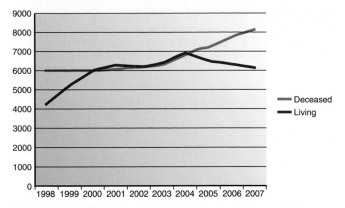

FIGURE 23-1. Total number of living and deceased donors of all organs recovered for transplant, 1998–2007. Source: 2008 OPTN/SRTR Annual Report.

TABLE 23-2	Criteria to Determine Cessation of Brain Function

Clinical Findings

In the absence of barbiturate use, hypothermia, or acute metabolic derangement:

- Absence of spontaneous respirations
- Absence of pupillary light reflex
- Absence of corneal reflex
- Sustained apnea when disconnecting respirator

Confirmatory Tests

- Cerebral angiography
- Electroencephalography
- Transcranial Doppler ultrasonography
- Cerebral scintigraphy (technetium Tc^{99m} hexametazime)

The recognition of a potential deceased donor is the initial step in organ donation. Solid organs can be transplanted if they remain perfused in situ until the time of retrieval. Therefore, any patient who has normal cardiac function and has been pronounced dead using **brain death** criteria is a potential donor. The diagnosis of **brain death** must be made before organ recovery is performed. The clinical neurologic examination remains the standard for the determination of brain death. The primary physician or a neurologic specialist usually makes

TABLE 23-1	U.S. Organ Donors by Organ and Donor Type, 1998–2007			
		1998	**2007**	**Percentage Change**
All Organs	Total	10,362	14,399	39%
	Deceased	5,793	8,091	40%
	Living	4,569	6,308	38%
Kidney	Total	9,761	13,281	36%
	Deceased	5,339	7,245	66%
	Living	4,422	6,036	36%
Pancreas	Total	1,464	1,927	32%
	Deceased	1,462	1,927	32%
	Living	2	0	–
Liver	Total	4,935	7,208	46%
	Deceased	4,843	6,942	43%
	Living	92	266	189%
Intestine	Total	80	206	126%
	Deceased	78	205	162%
	Living	2	1	
Heart	Total	2,447	2,289	–6%
	Deceased	2,447	2,289	–6%
	Living	–	–	–
Lung	Total	817	1,388	70%
	Deceased	764	1,382	81%
	Living	53	6	–9%
Donation After Cardiac Death	Total	75	793	957%

Source: OPTN/SRTR Data as of May 1, 2008.

this diagnosis. The President's Commission for the Study of Ethical Problems in Medicine and Biochemical and Behavioral Research defined brain death and endorsed criteria that are used as guidelines. These guidelines are separated into clinical criteria and confirmatory objective studies. Clinical criteria indicate that the individual is totally unresponsive to stimuli (Table 23-2). Clinical situations that mimic complete unresponsiveness (e.g., barbiturate or opiate overdose, profound hypothermia) must be excluded or corrected. Confirmatory studies support the diagnosis of brain death, but this diagnosis may be made by clinical criteria only. Evaluation of the potential donor requires serial observations over a period of 6 to 24 hours. During this time, referral by the primary hospital staff to the organ procurement organization is initiated.

The most rapid increase in the rate of organ recovery from deceased persons has occurred in the category of donation after "cardiac death," that is, a death declared on the basis of cardiopulmonary criteria (irreversible cessation of circulatory and respiratory function) rather than the neurologic criteria used to declare "brain death" (irreversible loss of all functions of the entire brain, including the brain stem). The United Network for Organ Sharing (UNOS), a private nonprofit group based in Richmond, Virginia, operates the Organ Procurement and Transplantation Network (OPTN) under contract with the federal government and is committed to increasing the number of donors. OPTN/UNOS, as the networks are collectively known, have developed rules for donation after cardiac death. According to these rules, finalized in March 2007, the process begins with the selection of a suitable candidate and the consent of the legal next of kin to the withdrawal of care and retrieval of organs. Subsequently, life-sustaining measures are withdrawn under controlled circumstances in the intensive care unit (ICU) or the operating room; organ donation after an unexpected fatal cardiac arrest is rare. When the potential donor meets the criteria for cardiac death, a physician unconnected with the transplant team pronounces the patient dead. The time from the onset of asystole to the declaration of death is generally 5 minutes. The organs most commonly recovered are the kidneys and liver but occasionally the pancreas, lungs, and, in very rare cases, the heart are recovered. To avoid obvious conflicts of interest, neither the surgeon who recovers the organs nor any other personnel involved in transplantation can participate in end-of-life care or the declaration of death.

The outcomes for organs transplanted after cardiac death are similar to those for organs transplanted after brain death. However, the length of time varies as to which organs can be subjected to cessation of circulation to the initiation of perfusion with cold preservation solutions and still be transplanted successfully. It is best to retrieve the liver <30 minutes after the withdrawal of life-sustaining measures; the kidneys and pancreas may often be recovered up to 60 minutes after such withdrawal. If a patient does not die in a suitable time frame to permit organ recovery, end-of-life care continues and donation is canceled. This may happen in up to 20% of cases.

Eligible donors are previously healthy people who have sustained irreversible central nervous system injury as a result of trauma, cerebrovascular accident, central nervous system tumors, or cerebral anoxia. Contraindications to donation include organ-specific chronic medical problems, malignancy other than primary brain tumors, cardiac arrest that causes prolonged warm ischemia of organs, uncontrolled infection, and HIV infection. Transplantation of livers (with normal biopsies) and kidneys from hepatitis B core (HBc) Ab+ donors into recipients with appropriate serologic and viral profiles poses minimal risk of posttransplantation morbidity and mortality from viral transmission or disease. Similarly, organs (even livers with normal biopsies) can be recovered and transplanted from donors who are hepatitis C virus (HCV) Ab+. The Federal Centers for Disease Control advise against using individuals as donors whose history or behavior makes them high risk for having transmissible disease, except in emergency situations. Individuals who indulge in risky sexual behavior, who use intravenous drugs, or who have been recently incarcerated in correctional institutions are considered high risk for harboring transmissible disease. Expanded criteria for kidney donors are those older than 60 years of age and with a history of hypertension, cerebrovascular accident as a cause of death, and a final preprocurement creatinine level of >1.5 mg/dL.

Age is a relative contraindication to donation. Acute or chronic diseases that affect certain organs may exclude them from consideration. Preexisting renal disease excludes kidney donation, and diabetes mellitus precludes pancreatic donation. Cardiac trauma, coronary artery disease, pneumonia, and advanced age exclude cardiac and heart–lung donation. Donors who are older than 35 to 40 years of age may require coronary catheterization to rule out significant cardiac disease. Pulmonary trauma, pneumonia, and respiratory compromise preclude lung donation. Bronchoscopy may be required to rule out infection. Minimal hypertension may not be a contraindication to kidney donation, although severe hypertension is an absolute contraindication to cardiac or renal donation. Laboratory studies and biopsy are useful to determine the acceptability of donor organs (Table 23-3). Organs (even livers) from donors with a history of hepatitis B may be used in selected cases where the recipient has antibody protection, or is in life-threatening need of an organ transplant.

Consent for organ or tissue donation is obtained through a signed donor card, the appropriate driver's license designation, a consent statement, or a will. The U.S. system of organ donation relies on obtaining written consent for donation from next of kin, in the absence of a signed donor card or driver's license. If a medical examiner is involved, permission may also be required from the medical examiner. Public education efforts emphasize the fact that the optimal situation for organ donation occurs when the family has previously discussed and agreed on organ donation.

TABLE 23-3	Laboratory Studies Used to Determine Acceptability of Organs for Transplantation
Laboratory Study	**Evaluated Organ**
Cardiac catheterization, echocardiogram	Heart, heart–lung
Electrocardiogram	—
Chest radiograph	—
Creatinine phosphokinase with MB bands	—
Bronchoscopy	Lung
BUN, creatinine	Kidney
Glucose	Pancreas
Liver Function Tests	Liver
Blood, urine, sputum culture	All
Hepatitis screen	—
Serologic test for syphilis	—
HIV	—
Blood group	—

Donor Management

After the donor is declared brain dead, treatment is directed toward optimizing organ function. Ventilation is maintained with a mechanical respirator, and arterial blood gases are monitored. Because many patients who have closed head injuries are purposefully dehydrated to decrease cerebral edema, vigorous rehydration may be necessary. Donors who have massive diuresis because of diabetes insipidus may require vasopressin. If vigorous hydration with crystalloid or colloid is inadequate to maintain end organ perfusion, a vasopressor (dopamine or dobutamine) is used. Vasoconstrictors are avoided because of their vasospastic effect on the renal and splanchnic beds. Monitoring of cardiac and pulmonary function is imperative when a heart, heart–lung, or lung donation is considered. Bone, skin, dura, fascia, and cornea donors do not need a functioning cardiovascular system, and the corresponding tissue can be procured 12 to 24 hours after the cessation of cardiac and respiratory function.

Organ Preservation

Effective preservation of whole organs after recovery enhances the success of deceased donor transplantation by providing time for distant transplant centers to retrieve the needed organs, perform precise tissue typing and cross matching between donor and recipient, prepare the recipient, and work with national and international organ sharing programs. The most critical steps in the preservation of solid organs are rapid organ cooling and sterile storage in a cold environment.

The kidney, heart, lung, liver, and pancreas are routinely flushed in situ with a cold solution to stop metabolism rapidly. Usually, hyperosmotic (325 to 420 mOsm/L) or hyperkalemic solutions are used. In some situations, a colloid is added. The organs are subsequently removed, individually packaged in sterile containers, and placed in ice. Hypothermic (7°C to 10°C) continuous pulsatile machine perfusion with a colloid solution is used to extend renal preservation time. Pulsatile machine preservation is sometimes administered with an apparatus that includes a pulsatile pump, a membrane oxygenator, and tubing connected to the renal artery. The colloid solution is continuously recirculated. Cryopreservation with cryoprotectants (e.g., glycerin, dimethyl sulfoxide) and lyophilization (freeze-drying) are useful in preserving skin, skeletal, and scleral tissues. Nutrient media and normothermic or hypothermic preservation are used with cornea, skin, cartilage, and bone.

Organ and Tissue Allocation

After organs and tissues are recovered from a deceased donor, UNOS, the national allocation system, distributes the organs appropriately. All donors are registered with UNOS. As organs become available, the computer listing process matches the patients on the waiting list and the organs according to ABO compatibility. In addition, kidneys and kidney–pancreas combinations are distributed according to human leukocyte antigen (HLA) match and waiting time. Hearts, livers, and lungs are primarily shared on the basis of ABO match. In addition, the Model for End Stage Liver Disease (MELD) score is used for liver allocation (see Chapter 18, Liver). However, the seriousness of the recipient's condition, distance from the donor center, size match, and waiting time are also used to determine which ABO-matched recipient has priority. The national program allows sharing of these scarce resources equitably while balancing medical and ethical issues.

Tissues and cornea are distributed through appropriate local and national banking systems. The allocation of musculoskeletal tissue is different because several tissues can be banked for long periods. Therefore, tissue allocation is managed through tissue banks that have a variety of tissues "on the shelf." Centers that perform tissue transplantation can obtain the necessary tissues as specific needs arise. There is no national computer system similar to UNOS for tissue allocation. However, standards for tissue procurement, processing, storage, and distribution have been established by the American Association of Tissue Banks and the Food and Drug Administration. Distribution of corneal grafts is based on local waiting lists. For bone marrow, there is a national computer network of living donors that allows volunteers to donate perfectly matched bone marrow to those in need.

IMMUNOLOGY

Transplantation involves a surgical procedure that transfers tissue from one site to another in the same individual or between different individuals. This tissue transfer can take a number of forms. An **autograft** is transplanted from one site of the body to another in the same individual (e.g., skin graft removed from the leg and placed on a wound elsewhere). An **isograft** is transferred between genetically identical individuals (e.g., renal transplant between monozygotic twins). An **allograft** is transplanted between genetically dissimilar individuals of the same species (e.g., deceased donor renal transplant). A **xenograft** is tissue that is transferred between different species (e.g., porcine skin grafted onto a human burn victim). An **orthotopic** graft involves placement of an organ in the normal anatomic position. An orthotopic graft usually necessitates removal of the native organ (e.g., cardiac or liver transplantation). A **heterotopic graft** involves placement of an organ at a site different from its normal anatomic position (e.g., kidney).

Components of the Immune System

The immune system is composed of cellular (T cells) and humoral (B cells/antibodies) components. T cells are derived from the thymus and play a central role in cellular immunity. They can be divided into CD4 and CD8 T cells and can recognize antigens presented by the major histocompatibility complex (also called HLA), through T cell receptors (TCRs) expressed on their cell surface. B cells express a highly specialized form of antigen receptors, known as surface immunoglobulins, and are the precursors of plasma cells, which can secrete a soluble form of immunoglobulin, the antibody.

The highly polymorphic HLA loci are the primary targets of the alloimmune response. These genetic loci are located on the short arm of the sixth chromosome and are responsible for two classes of histocompatibility molecules. Class I antigens are single chain glycoproteins and are cataloged as HLA, B, or C. These antigens are expressed on essentially all somatic cells and are recognized by CD8 T cells. Class II antigens are glycoproteins that have two polymeric chains, each with a common subunit. These antigens are present on B cells, dendritic cells, activated T cells, endothelial cells, and monocytes. Several series are found within this HLA locus, including the HLA–D locus and the HLA-Dr, Dq, and Dp loci. These Class II HLA molecules are recognized by CD4 T cells.

The subloci are genetically transferred as haplotypes on a single segment of chromosome. Thus, a recipient shares one of two haplotypes with each parent. According to Mendelian genetics, a recipient has a 25% chance of sharing two haplotypes (called HLA identical), a 50% chance of sharing one haplotype, and a 25% chance of not sharing a haplotype with a sibling. Unrelated individuals randomly share similar antigens.

Antibodies may be present at birth (e.g., ABO blood group antibodies), or they may be acquired. Successful transplantation requires transplantation of ABO blood group compatible organs. Unless transplantation occurs as part of a donor-incompatible protocol with recipient pretreatment, transplantation of incompatible organs that express ABO antigens (e.g., kidney, heart) results in antibody-mediated killing of the endothelium leading to thrombosis and organ necrosis, (**hyperacute rejection**). Donor-specific anti-HLA antibodies (DSAs) can be present in a patient before transplantation due to sensitization events (e.g. previously failed allograft, blood transfusion, or pregnancy). The presence of pretransplant DSAs can predispose kidney grafts to a higher risk of acute and chronic antibody-mediated rejection.

Cross Match

Sera from prospective transplant recipients are routinely screened for the presence of preformed anti-HLA antibodies to determine the extent of alloimmunization. The screening is performed against a panel of cells, representing most antigens encountered in the general population. A complement-dependent cytotoxicity assay (CDC) is utilized. Lymphocytes from a panel of donors are mixed with the sera of the recipient and complement is added to determine whether the recipient has antibodies that bind to the donor cells and thus activate complement. The results are reported as a percentage of panel cells that are killed by reacting with the anti-HLA antibodies in a patients' serum, thus the term Panel Reactive Antibody (PRA). The same technique has been used for cross-matching recipients against potential donors to determine their suitability.

The pretransplantation crossmatch test is the final immunologic screening step. Using the previously described HLA antibody screening assays, the potential donor's lymphocytes serve as the target cells for the patient's serum. There are two types of CDC crossmatch that depend on the type of donor lymphocytes that are used (T and B cells). A positive T-cell CDC crossmatch is an absolute contraindication to kidney transplantation. A more sensitive technique is the flow cytometry crossmatch, which can detect very low levels of circulating antibodies. Patient sera are incubated with donor lymphocytes and stained with fluorescence-labeled anti-CD3 (T cell marker) and anti-CD19 (B cell marker). Positive flow cytometry crossmatches have been associated with a higher rate of early acute rejection. If certain organs are transplanted in the presence of a positive crossmatch, circulating anti-HLA antibodies attach to the endothelium of the donor organ. The effects of circulating preformed antibodies may be neutralized with the use of plasmapheresis and infusion of IV immunoglobulin G (IgG). ABO matching and cross-matching are the most common tests performed before transplantation. Bone, skin, dura, and other cryopreserved or lyophilized tissues usually do not require ABO typing and cross-matching because their immunogenic activity is very weak after preservation.

Immunologic Events after Transplantation

Transplantation tolerance is defined as immune unresponsiveness to graft alloantigens in the absence of ongoing therapy, but not to other (third-party) antigens. The functional characteristics of tolerance are lack of demonstrable immune reactivity to donor graft alloantigens, presence of immune reactivity to other alloantigens, and absence of generalized immunosuppression for graft maintenance (Table 23-4).

Rejection is an immunologic attempt to destroy foreign tissue after transplantation. It is a complex and incompletely understood event. Four types of clinically identified rejection occur. The forms of allograft rejection are classified according to the time of occurrence and the immune mechanism involved.

Hyperacute rejection occurs soon (minutes to several hours) after graft implantation. The organ becomes flaccid, cyanotic, and, in the case of the kidney, anuric. Histologically, polymorphonuclear leukocytes are packed in the pericapillary area, and endothelial necrosis with vascular thrombosis occurs. Hyperacute rejection is associated with preformed antibodies in the recipient directed toward either ABO blood group or HLA antigens. It rarely occurs today because of the practice of cross-matching and blood group matching (Table 23-4).

Accelerated acute rejection occurs during the first several days after transplantation. In the kidney, it is characterized by oliguria and may be accompanied by disseminated intravascular coagulation, thrombocytopenia, and hemolysis. The organ becomes swollen, tender, and congested. Histologically, extensive arteriolar necrosis and perivasculitis are present. Monocyte/macrophage infiltration of renal allografts has been shown to adversely affect graft survival. Intense CD4 deposition in the glomerular basement membrane and peritubular capillaries can be found by immunofluorescence staining. This type of rejection is believed to represent an immunologic memory response to prior sensitization.

Usually, the antibody crossmatch is negative, but may become positive after rejection occurs. A preformed antibody may be present at a low or undetectable level that produces a negative pretransplant crossmatch. This type of rejection is rare, and is difficult to control with current immunosuppressive regimens and may contribute to early graft loss. Even with the use of modern immunosuppressive therapy, acute rejection can occur in all deceased organ transplants. It may even occur in well-matched living related donor kidney transplants. Microscopically, T cell infiltration occurs into vascular and interstitial spaces. The presence of dense clusters of B cells may be strongly associated with severe graft rejection, suggesting a pivotal role of infiltrating B cells in acute rejection. In the kidney, glomeruli are often spared relative to other regions. In the heart, the infiltrate is usually pericapillary and is associated with interstitial edema and myonecrosis. In the liver, the infiltrate is often seen in the area of the portal triad. In the lung, bronchiolitis occurs.

TABLE 23-4	Rejection: General Pathology		
Rejection Type	**Time**	**Pathology**	**Treatment**
Hyperacute	Immediately to hours	Swollen, edematous organ Antibody-mediated vascular thrombosis and necrosis Polymorphonuclear infiltrates	Usually prevented by cross-matching and blood group matching
Accelerated	2–5 days	Swollen, edematous organ Arterial necrosis Vasculitis Lymphocyte infiltration	No effective treatment
Acute	7–10 days; may recur during subsequent years	Mononuclear cell infiltration into vascular and interstitial spaces	Increased immuno-suppression or change to different regimen
Chronic	Years	Obliterative vasculopathy Relentless deterioration Glomerular sclerosis, tubular atrophy, and interstitial fibrosis (kidney)	No effective treatment
		Myocardial fibrosis and coronary obliteration (heart)	—
		Progressive bile duct loss (liver)	—
		Bronchiectasis, pleural thickening (lung)	—

TABLE 23-5	Clinically Available Immunosuppressive Agents and Techniques in Organ Transplantation

Pharmacologic	Biologic
Azathioprine	Polyclonal sera
Cyclosporine	Monoclonal sera
Tacrolimus	Daclizumab
Sirolimus	Basiliximab
Steroids	
Mycophenolate mofetil	

Acute rejection is treated with increased doses of immunosuppression. If it is reversed, the patient has an excellent chance of retaining the graft.

Chronic rejection is a slow, progressive immunologic process that occurs over a period of months to years. It is characterized by vascular intimal hyperplasia, lymphocytic infiltration, and atrophy and fibrosis of renal, cardiac, or hepatic tissue. Chronic rejection is mediated by both immune and nonimmune mechanisms through poorly understood mechanisms. The healing process after repeated episodes of acute rejection, chronic graft injury by a delayed type of hypersensitivity response, chronic ischemia, antibody formation, calcineurin-inhibitor toxicity, and enhanced transforming growth factor (TGF)-β production have been proposed as alternative stimuli for the development of chronic allograft dysfunction. In the kidney, this injury is now described as "interstitial fibrosis with tubular atrophy" (IFTA).

Immunosuppressive Drug Therapy

All recipients of allografts require immunosuppressive therapy. The sole exception is a patient who receives a transplanted organ from an identical monozygotic twin (isograft).

Because of their lack of lymphatic drainage, the eyes are an immune-privileged site. Thus, matching and systemic immunosuppression are rarely required for corneal transplants. However, when rejection occurs, topical steroids are used. The role of immunosuppression is twofold: (1) to provide maintenance suppression of the immune system to prevent rejection and (2) to treat episodes of rejection if the recipient "breaks through" the maintenance program. Immunosuppressive agents are classified as biologic or pharmacologic (Table 23-5).

Immunosuppressive agents are usually used in combination, because no single agent or technique provides adequate therapy. For this reason, agents are often chosen to modulate the immune system at various times after transplantation and to complement each other by suppressing the immune system at different levels or by different mechanisms. Multimodal therapy reduces the toxicity and side effects of individual drugs by enabling lower doses of each while still maintaining an adequate level of immunosuppression (Table 23-6).

Pharmacologic Agents

Pharmacologic agents can be classified as corticosteroids, calcineurin inhibitors, inhibitors of nucleotide metabolism, inhibitors of the protein TOR (target of rapamycin), or lymphocyte-trafficking modulators. The most commonly used immunosuppressive agents are corticosteroids (prednisone, methylprednisolone). These compounds are used to provide maintenance immunosuppression and, in higher doses, to treat rejection. Glucocorticoids bind to a cytosolic receptor that translocates to the nucleus, where the complex binds to DNA regulatory sequences. Glucocorticoids decrease the transcription of key cytokines. Steroids are lympholytic—they kill T and B cells and inhibit the release of interleukin-1 from macrophages. Prednisone is the most common steroid preparation used in transplantation. Steroids are initially given at high doses intravenously during the transplant surgery and then tapered to 5 to 10 mg/day at 2 to 3 months after transplantation. The complications of steroid use are variable

TABLE 23-6	Drugs Used for Immunosuppression

Name	Use	Mechanism of Action	Side Effects
Corticosteroids	Maintenance, rejection therapy	Lympholysis, inhibition of IL-1 release	Cushing's syndrome, dyspepsia, HTN osteonecrosis, post-transplant diabetes mellitus
Azathioprine (Imuran)	Maintenance	Inhibition of nucleic acid synthesis	Bone marrow depression, veno-occlusive hepatic disease, arthralgias, pancreatitis, red cell aplasia
Cyclosporine (Sandimmune, Neoral, Gengraf)	Maintenance	Inhibition of secretion and formation of IL-2 (by inhibiting calcineurin)	Nephrotoxicity, hypertension, hyperkalemia, hepatotoxicity, hirsutism, gingival hyperplasia, tremors
Tacrolimus (FK-506, Prograf)	Maintenance, treatment of refractory rejection	Inhibition of production of IL-2	Nephrotoxicity, glucose intolerance, neurotoxicity
Mycophenolate mofetil (CellCept)	Maintenance	Inhibition of inosine monophosphate dehydrogenase	Gastrointestinal intolerance, neutropenia
Sirolimus	Maintenance	Inhibitor TOR	Neutropenia, dyslipidemia, impaired wound healing
OKT3 (monoclonal antibody)	Treatment of rejection	Depletion of T cells Modulation of CD receptor from surface of T cells	Fever, chills, pulmonary edema, lymphoproliferative disorder
Polyclonal antilymphocyte	Induction therapy	Depletion of lymphocytes Treatment of rejection	Anaphylaxis, fever, leukopenia, thrombocytopenia, lymphoproliferative disorders, cytokine-20 release syndrome
Daclizumab, basiliximab	Induction therapy	Block IL-2 receptor	Minimal

and include dyspepsia, cataracts, osteonecrosis, Cushing's syndrome, acne, capillary fragility, and glucose intolerance. There are some protocols in effect that eliminate steroids after a period of posttransplant therapy.

Cyclosporine (CsA, Sandimmune, Neoral, and Gengraf) is a calcineurin inhibitor. It inhibits the expression of multiple genes involved in T cell activation and proliferation, including IL-2 and other lymphokines. CsA binds to a cytoplasmic immunophilin called cyclophilin, thereby producing a complex that inhibits the calcium-sensitive phosphatase calcineurin. It ultimately prevents the proliferation and maturation of cytotoxic T cells that cause graft rejection. This drug is a potent immunosuppressant and is used for maintenance therapy in combination with other agents. It is not effective in the treatment of rejection. Complications include dose-dependent nephrotoxicity, hyperlipidemia, hyperuricemia, hepatotoxicity, hyperkalemia, hypertension, gingival hyperplasia, tremors, and hirsutism. Whole blood levels of cyclosporine are routinely monitored to ensure maximal therapeutic benefit and minimize complications.

Since cyclosporine is metabolized in the liver by the cytochrome P_{450} system, liver disease and drugs that interact with or are metabolized competitively by that system should be monitored closely for effects on cyclosporine levels and toxicity as well as for their own toxicities. Examples of such drugs are barbiturates, phenytoin, imidazole antifungals, macrolide antibiotics, and rifampin.

Tacrolimus (FK506, Prograf) is a macrolide antibiotic. Its mechanism of action is similar to that of cyclosporine (inhibiting the production of interleukin-2 and other cytokines) except it binds to the FK-binding protein. It is more potent than cyclosporine and is now the predominantly used calcineurin inhibitor in the United States. It is used for maintenance immunosuppression in combination with steroids and azathioprine (or mycophenolate mofetil). Its side effects include dose-dependent nephrotoxicity, glucose intolerance, infections, and alopecia. As with cyclosporine, drug monitoring is essential, and P_{450} interacting drugs should be carefully scrutinized.

Azathioprine (Imuran) is an antimetabolite. It is metabolized to its active form, 6-mercaptopurine, by the liver. It acts principally to inhibit the synthesis of nucleic acid. Therefore, it is a relatively nonspecific agent, and it affects all replicating cells of the body. Its major side effect is bone marrow depression manifested by leukopenia and thrombocytopenia. These effects are dose dependent. Other side effects include veno-occlusive hepatic disease, arthralgias, pancreatitis, and red cell aplasia. It is used for baseline immunosuppression but never to treat rejection directly. It is always used with other immunosuppressants. Recently, it has been replaced by mycophenolate mofetil (MMF).

MMF (CellCept) was approved for clinical transplantation in 1995. Its mechanism of action differs from that of the other compounds; it is a noncompetitive, reversible inhibitor of inosine monophosphate dehydrogenase (the enzyme necessary to convert inosine monophosphate to guanosine monophosphate) and is a specific T- and B-cell antimetabolite. Because only lymphocytes require the de novo synthesis of guanosine monophosphate, MMF profoundly inhibits T- and B-cell function. This drug is used in combination with steroids and cyclosporine or tacrolimus for maintenance therapy. The compound is particularly effective in transplant populations that are at high risk for rejection (e.g., African Americans, children, previously transplanted patients). Its major side effect is gastrointestinal intolerance and bone marrow suppression.

Sirolimus or rapamycin (Rapamune) is a macrolide antifungal that interferes with the intracellular signaling pathways of the IL-2–dependent clonal expansion of activated T lymphocytes. Like the calcineurin inhibitors, it binds to a cytoplasm binding protein (FKBP). The ligand engages a protein, TOR, a key regulatory kinase, which, once inhibited, reduces cytokine-dependent cellular proliferation. Sirolimus is approved as an adjunctive agent in combination with prednisone and calcineurin inhibitors. The major side effects seem to be impaired wound healing, myelosuppression, and hyperlipidemia. There is also evidence of pulmonary toxicity, proteinuria, and painful oral ulcers.

Biologic Agents

Biologic agents are either polyclonal or monoclonal sera that are prepared by immunizing an animal (e.g., horse, rabbit, mouse, and rat) with human lymphocytes or thymocytes. The polyclonal sera antithymocyte globulin (Thymoglobulin) and antilymphocyte globulin (ATGAM) are beneficial when used as induction therapy during the first 1 or 2 weeks of therapy for solid organ transplant recipients or to treat acute cellular rejection. Induction agents are given in the early peritransplantation period to decrease the risk of acute rejection and possibly of delayed graft function. These agents are generally given to immunologically high-risk patients and those patients receiving early steroid withdrawal. These preparations are usually given intravenously and are never used for maintenance therapy. Monoclonal antibodies have been prepared against various cell surface receptors on the T cell and are directed against specific T-cell subsets, not against the entire T- or B-cell population. One of these antibodies, OKT3, is directed against the CD3 receptor on the T cell and is used for prophylactic induction therapy as well as for treatment of acute cellular rejection. The humanized anti-TAC (anti-CD25) monoclonal antibody preparations, daclizumab (Zenapax) and basiliximab (Simulect), block the IL-2 receptor, which is composed of upregulated inactivated T cells.

New Immunosuppressive Drugs

Several compounds are currently under development. Some modify currently used immunosuppressants, minimizing their side effects or improving their pharmacologic characteristics; others have a novel mechanism of action. Everolimus (SDZ-RAD) is a derivative of Sirolimus with improved oral bioavailability. Campath-1H (Alemtuzumab), a humanized anti-CD52 monoclonal antibody that depletes T and B lymphocytes, natural killer cells, and some monocytes and macrophages, has been tested in renal transplantation in humans in combination with cyclosporine monotherapy with good results. CTLA4-Ig, a fusion protein, blocks CD28-mediated costimulatory signals and prolongs graft survival or introduces long-term graft acceptance in several animal models.

Currently, six new agents, three small molecules (ISA247, a semi synthetic analogue of cyclosporine; AEB071, a protein kinase C isoforms inhibitor; CP 690,550, a selective Janus kinase inhibitor) are in phase II trials and three biologics (belatacept, a second generation CTLA4Ig; efalizumab, a humanized antiCD11a [LFA1] monoclonal antibody; and alefacept, a LFA3-IgG1 fusion receptor protein) are in phase II/III clinical trials.

The success of a graft depends on the degree of genetic similarity between the organ and the host, on the ischemia reperfusion injury induced by the cold storage, and on the effectiveness of the immunosuppressive means used to alter host response.

END-STAGE RENAL DISEASE AND KIDNEY TRANSPLANTATION

Dialysis

Treatment of end-stage renal failure often involves long-term hemodialysis or peritoneal dialysis to maintain life. Because of the availability of maintenance dialysis, kidney transplantation is usually a nonemergency procedure that allows tissue typing and matching, long-term survival without transplant and survival after transplant rejection. The principle of dialysis is simple: on one side of the semipermeable membrane is the extracellular fluid of the patient; on the other side of the membrane is the material that is to be discarded. Products of normal metabolism that are not excreted by the failed kidney accumulate in the extracellular fluid, pass through the semipermeable membrane to the dialysate solution, and are discarded. Hemodialysis requires connection of the patient's vascular space to a dialysis machine. In acute situations, large cannulae are inserted into the venous circulation through the femoral, jugular, or subclavian veins. For long-term hemodialysis, permanent access to the circulation is achieved by the creation of an autologous arteriovenous fistula, connecting an artery to a vein in an easily accessible and reusable area (e.g., radial artery and cephalic vein just above the anteromedial elbow joint). A vascular bridging conduit of polytetrafluoroethylene (PTFE) graft may be placed in a subcutaneous tunnel, with one end sewn to an artery and the other to a vein to provide a large caliber shunt for hemodialysis. In peritoneal dialysis, access to the peritoneal membrane requires a transabdominal-indwelling catheter that is used for infusion and drainage of dialysate fluid. Most procedures to place hemodialysis and peritoneal catheters are performed under local anesthesia.

Patients on dialysis who await a transplant for 2 years have a three times greater chance of losing their new kidneys than do those who wait <6 months. Those on dialysis the longest often are sicker at the time of the transplantation and thus will not do as well as those who are on dialysis for a short time. There is 22% mortality in the first year of dialysis and 60% mortality in 5 years. For patients on dialysis, the longer the wait, the more complications they develop. There are more than 88,000 people waiting for renal transplants. In 2008, there were 10,552 deceased donor renal transplants and 5,969 living donor renal transplants. Most patients who undergo kidney transplantation have to wait up to 3 to 7 years for transplant depending on their location. Renal transplantation is associated with a significantly improved survival compared with hemodialysis in patients with end-stage renal disease. This seems to be a result of a reduced incidence of cardiovascular complications after renal transplantation compared to those remaining on dialysis.

Indications for Transplant

Renal transplantation is regarded by most physicians as the preferred treatment for chronic renal failure. Transplantation is life saving and more cost-effective than other modalities of renal-replacement therapy. According to the UNOS, the 1-year graft survival rate for a living donor renal transplant is 96.4% and for a deceased donor transplant is 91.3%. The recipient mortality in the first year was <5%. Rejection and the donor shortage are the major obstacles to the routine application of renal transplantation. A patient who has end-stage renal failure from any cause may be a candidate for transplant, regardless of the type or duration of dialysis support required. The acceptable age range for kidney recipients is 1 to 70 years, although infants and patients who are older than 70 years of age can be successfully transplanted. The patient should be currently free of infections and free of cancer for at least 5 years. Patients with localized cancers (e.g., skin cancer) may undergo transplantation after successful excision of the lesion. Other chronic disease processes should be minor, self-limited, or under control (e.g., a patient with known coronary artery disease should be optimally treated and show cardiovascular stability before undergoing renal transplantation).

Transplant Procedure

The renal graft is usually transplanted heterotopically in the extraperitoneal iliac fossa of the pelvis (Figure 23-2). In most cases, the native kidneys are left intact. General endotracheal anesthesia is induced with the patient in the supine position on the operating table. A urinary balloon catheter is inserted. The bladder can be filled with antibiotic solution, which is left indwelling, or the Foley catheter can be attached to a Y-connector and irrigation system so the bladder can be filled. Intraoperative monitoring may include a central venous pressure catheter, pulse oximetry, and/or arterial blood pressure line. A curvilinear incision is made in either the right or left lower abdomen. The extraperitoneal iliac fossa is used because of the presence of the iliac vessels and its proximity to the urinary bladder. The transplant is protected by the iliac bone posterolaterally and the abdominal musculature anteriorly; yet the graft is superficial enough for percutaneous biopsy. The right side is generally preferred as the external iliac vessels are more superficial on this side. In theory, the renal graft can be transplanted anywhere that there is a suitable recipient artery, vein, and urine conduit or reservoir.

Three layers of the abdominal wall—the external oblique, internal oblique, and transversus abdominis—are divided to afford access to the iliac fossa. The inferior epigastric vessels are divided and a long stump of the inferior epigastric artery is preserved in case it may be necessary to use in a separate anastomosis to a lower pole renal artery. The spermatic cord is preserved in men, and in women, the round ligament is divided. The diaphanous peritoneal membrane is rolled medially off the external iliac vessels. Lymphatic channels that overlie the iliac vessels are divided to expose the artery and vein. These channels are ligated to prevent lymphatic leaks, lymphocele formation, and subsequent ureteral obstruction or iliac vein compression. It is common practice to anastomose the transplant artery end-to-side on the external iliac artery. If multiple arteries are present, they can be reconstructed in several ways. They can be syndactalized, the inferior epigastric artery can be utilized as mentioned earlier, or they can be sewn in on a common aortic patch. The renal vein is routinely sewn to the side of the external iliac vein. The left donor kidney is generally preferred because of its longer vein; however, a short right renal vein of a deceased-donor kidney can be extended using the attached inferior vena cava. In the case of multiple draining renal veins, the decision must be made as to whether to implant both veins separately, leave them on a common caval patch, or ligate the smaller of the veins. Since venous drainage is not segmental, unlike arterial inflow, it is usually safe to ligate smaller veins. The clamps are then removed and

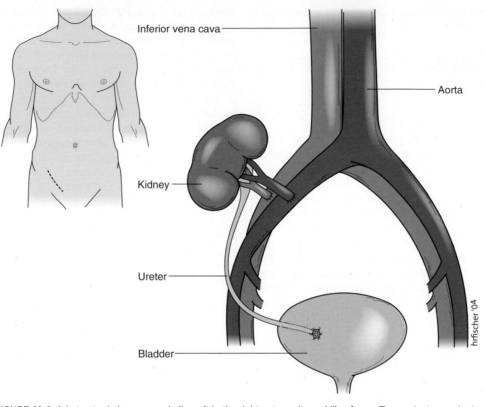

FIGURE 23-2. A heterotopic human renal allograft in the right extraperitoneal iliac fossa. The renal artery and vein anastomoses are end to side, respectively, to the common iliac artery and vein. A tunneled ureteroneocystostomy allows normal micturition.

reperfusion begins. The time that transpires between removing the graft from ice and reperfusion with oxygenated blood is known as the "warm ischemia time." This period ranges from 20 to 45 minutes. Warm ischemia time longer than 45 minutes is associated with increased incidence of delayed graft function and longer than 60 minutes may promote primary nonfunction.

Urinary drainage from the renal graft is established by surgically connecting the graft ureter to the bladder. The ureteroneocystostomy is usually accomplished via the extravesical approach, whereby the spatulated end of the transplant ureter is sewn to the bladder, mucosa to mucosa, after incision through the detrusor muscle. The detrusor muscle is then reunited to buttress the anastomosis and create an antireflux valve (an extravesical Lich-Gregoire ureteroneocystostomy). A double pigtail ureteral stent is sometimes placed to prevent ureteric complications. The stent is then endoscopically removed several weeks later. There are some complications associated with stents, for example, an increase in the incidence of urinary tract infections, calcification, and stent migration. As a result, studies now support a practice of selective stenting based on the surgeon's judgment (e.g., for anastomoses that are technically difficult, contracted bladder, or friable mucosa.)

Complications

Wound infection is the most common complication after renal transplantation (Table 23-7). Contributory factors include obesity, diabetes, uremia with protein malnutrition, and immunosuppression. Typically, the characteristic findings of fever, local erythema, swelling, and drainage present 4 to 7 days after surgery. The prevalence of thrombosis of the transplant artery or vein is 1%. Clinically, acute anuria raises the concern for the presence of graft thrombosis. Doppler ultrasonography or radionuclide scanning show greatly decreased or no flow to the graft. If the index of suspicion for thrombosis is high—for example, an uneventful live donor graft that does not diurese postoperatively—the patient should be taken back to the operating room for immediate exploration. Characteristically, "surgical" bleeding—requiring a return to the operating room—presents in the early postoperative period with tachycardia, hypotension, and, after volume resuscitation, a falling hematocrit. Bleeding is more likely in renal transplant recipients than normal patients because of decreased platelet adhesiveness secondary to uremia. The prevalence of urine leak is approximately 2%. A large urine leak at the ureter-to-bladder anastomosis due to a technical flaw results in a rapid fall-off in urine output in the early postoperative period. Ureteral necrosis and leak may be due to procurement errors (e.g., degloving) or ischemia from rejection-induced vasculitis and thrombosis of periureteral blood supply. Obstruction occurs in about 2% of renal transplants. Decompression can be accomplished by percutaneous, endourological, open operative approaches, or a combination of modalities. Nonrenal early complications include infections and cardiovascular events (e.g., postoperative myocardial infarction, cerebrovascular accident, deep vein thrombosis). Kidney transplant recipients are usually treated prophylactically for ulcer disease with an H_2 receptor blocker. Infections are the most common complications (see Figure 23-3 for timing of infections in relation to transplantation). They may be common (e.g., pneumococcal pneumonia) or unusual (e.g., necrotizing fasciitis from a rare fungus). Organisms that cause clinical infection in the

TABLE 23-7	Complications of Renal Transplantation	
Type	**Early**	**Late**
Renal	Massive diuresis	Ureteric stenosis
	Ureter anastomotic leak	Vascular anastomotic stenosis
	Hemorrhage	Recurrent primary renal disease
	Lymphocele	Rejection
	Rupture	Neoplasia
	Thrombosis	
Nonrenal	Infection	Infection
	Myocardial infarction	Progressive atherosclerotic vascular disorders, hypertension
	Diabetes mellitus	
	Steroid-induced acne	Hepatic disease
	Peptic ulcer disease	Thromboembolic disorders Cushing's syndrome
		Aseptic joint necrosis
		Cataract
		Posttransplant lymphoproliferative disorder

immunosuppressed host include cytomegalovirus (CMV), common bacteria, fungi, and protozoa such as *Pneumocystis (carinii) jiroveci*. For this reason, all patients receive antifungals and trimethoprim sulfamethoxazole (for *Pneumocystis* prophylaxis). CMV infection is one of the most common infections posttransplant. It is manifested by fever, malaise, weakness, gastrointestinal bleeding, and esophagitis. The disease results from the infection of a seronegative recipient by a positive donor or from reactivation of the recipient endogenous viral load by excessive immunosuppression, especially in the context of biologic agents. Prophylactic therapy with Valganciclovir is commonly used.

Prognosis

The results of kidney transplantation have improved since 1975. Functional graft survival rates of 80% to 88% for deceased kidneys and 95% for living related donor organs at 1 year are now common (Table 23-8). In addition, patient survival now exceeds 95% at 1 year. Rates of infection-related deaths have fallen drastically. These improvements are the result of better selection of patients with end-stage renal failure and recognition of the limits of antirejection therapy. Overuse of immunosuppressive therapy does not result in

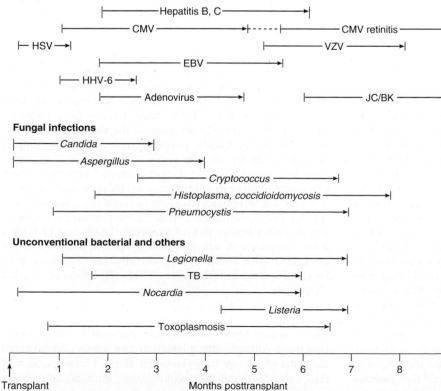

FIGURE 23-3. Timing of infections in relation to transplantation.

| TABLE 23-8 | One-Year Adjusted Graft Survival by Organ and Year of Transplant, 1997–2006 |

Organ	Year of Transplant									
	1997	1998	1999	2000	2001	2002	2003	2004	2005	2006
	(%)	(%)	(%)	(%)	(%)	(%)	(%)	(%)	(%)	(%)
Kidney: Deceased Donor	88.0	88.4	87.7	87.7	88.8	88.9	89.2	90.0	90.2	90.8
Kidney: Living Donor	94.0	94.6	94.4	94.2	94.4	95.0	95.4	95.2	95.2	96.2
Pancreas: Transplant Alone	71.3	78.9	83.8	74.8	77.6	80.4	68.7	76.4	86.4	76.3
Pancreas After Kidney	73.7	72.5	80.1	73.6	82.2	77.4	77.5	78.4	76.8	77.7
Kidney–Pancreas: Kidney	92.0	91.3	91.8	92.7	91.9	92.0	92.3	92.9	93.7	92.0
Kidney–Pancreas: Pancreas	85.8	83.6	84.2	84.4	85.6	87.1	86.6	85.7	87.8	84.2
Liver: Deceased Donor	78.2	79.5	79.2	80.4	80.2	82.1	81.7	82.9	81.5	83.2
Liver: Living Donor	83.0	67.9	72.7	77.2	80.4	80.0	84.1	84.4	84.2	85.9
Intestine	55.6	51.8	50.2	69.7	61.7	70.7	77.9	77.6	73.4	69.6
Heart	84.7	85.2	83.4	85.4	85.4	86.3	87.5	87.6	87.1	87.5
Lung	74.3	74.1	74.6	75.6	76.1	79.9	82.4	83.9	81.5	83.6
Heart-Lung	59.4	54.6	56.6	63.2	74.5	61.9	51.1	73.6	76.3	70.8

Source: OPTN Data May 2008.

better graft survival and is detrimental to patient survival. The loss of a renal allograft requires a return to dialysis, but second and subsequent renal allografts are often performed successfully.

Although complications occur, kidney transplantation is the model of solid organ replacement therapy. In the United States, more than 15,000 patients undergo this procedure annually.

PANCREAS AND ISLET CELL TRANSPLANTATION

Indications

Pancreatic transplantation is the only form of treatment of types I diabetes mellitus that establishes a long-term, insulin independent, normoglycemic state. To achieve this end, either whole organ, segmental, or islet cell transplantation is offered to patients who have this disease. In 2008, there were 435 pancreas-alone transplants and 837 simultaneous kidney–pancreas transplants. Although successful whole-organ or islet-cell-only transplantation affords the patient normoglycemia, the effect of pancreatic transplantation on the chronic complications of diabetes mellitus is less clear. However, peripheral neuropathy may improve, and diabetic retinopathy may stabilize. In patients who undergo simultaneous kidney–pancreas transplants, the kidney may be protected because glomerular and mesangial changes (signs of early diabetic damage) are absent from the kidney after simultaneous kidney–pancreas transplantation. Unfortunately, the effects of pancreatic transplantation on the main causes of morbidity and mortality in diabetic patients (e.g., vascular disease, infection) are missing. The last two decades of work in this field showed that patients who have diabetes and functioning pancreatic grafts could enjoy perfect metabolic control and the freedom from dietary restrictions.

Whole Organ Pancreas Transplantation

Procedure

The donor pancreas and duodenal C-loop are transplanted together in the pelvis of the recipient (Figure 23-4A, B). The operation is performed in an intraperitoneal location. The arterial supply of the pancreas, including the splenic and superior mesenteric arteries, is reconstructed using a donor iliac artery Y-graft, which is anastomosed to the recipient iliac artery. The pancreatic venous drainage (donor portal vein) is attached to the recipient iliac vein. The donor duodenal C-loop is used to drain the donor pancreatic exocrine secretions. Since 1995, many centers have switched from bladder to enteric drainage of the exocrine secretions in simultaneous kidney–pancreas transplantation. Enteric exocrine drainage may be performed with either systemic (systemic-enteric) or portal (portal-enteric) venous delivery of insulin. Although controversy exists regarding the optimal surgical technique, excellent survival rates are achieved with all three techniques. Portal–enteric drainage is not associated with a higher risk of pancreas thrombosis or with a lower incidence of acute rejection. Enteric drainage is not associated with a higher risk of infection. Pancreas graft function and readmissions are similar, regardless of surgical technique.

Complications

The postoperative course of combined whole-organ pancreatic–kidney transplantation is more complicated than that of kidney transplantation alone. More episodes of rejection occur, and they require more immunosuppression.

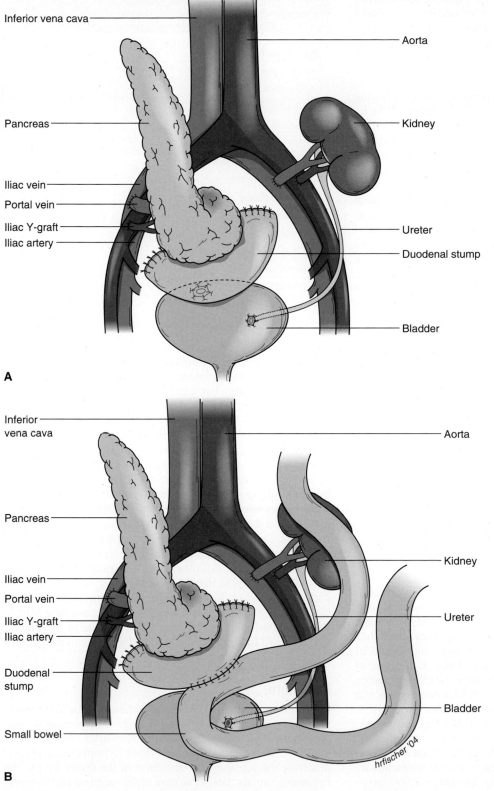

Inferior vena cava

Pancreas

Iliac vein
Portal vein
Iliac Y-graft
Iliac artery

Aorta

Kidney

Ureter

Duodenal stump

Bladder

A

Inferior
vena cava

Pancreas

Iliac vein
Portal vein
Iliac Y-graft
Iliac artery

Duodenal
stump

Small bowel

Aorta

Kidney

Ureter

Bladder

hrfischer '04

B

FIGURE 23-4. Pancreatic transplants using bladder A, or enteric B, drainage.

Subsequently, the patients have more infectious complications and longer hospital stays. The frequency of vascular complications is similar to that of renal transplant patients, but urinary complications (e.g., infection, leakage, minor bleeding) are greater in pancreas transplant patients if the anastomosis is performed to the bladder. Pancreas-alone transplants have similar complications, including anastomotic leak, vascular thrombosis, and urinary complications, but rejection episodes are more difficult to monitor.

Prognosis

The success rates for whole-organ pancreas transplantation approach those for other solid-organ transplantations. Some series report patient survival rates of 95% and graft survival rates of more than 80%. These rates are comparable to those for renal transplantation. Patients who undergo successful pancreatic transplants report an increased sense of well-being and better overall rehabilitation.

Islet Cell Transplantation

Islet cell transplantation offers the potential for long-lasting strict glucose control. Recent strides have been made by increasing the number of viable islets from a donor pancreas with the use of new, gentler digesting agents. Techniques to culture or freeze the islets may eventually provide an islet banking and distribution system for elective transplantation. The proper delivery system for islets is still debatable. Current options include injection into the portal vein, placement under the renal capsule, and encapsulation into immunoisolated chambers. The increased rejection rate, the need for large numbers of islets, and the small number of donors relative to the large potential recipient pool have held back the widespread implementation of islet cell transplantation. The initiative sponsored by the Immune Tolerance Network (ITN) and the National Institutes of Health has announced preliminary results from its 36-patient multicenter clinical trial of the Edmonton Protocol for islet transplantation (portal vein injection and steroid free immunosuppression). An early analysis confirms that the treatment for type 1 diabetes pioneered in Edmonton, Canada, can be successfully replicated at other clinical sites. Of the 15 patients able to complete their transplants, 12 (80%) are currently insulin free, in some cases for up to 1 year. Six graft failures were reported following initial transplant. The rate of insulin independence is 52%. Differences in success rates between individual clinical centers were noted, which underscore the challenges that lie ahead in the widespread adoption of the technique.

LIVER TRANSPLANTATION

Indications

Liver transplantation is indicated in patients with irreversible, progressive liver disease who have failed medical therapy. To be considered a candidate for liver transplantation, a patient should have no evidence of malignancy other than small incidental hepatocellular (HCC) tumors and should be free of infection and active substance abuse at the time of transplantation. Current recommendations for transplantation in the presence of incidental hepatocellular tumors are that liver transplantation is indicated in patients with limited HCC (Stage 1 to II, i.e., T1 or T2, NO, MO disease) and no evidence of invasion of large vascular structures or extrahepatic disease. The prognostic value of high α-fetoprotein (AFP) levels is controversial, although recurrence is more frequent with higher AFP values, especially values >1,000 to 2,000, probably because of either more extensive disease in the liver than noted on preoperative imaging or occult extra hepatic disease. The best results are obtained if transplantation is carried out before the onset of terminal events associated with end-stage liver failure. Table 23-9 lists diseases that are treated by liver transplantation.

Cirrhosis secondary to infection with hepatitis C is now the most common indication for liver transplantation in the United States. Waiting times before transplantation may be

TABLE 23-9	Diseases Treated with Liver Transplantation
Chronic Liver Failure	
Alcoholic liver disease	
Viral Disease	
Hepatitis B/hepatitis C	
Cholestatic liver disease	
Primary biliary cirrhosis	
Primary sclerosing cholangitis	
Metabolic liver disease	
Wilson's disease	
α_1-antitrypsin disease	
Vascular disease	
Budd-Chiari syndrome	
Benign tumors	
Acute Liver Failure	
Toxic liver injury	

1 year or longer, depending on the availability of organs and the condition of the recipient. Patients with cirrhosis are prioritized on the waiting list according to their MELD score. The MELD score is a numerical scale ranging from 6 to 40 (the higher the value the more severely ill the patient) calculated using the patient's serum bilirubin, international normalized ratio (INR), and creatinine (see Chapter 18, Liver).

Patients with acute or fulminant liver failure receive priority on the liver waiting list. Liver donor/recipients are matched by blood group only and a crossmatch is not required. The only priority exception to MELD is a category known as Status 1. Status 1 patients have acute (sudden and severe onset) liver failure and a life expectancy of hours to a few days without a transplant. Less than 1% of liver transplant candidates are in this category. All other liver transplant candidates age 12 and older are prioritized by the MELD system. A patient's score may go up or down over time depending on the status of his or her liver disease. Most candidates will have their MELD score assessed a number of times while they are on the waiting list. This will help ensure that donated livers go to the patients in greatest need at that moment.

Procedure

There are a number of possible techniques for liver transplantation. The classic orthotopic liver transplantation uses the whole liver from a deceased donor. After completion of the native hepatectomy, the new liver is implanted by anastomosing the suprahepatic vena cava of the donor liver to the remaining suprahepatic vena cava of the recipient and then performing an infrahepatic vena caval anastomosis (Figure 23-5). The donor hepatic artery is sewn to the recipient artery, and the donor portal vein is sewn to the recipient portal vein. Biliary drainage is commonly achieved either by duct-to-duct anastomosis or by Roux-en-Y choledochojejunostomy. A modification of the classic technique outlined above, "the piggyback operation," allows the liver to be dissected off the vena cava without division of the cava. This method is associated with improved intraoperative hemodynamic stability and

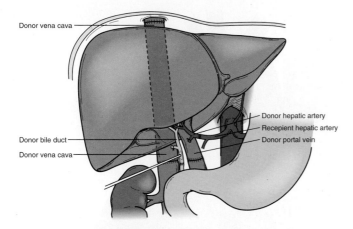

FIGURE 23-5. An orthotopic human hepatic allograft. End-to-end vascular anastomoses connect the donor and recipient hepatic artery, portal vein, and vena cava both suprahepatically and infrahepatically. The most commonly used common bile duct-to-duct anastomosis is shown.

TABLE 23-10	Postoperative Complications of Liver Transplantation
Immunologic	
Acute rejection	
Chronic rejection	
Technical	
Bleeding	
Hepatic artery thrombosis	
Portal vein thrombosis	
Biliary leak/stricture/sludge	
Graft function	
Primary nonfunction	
Graft dysfunction	
Infection	
Bacterial	
Fungal	
Viral	
Systemic	
Cardiac failure	
Respiratory failure	
Renal failure	
Drug related	
Nephrotoxicity	
Hypertension	
Recurrent disease	

a reduced incidence of posttransplant renal insufficiency. One requirement for hepatic transplantation is size match between the donor and recipient livers. This match is particularly difficult to obtain in a timely manner in small children. This problem led to the introduction of reduced size livers, usually the left lobe or lateral segment. The resulting segment of liver, its blood supply, and the bile duct are reimplanted into the recipient. The success rate with this procedure is equivalent to that of whole liver grafts, and it is even used for adult recipients. In fact, split livers are used to provide transplants to two recipients. In recent years, the demand for liver transplantation has exceeded the supply of cadaveric organs, leading to the introduction of living donor liver transplantation in adults as well as children. In adults, the right lobe of the liver is removed from a living donor and transplanted into the recipient (Figure 23-6). In children, the smaller left lobe is usually removed from the donor.

Complications

Complications of liver transplantation may be categorized as immunologic, technical, infective, drug related, systemic, or related to poor graft function (Table 23-10). Acute rejection

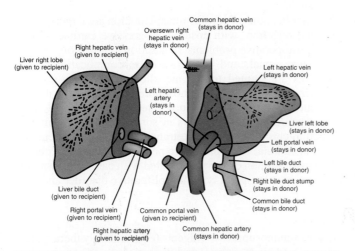

FIGURE 23-6. Living donor right hepatectomy. The right hepatic duct, hepatic artery, and right portal vein are divided after division of the liver.

may occur, but it is usually less common and milder than that seen in kidney transplantation. Chronic rejection may be an indication for retransplantation. Primary nonfunction is a condition in which the transplanted liver fails to function and is an indication for emergency retransplantation. Various degrees of graft dysfunction may occur and may usually be managed supportively. Untreated hepatic artery thrombosis occurring in the first week of transplantation is a devastating complication and is also an indication for urgent retransplantation. Unlike the native liver, the transplanted liver is almost totally dependent on blood supply from the hepatic artery in order to maintain the integrity of the biliary tree. Hepatic artery ischemia may therefore lead to biliary strictures. Cardiac, respiratory, and renal complications may occur after any major surgery, and liver transplantation is no exception. Late complications of liver transplantation include recurrent disease, chronic rejection, and toxicity from immunosuppressive drug therapy.

Prognosis

Patient and graft survival rates in liver transplantation approach 85% at 1 year for patients who are operated on before the terminal phase of their disease. In patients who are hospitalized in the ICU at the time of transplantation, survival statistics for both the operation and the postoperative period are poor. Many patients, particularly those transplanted for viral hepatitis, are at risk of developing recurrent disease.

HEART, HEART–LUNG, AND LUNG TRANSPLANTATION

Heart Transplantation

Indications

The indication for heart transplantation is end-stage cardiac disease not amenable to other medical or surgical therapy (Table 23-11). Patients who have N.Y. Heart Classification symptoms on optimal medical therapy whose prognosis for survival is <50% at 1 year are also suitable candidates.

Age, up to 65 years, is not a contraindication. Oxygen consumption at maximal exercise, a peak VO_2 of <10 mL/kg/minute, has been used as an objective criterion for candidacy for transplantation. The patient must be free of infection and neoplasm and have full potential for rehabilitation. Specific indications for heart transplantation include idiopathic cardiomyopathy, viral cardiomyopathy, ischemic cardiac disease, postpartum cardiomyopathy, terminal cardiac valvular disease, and hypertensive cardiomyopathy. Many patients are maintained on ventricular assist devices as a bridge to transplantation. Severe pulmonary hypertension with a fixed pulmonary vascular resistance of six Wood's units at rest (normal = 1.16 to 3) is a contraindication to heart transplantation, and heart–lung transplantation should be considered. Cardiac transplantation is most often performed in adults because many congenital cardiac defects can be corrected surgically. However, neonatal and pediatric cardiac transplantation is also performed successfully.

Procedure

The ideal cardiac preservation time is under 6 hours. Thus, donor and recipient surgeries are scheduled to coincide. Since the number of donors is far exceeded by the number of potential recipients, and cold time is an important consideration, hearts are distributed through the UNOS computer system to the sickest patients. These patients, who usually require mechanical or medical support in the ICU, are in a hospital that is close enough to the donor hospital to enable implantation within the prescribed cold ischemia limits.

The usual cardiac transplant is a size-matched ABO-matched orthotopic allograft. Tissue typing is usually not done preoperatively. The recipient heart is removed, and the donor heart is sewn into place by attaching the left and right atria of the donor heart to the left and right atria of the recipient. The pulmonary artery and aortic anastomoses are completed (Figure 23-7). The heart is resuscitated and allowed to take over support of the recipient.

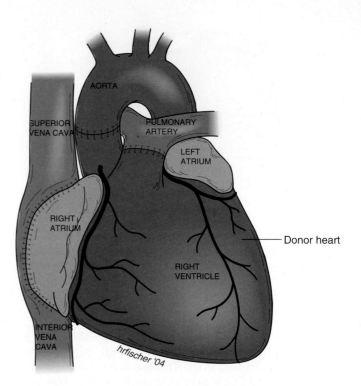

FIGURE 23-7. An orthotopic human cardiac allograft. The left and right atria of the graft are sutured to the posterior most atrial walls, which remain intact in the recipient. End-to-end anastomoses of the pulmonary artery and aorta are completed before the transplanted heart is resuscitated and cardiopulmonary bypass support is terminated.

Some centers use heterotopic grafts. These grafts allow the recipient's heart to remain as a safety net if the donor heart is rejected. In heterotopic grafts, the donor heart is placed alongside the recipient heart, and the donor and recipient atria and aorta are anastomosed. A graft is used to connect the donor pulmonary artery to the recipient pulmonary artery. In some instances of heterotopic transplants for cardiomyopathy, once the donor heart rejects the recipient heart, the native heart has recovered enough to be able to take over functionally. Heterotopic transplants may also be used if pulmonary vascular resistance is high or if there is a size mismatch between donor and recipient.

Complications

The complications of cardiac transplantation are largely infection and rejection, with ensuing progressive cardiac failure. Early postoperative problems, in addition to infection, include respiratory, renal, and cerebrovascular complications. Late problems are limited to chronic allograft rejection and the long-term effects of immunosuppressive therapy, including calcineurin-inhibitor–induced nephropathy. Accelerated coronary artery disease occurs in some patients and may be related to chronic rejection. Retransplantation and percutaneous transluminal angioplasty are performed for this problem. The most common cancers associated with cardiac transplants are skin, posttransplant lymphoproliferative disorder and lung cancer.

Prognosis

Newer immunosuppressive agents (e.g., antibody therapy, tacrolimus, and cyclosporine) and the serial use of endomyocardial biopsy to diagnose rejection have improved the outcome

TABLE 23-11	Indications for Cardiac Transplantation	
Adult		
	Cardiac ischemia/cardiac fatigue	45%
	Nonischemic cardiomyopathy	45%
	Valvular heart disease	4%
	Congenital heart disease (adult)	2%
Pediatric		
	Cardiomyopathy	60%
	Congenital heart disease	40%

of cardiac transplantation. The current 1-year graft and patient survival rate is 80% or higher, the 5-year rate is 60% to 70%, and the 10-year rate is 45%. The median survival is 9.3 years. In the first year, mortality associated with cardiac transplants is often due to graft failure, non-CMV infection, and multiorgan failure. Beyond 5 years cardiac allograft vasculopathy, cancer and non-CMV infection account for the majority of deaths.

Heart–Lung Transplantation

Heart–lung transplantation is performed when severe pulmonary hypertension accompanies cardiac disease. It is also performed for congenital heart disease such as Eisenmenger's syndrome. It may sometimes be used in a "domino procedure" where heart and lung are given to one recipient with cystic fibrosis and his normal heart is given to someone else who requires a heart transplant. In addition to the complications of cardiac transplantation, complications of heart–lung transplantation include restrictive fibrosis of the lung. Acute and chronic rejection of the lung may be manifested by bronchiolitis. The 1-year survival rate for heart–lung transplant recipients is 63%.

LUNG TRANSPLANTATION

Indications

Single-lung and sequential double-lung transplantations are performed for patients with α_1-antitrypsin deficiency, interstitial pulmonary fibrosis, primary pulmonary hypertension, and cystic fibrosis and emphysema (Table 23-12). Single- or double-lung transplantation can provide total pulmonary function to patients with end-stage pulmonary disease without suppuration and concomitant cardiac failure.

A forced expiratory volume (FEV_1) of <25%, partial pressure of carbon dioxide ($PaCO_2$) of >55 torr or an elevated pulmonary artery pressure in the presence of deteriorating clinical function are good indicators of the need for pulmonary transplantation. Lung cancer is a contraindication to lung transplantation. Recipients must be free of infection and are usually younger than 65 years of age. The donor and the recipient must be of equivalent height and weight. Living donor lobar donation is possible especially if the recipient is a child. Since the number of recipients is greater than the number of lungs available, a reasonably equitable system called the Lung Allocation Score (LAS) has been developed for potential recipients over 12 years. It takes into account patient disease, extent of diseased lung, functional status, and comorbidities to try to find a balance between urgency of need and likelihood of a favorable outcome.

Complications

Rejection is the most common complication. It is diagnosed by the appearance of infiltrates on chest x-ray and is confirmed with transbronchial or transthoracic needle biopsy and bronchioalveolar lavage, slowing infiltrating, mononuclear cells, endotheliitis, or alveolar necrosis. Breakdown of the bronchial anastomosis is a dreaded complication that occurs in 5% of transplants. For this reason, to enhance healing, the dose of steroids is kept as low as possible. The use of calcineurin inhibitors has enabled lower steroid use. In lung transplantation, acute and chronic rejection of the lung may be manifested by bronchiolitis. Obliterative bronchiolitis is the primary manifestation of chronic rejection and is the greatest cause of long-term mortality. It is diagnosed by biopsy. Early mortality is associated with unsuspected donor lung injury and reperfusion injury. Pulmonary infection with bacteria, fungi, or CMV is common in the postoperative period. Bronchioalveolar lavage is useful to direct antibiotic therapy.

Procedure

The surgery is performed through a posterolateral thoracotomy for single-lung transplants and through a transverse thoracotomy for double-lung transplants. The donor pulmonary veins are sewn to a left atrial recipient cuff after the sleeve bronchial anastomosis is performed. Finally, the pulmonary arteries are anastomosed. Care must be taken to avoid fluid overload to minimize lung edema in the postoperative period.

Prognosis

Patient survival rates for lung transplantation are 77% at 1 year and 45% at 5 years, and 25% at 10 years. Bilateral lung transplant patients have better survival than single-lung recipients. Double-lung transplantation is preferred in situations where there has been chronic lung infection in cystic fibrosis or bronchiectasis. In single-lung transplantation, residual infection may be transferred from the native to the transplant lung. Also, in extensive emphysema where there is the possibility of air trapping in the native lung and mediastinal shift compressing the transplanted lung, double-lung transplant is recommended.

INTESTINAL TRANSPLANTATION

Bowel transplantation was first attempted in humans during the 1960s. At that time, patients were dying of starvation after having a large portion of their bowel removed because of disease or trauma. Parenteral (intravenous) feeding was not yet available, and surgeons hoped that the transplanted bowel would function normally. These first intestinal transplant patients died, however, from technical complications, rejection, or infection. Successful intestinal transplants were not performed until the mid-1980s. Now, many patients have been able to stop total parenteral nutrition (TPN), resume a normal diet, and enjoy a healthy lifestyle after intestinal transplantation. From studies of TPN-dependent patients, the incidence of irreversible intestinal failure is estimated to be—two to three cases per million persons per year. The number of candidates listed for the various forms of intestine transplantation has steadily increased. As of December 2008, the UNOS database listed 224 patients awaiting intestinal transplantation.

Indications

Most candidates are younger than 60 years, white, and male. Short-gut syndrome, the prime indication for small intestinal transplantation, has an incidence of two to three per 1 million

TABLE 23-12	Indications for Lung Transplantation	
COPD		38%
Pulmonary fibrosis		17%
Cystic fibrosis		17%

population. The syndrome is the result of many intestinal disorders, including intestinal strangulation or infarction from midgut volvulus, obstruction, or internal hernias; trauma; and vascular accidents of the mesenteric vessels. Other associated diseases include Crohn's disease, low-grade tumors, and necrotizing enterocolitis. Candidates for transplantation must depend on parenteral nutrition. Some transplant centers perform cluster-graft transplantation, including liver, pancreas, and small bowel, after upper abdominal exenteration.

The median time to transplant for new list registrations is 261 days and is one of the longest of any solid organ transplant. The contraindications of intestinal transplantation are essentially the same as is seen in other types of transplants and include significant coexistent medical conditions that have no potential for improvement following transplantation, and active uncontrolled infection or malignancy that is not eliminated by the transplant process.

The number of intestinal transplants performed has been consistently growing and is expected to increase. From 1997 to 2006, the number of isolated intestinal transplants increased 171%. Still, major issues remain, such as the extremely high mortality in patients on the waiting list and the organ shortage. Another issue is the difficult balance between appropriate immunosuppression in order to avoid rejection and over immunosuppression with its devastating complications. This issue makes the development of markers to detect early rejection imperative. Many efforts have been placed in techniques to induce a state of microchimerism and tolerance by transplanting bone marrow along with the intestinal allograft. This ongoing research may change the future of transplantation of the small bowel and other organs.

Procedure

The donor bowel may come from a living relative or from a deceased donor. A segment of small bowel at least 100 to 150 cm long is necessary to provide an adequate absorptive surface. The allograft may be heterotopic or orthotopic. The ends of the bowel may be anastomosed to the recipient's remaining bowel or brought up to the abdominal wall as an ileostomy. The latter approach allows easy observation and biopsy to monitor rejection or ischemia. The intestinal graft implantation begins with the take down of adhesions, which are usually abundant in these patients secondary to previous surgeries. The aorta and cava are dissected in preparation for the vascular anastomosis and the proximal and distal ends of the remnant digestive tract are dissected free. The venous anastomosis to the graft is usually performed to the recipient cava but may be to the portal vein. The arterial anastomosis is performed to the abdominal aorta. A loop ileostomy is created for future endoscopic surveillance.

Complications

Complications include rejection, graft-versus-host disease, and sepsis from the translocation of bacteria through the bowel mucosal barriers.

Prognosis

Survival after intestinal transplantation has shown steady improvement over the last decade. The 1-year adjusted patient survival improved from 57 ± 6.5% in 1997 to 80 ± 3.3% in 2005. When analyzing the results for intestinal transplantation, separating results of intestine-alone transplants and liver–intestine transplants is essential. For recipients of intestine alone, unadjusted patient survival is 81% for 1 year, 67% for 3 years, 54% for 5 years, and 43% for 10 years. Patient survival for recipients of liver–intestine transplants is 76% for 1 year, 70% for 3 years, 58% for 5 years, and 38% for 10 years. Intestine graft survival for the same intervals is 75%, 69%, 56%, and 36%, respectively.

SAMPLE QUESTIONS

Questions

Choose the best answer for each question.

1. A 45-year-old man remains intubated and on mechanical ventilation following complications of myocardial infarction. He cannot be weaned from pressors and is expected to die. His past medical history is significant for hypertension, type II diabetes mellitus, and pneumococcal meningitis successfully treated 3 months ago. The family asks to withdraw support and agrees to organ donation once his heart stops beating. His heart stops before all retrieval arrangements are in place and he is rushed to the operating room. The transplant team arrives 30 minutes later to recover the organs. Which of the following is a contraindication to liver retrieval?

   A. History of pneumococcal meningitis

   B. Coronary artery disease

   C. Diabetes mellitus

   D. Hypertension

   E. Prolonged warm ischemia

2. A 28-year-old man is brought to the emergency department 25 minutes after he attempts suicide by shooting himself in the head with a .22 caliber pistol. He was recently diagnosed with a glioblastoma multiforme. His past history includes abuse of drugs and alcohol from which he has been abstinent for 2 years. He has positive serology for both hepatitis C and HIV. He is declared brain dead. Which condition prohibits organ donation?

   A. Brain tumor

   B. History of illicit drug and alcohol use

   C. Positive serology for HIV

   D. Positive serology for hepatitis C

   E. Irreversible CNS injury

3. A 26-year-old man is in the operating room undergoing a renal transplant. He has chronic renal failure secondary to post streptococcal glomerulonephritis. He is receiving a kidney transplant from his older brother. They have the same blood type, and HLA testing suggests a one-haplotype match. The recipient's kidneys are left in place and the donated kidney is placed in the right pelvis. This particular transplant is best termed a(n)

   A. isograft.

   B. allograft.

   C. orthotopic graft.

   D. autograft.

   E. xenograft.

4. A 30-year-old man had a deceased donor kidney transplant 2 years ago. His renal function is normal. He is currently maintained on an immunosuppressive regimen, which includes cyclosporine and prednisone. When used for immunosuppression in this man, cyclosporine

   A. induces the generation of an anti–T-cell antibody.

   B. can lead to a high incidence of ocular cataracts.

   C. induces the production of interleukin-1.

   D. permits the concurrent use of a lower dose of steroids.

   E. prevents hyperkalemia and hyperuricemia.

5. A 45-year-old man with chronic hepatitis C and cirrhosis is being considered for liver transplantation. In addition to serum bilirubin and creatinine levels, what other parameter is needed to calculate the model for end stage liver disease (MELD) score and thereby prioritize this man to receive a liver transplant?

   A. Prothrombin time/international normalized ratio (INR)

   B. Creatinine clearance

   C. Platelet count

   D. Aspartate aminotransferase

   E. Body mass index

Answers and Explanations

1. Answer: E

A. Only *active* infection is an absolute contraindication.

B. Coronary artery disease is not a contraindication to liver retrieval.

C. Diabetes is not a contraindication to liver retrieval.

D. Hypertension is not a contraindication to liver retrieval.

E. It is best to retrieve the liver <30 minutes after the withdrawal of life-sustaining measures; the kidneys and pancreas may often be recovered up to 60 minutes after such withdrawal. Therefore E is correct.

Refer to section on organ donation.

2. Answer: C

A. Malignancy *other than* primary brain tumors is a contraindication.

B. History of illicit drug and alcohol use is not an absolute contraindication if serologies are negative. These organs are frequently used in an emergency situation.

C. HIV positivity is an absolute contraindication to organ donation. Therefore, C is correct.

D. Positive serology for hepatitis C is not an absolute contraindication to organ donation as the risk of viral transmission is very low. Livers may be procured from hepatitis C–positive donors if the liver biopsy is normal.

E. Irreversible CNS injury is not a contraindication

Refer to section on organ donation.

3. Answer: B

A. An isograft is transferred between genetically identical individuals (e.g., renal transplant between monozygotic twins).

B. An allograft is transplanted between genetically dissimilar individuals of the same species (e.g., deceased donor renal transplant). Therefore, B is correct.

C. Kidney transplants are placed heterotopically, that is, at a site different from its normal anatomic position.

D. An autograft is transplanted from one side of the body to another in the same individual (e.g., skin graft removed from the leg and placed on a wound elsewhere).

E. A xenograft is tissue that is transferred between different species (e.g., porcine skin grafted onto a human burn victim).

Refer to section on Immunology.

4. Answer: D

A. Cyclosporine inhibits the expression of multiple genes involved in T-cell activation and proliferation, including IL-2 and other lymphokines.

B. Cataract development is a complication of steroid use but not the other commonly used immunosuppressive agents.

C. Cyclosporine inhibits the expression of multiple genes involved in T-cell activation and proliferation, including IL-2 and other lymphokines.

D. This is true. Therefore, D is correct.

E. Hyperkalemia is one of the side effects of cyclosporine therapy.

5. Answer: A

A. A is correct.

B. Serum creatinine and not creatinine clearance is used to calculate the MELD score.

C. The platelet count is not one of the parameters used to calculate the MELD score.

D. While the aspartate aminotransferase is frequently elevated, it is not a component of the MELD score.

E. Body mass index is not a component of the MELD score.

Refer to section on Liver Transplantation under Indications.

24

Surgical Oncology: Malignant Diseases of the Skin and Soft Tissue

D. SCOTT LIND, M.D. • MOHAMMED I. AHMED, M.B.B.S., M.S. (SURGERY) • CHRIS DE GARA, M.B.B.S., M.S. • JAMES WARNEKE, M.D.

Objectives

Surgical Oncology

1. Recognize that cancer represents a diverse group of diseases.
2. List the etiologic factors associated with cancer.
3. Discuss the contemporary multi-modal management of cancer.

Malignant Diseases of the Skin

1. Define the broad categories of skin cancer and their distinguishing features.
2. Discuss the etiologies and incidences of skin carcinomas.
3. List the signs and symptoms of skin cancer.

4. Compare and contrast the various methods used to diagnose skin cancer.
5. Describe the staging system for skin cancer.
6. Summarize the local, regional, and systemic therapies for skin cancer.

Malignant Diseases of the Soft Tissue

1. List the clinical features of soft tissue sarcomas.
2. Outline the methods for the diagnosis and staging of soft tissue sarcoma.
3. Discuss the treatment of sarcomas, including surgery, radiation therapy, and chemotherapy.

■ SURGICAL ONCOLOGY

Cancer is a diverse group of diseases collectively characterized by an unregulated proliferation of undifferentiated cells that invade local tissue and may spread or metastasize to other parts of the body.

EPIDEMIOLOGY

One in four deaths in the United States is due to cancer, second only to deaths from heart disease. In 2011, approximately 1,596,670 new cancer cases and 571,950 cancer deaths were projected in the United States. While the types and incidence of cancer differ in men and women (Table 24-1), it is the leading cause of death before age 65 in both genders (Table 24-2). In children between the ages of 1 and 14 years, cancer is second only to deaths by accidents.

CANCER BIOLOGY

According to a model proposed by Hanahan and Weinberg, malignant transformation is the result of cells acquiring four

functional capabilities: (1) the ability for self-sufficient growth, (2) an insensitivity to antigrowth signals, (3) the ability to evade apoptosis (programmed cell death), and (4) the capacity of limitless replication. Two other functional capabilities acquired by cancer cells include sustained angiogenesis and tissue invasion, but these changes occur not only within the cancer cell itself but also in its interaction and relationship with other elements.

ETIOLOGY OF CANCER

Most cancers are caused not by a single physical, chemical, or biological factor but by a complex combination of exogenous and/or endogenous factors (Table 24-3).

RISK ASSESSMENT

Cancer risk assessment involves estimating a person's susceptibility for developing cancer. Genetic counseling is the process of helping people understand consequences of an inherited risk for developing cancer. Estimating an individual's risk for developing cancer entails taking a detailed history about medical and environmental risk factors for cancer such as inflammatory

TABLE 24-1	The Most Common Cancers in Men and Women, by Incidence	
	Cancer Site	Incidence (%)
Men	Prostate	29
	Lung and bronchus	14
	Colon and rectum	9
	Urinary bladder	6
	Melanoma of the skin	5
Women	Breast	30
	Lung and bronchus	14
	Colon and rectum	9
	Uterine corpus	6
	Thyroid	5

bowel disease, hepatitis C, and radiation or chemical carcinogen exposure, together with lifestyle risk factors (i.e., smoking, diet, exercise, alcohol intake). In addition, a thorough family history including both maternal and paternal relatives is an essential part of cancer risk assessment. Patients are referred for testing for hereditary cancer syndromes (i.e., genetic testing) based on the information gathered from a detailed family history. Several models or tools are available to aid the clinician or genetics counselor to calculate an individual's risk of developing a particular type of cancer. For example, the Gail model is a tool used in breast cancer risk assessment. This tool calculates the probability of a woman developing breast cancer, taking into account risk factors such as age, age at menarche, age at first live birth, number of first-degree relatives with breast cancer, and number of previous breast biopsies and histology. Several other risk assessment models are currently available and are being developed for breast and other cancers.

SCREENING

Screening involves testing asymptomatic individuals who may be at higher risk for a particular medical condition to detect the condition early and improve outcomes.

Cancer screening is best performed in high-risk populations. The type of cancer that is being screened for should have (1) an asymptomatic phase of sufficient duration for the patient to benefit from any treatment, (2) the potential to produce significant morbidity and mortality if detected late, and finally (3) an effective treatment method. The screening test should be sensitive, specific, reliable, cost-effective, and

TABLE 24-2	Estimated Cancer Deaths by Sex in the United States (2011)	
	Cancer Site	Number of Deaths
Men	Lung and bronchus	85,600
	Prostate	33,720
	Colon	25,250
Women	Lung and bronchus	71,340
	Breast	39,520 (Men: 450)
	Colon	24,130

convenient. Examples of cancers in which screening is recommended appear in Table 24-4.

DIAGNOSIS

Biopsy

All cancer treatment is dependent upon an accurate diagnosis. Several biopsy methods are available to obtain an accurate diagnosis for solid tumors, including fine-needle aspiration biopsy (FNAB), core-needle biopsy, excisional biopsy, and incisional biopsy.

FNAB consists of removing cells from a suspicious mass using a thin or fine needle. After the cells are removed or aspirated they are stained for cytologic examination. FNAB is a safe, minor procedure; its accuracy depends on an experienced cytopathologist. FNAB has a higher false-negative rate (i.e., negative result when cancer is present) than core-needle, excisional, and incisional biopsy methods. Further, FNAB does not permit accurate grading (i.e., degree of differentiation) of the cancer because it does not show the tissue architecture. FNAB is used in the diagnosis of breast lumps, thyroid nodules, enlarged lymph nodes, lung, and other nodules.

Core-needle biopsy is removal of tissue from a suspicious mass using a larger needle (i.e., 14 gauge) than that used in FNAB. It is generally used for prostate, breast, liver, and other masses. This biopsy method provides more histologic information than FNAB because it involves removal of tissue rather than simply cells. The possibility of diagnostic errors with core-needle biopsy is much lower than with FNAB.

Excisional biopsy refers to the complete removal of a lesion, while incisional biopsy refers to partial removal of a lesion. The size, location, and surgical treatment plan all influence the decision to perform excisional versus incisional biopsy.

Imaging techniques, such as ultrasonography or computed tomography (CT), can direct the biopsy (i.e., image-guided biopsy) to improve accuracy and minimize patient morbidity. Of note, the selection of an inappropriate biopsy method can compromise subsequent definitive surgical therapy. As a general rule, the least invasive biopsy method that minimizes disruption of surrounding tissue and provides the most accurate diagnosis is optimal to facilitate definitive surgical resection.

Laboratory Evaluations

Laboratory evaluations for patients undergoing a diagnostic workup for cancer may include a complete blood count, electrolyte counts, liver function tests, and tumor markers, depending on the type of cancer.

Imaging Techniques

Imaging techniques to further establish a diagnosis and assist in staging include ultrasonography, plain radiographs, contrast examination of the gastrointestinal (GI) or genitourinary (GU) tracts, CT, CT colonography and virtual colonoscopy, magnetic resonance imaging (MRI), dynamic enhanced MRI (DEMRI), and positron emission tomography (PET).

Sampling Techniques

More invasive diagnostic methods include upper and lower GI tract endoscopy and endoscopic retrograde cholangiopancreatography (ERCP). Laparoscopy, thoracoscopy, and mediastinoscopy may be performed as well depending upon the type and location of the tumor.

TABLE 24-3	Etiological Factors Associated with Cancers

Etiological Factor	Cancer
Exogenous factors	
Physical	
Ultraviolet light	Basal cell carcinoma, malignant melanoma
Ionizing radiation	Skin cancers, leukemia
Chemical	
Benzene	Leukemia
β Napthylamine	Bladder cancer
Vinyl chloride	Angiosarcoma of the liver
Asbestos	Mesothelioma
Tar	Squamous cell carcinoma
Tobacco smoke	Lung cancer
Viral	
Hepatitis B virus (HBV)	Hepatocellular carcinoma
Epstein-Barr virus (EBV)	Burkitt's lymphoma, nasopharyngeal carcinoma, Hodgkin's disease, lymphomas
Human papilloma virus (HPV)	Cervical cancer, skin cancer, oropharyngeal cancer
Human T lymphotrophic virus (HTLV-1)	ATL
Hepatitis C virus (HCV)	Hepatocellular carcinoma (HCC)
Human herpes virus (HHV-8)(KSHV)	Kaposi's sarcoma (KS), primary effusion lymphoma (PEL), Castleman's disease
Simian virus 40 (SV 40)	Brain, bone, mesothelioma
Parasitic	
Schistosoma haematobium	Bladder cancer
Opisthorchis sinensis	Carcinoma pancreas, carcinoma bile ducts
Dietary carcinogens	
Aflatoxins	Esophageal cancer
Smoked foods	Stomach cancer
Alcohol	Oropharyngeal cancer, esophageal cancer
Chronic irritation	
Chronic dermatitis	Marjolin's ulcer (squamous cell carcinoma)
Endogenous factors	
Hormones	
Estrogen	Breast, endometrium, ovary
Testosterone	Testis, prostate
Immunity	
Bone marrow or solid organ transplantation	Hodgkin's disease. Kaposi's sarcoma, skin, oropharynx, bone
HIV and AIDS	Kaposi's sarcoma, non-Hodgkin's lymphoma, invasive cervical cancer
Genetic	
Retinoblastoma (Rb) gene	Childhood retinoblastoma
Wilms' tumor (WT) gene	Nephroblastoma
Familial adenomatous polyposis (FAP) gene	Colon carcinoma
BRCA1 and *BRCA2* gene	Breast, ovarian, colon, prostate cancers
MEN-1	Pancreatic islet cell cancer, parathyroid hyperplasia, pituitary adenoma
RET	Medullary thyroid cancer, pheochromocytoma, parathyroid hyperplasia
Mutations of p53	Li-Fraumeni syndrome
Autosomal recessive	Turcot syndrome

Additional Aids to Diagnosis

Newer aids to diagnosis include gene expression profiling, which is the measurement of the activity of thousands of genes at once to give a picture of cellular function. It can be used, for example, to differentiate between benign and malignant thyroid lesions. Proteomics is the study of how proteins are modified and expressed, how they interact with one another, and how they are involved in the metabolic pathways. Proteomics is just beginning to be applied clinically; for example, it is used in the staging of ovarian cancer.

TABLE 24-4	Cancer Screening Recommendations	
Test	**American Cancer Society Guidelines**	**U.S. Preventative Services Task Force Guidelines**
Physical examination	>20	—
Clinical breast examination	>20 q 3 years	Optional (not sufficient evidence to recommend)
	>40 yearly	
Mammogram	Female >40 yearly	Every 1–2 years 50–69
Breast MRI	Female >40 with >20% lifetime risk	Not discussed
Fecal occult blood test	Yearly >50	Yearly, >50 years and <75 years
Fecal immunochemical test	Yearly >50	—
Colonoscopy	At 50 and q 10 years	—
	Earlier if strong family history (1 first-degree relative <60 or 2 of any age)	
PSA and digital rectal examination	Discussion of screening at age >50 or >45 in patients with first-degree relative with prostate cancer	Not recommended
Pap smear	3 years after onset of intercourse or 21, then q 1 year with Pap test or q 2 year with liquid-based Pap test	Q 3 years after onset of intercourse until 65 if consistently normal

MRI, magnetic resonance imaging; PSA, prostate-specific antigen.

Source: Adapted from Scher LA and Weinberg G. General surgery board review, 4th ed. Philadelphia, PA: Lippincott Williams & Wilkins, 2012:112, with permission.

STAGING AND GRADING

Staging involves assigning cancers into various groups based upon features of the primary tumor and the presence or absence of regional or distant spread of the primary tumor. This grouping aids clinicians in predicting prognosis and in determining the correct treatment. The most widely used staging system for cancer is the American Joint Committee on Cancer (AJCC) Tumor, Node, Metastasis (TNM) staging system.

Staging for some cancers involves histological grading of the primary tumor into three grades: Grade 1 = well differentiated (low grade), Grade 2 = moderately differentiated (intermediate grade), and Grade 3 = poorly differentiated/anaplastic (high grade).

Tumor Markers

Tumor markers are substances that are produced by tumors or by the body in response to the tumor. Tumor marker secretion helps in diagnosis, staging, assessing response to treatment, and detecting tumor recurrence. Tumor markers may be classified into three broad categories, proteins, genetic mutations, and epigenetic changes. Protein tumor markers may be enzymes, hormones, or oncofetal antigens (Table 24-5).

MANAGEMENT

Contemporary cancer management requires a multimodal treatment approach involving surgery, chemotherapy, and radiation. Physicians from each discipline (surgery, medicine, and radiation oncology) must have a working knowledge of each other's specialty. Outcomes are optimized when representatives from all three cancer disciplines meet and discuss treatment plans for cancer patients at a multidisciplinary tumor board (i.e., breast cancer, head and neck, GI, and other tumor boards). Teamwork and communication among all cancer caregivers are essential.

Role of Surgery

Surgery is the oldest and for many centuries was the only form of cancer therapy. The introduction of antisepsis and anesthesia permitted safer, less painful cancer operations. The current roles of surgery in the management of cancer can be categorized as risk reducing, diagnostic, curative, or palliative. An improved understanding of tumor biology, advances in imaging and surgical techniques, together with evidence-based data from mature clinical trials have all produced a shift from radical resections to less morbid procedures for many solid tumors.

Prophylactic or risk-reduction surgery is increasingly being employed to remove tissue or organs at increased risk for the subsequent development of cancer. For some procedures, such as mastectomy, the term *risk-reduction* is preferred over prophylactic surgery, because the operation significantly reduces but does not eliminate the risk of breast cancer. Some breast tissue is left behind following mastectomy and the patient must be made aware of this fact. Other conditions where risk-reduction surgery is being utilized include mastectomy and oophorectomy in patients who have inherited the *BRCA* genes, thyroidectomy in patients with multiple endocrine neoplasia 2

TABLE 24-5	Tumor Markers
Tumor Marker	**Cancer**
Carcinoembryonic antigen (CEA)	Cancer of the colon and rectum
α-Fetoprotein (AFP)	Hepatocellular carcinoma
Carbohydrate antigen 19-9	Pancreas cancer
Prostate-specific antigen	Prostate cancer (only tissue specific)
Carbohydrate antigen 125	Ovarian cancer
α-Fetoprotein (AFP) and human chorionic gonadotrophin (hCG)	Testicular germ cell cancers
AFP	90%–95% of yolk sac tumors
	20% of teratomas
	10% of embryonal carcinomas
hCG	90% of choriocarcinomas
Calcitonin	Medullary thyroid cancer

TABLE 24-6	Conditions in Which Prophylactic Surgery Can Prevent Cancer	
Underlying Condition	**Associated Cancer**	**Prophylactic Surgery**
Cryptorchidism	Testicular	Orchiopexy
Polyposis coli	Colon	Colectomy
Familial colon cancer	Colon	Colectomy
Ulcerative colitis	Colon	Colectomy
Multiple endocrine neoplasia types 1 and 2	Medullary cancer of the thyroid	Thyroidectomy
Familial breast cancer	Breast	Mastectomy
Familial ovarian cancer	Ovary	Oophorectomy

Source: Paige M. Porrett et al. The surgical review, 3rd ed. Philadelphia, PA: Lippincott Williams & Wilkins, 2010:210.

Adapted from Rosenberg SA. Principles of cancer management: surgical oncology. In: DeVita VT, Hellman S, Rosenberg SA, eds. Cancer: principles and practice of oncology, 6th ed. Philadelphia, PA: Lippincott Williams & Wilkins, 2002:259, with permission.

(MEN-2) syndrome, and colectomy in patients with familial polyposis or ulcerative colitis (Table 24-6).

Surgeons are frequently asked to obtain tissue to provide a prompt and accurate diagnosis of cancer. Following diagnosis, surgeons may perform any number of staging procedures including sentinel node biopsy (i.e., breast cancer and melanoma), laparoscopy (i.e., stomach and pancreas cancer), and mediastinoscopy (i.e., lung cancer).

Surgery with curative intent varies with the type of cancer but generally consists of en bloc resection of the primary tumor. En bloc resection refers to removal of the entire tumor and any adjacent structures or organs that are involved by tumor in an effort to obtain tumor-free margins and minimize the risk of local recurrence. An adequately performed en bloc resection also incorporates any previous biopsy incision and does not violate the primary tumor or tissue immediately adjacent to tumor. In general, more aggressive (i.e., poorly differentiated, infiltrative) cancers necessitate a wider en bloc resection (i.e., wider margin of resection). Certain cancers (esophageal, gastric, pancreatic, and colorectal) may require en bloc removal of the contiguous regional lymph nodes (i.e., lymphadenectomy) in addition to removal of the primary tumor. In the absence of nodal metastases, sentinel lymph node biopsy can be performed with other cancers (i.e., breast cancer and melanoma) and spare node-negative patients the morbidity of a lymph node dissection.

Surgical therapy of metastatic disease (i.e., metastasectomy) is appropriate treatment in select patients. Important factors in determining the value of metastasectomy include: the disease-free interval (elapsed time from initial treatment to recurrence), the organ(s) of involvement, and the ability to render the patient tumor-free with an acceptable morbidity and mortality. Examples where surgical resection of metastatic disease can be effective include resection of hepatic metastases from colorectal cancer and pulmonary metastases from soft tissue sarcoma.

Surgeons are increasingly asked to perform palliative (i.e., noncurative) operations on cancer patients to improve quality of life. Examples of palliative operations include surgery to debulk tumors (i.e., cytoreductive surgery), alleviate pain, control hemorrhage, relieve obstruction, repair a perforated viscus, or to provide nutritional support. Surgeons may also be asked to perform vascular access procedures to facilitate the delivery of chemotherapy.

Chemotherapy

As antineoplastic drugs (Table 24-7) become more effective, more cancer patients are receiving chemotherapy as part of their treatment. Chemotherapy can be delivered in a primary, adjuvant, and neoadjuvant fashion. Primary chemotherapy refers to delivery of chemotherapy alone without any additional therapies such as surgery or radiation therapy. Primary chemotherapy is used in many of the hematologic malignancies such as leukemia and lymphoma. Chemotherapy is frequently administered in an adjuvant fashion to a patient who has undergone surgery with curative intent but who is at high risk for relapse (i.e., node-positive breast cancer). Finally, chemotherapy can also be given to patients before surgery (i.e., neoadjuvantly) to "downsize" the tumor to permit a less radical operation, such as delivering neoadjuvant chemotherapy to women with large breast cancers to allow breast-conserving surgery. Chemotherapy can also be given locally or regionally to a tumor or the organ containing the tumor to achieve much higher drug concentrations than can be delivered systemically. Examples of regional chemotherapy include intraperitoneal chemotherapy for some GI tract and ovarian tumors, isolated limb perfusion for extremity melanoma and sarcoma, and isolated hepatic artery infusion for the management of hepatic metastases from colorectal cancer.

Hormonal Therapy

The growth of some cancers, such as breast and prostate cancer, is dependent on sex hormones. Therefore, reductions in circulating hormone levels either by removal of the organs producing these hormones or the use of agents to block or antagonize a particular hormone can be useful in treating hormone-dependent cancers.

In prostate cancer, hormonal interventions include orchiectomy or the administration of stilbestrol (a synthetic estrogen), luteinizing-hormone-releasing hormone (LHRH) analogues (gonadorelins), or antiandrogen drugs (cyproterone or flutamide). In breast cancer, interventions include oophorectomy or administration of tamoxifen (antiestrogen), progestogens (megestrol), LHRH (gonadorelin) antagonists, or aromatase inhibitors.

Radiation Therapy

Radiation has been used in medicine for over a century since the discovery of x-rays by Wilhelm Roentgen in 1895 and the use of radioactive isotopes by Marie Curie in 1898. Since these pioneering efforts, ionizing radiation is now extensively used in the treatment of cancer. It can be used as the primary treatment of radiosensitive tumors such as seminoma and localized Hodgkin's disease. Radiation therapy can also be used in conjunction with other cancer therapies, and some chemotherapeutic agents can serve as radio-sensitizers, such as cisplatin and 5-fluorouracil. In some instances, radiation therapy is preferred over surgery as a cancer treatment when organ or tissue preservation is desired, such as in laryngeal cancer and basal cell carcinoma of the face.

Radiation may be delivered using several techniques including teletherapy, brachytherapy, or systemic radioisotope therapy. External beam radiotherapy or teletherapy is delivered with an external radiation source and it is the most

TABLE 24-7 Chemotherapeutic Agents and Their Indication

Chemotherapeutic Agent	Indication
Alkylating agents (bind to DNA)	
Nitrosoureas (carmustine [BCNU], lomustine [CCNU])	Brain tumors
	Lymphomas
	Hodgkin's disease
Cyclophosphamide	Hematologic malignancies
	Hodgkin's disease
	Non-Hodgkin's lymphoma
Chlorambucil	Chronic lymphocytic leukemia
Mechlorethamine	Lymphomas
	Hodgkin's disease
Decarbazine	Melanoma
	Hodgkin's disease
	Non-Hodgkin's lymphomas
	Sarcomas
Procarbazine	Hodgkin's disease
	Lymphomas
Platinum analogues (cross-link DNA)	
Cisplatin	Carcinoma ovary, testis, cervix
Carboplatin	Carcinoma ovary, bone-marrow transplantation
Oxaliplatin	
Antimetabolites (analogues of normal cellular nutrients)	
Methotrexate	Carcinoma breast, head and neck
6-Mercaptopurine	Acute lymphoblastic leukemia
5-Fluorouracil	Carcinoma breast, cervix, head and neck, GI tract
Antimicrotubule (disrupt the mitotic spindle/microtubule inhibitor)	
Vinca alkaloids (vincristine, vinblastine)	Hematologic malignancies, breast, kidney, testis, head and neck cancers
Topoisomerase inhibitors (bind to and inhibit topoisomerase enzyme: etoposide, teniposide, topotecan)	Hematologic malignancies, lung, bladder, prostate, and testicular cancers
Antibiotics (interfere with the synthesis of nucleic acids: doxorubicin, dactinomycin, plicamycin, mitomycin, bleomycin)	Various solid tumors

commonly used form of radiation for the treatment of cancer. In contrast to external beam radiotherapy, brachytherapy is delivered with the radiation source near or within the target tissue. Brachytherapy is used to treat cervical, breast, prostate, and other cancers. Radioactive iodine (Iodine-131), which is used for the treatment of thyroid cancer, is an example of systemic radioisotope therapy. Advances in imaging techniques have improved the targeting of radiation treatments such that tumors can be treated with less toxicity to surrounding tissues. Stereotactic radiation is a specialized, highly focused type of external beam radiation therapy in which the tumor is precisely targeted using detailed imaging scans. Stereotactic radiation

can be used to treat brain and spinal cord tumors. Radiotherapy injures or destroys cells by damaging their genetic material through the production of free radicals. Although both cancer cells and normal cells are affected, most of the normal cells recover and continue to function. Complications of radiation therapy include lethargy, skin rashes, desquamation, nausea, vomiting, anorexia, urinary frequency, dryness of mouth, impaired blood supply, and delayed healing.

Targeted Therapy

Targeted therapy uses drugs or other agents that block the growth and spread of cancer by interfering with specific molecules involved in tumor growth. Such agents can inhibit growth factor receptors, intracellular signal transduction, or the cell cycle. Some therapies are apoptosis based, while others use antiangiogenic compounds. Examples are shown in Table 24-8.

Immunotherapy

Cancer immunotherapy is the use of the immune system to kill tumor cells. Immunotherapy may be active or passive. Examples of each appear in Table 24-9.

Gene Therapy

Gene therapy aims at altering the genetic program of cancer cells. Strategies used for this purpose include the following:

1. Mutation compensation
2. Molecular chemotherapy
3. Immunopotentiation
4. Antiangiogenic therapy
5. Viral-mediated oncolysis
6. Nonviral gene delivery: Injection of naked DNA and DNA complexed to cationic carriers
7. Gene therapy combined with radiation therapy and/or chemotherapy

Unfortunately, clinical trials to date have demonstrated only limited responses with gene therapy.

Photodynamic Therapy

Photodynamic therapy (PDT) is a method of cancer treatment that uses a photosensitizer, a light source, tissue oxygen, and, generally, lasers. The singlet oxygen that is created is a very aggressive chemical that can kill cells through apoptosis or necrosis.

TABLE 24-8 Examples of Targeted Therapy

Type of Agent	Specific Agent	Cancer
Tyrosine kinase inhibitors	Imatinib	Chronic myelogenous leukemia
	Gefitinib	GIST
Monoclonal antibody	Anti-HER2/neu antibody—trastuzumab	Breast cancer
	Anti-CD20 antibody—rituximab	B-cell malignancies
Peptides	Radionuclides	Hemopoietic tumors

TABLE 24-9	**Examples of Immunotherapy Used to Treat Cancer**		
Type of Immunotherapy	**Class of Agent**	**Agent**	**Cancer**
Active immunotherapy			
	Nonspecific stimulants	Bacille Calmette-Guerin (BCG)	Superficial bladder cancer
			Metastatic melanoma
		Levamisole	Colon cancer (with 5-fluorouracil)
		Cytokines/interferons	Hematologic malignancies
			Some epithelial carcinomas
		IL-2	Metastatic melanoma
			Renal cell carcinoma
			Non-Hodgkin's lymphomas
	Specific active immunotherapy	Vaccines derived from tumor cells or antigen presenting cells (APCs)	
Passive immunotherapy			
	Monoclonal antibodies		
	Immune cells	Nonspecific lymphokines-activated killer (LAK) cells + IL-2	Metastatic melanoma
		Specific tumor infiltrating lymphocytes (TILs) + IL-2	Metastatic melanoma

PREVENTION

Cancer prevention can be primary (taking care of healthy persons), secondary (taking care of those who have premalignant conditions), or tertiary (taking care of those have been cured of their original disease). It can be achieved by chemoprevention through the use of chemotherapeutic agents. Examples include tamoxifen to prevent breast cancer, celecoxib to prevent polyps in familial adenomatous polyposis, and 13-*cis*-retinoic acid to prevent leukoplakia. Prevention can also be achieved surgically, as described in Table 24-6.

THE FUTURE OF CANCER MANAGEMENT

Tremendous progress has been made in our basic understanding of cancer, and undoubtedly continued research advances will translate to further improvements in cancer management. Timely translation of research findings to clinical practice is essential to accelerate our progress against cancer. With advances in imaging techniques, many cancers will be detected earlier, permitting more effective therapy. The identification of new tumor markers will also result in improvements in the detection and treatment of cancer. Innovative techniques that will be increasingly used in cancer management include minimally invasive procedures, ablative techniques, the application of proteomics and transcriptional and gene expression profiling. Technologies for the detection of somatic mutations will also come into use in clinical decision making. Finally, developments will continue in the fields of molecular oncology and personalized cancer therapy.

■ MALIGNANT DISEASES OF THE SKIN

The skin is the largest organ in the human body and skin cancer is the most common malignant tumor. There are over 1 million new cases of skin cancer annually in the United States, accounting for approximately 35% to 40% of all new cancers. Cutaneous malignancies are typically divided into two broad categories: melanoma and nonmelanoma skin cancers. Ultraviolet (UV) radiation is the primary risk factor for most skin cancers and the sun is the predominant source of UV radiation. Therefore, avoidance of the sun and protection from its harmful effects can prevent skin cancer. Most skin cancers arise in the outermost layer of the skin, the epidermis, and consequently they are visible at an early, highly curable stage. Therefore, all physicians must recognize the early signs and symptoms of skin cancer, and they should also be familiar with the preferred diagnostic methods.

BASAL CELL AND SQUAMOUS CELL CARCINOMA

Incidence and Etiology

Convincing evidence exists that UV radiation causes skin cancer. Skin cancer is more common in fair-skinned, sun-sensitive individuals. The incidence of skin cancer is also higher as solar radiation increases at higher elevations and decreasing latitudes. In addition, those individuals who are subject to occupational (i.e., farmers or fishermen) or recreational (i.e., sun-bathers) sun exposure have a higher incidence of skin cancer. Finally, skin cancers are more commonly seen on sun-exposed parts of the body (i.e., face, dorsum of hands, and forearms) and less frequently on the least exposed areas (i.e., trunk and legs).

UV light is electromagnetic radiation with a wavelength in the range 10 to 400 nm. Sunlight consists of two main types of UV radiation, UVA and UVB. Both UVA and UVB radiation contribute to freckling, skin wrinkling, and the development of skin cancer. UVB radiation (290 to 320 nm) has more energy than UVA radiation and it causes the most skin damage. UVA radiation (320 to 400 nm) is less powerful than UVB, but it penetrates deeper into the skin. UVA light is used in tanning booths. Overexposure to UV radiation may cause skin cancer via direct

or indirect damage to DNA. UV radiation causes point mutations in the p53 tumor suppressor gene. The cumulative effect
of solar radiation causes irreversible skin damage. Skin cancers
are often seen in association with other solar radiation–induced
skin damage, including wrinkling, telangiectasias (dilated
blood vessels), actinic keratosis (erythematous, rough-surfaced
lesions), and solar elastosis (yellow papules). Since exposure to
the sun is modifiable behavior, there is an opportunity for the
primary prevention of skin cancer by educating patients about
the hazards of sun exposure and tanning beds. Unfortunately,
current social values in the United States regard a suntan as
healthier and more physically attractive than fair or untanned
skin. Consequently, the popularity of sun bathing and a significant increase in the use of tanning beds have caused a dramatic
increase in skin cancer. In fact, there has been a 15% to 20%
increase in skin cancer incidence in the last decade alone.

Basal cell carcinoma (BCC) and **squamous cell carcinoma** (SCC) account for 70% of cases and SCC for 25% of
nonmelanoma skin cancers, respectively. The incidence of
nonmelanoma skin cancer increases with age, probably as a
result of cumulative exposure to UV radiation over one's lifetime. Most patients with BCC and SCC are older than 65 years
of age at the time of diagnosis. There is a 3:1 predominance
of these tumors in men; partly because of male employment
patterns men receive greater sun exposure. Fortunately, the
cure rate for nonmelanoma skin cancers is high when they are
detected early, and skin cancer is amenable to early diagnosis
since most early lesions are visible and accessible for biopsy.
For these reasons, all physicians must recognize these tumors
at an early stage and any suspicious lesions should be biopsied.
Delayed diagnosis of skin cancer requires wider resections
with complex reconstructions producing greater cosmetic and
functional deformities (Figures 24-1 and 24-2). Furthermore,
although BCCs rarely metastasize, large, poorly differentiated
SCCs can spread locally, regionally, and distantly. SCCs most
commonly spread to the regional lymphatic basin and less
commonly to distant sites such as the lungs and liver. Despite
early detection efforts, approximately 2000 individuals die
from nonmelanoma skin cancers annually.

Chemical exposure is also implicated in the development of
skin cancer. In the late 1700s, Sir Percivall Pott, an English surgeon, was the first person to show that cancer could be caused
by an environmental carcinogen. Pott demonstrated the relationship between soot and carcinoma of the skin of the scrotum
in chimney sweeps. Other examples of chemical substances that
can produce skin cancer used with prolonged exposure include
arsenic, paraffin oil, creosote, pitch, fuel oil, coal, and psoralens
with UVA photochemotherapy. Cigarette smoking is also associated with SCC of the lip, mouth, and nonmucosal skin.

Skin cancer can also arise in areas of chronic inflammation
such as burns, scars, ulcers, and sinus tracts (e.g., at the site of a
chronic osteomyelitis infection, chronic pilonidal sinus, hidradenitis suppurativa). SCC arising in a chronic nonhealing wound
is referred to as a Marjolin's ulcer because it was first described
in 1828 by the French surgeon, Jean Nicholas Marjolin. Skin
cancers that develop in chronic wounds are more aggressive,
and they have an increased risk of local recurrence, distant
spread, and poor outcome. Any chronic wound that fails to heal
or undergoes a recent change should be biopsied (Figure 24-3).

Virus infections also play a role in the development of some
skin cancers. For example, human papilloma virus (HPV)
is the virus that can cause condyloma acuminata or genital
warts. In 1925, Buschke and Löwenstein first described a

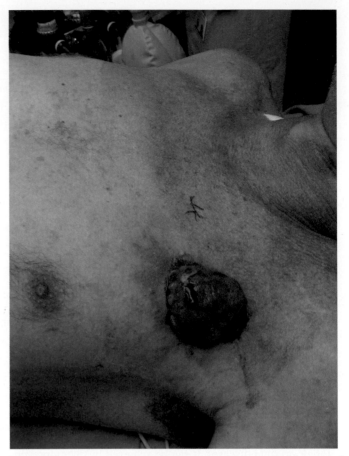

FIGURE 24-1. **Large, neglected BCC of the left chest in an elderly man.** The deep margin of the tumor involved the pectoralis major muscle.

large, cauliflower-like, verrucous cancer that develops in a
giant condyloma acuminata (Figure 24-4). HPV type 6 or 11
is regularly found in association with this destructive tumor.
Risk factors for these tumors include immunosuppression,
chronic irritation, and poor personal hygiene in the anogenital
area. Large cauliflower-like genital warts should be biopsied in
multiple areas to determine whether SCC is present. Patients
with giant condyloma acuminata and multiple fistulous tracts,

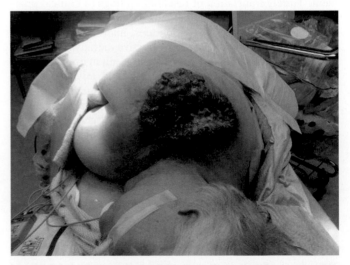

FIGURE 24-2. **Large, neglected BCC of the right shoulder in an elderly woman.** The lesion involved a significant amount of skin and the deep margin of the tumor involved the deltoid and trapezius muscles.

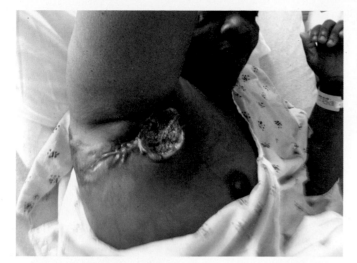

FIGURE 24-3. Squamous cell cancer arising in an area of longstanding hidradenitis suppurativa in the axilla of an African American woman.

purulent discharge, or involvement of the anal sphincter may require a colostomy to prevent fecal soilage. The definitive treatment for giant condyloma acuminata is radical surgical excision often requiring tissue flap reconstruction. Unfortunately, despite radical surgery, there is still a high rate of local failure for these aggressive skin cancers.

Genetic and ethnic factors play an important predisposing role in the development of SCC and BCC. Caucasians with light hair and blue eyes are at greater risk than those ethnic groups with darker skin pigmentation such as Blacks and Asians. The increased melanin in ethnic groups with darker skin pigmentation may afford protection against the damage caused by solar radiation. A few rare genetic conditions result in a high risk for skin cancer. Xeroderma pigmentosum is a rare, inherited disease that is characterized by faulty DNA repair of UV damage. All patients who have this genetic abnormality eventually develop numerous cutaneous neoplasms (Figure 24-5). Albinism is another inherited disorder that results in little or no production of the photoprotective pigment melanin. Albinos have severe intolerance to sunlight and increased susceptibility to skin cancer in exposed areas. Familial basal cell nevus

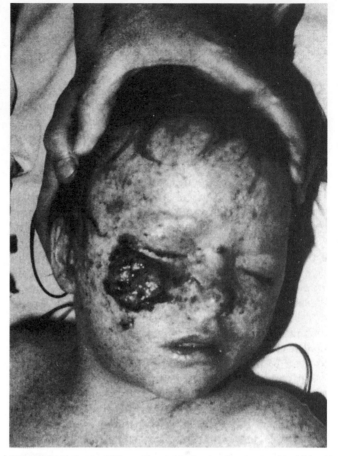

FIGURE 24-5. Large SCC on the right cheek of a 4-year-old child with xeroderma pigmentosum.

syndrome, also known as Gorlin's syndrome, is a rare autosomal dominant disorder with germ-line mutation in human patched gene (PTCH) that results in developmental abnormalities and numerous BCCs early in life. Finally, epidermodysplasia verruciformis is an extremely rare hereditary skin disorder characterized by abnormal susceptibility to HPVs; it is associated with a high risk of carcinoma of the skin.

Chronically immunosuppressed individuals, such as patients who have undergone solid organ transplantation, or who have HIV, or who are long-term steroid users, are at increased risk for the development of skin cancers. These cancers tend to be more aggressive with a greater risk of local recurrence, distant spread, and death. Therefore, sun protective measures are extremely important in this high-risk group of patients.

Although less commonly used today for benign conditions, therapeutic radiation is another physical agent that is responsible for the development of malignant skin tumors, usually SCC. This phenomenon is particularly true for dentists and physicians who used x-ray equipment without appropriate protection and in patients who receive radiation treatment for benign skin conditions such as acne.

BASAL CELL CARCINOMA

Clinical and Histopathologic Characteristics

BCC arises from the basal layer of the epidermis and its appendages such as hair follicles and sebaceous glands. These cancers

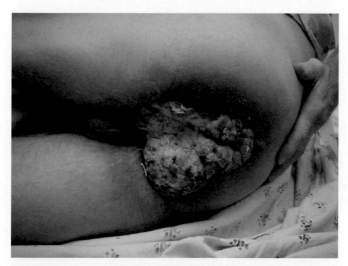

FIGURE 24-4. Verrucous squamous cell cancer arising in a giant condyloma acuminata in the anogenital area (Buschke-Löwenstein tumor).

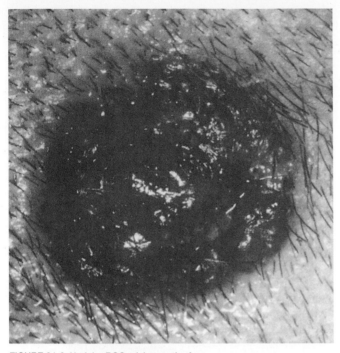

FIGURE 24-6. Nodular BCC arising on the face.

typically grow slowly and almost never metastasize. If BCCs are left untreated, however, they can produce considerable morbidity through local invasion and destruction of surrounding normal tissue. These cancers spread microscopically a significant distance beyond the grossly visible tumor. Approximately 70% of BCCs occur on the face secondary to the sun exposure. The clinical presentation of BCC is divided into three main groups: nodular, superficial, and morhpeaform.

Nodular BCC is the most common type and generally appears on the face as a smooth, dome-shaped, round, waxy, or pearly papule (Figure 24-6). This BCC subtype is slow growing and it may take as long as 1 year to double in size. Nodular BCC may have telangiectasias or small dilated blood vessels on the surface that bleed when traumatized. As the tumor outgrows its blood supply, the center of the lesion undergoes necrosis, forming an ulcer with the potential to invade deeply into adjacent structures (rodent ulcer). Pigmented BCC is similar to the nodular form, except that it contains melanocytes that give it a dark brown or a blue-black color and sometimes it may be confused with melanoma.

Approximately 30% of BCCs are the superficial subtype and they occur more frequently on the trunk. Superficial BCCs frequently present as a shiny, scaly papule, or erythematous patch that may be atrophic in the center. These tumors may also appear multicentric with areas of normal appearing skin between areas of involved skin.

Morpheaform or sclerosing BCC is less common accounting for approximately 5% to 10% of BCC. It typically appears as a smooth, indurated, yellow plaque with ill-defined borders. The overlying skin may remain intact leading to a delay in diagnosis. The skin looks shiny and taut because the tumor causes an intense fibroblastic response that gives it a scar-like appearance (Figure 24-7). The true margin of this form of BCC is difficult to determine because the tumor cells invade normal tissue well beyond the visible margins. Therefore, sclerosing BCC should be treated with a wider excision with careful attention to the margins of excision.

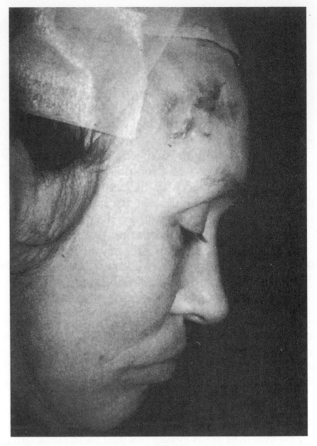

FIGURE 24-7. Large morphea-type BCC of the forehead.

Other less common subtypes of BCC include basosquamous cell carcinoma, an aggressive variant and polypoid BCC, which is a cutaneous condition characterized by exophytic nodules on the head and neck.

Histologically, BCC consists of masses of darkly stained tumor cells that grow from the basal layer of epithelium and into the dermis and subcutaneous tissue. BCC causes no pain or discomfort and the patient may defer seeking medical attention until the lesion is well advanced. Alternatively, the patient may first seek care because of troublesome bleeding from the tumor when it is traumatized, such as by shaving.

Treatment

Excision is the preferred management for BCC. The surgical goal is complete removal of the tumor with minimal functional deformity and optimal cosmetic outcome. There are no evidence-based guidelines for margins of excision for BCC but, if possible, a 1.0-cm margin of normal tissue is recommended. Wider margins of resection are suggested for morphea-like or fibrosing tumors. On the other hand, narrower margins of excision may be necessary if the lesion is located near a critical anatomic feature such as an eyelid. Cryotherapy (freezing the tumor) or electrodessication and curettage (using a sharp spoon-like instrument or curette with electrocautery) can be used to treat small BCCs (≤0.5 cm). Cryotherapy causes cellular destruction by freezing and thawing. Electrodessication uses high-frequency current to destroy the lesion. Both methods are fast, cost effective, and can be performed in an office setting with local anesthesia. Both of these treatments take several weeks to heal and may result in hypopigmentation and scarring. Another disadvantage of these destructive therapies is that they do not permit histologic analysis of the lesion and assessment of the margins of excision.

Moh's micrographic surgical technique may be used to remove BCCs that arise or recur in cosmetically sensitive areas, such as face, where there is a need to preserve normal tissue. This method of excision is usually performed by a specialist who has completed training in Moh's surgery. Moh's surgery consists of carefully labeling and orienting the specimen at the time of excision (e.g., superior margin, anterior) and creating a diagram (Moh's map) of the position of the specimen in relation to the surrounding structures. Moh's surgeon then carefully examines frozen sections to determine proximity of the tumor to the resection margin. When the margins are determined to be clear of tumor, the surgical wound is either closed primarily, skin-grafted, or covered with a tissue flap. If there is uncertainty about the margin of the specimen, additional tissue is sent for frozen-section examination until tumor-free margins are achieved. If the wound is large, it is covered with a sterile dressing until the results are obtained, at which point the patient is referred to a plastic surgeon to provide definitive wound coverage. This careful, stepwise excision with immediate pathologic assessment of margins ensures that all margins are free of residual tumor and preserves normal skin.

Topical chemotherapy using 5-fluorouracil (5-FU, Efudex) cream can be useful in patients with too many superficial BCCs to excise or patients with extensive skin damage. The treatment requires application of a lotion or cream once or twice per day for approximately 1 month. The dosage is adjusted (1%, 2%, or 5% 5-FU concentration) to achieve moderate erythema. The discomfort of the inflammatory reaction and erythema causes some patients to discontinue treatment.

Finally, radiation therapy is a treatment option for elderly patients with BCC who are not good surgical candidates. Similar to other ablative therapies, primary radiation therapy permits no histologic assessment of the tumor and the margins.

Prognosis

Surgical excision cures the majority of patients with BCC. Incomplete excision (i.e., tumor cells left at the margins) usually causes recurrence at the site of tumor removal. Approximately 20% of patients who have a single BCC develop a new primary lesion within 1 year, while patients with multiple tumors have a 40% risk of developing a second BCC within 1 year. Therefore, long-term skin surveillance at 6-month to 1-year intervals is imperative after tumor resection in all patients with BCC. These patients must also be educated about the hazards of UV radiation and the importance of sun-safe behaviors.

SQUAMOUS CELL CARCINOMA

Clinical and Histopathologic Characteristics

SCC arises from the keratinocytes of the epidermis. Unlike BCC, SCC has the potential for metastatic spread, and the risk of metastasis of SCC correlates with size and the grade (i.e., percentage of undifferentiated cells) of the lesion. The most common site of metastasis for SCC is the regional lymph nodes, while distant sites include the lung, liver, and brain. SCC has a varied presentation, but most commonly presents as an ulcerated, erythematous nodule or erosion with indistinct borders (Figure 24-8). It is most commonly found on

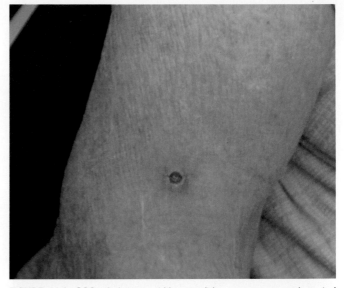

FIGURE 24-8. SCC of the arm with a nodular appearance and central ulceration.

the lower lip and elsewhere in the head and neck as well as in other areas of sun-damaged skin, such as the back of the hands and forearms. The tumor may arise *de novo* or from an area with preexisting skin damage, burn scars, chronic ulcers, osteomyelitic sinuses, or chronic granulomas. SCC is also seen in scars in patients with chronic discoid lupus erythematosus (Figure 24-9). Multiple biopsies should be performed on any chronic nonhealing ulcer that is increasing in size and is not responding to appropriate therapy. SCC *in situ* or Bowen's disease is characterized by tumor cells that have not yet broken through the epidermal–dermal junction. Bowen's disease clinically resembles a red patch or crusting plaque, and without treatment it can progress to invasive SCC with the potential for metastatic spread. The overall rate of metastasis for SCC is low (approximately 1% to 2%). However, tumors that arise in burns, draining osteomyelitic sinuses, chronic ulcers, and Bowen's disease tend to metastasize more often than tumors that arise in sun-damaged skin.

Most SCCs appear clinically as an erythematous firm papule on normal or sun-damaged skin. SCC may initially be difficult to distinguish from a hyperkeratotic lesion but as the tumor enlarges, it forms a nodule with central ulceration with

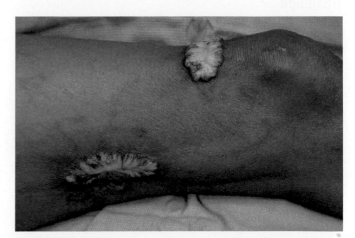

FIGURE 24-9. Multiple SCCs arising in an immunosuppressed patient with discoid lupus.

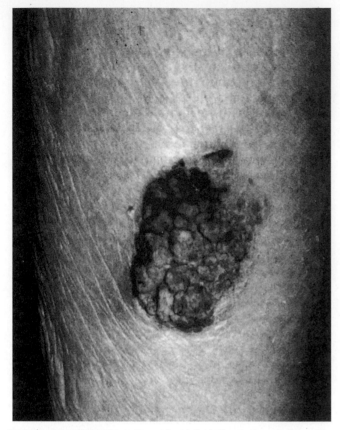

FIGURE 24-10. SCC with crusting and scab formation as a result of repetitive trauma and bleeding.

a white or yellow necrotic base. When this base is removed, a crater-like defect remains. Typically SCC does not have the pearly, raised margins of BCC. SCCs often have crusts or scabs as a result of repetitive trauma and bleeding (Figure 24-10). As with BCC lesions, SCC lesions may enlarge and destroy adjacent normal tissue.

Microscopically, the tumors are irregular nests of epidermal cells that infiltrate the dermis to varying depths and show varying degrees of differentiation. The more differentiated the tumor is, the greater is the number of epithelial pearls (keratinous material) seen in the depths of the tumor.

Treatment

Like BCC, surgical excision is the preferred treatment for SSC. The recommended margin of resection is 1.0 cm, and the same criteria apply for closure of the defect resulting from excision of SCC as with BCC. Since SCC has the potential to spread to the regional lymphatics, sentinel node biopsy is an option for patients with lesions at risk for occult nodal metastases, such as those larger than 2.0 cm in diameter. For details of the technique of sentinel node biopsy, see the treatment subsection of the melanoma section below. Patients with histologically proven metastases to the draining lymphatic basin (i.e., neck for lesions of the face, axilla for lesions of the upper extremity, groin for lesions of the lower extremity) require lymphatic dissection. Patients at high risk for recurrence in the lymphatic basin after lymphadenectomy (i.e., four or more nodal metastases, extracapsular tumor extension) may also require radiation therapy to the regional lymphatics.

In addition to cryotherapy, electrodessication, and topical 5-FU, other nonsurgical treatments for SCC *in situ* include photodynamic therapy and the topical immune response modifier, Imiquimod. Photodynamic therapy uses porphyrins to produce tumor cell cytoxicity after stimulation by light of a certain wavelength. Imiquimod takes advantage of the antitumor properties of immune cells and local cytokine production. Both of these nonsurgical therapies do not permit histologic analysis of margins and may require a high number of treatments to ensure complete removal of the lesion.

Prognosis

As with BCC, the prognosis for small SCCs is excellent, with a cure rate of 95%. In larger lesions that penetrate the subcutaneous tissue, the risk of nodal metastasis increases substantially. After lymph node involvement occurs, the prognosis is poor. Two-thirds of patients with SCC that has penetrated into the subcutaneous tissue may ultimately die from metastatic disease. The majority of patients with lymph node involvement eventually die of their disease. Follow-up in patients with excised SCC lesions should be as rigorous as in patients with BCC. The patient is examined every 6 months for local recurrence, evidence of regional nodal metastasis, or new lesions.

MELANOMA

Incidence and Etiology

The incidence of melanoma is increasing at an exponential rate (Figure 24-11). Over the last half of the twentieth century, diagnosis of melanoma has increased over 600% while the death rate has risen over 160%. While this increase in incidence may, in part, be the result of an increasing number of skin biopsies performed, it does not appear to be the result of more complete reporting or an alteration in the pathologic criteria for the diagnosis of melanoma. In fact, the incidence of melanoma may even be higher than the aforementioned rate because some melanomas are treated by destructive methods (i.e., cryotherapy) and, therefore, no specimen is sent for histologic examination. Furthermore, many hospital-based tumor registries do not capture patients with melanoma diagnosed and treated in small outlying clinics.

While melanoma only accounts for 4% of cutaneous malignancies, it accounts for 80% of all deaths from skin cancer. There are an estimated 60,000 new cases of melanoma and 8000 deaths from melanoma yearly in the United States. Currently, melanoma is the fifth most common cancer in men and the seventh most common in women, but it is the most common cancer in women of ages 20 to 29. The incidence of melanoma increases with age from 0.4 cases per 100,000 people aged 10 to 19 years to 35 cases per 100,000 people older than 80 years. In addition, the lifetime risk of developing melanoma is currently estimated to be one in 50.

UV radiation is a primary cause of melanoma and the primary source of UV radiation is sunlight. The pattern, timing, and duration of exposure to UV radiation are all important in melanoma development. Intense episodic exposure to sunlight in areas that are infrequently exposed to sunlight, such as the back, is associated with melanoma. Several studies in Australia, New Zealand, and the United States show an increased incidence of melanoma near the equator. Melanomas occur with increased incidence on the legs in women and on the

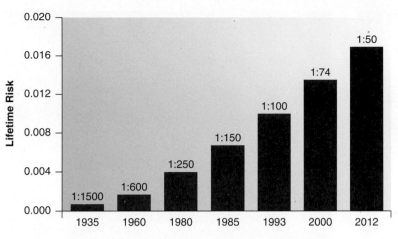

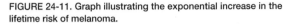

FIGURE 24-11. Graph illustrating the exponential increase in the lifetime risk of melanoma.

trunk in men. These data suggest that exposure to sunlight has a role in the etiology of melanoma, but they do not explain the occurrence of melanoma in areas of the body that have minimal exposure to sunlight.

Sunburn is a marker of excessive episodic exposure to UV radiation. Sunburns in childhood and adolescence appear to do the most damage leading to subsequent development of melanoma. Therefore, efforts to educate the public about the hazards of UV radiation and the importance of sun-safe behaviors should begin in childhood. It is much easier to learn healthy habits in life than to break bad habits later in life. The American Cancer Society guidelines for skin cancer prevention include:

1. Avoid the sun, particularly during the peak times of UV radiation from 10 AM to 4 PM.
2. When in the sun, wear protective clothing including sunglasses with UV protection and a wide-brimmed hat.
3. When in the sun, use sun screen with a sun protective factor of 15 or greater and apply it 30 minutes before, apply it liberally, and reapply if sweating or if you come out of the water.
4. Avoid tanning beds.

Unfortunately, many people fail to apply enough sunscreen per unit area of skin. In addition, many people get a false sense of protection when using sunscreen and they mistakenly spend more time in the sun, which then increases their risk for subsequent skin cancer.

The incidence of melanoma is influenced by skin pigment, with the lowest rates (0.8 per 100,000 population) occurring among blacks. On the other hand, incidence rates among the Celtic population in Australia and New Zealand are the highest in the world (40 per 100,000). The so-called melanoma phenotype consists of fair-complexioned individuals with blue eyes and red or blonde hair who freckle and burn easily upon brief sun exposure.

Approximately one-fourth of all cutaneous melanomas occur in the head and neck area. Of these, the majority occurs outside the hair-bearing scalp. The site distribution of malignant melanoma in blacks is strikingly different from that in whites. In blacks, approximately 70% of melanomas are found on the palmar surface of the hands and plantar surface of the feet, compared with <5% in whites. Approximately 50% to 60% of melanomas arise from or near-benign nevi. The triggering event for malignant transformation of benign nevi remains unknown. Benign nevi are extremely common, and very few become malignant. The one exception is **congenital**

giant hairy nevus (bathing trunk nevus), which undergoes malignant transformation to melanoma in 10% to 30% of untreated lesions.

Familial malignant melanomas account for approximately 10% of all melanomas, but almost half of patients who have multiple primary melanomas have a family history of melanoma. Familial melanomas tend to occur at a younger age than sporadic tumors. In addition, any patient who has experienced a melanoma is at risk for a second melanoma.

A third recognized risk factor for hereditary melanoma is **familial atypical mole and melanoma syndrome (FAM-M)**, previously called dysplastic nevus syndrome. Patients with familial melanoma have large premalignant nevi, predominantly over the shoulders, upper chest, and back. Hereditary melanoma and FAM-M are associated with genetic alterations in chromosomes 1p, 6q, 7, and 9. Genetic predisposition to malignant melanoma is also associated with the hereditary syndrome **xeroderma pigmentosum**, which is an autosomal recessive disorder characterized by defective DNA repair mechanisms required to repair damage caused by UV radiation.

Embryology of Melanocytes

Melanocytes are cells derived from neural crest tissue. During early gestation, the cells migrate to the skin, uveal tract, meninges, and ectodermal mucosa. Melanocytes reside in the basal layer of the epidermis and produce melanin pigment. The density of melanocytes in Caucasians and African Americans is approximately the same for any skin site. The differences in skin pigmentation are the result of the melanosome-pigment package that is passed out of the melanocyte, by way of its dendritic processes, and phagocytized by surrounding keratinocytes. These cells then migrate up to the epidermis, where they cause the phenotypic patterns and degrees of skin coloration observed in people.

Clinical and Histopathologic Characteristics

Melanoma is classified into four main morphologic subtypes: **superficial spreading melanoma, nodular melanoma, lentigo maligna melanoma,** and **acral lentiginous melanoma.** None of these subtypes however, is a predictive of outcome independent of the T stage (i.e., tumor thickness and presence of ulceration). Melanoma has two distinct growth patterns: **horizontal and vertical.** The horizontal, or lateral, growth phase results in increasing lesion size, but less risk of distant

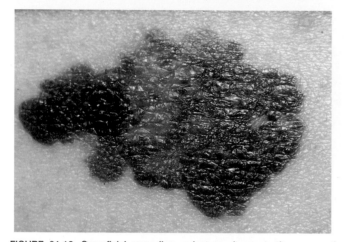

FIGURE 24-12. Superficial spreading melanoma demonstrating areas of regression.

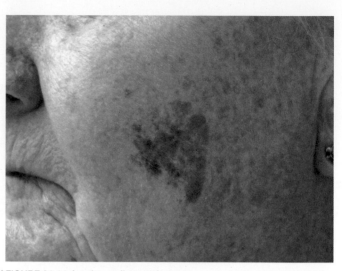

FIGURE 24-14. Lentigo maligna melanoma.

spread. The vertical growth phase is more dangerous because of increased likelihood of invasion, access to the lymphatics and/or blood vessels, and the potential for metastatic spread.

Superficial spreading melanoma is the most morphologic common subtype of melanoma accounting for approximately 70% of all cutaneous melanomas. It is most commonly found on the legs in women, while the back is most common site in men. The peak incidence of superficial spreading melanoma occurs in the fifth decade. This tumor has both radial and vertical growth phases. Early superficial spreading melanoma lesions are of many colors (usually tan, brown, blue, and black). More advanced lesions have palpable nodularity, which indicates the development of a vertical growth phase. Some of these tumors have depigmented areas that represent areas of spontaneous regression (Figure 24-12).

Nodular melanoma accounts for approximately 10% to 15% of all cutaneous melanomas and is the most malignant subtype because of a dominant vertical growth phase. Nodular melanoma occurs twice as often in men as in women (Figure 24-13). The host cellular response is usually less than that seen with other types of melanoma. Nodular melanoma is blue-black in color with less variability in color and margins than superficial spreading melanoma.

Lentigo maligna melanoma (Hutchinson's freckle) is a subtype of melanoma characterized by slow, but insidious growth and by its tendency to occur on the sun-exposed areas of the face, head, and neck of older people. This type of melanoma constitutes 5% to 10% of cutaneous melanomas and is the most benign type of cutaneous melanoma. It usually begins as a circumscribed macular patch of mottled pigmentation, showing shades of dark brown, tan, or black (Figure 24-14). It is often referred to as "a stain on the skin." The median age at diagnosis is approximately 70 years and women are affected more often than men. While lentigo maligna melanoma has a slow, benign-appearing growth pattern, the margins are ill defined, and therefore achieving a tumor-free margin can be challenging. A staged surgical approach to lentigo maligna involves performing the wide excision and temporary wound coverage with a biologic dressing. If the margins are tumor free, then the definitive reconstruction can be performed. If tumor is present at a margin, then additional resection can be performed to achieve tumor-free margins before a definitive reconstructive procedure.

Acral lentiginous melanoma occurs on the palmar surface of the hands and the plantar surface of the feet (Figure 24-15) and in subungual (i.e., beneath the nail plate) sites (Figure 24-16).

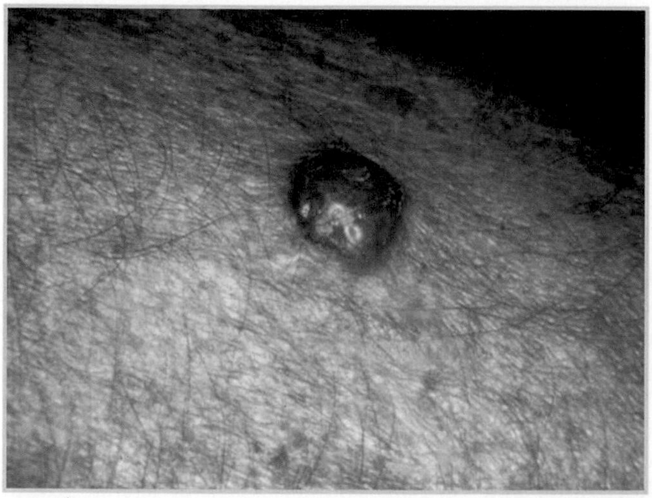

FIGURE 24-13. Nodular melanoma.

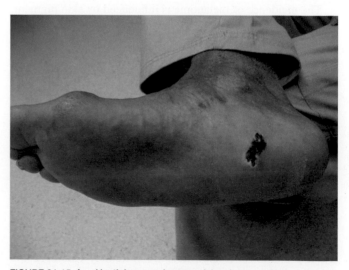

FIGURE 24-15. Acral lentiginous melanoma of the plantar surface of the foot.

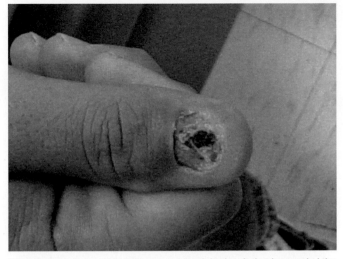

FIGURE 24-16. Subungual melanoma of the right thumb that has eroded the overlying nailplate.

Acral lentiginous melanoma has both a radial and a vertical growth phase and in the subungual location, the radial growth phase may simply be a streak in the nail associated with irregular tan-brown staining of the nail bed. Subungual melanomas frequently distort the nailplate and are often misdiagnosed as a fungal infection resulting in a delay in diagnosis.

Desmoplastic melanoma is a subtype of melanoma that is more common in the head and neck, and it has sarcoma-like features and behavior. Desmoplastic melanoma has a high risk for local recurrence and radiation therapy may be indicated to reduce this risk.

Melanoma occasionally occurs as a metastatic lesion without a demonstrable primary site, suggesting complete regression of the primary site. Finally, there is a rare subtype of melanoma with a complete absence of pigment called amelanotic melanoma that is extremely difficult to detect at an early stage.

Diagnosis

Since the skin is accessible to direct visual inspection, cutaneous melanoma is amenable to early detection and diagnosis. The majority of melanomas "write their message with ink in the skin." Patients with early stage "thin" melanomas (thickness <1.0 mm) have a 5-year survival rate of 90%. Therefore, all health care providers must be able to recognize the signs of melanoma. A complete skin exam in a well-light room is an essential part of any physical examination. A magnifying glass can be of value, and the clinician must inspect the scalp, palms, soles, and mucosa. A convenient mnemonic for the recognition of melanoma is the ABCDE rule, which includes:

A = Asymmetry: One-half of the skin lesion does not match the other half.

B = Border: The edges are ragged, irregular, or blurred.

C = Color: There is variation in the color with differing shades of brown, black, or blue.

D = Diameter: The lesion is larger than 6 mm (the size of a pencil eraser).

E = Evolution: The lesion has grown or changed since the last evaluation.

Any lesions exhibiting the above criteria should be biopsied. Although melanoma can develop anywhere on the skin, the most common location are the legs of women and the trunks of men. Lesions that are occasionally confused with cutaneous melanoma include **junctional nevi, compound nevi, intradermal nevi, blue nevi, BCCs, seborrheic keratoses, dermatofibromas,** and **subungual hemorrhage**. Characteristics that help with the differentiation of these lesions from melanoma are listed here. Junctional nevi usually appear during the early years of life and are particularly apparent during adolescence. They vary in size from a few millimeters to several centimeters. They are light to dark brown, with a flat, smooth surface and irregular edges. Compound nevi are usually brown or black, with a raised nodular surface that often contains hair. They are usually smaller than 1 cm and occur in all age groups. Intradermal nevi can be very large, although they are usually <1 cm in diameter. Their color varies from light to dark brown, and they may have a raised warty or smooth surface. The presence of coarse hairs distinguishes them from other nevi. Blue nevi are smooth blue-black lesions that are smaller than 1 cm, with well-defined, regular margins. They usually occur on the face, the dorsum of the feet and hands, and the buttocks. They are rarely associated with malignant melanoma. BCCs are most common in middle-aged people. A pigmented BCC tumor is usually blue-black, with raised edges and capillary neovascularity. Initially, the lesion is smooth, but it can become ulcerated. Seborrheic keratoses are occasionally black. They are usually 1 cm or larger and typically appear as raised and warty, with a greasy consistency. They appear to be stuck onto the skin. Dermatofibromas are occasionally dark brown. They are usually smooth, slightly raised, and without hairs. They typically grow very slowly and never become malignant. A malignant version of this tumor, dermatofibrosarcoma protuberans (DFSP), also occurs as a slow-growing tumor that may rarely be pigmented. Subungual hemorrhage is usually sudden in onset and is sharply defined beneath the nail bed. By comparison, subungual melanoma has a gradual onset and has poorly demarcated streaks that extend along the axis of the nail. The diagnosis of hemorrhage is confirmed by puncturing the nail and evacuating the blood. In time, the entire subungual hemorrhage migrates distally, and the nail bed clears. Subungual melanoma, however, is a persistent lesion. However, if there is any question about a lesion, histologic examination provides the necessary confirmatory evidence.

Excisional Biopsy

Excisional biopsy consisting of complete excision of the lesion, down to subcutaneous tissue with a narrow margin of normal-appearing skin, is the preferred method of biopsy. Excisional biopsy permits histopathologic analysis of the entire lesion to determine the depth of penetration. Accurate staging is critical for further management of melanoma. Before infiltrating local anesthesia, the physician outlines an ellipse around the lesion with narrow (i.e., 2- to 4-mm) margins. On the extremity, the incision is placed parallel to the long axis to facilitate primary closure upon reexcision should the excised lesion prove to be melanoma. After the ellipse is outlined, local anesthesia is infiltrated into normal tissue around rather than directly into the lesion. Full-thickness skin and subcutaneous tissue are excised and the skin is reapproximated (Figure 24-17). If the size or location of the primary site prevents excisional biopsy, then an incisional or punch biopsy is performed.

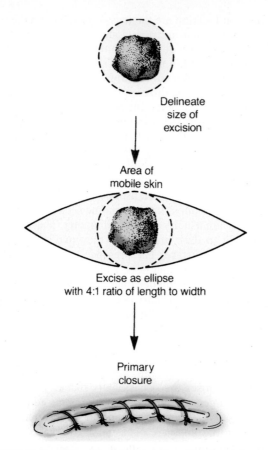

Delineate
size of
excision

Area of
mobile skin

Excise as ellipse
with 4:1 ratio of length to width

Primary
closure

FIGURE 24-17. Surgical excision of a skin lesion with primary closure.

Incisional Biopsy

When a lesion is too large for excisional biopsy, incisional biopsy may be performed without compromising cure rates as long as definitive surgical therapy is initiated promptly. However, the possibility of sampling error must be considered when incisional or punch biopsy is performed. Punch biopsy is performed with a disposable device that has a hollow sharp tip of varying diameters (i.e., 3, 4, and 5 mm). Shave biopsy is not the preferred method of biopsy because it fails to provide an accurate depth of invasion. In addition, shave biopsy can result in inflammatory cells at the base of the lesion that make precise determination of depth of invasion difficult when an excisional biopsy follows a shave biopsy.

Staging

The characteristics of melanoma that are important in determining subsequent management and prognosis are tumor thickness, ulceration, nodal metastases, and distant metastases. Two systems are used to determine tumor depth of invasion of melanoma. The **Clark system** for primary melanoma is based on the histologic level of invasion of the tumor. Level I lesions are confined to the epidermis, level II lesions invade the papillary layer of the dermis, level III lesions reach the junction of the papillary and reticular layers, level IV lesions invade the reticular dermis, and level V lesions invade the subcutaneous fat. A disadvantage of the Clark system is that different pathologists may interpret the levels of invasion variably. In addition, the Clark level is only used for staging when the Breslow tumor thickness is <1.0 mm.

The **Breslow system** is the other method for assessing melanoma thickness. Breslow staging uses an ocular micrometer to measure the thickness of the tumor in millimeters from the granular layer of the epidermis to the deepest point of vertical growth. The Breslow system allows more objective evaluation and easier comparison among pathologists. The Breslow thickness predicts the risk of metastasis and determines the margin width required for reexcision.

The American Joint Committee on Cancer (AJCC) TNM (tumor, node, metastasis) system combines information from the Breslow system, whether the lesion is ulcerated, and information about the status of lymph nodes and distant metastases to provide a comprehensive staging system (http://www.cancerstaging.org/index.html).

Malignant melanoma can spread through both the lymphatic and blood routes. Lymphatic spread can present clinically as in-transit metastases or as enlarged nodes. In-transit metastases occur when melanoma cells are trapped between the primary tumor and regional lymph nodes and produce a region of subcutaneous metastases more than 3 cm from the primary site. Distant metastasis from melanoma may occur in any tissue, with skin, subcutaneous tissue, and distant lymphatic sites being most common. Lung, brain, liver, and bone are less frequent sites. Evaluation of large numbers of patients has led to the recognition that within the group with distant metastatic disease, those with spread to skin, subcutaneous tissue, or lymphatic sites fare better than those with spread to lung or to all other visceral sites.

Treatment

Definitive surgical treatment of primary melanoma involves a wide excision of the surrounding normal skin and subcutaneous tissue. The goal of wide local excision is to completely excise all melanoma cells while minimizing morbidity, cosmetic disfigurement, functional impairment, and cost. In the early half of the 20th century, all melanomas were treated using a 5.0-cm margin requiring a skin graft for coverage and leaving a significant cosmetic deformity. The recommended width of excision of a melanoma has declined over the last 20 to 30 years, and there are now evidence-based guidelines for margins of excision dependent on the tumor thickness. A margin of 1.0 cm is generally recommended for thin melanomas ≤1.0 mm in depth. For intermediate-thickness melanomas (1 to 4 mm), 2-cm margins of excision are adequate. Melanomas deeper than 4 mm require a 3.0-cm margin. In general, most wide excisions can be closed primarily and skin grafts avoided.

If regional lymph nodes are palpable on physical examination, regional node dissection is performed. In the absence of lymphadenopathy, sentinel lymph node (SLN) biopsy can accurately stage patients by determining the histological status of the draining nodes. The SLN is the principal node that drains that skin where the melanoma is located. By examining the SLN, a decision can be made to leave the node basin intact if the SLN is tumor free (i.e., negative) or to remove the nodes because the SLN contains melanoma cells (i.e., positive). The technique of SLN biopsy involves the use of a dye, such as isosulfan blue, a radiolabeled material (i.e., ^{99m}Tc sulfur colloid), or a combination of the two injected intradermally around the site of the melanoma or on either side of the biopsy scar. The best results occur when the vital blue dye and lymphoscintigraphy methods are combined. An incision is made over the draining regional lymph basin. All clinically suspicious, radioactive, and/or blue lymph nodes are removed. The SLN is identified and examined outside the draining basin (i.e., *ex vivo*) with a handheld gamma counter. If the counts are elevated, the node is removed and submitted for histologic examination and immunohistochemical studies. If the sentinel node is negative, there is >95% chance that the remaining lymph nodes are tumor free. If the sentinel node is positive, then a complete node dissection is required because the probability of finding other positive lymph nodes is significant. The sensitivity and predictive value of SLN biopsy can be improved by the use of immunohistochemistry methods that identify proteins unique to melanoma cells and by the use of reverse transcriptase-polymerase chain reaction to identify genes unique to melanoma cells. While these methods increase the sensitivity of melanoma detection, the routine use of reverse transcriptase-polymerase chain reaction in staging melanoma is still under evaluation to determine its utility and predictive value.

Adjuvant treatment is treatment that is given in addition to the primary surgical therapy when all detectable disease has been removed, but where there remains a high risk of relapse due to occult disease. Interferon-α, a proinflammatory cytokine, is the only beneficial adjuvant therapy for melanoma patients. Unfortunately, the overall survival benefit from interferon is small and it has significant toxicity and cost.

The majority of distant metastases develop within 5 years of diagnosis, but delayed recurrences of melanoma may occur even decades after diagnosis. Surgery is the main treatment for metastatic melanoma. While resection of isolated distant metastasis may improve survival, the management of distant disease is rarely curative and is determined primarily by its location and symptoms. Metastatic disease to the brain is usually treated with either stereotactic radiosurgery alone or resection. Pulmonary and liver metastases may be resected depending upon the disease-free interval, location, and number of metastases. Hepatic metastases may be ablated by nonresectional methods such as radiofrequency ablation. Patients with distant metastases may undergo palliative chemotherapy, or immunotherapy. Recent trials using Ipilimumab, a monoclonal antibody that binds to cytotoxic T lymphocyte-associated antigen 4 (CTLA-4), and Vemurafenib, another antibody that targets the *BRAF* gene, have shown significant activity in metastatic melanoma. In addition, all patients with metastatic melanoma should be considered for enrollment in a clinical trial. Distant spread to an extremity that involves in-transit metastases may be managed by regional limb perfusion with a chemotherapeutic agent (e.g., L-phenylalanine mustard) and hyperthermia. This treatment is beneficial only if the disease is confined to that extremity; there are no data indicating that it prolongs patient life. Regardless of the protocol, the response rate is low (20%), even when partial and complete responses are combined.

Immunotherapy as an adjuvant to surgical treatment remains an important but incompletely achieved goal. Trials underway are testing a variety of vaccines, dosages, and routes of administration. Access to these agents in most cases requires participation in a clinical trial.

Radiation is rarely used as the single treatment for melanoma. It may have a role for special types of melanoma such as desmoplastic melanoma, which is characterized histologically by spindle cells and behaves somewhat like a sarcoma. Radiation therapy may also be of value to reduce local recurrence of melanoma in nodal basins with four or more lymph nodes containing melanoma.

■ MALIGNANT DISEASES OF THE SOFT TISSUE

SARCOMA

Adult soft tissue sarcomas are rare tumors derived from embryonic mesoderm. Unlike more common solid tumors, such as breast, lung, and colorectal cancer, they are not derived from epithelial tissues. Less than 1% of all cancers are sarcomas. Of sarcomas, 66% occur in the extremity, 20% on the trunk, and 13% in the retroperitoneum. There are over 50 subtypes, the most common being undifferentiated high-grade pleomorphic sarcoma (malignant fibrous histiocytoma (24%), leiomyosarcoma (21%), and liposarcoma (19%) (Figure 24-18). As with other malignancies, the stage of the tumor determines patient outcome, and, somewhat peculiar to sarcoma, stage is largely determined by grade. Sarcoma is particularly prone to local recurrence if incompletely excised in the first instance. The complex nature and rarity of the tumor means that it is best managed by a multidisciplinary team of oncologists (surgical, radiation, and medical), supported by a dedicated sarcoma pathologist.

Incidence and Etiology

There are approximately 9000 new cases and 4000 deaths from sarcoma annually in the United States. Patients with sarcoma may present with a history of trauma to the area; however, a causal relationship has never been established. It is more likely that injury calls attention to the preexisting tumor. Risk factors that have been associated with sarcoma occurrence include occupational exposure, radiation, chronic lymphedema, and both germline and somatic mutations in oncogenes and tumor suppressor genes.

A variety of chemical agents and carcinogens have been linked to the development of sarcoma. Asbestos (hydrated

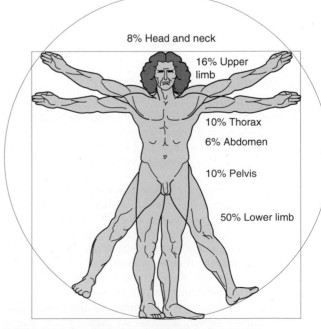

FIGURE 24-18. Site distribution of adult soft tissue sarcoma.

silicate) is associated with the development of pleural mesothelioma. Exposure to phenoxyacetic acid herbicides (lawn pesticides) and their byproducts, dioxin and Agent Orange, has been associated with increased incidence of sarcomas, most notably in soldiers who fought in the Vietnam War. The manufacture of polyvinyl chloride (PVC) has been associated with the development of the particularly aggressive sarcoma, hepatic angiosarcoma.

There is an 8- to 50-fold increase in incidence of sarcoma reported in patients treated with radiation for carcinoma of breast, cervix, ovary, testes, and lymphatic system. To be diagnosed as a radiation-associated sarcoma, the lesion must be in the radiated field, be of different histology to the tumor originally treated with radiation, and develop after a latency period of at least 3 years.

Lymphangiosarcoma can occur in chronic lymphedema. Angiosarcoma in the context of lymphedema from a radical axillary dissection for a carcinoma of the breast is known as Stewart-Treves syndrome.

Gene rearrangements have been found in Ewing's sarcoma, clear-cell sarcoma, myxoid/round-cell liposarcoma, alveolar rhabdomyosarcoma, desmoplastic small round-cell tumors, and synovial sarcoma. Oncogenes implicated so far include MDM2, N-myc, c-erB2, and ras oncogenes. But majority of soft tissue sarcomas harbor multiple oncogene and tumor suppressor gene mutations as well as chromosomal aberrations.

Germ-line mutations in the tumor suppressor gene p53 cause the Li-Fraumeni syndrome and increase the risk of rhabdomyosarcoma, osteosarcoma, and some other soft tissue sarcoma, as well as early-onset breast carcinoma and other neoplasms. Germ-line mutations in the neurofibromatosis type 1 gene *NF1* produce Von Recklinghausen syndrome and increase the incidence of malignant peripheral nerve sheath rumor (neurofibrosarcoma, malignant peripheral nerve sheath tumor [MPNST]). Gardner's syndrome (a subset of familial polyposis patients) is associated with an increased incidence of desmoid tumors (aggressive fibromatosis). The familial polyposis syndromes are due to a mutation in the *APC* gene. In addition, somatic mutations in the p53 tumor suppressor gene have been reported in 30% to 60% of soft tissue sarcomas. Mutations or deletions in the Rb gene can lead to the development of retinoblastoma as well as osteosarcoma.

Clinical Presentation and Evaluation

Soft tissue sarcomas arise from a variety of cell types and are difficult to diagnose. Using panels of immunohistochemical stains, a pathologist can more accurately identify the more common histologic types (Figure 24-19 and Table 24-10). Tumor grade (Table 24-11) also provides important prognostic information.

In addition to histologic subtype, sarcomas can be divided into those with limited metastatic potential and those with significant metastatic potential (Table 24-12). Lymph node metastases are not a common feature of sarcoma, occurring in <5% of tumors, except specific histologic subtypes such as epithelioid sarcoma, rhabdomyosarcoma, clear-cell sarcoma, and angiosarcoma. As with other cancers, sarcoma is staged according to the American Joint Committee on Cancer (AJCC) staging criteria (http://www.cancerstaging.org/index.html). The stage assigned depends on tumor grade, tumor size, and the presence of metastases and nodes.

Patient outcome is influenced by tumor size, with smaller lesions (≤5 cm T1 lesions) having a better prognosis. Tumor grade also influences outcome, with higher-grade lesions being more likely to spread or to recur. In addition, T staging is further divided into tumors that are above (a) or below (b) the superficial fascia. This staging system not only has major prognostic significance, but also guides the multidisciplinary sarcoma team in patient management.

The overall clinical behavior of most sarcomas is similar and is determined by anatomic location, grade, and size of tumor. The metastatic tumor spread is hematogenous, the primary site being the lung; however, in advanced disease, subcutaneous metastases are not uncommon. For intra- and retroperitoneal disease, liver metastases and eventual sarcomatosis (extensive sarcoma tumor nodules within the peritoneal cavity) are common in the terminal phases of the disease.

Sarcoma is predominantly treated with surgery. The surgical goal is to resect the tumor with at least a 2-cm margin of normal tissue surrounding the lesion. Where the ability to achieve a 2-cm margin is in doubt, owing to close proximity of vital structures (e.g., major nerves or arteries), adjuvant (in addition to, but after surgery) or neoadjuvant (in addition to, but before surgery) radiotherapy is employed. This strategy not only improves the limb-sparing rate (fewer amputations), but also improves local control. Administering neoadjuvant radiotherapy for retroperitoneal tumors can be problematic given the limited tissue tolerances of certain organs (e.g., liver, 2000 rads). When margins are positive or very close (<2 mm), the local recurrence rate approaches 100%.

Sarcoma is notable in that approximately one-third of patients are asymptomatic at the time of presentation. As a consequence, some of these tumors may grow extremely large (20 to 30 cm). Sarcoma tends not to invade other structures, but rather to have a pushing type of growth. In addition, these tumors tend not to compress luminal structures such as the gut or vessels. The presence of significant neurovascular or gastrointestinal compressive or obstructive symptoms implies locally advanced disease. Additional worrisome clinical features are a history of a rapid growth of tumors and the presence of lymphadenopathy.

Treatment

When a patient presents with a clinically suspicious mass, appropriate imaging and staging studies are carried out to determine the extent of local disease and whether there is any metastatic disease (Figure 24-20). Next, a core biopsy is undertaken after discussion in multidisciplinary setting, including radiology, to ensure the biopsy is done at the region of viable tumor. Multiple cores are encouraged to rule out tumor heterogeneity and to ensure detailed histological and immunohistochemistry studies can be performed, and if this yields inadequate tissue for diagnosis, then an open biopsy is performed in the axial plane that would be used for excision of the lesion. Resection with adequate margins of normal tissue will be sufficient for the management of small (≤5 cm), superficial, well-differentiated lesions. All other tumors require multidisciplinary management, with many of the components of treatment decided by a team prior to resectional surgery.

Superficial

Superficial extremity sarcomas are defined by the AJCC staging system as those superficial to the deep fascia.

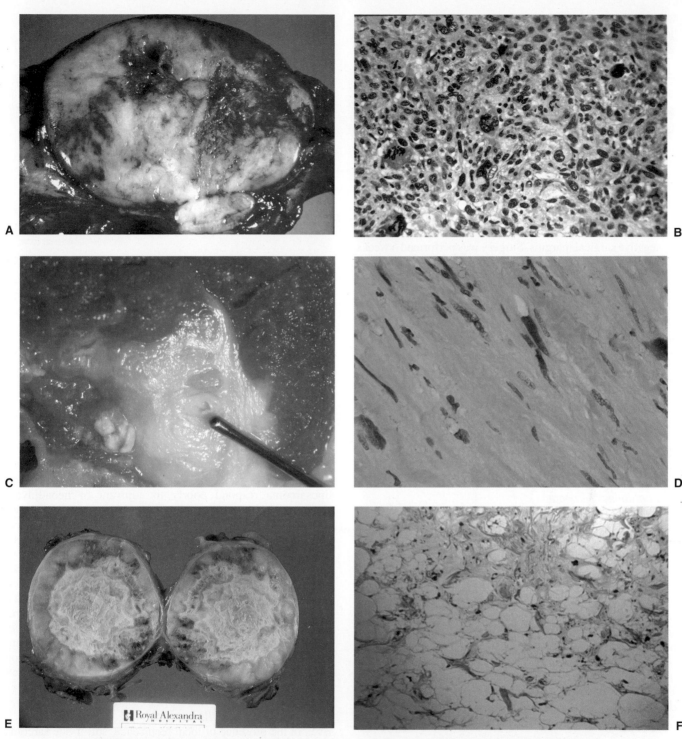

FIGURE 24-19. Common sarcoma histology types. A, Mixofibrous histiocytoma (previously called malignant fibrous histiocytoma) growth appearance of sectioned tumor. **B,** Microscopic appearance Mixofibrous histiocytoma. **C,** Leiomyosarcoma growth appearance of sectioned tumor. **D,** Microscopic appearance of leiomyosarcoma. **E,** Liposarcoma growth sectioned. **F,** Microscopic appearance of liposarcoma.

Figure 24-21A shows an example of a young woman with type 1 neurofibromatosis in whom a single neurofibroma degenerated into an MPNST (neurofibrosarcoma). Figure 24-21B shows neovascularization of the skin overlying the tumor as well as café-au-lait spots visible on the anterior abdominal wall. Wide resection, including 2-cm margins of skin and subcutaneous tissue plus the deep fascia, was performed, followed by rotation flap and skin graft of the resultant defect. The lesion

was low grade and did not require any adjuvant chemotherapy or radiotherapy.

Deep
Figure 24-22 shows a sarcoma in a 56-year-old man who presented with a 3-month history of a rapidly expanding mass involving the adductor compartment of the thigh. The skin overlying the lesion was warm to the touch. Radical external-beam radiotherapy (6500 rads over 6 weeks) was

TABLE 24-10	Immuohistochemical Stains Utilized for Subclassifying Sarcomas
Stain	**Cell of Origin**
5100	Nerve, fat
Smooth muscle action	Smooth muscle
Desmin	Mature and immature skeletal muscle
Myogenin	Immature skeletal muscle (i.e., rhabdomyosarcoma)
CD31	Blood vessel (endothelial cells)

TABLE 24-12	Metastatic Potential of Various Sarcoma Histologies	
Low Metastatic Potential	**Intermediate Metastatic Potential**	**High Metastatic Potential**
Desmoid tumor	Myxoid liposarcoma	Alveolar soft part sarcoma
Atypical lipomatous tumor	Myxoid malignant fibrous histiocytoma	Angiosarcoma
Dermatofibrosarcoma protuberans (DFSP)	Extraskeletal chondrosarcoma	Clear-cell sarcoma ("melanoma of soft parts")
Hemangiopericytoma		Epithelioid sarcoma
		Extraskeletal Ewing's sarcoma
		Extraskeletal osteosarcoma
		Undifferentiated high-grade pleomorphic sarcoma (malignant fibrous histiocytoma)
		Liposarcoma (pleomorphic and dedifferentiated)
		Leiomyosarcoma
		MPNST (neurofibrosarcoma)
		Rhabdomyosarcoma
		Synovial sarcoma

administered to arrest the rapid growth and to assist in achieving negative surgical margins. Surgery was performed 6 weeks following completion of radiotherapy. A wide resection of the tumor was not possible because of close proximity to the neurovascular bundles. Therefore, a "marginal" resection (close or narrow margins) was performed to save the patient's limb. As a result of the high grade and aggressive nature of this lesion, the patient received six cycles of adriamycin-based chemotherapy postoperatively.

However, adjuvant chemotherapy for sarcoma remains controversial, as recent clinical trials and meta-analyses have produced conflicting results. In a meta-analysis first published in 2002 and updated in 2008, there was only a 4% absolute survival benefit for adjuvant chemotherapy at 10 years, at the expense of treatment-related toxicity. The benefits were observed in those with high-grade tumors, >5 cm, deep location, and in the extremity.

Retroperitoneal Sarcoma

Figure 24-23 demonstrates a large right retroperitoneal liposarcoma, which has pushed the right kidney out from the retroperitoneal space and is now palpable anteriorly. Two components of the tumor are visible: the darker area more consistent with simple fat laterally, and a more solid central component compressing the aorta. A thoracoabdominal incision is necessary to completely excise this tumor. An on-block resection is required involving not only resecting the tumor, but also the right kidney and adrenal gland and right colon. For large lesions high in the left retroperitoneum, the spleen, portions of the stomach, diaphragm, pancreas, and duodenal jejunal flexion may also need to be resected to completely remove the tumors. The ability to achieve a wide resection margin with such large tumors within the

peritoneum or retroperitoneum is impossible owing to vital structures. Liposarcomas except for myxoid/round-cell liposarcoma respond poorly to adjuvant or neoadjuvant chemoradiotherapy. Given the size and location of the tumor, it is anticipated that there is a 60% to 80% chance of local recurrence, and ultimately the development of sarcomatosis within the peritoneal cavity.

Figure 24-24A shows a computed tomography (CT) scan of a large pelvic sarcoma. The rectum, prostate, urethra, and bladder are intimately related to this 12-cm tumor, and, as a consequence, an anterior and posterior total pelvic exenteration (i.e., removal of the tumor, rectum, and bladder with permanent colostomy and ileoconduit) was necessary to completely resect this tumor. Figure 24-24B is the postresection CT scan, showing loops of small bowel filling the space left by the pelvic organs and tumor.

Management of Local Recurrence

Even in the presence of local recurrence, soft tissue sarcoma remains primarily a surgical disease. Typically, these sarcomas will recur within 2 years (80%) of the original tumor presentation. Confirmation of the diagnosis of local recurrence is best made by image-guided core biopsy. Imaging studies (CT and/or magnetic resonance imaging [MRI]) are required to delineate the extent of local recurrence and determine further resectability. Additional imaging studies are carried out (CT thorax) to restage the patient for metastatic disease. Local excision of local recurrence is always attempted; however, the need to obtain wide margins is of less paramount importance. The outcome of patients who develop local recurrence is poorer than that of those who do not, and further local recurrence and subsequent development

TABLE 24-11	Histologic Grading of Sarcoma		
Parameter	**Low (G1)**	**Intermediate (G2)**	**High (G3)**
Cellularity	+	++	+++
Differentiation	+++	++	+
Pleomorphism	+	++	+++
Mitotic Rate	+	++	+++
Necrosis	–	+	++
Hemorrhage	–	–	++

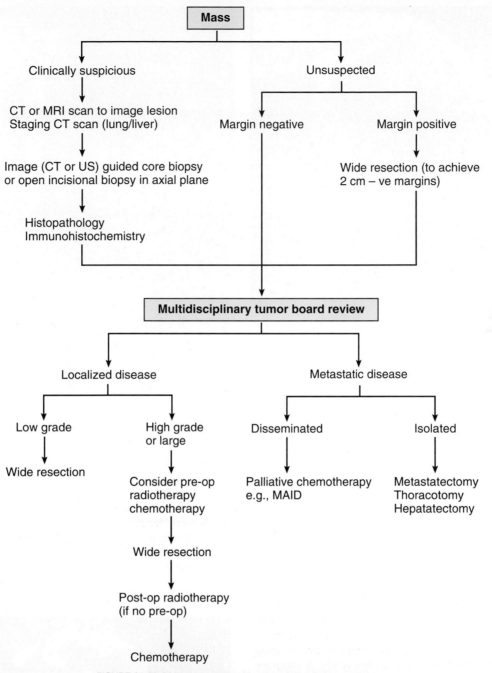

FIGURE 24-20. Management algorithm for adult soft tissue sarcoma.

of metastatic disease is heavily dependent on the adequacy of the original surgery, grade of the original tumor, and subsequent recurrences. Dedifferentiation from low to high grade is uncommon, but may occur in liposarcoma. If not previously administered, radiotherapy may be of value in controlling further local recurrence or making unresectable local recurrence resectable.

Management of Distant Disease

Isolated lung metastases can be treated with thoracotomy and metastasectomy, especially those patients with a disease-free period of more than 1 year, and <10 lesions within both lungs. Of these patients, 15% to 30% remain disease free in 5 years or are cured. Generally, however,

metastatic disease implies an inability to cure the patient, who will be offered palliative therapy. Response rates to chemotherapy are poor: 20% to 40% partial response and rare complete response. The benefits of single agent versus multi-agent chemotherapy for metastatic sarcoma remain to be established. In a recent meta-analysis (*Sarcoma.* 2000;4:103–112), although combination chemotherapy yielded a higher overall response rate, and progression-free survival, no overall survival benefit has been observed at the expanse of toxicity. The benefit seemed to be observed in patients younger than 40 years old. Currently, the EORTC has an ongoing study comparing high-dose doxorubicin with high-dose doxorubicin and ifosfamide with G-CSF support. All these chemotherapy regimens are

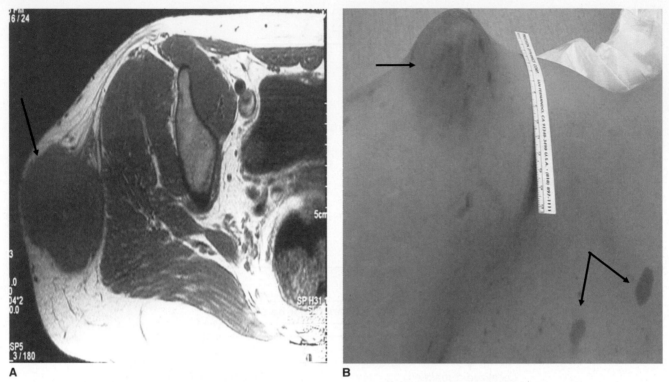

FIGURE 24-21. MPNST (neurofibrosarcoma) in a patient with type 1 neurofibromatosis (G1T2N0M0). A, MRI of PNET tumor of right hip; arrow indicates tumor. B, PNET tumor: Clinical view. Upper arrow shows area of neovascularization over the tumor; lower arrows shows café-au-lait spots typical of Von Recklinghausen syndrome.

given every 3 weeks and CT scanning is being done after each—two to three cycles, for a maximum of six cycles, at which the lifetime maximum dose of doxorubicin will be administered.

Prognosis

Overall, patient 5-year survival rate ranges from 90% for superficial low-grade tumors to 20% for advanced (metastatic disease, large, deep, or high-grade local) disease. In addition, resection margin involvement is an unfavorable survival factor (Table 24-13). No blood tests are of value in the follow-up of soft tissue sarcoma. For patients with superficial low-grade sarcomas excised for cure, clinical examination every 6 months (for the first 2 years), then yearly, is adequate

follow-up. For deep-extremity or retroperitoneal sarcomas, imaging with CT or MRI will detect local recurrence. Because these tumors have a risk of metastasizing, a CT of the thorax is commonly used, beginning every 6 months for 2 years, followed by yearly exams. However, data from the National Cancer Institute suggest that chest radiography is adequate.

(See Table 24-14 for a useful Adult Soft Tissue Sarcoma Fact Sheet.)

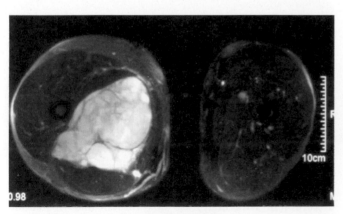

FIGURE 24-22. Sarcoma of the thigh (G3T2N0M0).

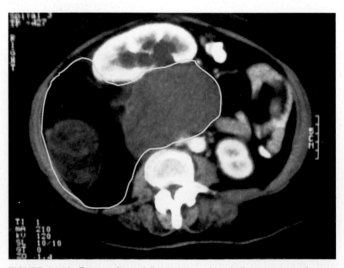

FIGURE 24-23. Retroperitoneal liposarcoma. Line indicates extent of tumor with denser liposarcoma being the more dedifferentiated parts. Note how the right kidney has been pushed from its normal location to lie just under the anterior abdominal wall.

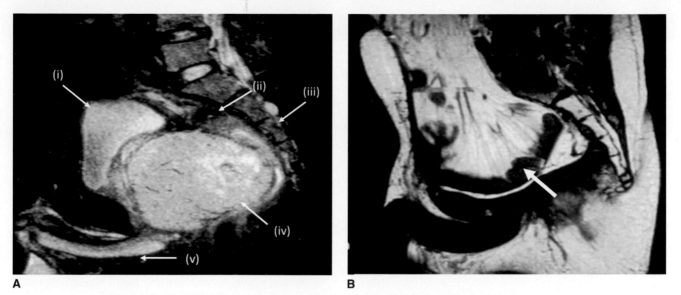

FIGURE 24-24. Pelvic sarcoma. A, Preoperative MRI: (i) Bladder; (ii) Rectum; (iii) Sacrum; (iv) Tumor; (v) Corpora caversarcoma. **B,** Postoperative MRI following pelvic exenteration. Note how a loop of small bowel and its mesentery have now filled the pelvis where the tumor, bladder, and rectum used to be.

SPECIFIC SARCOMAS AND SARCOMALIKE LESIONS

Gastrointestinal Stromal Tumor

Gastrointestinal stromal tumor (GIST) represents a subgroup of sarcoma arising from the cell of Cajal in the myenteric plexus in the muscularis mucosa of gastrointestinal neural origin (Figure 24-25). These tumors are unique in that they have a specific genetic makeup and may express CD34 (hematopoietic progenitor cell antigen) and CD117 (C-kit protein, a membrane receptor with a tyrosine kinase component) antigens. GIST is characterized by the presence of somatic mutation of c-kit (80% to 85%) or platelet-derived growth factor receptor-A (PDFGR-A) gene (10%), while 5% to 10% harbor none of these gene mutations. Unlike other soft tissue sarcomas, GIST uncommonly metastasizes to the lungs but almost always recurs in the liver and/or peritoneal surface. In the past, this tumor had a poor prognosis; however, the recent development of targeted chemotherapy in the form of tyrosine kinase inhibitor targeting c-kit and PDGFRA, such as imatinib mesylate, has shown impressive results in reversing and stabilizing metastatic disease. Hepatectomy can be a treatment option for those patients with isolated liver metastases (<4) and with long disease-free interval. Discussion with medical oncology and surgical oncology or hepatobiliary surgeon is advised prior to resection. Treatment consists of resection of the tumor with negative margins, and clinical trials are ongoing to determine the long-term results of tyrosine kinase inhibitors in metastatic as well as in the adjuvant setting.

Dermatofibrosarcoma Protuberans

Dermatofibrosarcoma protuberans (DFSP) is a low-to-moderate malignant potential soft tissue sarcoma arising from the skin. It is characterized by the presence of chromosomal translocation between 17 and 22, resulting in the formation of fusion gene COL1A1-PDGFB in 50% to 75% of DFSP. The fusion PDGFB is functional and will activate PDGFRB, leading to proliferation of the tumor. This unusual skin and subcutaneous lesion has limited, if any, metastatic potential (<5%). However, if completely excised with positive margins, local recurrence is guaranteed. These lesions typically have a long time course and may recur over a 25-year time period. The local recurrence potential is easy to underestimate, but with wide resection margins and appropriate reconstruction, a cure can be assured. Figure 24-26 shows the obvious nodularity of this subcutaneous lesion of the thigh. A wide resection was taken incorporating the vastus medialis muscle. The defect was covered with meshed split-thickness skin graft. Figure 24-26E shows the results 1 month postoperatively.

Desmoid (Aggressive Fibromatosis)

Desmoid represents an intermediate-grade malignancy of fibrous tissue. An example of the MRI appearance of this lesion is seen in Figure 24-27. Typically, these lesions have a propensity for local recurrence and infiltration within muscle

TABLE 24-13	Prognostic Factors for Soft Tissue Sarcomas	
	Prognosis	
Factor	**Favorable**	**Unfavorable**
Grade	Low	High
Size	<5 cm	>5 cm
Primary site	Superficial	Deep
Surgical margin	Clear	Involved

TABLE 24-14	Adult Soft Tissue Sarcoma Fact Sheet

Rare tumors <1% of all cancers	NEVER "SHELL-OUT"
In Alberta—50 new cases per year	Easy to do as tumors appear to have a (pseudo)capsule
Derived from mesoderm (mesenchyme)	Local recurrence virtually 100%
Cf. adenocarcinoma (breast, colon, lung) endoderm	Surgery for recurrent disease common
Nonepithelial	Cf. lung, pancreas, etc.
Cf. adenocarcinoma (breast, colon, lung)	Chemotherapy
PVC (hepatic angiosarcoma), Agent Orange, and radiation associated	Limited currently
Genetics	5% survival advantage in adjuvant setting
Neurofibromatosis (von Recklinghausen)	Only certain tumors respond, e.g., not liposarcoma
Gardener's syndrome	No real affect in low grade
Li-Fraumeni	Is used in metastatic palliative setting
Majority occur in limbs mainly lower (most muscle)	New genetic designer drugs (e.g., imatinib) promising
15% retroperitoneal	Radiotherapy
15% trunk	Often used in conjunction with surgery either preop to make tumor resectable or postop to reduce local recurrence rate
May grow large as they do not tend to obstruct or invade	Limited value in low-grade tumors and retroperitoneum
Over 30 subtypes	High doses (50 Gy pre-op or 60–70 Gy/6–7000 rads) required, cf. breast 45–50 Gy
Commonest: liposarcoma, leiomyosarcoma, and malignant fibrous histiocytoma	Wound complications as a consequence
Prognosis dependent on stage and grade	5-year survival
Best—low grade, superficial, <5 cm, negative resection margins	50% overall
<10% metastasize to nodes—if present indicates poor prognosis	Low-grade superficial up to 90%
Synovial, epitheloid, rhabdomyosarcoma—rest vs. rare	High-grade retroperitoneal 30%
Grade is a histologic assessment (low, moderate, and high)	Complex disease
More necrosis, hemorrhage, pleomorphism, >10 mitoses per HPF = high grade	Ideal results if managed by multidisciplinary team
Complex diagnosis involving multiple stains requires expert pathologist	Medical, radiation, orthopedic, and general surgical oncologists and dedicated pathologist
Metastasize	Follow up of value (cf. breast, gastric, pancreas, etc.)
Lung initially and liver and other organs later	6 monthly CT or MRI ± CXR if deep
If isolated metastasectomy	If superficial, clinical examination sufficient
Diagnose by biopsy	As reoperation definite role occasional cure, but mainly QOL and longer survival
Percutaneous core by radiologist (after CT or MRI)	No screening lab work
Or open in AXIAL NEVER TRANSVERSE direction	
Surgical disease	
Aim to remove tumor with 2-cm margin	
Often not possible as close relation to vital structures, e.g., sciatic nerve, aorta, vena cava	
Need to be radical (en bloc resection of adjacent organ—e.g., kidney, adrenal, colon, spleen) to give best chance of cure	
Limb-sparing surgery plus radiotherapy as good as amputation	
Do margin biopsies in OR and Weck (surgical) clip suspicious areas	
Frozen section rarely of value as difficult for pathologist	

and soft tissue. Treatment consists of a wide resection. When this is not possible, radiotherapy may provide a reasonable chance of reducing the risk of local recurrence. More recently, evidence has emerged that these tumors may respond to nonsteroidal anti-inflammatory drugs, tamoxifen, or some combination of these agents. Response to these agents is typically slow, but continues for months or years. For advanced or recurrent lesions, radiation and chemotherapy are also important treatment modalities. Imatinib is currently licensed by the U.S. Food and Drug Administration for the treatment of unresectable, recurrent, and/or metastatic DFSP. Response

rate was reported to be 50% to 65% for all patients, especially for those with the characteristic chromosomal translocation. In cases of extensive local disease, imatinib can be used neoadjuvantly, which can render the tumor resectable after months of therapy.

Kaposi's Sarcoma

In the past, Kaposi's sarcoma (KS) was largely limited to elderly Jewish men of Mediterranean descent and to people from sub-Saharan Africa. With the AIDS epidemic, the

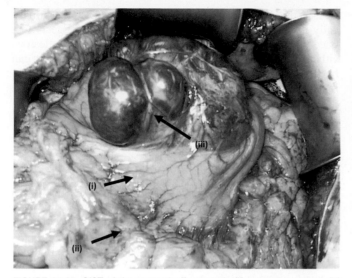

FIGURE 24-25. GIST of the stomach: (i) stomach; (ii) greater omentum; (iii) tumor—note the "encephaloid" (looping-like brain substance) appearance.

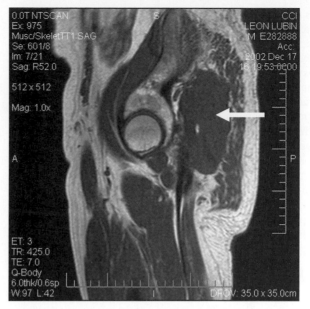

FIGURE 24-27. Aggressive fibromatosis of the buttock.

incidence of KS has increased. There are now four subtypes of KS based on epidemiologic variations: classic KS, African endemic KS, iatrogenic KS, and epidemic, AIDS-associated KS. KS is the most common neoplastic complication of AIDS. Homosexual and bisexual men are much more likely to have KS than others with AIDS. This finding suggests a sexually transmitted etiology in this patient population, and the causative agent appears to be human herpesvirus 8 (HHV8).

Iatrogenic KS occurs in patients immunosuppressed by drug therapy. These lesions may regress if the immunotherapy can be stopped.

Kaposi's sarcoma lesions initially appear as flat, blue patches that resemble a hematoma. Later, they become raised, rubbery nodules. Non-AIDS KS is typically found on the lower extremities. AIDS-related KS often begins in the perioral mucosa. The palate is the most common site. AIDS-related

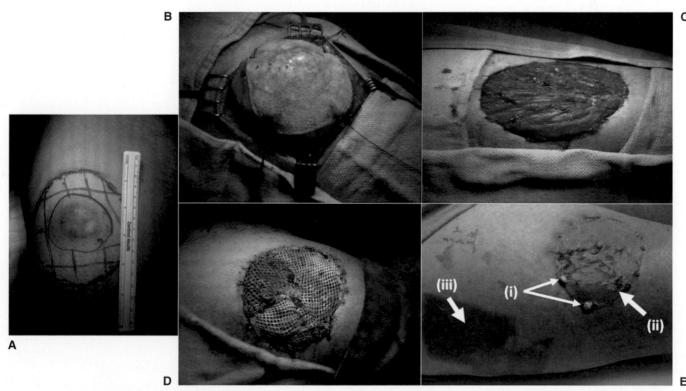

FIGURE 24-26. MRI image of DFSP of right thigh. A, Tumor with 3-cm resection margin marked out. B, Wide resection of tumor including deep fascia of vastus medialis muscle to achieve negative resection margins. C, Vastus medialis. D, Meshed skin graft applied to resection site. E, 1 month postop: (i) areas of overgranulation treated with silver nitrate; (ii) 100% "take" of skin graft; (iii) skin graft donor site.

KS is often multifocal, with rapid spread to the lymph nodes. It often involves the gastrointestinal tract, presenting as GI bleed, obstruction, and dysphagia. Other mucosal surfaces can be involved including respiratory, GU, and even CNS. Biopsy shows endothelial cells, with fibroblasts, spindle cells, and increased capillary growth. These malignancies are considered angiosarcomas.

Surgical excision or local radiation is effective for small, localized lesions. Liposomal doxorubicin is the licensed agent for the treatment of disseminated or unresectable KS. Patients with AIDS-related KS should also be treated concurrently with multiple antiretroviral therapy through consultation with an infectious disease specialist. The tolerability of liposomal doxorubicin can be poor in this population due to their poor performance status, concurrent opportunistic infections, and the toxicities from antiretroviral therapy. Responses to liposomal doxorubicin can be observed rapidly and dramatically after a few treatments. Recent literature suggests that once the CD4 count is 400 or above and most of the lesions either regress or are asymptomatic, liposomal doxorubicin can be stopped. Further regression occurs, which is likely due to reconstitution of the immune system. Local radiation shrinks these lesions and provides palliation. Treatment includes single-drug regimens with vinblastine or VP-16.

ACKNOWLEDGMENT

The authors wish to acknowledge the editorial comments and inputs from Dr. Quincy Chu, Medical Oncologist, Alberta Cancer Board; Dr. Carolyn O'Hara, Sarcoma Pathologist, Alberta Health Services; and Miss Amanda Beaulieu, 3rd year Medical Student, University Saskatchewan.

thePoint ☀ Go to http://thePoint.lww.com/activate and use your scratch-off code on the inside cover of this book to access bonus chapters, question bank, videos, and more.

SAMPLE QUESTIONS

Questions

Choose the best answer for each question.

1. A 42-year-old woman complains of a mole on her left forearm that has recently changed. She states that the mole has been there since "as long as she can remember" but over the last 6 months, it has gotten larger and darker. She has no other medical problems and takes no medication. She has two children ages 12 and 14. She works part-time in a physician's office. She also worked as a lifeguard during the summers as a teenager. Her 75-year-old father had some skin cancers removed from his face last year that she says "were not the bad kind of skin cancer." She has no other family history of skin or other cancers. Her physical examination is unremarkable except for a 1.5-cm asymmetrical mole with blue-black colors and irregular borders on the anterior surface of her left forearm. Complete skin examination shows no other suspicious skin lesions and she has no lymphadenopathy. The next most appropriate step in management of the forearm lesion is
   A. repeat skin examination in 1 year.
   B. superficial shave biopsy.
   C. excisional biopsy.
   D. needle biopsy.
   E. Moh's micrographic surgery.

2. A 57-year-old man recently underwent a biopsy of a mole on his back below the tip of his left scapula that revealed a 1.5-mm maximum thickness, nonulcerated melanoma. He has a history of hypertension for which he takes a diuretic but has no other medical problems. His physical examination reveals a 2-cm healing back incision without evidence of infection. He has no other suspicious skin lesions or lymphadenopathy. The next most appropriate step in management is
   A. follow-up in clinic in 3 months.
   B. PET/CT scan.
   C. wide excision alone.
   D. wide excision and sentinel lymph node biopsy.
   E. Moh's micrographic surgery.

3. A 65-year-old woman presents with an enlarging nontender mass in her right inguinal area. She states that the mass has been present for 3 months and has been growing. She denies any history of trauma or recent infections. Physical examination reveals a 3-cm firm mass in her right groin over the femoral artery with no overlying skin changes. The rest of her exam is unremarkable. Chest radiograph and CBC are normal. A fine-needle aspiration (FNA) of the mass reveals atypical lymphocytes but no obvious malignancy. The most appropriate next step in diagnosis is
   A. excisional biopsy.
   B. bone marrow aspiration.
   C. bronchoscopy.
   D. TB skin test.
   E. repeat needle aspiration of the mass.

4. A 73-year-old man presents with a mass in his anterior right thigh for the past 4 months. The mass is not tender and he denies any history of trauma to the area. He denies any prior exposure to chemical agents, prior radiation therapy, or family history of cancer. His physical examination reveals an 8-cm firm mass deep in the anterior compartment of his proximal thigh. There are no overlying skin changes. In addition to MRI of the extremity, the most appropriate next step in management is
   A. excisional biopsy.
   B. fine-needle aspiration.
   C. bone scan.
   D. core biopsy.
   E. genetic testing for p53.

5. A 53-year-old man who underwent a partial gastrectomy for a gastrointestinal stromal tumor (GIST tumor) 4 years ago complains of weakness and fatigue for the past 3 months. A CT scan reveals multiple bilobar liver masses, and CT-guided biopsy shows recurrent GIST tumor. Immunohistochemical staining for which of the following is essential for the patient's subsequent treatment?
   A. p53
   B. CD117
   C. Her2-*neu*
   D. CEA
   E. N-*myc*

Answers and Explanations

1. Answer: C

The patient presented in this question has a mole that fulfils several criteria (i.e., A, Asymmetry; B, Borders; C, Color; D, Diameter; E, Evolution) to be sufficiently suspicious for melanoma to merit biopsy. There are multiple methods for biopsy of skin lesions and each has its own limitations. The most appropriate next step in diagnosis of a suspicious mole is excisional biopsy with removal of the entire lesion with a small rim (1 to 2 mm) of normal skin. Superficial shave biopsy is not the most appropriate method of biopsy of a skin lesion that is suspicious for melanoma because it fails to provide accurate information related to the depth of invasion should the lesion prove to be a melanoma. Microscopic tumor depth of invasion in the skin is an important prognostic factor in the staging of melanoma. Needle biopsy would not be an appropriate method of biopsy of a mole because it does not yield sufficient tissue for the pathologist to determine if the mole is a melanoma. Pathologists prefer removal of the entire lesion so they can examine it in its entirety. Moh's micrographic surgery is a specialized surgical technique to precisely remove a skin cancer with complete margin control while healthy tissue is spared. Moh's surgery is relatively expensive but may be indicated in anatomically important areas (eyelid, nose, lips) where sparing normal tissue and local control are important. Moh's is not appropriate in the patient presented in the question because no diagnosis has been made yet and preservation of normal tissue is not as important on the forearm as it might be on the face. Cryotherapy refers to freezing a skin lesion, but it should never be used to treat a suspected melanoma because no tissue is sent for pathologic examination with this form of therapy.

2. Answer: D

Once a diagnosis of melanoma is made, the next steps in treatment involve (1) addressing the local disease to reduce the risk of local recurrence and (2) determining which patients are at risk for tumor spread to the regional lymph nodes. In the absence of any known metastatic disease, both of these steps are predicated on an accurate depth of invasion of the primary melanoma. Wide excision is indicated following excisional biopsy, even if the margins of excision are free of tumor, to ensure removal of tumor cells outside the borders of the lesion. The recommended margins of excision are based on data from prospective randomized trials, but the fundamental principle is that the deeper the lesion the wider the recommended margins of excision. In addition to addressing the local tumor, the next step in treatment or staging involves determining the status of the regional nodes by sentinel lymph node biopsy. The sentinel node is the principal node of tumor spread for that part of the skin. Similar to the risk of local recurrence, the deeper the primary melanoma, the more likely the chance of occult nodal metastasis. Patients with melanomas thicker than 1 mm in depth are candidates for sentinel node biopsy. The patient in the question has a melanoma of his back with ambiguous lymphatic drainage. He would benefit from lymphatic mapping to determine the draining nodal basin. Lymphatic mapping is best performed in a nuclear medicine suite, where patients undergo an intradermal injection of a radionuclide (technetium-99m filtered sulfur colloid) followed by scanning with an external gamma camera to determine the lymphatic drainage. Then, intraoperatively at the time of the wide excision and sentinel node biopsy, the surgeon injects a vital dye intradermally and then uses a handheld gamma probe to locate and remove all radioactive and/or blue-staining lymph nodes. Follow-up alone would not be appropriate in a patient with a melanoma 1.5 mm in depth. PET/CT is used for staging, but the yield is not high enough to justify its use unless the tumor is >4 mm in depth or has metastasized to the regional nodes. Adjuvant interferon is also not indicated unless the tumor is >4 mm in depth or has metastasized to the regional nodes. Moh's surgery is not indicated for a back melanoma because preservation of normal tissue is not as important as it might be on the face.

3. Answer: A

The presence of a 3-cm firm groin mass in a 65-year-old woman requires a thorough evaluation. She has already undergone a fine-needle aspiration (FNA) of the mass demonstrating atypical lymphocytes; therefore, the next most appropriate step is complete removal of the lymph node for pathologic examination (lymphoma is suspected). While FNA is simpler and less invasive than excisional biopsy, it only provides cells and the entire node is usually required by the pathologist to determine the type of lymphoma. Repeat FNA is unlikely to yield any additional information given the first FNA result showing atypical lymphocytes. Bone marrow aspiration may be indicated after a diagnosis of lymphoma is made. Bronchoscopy and a tuberculin skin test are not indicated in this patient.

4. Answer: D

Soft tissue sarcomas arise from the mesenchymal tissue and the most common sites in adults are the extremities. The most common presentation is a mass that is increasing in size and delays in diagnosis are common. Adequate tissue can be obtained by core or incisional biopsy. Core biopsy involves removal of a core of tissue about 1 to 2 mm in diameter using a large needle. This procedure is best performed using image guidance and it can be done under local anesthesia. Incisional biopsy is best done by the surgeon who will perform the definitive tumor resection so that the incision can be placed appropriately. Fine-needle aspiration (FNA) biopsy will not yield enough tissue to make an accurate diagnosis and to determine the histologic type and tumor grade. A poorly planned biopsy may compromise subsequent curative resection. Excisional biopsy of soft tissue sarcomas disturbs tissue planes and may produce hematomas that require larger definitive resections and may even lead to amputation. Bone scan and chemotherapy would not be appropriate prior to a tissue diagnosis. In the absence of a family history suggestive of Li-Fraumeni syndrome, genetic testing is not indicated.

5. Answer: B

Gastrointestinal stromal (GIST) tumors are the most common sarcomas of the gastrointestinal (GI) tract and the most common site of GIST tumors is the stomach. Unlike other soft tissue sarcomas, GIST tumors uncommonly metastasize to the lungs but more frequently spread to the liver and/or peritoneal surfaces. Liver resection or hepatectomy is a treatment option for those patients with resectable liver metastases, but the patient has multiple bilobar liver metastases. GIST tumors are frequently associated with a mutation in the *c-kit* gene, which encodes for expression of CD117 (c-kit protein, a membrane receptor with a tyrosine kinase component) antigen. Recently, a tyrosine kinase inhibitor targeting *c-kit* (imatinib or Gleevec) has been found to be effective in treating metastatic GIST tumors. Therefore, all patients with GIST tumors should have their tumors checked for *c-kit* staining. People who inherit only one copy of the tumor suppressor gene, p53, have Li-Fraumeni syndrome, which is associated with several tumors including breast cancer, brain tumors, adrenal cortical carcinoma, acute leukemia, and bone and soft tissue sarcomas. Amplification of the Her2-*neu* oncogene gene or overexpression of its protein product is associated with poor prognosis in breast cancer. Carcinoembryonic antigen (CEA) is an oncofetal antigen associated with colorectal and other cancers, while N-*myc* is an oncogene that is amplified in neuroblastoma.

Appendix
Figures from Chapter 10, Burns

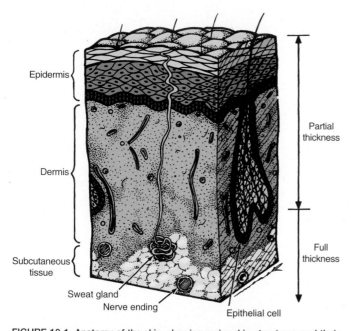

FIGURE 10-1. Anatomy of the skin, showing major skin structures and their relation to partial- and full-thickness burns. Epithelial cells make up the lining of hair follicles and sweat glands, and these structures penetrate deeply into—sometimes through—the dermis. Even very deep partial-thickness burns can heal if these "epidermal appendages" survive. Dermal capillaries and nerve endings also reside in the deep dermis and survive most partial-thickness burns.

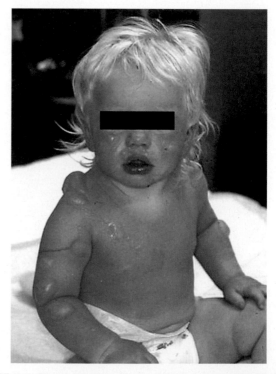

FIGURE 10-2. This small child suffered extensive sunburn when his mother left him in a stroller at a softball game. There are scattered areas of superficial blisters on the arms and face—these are partial-thickness dermal ("superficial second-degree") burns. The majority of the torso, forearms, and forehead demonstrate erythema without blistering typical of epidermal ("first-degree") burns. These areas will fade back to normal color within a few hours without blistering and will heal without scars. Although most epidermal burns require little specific treatment, a patient with a wound this extensive—especially in a very young or old person—could require short-term admission for fluids and pain control.

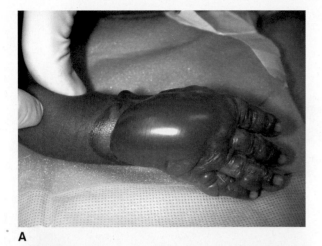

A

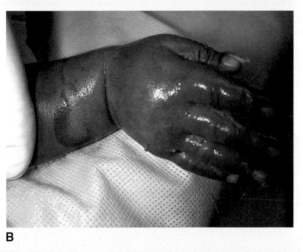

B

FIGURE 10-3. Superficial partial-thickness burn that occurred when this child reached into a pot of hot water. Figure 10-3A shows distended, fluid-filled blisters that are characteristic of superficial injuries (deeper burns will form blisters, but usually don't contain much fluid). After debridement of blisters (Fig. 10-3B), the underlying dermis is bright red, moist, painful, and blanches readily with direct pressure. Removing blisters from these wounds is uncomfortable, but facilitates wound care. In addition, removal of blistered skin permits more accurate assessment of burn extent and depth.

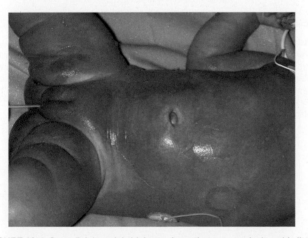

FIGURE 10-4. Superficial partial-thickness burn that occurred when this little girl pulled a cup of coffee off a table into her lap. Blisters have already been debrided. The wound is bright red, moist, and painful, and blanches with direct pressure. Although such wounds are often very frightening to patients and families, they can be reassured that with appropriate topical therapy and pain control the wound will heal within 7-10 days, and is unlikely to result in scarring. As these photos illustrate, injuries from scalding water are often superficial, although they can be much deeper. Remember that the *appearance* of the wound, rather than the etiology, is the best guide to the depth of injury!

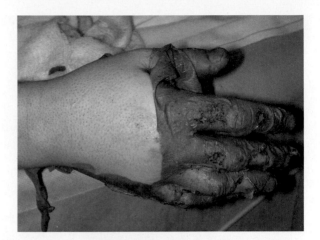

FIGURE 10-5. The following several figures illustrate deep partial-thickness injuries, which can vary greatly in appearance depending on the etiology, duration of exposure, and exact depth of the injury. Figure 10-5 shows a quite deep burn of the dorsal hand from an electrical flash injury. The epidermis is loose and slides off almost like a glove, revealing waxy white dermis, which has relatively little remaining sensation. Note that there is no fluid beneath the blistered epidermis.

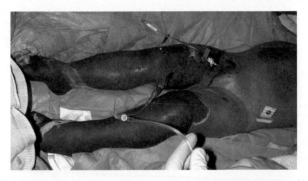

FIGURE 10-6. This shows a child who was immersed in hot bath water. Note that although the legs are red, the skin surface is dull and dry. These wounds show almost no blanching with direct pressure. Although many scald injuries are superficial, immersion burns in small children can be very deep. This child required skin grafting of almost the entire area.

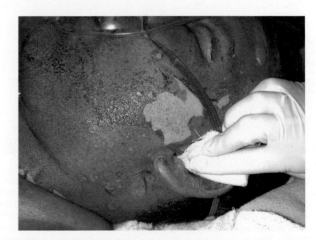

FIGURE 10-7. This shows a flash burn to the face. The epidermis is discolored, dry, and fairly adherent. However, it comes off easily when rubbed gently with gauze, revealing waxy white, dry, relatively anesthetic dermis beneath. In evaluating burn wounds, attempting to remove discolored epidermis will often help reveal the true depth of injury, and may also show that the burn extends farther than is apparent on cursory examination.

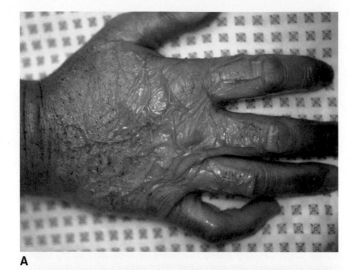

A

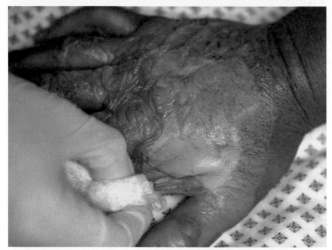

B

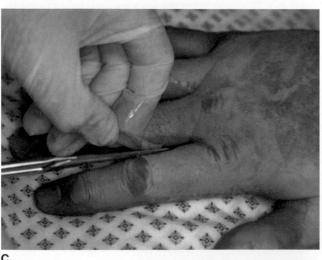

C

FIGURE 10-8. This man burned his dorsal hand with hot grease while cook-ing. In Figure 10-8**A** the epidermis is loose and discolored, but dry. With aggressive debridement (Figs. 10-8**B**, 10-8**C**) the epidermis is removed, revealing pale, dry dermis beneath. Compare this hand to that in Figure 10-3. Although the child's hand is a more dramatic-appearing injury (and probably caused far more anxiety in the family), it is much less severe, and far more likely to heal with simple dressings.

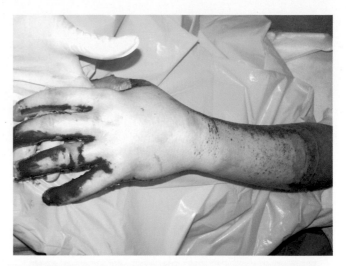

FIGURE 10-9. Deep partial-thickness burn of the hand and forearm from a propane flash. The wound has already been debrided. The dorsal hand and fore-arm are waxy white, dry, and relatively insensate. Note that the margins of the burn wound—particularly around the fingers—are red and appear more superficial. The exact depth of this wound is difficult to determine, but it will clearly benefit from skin grafting.

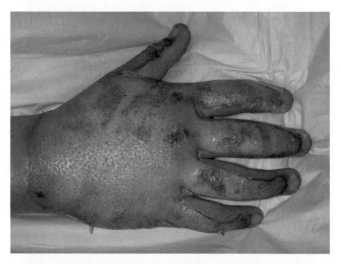

FIGURE 10-10. This burn of the dorsal hand is about 10 days old. Areas of different burn depth are apparent. There is still some fairly solid eschar over the dorsal hand and fingers, but eschar has separated over the proximal (wrist) edge, revealing pink healing tissue. Regularly spaced, small darker-red spots are epi-dermal appendages ("skin buds"), where epidermis is growing upward from hair follicles. The appearance of uniform skin buds indicates that the wound will heal reliably within about 14 days.

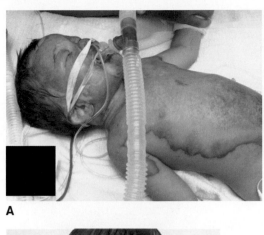

A

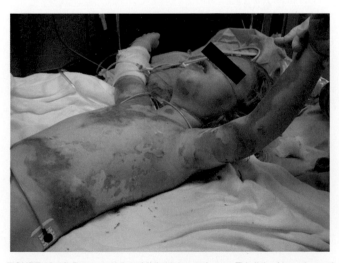

B

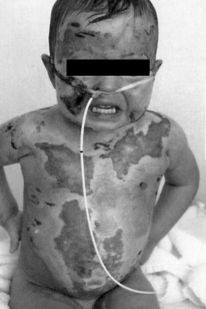

C

FIGURE 10-11. **This series of old photos illustrates some of the challenges encountered when treating large burns of indeterminate depth.** Figure 10-11**A** shows a two-year old girl who pulled a frying pan off a counter, scalding her face, torso, and shoulders. The burn is about 48 hours old. She initially required endotracheal intubation because of facial swelling, but facial edema is now resolving. The wounds are largely covered with pale, dry eschar, suggesting a deep injury. However, the margins of the wound look pinker and somewhat more superficial. Figure 10-11**B** was taken at 5 days. The solid eschar over her chest and abdomen looks deeper, with areas of brownish discoloration. The margins of the wound are pink and beginning to separate. Figure 10-11**C** was taken at 14 days following injury. Her shoulders, cheeks, and abdomen have largely epithelialized, but solid eschar remains on her chest and central abdomen. These areas were skin-grafted the following day. These photos show how burn wounds can change in appearance as they heal. Only experience in burn wound assessment can permit accurate diagnosis of these different stages of healing.

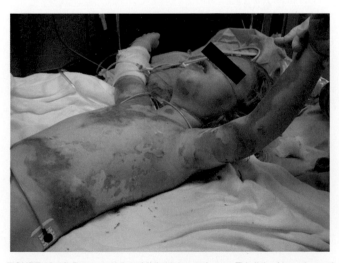

FIGURE 10-12. **Deep partial and full-thickness burns.** This little girl was burned when her clothing caught fire while she was cooking over the stove. She has extensive burns of the torso and arms which appear deep centrally, with white, dry eschar. The margins look more superficial, but they are also dry and do not blanch with pressure. Almost this entire wound required skin grafting.

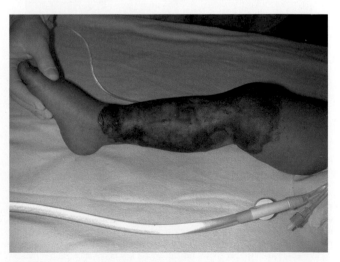

FIGURE 10-13. **Full-thickness burn of the leg.** This little boy was playing with matches and gasoline, and ignited his pant leg. The wound is a variety of colors, from dull white to black, but almost the entire wound is dry, leathery, and insensate. The contraction of dermal proteins, causing a tourniquet-like effect, is apparent.

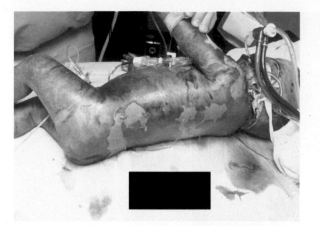

FIGURE 10-14. This horrifying photo shows a child who sustained full-thickness burns of 100% total body surface area when his mother left him unattended in the bathtub. He turned on the hot water and was unable to climb out. The wounds are dry, tensely swollen, and show no capillary perfusion. This child died shortly after the photo was taken. This is a grim reminder that tap water can be a lethal danger to children, the elderly, and disabled, and that the etiology of injury does not define its depth.

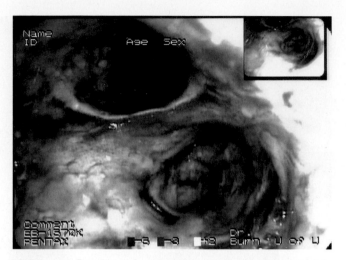

FIGURE 10-16. Bronchoscopic appearance of the trachea following inhalation injury. Extensive carbonaceous deposits can be seen throughout the trachea and mainstem bronchi. Other characteristic findings can include sloughing of the tracheal mucosa, erythema, and swelling.

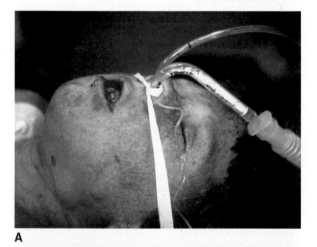

A

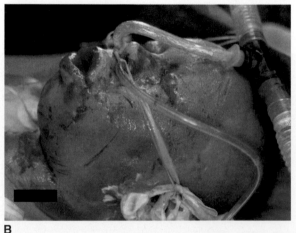

B

FIGURE 10-15. This young man suffered an extensive burn injury from a gas explosion. Figure 10-15**A** was taken about 45 minutes after injury. He has extensive deep burns of the face, which are indicated by the grayish, dry skin and charring about the lips. Though he was breathing normally, prophylactic intubation was performed. Figure 10-15**B** shows his face just a few hours later. He has massive facial edema affecting his lips, eyelids, and neck. Without an endotracheal tube it is likely that his airway would occlude. In treating extensive burns of this nature it is important to consider intubation early, before evidence of airway compromise develops. Also note that this patient has been nasally intubated. These are old photos; nasal intubation is rarely used today.

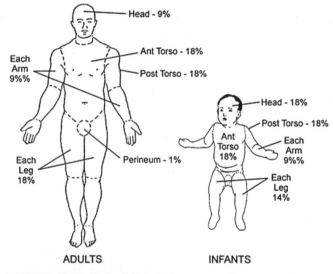

THE RULE OF NINES
FOR ESTIMATING BURN SIZE

ADULTS INFANTS

FIGURE 10-17. The "Rule of Nines." This method permits estimation of burn size by dividing the body into parts, each of which comprises nine percent total body surface area. Users should estimate what *fraction* of each body area is burned (for example, half of the right arm is 4.5% TBSA). These areas are then added to produce a total burn size. A separate diagram is used for small children because of their proportionally larger heads and smaller legs.

BURN ESTIMATE AND DIAGRAM
AGE vs AREA

Area	Birth 1 yr.	1-4 yr.	5-9 yr.	10-14 yr.	15 yr.	Adult	2°	3°	Total	Donor Areas
Head	19	17	13	11	9	7				
Neck	2	2	2	2	2	2				
Ant. Trunk	13	13	13	13	13	13				
Post. Trunk	13	13	13	13	13	13				
R. Buttock	2½	2½	2½	2½	2½	2½				
L. Buttock	2½	2½	2½	2½	2½	2½				
Genitalia	1	1	1	1	1	1				
R. U. Arm	4	4	4	4	4	4				
L. U. Arm	4	4	4	4	4	4				
R. L. Arm	3	3	3	3	3	3				
L. L. Arm	3	3	3	3	3	3				
R. Hand	2½	2½	2½	2½	2½	2½				
L. Hand	2½	2½	2½	2½	2½	2½				
R. Thigh	5½	6½	8	8½	9	9½				
L. Thigh	5½	6½	8	8½	9	9½				
R. Leg	5	5	5½	6	6½	7				
L. Leg	5	5	5½	6	6½	7				
R. Foot	3½	3½	3½	3½	3½	3½				
L. Foot	3½	3½	3½	3½	3½	3½				
						TOTAL				

Cause of Burn_____

Date of Burn_____

Time of Burn_____

Age_____

Sex_____

Weight_____

BURN DIAGRAM

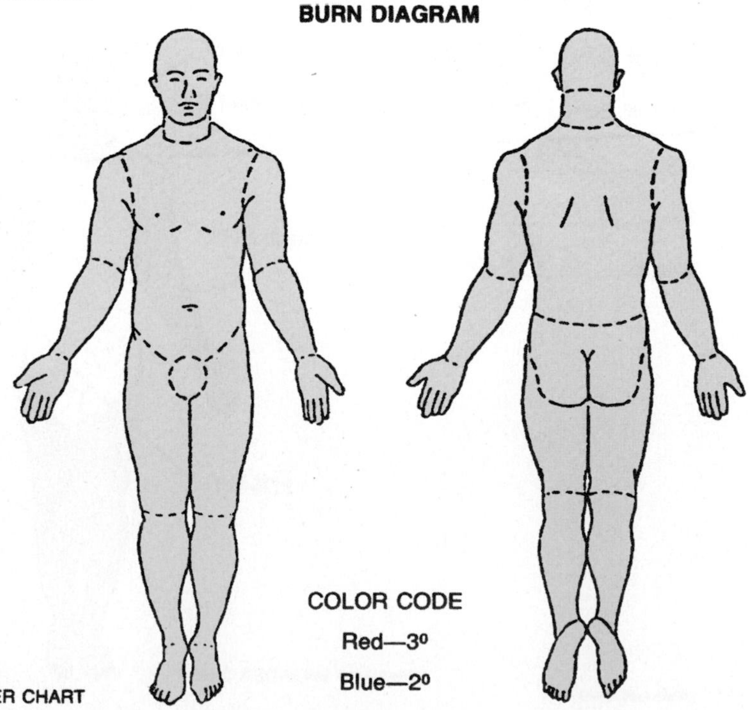

COLOR CODE

Red—3°

Blue—2°

LUND AND BROWDER CHART

FIGURE 10-18. Lund and Browder Chart. This diagram was developed during World War II to help document and estimate the extent of burn injuries. Following initial debridement, the examiner should draw the burn injuries on the figure, calculate how much of each body area is burned, then add all areas to produce a total burn size. Inexperienced providers tend to overestimate burn size, and underestimate depth. We hope that the figures included with this chapter will help readers evaluate burn wounds more accurately.

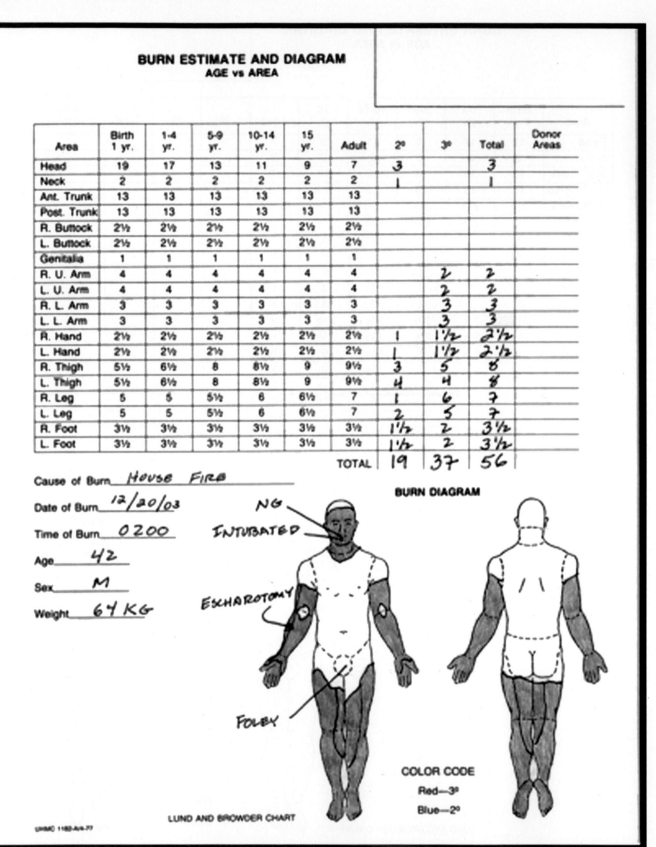

BURN ESTIMATE AND DIAGRAM
AGE vs AREA

Area	Birth 1 yr.	1-4 yr.	5-9 yr.	10-14 yr.	15 yr.	Adult	2°	3°	Total	Donor Areas
Head	19	17	13	11	9	7	3		3	
Neck	2	2	2	2	2	2	1		1	
Ant. Trunk	13	13	13	13	13	13				
Post. Trunk	13	13	13	13	13	13				
R. Buttock	2½	2½	2½	2½	2½	2½				
L. Buttock	2½	2½	2½	2½	2½	2½				
Genitalia	1	1	1	1	1	1				
R. U. Arm	4	4	4	4	4	4		2	2	
L. U. Arm	4	4	4	4	4	4		2	2	
R. L. Arm	3	3	3	3	3	3		3	3	
L. L. Arm	3	3	3	3	3	3		3	3	
R. Hand	2½	2½	2½	2½	2½	2½	1	1½	2½	
L. Hand	2½	2½	2½	2½	2½	2½	1	1½	2½	
R. Thigh	5½	6½	8	8½	9	9½	3	5	8	
L. Thigh	5½	6½	8	8½	9	9½	4	4	8	
R. Leg	5	5	5½	6	6½	7	1	6	7	
L. Leg	5	5	5½	6	6½	7	2	5	7	
R. Foot	3½	3½	3½	3½	3½	3½	1½	2	3½	
L. Foot	3½	3½	3½	3½	3½	3½	1½	2	3½	
						TOTAL	19	37	56	

Cause of Burn __HOUSE FIRE__

Date of Burn __12/20/03__

Time of Burn __0200__

Age __42__

Sex __M__

Weight __64 KG__

BURN DIAGRAM

NG
INTUBATED
ESCHAROTOMY
FOLEY

LUND AND BROWDER CHART

COLOR CODE
Red—3°
Blue—2°

UHMC 1182-A/4-77

FIGURE 10-19. A completed Lund and Browder Diagram of a man injured in a house fire. Partial-thickness ("second-degree") and full-thickness ("third-degree") burns are colored separately. Note that if the "rule of nines" had been used to estimate this burn, approximately the same total burn size would have been obtained:

RIGHT ARM = 9%
LEFT ARM = 9%
RIGHT LEG = 18%
LEFT LEG = 18%
HALF THE HEAD = 4.5%
TOTAL = 58.5% TBSA

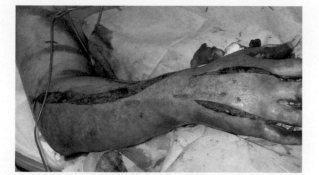

FIGURE 10-20. Escharotomy of the upper extremity. This extensively burned arm and hand developed progressive tense edema, numbness and tingling, and deep throbbing pain. Intramuscular pressures were measured using a sterile needle connected to a pressure transducer, and were in excess of 30 cm/H₂O. Escharotomies were performed at the bedside using deep sedation and electrocautery. The wound edges have separated markedly due to the underlying edema. It should be remembered that escharotomy does not reduce the *swelling* associated with the burn injury, but is done to relieve the *compression* produced by edema accumulation beneath the unyielding surface of a deep burn injury.

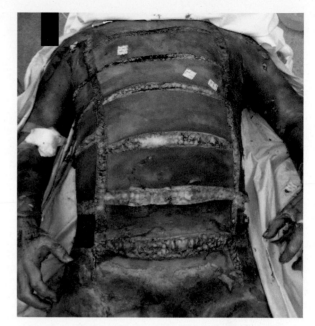

FIGURE 10-22. This man suffered massive full-thickness burns in an auto crash. During initial evaluation at a community hospital, he developed sudden respiratory compromise and rigid edema of the torso. The emergency physician, in consultation with the burn center, made a series of escharotomy incisions on his chest and abdomen to relieve this compression and permit adequate ventilation. Each incision resulted in 1–2 additional inches of expansion of his torso. The edema of his upper extremities is also apparent—these will require emergency decompression as well. However, extremities will tolerate limited periods of compression, while respiratory compromise from chest wall edema requires immediate surgical intervention. Because these wounds are all full-thickness, they will be excised and skin grafted, so no scarring will result from the escharotomies themselves.

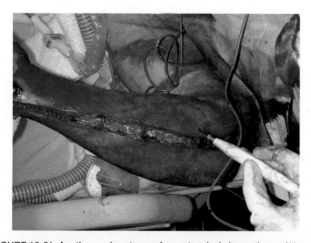

FIGURE 10-21. Another escharotomy of an extensively burned arm. Although this burn appears to be relatively superficial, a circumferential injury of this nature can still lead to compartmental compression. Remember that edema formation is progressive over the 24 hours following injury; an arm that is initially soft can become tensely swollen as resuscitation proceeds, so *serial* evaluation for evidence of circulatory compromise is essential!

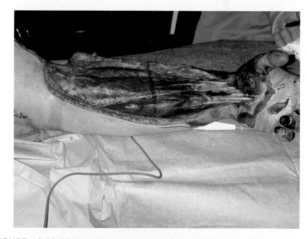

FIGURE 10-23. High-voltage electrical injury of the hand. Charring and full-thickness injury of the base of the palm is apparent. The fingers and wrist are "fixed" in flexion because of coagulation necrosis of the flexor muscles of the forearm. Brownish necrosis of the flexor tendons and distal muscles are apparent. Note the dramatic separation of the skin edges following fasciotomy. The hand is unsalvageable; the blue line indicates the approximate level of amputation to be performed.

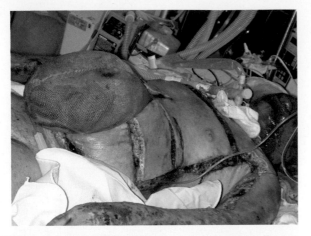

FIGURE 10-24. Total body edema following a massive burn injury. This man suffered burns to over 65% TBSA. In this photo, taken 48 hours post-injury, all of the complications of edema formation can be seen: massive facial swelling, with tracheostomy to provide airway support; extremity escharotomies; and abdominal compartment syndrome. Despite torso escharotomies, progressive abdominal swelling and hypertension developed, leading to respiratory compromise, oliguria, and hypotension. He underwent emergency laparotomy and evisceration. Because of this massive edema, his abdomen could not be closed. His viscera are contained within a silo constructed from Dexon mesh. Over time, this edema will resolve. Return to the OR will be planned daily to gradually reduce his viscera within his abdomen and close his fascia.

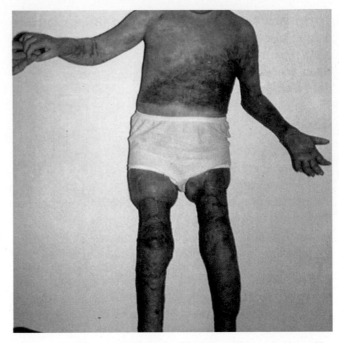

FIGURE 10-26. The long-term result of fascial excision and skin grafting. Fascia is well vascularized, and will "take" skin grafts well. However, the resulting wound is stiff, and the lack of subcutaneous padding results in chronic discomfort and poor joint mobility, as well as the obvious problems with appearance.

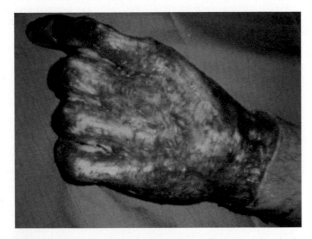

FIGURE 10-25. Fascial excision of a burned hand. Burns can be excised to the level of underlying fascia relatively easily, because of the natural tissue plane that exists at this level. Fascial excision is relatively bloodless, quick, and requires less skill than tangential excision. Very deep burns may require excision to this level. However, as this figure illustrates, fascial excisions remove all of the subcutaneous "padding" from the area, resulting in an obvious "step-off" transition to normal tissue.

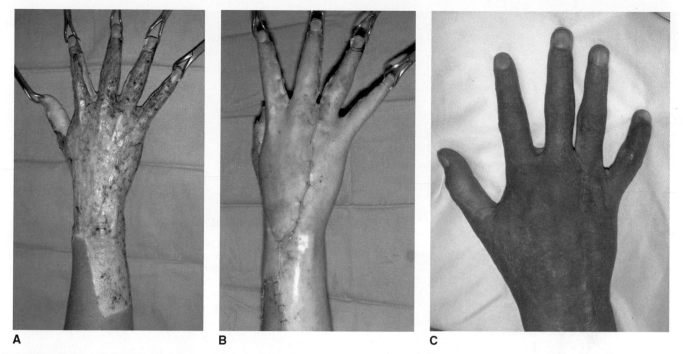

A   **B**   **C**

FIGURE 10-27. Tangential excision and sheet grafting. The man presented with a deep partial-thickness burn of the dorsal hand and forearm. Figure 10-27**A** shows the hand following tangential excision and hemostasis (towel clips are used to suspend the hand for grafting). Some subcutaneous fat and capillaries can be seen. Figure 10-27**B** shows the hand following coverage with split-thickness skin grafts harvested from the thigh and applied as sheets. Figure 10-27**C** shows the hand approximately 6 months later. Skin texture, contour, color, and function are excellent. This type of result is the goal of all skin-grafting surgery.

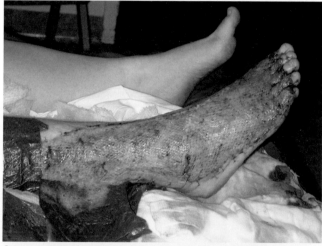

A

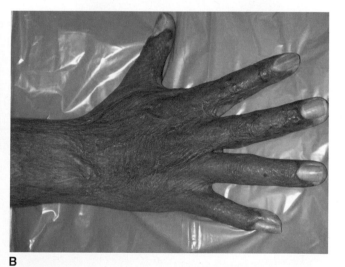

B

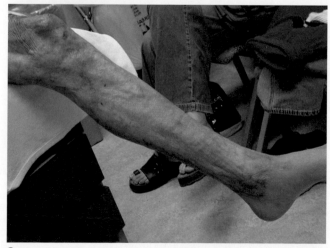

C

FIGURE 10-28. Typical results from tangential burn excision and coverage with meshed skin grafts. Meshing grafts "narrowly" produces multiple slits in the graft, which facilitates graft "take," prevents fluid collections beneath the skin, and speeds durable healing. Figure 10-28**A** shows a recent skin graft at the first dressing change (the black sheet is Acticoat, a topical antibiotic dressing). The mesh pattern is "closed" and the graft is uniformly pink and adherent. Figures 10-28**B** and **C** show long-term results. The mesh pattern is always visible, but the functional results of these grafts are usually good. Mesh grafts take more easily and reliably than sheet grafts, which can remain fragile for prolonged periods.

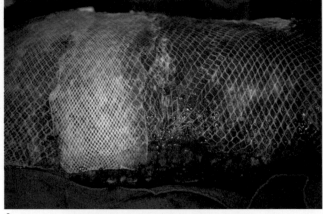

A

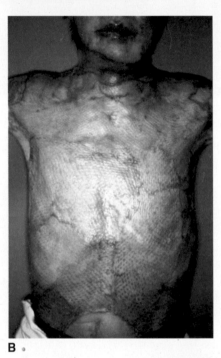

B .

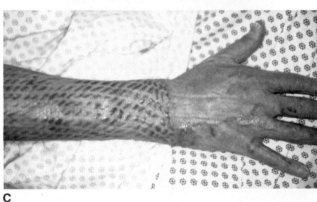

C

FIGURE 10-29. Widely meshed skin grafts. This patient suffered extensive deep burn injuries. To cover the torso, limited donor sites were harvested and widely meshed to permit them to be expanded and cover a larger area. Narrowly meshed human cadaver allografts (partially applied on the left) are used to cover these fragile autografts until epithelialization is complete. Figure 10-29**B** shows the final result. The meshed pattern is apparent but the skin is flexible and of good quality. Figure 10-29**C** shows another example. In this case, limited donor skin has been used to sheet graft the hand to maximize functional and cosmetic results, while widely meshed grafts have been placed on the forearm.

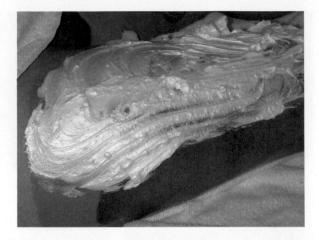

FIGURE 10-30. Application of silver sulfadiazine cream. This topical antibiotic is effective against a wide range of pathogens, and is extensively used to treat large burn injuries. Today, a wide variety of topical agents is available for burn wound care.

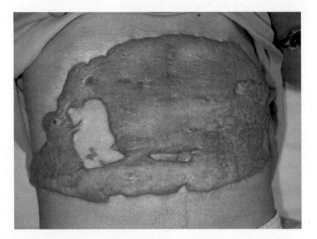

FIGURE 10-31. Severe hypertrophic scarring of the abdomen following a deep partial-thickness burn that healed spontaneously. Such severe hypertrophic scarring can be treated with compression therapy, injection of topical steroids, and even radiation therapy, but is best prevented by appropriate excision and skin grafting, which will usually result in a much better cosmetic and functional appearance.

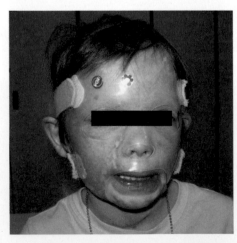

FIGURE 10-32. Compressive face mask. This child was burned in an automobile fire and required extensive skin grafting to her face. Long-term use of elastic face masks tends to produce deformities of the mandible in children, and are unattractive and socially stigmatizing. Instead, a rigid mask of clear plastic was custom-made, which the patient wears for most of every day. This compresses the skin grafts as they remodel, resulting in a smoother result with fewer contractures. Such masks are typically worn for at least a year following injury.

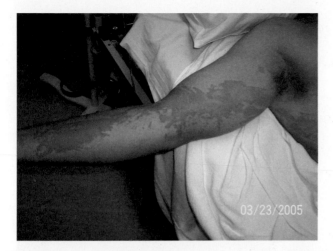

FIGURE 10-33. Chemical injury to the arm and forearm. Caustic chemicals including acids, alkalis, and petroleum products cause coagulation necrosis of the skin without heat. This wound has some elements that are erythematous and appear to be partial-thickness in depth, but the brownish central areas are probably deep. Chemical burns are frequently deeper and more serious than they initially appear.

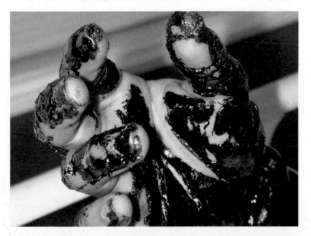

FIGURE 10-34. Tar injury of the hand. Tar is an organic compound that can cause skin irritation, but most tar burns are primarily thermal burns. Tar can be difficult to remove; cooling it rapidly with water will minimize the injury, after which tar can be left in place until it can be removed safely with specific solvents or mineral oil. Do not attempt to remove tar with gasoline, which can cause a much more severe chemical injury.

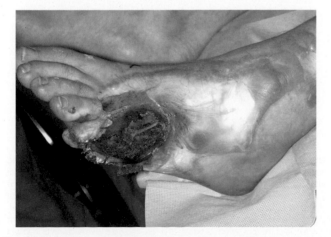

FIGURE 10-35. High-voltage electrical injury of the foot. Physicians often use the term "entrance" wound to denote the site of contact with current, and "exit" wound to denote the site of contact with ground. However, with alternating current injuries these two cannot be distinguished on clinical examination. This photo shows obvious full-thickness charring of the small toe down to bone (a "fourth-degree") injury, and extensive surrounding full-thickness injury. This patient required trans-metatarsal amputation and skin grafting.

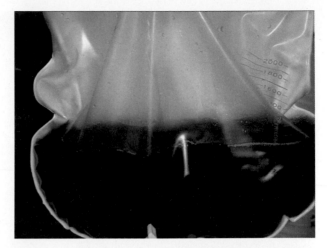

FIGURE 10-36. Myoglobinuria. With severe electrical injuries, destruction of skeletal muscle releases myoglobin, which is excreted in the urine. Although urine can be tested specifically for this pigment, the gross appearance of the urine is enough to make the diagnosis. Remember that major thermal burns can cause sufficient destruction of red cells to cause hemoglobinuria, which has the same appearance. Both myoglobin and hemoglobin can cause pigment-induced acute renal failure. Aggressive fluid resuscitation—aimed at maintaining urine output of 50–100 mL/hr in adults—will usually resolve this problem within 12–24 hours.

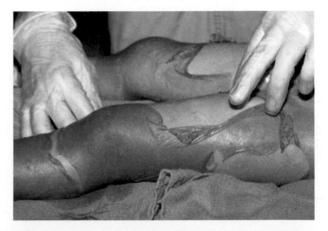

FIGURE 10-37. Severe Toxic Epidermal Necrolysis (TEN). This child demonstrates confluent epidermal sloughing, which is readily removed with gentle pressure (Nikolsky sign).

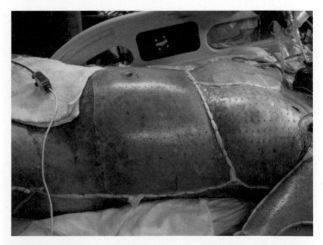

FIGURE 10-38. This young woman with toxic epidermal necrolysis after taking trimethoprim-sulfa for acne. She developed extensive blistering of her torso, arms, face, scalp, and thighs, totaling about 75% TBSA. After initial evaluation in the burn center, she was taken to the operating room where her blistered skin was removed, and the wounds covered with Biobrane, a collagen-impregnated fabric that adheres tightly to the wound, effectively "sealing" it off until epidermal regeneration occurred spontaneously in about 10 days. She made an uneventful recovery.

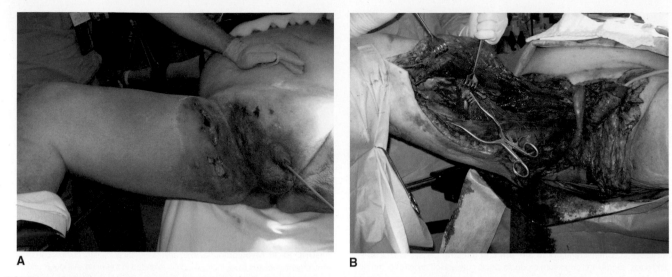

A

B

FIGURE 10-39. Severe necrotizing soft-tissue infection. This diabetic man presented with a several-day history of swelling and pain in the right groin, associated with fever, confusion, hypotension, and severe hypoglycemia. Figure 10-39**A** shows the initial presentation. There is an obvious necrotic wound of the groin with foul-smelling, purulent drainage, and extensive erythema and swelling of the medial thigh. Figure 10-32**B** shows the result of surgical debridement. Purulent, necrotic material was removed from the entire medial thigh, including the scrotum. Grey-brown necrotic exudates can be seen at the distal extent of the wound.

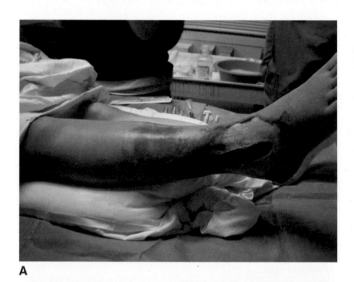

A

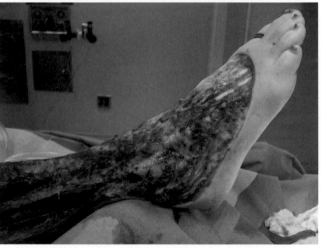

B

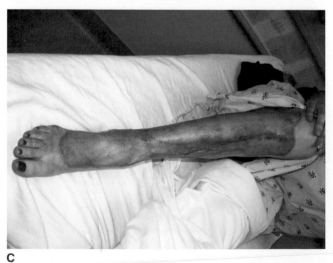

C

FIGURE 10-40. Necrotizing group A streptococcal infection. This young woman "sprained" her ankle while skiing. Two days later she developed fever, chills, and a progressive necrotic wound over the lateral ankle. Figure 10-40**A** shows the leg on presentation, with dusky erythema, swelling, and pain extending proximal to the area of obvious necrosis, which had been incised at an outside hospital. Following debridement, Figure 10-40**B** shows shaggy, fibrinous exudates adherent to the fascia of the foot, which is viable. She required extensive excision of involved tissue, antibiotics, and fluid support. Several days later she underwent skin grafting to the open wound. The result is shown in Figure 10-40**C**. She made a full recovery and has returned to skiing.

Glossary

abrasion wound that has superficial loss of epithelial elements; dermis and deeper structures remain intact.

absorbable sutures surgical suture material prepared from a substance that is digested by body tissues and therefore is not permanent; available in various diameters and tensile strengths; can be treated to modify its resistance to absorption; can be impregnated with antimicrobial agents.

achalasia esophageal motility disorder characterized by failure of the circular esophageal muscle in the distal 2 cm of the esophagus to relax.

acidemia elevation of blood hydrogen ion.

acidosis primary increase in PCO_2 or primary decrease in HCO_3.

acral lentiginous melanoma malignant melanoma that occurs in areas with no hair follicles (e.g., palms, nail beds, soles of feet).

activated partial thromboplastin time (APTT) clotting test used to detect deficiencies in the intrinsic coagulation pathway; a prolonged APTT indicates deficiencies in factor I, II, V, VIII, IX, X, XI, or XII.

adenoma mucosal tumor of the small and large intestine; tubular, villous, and mixed cell types are seen.

adenoma, hepatic benign tumor that consists of unencapsulated sheets of hepatocytes without ductular elements; apparently hormonally responsive; risk of spontaneous rupture.

adenoma, parathyroid benign tumor of a parathyroid gland.

adenoma, toxic solitary autonomous hyperactive thyroid nodule.

adenoma, villous polyp characterized by sessile morphology; relatively high incidence of malignant degeneration.

adhesion fibrous tissue that often occurs after abdominal surgery; can lead to bowel obstruction.

adhesion, platelet sticking of platelets to surfaces other than another platelet; collagen is the common in vivo surface to which platelets adhere.

adrenal incidentaloma incidentally discovered adrenal mass that is not associated with any symptoms that overtly suggest adrenal abnormality.

adrenal insufficiency (Addisonian crisis) result of inadequate circulating glucocorticoids; common signs and symptoms are postural hypotension, dizziness, nausea, vomiting, abdominal pain, weakness, fatigability, hyperkalemia, and hyponatremia; if not treated promptly, causes complete cardiovascular collapse and death.

adrenocorticotropic hormone (ACTH) stimulation test administration of synthetic ACTH to stimulate the secretion of cortisol and evaluate the adequacy of adrenal reserve and the integrity of the hypothalamic–pituitary–adrenal axis.

advance directive a mentally capable patient's instructions regarding his or her medical care if he or she becomes incapacitated and unable to make decisions.

afterload resistance to ventricular ejection; may be increased by obstruction (i.e., aortic stenosis) or vascular constriction (i.e., increased systemic vascular resistance).

aggregation, platelet platelet-to-platelet sticking; a white clot is formed that is composed almost exclusively of platelets.

airway, nasopharyngeal (nasal) device, usually made of rubber, designed to prevent the tongue from obstructing the nasopharynx; placed through a nostril into the nasopharynx; well tolerated in the patient with an intact gag reflex.

airway, oropharyngeal (oral) device, usually made of plastic, designed to prevent the tongue from obstructing the oropharynx; placed through the mouth and over the tongue; should not be used in a conscious patient with an intact gag reflex because it can cause gagging, vomiting, and aspiration.

aldosterone hormone produced by the zona glomerulosa in the adrenal gland; secreted as part of the renin–angiotensin system in response to decreased blood flow in the kidneys; causes sodium retention and potassium and hydrogen loss in the distal tubule.

alkalemia depression of blood hydrogen ion.

alkalosis primary decrease in PCO_2 or primary increase in HCO_3.

allograft (homograft) tissue transferred between genetically dissimilar members of the same species (e.g., most human transplants).

alpha$_1$-antitrypsin deficiency inherited autosomal dominant disorder that causes varying degrees of liver and lung injury over a patient's lifetime; some patients have predominantly pulmonary dysfunction; others have liver disease that leads to cirrhosis and the need for liver transplantation.

amaurosis fugax transient monocular blindness as a result of emboli to the ipsilateral ophthalmic artery; classically described as a curtain of blindness being pulled down from the superior to the inferior aspect of the affected eye.

anal fissure painful linear tear in the lining of the anal canal below the dentate line.

aneuploid having an abnormal number of chromosomes, not an exact multiple of the haploid number, in contrast to having abnormal numbers of complete haploid sets of chromosomes (e.g., diploid, triploid); prognostic factor used to estimate the risk of recurrence of breast cancer; ploidy is measured with flow cytometry, which permits analysis of DNA content per cell and allows determination of ploidy levels within a tumor cell population; diploid indicates a good prognosis; aneuploid indicates a poorer prognosis.

aneurysm dilation of an artery to greater than one and a half to two times its normal size; may be saccular (sac-like bulging on one side of the artery) or fusiform (elongated, spindle-shaped diffuse dilation of the arterial wall).

angioplasty reconstruction of a blood vessel, either surgically or by balloon dilation; surgical angioplasty entails reconstruction of the artery, usually with a patch; balloon angioplasty involves percutaneous placement of an intra-arterial balloon; the balloon is then inflated, thereby disrupting the arterial plaque as well as a portion of the media and consequently enlarging the artery.

ankle–brachial index comparison of the systolic blood pressure at the level of the ankle divided by the brachial arterial pressure; this ratio provides an assessment of the degree of lower extremity arterial occlusive disease, with the brachial arterial pressure used as a control.

annular pancreas ring of pancreas encircling the duodenum; caused by a failure of the embryonic primordia to unite completely; each portion has its own duct.

antibiotic resistance resistance to a previously effective antibiotic by a microbial pathogen through changes in its DNA structure.

antidiuretic hormone (vasopressin) hormone produced by the supraoptic and paraventricular nuclei of the hypothalamus; secreted in response to increased osmotic pressure and decreased effective plasma volume; also released in response to stress; regulates water balance by stimulating resorption in the distal renal tubule.

antisepsis prevention of infection by inhibiting the growth of infectious agents.

antrectomy distal gastric resection that removes the gastrin-producing cells of the stomach.

aponeurosis flat tendon; broad, fibrous sheet of tendinous fibers that provides attachment to broad muscles (e.g., oblique muscles of the abdominal wall).

appendicitis inflammation of the appendix.

asepsis absence of living pathogenic organisms; state of sterility.

asplenism complete loss of splenic function.

atherosclerosis degenerative change of the arterial wall; characterized by endothelial dysfunction, inflammatory cell adhesion, and infiltration and accumulation of cellular and acellular elements within the arterial wall; lipid deposition is associated with fibrosis and calcification and can lead to severe arterial occlusive disease.

autograft graft (e.g., skin) that consists of the patient's own tissue.

avulsion tearing away or forcible separation of tissue; may be partial or total.

B cells immunocytes derived from bone marrow stem cells; commonly, B cells produce circulating antibodies and are responsible for the humoral response to foreign tissues.

bacteremia presence of viable bacteria in the blood.

Ballance's sign percussion dullness of the left flank; occurs with a ruptured spleen.

Barrett's esophagus presence of columnar epithelium in the esophagus; results from a metaplastic change caused by repeated inflammation of normal squamous epithelium; small, but significant tendency toward the development of cancer.

basal cell carcinoma carcinoma of the skin that arises from the basal cells of the epidermis or hair follicles.

basal cell carcinoma, morphea-like tumor with an indurated, yellow plaque with ill-defined borders; overlying skin remains intact for a long period; less common than nodular basal cell carcinoma.

basal cell carcinoma, nodular most common variant of basal cell carcinoma; characterized by a central depression and a rolled border; usually located on the head and neck.

basal cell carcinoma, pigmented similar to nodular basal cell carcinoma, except that tumors contain melanocytes; may be confused with melanoma.

Beck's triad three classic clinical signs of cardiac tamponade: (1) muffled (distant) heart sounds, (2) elevated central venous pressure (jugular venous distension), and (3) hypotension.

bezoar accumulation of a large mass of undigested material in the stomach.

biliary colic episodic epigastric or right upper quadrant abdominal pain; associated with nausea and vomiting; secondary to transient cystic duct obstruction with a gallstone; tends to occur postprandially; usually lasts 1 to 4 hours.

Billroth I procedure gastrointestinal reconstruction that creates an anastomosis between the distal end of the stomach and the duodenum (gastroduodenostomy).

Billroth II procedure gastrointestinal reconstruction that creates an anastomosis between the stomach and a loop of jejunum (gastrojejunostomy).

bleeding disorder, acquired hemostatic defect caused by a nongenetic factor (e.g., liver disease, anticoagulation therapy); more common than congenital bleeding disorders.

bleeding disorder, congenital inherited hemostatic defect (e.g., hemophilia, von Willebrand's disease); fairly uncommon.

bleeding history important part of the presurgical evaluation; a personal or a familial bleeding problem is the most important predictive factor of operative and perioperative bleeding complications.

bleeding time test interval between the appearance of the first drop of blood and the removal of the last drop after incision of the forearm or puncture of the ear lobe or finger; bleeding time is prolonged in cases of thrombocytopenia, diminished prothrombin, abnormal platelet function, phosphorus or chloroform poisoning, and in some liver diseases; it is normal in hemophilia.

blood cell, red (erythrocyte) cellular portion of the blood that contains hemoglobin; responsible for carrying oxygen to the tissues.

blood cell, white (leukocyte) cellular portion of the blood that does not contain hemoglobin; classified as granular (i.e., neutrophils, eosinophils, basophils) and nongranular.

Boerhaave's syndrome full-thickness rupture of the esophagus (in contrast, Mallory-Weiss syndrome is a bleeding mucosal rupture at the same site); associated with loss of gastroesophageal contents (typically into the left side of the chest) and acute sepsis; may cause a syndrome similar to myocardial infarction.

Bowen's disease skin condition characterized by chronic scaling and occasionally a crusted, purple, or erythematous raised lesion; may become invasive squamous cell carcinoma.

brain death irreversible cessation of all brain function.

BRCA-1 gene BRCA-1 and BRCA-2 are the two major genes responsible for the inherited predisposition to breast cancer; BRCA-1 is also related to ovarian cancer; in patients who have mutations in either gene, the risk of breast cancer is approximately 80% by age 70; in contrast, the lifetime risk is approximately 12% in the general population.

Breslow system system for microstaging malignant melanomas based on the thickness of the tumor in millimeters; survival is related to tumor thickness.

bruit auscultatory sound over an artery; produced by turbulent flow.

burn center specialized care unit with facilities, personnel, and resources devoted to the care of patients with serious burn injuries.

burn, epidermal first-degree burn injury that involves only the epidermal layer of the skin; does not blister; has relatively minor physiologic effects; heals without scarring.

burn, first-degree see *burn, epidermal.*

burn, full-thickness third-degree burn injury that involves the entire epidermis and dermis; usually requires skin grafting.

burn, partial-thickness second-degree burn injury that involves some, but not all, of the dermis; variable in appearance, but because epidermal appendages are intact, heals if followed long enough; deep partial-thickness burns are usually treated with skin grafting.

burn, second-degree see *burn, partial-thickness.*

burn, third-degree see *burn, full-thickness.*

carcinoembryonic antigen antigen produced by many gastrointestinal tumors; measured in the blood; used in surveillance for cancer recurrence.

carcinoid syndrome carcinoid tumor that causes a syndrome of signs and symptoms that include cutaneous flushing, diarrhea, bronchospasm, skin lesions, and vasomotor instability.

cardiac output quantity of blood pumped by the heart into the pulmonary and systemic circulation each minute.

cardiac tamponade compression of the heart from accumulation of fluid or blood within the pericardial sac; ventricular filling is restricted; the increased pressure within the pericardial sac is transmitted to each cardiac chamber; results in equalization of the right atrial, right ventricular diastolic, pulmonary artery diastolic, pulmonary capillary wedge, left atrial, left ventricular diastolic, and intrapericardial pressures.

cardiogenic state decreased cardiac output from inadequate function of the heart itself, rather than deficiencies in venous return.

cerebral blood flow cerebral perfusion pressure divided by cerebrovascular resistance.

cerebrovascular accident (stroke) region of cerebral infarction secondary to arterial atheroembolism or hypoperfusion.

Charcot's triad triad of clinical findings that includes right upper quadrant abdominal pain, fever and chills, and jaundice; associated with cholangitis.

Child's classification series of five parameters (serum bilirubin, serum albumin, presence of ascites, encephalopathy, and nutrition) used to grade the status of liver disease.

chin-lift maneuver maneuver used to open the mouth so that the oral cavity can be inspected and patency assured; accomplished by placing the fingers of the left hand under the chin while the thumb is placed anteriorly below the lips; the chin is grasped and lifted forward and downward; the mouth is opened for inspection; a more secure grip on the jaw is accomplished by placing the thumb inside the mouth and behind the lower incisors.

cholangiocarcinoma adenocarcinoma that has two types: infiltrating bile duct tumor that usually arises at the level of the bile duct bifurcation and, less commonly, solid intraparenchymal tumor within the substance of the liver.

cholangiogram radiographic image of the bile ducts; obtained by injecting contrast material through a needle or catheter.

cholangiogram, percutaneous transhepatic radiologic imaging of the biliary tree; obtained by inserting a needle through the abdominal wall into the liver parenchyma and injecting contrast material directly into the intrahepatic bile ducts; used to extract stones, obtain a cytology specimen, or place a catheter.

cholangitis, acute acute infection of the bile ducts; caused by a stone, stricture, or neoplasm.

cholangitis, acute suppurative acute infection of the bile ducts; complicated by the finding of pus; requires urgent drainage.

cholecystectomy, laparoscopic removal of the gallbladder with a laparoscopic approach; preferred approach for most elective and many emergency situations.

cholecystitis, acute acute infection of the gallbladder; usually caused by calculus obstructing the cystic duct.

cholecystitis, acute acalculous acute infection of the gallbladder without underlying gallstone disease; usually occurs in patients who are being treated in intensive care units for other medical problems.

cholecystitis, acute emphysematous acute infection of the gallbladder; caused by gas-forming bacteria; characterized by air in the wall or lumen of the gallbladder or in the bile ducts; often associated with diabetes mellitus; requires emergency cholecystectomy.

cholecystitis, acute gangrenous acute infection of the gallbladder that progresses to gangrene; requires emergency cholecystectomy.

choledocholithiasis presence of a stone(s) in the common bile duct; stones usually originate in the gallbladder and pass through the cystic duct into the common bile duct.

circulating nurse usually a registered nurse; a member of the operating room team who does not directly participate in the surgical procedure, but manages activities outside the sterile field; duties include opening sterile supplies, counting sponges, making and answering calls, delivering specimens, maintaining records, and other vital tasks.

Clark system system for microstaging malignant melanomas based on the anatomic level (I through V) of invasion of the tumor; survival is related to the depth of invasion.

claudication reproducible pain that occurs in a major muscle group; precipitated by exercise and relieved by rest; classically, pain occurs in the posterior calves after mild to moderate exercise.

closed-gloving technique method of donning surgical gloves in which the hands are not pushed fully through the cuffs of the surgical gown; usually practiced by surgical technicians as a self-gloving technique.

coagulation factor substance in the blood that is necessary for clotting; numbered with Roman numerals.

coagulation pathway, common final steps that lead to the generation of a clot; includes factors I (fibrinogen), II (prothrombin), V, and X; the end product is fibrin.

coagulation pathway, extrinsic part of the first stage of coagulation; requires the interaction of factor VII with tissue thromboplastin to convert factor X to factor X^a.

coagulation pathway, intrinsic part of the first stage of coagulation; initiated by the interaction of factor XII with negatively charged surfaces; other coagulation factors in this pathway are factors VIII, IX, and XI; the eventual product converts factor X to factor X^a.

collagen principal structural protein of the body; its production, remodeling, and maturation define the second and third stages of wound healing.

colloid fluid for intravenous administration; consists of water, electrolytes, and protein or other molecules that are of sufficient molecular weight to exert a colloid oncotic pressure effect similar to that of endogenous albumin; packed red cells are often considered colloid, but do not meet this definition.

colonoscopy flexible diagnostic instrument that uses light-transmitting fiber optics; allows visualization of the entire colon and terminal ileum.

colostomy surgical procedure in which the colon is divided and the proximal end is brought through a surgically created defect in the abdominal wall and sewn to the skin.

compartment syndrome elevation of the pressure within a fascial compartment of the upper or lower extremity; interstitial tissue pressure becomes higher than capillary perfusion pressure, resulting in ischemia to the muscles and nerves within the fascial compartment.

complement system of 20 or more proteins present in the serum; when activated, these proteins stimulate lymphocytes, macrophages, and reticuloendothelial cells as part of the host defense against bacterial pathogens.

consensus formula for burn resuscitation widely used formula for resuscitation from burn shock: 4 mL lactated Ringer's solution Ñ body weight (kg) × burn (percentage of total body surface area).

contractility the force of cardiac muscle contraction under conditions of a predetermined preload or afterload.

contusion soft tissue swelling and hemorrhage without violation of the skin elements.

contusion, pulmonary injury to the lung parenchyma that causes interstitial hemorrhage, alveolar collapse, and extravasation of blood and plasma into the alveoli; causes a ventilation–perfusion mismatch that results in hypoxemia; physical examination may show blunt or penetrating injury to the chest; radiographic studies show a poorly defined infiltrate that develops over time.

Cooper's ligament strong fibrous insertion of transversus abdominis muscle on the pectineal line of the pelvis.

Courvoisier's law obstruction of the common bile duct by carcinoma of the pancreas or other malignancies of the distal common bile duct may lead to an enlarged palpable, nontender gallbladder; contrariwise, obstruction by stones in the common bile duct does not lead to a palpable, nontender gallbladder because scarring from chronic gallbladder inflammation prevents enlargement of the gallbladder.

Courvoisier's sign in a small percentage of cases, obstruction of the common bile duct by carcinoma of the pancreas causes enlargement of the gallbladder; obstruction caused by stones in the common bile duct does not cause enlargement because scarring from infection prevents the gallbladder from distending.

crepitus crackling; the sensation felt or sound heard when palpating soft tissue that contains gas or when moving fractured bones.

cricothyroidotomy incision through the skin and cricothyroid membrane through which a small tracheostomy tube is inserted to relieve airway obstruction.

Crohn's disease inflammatory process of the small intestine and colon; usually causes transmural involvement of the small intestinal wall; occasionally similar to acute appendicitis.

crossmatch in vitro process of mixing donor leukocytes with recipient serum and complement; used to determine whether the recipient produces antibodies that are cytotoxic to the leukocytes, thus predicting rejection of a potential allograft.

crystalloid fluid for intravenous administration; consists of water, electrolytes, and sometimes glucose in isotonic or hypertonic concentrations.

Cushing reflex increase in systemic blood pressure associated with bradycardia and a slowed respiratory rate; caused by increased intracranial pressure.

Cushing's disease Cushing's syndrome (see below) caused by excess production of adrenocorticotropic hormone by an adenoma of the anterior pituitary gland; first defined in 1932.

Cushing's syndrome constellation of clinical findings that result from excessive circulating glucocorticoids.

cytopenia decreased number of cells, usually hematologic cells; anemia is decreased red cell count; leukopenia is decreased white cell count; thrombocytopenia is decreased platelet count.

dead space potential or real cavity that remains after closure of a wound and is not obliterated by the operative technique.

debridement technique to remove dead skin, other nonviable tissue, and debris from a wound surface; some surgeons use this term to describe excision of burns, but it usually refers only to treatment provided at the bedside, without anesthesia.

deep-space compartment confined anatomic space; increased pressure within such a space (e.g., from edema) limits circulation and threatens tissue function and viability.

dentate line anatomic line that delineates the conversion of squamous epithelium to cuboidal and columnar epithelium in the anal canal.

dermatofibroma slowly growing benign skin nodule; poorly demarcated cellular fibrous tissue encloses collapsed capillaries, with scattered hemosiderin-pigmented and lipid macrophages.

dexamethasone suppression test dexamethasone is administered to suppress cortisol secretion; in Cushing's syndrome, this suppression does not occur.

diagnostic peritoneal lavage surgical procedure used to identify an intraperitoneal injury; under local anesthesia, a peritoneal catheter is inserted into the peritoneal cavity through a small midline incision; a syringe is attached to the catheter and aspirated; if 10 mL blood is aspirated, the test result is positive; if <10 mL blood is aspirated, then 1000 mL or 10 mL/kg warm lactated Ringer's or normal saline solution is infused into the peritoneal cavity; after 5 to 10 minutes, the lavage fluid is retrieved by gravity siphon technique; a 50-mL portion is sent to the laboratory for microscopic analysis, cell count, and bile and amylase analysis; the result is positive for blunt trauma if the red blood cell count is 100,000 cells/mm^3 or greater, if the white blood cell count is more than 500 cells/mm^3, if bacteria, bile, or food particles are present, or if amylase is greater than serum amylase; a negative study does not exclude retroperitoneal injury to the duodenum, pancreas, kidneys, diaphragm, aorta, or vena cava.

disseminated intravascular coagulation hemorrhagic syndrome that occurs after the uncontrolled activation of clotting factors and fibrinolytic enzymes throughout the small blood vessels; fibrin is deposited, platelets and clotting factors are consumed, and fibrin degradation products that inhibit fibrin polymerization and clot formation are created, resulting in bleeding.

Dripps-American Surgical Association Classification system of patient classification (I to IV); based on chronic health status; used to estimate perioperative risks.

duct of Santorini accessory pancreatic duct.

duct of Wirsung main pancreatic duct.

dumping syndrome complex myriad symptoms; may include crampy abdominal pain and diarrhea; secondary to ablation of the pyloric sphincter mechanism.

durable power of attorney for health care formal advance directive that names a specific person to make health care decisions for the patient if the patient becomes unable to do so.

dysphagia difficulty in swallowing.

elemental diet chemically defined enteral diet of high osmolarity and low viscosity; designed to meet specific nutritional and metabolic needs that cannot be achieved naturally.

embolism occlusion or obstruction of an artery by a transported thrombus, atherosclerotic plaque, bacterial vegetation, or foreign body.

endarterectomy surgical excision of the intima, atherosclerotic plaque, and a portion of the media of an atherosclerotic blood vessel.

endoscopic retrograde cholangiopancreatogram (ERCP) radiologic imaging of the biliary tree and pancreatic duct by retrograde injection of contrast material through a cannula placed endoscopically in the ampulla of Vater; used to extract stones, obtain a cytology specimen, or place a catheter.

eschar coating of dead skin, serum, and debris that forms on the surface of a burn wound.

escharotomy incision made through burned tissue to relieve compression caused by edema formation beneath rigid eschar.

esophageal diverticulum outpouching of all layers of the esophagus; typically located in the cervical, midthoracic, or epiphrenic region; associated with dysfunction of the cricopharyngeus muscle and lower esophageal sphincter complex; in Zenker's diverticulum, only the mucosa projects through the esophageal wall.

esophageal myotomy incision in the muscular portion of the esophagus; performed for achalasia or another esophageal motility disorder; converts the esophagus into a larger, but passive tube.

esophageal stricture stenosis of the esophagus; typically occurs from gastric acid reflux, from neglected reflux esophagitis, or after corrosive materials are swallowed.

excision, early technique of burn wound treatment; burned tissue is surgically removed before spontaneous eschar separation occurs.

excision, fascial technique of burn wound excision; the skin and subcutaneous tissue are removed to the level of the fascia.

excision, tangential technique of burn wound excision; only burned tissue is removed with a dermatome, leaving viable dermis and subcutaneous tissue behind.

extracorporeal shock wave lithotripsy (ESWL) fragmentation of gallstones with a shock wave; performed ultrasonographically; limitations include strict eligibility criteria, high failure rate, high recurrence rate, and the need for an expensive solvent (ursodeoxycholic acid) and expensive equipment.

false diverticulum diverticulum characterized by mucosal outpouching through a weakened portion of the colon wall.

familial atypical mole and melanoma (FAM-M) syndrome risk factor for hereditary melanoma; associated with mutations on chromosomes 1p and 9p.

familial medullary thyroid carcinoma autosomal dominant condition caused by a mutation of RET; associated with medullary thyroid carcinoma, but no other endocrine abnormalities.

fasciotomy incision through the fascia to relieve increased pressure; used to treat compartment syndrome.

feeding, postpyloric feeding into the gastrointestinal tract distal to the pyloric valve, usually with a nasoduodenal or gastroduodenal tube.

feeding, prepyloric feeding into the gastrointestinal tract proximal to the pylorus with a nasogastric or gastrostomy tube.

felon infection of the pulp space of the digits in the hand.

Felty's syndrome leg ulcers or chronic infection associated with splenomegaly and neutropenia in patients with rheumatoid arthritis.

fibrin essential portion of a blood clot; white, fibrous protein formed from fibrinogen by the action of thrombin.

fibrinogen factor I; globulin produced in the liver and converted to fibrin during blood clotting.

fibromuscular dysplasia idiopathic nonatherosclerotic hyperplastic and fibrosing lesion of the intima, media, or adventitia; the most common form is medial fibroplasia.

fine-needle aspiration biopsy cytology cytologic examination of cells aspirated from the thyroid; also the most commonly used technique to diagnose palpable breast masses; a small-gauge needle is used to extract three random samples of the breast mass; the contents of the needle are smeared on a glass slide using a technique similar to that used with a Pap smear.

fistula abnormal connection between two epithelial-lined structures.

fistula, aortoenteric abnormal communication between the abdominal aorta and the third portion of the duodenum where it overlies the aorta; usually associated with breakdown of a previous aortic bypass graft anastomosis, although primary aortoenteric fistulae occur.

fistula-in-ano abnormal communication between the anus at the level of the dentate line and the perirectal skin through the bed of a previous abscess.

flail chest result of fracture of consecutive ribs in multiple places (i.e., each rib is fractured in at least two places); the free-floating, or flail, segment of the chest wall moves paradoxically with inspiration and expiration.

follicle extracellular space within the thyroid; contains colloid; bordered by follicular cells; triiodothyronine (T_3) and thyroxine (T_4) are stored bound to thyroglobulin.

follicular cells thyroid cells that process iodine into thyroid hormone.

fulminant hepatic failure hepatic failure associated with massive hepatocyte necrosis or severe impairment; occurs within 8 to 12 weeks of the onset of symptoms; findings are not associated with chronic liver disease; unless liver transplantation is performed, may progress to coma and brainstem herniation from increased cerebral pressure.

fundoplication operation to restore competence to the esophagogastric junction as part of the treatment of sliding hiatal hernia and reflux esophagitis; the most common is the Nissen fundoplication, in which the gastric fundus is wrapped around the lower and intra-abdominal segment of the esophagus to produce an acute angle of His and other functional changes.

gallstone ileus mechanical obstruction of the intestine caused by a large gallstone that erodes through the gallbladder into the duodenum; may be associated with pneumobilia; the point of obstruction is often in the distal ileum.

gas-bloat syndrome abdominal bloating associated with inability to vomit; may occur after gastric fundoplication.

gastric outlet obstruction obstruction in the pyloric area of the stomach secondary to repeated bouts of acute duodenal ulcerations with subsequent scarring.

gastrin hormone produced by the G cells of the stomach; stimulates acid secretion by the parietal cell.

gastritis diffuse erythema and disruption of the mucosa of the stomach; associated with the ingestion of irritating agents.

Glasgow Coma Scale method used to classify the severity of head injuries; eye opening score 1 to 4, verbal response score 1 to 5, and motor response score 1 to 6.

globus hystericus subjective sensation of a lump in the throat.

goiter thyroid enlargement.

graft, heterotopic graft placed at a site different from the normal anatomic position (e.g., renal transplant).

graft, orthotopic graft placed in the normal anatomic position (e.g., cardiac transplant).

granulocyte colony stimulating factor similar to erythropoietin for red cells; stimulates the maturation of white blood cells; dramatically decreases the sequelae of leukopenia after chemotherapy.

Graves' disease autoimmune thyrotoxicosis.

H₂ blockade most common modality used to treat duodenal ulcer disease; blocks the histamine receptor of the parietal cell; one-half of the total is given in the first 8 hours postburn; the rest is given over the next 16 hours.

hamartoma benign tumor; normal tissues grow rapidly compared with surrounding normal tissues.

Harris-Benedict equations pair of regression equations based on sex, age, height, and weight; used to estimate resting metabolic expenditure.

Hartmann's pouch A spheroid or a conical pouch at the junction of the neck of the gallbladder and the cystic duct.

Hartmann's procedure stapling or oversewing of the distal end of a sigmoid colon resection, leaving a blind rectal stump in the peritoneal cavity.

Hashimoto's thyroiditis autoimmune thyroiditis; first described by Japanese surgeon Hakuru Hashimoto (1881 to 1934).

healing, primary primary adhesion of tissue after a wound is closed by direct approximation of the edges; no granulation tissue is formed.

healing, secondary closing of a wound by secondary adhesion; the wound is left open and allowed to heal spontaneously.

healing, tertiary active closing of a wound after a delay of days to weeks; an open wound is closed with sutures or sterile tape before it heals; the secondary healing process is interrupted.

Heinz bodies erythrocyte inclusions that consist of denatured hemoglobin.

Helicobacter pylori Gram-negative bacterium associated with the pathogenesis of gastritis, gastric ulcers, and duodenal ulcers.

hemangioma tumor composed primarily of blood vessels; can involve the small and large intestine and liver.

hemangioma, cavernous benign, often incidentally found, tumor; consists of endothelial vascular spaces separated by fibrous septa; spontaneous rupture is rare; most patients require no specific treatment.

hemochromatosis autosomal recessive disease; characterized by excessive absorption of iron from the intestinal tract; affects the liver, heart, pancreas, and spleen.

hemoglobinopathy abnormality in hemoglobin structure; may lead to anemia and red cell structural abnormalities.

hemolytic anemia anemia caused by destruction of red blood cells.

hemophilia, type A X-linked recessive disorder of the blood; occurs almost exclusively in men; marked by a permanent tendency to hemorrhage as a result of factor VIII deficiency; characterized by prolonged clotting time, decreased formation of thromboplastin, and diminished conversion of prothrombin to thrombin.

hemothorax blood in the pleural cavity.

hemothorax, massive rapid loss of more than 1500 mL of blood into the pleural cavity; class III or greater hemorrhage into the pleural cavity.

hepatic encephalopathy poorly understood neuropsychiatric disorder; associated with advanced liver disease and portosystemic shunting; suspected etiologies include altered amino acid levels in the systemic circulation.

hepatocellular carcinoma (hepatoma) tumor, usually in the setting of cirrhosis (70% to 80%); accounts for 90% of all primary liver malignancies; most are advanced at presentation; fewer than 20% of patients are candidates for standard surgical resection.

her-2-neu oncogene oncogene whose expression indicates a poor prognosis, particularly in patients with node-positive breast cancer.

hereditary spherocytosis inherited condition that can lead to hemolytic anemia because of rigid, abnormally shaped erythrocytes that are sequestered and destroyed in the spleen.

hernia protrusion of all or part of a structure through the tissues that normally contain it.

hernia, direct groin hernia that results from protrusion through the attenuated posterior inguinal wall.

hernia, femoral protrusion of intraabdominal structures through the femoral canal.

hernia, indirect groin hernia into a patent processus vaginalis.

hernia, Richter's hernia at any site through which only a portion of the circumference of a bowel wall, usually the jejunum, incarcerates or strangulates.

hernia, sliding hernia in which a portion of the wall of the protruding peritoneal sac is made up of some intra-abdominal organ; as the sac expands, the organ is drawn out into the hernia.

hernia, umbilical protrusion of bowel or omentum through the abdominal wall under the skin at the umbilicus.

Hesselbach's triangle triangular area in the lower abdominal wall bounded by the inguinal ligament below, the border of the rectus abdominis medially, and the inferior epigastric vessels laterally; site of direct inguinal hernias.

Hodgkin's disease malignant lymphoma marked by chronic enlargement of the lymph nodes that is often local at onset and later generalized, together with enlargement of the spleen and often of the liver, no pronounced leukocytosis, and often anemia and continuous or remittent fever; associated with inflammatory infiltration of lymphocytes and eosinophilic leukocytes and fibroses.

Howell-Jolly bodies erythrocyte inclusion of nuclear remnants; usually found on peripheral blood smears after splenectomy.

human leukocyte antigens (HLA) antigens expressed by all nucleated cells; used to determine histocompatibility; the genetic loci that determine these antigens are located in the sixth human chromosome.

hyperparathyroidism, primary condition caused by excess secretion of parathyroid hormone, usually from a parathyroid adenoma.

hyperparathyroidism, secondary overactivity of the parathyroid glands in response to physiologic changes caused by chronic renal failure.

hyperparathyroidism, tertiary autonomous overactivity of the parathyroid glands; causes hypercalcemia; usually caused by chronic renal failure.

hyperplasia, atypical increased number of abnormal-appearing cells in the milk ducts; precedes ductal carcinoma in situ on the continuum from cells lining a normal milk duct, to ductal carcinoma in situ, to invasive cancer.

hyperplasia, focal nodular benign tumor that usually contains a central scar with both ductal elements and hepatocytes; spontaneous rupture is rare; most require no specific therapy.

hyperplasia, parathyroid diffuse enlargement and overactivity of the parathyroid glands.

hypersplenism excess splenic function manifested by cytopenia; may be unrelated to spleen size.

hypoperfusion inadequate blood flow to tissues.

hyposplenism diminished splenic function; usually increases susceptibility to infection, particularly with encapsulated bacteria.

hypovolemia decreased intravascular volume; causes decreased venous return.

ileoanal pullthrough operative procedure of choice for ulcerative colitis; consists of total colectomy, mucosal proctectomy, creation of a storage reservoir, and anastomosis to the dentate line; obviates a permanent ileostomy.

ileocecal valve termination of the small intestine; regulates the passage of intestinal contents into the large intestine.

immune thrombocytopenic purpura thrombocytopenia caused by antibodies directed at platelets; leads to platelet sequestration in the spleen.

incarceration confinement of a herniated structure to its protruded position.

indirect calorimetry method to measure precisely the resting metabolic rate by analysis of inspired and expired gases for O_2 and CO_2; when coupled with urine urea nitrogen, can be used to compute the proportion of protein, carbohydrate, and fat substrates being oxidized.

infection microbial phenomenon characterized by an inflammatory response to the presence of microorganisms or the invasion of normally sterile host tissue by organisms.

infection, nosocomial infection that occurs because of or during hospitalization and treatment.

infection, overwhelming postsplenectomy highly lethal infection (75% mortality rate) caused by encapsulated bacteria (*Streptococcus pneumoniae* is the most common); loss of the spleen increases susceptibility to these bacteria.

infection, polymicrobial infection that is difficult to treat because it involves multiple bacterial species.

inflammation cellular processes that are activated by a variety of cellular and tissue injuries; necessary for tissue repair and wound healing.

inflammation, severe inflammation stimulated by cellular or tissue injury; causes total body cellular or organ malfunction.

informed consent transfer of information between physician and patient that allows the patient to make a knowledgeable decision about a particular treatment.

inhalation injury injury that occurs from inhaling smoke or the products of combustion; occurs as carbon monoxide poisoning, upper-airway injury, or pulmonary parenchymal injury.

injury, reperfusion myocardial impairment, usually with arrhythmia, following the opening of arterial blockage and considered to be due to oxygen-derived free radicals.

inotropic drug agent that increases the contractility of heart muscle.

internal hemorrhoids vascular venous cushions that arise above the dentate line; often associated with swelling, bleeding, and discomfort.

iodine element concentrated and complexed exclusively by thyroid tissue.

isograft tissue transferred between genetically identical individuals (e.g., monozygotic twins).

jaw-thrust maneuver maneuver used to open the mouth so that the oral cavity can be inspected and patency assured; accomplished by standing behind the patient's head, placing the fingers behind the angle of the jaw, grasping the jaw on both sides, and then lifting it forward; the thumbs are used to open the mouth by drawing the mouth and chin downward.

Kehr's sign/omalgia pain at the top of the left shoulder referred from diaphragmatic irritation (e.g., from blood from a ruptured spleen).

Kupffer cell liver-based macrophage that accounts for 80% to 90% of the body stores of fixed macrophages; responsible for hepatic clearance of toxins, including endotoxin and specific infectious organisms; also responsible for the generation of cytokines and other inflammatory mediators.

Kussmaul's sign increase in central venous pressure with inspiration; seen in severe cardiac tamponade.

laceration torn or jagged wound or accidental cut wound.

leiomyoma tumor that involves the small or large intestine or any other smooth muscle.

leiomyosarcoma malignant tumor of smooth muscle.

lentigo maligna melanoma (Hutchinson's melanotic freckle) malignant lesion of the elderly; arises in sun-damaged skin; occurs primarily on the face and neck.

ligament of Treitz area of the small intestine where the duodenum meets the jejunum; located to the left of the midline in the left upper quadrant.

lower esophageal sphincter complex of anatomic structures that acts as a sphincter and keeps gastric acid in the stomach, yet allows swallowing, belching, or vomiting.

lymphedema swelling caused by the obstruction of lymphatic vessels or lymph nodes and the accumulation of large amounts of lymph; lymphedema of the arm, one of the most disabling complications of axillary dissection, occurs in 2% to 3% of cases after a level I or level II axillary dissection; usually occurs 6 months to many years after the surgical procedure.

lymphoma lymphatic malignancy that arises in the lymphoreticular components of the reticuloendothelial system.

lymphoma, non-Hodgkin's lymphoma other than Hodgkin's disease; classified by Rappaport according to pattern (nodular or diffuse) and cell type; a working or international formulation separates lymphomas into low, intermediate, and high grades and into cytologic subtypes that reflect follicular center cell or other origin.

lyophilization process of preserving tissue by removing its water content through freezing and rewarming in a vacuum.

magnification, compression views special mammographic techniques used to evaluate an abnormal density seen on a routine two-view screening mammography; if a density is real, magnification and compression of the breast tissue make the lesion more discrete; if the lesion represents an area of breast parenchyma that is more dense than surrounding tissue, compression usually causes the area to appear normal and diminishes clinical concern.

mass contractions contraction pattern that is unique to the colon; characterized by contraction of long segments of colon and resulting in mass movement of stool.

McBurney's point point on the anterior abdominal wall; located between the middle and outer thirds of a line drawn between the anterior iliac spine and umbilicus; represents on the anterior abdominal wall the location of the appendix.

Meckel's diverticulum true diverticulum of the ileum; occurs in 1% to 3% of the population; associated with bleeding, inflammation, and bowel obstruction.

medullary thyroid carcinoma carcinoma that originates from the C cells (calcitonin-secreting cells) of the thyroid; part of the multiple endocrine neoplasia types 2A (MEN-2A) and 2B (MEN-2B), and familial medullary thyroid carcinoma syndromes.

melanoma malignant neoplasm of the skin; derived from the cells that form melanin.

menin gene associated with multiple endocrine neoplasia type 1.

microcalcifications, mammographic breast calcifications that are classified as benign, indeterminate, or pleomorphic; benign microcalcifications are isolated, smooth, round densities that need no further evaluation; pleomorphic microcalcifications are irregularly shaped and resemble broken glass; they suggest ductal carcinoma in situ and require biopsy; microcalcifications that exhibit both benign and pleomorphic characteristics are called indeterminate; they require either biopsy or mammographic reevaluation in 6 months; if not associated with ductal carcinoma in situ, these microcalcifications are seen in fibrocystic conditions.

mitotane adrenolytic agent used to treat adrenocortical adenocarcinoma.

multiple endocrine neoplasia (MEN) familial endocrine tumor syndromes inherited as autosomal dominant conditions; three types: MEN-1, MEN-2A, and MEN-2B.

multiple endocrine neoplasia type 1 (MEN-1) autosomal dominant condition associated with primary hyperparathyroidism, pituitary adenomas, pancreatic islet cell tumors, carcinoid tumors of the thymus or bronchus, and lipomas.

multiple endocrine neoplasia type 2A (MEN-2A) autosomal dominant condition caused by a mutation of RET; associated with medullary thyroid carcinoma, pheochromocytoma, and parathyroid hyperplasia.

multiple endocrine neoplasia type 2B (MEN-2B) autosomal dominant condition caused by a mutation of RET; associated with a characteristic phenotype, medullary thyroid carcinoma, and pheochromocytoma.

multiple organ system failure altered organ function in an acutely ill patient; homeostasis cannot be maintained without intervention.

Murphy's sign sharp pain on deep inspiration during palpation in the right upper quadrant; associated with acute cholecystitis.

necrotizing fasciitis soft tissue infection that spreads along the fascia and causes necrosis; often caused by mixed aerobes and anaerobes; when the male genitalia are involved, called Fournier's disease.

Nelson syndrome development of an adrenocorticotropic hormone–producing pituitary tumor after bilateral adrenalectomy in Cushing's syndrome; causes aggressive growth and hyperpigmentation of the skin.

nevus, blue dark blue or blue-black nevus covered by smooth skin; formed by melanin-pigmented spindle cells in the lower dermis.

nevus, compound common nevus caused by nests of cells in the dermis and epidermal–dermal junction.

nevus, congenital giant hairy large, hairy congenital pigmented nevus that often involves the entire lower trunk; high risk for melanoma.

nevus, intradermal most common benign nevus in adults; caused by nests of melanocytes in the dermis.

nevus, junctional slightly raised, flat, pigmented tumor; caused by nests of nevus cells in the basal layer at the epidermal–dermal junction.

nitrogen balance nitrogen intake (g/day) minus nitrogen excretion (24-hour urine urea nitrogen plus 3 g for unmeasured nitrogen losses); crucial goal in nutritional support.

nodular melanoma most malignant melanoma tumor; grows vertically, is blue-black, has a palpable nodular component in its earliest development, and develops quickly.

normal serum laboratory values (in commonly used units and Système Internationale [SI] units)

Serum	Common Units	SI Units
K$^+$	3.5–5.0 mEq/L	3.5–5.0
Na$^+$	135–145 mEq/L	135–145
Ca^{2+} (total)	8.9–10.3 mg/dL	2.23–2.57
Ca^{2+} (ionized)	4.6–5.1 mg/dL	1.15–1.27
Mg^{2+}	1.3–2.1 mEq/L	0.65–1.05
Cl$^-$	97–110 mEq/L	97–110
CO$_2$ (serum, not PaCO$_2$)	22–31 mEq/L	22–31
PO$_4$$^=$	2.5–4.5 mg/dL	0.81–1.45
Blood urea nitrogen	8–25 mg/dL	2.9–8.9
Creatinine	0.6–1.5 mg/dL	53–133 mmol/L
Fasting glucose	65–110 mg/dL	3.58–6.05

obturator sign clinical sign elicited during acute appendicitis by passive rotation of the flexed right thigh; an acutely inflamed appendix irritates the obturator internus.

odynophagia pain on swallowing.

oliguria in an adult, urine output of <500 mL/day.

omeprazole potent inhibitor of hydrochloric acid production; acts by blocking the proton pump of the parietal cell.

open-gloving technique method of donning surgical gloves when a gown is not required or when the hands have been passed fully through the cuffs of the surgical gown; usually requires an assistant because it is difficult to accomplish individually without contaminating the outside of the glove.

opsonins proteins that bind to particulate and bacterial antigens and facilitate phagocytosis.

orthostatic (postural) hypotension excessive decrease in blood pressure on assuming the erect position; usually marked by an increase in heart rate.

osmolality number of osmoles per kilogram of water; total volume is 1 L plus a relatively small volume occupied by the solute.

osmolarity number of osmoles per liter of solution; volume is <1 L by an amount equal to the solute volume.

pancreas divisum congenital abnormality of the pancreas; the duct of Santorini is not fused to the duct of Wirsung because of failure of the dorsal and ventral pancreatic buds to fuse during embryonic development.

pancreatic magna largest branch of the splenic arteries; supplies the body of the pancreas.

pancreaticoduodenectomy (Whipple procedure) removal of the head of the pancreas, duodenum, and distal common bile duct; performed for carcinoma of the pancreas, duodenum, or distal common bile duct, and for trauma.

pancreatitis, acute single episode of diffuse pancreatitis in a previously normal gland.

pancreatitis, acute biliary (gallstone) acute inflammation of the pancreas secondary to gallstones; usually caused by passage of small gallstones and sludge through the ampulla of Vater.

pancreatitis, chronic chronic inflammatory process in the pancreas that destroys its functional capabilities; characterized by endocrine and exocrine deficiency and constant pain.

pancreatitis, gallstone acute inflammation of the pancreas caused by gallstones occluding the ampulla of Vater.

Pappenheimer bodies iron inclusions in erythrocytes.

paradoxical aciduria aciduria in the late stages of hypokalemic metabolic alkalosis; the urine becomes acidic as the kidney, in an attempt to retain potassium, excretes hydrogen ions despite the overlying metabolic alkalosis (in which case hydrogen ions would be retained).

parafollicular cells cells of neuroendocrine origin within the thyroid that secrete calcitonin.

paraganglionoma pheochromocytoma located outside the adrenal medulla (extraadrenal pheochromocytoma).

parathyroid glands endocrine glands in the neck that secrete parathyroid hormone.

parathyroid hormone (parathormone) peptide hormone secreted by the parathyroid glands; primarily responsible for maintaining calcium homeostasis.

parenteral nutrition, peripheral 3% amino acid and 10% dextrose solution with lipid emulsion; delivered into a peripheral or central vein to satisfy the nutritional needs of a nonstressed patient.

parenteral nutrition, total high-osmolarity solution of amino acids, dextrose, and often lipid emulsion; delivered into a central vein to satisfy all of a patient's nutritional needs.

parietal cell cell found in the fundus of the stomach; produces hydrochloric acid and intrinsic factor.

paronychia local infection of the skin over the mantle of the fingernail and lateral nail folds.

PEG/PEJ percutaneous endoscopic gastrostomy, alone or with accompanying percutaneous jejunal tube placement; feeding tube placement performed in the intensive care unit or endoscopy suite rather than with laparotomy in the operating suite, which would require a general anesthetic.

pericardiocentesis needle puncture of the pericardium to aspirate fluid or blood to relieve cardiac tamponade.

peristaltic waves waves of alternate circular contraction and relaxation in the gastrointestinal tract that propel food and fluids onward.

peritonitis inflammation of the surfaces of the peritoneal cavity.

Peyer's patches aggregates of lymphoid cells in the lymph nodes in the gastrointestinal tract; concentrated in the ileum.

phase, proliferative second stage of wound healing; characterized by the laying down of collagen by fibroblasts.

phase, remodeling third stage of wound healing; characterized by the maturation of collagen and flattening of the wound scar.

phase, substrate (inflammatory, lag, exudative) first phase of wound healing; characterized by inflammation, macrophage formation, and appearance of substrates for collagen synthesis.

pheochromocytoma neoplasm of the adrenal medulla; arises from chromaffin tissue of neural crest origin; secretes excess epinephrine, norepinephrine, dopamine, or other vasoactive amine; causes a constellation of signs and symptoms as a result of catecholaminemia; associated with the familial endocrine syndromes multiple endocrine neoplasia types 2A (MEN-2A) and 2B (MEN-2B).

plasma fluid (noncellular) portion of the circulating blood; distinguished from serum, which is obtained after coagulation.

plasma, fresh frozen separated plasma, frozen within 6 hours of collection; used to replenish coagulation factor deficiencies (e.g., liver failure, excessive warfarin [Coumadin] effect).

platelet irregularly shaped disk in the blood; has granules, but no definite nucleus; approximately one-third to one-half the size of an erythrocyte; contains no hemoglobin; known chiefly for its role in hemostasis.

platelet count calculation of the number of platelets in 1 mm^3 of blood by counting the cells in an accurate volume of diluted blood; normal = 150,000 to 400,000 mL.

Plummer's disease toxic multinodular goiter.

pneumonia active infection within the lung parenchyma.

pneumoperitoneum free intraperitoneal air caused by perforation of the stomach, duodenum, or other part of the intestinal tract.

pneumothorax air or gas in the pleural cavity.

pneumothorax, open (sucking chest wound) large chest wall defect that permits equilibration of intrapleural and atmospheric pressures; leads to lung collapse; if the defect is at least two-thirds the diameter of the trachea, resistance to flow is lower through the defect than through the trachea; air moves into and out of the pleural space instead of through the trachea, and effective ventilation is prevented.

pneumothorax, tension air leaks out of the lung or bronchi into the pleural cavity and is trapped; intrapleural pressure rises and can exceed atmospheric pressure; the ipsilateral lung collapses; the mediastinum and trachea are pushed to the contralateral side, causing compression, distortion, and kinking of the superior and inferior vena cavae; venous return to the heart is significantly decreased; oxygen delivery is compromised; without rapid treatment, death ensues.

polycystic liver disease autosomal dominant disorder that causes progressive formation of multiple cysts; rarely leads to hepatic failure, but can cause significant symptoms associated with the mass effect of hepatic cysts.

polyp small mucosal excrescence that grows into the lumen of the colon and rectum.

polyp, pedunculated polyp that is rounded at the end and attached to the mucosa by a long, thin neck.

polyp, sessile flat polyp that is intimately attached to the mucosa.

polyvalent pneumococcal polysaccharide vaccines vaccines that contain polysaccharide antigens from many pneumococcal types; current vaccines contain 23 common types that cause infection in humans.

portal hypertension abnormally elevated pressure within the portal vein or its tributaries; causes gastroesophageal varices, variceal hemorrhage, and ascites.

portosystemic shunts large-caliber connections between the portal and systemic circulatory systems; reduce portal pressure; effectively control varices and ascites, but may be associated with hepatic encephalopathy.

position, reverse Trendelenburg positioning of a patient so that the head is elevated and the feet are lower than the heart.

position, Trendelenburg positioning of a patient so that the head of the table is tilted at a 45° angle; the feet are elevated and the head is kept below the level of the heart.

prealbumin plasma protein with a 4-day half-life; used to reflect visceral protein status and the effectiveness of nutritional support when measured weekly.

preload magnitude of myocardial stretch; the stimulus to muscle contraction described by the Frank-Starling mechanism.

pressure, central venous blood pressure measurement taken in the superior vena cava; reflects right ventricular end-diastolic pressure (preload).

pressure, cerebral perfusion difference between mean arterial pressure and intracranial pressure.

pressure, colloid osmotic difference in pressure between intravascular and interstitial fluid; mostly caused by albumin in the plasma, but not in the interstitium.

pressure, pulmonary artery occlusion (pulmonary capillary wedge pressure, wedge pressure) left atrial pressure measured by advancing a balloon-tipped catheter into the pulmonary artery until it goes no further; normal pressure is 8 to 12 mm Hg.

primary aldosteronism (Conn's syndrome) excessive, autonomous production of aldosterone by a benign adrenocortical adenoma; rarely caused by adrenocortical carcinoma; first described in 1955 by Jerome Conn at the University of Michigan.

primary biliary cirrhosis progressive small bile duct obstruction that leads to cirrhosis, likely from cytotoxic T cells; predominantly affects middle-aged women.

primary sclerosing cholangitis idiopathic disease that causes a chronic fibrotic stricturing process; can involve both the intrahepatic and extrahepatic biliary tree; the only effective long-term treatment is liver transplantation.

prophylactic antibiotics antibiotics administered to prevent infection.

prothrombin time (PT) time required for clotting after thromboplastin and calcium are added in optimal amounts to plasma with normal fibrinogen content; if prothrombin is diminished, the clotting time increases; PT is sensitive to levels of clotting factors V, VII, and X, prothrombin, and fibrinogen.

proximal gastric vagotomy antiulcer operation; selectively denervates vagal stimulation to the parietal cells; maintains the function of the pyloric sphincter.

pseudoaneurysm dilation of the artery wall that does not contain all three layers; usually forms at areas of trauma or regions of weakened arterial graft anastomosis.

pseudocyst, pancreatic cyst (without an epithelial lining) of the pancreas or of the pancreas and adjacent structures; often the result of pancreatitis.

pseudopolyp small island of normal mucosa surrounded by deep ulceration; creates the appearance of a polyp.

psoas sign clinical sign used in acute appendicitis; elicited by extension of the right hip, which causes the inflamed appendix to irritate the iliopsoas muscle.

pulse oximetry photoelectric measurement of the oxygen saturation of capillary blood.

pulsus paradoxus decrease in systolic blood pressure, during inspiration, >10 mm Hg; seen in cardiac tamponade.

pus collection of dead phagocytic cells, fibrin, and plasma proteins; densities of both dead and viable microorganisms and bacterial products that form in a closed area at the site of bacterial invasion.

pyrosis substernal pain or burning; usually associated with regurgitation of gastric juice into the esophagus.

radioactive iodine isotope (^{131}I) of iodine used to evaluate or treat thyroid disease.

radionuclide biliary scan (HIDA scan) diagnostic test in which a ^{99m}Tc-labeled derivative of iminodiacetic acid is injected intravenously; the radionuclide is excreted into the bile ducts and enters the gallbladder through the cystic duct; absence of gallbladder filling in 4 hours, along with filling of the common bile duct and passage of radionuclide into the duodenum, strongly suggests acute cholecystitis.

Ranson's criteria in patients with pancreatitis, a group of risk factors that are present on admission or within 48 hours and aid in the prediction of major complications and death.

red pulp anatomic portion of the spleen; contains the cords; site of removal of antibody-sensitized cells and particulate material.

reduced-size liver transplant use of only the left lobe or the left lateral segment of a living or cadaver liver as a transplant, especially in children.

reflux esophagitis inflammation of the lower esophagus; related to reflux of gastric acidity; contact burn related to the duration and degree of gastric acid contact.

regurgitation flow of material in the opposite direction of normal (e.g., return of undigested food from the stomach into the mouth).

rejection, accelerated acute destruction of a graft in the first few days after transplantation by a second set of anamnestic responses of preformed antibodies and lymphocytes.

rejection, acute reversible attack on a transplanted organ mediated by T lymphocytes; causes organ dysfunction.

rejection, chronic slow, progressive immunologic destruction of a transplanted organ over years; mediated by both humoral and cellular elements.

rejection, hyperacute destruction of a graft by the recipient through preformed antibodies (e.g., ABO, HLA, or species-specific antibodies); occurs within hours of transplantation.

resection, abdominoperineal removal of the lower sigmoid colon, rectum, and anus, leaving a permanent proximal sigmoid colostomy.

resection, low anterior removal of the distal sigmoid colon and upper one-half of the rectum with primary anastomosis of the proximal sigmoid to distal rectum.

respiratory quotient (RQ) ratio of CO_2:O_2 consumption; reflects whether the patient's energy supply is inadequate (RQ < 1), balanced (RQ = 1), or excessive (RQ > 1).

rest pain pain in the distal extremities, especially the toes and metatarsal heads, when the extremity is elevated; elevation decreases the hydrostatic perfusion pressure of the lower extremities; they become ischemic, and pain occurs; symptoms are usually relieved with "dangling" of the affected extremities.

resting metabolic expenditure energy needed by a resting, supine person after an overnight fast.

resuscitation restoration from potential or apparent death; the airway is secured, ventilation is assured, and oxygen is administered; external blood loss is controlled with direct pressure; intravenous lines are established with a balanced electrolyte solution; Ringer's lactate is preferred in patients with traumatic injury; intravascular volume is restored; hypothermia is combated with high-flow fluid warmers; aspiration and gastric distension are reduced with the placement of a gastric tube; pulse oximetry, blood pressure, electrocardiographic readings, and urine output are monitored; in patients with traumatic injury, these measures are begun simultaneously with the primary survey.

RET proto-oncogene tyrosine kinase receptor oncogene; used as a gene marker for multiple endocrine neoplasia types 2A (MEN-2A) and 2B (MEN-2B) and familial medullary thyroid carcinoma.

Reynold's pentad right upper quadrant abdominal pain, fever and chills, jaundice, hypotension, and mental confusion; associated with acute suppurative cholangitis.

ring sign (target sign) pattern produced when a drop of bloody cerebrospinal fluid is placed on filter paper; because cerebrospinal fluid diffuses faster than blood, the blood remains in the center and one or more concentric rings of clearer (pink) fluid form around the central red spot; used to test bloody otorrhea and rhinorrhea for the presence of cerebrospinal fluid.

Rovsing's sign clinical sign of pain seen in acute appendicitis; pressure applied to the left lower quadrant of the abdomen creates pain in the right lower quadrant.

S phase phase in the growth cycle of a cell; a finding of more than 6% or 7% of cells in the S phase in a tissue sample, as measured by flow cytometry, suggests a rapidly growing tumor.

SCALP mnemonic for remembering the five layers of the scalp; Skin, subCutaneous tissue, galea Aponeurotica, Loose areolar tissue, and Periosteum (pericranium).

scrub nurse member of the surgical team who participates directly in the surgical procedure; manages the sterile instruments and supplies; often assists with the procedure.

Seagesser's sign neck tenderness produced by manual compression over the phrenic nerve; caused by diaphragmatic irritation (e.g., by blood from a ruptured spleen).

seborrheic keratosis superficial, benign, verrucous lesion; consists of proliferating epidermal cells; usually occurs in the elderly.

secretin duodenal hormone that inhibits gastric acid secretion and gastric emptying.

selective shunts shunts that decompress gastroesophageal varices, but maintain prograde portal profusion to the liver; best known is the distal splenorenal shunt.

Sengstaken-Blakemore tube tube placed through the esophagus for balloon tamponade of gastric and esophageal varices; provides temporary occlusion.

sepsis systemic response to infection as manifested by two or more of the following conditions:

1. Temperature > 37°C or <36°C
2. Heart rate > 90 beats/min
3. Respiratory rate > 20 breaths/min or $PaCO_2$ < 32 mm Hg
4. White blood cell count > 12,000 cells/mm^3, < 4000 cells/mm^3, or > 10% immature (band) forms

sepsis, burn wound invasive infection of a burn wound; bacteria penetrate beneath the burned surface and invade viable tissue and blood vessels.

shock inadequate organ perfusion; types include anaphylactic, cardiogenic, hemorrhagic, hypoadrenal, hypovolemic, neurogenic, and septic; total body cellular metabolism is malfunctional.

shock, burn severe loss of intravascular volume caused by fluid sequestration in and beneath burn wounds.

shock, spinal neurologic condition that occurs after spinal cord injury; caused by acute loss of stimulation from higher levels; this "shock" or "stun" to the injured cord makes it appear functionless; there is complete flaccidity and areflexia instead of the predicted spasticity, hyperreflexia, and positive Babinski sign that are seen in the classic upper motor neuron lesion; not a synonym for neurogenic shock, which is inadequate organ perfusion.

silver sulfadiazine (Silvadene, SSD, Thermazene) topical antibiotic widely used in burn treatment; active against a wide range of Gram-positive and Gram-negative organisms and yeast; many other topical agents are also available.

singultus hiccup.

Sister Mary Joseph's node hard nodule at the umbilicus; associated with metastatic gastric carcinoma.

skin graft, full-thickness graft obtained by excising an ellipse of skin and subcutaneous tissue, usually from the groin or flank; donor site is closed with sutures.

skin graft, split-thickness graft obtained by excising tissue at the level of the dermis, leaving a base that heals spontaneously.

somatostatin pharmacologic agent that reduces variceal bleeding by inducing mesenteric vasoconstriction; diminishes variceal bleeding in at least 50% of patients.

splenectomy removal of the spleen.

splenic cords (of Billroth) reticular portion of the spleen in the red pulp that lacks endothelium; blood percolates slowly and comes in contact with numerous macrophages.

splenomegaly, congestive enlargement of the spleen as a result of vascular engorgement (e.g., portal hypertension).

splenomegaly, infiltrative enlargement of the spleen because of accumulation of materials within the splenic reticuloendothelial cells (e.g., Gaucher's disease with accumulation of glucocerebrosides).

spontaneous nipple discharge discharge on clothing in the absence of breast stimulation; in contrast, elicited discharge is noted after the nipple or breast is squeezed, or after vigorous mammography; only spontaneous discharge requires evaluation.

squamous cell carcinoma malignant neoplasm derived from stratified squamous epithelium; variable amounts of keratin are formed in relation to the degree of differentiation; if the keratin is not on the surface, a "keratin pearl" is formed.

sterile field operative area that is covered with sterile drapes and prepared for the use of sterile supplies and equipment; classically, includes the instrument table, Mayo stand, and operative area.

sterile technique moving, working, or functioning in a sterile environment with sterile equipment to prevent contamination of the incision site.

sterilization physical or chemical process by which all pathogenic and nonpathogenic microorganisms are destroyed.

sterilization, dry-heat killing of microorganisms through heat absorption.

sterilization, ethylene oxide gas sterilization technique used for instruments or objects that are sensitive to heat or moisture; ethylene oxide is cidal to all microorganisms, but requires a longer exposure time (3 to 6 hours) than heat sterilization.

sterilization, moist-heat sterilization technique that uses saturated steam under pressure (autoclave); easiest, fastest, and least expensive method of sterilization.

strangulation vascular compromise of an incarcerated organ.

Sturge-Weber syndrome facial hemangioma (causing a port wine stain) occupying the cutaneous distribution of the trigeminal nerve, angiomatous malformations of the brain and meninges, and occasionally pheochromocytoma.

surrogate decision maker person empowered to make decisions for a patient who is not competent to do so.

survey, primary rapid initial evaluation of a patient with traumatic injury; involves the diagnosis and treatment of all immediately life-threatening injuries; the essence of the "ABCDEs" of trauma management; sequentially, the physician protects the cervical spine while assessing the injured patient's Airway, Breathing, Circulation, and neurologic Disability; Exposure of the patient and prevention of hypothermia are the last steps; all immediately life-threatening injuries are treated in sequence before proceeding to the next phase.

survey, secondary detailed, head-to-toe evaluation of a trauma patient; includes a history and physical examination to identify all injuries; begins after the primary survey is completed, resuscitation is initiated, and the airway, breathing, and circulation are reassessed; tubes or fingers are placed in every orifice; baseline laboratory studies are drawn if they were not drawn when the intravenous lines were started; portable radiographs are taken; special procedures (e.g., peritoneal lavage) are done during this phase.

syndrome of inappropriate secretion of antidiuretic hormone (SIADH) syndrome associated with physiologically uncontrolled production of antidiuretic hormone by malignant tumors or disturbances from intracranial injury disorders.

systemic inflammatory response syndrome syndrome that indicates systemic inflammation; caused by a variety of cellular and tissue injuries (see Chapter 5 for the criteria-based definition).

T cell thymus-derived cell; involved in the cellular response to foreign tissue; produces cytokines, recruits other cells, and differentiates into helper, suppressor, and cytotoxic cells.

target sign see *ring sign*.

tenosynovitis infection of the tendon sheath, usually of the hand.

thalassemia deficit in the synthesis of one or more subunits of hemoglobin; leads to erythrocyte abnormalities and anemia; many types are seen, but β-thalassemias are the most common.

therapy, hormone replacement therapy, often initiated after surgical or natural menopause, to prevent the perimenopausal and postmenopausal symptoms of estrogen withdrawal (e.g., hot flashes, vaginal atrophy, urogenital deterioration); also seems to significantly diminish osteoporosis and cardiac disease.

therapy, protein-sparing 3% amino acid and 5% dextrose solution delivered by peripheral veins; minimizes proteolysis in a nutritionally fit, fasting patient.

thionamides class of antithyroid drugs (e.g., propylthiouracil, methimazole); inhibit iodide organification and iodotyrosine coupling; reduce the rate of peripheral conversion of thyroxine (T_4) to triiodothyronine (T_3).

third-space fluid accumulation accumulation of extracellular and intracellular fluid in response to regional or total body cellular or tissue injury; accumulation in excess of the volume of fluid that normally occupies these regions; sequestration decreases intravascular fluid volume.

thrill palpable turbulence within an arterial vessel as a result of disturbed flow.

thrombin time time needed for a fibrin clot to form after thrombin is added to citrated plasma; prolonged thrombin time is seen in patients who are receiving heparin therapy, those who have factor I (fibrinogen) deficiency, and those with elevated levels of fibrin or fibrinogen split products.

thrombocytosis platelet count >400,000/mm³.

thrombosis formation of an occlusive or nonocclusive blood clot within a blood vessel or cavity of the heart.

thrombotic thrombocytopenic purpura disease of arteries and capillaries; characterized by thrombosis and thrombocytopenia.

thrombus blood clot that forms within a blood vessel and remains in place, often causing an obstruction.

thyroglobulin molecule on which iodine is complexed to form triiodothyronine (T_3) and thyroxine (T_4).

thyroid carcinoma (papillary, follicular, medullary, or anaplastic) types of thyroid cancer; papillary and follicular carcinomas are well-differentiated carcinomas of follicular cells; medullary carcinomas are of parafollicular cell origin; anaplastic carcinomas dedifferentiate from follicular cells.

thyroid-stimulating hormone (TSH, thyrotropin) hormone secreted by the pituitary to regulate thyroxine (T_4) production and secretion by the thyroid.

thyroidectomy surgical excision of the thyroid gland.

thyrotoxicosis (hyperthyroidism) overactive thyroid.

thyroxine (T_4, tetraiodothyronine) major hormone secreted by the thyroid in response to thyroid-stimulating hormone; feeds back to regulate thyroid-stimulating hormone.

tonicity "effective" osmolality; often used to describe intravenous fluid replacement or body fluids (e.g., hypotonic, isotonic, or hypertonic solutions or fluids mean, respectively, less effective, same, or more effective osmolality).

total body water portion of body weight composed of water and fluids; in a typical 70-kg man, 60% of body weight is water and fluids; in women and the elderly, it is 50% to 55%.

toxic multinodular goiter thyroid enlargement from multiple nodules that may cause compression symptoms.

transient ischemic attack reversible changes in mentation, vision, and motor or sensory function; usually lasts seconds to minutes; completely resolves within 24 hours.

transjugular intrahepatic portacaval shunt (TIPS) radiologically placed intrahepatic shunt; connects the portal vein with the hepatic vein; bypasses the increased hepatic resistance.

triangle of Calot hepatocystic triangle bounded by the inferior margin of the liver, common hepatic duct, and cystic duct; traversed by several important normal and anomalous structures.

triiodothyronine (T_3) thyroid hormone that acts at the tissue level where it is formed by deiodination of thyroxine (T_4).

truncal vagotomy complete transection of both vagal trunks at the gastroesophageal junction; eliminates vagal stimulation of the parietal cell.

tumor, carcinoid most common tumor of the appendix; may cause carcinoid syndrome; often malignant.

tumor, phyllodes breast tumor seen in younger women; usually a large, smooth, nontender mass; clinically similar to fibroadenoma, but larger; most are benign, but a small percentage are malignant; treatment involves wide excision.

ulcer, duodenal ulcer that usually occurs in the first portion of the duodenum as a result of acid hypersecretion.

ulcer, gastric ulcer that typically occurs on the lesser curvature of the stomach; usually secondary to mucosal breakdown of the stomach.

ulcer, Marjolin's squamous cell cancer that arises in the inflammatory scar of a nonhealing ulcer (e.g., chronic wound, fistula-in-ano, osteomyelitis).

ulcerative colitis mucosal disease of the colon; causes significant diarrhea and bleeding; tends to become malignant.

United Network for Organ Sharing (UNOS) organization of transplant centers, organ procurement agencies, and professional and patient groups; regulates organ allocation and procurement in the United States.

urine urea nitrogen 24-hour urine collection assayed for urea; used to measure nitrogen loss and calculate nitrogen balance.

vasoconstriction reduction in the caliber of blood vessels; leads to decreased blood flow.

venous return quantity of blood that returns to the right atrium from the systemic veins each minute.

volvulus rotation of a segment of the intestine on the axis formed by the mesentery; causes obstruction of the bowel.

vomiting forcible expulsion of stomach contents through the mouth.

von Hippel-Lindau disease neuroectodermal dysplasia associated with cystic cerebellar hemangioblastoma and angiomatous malformation of the retina and pheochromocytoma.

von Recklinghausen's disease common neuroectodermal dysplasia; multiple neurofibromas of peripheral nerves; associated with pheochromocytomas.

von Willebrand's disease hemorrhagic diathesis characterized by a tendency to bleed, primarily from the mucous membranes; laboratory abnormalities include prolonged bleeding time, variable deficiency of factor VIII clotting activity, prolonged activated partial thromboplastin time, reduced von Willebrand's antigen and activity, and reduced ristocetin-induced platelet aggregation; inheritance is autosomal dominant, with reduced penetrance and variable expressivity.

water brash heartburn with regurgitation of sour fluid or almost tasteless saliva into the mouth.

Wernicke-Korsakoff syndrome syndrome caused by excessive alcohol intake; bilateral sixth cranial nerve palsy, nystagmus, diplopia, disconjugate gaze, and strabismus; ataxia is typical; mental changes include generalized apathy and lack of awareness; delirium is a late manifestation.

white pulp anatomic portion of the spleen where lymphocytes and lymphatic follicles reside; probably site where soluble antigens are processed.

Wilson's disease autosomal recessive disorder caused by excess copper; causes markedly diminished copper excretion into the biliary tree; correctable with liver transplantation.

wound, clean surgical wound, made under sterile conditions, that does not enter the gastrointestinal, respiratory, or genitourinary tract; wound in which there is a break in sterile technique; wound that is not exposed to a significant bacterial population.

wound, clean-contaminated surgical wound that enters the gastrointestinal, respiratory, or genitourinary tract without significant spillage; wound in which there is a break in sterile technique; wound that is initially clean, but is exposed to endogenous colonization during the procedure.

wound, contaminated surgical wound in which extensive spillage from the gastrointestinal tract occurs; fresh traumatic wound; wound in which a major break in sterile technique occurs; wound in which gross contamination occurs during the procedure.

wound, dirty wound that contains dirt, fecal material, purulence, or other foreign material; high risk of infection.

wound, infected wound with a bacterial count of more than 10^5 organisms/g tissue.

xenograft tissue transferred between members of different species.

xeroderma pigmentosum eruption of exposed skin that occurs in childhood; characterized by numerous pigmented spots that resemble freckles; larger atrophic lesions eventually cause glossy, white thinning of the skin.

Zollinger-Ellison syndrome severe variant of duodenal ulcer disease; results from the independent production of gastrin by a tumor (gastrinoma) that arises in the pancreas or paraduodenal area.

Index

Note: Page numbers followed by an f denote figures; those followed by a t denote tables.